BAILEY'S TEXTBOOK OF
MICROSCOPIC ANATOMY

EIGHTEENTH EDITION

BAILEY'S TEXTBOOK OF
MICROSCOPIC ANATOMY

EIGHTEENTH EDITION

Douglas E. Kelly, Ph.D.

Professor and Chairman, Department of Anatomy and Cell Biology
University of Southern California
School of Medicine
Los Angeles, California

Richard L. Wood, Ph.D.

Professor, Department of Anatomy and Cell Biology
University of Southern California
Los Angeles, California

Allen C. Enders, Ph.D.

Professor and Chairman, Department of Human Anatomy
University of California, Davis
Davis, California

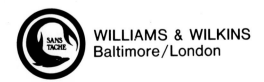

WILLIAMS & WILKINS
Baltimore/London

Editor: Toni M. Tracy
Associate Editor: Carol-Lynn Brown
Copy Editor: Leilani Ellison
Design: Joanne Janowiak
Illustration Planning: Lorraine Wrozsek
Production: Raymond E. Reter

Accurate indications, adverse reactions, and dosage schedules for drugs are provided in this book, but it is possible that they may change. The reader is urged to review the package information data of the manufacturers of the medications mentioned.

Made in the United States of America.

Previous editions copyrighted in 1904, 1906, 1910, 1913, 1916, 1920, 1925, 1932, 1936, 1940, 1944, 1948, 1953, 1958, 1964, 1971

Seventeenth edition, 1978
Reprinted 1979, 1980, 1981, 1982, 1983

Foreign editions:
  Spanish, 1948, 1962
English language co-edition:
  Indian, 1967

Library of Congress Cataloging in Publication Data

Bailey, Frederick R. (Frederick Randolph), 1871–1923.
  Bailey's textbook of microscopic anatomy

  Bibliography: p.
  Includes index.
  1. Histology. I. Kelly, Douglas E., 1932– . II. Wood, Richard L. (Richard Lyman), 1929– . III. Enders, Allen C. IV. Title. V. Title: Textbook of histology. [DNLM: 1. Histology. QS 504 B154t] QM551.B24 1984   611'.018   83-19838
ISBN 0-683-04568-7

Composed and printed at the
Waverly Press, Inc.
Mt. Royal & Guilford Aves.
Baltimore, MD 21202, U.S.A.

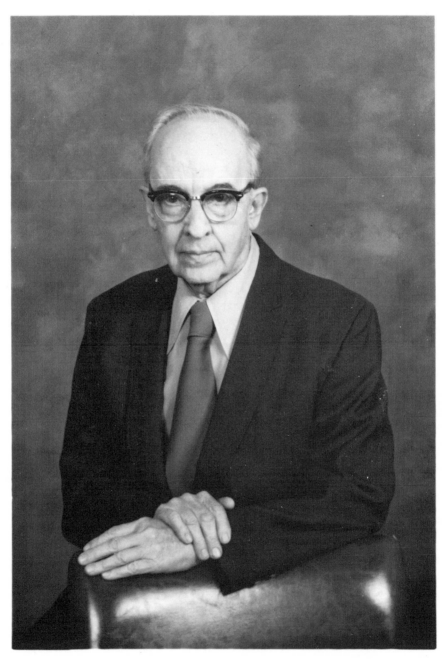

DEDICATION
To
Wilfred M. Copenhaver, Ph.D.

v

Preface to the Eighteenth Edition

1984 marks the 80th anniversary of *Bailey's Textbook of Histology.* At the hands of many individuals and teams, the book has served several generations of biomedical students and their mentors. It has portrayed the maturing of paraffin section-based light microscopic histology, the advent and development of histochemistry and cytochemistry, the perfection of techniques to study cells and tissues in culture, and the explosion of new structural insight occasioned by the introduction of transmission and scanning electron microscopy. Even today, structural biology is expanding rapidly, largely at molecular levels of organization and interaction, through the development of freeze-fracture methods, immunocytochemical techniques, and correlated biochemical identification.

The science of histology has matured into far more than the study of living tissues— which is the definition of histology. Therefore, the 18th edition of this textbook carries a new title which appropriately recognizes that maturation and growth. Revisions to the text and additions of much new illustrative material have been accomplished with a central objective of emphasizing newer findings and fitting them into a conceptual framework which continues to emerge with increasing clarity. Discussions of the cellular and molecular basis of organization, connective tissues, contractile systems, blood and lymphatic organs, the integument, the digestive, urinary, and reproductive systems, endocrines, and the organs of special sense have received thorough revisions along these lines.

Yet, some of the principal lessons of this textbook deal not with new findings, but with new or remaining questions. We have tried to present current information in a manner which also emphasizes remaining puzzles and some of the newly apparent concepts.

At the University of Southern California, we have found it advantageous to teach human embryology in a closely integrated fashion with microscopic anatomy and cell biology. Students learn the embryonic body plan and emergent organ systems as arenas in which the differentiation of the basic cells and tissues is occurring. They learn organelles, cells, and tissues as products of developmental processes and recognize thereby both essential differences and similarities among differentiated cellular populations. In this spirit, we have departed somewhat from the usual histology textbook format to include an expanded chapter on early human development, and to include added embryological insight into most discussions of tissues and organs. We hope this will prove helpful to the wide variety of patterns in which courses in microscopic anatomy are taught.

Important artistic illustrations have graced the pages of *Bailey's Textbook* for many years. Some of the earlier works of Robert Demarest and Carl Kellner still remain in this edition. In recent years Peter Mendez and several of his students (Susan Weiner, Davi Grossman, Eric Reese, and Peter MacIver) have provided many new and informative interpretations of embryonic and cytological details which, because of three-dimensional complexity, are difficult for students to learn from text alone.

Deborah Davies deserves special mention for the half dozen new illustrations she provided related to muscle and sense organs. Dr. Joel Schechter was responsible for new three-dimensional renditions of muscle ensheathment, spleen, and lung.

The authors are grateful to Dr. Michael Cullen who provided expertise on neural tissue, Dr. Mikel Snow who provided a brief section on muscle regeneration, and many colleagues who graciously allowed the use of figures from their own scientific investigations. Each of these is cited in captions for the figures. The devoted editorial and technical help of Aileen Kuda, Sandra Schlafke, and Rick Welsh, and the expert secretarial services of Delcina McMillan, Nancy Polito, and Colleene Kiley are also greatly appreciated.

Finally, we wish to express our appreciation to the publishers for their cooperation and assistance in the production of this book and for their patience in awaiting its completion.

A brief resume of the history of this textbook seems appropriate on this 80th anniversary. The first edition was written by Professor Frederick R. Bailey at the College of Physicians and Surgeons and was published by William Wood and Company in 1904. Professor Bailey, with assistance from Professor Oliver Strong on the nervous system, continued the book through the sixth edition, published in 1920. Although the text has been rewritten by a number of authors since the time of Professor Bailey, it has adhered to his objective of emphasizing fundamentals. Remarkably, the current edition still carries a few of the original passages and illustrations.

Professors Strong and Adolph Elwyn revised the seventh edition (1925) and a part of the eighth edition (1932). Professors R. L. Carpenter, C. M. Goss, and A. E. Sev-eringhaus participated with Professors Philip E. Smith and Wilfred M. Copenhaver in completing the eighth (1932), ninth, and tenth editions. The current text retains some valuable contributions made by them.

Professor Smith served as editor of the ninth and tenth revisions and as coauthor of the eleventh, twelfth, and thirteenth editions. His contributions of material plus his sound editorial judgment had an important role in the success the textbook achieved during editions eight to thirteen inclusive. Professor Dorothy D. Johnson assisted with the thirteenth edition and became coauthor in the fourteenth edition. She made particularly valuable contributions to the chapters on the digestive system, respiratory system, and endocrine glands.

The fifteenth edition was almost entirely the editorial product of Professor Copenhaver. Professors Mary and Richard Bunge took part in authorship of the sixteenth edition along with Professor Copenhaver. In 1976, Professor Copenhaver was joined by Professors Douglas E. Kelly and Richard L. Wood in preparation of the seventeenth edition.

The eighteenth edition incorporates the first contributions of Professor Allen C. Enders, in collaboration with Professors Kelly and Wood. Regrettably, it also marks the departure of Professor Copenhaver from the project. Yet this eighteenth edition bears the unmistakable imprint of Professor Copenhaver's contributions, his many years of devoted leadership, and his wise, continuing counsel. It is therefore fitting that *Bailey's Textbook of Microscopic Anatomy*, eighteenth edition, is dedicated to Professor Wilfred M. Copenhaver.

Douglas E. Kelly, Ph.D.
Richard L. Wood, Ph.D.
Allen C. Enders, Ph.D.

Introduction

All living organisms consist of *cells*. These are the smallest structural units possessing those properties which we commonly associate with life. They are able to nourish themselves, to grow, to respond to stimuli, and to reproduce. Some organisms, the *protozoa*, consist of one cell only; more complex types, *metazoa*, may consist of infinite numbers of cells varying greatly in structural characteristics. Each of these multicellular organisms starts its existence as a single cell, a fertilized ovum, which by proliferation and differentiation gives rise to the adult body. At first the cells of the developing embryo are similar in shape and structure. As growth continues, differentiation leads to the formation of groups of specialized cells, each group differing in structure from the others, each group adapted to subserve one or more specific functions. These specialized groups form the *tissues* of the adult body. At a very early period the cells of the embryo become separated from each other by the formation of varying amounts of *intercellular* substance, which may be the result of cellular secretion or actual modifications of cellular substance. In some of the tissues this intercellular material assumes enormous proportions. Thus the adult body is composed of cells *and* intercellular material, all elements so interrelated as to form a normally functioning machine.

Cytology is the study of cells and their contents. *Histology* is the study of the tissues of the body. *Microscopic anatomy* is the integrated exploration of cells, intercellular materials, and tissues, since all of these require microscopic tools. The first two chapters of the book are devoted to a discussion of cells and the microscopic

techniques useful in their examination; the first chapter dealing with cells after fixation and the second with living cells. Chapter three places the properties of cells and tissues into an embryological context. Succeeding these discussions, the structure of the various tissues, and then the microscopic anatomy of principal organs is presented.

Over the years, histologists have tended to categorize the various cells and tissues of the body. They have classified them largely according to apparent differences, somewhat more than according to similarities. Textbooks of histology have tended to emphasize the categorizations, and students often dismiss their study of histology once they have memorized the essential differences that distinguish the categories under scrutiny. Yet we now understand ever more clearly that the similarities and common properties are as important as the differences. Nature has, in fact, not designed separate, distinct categories, but rather has evolved a spectrum of structural and functional possibilities around which the living organism is fabricated. Thus, in a broader consideration of microscopic anatomy it is ultimately more important to interrelate and compare the properties of cells and tissues than it is simply to separate and name them.

Whereas microscopic anatomy is a structural science and complements at finer levels of resolution anatomical knowledge gained from dissection, its intimate relation to biochemistry, physiology, and pathology must be emphasized. The cell is a unit not only of structure, but also of physiological activity. The formation of the specialized tissues is the structural expression of a physiological division of labor. The structures seen under any of the various types of light and electron microscopes assume meaning only in terms of their functional significance. Thus, the structure of muscles and glands, for example, can most profitably be studied by constant reference to contraction and secretion. Normal physiological processes are associated with normal structure; abnormal processes are usually expressed in the altered structure and relationship of the cells and intercellular substance.

Recognition of these considerations, then, implies an awareness of increased breadth in the term microscopic anatomy. To understand cells and tissues is to appreciate the common properties they have shared since their embryonic ancestry, the subtle and dramatic special propensities they have acquired during maturation, the minuteness of their most important parts, the delicate metabolic balance within which they normally operate, and the ease with which all of this can be altered to give conditions we define as disease. Understanding cells and tissues is not unlike understanding people and societies.

CONTENTS

CHAPTER 1

CELLS, TISSUES, AND MICROSCOPES

Cells are the fundamental structural units of living organisms. In multicellular animals (the metazoans) populations of similar cells and some of their products are aggregated to form *tissues*. These in turn are appropriately combined in the architecture of each *organ* of an organism. The first two chapters of this textbook explore the elementary properties of cells with the aim of gaining some understanding of the *cellular level of organization*. Some preliminary insight will also be presented regarding the *tissue level of organization*, and a variety of microscopic and other technical tools will be described as a basis for understanding the way in which structure of cells and tissues has been elucidated to date.

Recognition of the universal role of cells in the structure of virtually all living systems emerged during the 17th century. The resulting "cell doctrine" evolved coincident with the development of the earliest microscopes. Refinement of our understanding of the structure of cells and tissues has directly paralleled the increasingly efficient utilization of both visible and shorter wavelength optics for visualization of cells and their parts.

The goal of anatomical study is not just the acquisition of an accurate, static visualization of the structural elements of living systems. Rather, such visualization must lead eventually to an appreciation of those elements as dyamic, changing entities in the flux of activity that is life. Living *structure* is the fabric upon which *function* is organized; neither can be understood without reflection upon the other. Anatomists have traditionally striven to visualize and describe as directly as possible the struc-

tural components of cells, tissues, and organs in a manner which is most representative of the living state. It is a difficult task, for important structure is often not rendered visible unless the cell or tissue is killed, and the anatomist must try somehow to be assured that death has not rendered a distorted image of the living state. Moreover, anatomists have found repeatedly that the most challenging aspects seem to lie just beyond the resolution of the naked eye or microscopic tools at hand. Hence, the major challenge has been to develop better methods for accurate visualization of ever smaller parts.

We have recently seen an enormous expansion of cytology and histology, the studies of cells and tissues, respectively. Utilizing the methods of histochemistry, immunocytochemistry, various forms of light and electron microscopy, and tissue culture, cytological studies have clarified much of the structure of subcellular elements. These revelations, combined with new knowledge from biochemistry and cell physiology, have led to a firmer basic understanding of many of the ongoing processes of the living cell.

Neither the term "cell" nor the term "cell concept" will be new to readers of this text. The 19th century histologist Leydig defined a cell as "a mass of protoplasm containing a nucleus." This simple and useful description is still appropriate for animal cells today, for the minimal living structural unit is one having available the genetic material (within the *nucleus*) which allows it to carry out, relatively independently, all of the vital functions necessary to sustain life. Although cells in higher organisms may develop considerable dependence on one another, each retains within its nucleus identical sets of genetic information necessary to carry out all cell functions. Cells which lose their nuclei may continue to function for some time because the nucleus previously made provision for the manufacture of all the substances needed during the remaining life of the cell.

The substance of the cell outside the nucleus is called *cytoplasm*; the substance of the nucleus is *karyoplasm* or *nucleoplasm*. The entire cell is circumscribed by a membrane termed the *plasma membrane* or *plasmalemma*. As will be seen, the nucleus is separated from the cytoplasm by an envelope consisting of two membranes, and much of the volume of the cytoplasm is occupied by compartments which are each membrane-bounded.

METHODS OF STUDY

Our present knowledge of cell structure has been gained from an expanding variety of methods which fall logically into two groups; (*a*) methods employed with living cells and (*b*) methods involving dead cells (fixed or preserved). It should be emphasized that no single method should be used to the exclusion of all others. Studies on the living cell and those on preserved material yield complementary data and, by their different approaches, corroborate or question the other's findings. This chapter deals with preserved cells and Chapter 2 summarizes important findings from studies on living cells.

Preparation of Material

Some types of cells can be satisfactorily studied by placing them directly on slides for staining and for microscopic observation (e.g., Wright's stained blood smears). However for most cytological work it is necessary to cut tissues into thin, translucent slices only a few micrometers (microns, µm) thick. This process, termed sectioning, is done on instruments called microtomes and is facilitated by freezing the tissue or by embedding it in a supporting medium such as paraffin, celloidin, or plastics.

Most commonly, the first step in the preparation of histological sections is *fixation*. Numerous chemicals and their mixtures are used as fixatives (formalin, alcohol, etc). Fixation stabilizes the molecular structure (especially proteins) of tissue, begins a hardening which facilitates sectioning, and may promote affinity of certain tissue elements for particular dyes. In the process of fixation, proteins are denatured and may be cross-linked or otherwise rendered insoluble; lipids and carbohydrates may or may not be preserved, depending on the nature of the fixative. For example, many fats are removed from tissues immersed in alcoholic or other organic solvent fixatives. Therefore, it has often been necessary to use different technical procedures to study the various constituents of a cell.

For sectioning, the tissue is commonly infiltrated with *paraffin*. Because paraffin does not mix with water, the former will not penetrate into tissues until the latter is removed. *Dehydration* is accomplished by passing the tissues through a series of graded alcohols, up to 100%. Now, because paraffin is also insoluble in alcohol, the latter must be replaced by an agent miscible with both alcohol and paraffin, e.g., xylene or cedar wood oil. These agents also render the tissue translucent, and therefore this step in technique is known as *clearing*. The tissue is then placed in melted paraffin, which replaces the clearing agent; this step is referred to as *infiltration*. Next, the tissue is *embedded* in paraffin by allowing the latter to harden, and then the material is ready for sectioning and subsequent staining. Figure 1.1 shows photomicrographs of cells prepared by this method. Sections are usually 3 to 10 µm thick. Celloidin is an alternative embedding medium which is particularly useful for cutting large objects (e.g., brain) and for hard and brittle material (e.g., cartilage). Plastics, particularly *epoxy resins*, are increasingly being employed as the embedding medium for both light and electron microscopy. They pro-

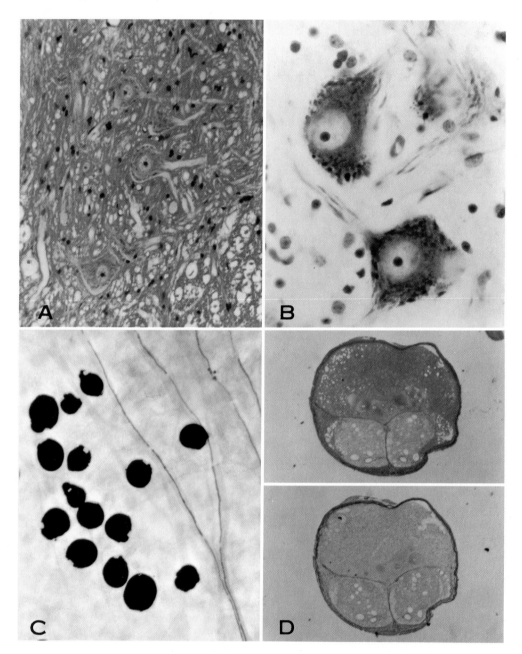

Figure 1.1. Staining of various components. *A*, hematoxylin and eosin-stained spinal cord. Four nerve cell bodies are stained blue to purple by hematoxylin because of their high content of basophilic nucleic acid. Much of the remaining tissue is stained magenta by eosin because of the preponderance of acidophilic protein components (×225). *B*, staining of nucleic acid by cresyl violet. In these two nerve cell bodies from spinal cord, the ribonucleic acid in the cytoplasm and in the nucleolus is heavily stained. The deoxyribonucleic acid of the nerve cell nucleus remains largely unstained because it is in a dispersed state. Smaller nuclei in which the nucleic acid is more condensed do stain with this dye (×440). *C*, the lipid stores of these 15 fat cells are revealed by staining with Sudan black. The small indentations in some of the black deposits are the unstained nuclei. The slender strands are myelin sheaths, which also stain because of the high lipid content. Nervous tissue in culture (×175). *D (upper figure)* Cross section of a lobster ganglion (collection of nerve cells) demonstrating a high glycogen content. The glycogen is stained pink by the periodic acid-Schiff reaction. If the tissue is first treated with amylase, which digests glycogen, the pink staining is not seen (*lower figure*). Nonglycogen components of the sheath surrounding this ganglion are stained purple with or without amylase treatment (×20).

duce less tissue and cellular damage than paraffin and allow the production of much thinner sections (down to 0.02 μm).

It is obvious that structures seen in sections may be altered by chemical fixation, dehydration, or the embedding process. Again and again, the description of features in the fixed cell has brought forth the objection that they are not true features of the living cell, but *artifacts* of technique. One gains confidence as to the faithfulness of images if they eventually compare favorably with direct observations of living cells or of similar cells prepared by a variety or techniques. In this way, cell biologists and histologists have gradually built an increasingly wide and accurate knowledge base of structural information.

The *freeze drying technique* seems in some instances to cause less alteration of the living tissue than do the standard methods. In this technique, fresh tissue is preserved by placing it in isopentane chilled to −170°C with liquid nitrogen. The frozen tissue is dehydrated in a vacuum and embedded without previous chemical fixation and dehydration in alcohols. This method is useful for localization of certain enzymes which are destroyed by the standard methods.

In the *frozen section technique*, a piece of tissue is placed directly on the stage of a special microtome equipped with an outlet for compressed carbon dioxide gas which cools the stage and freezes the tissue sufficiently for the cutting of sections. This method is widely used in clinical work for sectioning biopsy material when speed is important. In cytological work, the freezing method is particularly useful for studying the lipid content of cells because it avoids the use of fat solvents. It may be used for either fresh or mixed material; in the former case, it is useful for studying cell enzymes which are inactivated by chemical fixation.

The list of chemicals used for *staining* is even longer than that of those used for fixation. Most stains are classified as acids or bases. Actually, they are neutral salts

having both acidic and basic radicals. When the coloring property is in the acid radical of the neutral salt, the stain is spoken of as an acid dye, and the tissues which stain with the dye are called *acidophilic*. Eosin is an acid dye with such general usage that the terms *eosinophilic* and acidophilic are often used synonymously. In some cases, it is clear that *basophilic* substances which attract basic dyes are themselves acids, as in the staining of nucleic acids with methylene blue. It has long been realized that special methods and stains are frequently necessary to demonstrate different structures, but the nature of the reaction between tissue and dye is often poorly understood.

Histochemical methods for the study of chemically recognizable substances within tissues began many years ago with the iodine test for starch. Since that time, numerous correlated techniques have been developed for the identification and localization of specific molecules within cells. For example, in applying *spectrophotometry* to cytology, ultraviolet light is useful because nucleic acids absorb light more strongly in the ultraviolet region than in other regions of the spectrum. When a basophilic material such as RNA stains with a basic dye (such as pyronine or toluidine blue) but is unstainable after the section has been treated with pure ribonuclease which selectively removes RNA, it may be concluded that the stained material was RNA. This information may be correlated with the spectrophotometric data. A similar principle is used in the histochemical study of glycogen. In this case, the control slides are treated with saliva; the salivary enzyme amylase removes the glycogen.

The histochemical localization of the enzyme *acid phosphatase* is widely used to identify areas of lytic (digestive) activity in the cytoplasm (see below under "Lysosomes"). The section is placed in a fluid containing a phosphate compound and lead ions. The enzyme in the tissue frees the phosphate, which combines with the lead to form an insoluble precipitate which is visible in the electron microscope (see Fig. 1.40C). To make this visible in the light microscope, sulfide ions are added to form the coarser precipitate lead sulfide. Thus, the sites of dense reaction product may reveal the location of the enzyme.

Recently, very precise localizations of specific molecules have been possible through the use of *immunocytochemical* techniques. Here antibodies are prepared against specific molecules. The antibodies bind selectively to those molecules when exposed to them in a frozen or other type of section. If the antibody is combined directly or indirectly with a molecule which can be rendered visible by light or electron microscopy, the complex can be localized within the tissue section. Detection is often accomplished by combining the antibody to a molecule which glows when viewed in a light microscope under fluorescent light (*fluorescence microscopy*) (Fig. 1.2), or by combining the antibody with a heavy metal

such as gold which is visible by electron microscopy.

Radioautography is a technique whereby a radioactive form of a substance normally taken up by cells is supplied to living tissue. After incorporation, its intracellular location is detected by exposure to a coating of photographic emulsion applied to the specimen. The radioactivity lodged in the tissue activates the silver halide crystals in the emulsion, and with photographic development metallic silver grains are formed. They are visible in both the light (Fig. 1.3) and electron microscopes, depending upon the preparation. Again, more precise localization of activity results from the combined use of radioautography and electron microscopy. Electron microscopic radioautography has proven extremely useful in tracing the path of protein synthesis in the cell cytoplasm (see "Rough Endoplasmic Reticulum"). The use of radioactive thymidine, incorporated only into replicating

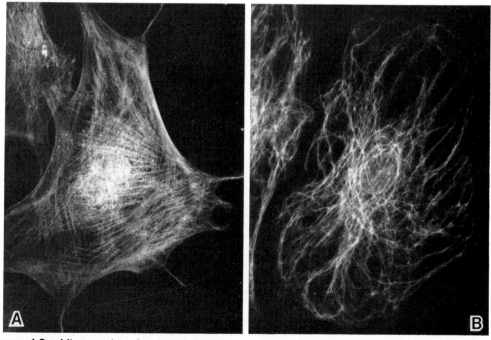

Figure 1.2. Micrographs of cultured fibroblastic cells (gerbil fibroma) prepared by the indirect immunofluorescence technique. *A*, reacted with antibody to actin, showing bundles of actin-containing microfilaments; *B*, reacted with antibody to tubulin, showing cytoplasmic microtubules (×150). (Courtesy of Dr. Lincoln Johnson).

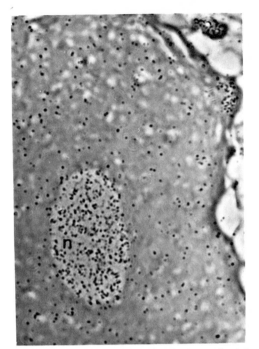

Figure 1.3. Radioautograph photographed in the light microscope. The black dots overlying the tissue are silver grains which mark the sites of incorporation of radioactive uridine into newly formed ribonucleic acid. The silver grains are more concentrated over the nucleus (*n*) than over the cytoplasm of this large lobster nerve cell (×500).

DNA, has been helpful in identifying dividing cells and in tracing cell migration in developing tissues.

The *preparation of sectioned tissue for examination in the electron microscope* must be done with extreme care. Fixatives are chosen to preserve structure in as life-like a form as possible; inferior preservation is far more apparent in the electron microscope than in the light microscope. A primary aldehyde fixation (glutaraldehyde or formaldehyde) coupled with a postfixation with osmium tetroxide is most commonly employed. Buffering to slightly above neutrality is beneficial for most tissues. A highly cross-linked embedding medium (such as the epoxy resins Araldite or Epon) is required in order to obtain the extremely thin sections that are examined in the elec-

tron microscope. Glass or diamond knives and specially designed microtomes are mandatory for such thin sectioning. Heavy metal "stains" (such as osmium, uranyl acetate, and lead citrate) are chosen for their ability to scatter electrons rather than to impart color. Because these techniques also yield preparations of superior quality for light microscopy, tissues prepared for electron microscopy are often sectioned at 1 or 2 μm, stained with a dye such as toluidine blue, and utilized for light microscopic study. Figure 1.4 is a semithin section prepared in this way.

The above methods provide information in direct association with a visible image of a cell or its parts. Many other important methods rely upon biochemical procedures in which cells are fractionated to isolate various components, and these in turn identified and characterized chemically. When such information can be correlated with the localization within intact cells as described above, an increasingly accurate understanding of cellular constituents and their interactions begins to emerge.

Major Microscopic Tools

An understanding of the observations made with different types of microscopes requires familiarity with the units of measurement in common usage and an appreciation of the dimensions of some structures commonly studied by biologists (Tables 1.1 and 1.2).

The usefulness of any type of microscope is dependent not merely upon its ability to magnify but, more importantly, upon its ability to resolve detail. The useful magnification of an ordinary light microscope is only about 1200×. The *resolving power* of a lens is its capacity to give separate images of objects close together. It is measured as the least distance between two points which can be seen as two instead of one. The resolving power is governed by the *numerical aperture* (NA) or light-gathering capacity of the objective lens and by the wavelength of light. Hence, in the light micro-

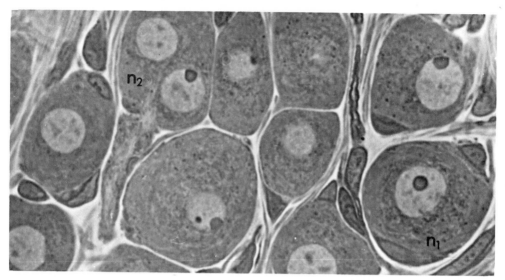

Figure 1.4. Nerve cells fixed and embedded in plastic for electron microscopic study and then sectioned at 1 μm and stained with toluidine blue for observation in the light microscope. This type of preparation is often termed a semithin section. At *lower right*, a typical neuron (n_1) is seen to contain a large pale nucleus with a dense nucleolus. A binucleate neuron (n_2) is also shown (×1100). (Reprinted with permission from M. B. Bunge, et al.: *J Cell Biol* 32:439, 1967.)

Table 1.1.
Measurements

Unit	Symbol and Definition
Micrometer (micron)	1 μm = 0.001 mm = 10,000 Å 1 μm = 1 × 10^{-3} mm
Nanometer (millimicron)	1 nm = 0.001 μm = 10Å 1 nm = 1 × 10^{-6} mm
Angstrom	1 Å = 0.1 nm = 0.0001 μm 1 Å = 1 × 10^{-7} mm

Table 1.2.
Dimensions of Some Elements Studied by Biologists

Structure	Dimension
Human ovum	100 μm 1,000,000 Å
Skeletal muscle cells (cross section)	10–100 μm 100,000–1,000,000 Å
Cardiac muscle cells (cross section)	9–20 μm 90,000–200,000 Å
Lymphocytes	6–10 μm 60,000–100,000 Å
Erythrocytes	7.7 μm 77,000 Å
Bacteria	0.1–10 μm 1,000–100,000 Å
Viruses	0.05–0.5 μm 500–5,000 Å (50–500 nm)
RNP granules (ribosomes)	0.015 μm 150 Å (15 nm)

scope, the resolution limit may be computed from the formula $R = 0.61\ \lambda/NA$, where R is the minimum distance between two resolvable points (in micrometers), λ is the wavelength of the light utilized (in micrometers), and NA is the numerical aperture of the objective lens in use. In practice, a yellow-green light with a wavelength of about 5400 Å is generally used, because the eye is more sensitive to this part of the spectrum, and with this light the limit of resolution of a 1.40-NA objective is 0.24 μm when a condenser with a comparable 1.40-NA is used to illuminate the specimen. With a 1.25-NA oil immersion objective, used on most student microscopes, the limit of resolution with a yellow-green light is 0.28 μm. A resolution of 0.17 μm can be achieved by using an oil immersion objective of 1.50 NA, but the refractive index of

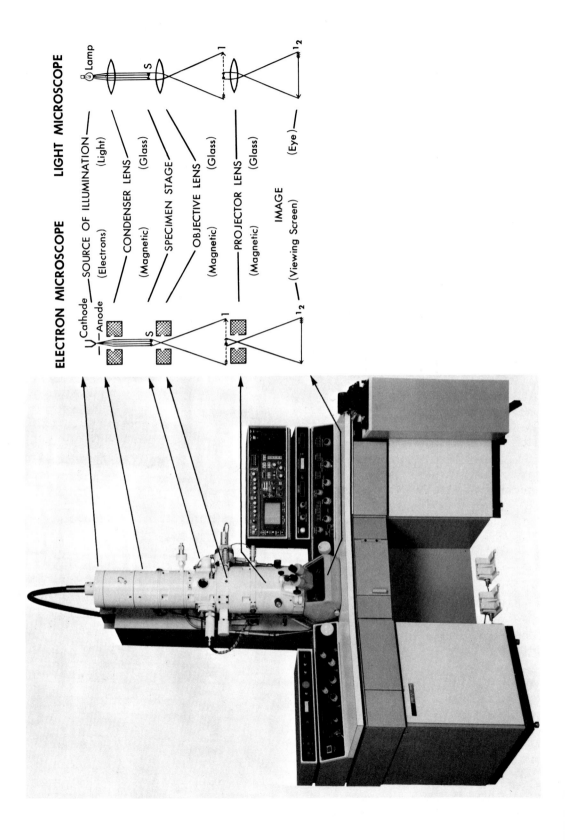

most optical material makes it impossible to increase the NA much further. It is evident that the way to increase resolving power is to use smaller wavelengths. However, glass lenses are not transparent to the wavelengths lower than 4000 Å, and it becomes necessary to use other refractive media. By using ultraviolet radiation having a wavelength of 2000 to 3000 Å and quartz lenses, resolving power can be increased to about 0.1 μm (100 nm, 1000 Å), but the main value of the ultraviolet microscope is for fluorescence labeling studies.

The chief advance in increasing resolving power has been made with the *transmission electron microscope*, which uses electrons in place of light, and electromagnetic fields as lenses (Figs. 1.5 and 1.6). The final image is visualized on a fluorescent screen and recorded on a photographic plate. The wavelength of a stream of high velocity electrons is so short that the resolving power of an electron microscope can be less than 3 Å (0.0003 μm) with test specimens and 5 to 10 Å with biological specimens. With this resolution, the electron microscope can be used profitably at very high magnifications. In common practice, the image is recorded at 1,000 to 100,000× and the photographic negative is enlarged 2 to 6× when the positive print is made, thus giving final magnifications to about 600,000×. The appearance of a typical cell by transmission electron microscopy is shown in Figure 1.7.

One limitation in transmission electron microscopy is the necessity of having extremely thin preparations (0.1 μm or less) because of the low penetration of the electrons. Another disadvantage stems from the fact that the tissues must be viewed in a high vacuum. Thus the study of living cells has not been possible with conventional specimens and instrumentation.

Current experimentation with ultrahigh voltage instruments (1,000,000 to 2,000,000 V) and special wet specimen chambers shows little promise of alleviating this limitation. Currently, the greatest advantage in using ultrahigh voltage instruments comes from the production of stereo images of much thicker (up to 1.0 μm) specimens. These aid visualization of intracellular components in three dimensions at high resolution.

The *scanning electron microscope* offers less resolution, but allows direct visualization and three-dimensional rendition of the surfaces of fixed and dehydrated cells, organs, or small organisms. The specimen, usually coated with a conductor such as gold, emits secondary electrons when struck by a focused scanning primary electron beam. The secondary electron emission for each point of the scanned specimen surface is amplified and synchronously displayed on a cathode ray tube, thus providing an electronic image such as is seen in Figure 1.8).

The desire to view cells and tissues without chemical fixation and without dehydration has led to another approach for preparing material for electron microscopy, called *freeze-fracturing* or *freeze-etching*. After rapid freezing of the tissue, a break is made directly through the frozen cells, and a delicate metal shadow cast is made of the fractured surface. This metal cast, called a *replica*, is then observed in the transmission electron microscope. The technique is especially used in the study of membranes, for the fracture frequently occurs in such a manner that it splits the leaflets of the membranes of cells and organelles. Thus, not only are the contours of membranous components revealed in the replica, but the technique also provides the first fairly direct method of visualizing the

Figure 1.5. Photograph of a modern electron microscope. The instrument shown may be used as a conventional transmission microscope (for viewing sections) or as a scanning electron microscope. Separate instruments of both types are also available. (Courtesy of JEOL (USA), Inc.)

Figure 1.6. Comparison of optical paths in an electron microscope (*left*) and a light microscope (*right*). The light microscope diagram is inverted to facilitate comparison. (Courtesy of RCA.)

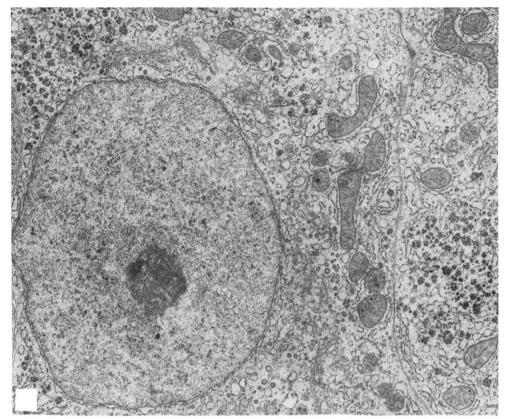

Figure 1.7. A transmission electron micrograph of a developing liver cell. Note the clarity of detail (resolution) as compared to that of even the best light microscope preparations (see Fig. 1.4). The cytoplasm contains organelles and inclusions that are considered in detail later in this chapter (×9950).

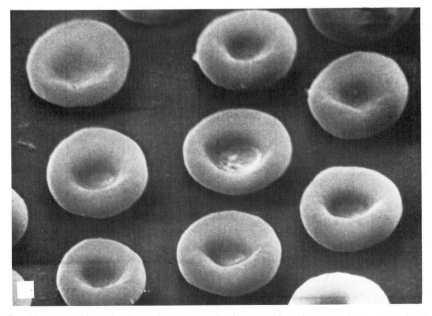

Figure 1.8. Human red blood cells as they appear in the scanning electron microscope. As illustrated here, this instrument allows unsectioned objects to be visualized in three dimensions (×3700). (Courtesy of Dr. Sarah Luse.)

interiors of individual membranes. Figure 1.9 is an electron micrograph from a freeze-fractured specimen.

The *phase microscope* is a modification of the light microscope particularly useful for the study of unstained cells, either living or fixed. Components of unstained cells usually appear indistinct with the ordinary microscope because they are fairly transparent and produce very little change in the intensity of transmitted light (Fig. 1.10*A*). On the other hand, the different proto-

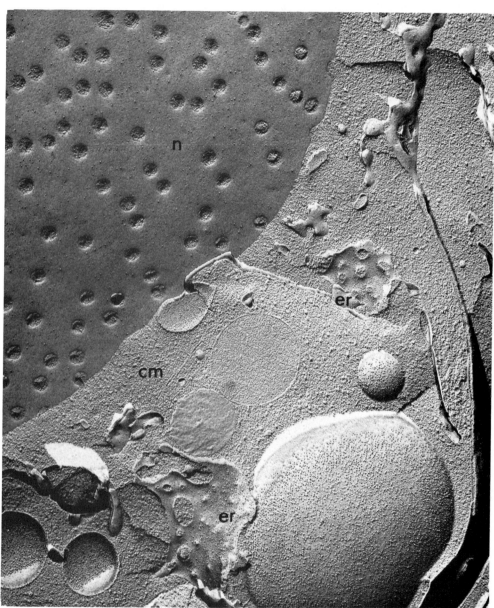

Figure 1.9. Electron micrograph of a platinum replica of a cell which was frozen without fixation and then fractured to enable visualization of the cell interior, especially membrane faces. After freeze-fracturing pores in the otherwise smooth nuclear envelope (*n*), sheets of fenestrated endoplasmic reticulum (*er*), the cytoplasmic matrix (cytosol) (*cm*), and a variety of cytoplasmic vacuoles are all clearly visible. Onion root tip (×36,000). (Reprinted with permission from D. Branton: *Proc Natl Acad Sci USA* 55:1048, 1966.)

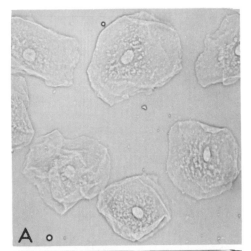

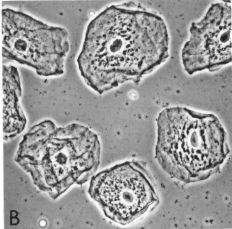

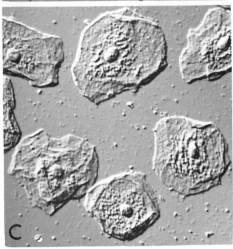

Figure 1.10. Epithelial cells from human oral mucosa as they appear in *A*, the bright field light microscope, *B*, the phase contrast microscope, and *C*, the Nomarski optical system (×250). (Courtesy of Carl Zeiss, Inc., New York.)

plasmic constituents produce phase changes because they vary in thickness and refractive index. The phase microscope converts phase variations into intensity variations and thereby enables the eye to detect more contrast between different structures (Fig. 1.10*B*).

The *interference microscope* utilizes the principles of the phase microscope more precisely. A light beam passing through the tissue is recombined with a separate light beam which has passed through the same optical apparatus without passing through the tissue. The manner in which these beams interfere with one another gives an index of the mass of the specimen, and it is thus possible to obtain precise information on the density of cellular regions, even in the living state. *Differential interference (Nomarski)* optics use similar principles and provides remarkable three-dimensional images of living cells and cell components (Fig. 1.10*C*).

The *fluorescence microscope* has recently come into common use. Selected wavelengths of light are used to illuminate the biological specimen. Specific molecules within the tissue absorb the light and emit light at other wavelengths. The exciting wavelength is absorbed with filters, and the emitted wavelength is viewed in the microscope objective. Because it is possible to label antibodies with molecules (such as fluorescein) that fluoresce under these conditions, it becomes possible to localize antigen-antibody complexes within tissues. This can be a most precise method of localizing specific proteins within tissues.

The resolution of these phase, interference, and fluorescence optics is, of course, limited to that of all light microscopes.

ORGANIZATION OF CELLS

Cells are the fundamental structural units of living organisms. Two essential features, revealed only with the advent of electron microscopy, characterize their structural organization. These are: (*a*) *compartmentation*, usually accomplished by the arrangement of systems of intracellular membranes; and (*b*) *cytoskeletal support* and *contractility*, performed by intracellular systems of various filaments acting upon the membrane systems. The basic medium which surrounds the cytoplasmic membrane and cytoskeletal components, as well as other structures to be discussed is sometimes termed the "*cytosol.*" Biochemists generally use the term cytosol for the component of fractionated cells that remains in suspension after prolonged high speed centrifugation. In this text we use the term to indicate the soluble components and otherwise unidentified constituents in which the organelles and inclusions are situated. Its main constituent is water. In combination with soluble organic molecules and salts, this cytosol forms a semifluid or viscid substance whose consistency varies in different cells or in the same cell under different conditions of physiological activity. The basic medium of the nucleus, termed *karyoplasm*, contains the dispersed chromosomal components and is ordinarily more viscous than the cytoplasm.

The chief ion of positive charge (cation) in solution in cell cytoplasm is K^+. The chief cation outside cells, in the general body fluids, is Na^+. Extracellular fluids contain about 120 meq/liter of Na^+ but less than 5 meq/liter of K^+; inside the cell a typical value is 10 meq/liter Na^+ and 140 meq/liter K^+. The tendency for Na^+ to leak into the cell and for K^+ to diffuse out to regions of lower concentration is counteracted by special properties of the cell membrane. The chief extracellular ion of negative charge (anion) is Cl^-; intracellularly, the important negatively charged molecules are HCO_3^-, HPO_4^{2-}, SO_4^{2-}, and certain proteins. The membrane surrounding most cells is quite impermeable to certain of these intracellular anions (which are osmotically active), and when membrane properties are altered and metabolic processes cease after death, the intracellular molecules tend to attract water and cells may swell.

The difficulties in understanding the life processes occurring within the cell derive in large part from their profound complexity and their remarkable miniaturization. The nucleus of human cells, which may be only a few micrometers in diameter, contains information (according to one estimate) for the manufacture of approximately 30,000 different proteins. A single cell may utilize 1000 or more different enzymes in the course of its day to day activities.

Early chemical analyses showed that the cell contains a high percentage of water and a host of small molecules, both organic and inorganic. The most characteristic components of the living cell, however, are the *macromolecules*: *nucleic acids*, *proteins*, and *complex carbohydrates*.

Biochemical fractionation and analysis indicate that many metabolic processes within the cell do not occur among constituents free in the cytosol. They occur instead within the framework of macromolecular formed elements called cell *organelles*. Many of these organelles are themselves membrane-bounded compartments, comprised of a complex of nucleic acids, proteins, and lipids. Each organelle is involved with discrete, though sometimes overlapping, metabolic and functional processes. In other words, *the contents of cells, collectively the protoplasm, are not a random biological broth but a collection of highly organized components distributed within the cell in a pattern suitable for their functional activities.*

Despite the fact that cellular components are a combination of materials, it is useful for the histologist to stain for specific components because such staining can indicate regions of exceptional concentration. For example, a lipid stain will clearly delineate the nerve myelin sheath (Fig. 1.1*C*). Myelin also contains protein and carbohydrate, but the exceptional concentration of lipids in myelin allows its differential staining. Thus, it is useful to discuss the major macromolecular components of cells in relation to methods for their histological demonstration.

Nucleic Acids

Nucleic acids provide the genetic blueprint for the most important products of the cell, the proteins, and the kinds and proportions of protein present give each cell its individuality.

Nucleic acids are complex compounds consisting of polymers of *nucleotides*. Each nucleotide contains a pentose sugar combined with phosphoric acid and with a nitrogen-containing base, either a purine (adenine, guanine) or a pyrimidine (thymine, uracil, cytosine). The phosphoric acid component gives the nucleic acids their marked affinity for basic dyes in stained preparations. On the basis of the type of pentose sugar, the nucleic acids fall into two groups: (*a*) *deoxyribonucleic acid* (DNA, containing the sugar deoxyribose) and (*b*) *ribonucleic acid* (RNA, containing the sugar ribose). The nucleic acids combine with the basic proteins, protamine and histone, to form nucleoproteins. The DNA molecule is composed of two long polynucleotide chains coiled around each other in the form of a double helix. Certain forms of viral RNA are known to be double-stranded, as is DNA; the conformation of native RNA molecules in animal cells is presently under active investigation.

DNA is found chiefly in the nucleus, confined to *chromosomes* which contain the genetic units called genes. DNA is the chief informational macromolecule of heredity. In the cytoplasm, small amounts of DNA are present within mitochondria (see below). The quantity of DNA in the nuclei of different cells of any given species is relatively constant, with the exceptions of mature germ cells, which have a reduced (*haploid*) number of chromosomes, and certain other cells, which may have a multiple (*polyploid*) number of chromosomes (some liver cells, for example). Naturally, there must be an increase in chromosomal DNA before chromosome division at mitosis; otherwise the DNA of the daughter cells would soon be depleted. Although the amount of DNA in the chromosomes of different cells is relatively constant, the amount of DNA-associated protein varies greatly. The latter is usually high in cells which have high metabolic activity in their cytoplasm (e.g., liver and kidney cells).

Ribonucleic acids are found both in the nucleus and the cytoplasm. This is because RNA is responsible for transcribing the genetic code stored in the structure of DNA, conveying it to the cytoplasm and then translating the code into the specific sequence of amino acids that make up the different proteins.

There are three major types of RNA in the cell, with differences in function. All are formed within the nucleus. *Messenger RNA* carries the transcribed genetic code in its linear sequence of bases and provides the actual template for protein synthesis. *Transfer RNA* serves to interpret the code provided by messenger RNA and simultaneously binds the amino acid the code specifies. As its name suggests, transfer RNA positions the attached amino acid in the forming polypeptide chain. However, for the transfer to occur properly, the messenger and transfer RNAs must interact with *ribosomal RNA*. Ribosomal RNA is the most prevalent form of RNA, and in the cytoplasm it occurs in combination with protein as discrete granules called *ribosomes*. Ribosomes provide the physical site at which assembly of the amino acids into protein takes place. They are synthesized as two subunits of different sizes that subsequently join to form the definitive ribosomes. The smaller subunit has a binding site for messenger RNA, and the larger subunit has two binding sites for transfer RNA. The latter are necessary for maintaining the proper topography for peptide bond formation and subsequent polypeptide chain elongation. The larger subunit also contains *peptidyl transferase*, the enzyme involved in formation of the peptide bond.

Ribosomes nearly always occur in clusters called *polyribosomes* or *polysomes*. Polysomes either lie free in the cytoplasm or may be attached to membranes of the endoplasmic reticulum. Attachment of ribosomes to the membrane of endoplasmic reticulum involves a separate binding site located on the large subunit.

Ribosomal staining in the cytoplasm is due almost entirely to ribosomal RNA; whether or not the ribosomes are attached to endoplasmic reticulum is irrelevant, and the protein of the ribosome contributes little to its staining properties. Ribosomes and endoplasmic reticulum are discussed further later in this chapter.

Reference has already been made to the fact that the identity of RNA can be confirmed by the use of a specific enzyme, *ribonuclease*. Although basophilia in itself is not a specific test for nucleic acids (other acids in the protoplasm attract basic dyes), it is true that many basophilic structures contain nucleic acids. It may be pointed out again that the nucleic acids occur in combination with proteins as nucleoproteins. The nucleoprotein reaction seen in sections stained with both basic and acidic dyes varies with the proportion of the different substances present. For example, the chromatin of the nucleus is very basophilic by reason of its high proportion of nucleic acid, whereas the nucleoprotein of the nucleolus is often acidophilic by reason of its proportion of certain basic proteins.

Amino Acids and Proteins

Proteins are indispensable for metabolic processes and structural organization of the cell. All enzymes, the vital catalysts of the chemical reactions in the cell, are proteins. Filament systems are almost entirely proteinaceous, and cellular membranes, while largely lipidic, contain many *integral proteins* and are coated with a wide variety of *glycoproteins* (discussed in detail later). Each type of protein is made up of a particular number and variety of amino acids joined in a precise sequence. Living systems contain about 20 different amino acids, each a single letter in the alphabet of protein structure. They have a characteristic capacity for combining with each other to form long chains. This property results

from the presence of a carboxyl group ($-$COOH) and an amino group ($-$NH$_2$) in each molecule. Condensation occurs when the acid group of one amino acid molecule combines with the basic group of another, with the loss of one molecule of water. This is known as peptide linkage, or a *peptide bond*. Chains of amino acids connected by peptide bonds are known as *polypeptides*. The sequence of amino acids in the peptide chain is very important. For instance, the hemoglobin of patients with sickle cell anemia differs from normal hemoglobin only in the substitution of a molecule of valine in the place of a molecule of glutamic acid.

Protein molecules consist of one or more peptide chains, and they have molecular weights ranging from 10,000 to 1,000,000 or more. These large molecules are generally described as having three levels of organization. The *primary structure* is provided by the amino acid sequence. The primary structure of a substantial number of protein molecules is known. Insulin, for example, is known to be composed of two polypeptide chains (with a total of 51 amino acids) bound together at two points by disulfide bonds between sulfur-containing amino acids within the chain. The *secondary structure* of proteins is formed when peptide chains spontaneously coil as a result of secondary bonding (such as hydrogen bonding) between their constituent amino acids. This secondary coiling produces the helical arrangement of the protein molecules. Sometimes these helical arrangements involve a number of polypeptide chains coiled together.

A *tertiary structure* of proteins may be formed when relatively straight sections of the polypeptide chain are bent at a number of points to fold the molecule up into a globular configuration. Many biologically active proteins (such as enzymes and hormones) are globular and are found in solution in the cytosol or in general body fluids. These globular proteins become partly unfolded in the presence of heat; this *denaturation* accounts for egg albumin's turning white upon heating. Histological *fixatives* are chemicals selected to stabilize the structural components of cells and tissues while causing as little change in protein conformation as possible.

Many proteins contain chemical entities in addition to amino acids; this forms the basis for another method of protein classification. The *simple proteins* yield only amino acids on hydrolysis. This group includes albumins, globulins, protamines, and histones. *Conjugated proteins* consist of a simple protein combined with another organic substance called the *prosthetic group*. The conjugated proteins yield amino acids plus the prosthetic group on hydrolysis. The conjugated proteins include nucleoproteins (proteins combined with nucleic acid), glycoproteins or mucoproteins (proteins combined with a carbohydrate), lipoproteins (proteins with fatty acids), and chromoproteins (e.g., hemoglobin).

The amino acids which form proteins contain groupings which ionize to form acids in some cases and bases in others. Thus, proteins may be predominantly acidic or basic and take up dyes which bind either to acid groups (basic or cationic dyes, such as methylene blue) or to basic groups (acid or anionic dyes, such as eosin). A commonly used stain, hematoxylin, contains components which together stain basophilic material (nucleic acids and acid proteins) blue and eosin colors acidophilic material (primarily basic proteins) pink or red (Fig. 1.1*A*).

Lipids

Lipids form a diverse group of compounds (including fats, phospholipids, glycolipid, and sterols) which are generally insoluble in water. They provide the most concentrated energy reserves of the cell. Fats, which contain fatty acids linked to glycerol, are generally stored within cells in droplets of varying size. These fats can be hydrolyzed to fatty acids and glycerol, and the fatty acids can then be oxidized for energy production. Further energy is derived as the 2-carbon fragments resulting from oxidation are used to fuel the citric acid cycle (see below).

Certain lipids, particularly *phospholipids* and *cholesterol*, form important components of cell membranes. The phospholipids are key compounds, for they have the important property of having a *hydrophobic end*, which repels water, and a *hydrophilic end*, which attracts water; this property contributes to the ability of the membrane to partition cellular regions of differing function. It should be noted that the steroid hormones are structurally very similar to the membrane component cholesterol, and one of their important effects is to alter the permeability of the cell membrane.

Some lipids, called *glycolipids*, are found in combination with sugar molecules, e.g., cerebrosides and gangliosides. These are also utilized in the construction of the cell membrane; it is believed that the lipid components form a major part of the membrane itself, with the carbohydrate component contributing to the surface hydrophilic coat of the membrane (see below under "Cell Membrane").

A substantial amount of lipid is extracted by the standard preparative techniques for histological sections. Lipids can be demonstrated either by the use of a lipid stabilizing fixative such as osmium tetroxide, or by freezing the tissues for sectioning, thus avoiding lipid solvents (Fig. 1.1*C*).

Carbohydrates

Many macromolecular compounds composed primarily of polymers of sugars, or which are protein-carbohydrate complexes, are exported from cells. Some become important constituents of the supportive and connective tissues of the organism. Others are components of body lubricants such as the mucus covering the surfaces of cells lining the gastrointestinal tract. Still others are stored within cells, as the most readily available energy reserve in the body. Carbohydrate compounds have been classified in many different ways. It is convenient to divide them into four general categories (*a*) polysaccharides, (*b*) polysaccharide-protein complexes, (*c*) glycoproteins, and (*d*) glycolipids (discussed above).

Polysaccharides are polymers of sugars.

The simplest polysaccharides are constructed from one repeating hexose unit. Their individuality is imparted by the types of chemical linkages within the polymer and the pattern of branching. The animal polysaccharide *glycogen* is a complexly branched polymer of glucose, as is plant starch. Both are stored within cells and are readily available for use when needed (Fig. 1.1*D*). Polysaccharides secreted by cells generally contain two or more monosaccharide components, one of which is an amino sugar. These are now referred to as *glycosaminoglycans*. Among these are *hyaluronic acid* (which is a copolymer of glucuronic acid and N-acetyl glucosamine) and *chrondroitin sulfate* (which is a copolymer of glucuronic acid and N-acetyl hexosamine sulfate). These molecules fom critically important extracellular lattices in connective and supportive tissues, where they impart appropriate degrees of viscosity and rigidity. They are commonly associated with protein by covalent bonds to form *proteoglycans* and these in turn many be linked to hyaluronic acid by noncovalent bonds to form proteoglycan aggregates. Proteoglycans are composed of 90 to 95% polysaccharide and only 5 to 10% protein.

Compounds containing substantial amounts of protein strongly (covalently) bound to smaller amounts of carbohydrate are usefully termed *glycoproteins*. These compounds are frequently found on the surfaces of cells. Glycoproteins are especially important in immunological reactions in the body.

STRUCTURAL AND FUNCTIONAL ORGANIZATION OF CELLS

Cells vary greatly in size, shape, and internal structure, as shown in Figures 1.11 and 1.51. These variations are adaptations for the different functions which the cells perform in different tissues and organs, and they are considered in more detail in succeeding chapters. Regardless of specialization, most cells retain a number of general characteristics in common (Fig. 1.12). The most obvious of these is the presence of many *organelles* and *inclusions* in common. Organelles are defined as cellular entities identifiable as distinct units with essential functions. Inclusions are variable in their presence and are not essential for the normal functioning of the cell. Examples of inclusions are secretory granules, fat globules and glycogen.

The Membranes of Cells

A *plasma membrane* or *plasmalemma* surrounds each cell, separating its contents from the external environment. In this important position it regulates the passage of materials into and out of the cell. This membrane, 7 to 11nm in thickness, is too thin to be resolved by the light microscope. However, it may be visualized if in an histological section it slants (and is thereby obliquely sectioned) and thus occupies an area wider than its true thickness. In addition, stain taken up by an exterior adherent coating on the membrane may enhance its visibility. Even when a cell membrane is not directly visualized, its presence can be inferred from observations on cells during micromanipulation, when cytoplasm spills out if the membrane is ruptured, and after alterations of the environmental tonicity. When red blood cells are placed in a hypotonic fluid or in water, they swell as a result of the action of osmotically active components of the cytoplasm. They may in fact burst, losing their contents (in this case, hemoglobin).

By treating red blood cells in the manner just described, it is possible to obtain a relatively pure preparation of plasma membrane for biochemical analysis. Such preparations contain about 35% lipid, including phospholipids and cholesterol, 60% protein, and a small amount of carbohydrate. From these data and from estimates of the surface areas of red cells, it is possible to calculate that there are enough lipid molecules to cover each cell twice. This observation, as well as physical measurements of membrane thickness, birefringence, X-ray diffraction, and surface tension, lent support to a model of membrane structure

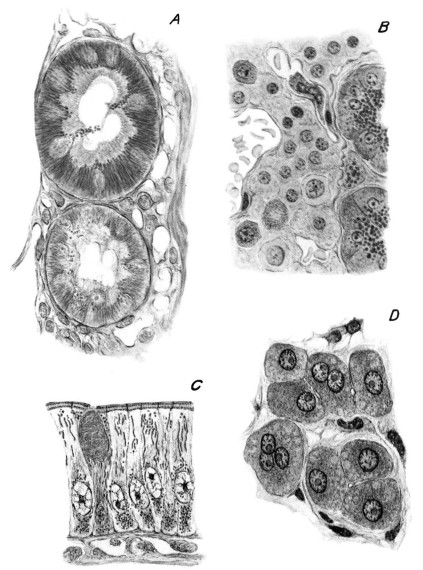

Figure 1.11. Staining of tissues by various techniques. *A*, kidney of mouse. Contrast the prominence of parallel red mitochondria in the proximal convoluted tubule *above* with the distal convoluted tubule *below*. Regaud, Altmann acid fuchsin. *B*, island of Langerhans from human pancreas, bordered at *right* by acinar cells, which show bluish basophilia and apical red secretion granules. In the island tissue are many B cells (orange), three red granular A cells, and two blue D cells. Helly, modified Masson. *C*, intestinal epithelium of cat, showing one goblet cell among absorbing cells. Note elongated red mitochondria and the striated cell border (*top*). Champy, modified Masson. *D*, liver cells from rhesus monkey filled with evenly distributed pinkish glycogen granules. One cell has two nuclei, another three, which is not uncommon. Biopsy, alcohol, Best's carmine. Camera lucida drawings. (Preparations by Dr. A. E. Severinghaus.)

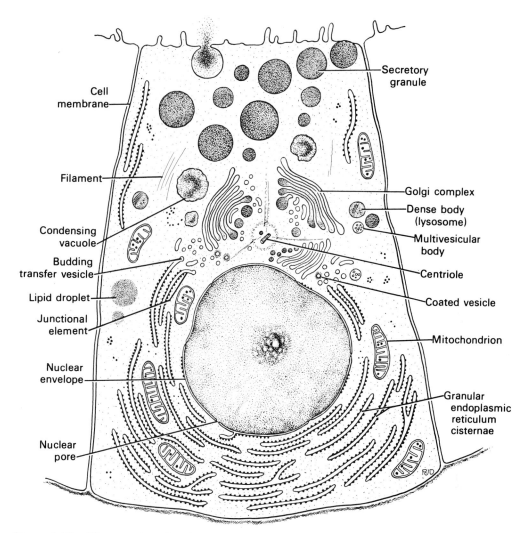

Figure 1.12. Diagram of a cell as it would appear in a thin section viewed in the electron microscope. All of the organelles depicted here are described in the text. The cell components and their organization indicate that this is a secretory cell. The secretory product is synthesized near the base of the cell in the region of the granular endoplasmic reticulum and is transported to the Golgi region, where it is packaged for release from the upper (apical) surface of the cell.

proposed by Danielli and Davson in 1935. This model depicts the plasma membrane as a double layer or bimolecular leaflet of lipids sandwiched between two protein coats (Fig. 1.13*B*). Although the location of protein in the model proved to be erroneous, the basic concept of phospholipid bilayers appears sound. The phospholipid molecules of the membrane have both hydrophobic ends, where the fatty acids are located, and hydrophilic ends, where the phosphate groups are attached. It is as-

sumed that the hydrophobic ends appose each other in the middle of the membrane, whereas the hydrophilic ends lie next to the enveloping protein layers. The presence of a continuous hydrophobic region could explain the low permeability of many membranes to water-soluble compounds and their high permeability to lipid-soluble materials. It is also consistent with the freeze-fracture data (see below).

When the cell membrane is sectioned at right angles to its surface and examined in

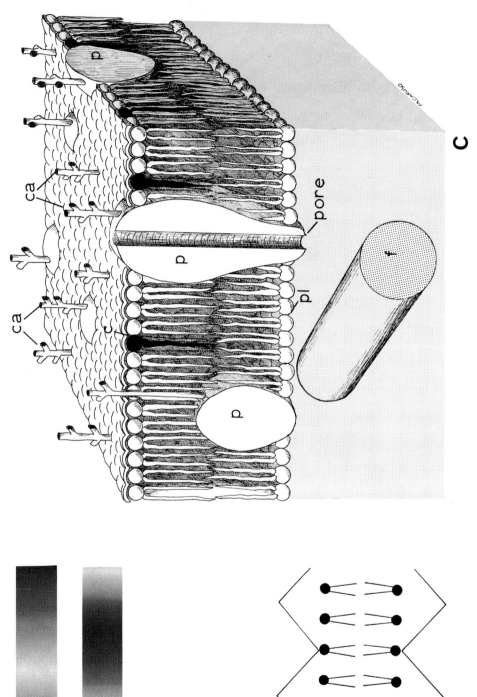

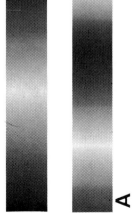

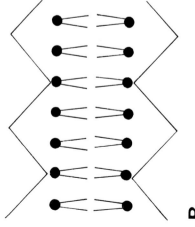

the electron microscope at lower magnifications, it appears as a dense line. High magnifications and staining make it possible to demonstrate that this line is, in fact, a pair of thinner dense lines separated by a light inner zone, all roughly of similar thickness (Fig. 1.13A). This triparite or *trilaminar* structure seemed to fit the Danielli-Davson model very well; the dense laminae correspnded to the two protein layers and the light intermediate stratum represented the bimolecular leaflet of lipid (Fig. 1.13C). The fact that many of the intracellular membranes also exhibited this trilaminar structure suggested that this was a basic design common to all membranes. Results of freeze fracture studies also support this concept. The fracture planes of rapidly frozen fixed or unfixed cells travel along pathways of lowest resistance, and typically such fractures tend to split membranes midway through their thickness. The splitting of membranes internally indicates an area of weak chemical interactions consistent with lipid hydrocarbon chains.

It seems clear, however, that a membrane with continuous lipid leaflets could not provide for all of the diverse functions that membranes are known to perform. It is now generally believed that, within the basic membrane structure described above, there are scattered sites whch provide for special membrane activities as, for example, the attachment of cytoplasmic filaments or the transport of sugars and amino acids across the membrane. At these sites, protein components apparently penetrate the lipid interface of the membrane (Fig. 1.13C).

Membranes are known to vary in protein content. In fact, the suggestion has been made that the protein content of membranes provides a rough index of their overall metabolic activity. Membranes, such as those comprising myelin, (a membranous wrapping around axons), that have a low protein content (about 20%) have little associated enzymatic activity and function passively in influencing electrical properties of nerve fibers. Mitochondrial membranes, on the other hand, contain dozens of enzymes and are composed of about 65% protein.

Gradually, it is being realized from newer analytical approaches to the study of cell membranes (especialy correlated biochemical and freeze-fracturing techniques), that a given cell membrane or territory of membrane is not likely to be a static mosaic in life. Rather, the evidence strongly suggests a "fluid" nature of membranes in which enzymes, attachment points, and reactive or permeability sites can be sequestered or dispersed in patterns or concentrations commensurate with physiological activity. Although the patterns of flux await further elucidation, one should consider the plasmalemma and other cell membranes in an often dynamic rather than static sense, displaying varying rates of renewal and the capability to mobilize appropriate molecular components at foci of specified activity.

Freeze-fracture techniques have provided a wealth of new information and hold con-

---

Figure 1.13. The appearance of the plasma membrane in electron micrographs is portrayed at *A*. At *B*, the Davson-Danielli bilayer model is shown. The central region of hydrocarbon chains of the phospholipid layers corresponds to the central light space in electron micrographs. *C* depicts the fluid mosaic model of membrane structure. The bimolecular leaflet contains phospholipids (*pl*), cholesterol (*c*), and proteins (*p*). Carbohydrate moieties (*ca*) extend from the external surface, some attached to protein and some to lipid. Some proteins (perhaps most) span the bilayer. Some are thought to form aqueous channels (pores) and some are involved with facilitated transport of certain ions or metabolites. Cytoplasmic filaments (*f*) may be closely associated with the membrane, and some microtubules (not illustrated) terminate near the membrane as well. The membrane bilayer exhibits fluidity, permitting integral proteins to move laterally, thus changing the sites of surface active areas, aqueous channels, and membrane interactions with microfilaments and microtubules.

siderable promise for further elucidation of membrane organization. It will be recalled that this method can be applied to unfixed and nondehydrated cells and tissues (as well as to fixed ones), and that it splits individual membranes so that the internal aspects of the cell membrane leaflets can be studied as well as the general contours and interrelationships of various membrane-bounded organelles (Figs. 1.9 and 1.14). Freeze-fracture methods reveal characteristic particles on the two exposed internal surfaces of a split membrane. It appears that these represent *integral proteins* or lipid-protein complexes and are related to the sites of localized enzymes, foci of attachment, or points of transmembrane transport. The composition and function of these *"intramembrane particles"* differ in different kinds of membranes, and these features are being intensively investigated by correlated biochemical and ultrastructural approaches.

On the exterior of the cell, appended to the surface of the cell membrane, is a layer of material containing substantial amounts of carbohydrates which are usually associated with lipids (glycolipids) or proteins (glycoproteins). This coat or *glycocalyx* may be very thick, as over the microvilli of epithelial cells of the intestinal mucosa (Fig. 1.15), or extremely thin, as that surrounding the membranes of the myelin sheath, but nevertheless it appears to be universally

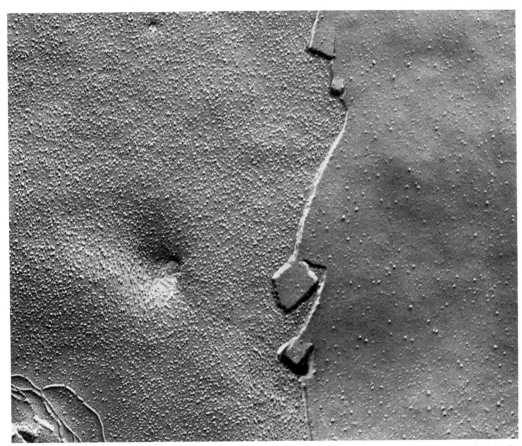

Figure 1.14. High magnification electron micrograph of a freeze-fracture replica showing split membranes of two neighboring cells viewed face-on. On the *right side* of the figure the fracture has split the membrane of one cell, exposing the outer face (E-face), whereas the *left side* shows the inner face (P-face) of the closely neighboring cell. Note the difference in numbers of intramembranous protein particles on the two faces (×59,250).

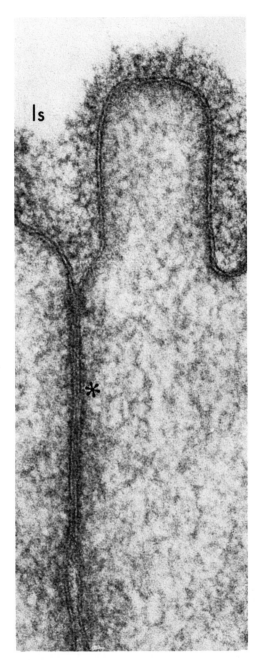

Figure 1.15. In the digestive tract the luminal surface (*ls*) of the absorbing cells is covered with highly regular finger-like protuberances called microvilli, one of which is pictured here. This electron micrograph clearly illustrates the trilaminar nature of the bounding cell membrane and shows the largely amorphous, "fuzzy" material coating the luminal surface of the cell. Along the lateral cell surfaces the bounding membranes may be more closely apposed than usual (as at *asterisk*) (×180,000). (Reprinted with permission from K.

present. Ionized groups on the terminal units of the saccharide chains (e.g., sialic acid) give many cell surfaces a negative charge. The presence of the glycocalyx and the negative charges undoubtedly contribute to the consistent and regular spacing of about 20nm which occurs between membranes of adjacent cells.

From the above discussion it will be apparent that there may well be as many different kinds of membrane as there are different kinds of cells and membrane-bounded organelles, endoplasmic reticulum, Golgi apparatus, lysosomal bodies, mitochondria and the nuclear envelope, and each may be capable of considerable change in life. *The intracellular membranes segregate the cytoplasm into compartments. These function in the storage of formed products, the control of interactions of substances in their proper order, the attachment of contractile and cytoskeletal proteins, and in increasing the surface area participating in metabolic processes.*

At the cell surface, the plasma membrane provides for the selection of what enters and what leaves the cell. In addition, in nerve and muscle cells the plasma membrane contains mechanisms to allow for sudden changes in ion permeability in response to changes in its electrical potential or configuration. It also has receptor sites for different kinds of chemcials such as hormones and neurotransmitters. Its surface characteristics determine how it relates to the surface on which it rests, and how it reacts (by adhesion, repulsion, or fusion) with other cells. The content and the configuration of the surface molecules are important factors in the immunological properties of the cell. These properties are maintained despite turnover of membrane constituents and exchanges of surface membrane with some of the intracellular compartments. The membrane may, in fact, be the most complex macromolecular

R. Porter and M. A. Bonneville: *Fine Structure of Cells and Tissues*, ed 3. Philadelphia, Lea & Febiger, 1968.)

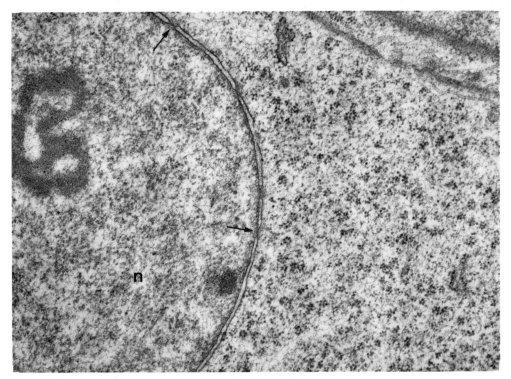

Figure 1.16. The envelope around the nucleus (*n*) of this sectioned developing cell displays a number of pores (*arrows*). The cytoplasm (*right*) is dominated by a high content of free ribosomes, many arranged in polysomal aggregates (×32,000). (Courtesy of Dr. Virginia Tennyson.)

aggregate in the cell, and the understanding of its structure and function is the key to understanding much of cell biology.

The Nucleus

The nucleus varies in shape and size in different types of cells. In rounded or cuboidal cells, it usually assumes a spherical form (Fig. 1.11*D*). In tall columnar or spindle-shaped cells, the nucleus is usually elongated, with its long axis corresponding to that of the cell (Fig. 1.11*C*). In cells whose cytoplasm becomes filled with inclusions, as in mucus-secreting and fat cells, the nucleus is generally flattened against the cell membrane (Fig. 1.1*C*). It usually reverts to a rounded form after such cytoplasmic constituents have been extruded.

In some cells, the nucleus becomes lobated, as in neutrophilic leukocytes and megakaryocytes. Cells with a lobed nucleus are often, although not always, in a highly differentiated stage and lack the ability to divide by mitosis (e.g., polymorphonuclear leukocytes). However, not all highly differentiated cells lacking mitotic ability have lobed nuclei. Although a cell usually has only one nucleus, some types, (e.g. parietal cells of the stomach, liver cells) often have two or more. Osteoclasts of bone usually have five or more nuclei.

Structure of the Nucleus

The interphase (nondividing) nucleus is bounded by a *nuclear envelope* and contains one or more *nucleoli*. Particles or clumps of *chromatin* are suspended in the nuclear ground substance.

The nuclear "membrane" described by earlier light microscopists is actually a unit of *two* closely apposed concentric membranes, the *nuclear envelope*. At intervals the two membranes curve together and join to form an opening, a *nuclear pore* (Figs.

1.16 to 1.18). The *inner* and *outer nuclear membranes* form a narrow enclosed space, the *perinuclear space*. It is isolated from the *nucleoplasm* within and from the *cytosol* without. The nuclear pores form channels which provide communication between nucleoplasm and cytosol. When the nuclear envelope is sectioned in a perpendicular plane, the pores appear to be spanned by a septum thinner than a regular membrane (Fig. 1.16), but when the pores are viewed face-on in tangential sections of the envelope their structure is seen to be complex (Fig. 1.18). The edge of the pore has an octagonal symmetry and the pore contents display a variable structure. A similar impression is gained from freeze-fracture images of the nuclear envelope, in which the pores are quite distinct (Fig. 1.9). The organization of the pores is of considerable interest because pores are known to play an important role in the exchange of materials between the nucleus and the cytoplasm. The nuclear envelope is related to the cytoplasmic endoplasmic reticulum because ribosomes may be attached to the membrane surface facing the cytoplasm (Fig. 1.17), continuities between the outer membrane and the sacs of endoplasmic reticulum are frequent, and the envelope is reformed from endoplasmic reticulum elements near the end of each cell division (all aspects to be discussed in detail below).

The *nucleoli* are round, dense, well defined bodies, although they do not have a limiting membrane. In general, there may be from one to four per nucleus, although they vanish temporarily during part of the division cycle. They are composed of RNA and associated proteins. Nucleoli usually stain intensely, but they exhibit a variable basophilia and acidophilia in different cells and at different times, depending on the relative proportions of RNA and basic protein.

The nucleolus contains fibrogranular and filamentous forms of ribonucleoprotein associated with the DNA of particular regions of certain chromosomes (Fig 1.19). After cell division the nucleoli are reformed at these *nucleolus organizer* sites. The nucleolus is important functionally as a factory for the assembly of the two subunits of cytoplasmic ribosomes. This accounts for their special prominence in nuclei of cells active in the synthesis of large quantities of secretory products.

Dispersed throughout the nucleus is DNA, the carrier of the hereditary code. The DNA double helix is about 2nm in diameter; the proteins adhering to this strand increase the diameter to 4 to 5 nm. Histone proteins have a primary structural role and nonhistone proteins are involved mainly with the regulation of gene expression. Thus, proteins play a role in the expression of activity of DNA, and they lend support to the helix as well. The DNA strands are intimately associated with certain histones to form repeating units, the *nucleosomes*. A supercoiling of this complex results in the appearance of threads that stain with basic dyes; these are termed *chromatin* (from the Greek *chroma*, color). Masses of these extremely long threads intertwine throughout the nucleus; it has been reported that an individual strand may be as long as 22,000 μm in human lymphocyte nuclei. Chromatin threads are too thin to be resolved in the light microscope, thus explaining why many nuclei appear nearly empty (Fig. 1.1*A* and *B*). Collectively, the networks of these diffuse thin nucleoprotein threads are termed the *euchromatin*. They represent potentially active regions along the DNA strands where *transcription* of the genetic code can take place.

At certain intervals along the thread, however, the DNP is additionally coiled, forming condensed clumps which can be seen in the light microscope (Fig. 1.20). These clumps, scattered throughout the nucleoplasm, but especially common along the nuclear envelope, are called *heterochromatin*; they stain brilliantly with basic dyes. Heterochromatin is believed to contain relatively inactive DNA, and when present in

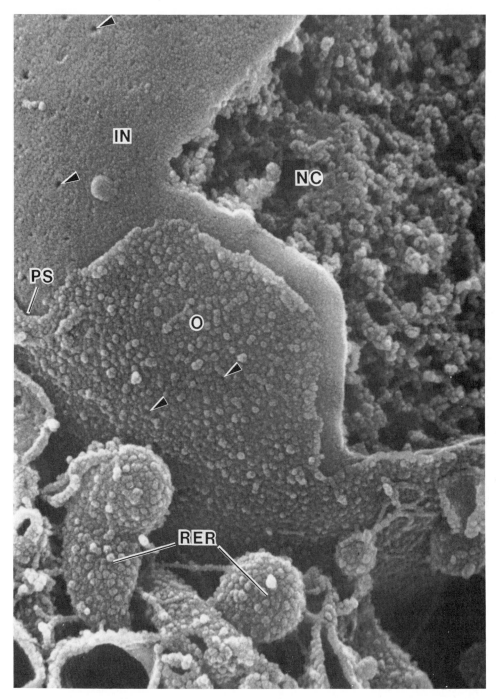

Figure 1.17. High resolution scanning electron micrograph of the nucleus of a cell (*upper two thirds of field*) and some nearby cytoplasmic territory. The inner (*IN*) and outer (*O*) nuclear membranes have been cracked away to reveal nucleoplasm and chromatin (*NC*) as well as the perinuclear space (*PS*) of the nuclear envelope. Note nuclear pores (*arrowheads*) and cisterns of rough endoplasmic reticulum (*RER*). Ribosomes are seen on the surface of the rough endoplasmic reticulum and the outer nuclear membrane (×100,000). (Reprinted with permission from K. Tanaka, et al: *Arch Histol Jpn* 39:165–175, 1976.)

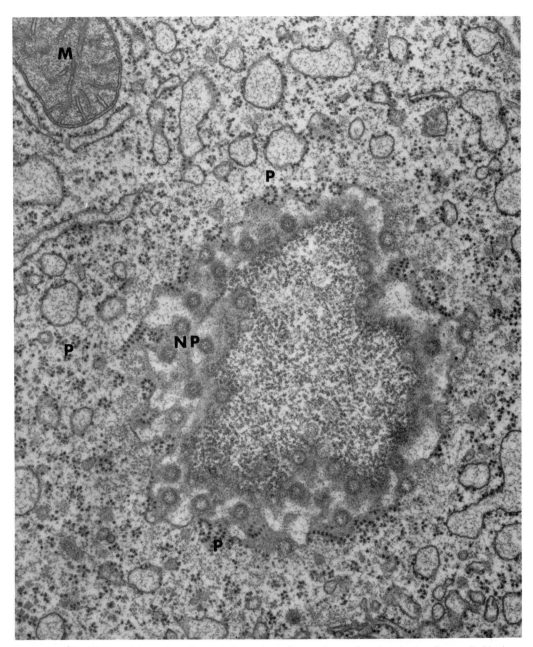

Figure 1.18. Tangential section through the edge of a nucleus of a developing liver cell. Nuclear pores show internal structure. Polyribosomes are associated with the cytoplasmic surface of the nuclear envelope and also occur free in the cytoplasm. *M*, mitochondrion; *NP*, nuclear pores; *P*, polyribosomes (×33,800).

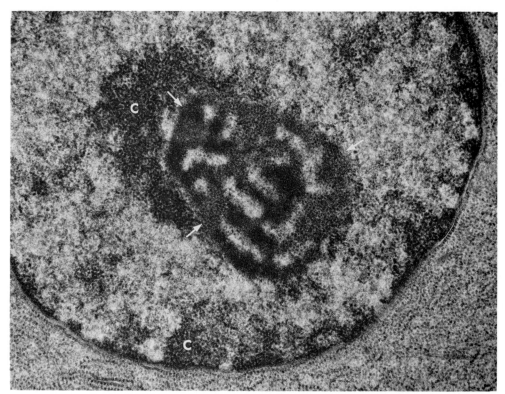

Figure 1.19. Electron micrograph, showing nuclear heterochromatin and a nucleolus. The nucleolus, indicated by *arrows*, contains granular and fibrillar elements which may be organized into a dense, meandering strand or network called the nucleolonema. Clumps of heterochromatin (c) abut on the nucleolus and the nuclear envelope. Acinar cell from bat pancreas (×25,000). (Reprinted with permission from D. W. Fawcett: *The Cell: Its Organelles and Inclusions.* Philadelphia, W. B. Saunders, 1966.)

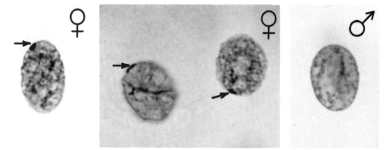

Figure 1.20. Photomicrograph of four isolated nuclei in a smear of oral mucosa cells from normal adult subjects. The dark areas in each are clumps of heterochromatin. The three nuclei on the *left*, obtained from females, each contain a small dense body situated near the nuclear envelope. These Barr bodies are not found in nuclei from males, as shown on the *right*. Thionin staining (×1800). (Reprinted with permission from M. L. Barr: In Overzier C (ed): *Intersexuality.* New York, Academic Press, 1963, p 48.)

prominent clumps is indicative of a cell quiescent from the standpoint of transcribing genetic information. In young cells where genetic transcription and protein synthesis are intense, the euchromatin predominates. But with maturity, increasing amounts of heterochromatic clumps become obvious near the end of the cell's life cycle. The whole nucleus may become small, very darkly staining, and homogeneously dense, a state termed *pycnosis*.

During mitotic cell division, (discussed fully in Chapter 2) the chromatin threads become condensed into *chromosomes* (Fig. 1.21). Division is the only time when the entire length of each chromatin thread is condensed into a unit that is visible by light microscopy. The configurations, as well as the number, of the mitotic (metaphase) chromosomes are constant, thus allowing their individual identification and analysis.

One of the sex chromosomes remains condensed in the nondividing or interphase cell and is known as the *Barr body*. First described in 1949 by Barr and Bertram, it is the second X chromosome, present normally only in females. Males normally contain one X and one Y chromosome in each cell of the body. Apparently, one X chromosome (but not more than one) must exist in an extended state because it participates in a number of metabolic activities other than sex determination. The Barr body constitutes a cytological marker for female

cells (Fig. 1.20) and is an aid in the clinical determination of sex in intersexual states as well as in studies of certain congenital diseases.

Considering the widely dispersed and/or coiled nature of chromatin, it is not surprising that electron microscopic observations of nuclei in thin sections reveal only a wealth of granules and very short filaments (Fig. 1.19). If chromosomes of the dividing cell are processed for electron microscopy without sectioning, their overall configurations can be appreciated (Fig. 1.21). Visualization of regionally active loci or *genes* on the chromatin threads is now beginning to be realized. (Fig. 1.22).

Functions

The standard histological section offers clues regarding nuclear activity. As has been discussed above, the degree of condensation of the chromatin is an inverse index of the amount of genetic material that is involved in synthetic activities. Cells with large, pale nuclei containing little condensed heterochromatin (such as neurons,

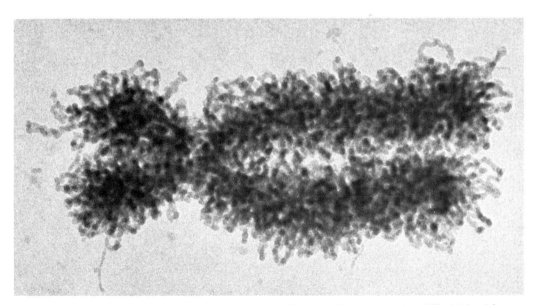

Figure 1.21. Electron micrograph of an unsectioned human chromosome (no. 12) obtained from a dividing cell. The chromosome is divided in half along its length (into two chromatids) except at the centromere. This chromosome weighs 13.2×10^{-13} g and contains about 4 cm of DNA double helix per chromatid. Some of the looping and coiling which allows the packing of all of this DNA into a chromosome 3 μm in length is visible ($\times$40,200). (Reprinted with permission from E. J. DuPraw: *DNA and Chromosomes.* New York, Holt, Rinehart and Winston, 1970.)

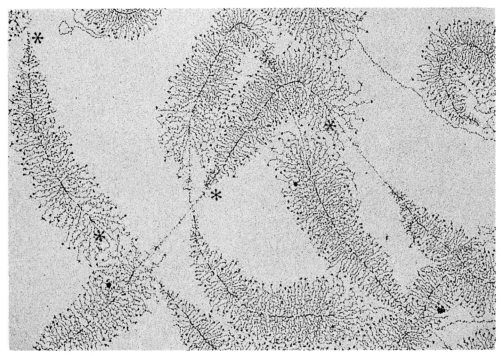

Figure 1.22. During the development of amphibian oocytes, the DNA increases sharply in amount and is contained within the 1000 or so forming extrachromosomal nucleoli. When this DNA is maximally unwound, it is seen in the electron microscope to be an extremely slender strand with periodic adherent material arranged in a feather-like pattern. Each "feather" (as indicated between *asterisks* in two areas here) is about 2.5 μm long and results from the attachment to the DNA axis of 100 forming ribonucleoprotein molecules in progressive stages of completion. Thus it is shown that about 100 precursor molecules of ribosomal RNA are being formed simultaneously at each gene. ×25,000. (Reprinted with permission from O. L. Miller, Jr., and B. R. Beatty: *Science* 164:955, 1969.)

Fig. 1.1*A* and *B*) are metabolically very active cells. Nucleoli are small (or absent) in cells which are not actively forming proteins (e.g., mature leukocytes) and generally large in cells which are actively synthesizing proteins (e.g., nerve cells, cells of regenerating tissues, and embryonic cells which must continually replenish their proteins).

One aspect of an abundant literature concerning nuclear cytoplasmic relationships has involved bisecting unicellular organisms so that only one part retains a nucleus. The part without the nucleus gradually dies, whereas the nucleated portion survives. With the removal of the nucleus, the DNA-RNA-protein production sequence is stopped, and the anucleate part lives only as long as survival time of its already available RNA and protein molecules permits. The overall importance of the nucleus has been nicely stated by Allfrey: *"The cell nucleus, central and commanding, is essential for the biosynthetic events that characterize cell type and cell function; it is a vault of genetic information encoding the past history and future prospects of the cell, an organelle submerged and deceptively serene in its sea of turbulent cytoplasm, a firm and purposeful guide, a barometer exquisitely sensitive to the changing demands of the organism and its environment."*

Cytoplasmic Organelles

Cytoplasm contains a number of organelles suspended in a background matrix which has been termed the *"cytosol."* The cytoplasmic organelles include ribosomes, endoplasmic reticulum (with and without ribosomes), Golgi apparatus, lysosomes, peroxisomes, centrosome and centrioles, mitochondria, filaments, and microtubules.

Ribosomes

As noted earlier in this chapter, the cytoplasm contains RNA, the nucleic acid involved with translation of the genetic code and formation of the myriad of specific cellular proteins. The major part of cytoplasmic RNA is combined with protein to form *ribosomes*, recognizable in electron micrographs as dense granules averaging 15 nm in diameter (Figs. 1.23 and 1.24). By light microscopy, areas rich in ribosomes are intensely basophilic, as is nuclear chromatin. Early cytologists correlated the cytoplasmic basophilia with the production of secretory granules and termed the basophilic substance *ergastoplasm* (from the Greek *ergastic*, a workman).

Highly basophilic cells include those engaged in synthesizing secretory proteins, such as pancreatic and salivary acinar cells, and cells in active growth stages, such as lymphoblasts, myeloblasts, and osteoblasts. Ribosomes occur freely in the cytoplasm *or* are lined up on flattened sacs of endoplasmic reticulum membrane (Figs. 1.23 and 1.24). *Ribosomes associated with endoplasmic reticulum are involved mostly in the formation of proteins for export from the cell or proteins to be incorporated into the membranes of the cell itself* (so-called *integral proteins*). When the ribosome is attached to endoplasmic reticulum, the *exportable* proteins produced are delivered into the reticulum cavities rather than into the cytosol (Figs 1.23, 1.25, and 1.26). *The free ribosomes, on the other hand, are involved primarily in the formation of proteins, including enzymes, for intracellular use.* In rapidly growing and dividing cells, which are increasing in cytoplasmic volume, free ribosomes are the most prominent of the cytoplasmic organelles (Fig. 1.16).

The present understanding of how ribosomes function in protein synthesis has been provided by a combination of biochemical and cytological techniques. The use of radioactive tracers has been particularly important in delineating the steps involved. By utilizing isolated ribosomes it has been demonstrated that if appropriate messenger and transfer RNAs are present, these organelles have the unique ability to incorporate amino acids into proteins.

Each ribosome is composed of approximately 60% RNA and 40% protein. The

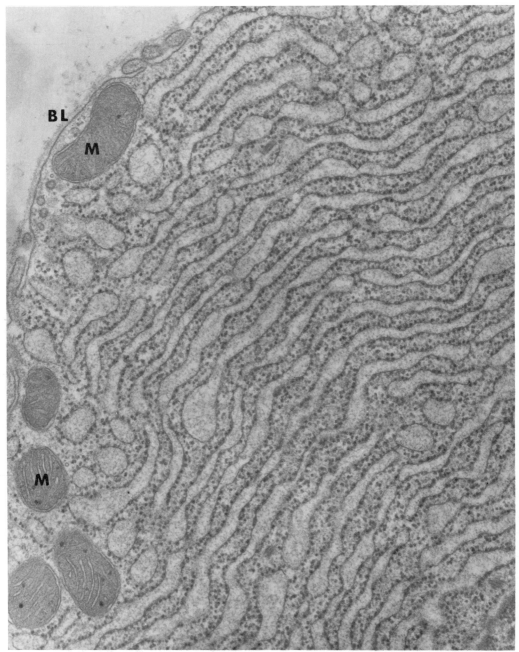

Figure 1.23. Ribosomes, the majority of which are associated with endoplasmic reticulum membranes in a pancreatic secretory cell. The base of the cell with its basal lamina appears at the *upper left*. *M*, mitochondria; *BL*, basal lamina (×42,000).

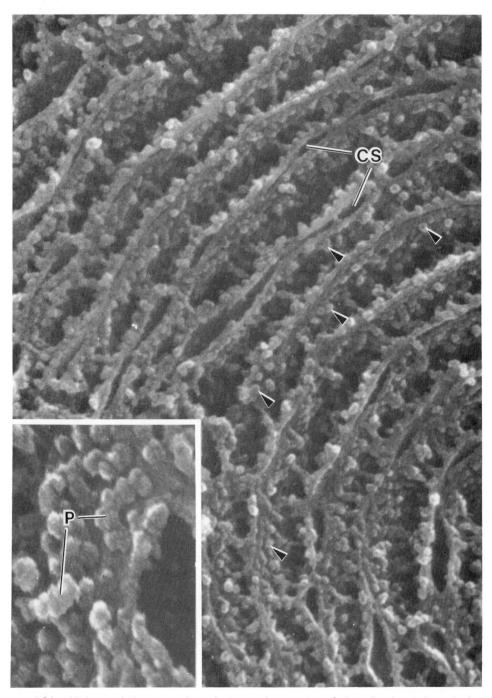

Figure 1.24. High resolution scanning electron micrographs of the sliced rough endoplasmic reticulum of a pancreatic acinar cell. Ribosomes (*arrowheads*) are arranged along the cytosol-facing surfaces of the cisternae. Cisternal spaces (*CS*) are narrow. *Inset*, high magnification view of a cisternal wall showing details of several polysomes (*P*) (×68,000; inset ×265,000). (Courtesy of Dr. K. Tanaka.)

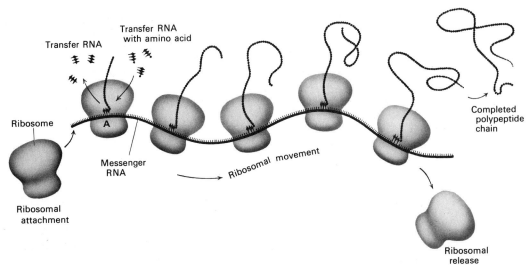

Figure 1.25. This diagram depicts the role of ribosomes in synthesis of protein for intracellular use. A polysome is formed as ribosomes attach, one by one, to one end of a strand of messenger RNA (mRNA). The binding to mRNA takes place on the smaller of the two ribosomal subunits. A molecule of transfer RNA (tRNA) becomes activated by linking with a specific amino acid; there are some 20 different tRNA molecules, one for each amino acid. The nature of the mRNA sites present in the receiving area of the ribosome (*A*) determines which tRNA, and thus which amino acid, is used. Thus, as the ribosome progresses along the mRNA strand, the code is translated by the tRNAs, which deposit in correct order the amino acids required for the production of a specific protein. The longer the mRNA strand, the farther the ribosome must travel and the greater the number of amino acids assembled. Each ribosome makes a complete chain. That there are five ribosomes in a polysome at a given time, as drawn here, is determined by the mRNA molecule. When the ribosome reaches the end of the strand, it is released and is available for reuse with the same or a different species of mRNA, and the completed polypeptide chain is liberated. (Diagram based upon drawings and descriptions by A. Rich.)

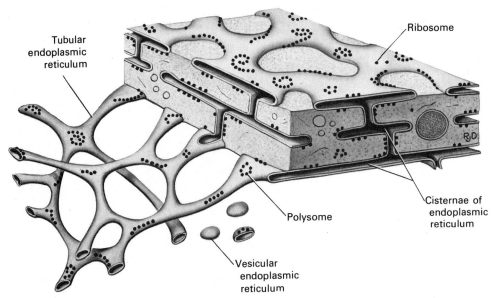

Figure 1.26. Diagram illustrating the interconnected cisternae and tubules of granular endoplasmic reticulum.

protein is extremely heterogeneous; over 75 different proteins with specific positions have been described for each ribosome. As explained earlier, the ribosome is made up of subunits of different sizes. The subunits are synthesized separately and only join together at the time protein synthesis is actually occurring. During this active phase of their life cycle they are associated in clusters (*polysomes*, Fig. 1.27) that vary in size according to the size of the polypeptide strand being synthesized and the length of the messenger RNA coding for that polypeptide. In the immature red blood cell which is synthesizing hemoglobin, polysomes contain an average of five ribosomes, and the polypeptide chains formed contain about 150 amino acids. In developing muscle cells which are producing myosin, an average of 56 ribosomes constitute a polysome involved with assembly of more than 1800 amino acids into the polypeptide

chain. The longer mRNA strand has spaces for more ribosomes and requires each ribosome to travel farther, thus providing for the assembly of a greater number of amino acids (as explained in Fig. 1.25). This assembly process is rapid: the entire globin chain of 150 amino acids requires about one minute.

Rough Endoplasmic Reticulum

The *endoplasmic reticulum* was first seen in 1945 by Porter, Claude, and Fullam, who were able to examine very thinly spread, cultured fibroblasts in one of the early electron microscopes. The presence of this lace-like network (or reticulum) in the inner or endoplasmic region of the cytoplasm (although it is not always so distributed) led to its name. Endoplasmic reticulum exists in the form of tubules and broad, flattened sacs (*cisternae*) of membrane in sheets in-

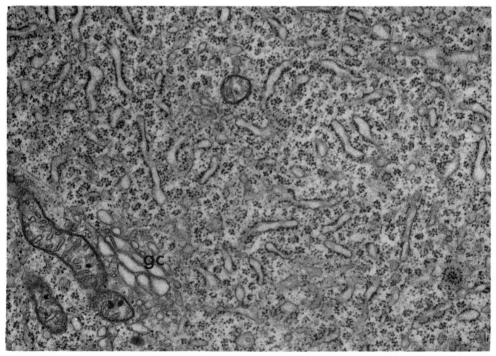

Figure 1.27. This electron micrograph shows a region containing free ribosomes and granular endoplasmic reticulum in the cytoplasm of a mature neuron. Compare this with the immature nerve cell shown in Fig. 1.16. Where the cisternae are cut *en face* (as at *lower right*), the coiled, looped, or curved arrangement of attached ribosomes in the polysome is clearly seen. Part of a Golgi complex (*gc*) and mitochondria appear at *lower left* (×29,000).

terconnected by branchings and anastomoses (Figs. 1.23, 1.24, and 1.26). Ribosomes may cover much of the endoplasmic reticulum surface; this association of ribosomal granules and endoplasmic reticulum is termed *rough* or *granular endoplasmic reticulum.*

Ribosomes attach both to endoplasmic reticulum membrane and to the outer membrane of the nuclear envelope, with which the endoplasmic reticulum is continuous, and to no other membranes of the cell (Fig. 1.17). When the reticulum membrane is sectioned perpendicular to its surface, the ribosomes dot the surface at more or less regular intervals (Fig. 1.23); when the membrane is sectioned such that patches of its cytoplasmic surface are visible, many of the ribosomes are seen to occur in circle, loop, spiral or rosette arrays which are the membrane-associated polysomes (Figs. 1.26 and 1.27). Occasionally, the proteins synthesized on the ribosomes are visible as dense or filamentous material within the lumina of the reticulum elements (Fig. 1.23).

The amount and configuration of the granular endoplasmic reticulum depend upon the cell type and the physiological state of the cell. The pancreatic acinar cell, which synthesizes and secretes exported packets of proteinaceous digestive enzymes (zymogen granules), is highly basophilic in its basal region. Such an area is filled with numerous granular endoplasmic reticulum cisternae which are regularly packed in parallel rows (Figs. 1.12, 1.23, and 1.24). Relatively few of the ribosomes lie free in the cytosol.

The pancreatic acinar cell is a good system for tracing newly synthesized exportable proteins through the cell, partly because different organelles involved at different times are concentrated in different regions of the cytoplasm. The ribosome-encrusted cisternae of endoplasmic reticulum are located chiefly in the basal portion of the cell, along with the nucleus and mitochondria (an energy source). The apical region of the cell, nearer to the lumen into which the product will be emptied, contains

numerous *zymogen granules* (Fig. 1.11*B*), interspersed with a few granular reticulum elements. In between these two regions (above the nucleus) there is a well developed network of *Golgi apparatus* oriented around two centrioles (see diagram, Fig. 1.12). The synthesis, intracellular transport, storage, and discharge of the digestive enzymes have been examined extensively by administering the radioactive amino acid leucine to an animal and later examining its pancreatic acini by means of light and electron microscopic radioautography (Figs. 1.28 to 1.31). The path of the exportable protein through the cell can be detected by looking for radioactive sites at various time intervals. Such sites indicate the presence of the leucine as it is used in the synthesis of new exportable proteins. These studies show that the proteins are synthesized on the ribosomes attached to endoplasmic reticulum and are transported within the reticulum to the Golgi zone, where they become concentrated and packaged into zymogen granules for temporary storage. In this manner the contents remain isolated from the remainder of the cytoplasm.

Two major questions remain: (*a*) How do proteins being synthesized on ribosomes attached to the cytosol side of the endoplasmic reticulum membrane gain access to the cisternal space? (*b*) How is the newly sequestered protein transferred from the reticulum cisternae to the Golgi cisternae, since continuities between the two membrane compartments are seldom seen?

The most widely accepted explanation for the first question is the so-called *signal hypothesis.* According to this hypothesis (for which there is a fair amount of supportive evidence), an initial segment of the forming peptide chain of secretory or integral membrane proteins contains a sequence of amino acids that signals the large ribosome subunit to attach to the reticulum membrane. Attachment is thought to occur at specific sites that are then triggered to interact with the ribosome in some unknown way to permit vectorial transit of

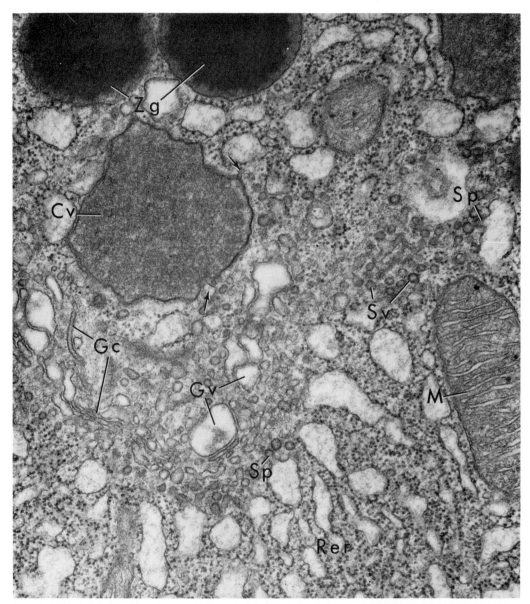

Figure 1.28. Electron micrograph of a portion of a pancreatic exocrine cell from a slice of a guinea pig pancreas incubated for 3 hr in vitro. The ultrastructure of the incubated cell is approximately the same as that of pancreatic cells fixed at biopsy. Note that the rough-surfaced endoplasmic reticulum (*Rer*) is composed partly of rough-surfaced and partly of smooth-surfaced cisternae. The latter have projections (*Sp*) into the Golgi complex, toward clusters of smooth-surfaced vesicles (*Sv*). Some of the latter are in contact (*arrows*) with the limiting membrane of a condensing vacuole (*Cv*). *Gc*, Golgi cisternae; *Gv*, Golgi vacuoles; *M*, mitochondrion; *Zg*, zymogen granules. This is a control specimen for comparison with pancreatic slices that were pulse-labeled with radioactive [³H]leucine and then postincubated for varying periods in order to study the secretory cycle by electron microscopic radioautographs. See next three figures (×43,400). (Reprinted with permission from J. D. Jamieson and G. E. Palade: *J Cell Biol* 34: 1967.)

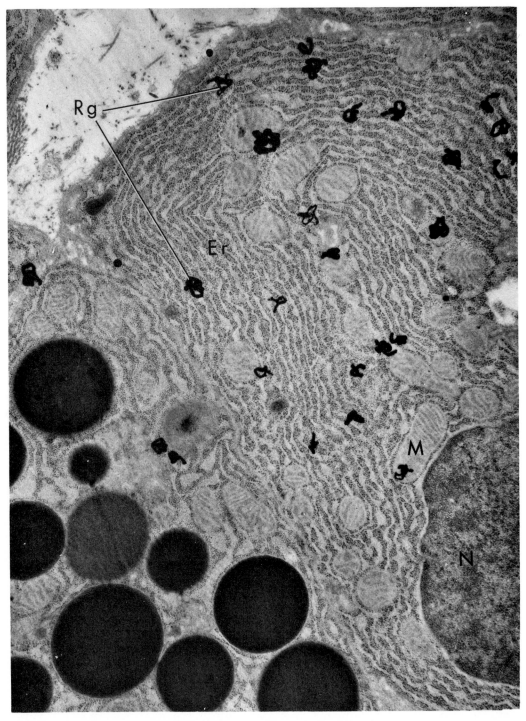

Figure 1.29. Electron microscopic radioautograph of a pancreatic exocrine cell from a slice of pancreatic tissue that was pulse-labeled in vitro for 3 min with L-[³H]leucine. Note that the radioautographic grains (*Rg*) are present chiefly over the rough surfaced endoplasmic reticulum (*Er*). *M*, mitochondrion; *N*, nucleus (×17,500). (Reprinted with permission from J. D. Jamieson and G. E. Palade: *J Cell Biol* 34: 1967.)

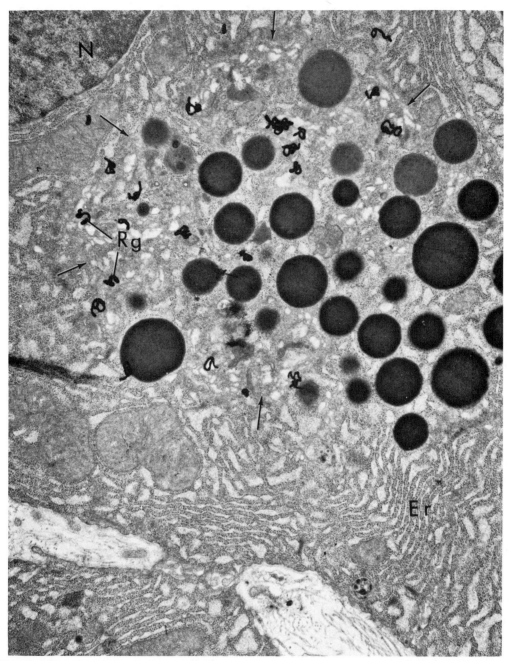

Figure 1.30. Electron microscopic radioautograph of a pancreatic exocrine cell after 3 min of pulse labeling, similar to that used for the cell shown in Figure 1.28, plus 7 min of postincubation. Note that most of the radioautographic grains (*Rg*), indicating the position of the labeled leucine, are present at the periphery of the Golgi complex (marked by *arrows*). *Er*, endoplasmic reticulum. (×16,700). (Reprinted with permission from J. D. Jamieson and G. E. Palade: *J Cell Biol* 34: 1967.)

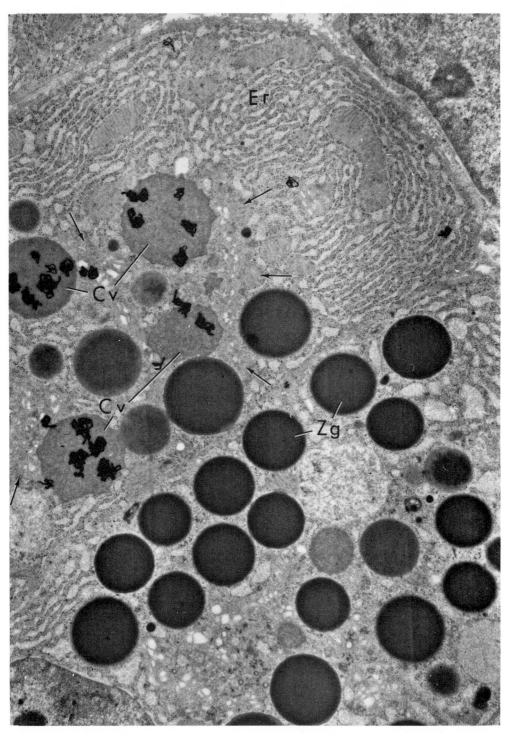

Figure 1.31. Electron microscopic radioautograph of a pancreatic exocrine cell after 3 min of pulse labeling, as shown in Figure 1.28, plus 37 min of postpulse incubation. The periphery of the Golgi complex is indicated by *arrows*. Note that most of the radioautographic grains are present over condensing vacuoles (*Cv*). This series of radioautographs shows that the secretory material, synthesized from leucine and other amino acids at the sites of ribosomes of the rough-surfaced endoplasmic reticulum, *Er*, is transported via cisternae to the Golgi region, where is is concentrated within condensing vacuoles which become zymogen granules (*Zg*) (×12,500). (Reprinted with permission from J. D. Jamieson and G. E. Palade: *J Cell Biol* 34: 1967.)

the nascent peptide chain through the reticulum membrane. The signal sequence, being first to enter the cisternal space, is then cleaved off by a signal peptidase, leaving the intact protein in the lumen.

As to the mechanism of transfer of the luminal protein in the endoplasmic reticulum to the Golgi elements, there are areas of endoplasmic reticulum bordering the Golgi zone, that may be part rough and part smooth; these cisternae are called *transitional elements*. Interspersed among them are swarms of small vesicles (about 50 nm in diameter) which occasionally appear continuous with, or budding from, the cisternae (Figs. 1.28 and 1.32). There is substantial evidence that these vesicles, termed *transfer vesicles*, ferry the synthesized product to the Golgi elements. The newly synthesized proteins are later visualized in *condensing vacuoles* (Fig. 1.31). These vacuoles, found in the Golgi zone,

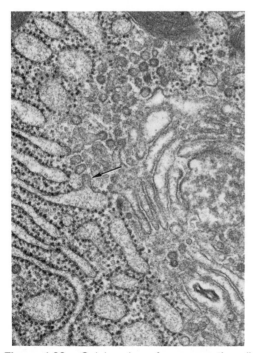

Figure 1.32. Golgi region of a pancreatic cell showing transfer vesicles between the endoplasmic reticulum and the Golgi membranes. At the *arrow* a transfer vesicle is pinching off from a cisterna of endoplasmic reticulum (×34,000).

are the sites of progressive accumulation and concentration of protein; they will become the spherical, more dense zymogen granules (see discussion below).

Smooth Endoplasmic Reticulum

Endoplasmic reticulum devoid of ribosomes (*smooth endoplasmic reticulum*) is primarily in the form of tubules which are often interconnected, tortuous, and very closely packed (Fig. 1.33). Although smooth endoplasmic reticulum elements may be continuous with rough reticulum, the constituent membrane appears thinner and is more difficult to preserve. The occurrence of smooth reticulum in cells was not recognized before the use of the electron microscope because it lacks distinctive staining properties.

The smooth endoplasmic reticulum is known to perform a variety of functions depending upon the cell type in which it resides. In liver cells, this organelle is considered to function in lipid and cholesterol metabolism. (The liver cell is exceptional in that it contains numerous arrays of smooth as well as rough reticulum, reflecting the manifold activities of these cells.) Smooth reticulum also aids in detoxification processes, e.g., by hydroxylation. When lipid-soluble drugs such as barbiturates or certain carcinogens are given to animals, greatly enlarged arrays of smooth reticulum appear in the hepatic cells. There is a concomitant increase in drug-metabolizing enzymes in smooth membrane fractions isolated from these cells. Investigators speculate that the toxic agent is taken up in the lipid portion of the induced membrane and is thereby brought into contact with the detoxifying enzymes associated with the same membrane. Glycogen particles often are enmeshed between the channels of liver smooth reticulum, suggesting a functional relationship.

In the interstitial cells of the testis, and in the cells of the ovarian corpus luteum and adrenal cortex, the extensive smooth

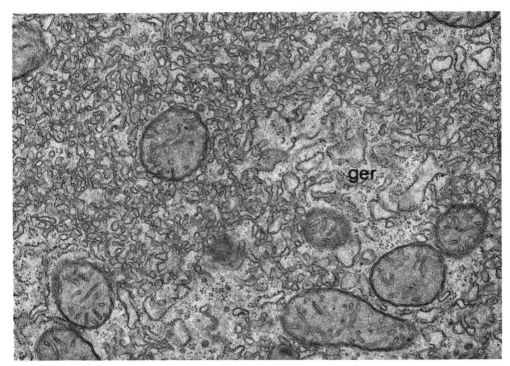

Figure 1.33. Interspersed among the mitochondria and elements of granular (rough) endoplasmic reticulum (*ger*) of this liver cell are slender anastomosing tubules of agranular endoplasmic reticulum. The agranular reticulum is increased in response to the administration of phenobarbital (which is detoxified in these regions) (×26,000). (Courtesy of Dr. Don W. Fawcett.)

reticulum is considered to participate in cholesterol synthesis and in the production of steroid hormones. The smooth reticulum contained within cells lining the intestine is involved in the metabolism and transport of lipids from components absorbed from the intestinal lumen. The prominent smooth endoplasmic reticulum in the gastric parietal cells is thought to participate in the secretion of chloride ions. Finally, the elaborate tubular network of smooth reticulum in muscle (sarcoplasmic reticulum) functions in sequestration of calcium (see Chapter 8).

The Golgi Apparatus

The *Golgi apparatus*, discovered by Golgi in 1898, is one of the organelles involved in secretory activity. It is either distributed throughout the cytoplasm or confined to a zone near the nucleus, depending upon the cell type. In elongated cells which border on an enclosed space, the Golgi complex lies betweeen the nucleus and the free surface border of the cell. In the light microscope, the Golgi apparatus is visualized after treatment with silver or osmium tetroxide, which is reduced to a black deposit (Fig. 1.34). In cells which synthesize a carbohydrate product, the Golgi region is stained magenta by the periodic acid-Schiff (PAS) technique. Vigorous controversy about the reality of this cell organelle persisted until the era of the electron microscope, when the Golgi apparatus was recognized as a ubiquitous cell structure of consistent form. The Golgi apparatus is composed of closely packed stacks of agranular membrane cisternae with associated vacuoles and vesicles (Figs. 1.28 and 1.35 to 1.37). Each stack may be curved; those cisternae on the convex or "outer" face often are more flattened than those on the concave or "inner" face.

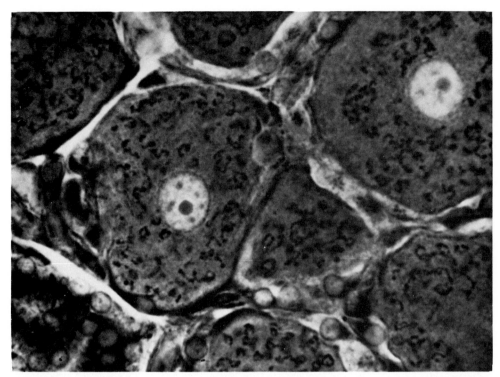

Figure 1.34. Scattered throughout the cytoplasm of these large neurons are dense ribbon-like deposits revealing the distribution of the Golgi apparatus. Light micrograph of a 5-μm section; Nassonow-Kolatschew technique (×914). (Reprinted with permission from W. Hild: Nervensystem. In von Möllendorff (ed): *Handbuch der Mikroskopische Anatomie des Menschen*, part 4. Vienna, Springer-Verlag, 1959, p 116.)

The role of the Golgi apparatus in concentrating and packaging secretory products has been firmly established. The protein moiety formed by the ribosomes associated with endoplasmic reticulum becomes contained *within* the reticulum cisternae. Post-translational processing begins immediately with the addition to the new protein of core carbohydrate components. Almost all proteins exported by the cell contain some carbohydrate. The product is then transported via small vesicles (*transitional vesicles*) to the Golgi apparatus where post-translational modifications are continued. In the Golgi cisternae, terminal glycosylation is accomplished, and sulfation occurs for those secretion products where this is a part of the synthetic sequence.

Early electron microscope studies reported a typical cupshaped organization of the Golgi apparatus with the convex aspect more closely associated with the endoplasmic reticulum and the concave portion displaying secretion droplets in various stages of formation and maturation (e.g., see Figs. 1.35, 1.36, and 1.37). This gave rise to the concept of a *"forming" ("cis") face* and a *"maturing" ("trans") face* for the organelle. More recent evidence has shown, however, that this is an overly simplistic view of the organization and function of the Golgi apparatus. In fact, the Golgi region is a major metabolic center in the cell. It serves to direct the traffic of most membranous organelles and their products in terms of secretion, uptake, and intracellular shuttling. Because of the multitude of functions, it is now clear that the polarization is not constant, and that there is a continual flux of membrane and various segregated products at the periphery of the cisternal stacks (Fig.

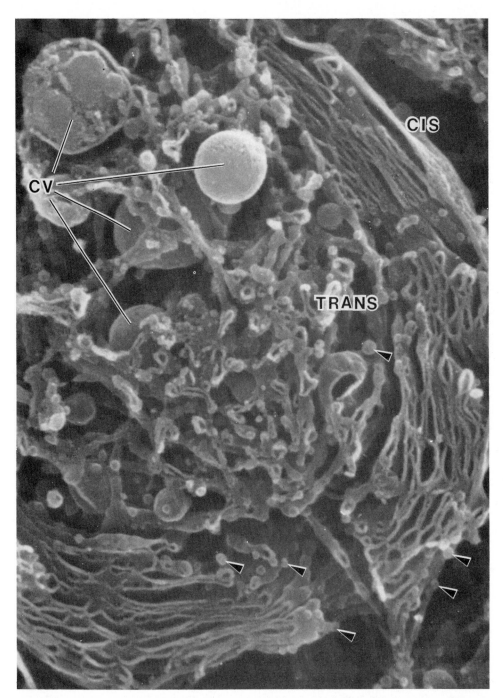

Figure 1.35. High resolution scanning electron micrograph of a sliced Golgi complex. The convex "forming" face (*CIS*) as well as the concave "maturing" face (*TRANS*) are visible. Note the abundant transfer vesicles (*arrowheads*) and larger condensation vacuoles (*CV*) (×42,000). (Reprinted with permission from K. Tanaka and T. Kinose: In Allen R, et al (eds): *Three Dimensional Microanatomy of Cell and Tissue Surface.* Netherlands, Elsevier-North Holland, 1981, pp 21–32.)

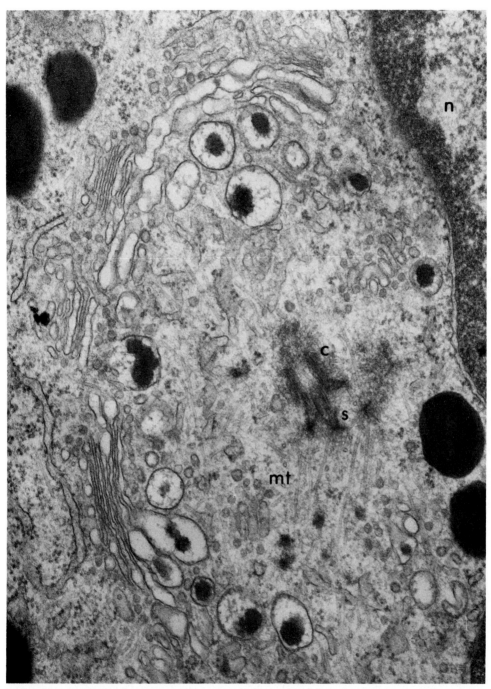

Figure 1.36. This electron micrograph is dominated by Golgi complex cisternae, which are curved around the centrioles (one of which is indicated at *c*) and toward the nucleus (*n*). Microtubules (*mt*) radiate from densities associated with the centrioles (pericentriolar satellites, *s*) and may be seen as circles (when sectioned transversely) or as double lines (when longitudinally sectioned). The largest dense inclusions here are azurophil granules, typical components of this cell, a polymorphonuclear leukocyte. They arise from the inner (or concave) surface of the Golgi complex by budding off the cisternae. They first appear as dense-centered vacuoles and gradually change into large, dense granules (×50,000). (Reprinted with permission from D. F. Bainton and M. G. Farquhar: *J Cell Biol* 28:277, 1966.)

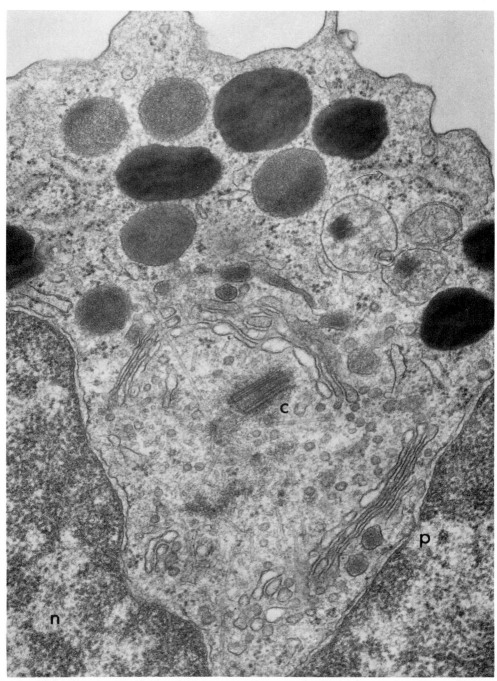

Figure 1.37. This electron micrograph shows other polymorphonuclear leukocyte granules, the specific granules, in various stages of formation from the outer or convex face of the Golgi complex at a later stage of development than that represented in Figure 1.36. Beneath the Golgi complex, in the cell center, is a longitudinally sectioned centriole (*c*). Extending from this region are straight profiles of microtubules. In the envelope surrounding the nucleus (*n*) are several pores, one of which is designated *p* (×50,000). (Reprinted with permission from D. F. Bainton and M. G. Farquhar: *J Cell Biol* 28:277, 1966.)

1.38). Thus, although the *cis-* and *trans* faces are usually recognizable morphologically, the directionality of flow of components being processed by the Golgi apparatus cannot be inferred with certainty from the morphology alone.

One of the important functions of the Golgi apparatus is to package products for secretion with a membrane that is plasma membrane-like. This presumably permits fusion of secretion droplets with the plasma membrane without grossly disturbing its normal polarity and permeability characteristics. However, the membrane added to the cell surface in this manner does not seem to be identical with that already present, and there is considerable evidence that much, if not all, of this membrane is promptly recycled by being taken back into the cell as small vesicles. The vesicles move

back to the Golgi region where the membrane appears to be re-utilized in the formation of other secretion droplets. A further discussion of membrane recycling appears below relative to other organelles and overall "*membrane traffic.*"

In addition to the functions already enumerated, the Golgi apparatus is involved with the assembly of the glycoprotein complexes characteristic of the outer surface of the plasma membrane and has a role in the formation of at least one other membranous organelle, the lysosome.

Lysosomes

By centrifuging the mitochondrial fraction in graded concentrations of sucrose, a class of organelles different in enzymatic content from mitochondria was discovered by de Duve in 1955. Enzymatic activity was

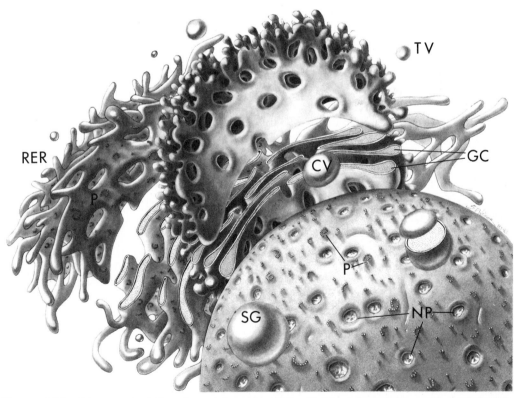

Figure 1.38. Diagram depicting the relationship of the Golgi apparatus to rough endoplasmic reticulum (*RER*) and the nucleus. *CV*, condensing vacuole; *GC*, dilated Golgi cisternae; *NP*, nuclear pores; *P*, polyribosomes; *SG*, secretory granule; *TV*, transitional vesicle.

not fully evident until the membrane bounding the particle became more permeable or was broken—a characteristic of importance for the cell, as discussed below. The dozen or more enzymes associated with these organelles, the *lysosomes*, are *hydrolases*. They function in the breakdown of proteins, carbohydrates, and nucleic acids at acid pH (e.g., cathepsins, glycosidases, sulfatases, phosphatases, ribonuclease, deoxyribonuclease).

The search for lysosomes in intact cells led to the realization that they are present in nearly all animal cell types (Fig. 1.39).

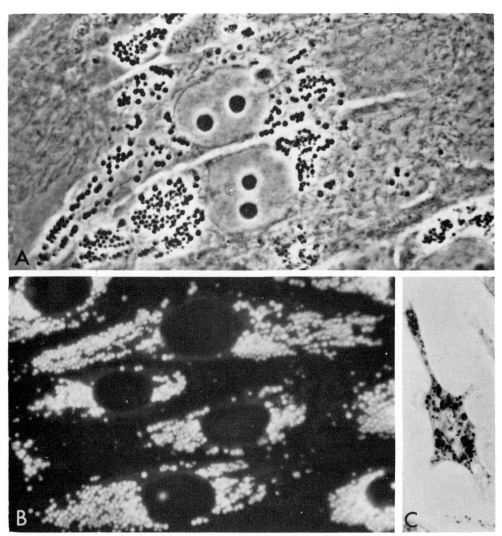

Figure 1.39. Lysosomes. *A*, as they appear in the phase contrast microscope in living monkey kidney cells. The lysosomes are the small black granules near the nuclei and may be compared to the light gray filamentous mitochondria in the more peripheral cytoplasm (×1200). *B*, as they appear in the fluorescence microscope. The brightly fluorescing granules are lysosomes which have taken up the fluorescent compound methylcholanthrene administered to similar cells in culture. Nuclei and mitochondria do not fluoresce (×550). *C*, after the Gomori method, the lysosomes appear as blackened granules in the light microscope. They are "stained" black by the deposition of a reaction product, lead sulfide, which results from the presence of an enzyme (acid phosphatase) characteristic of lysosomes. Mouse macrophage (×1130). (Reprinted with permission from A. Allison: *Sci Am* 217:62, 1967.)

Lysosomes are heterogeneous in size and content but are always bounded by a single membrane (Fig. 1.40). A lysosome may be identified in tissue sections on the basis of its acid phosphatase content. Acid phosphatase activity is revealed by the presence of a lead product resulting from enzymatic breakdown of an exogenous substrate in the presence of lead ions, the entire reaction occurring at pH 5.0 (Figs. 1.39C and 1.40C). Lysosomes are also identified by their ability to take up vital dyes (such as acridine orange) or drugs which can be traced intracellularly by fluorescence microscopy (Fig. 1.39B).

The lysosomes perform a variety of important roles for the cell. *Intracellular digestion* is one of the most important (see Fig. 1.41). Lysis takes place within the confines of membrane-enclosed digestion vacuoles, with no visible damage to the cytoplasm outside because the lysosomal membrane prevents enzyme release. An example of intracellular digestion is provided by the polymorphonuclear leukocyte. Its numerous specific granules are in fact lysosomes. When this white cell engulfs bacteria, the granules cluster around the newly formed vacuole, fuse with its limiting membrane, and discharge their content of destructive enzymes into the vacuole.

During starvation the lysosomal system may aid cell survival by the sequestration and digestion of a given cell's own organelles (*autophagy*), thus providing reserve nutrients for continued life. Autophagy is also involved with normal turnover of organelles and removal of damaged organelles. Substances in excess are digested by the lysosomal system as well; for example, vacuoles or vesicles of excess stored hormone are eventually broken down by lysosomes of the same cell.

Injurious substances which may or may not be digestible are sequestered within the lysosomal system. Cells exposed to silica or asbestos particles, for instance, are seen in the electron microscope to have lysosomes filled with the dense spheres or rods characteristic of these substances.

The list of compounds known to alter the permeability of the lysosomal membrane is extensive. Cortisone decreases the permeability, whereas vitamin A has the opposite effect. When a cell is deprived of oxygen or is damaged in some other way, the lysosomal membrane becomes more permeable or ruptures, thus allowing enzyme release with ensuing digestion of the cell (*autolysis*). Important questions under investigation are whether mitosis might be triggered by lysosomal digestion of a substance which normally represses division and whether certain types of cancer could result from chromosomal breakage by the lysosomal enzyme, deoxyribonuclease.

Related to the lysosomal population are *multivesicular bodies*, membrane-bounded bodies containing smaller membrane-bounded vesicles. Transitional forms between these organelles and regular lysosomes are often seen. Histochemical procedures have demonstrated that multivesicular bodies contain some acid hydrolases, notably acid phosphatase.

Lysosomes are formed in the cell by a similar sequence to that for production of secretory droplets. The constituent enzymes are synthesized on rough endoplasmic reticulum, transported to the Golgi region where they are sorted from other components, and sequestered into separate membrane-bounded bodies. The sorting appears to be accomplished by the addition of mannose-6-phosphate to lysosomal enzymes, which directs them specifically to a lysosome. At this stage of first appearance they are called *primary lysosomes*. Primary lysosomes can be stored in the cell for considerable time periods (for example, the primary granules in white blood cells), but more frequently, they soon fuse with a phagocytic vacuole and the released hydrolytic enzymes commence their degradative activity. Once lytic activity is initiated, the bodies are termed *secondary lysosomes*; the multivesicular body is one form of secondary lysosome (Fig. 1.41). Secondary lysosomes are extremely heterogeneous in structure and content. This stems from the

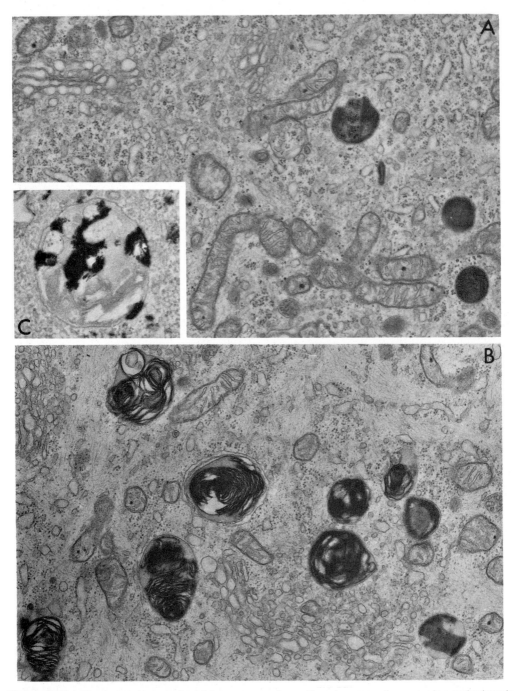

Figure 1.40. Electron micrographs of lysosomes. *A*, scattered among the granular endoplasmic reticulum, mitochondria, and Golgi complex. In normal tissue, lysosomes appear homogeneous or contain particles and stacked membrane-like structures. If the cultured nervous tissue illustrated here is given a tranquilizer, chlorpromazine, the lysosomes increase in number and size and take on a more heterogeneous appearance (*B*), as is typical for lysosomes after a variety of treatments. *C*, a chlorpromazine-induced lysosome after staining for acid phosphatase. The presence of dense patches of reaction product allows positive identification as a lysosome (*A* and *B*, ×24,000; *C*, ×34,500. *B* and *C* reprinted with permission from C. F. Brosnan, et al.: *J Neuropathol Exp Neurol* 29:337, 1970.)

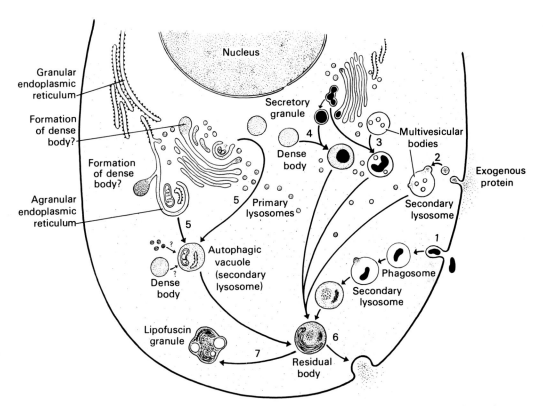

Figure 1.41. Summary of pathways in the lysosomal digestive system. A foreign body such as a bacterium is taken into the cell by invagination of the surface membrane, which then pinches off (endocytosis) (1). A *phagosome* thus formed acquires lytic enzymes by fusion with *primary lysosomes*, i.e., lysosomes which have not yet engaged in enzymatic activity. The resulting body is a *secondary lysosome*, i.e., a lysosome in which lytic activity is in progress or has occurred. Exogenous protein macromolecules may be taken up by the cell by means of small pinocytotic vesicles, which form from surface membrane, break away, and flow into the cytoplasm to merge with multivesicular bodies (2). Again, necessary enzymes for processing this material are brought to the multivesicular bodies by primary lysosomes. The digestion of endogenous protein (such as excess secretion granules) may occur in multivesicular bodies or dense bodies (3, 4). Bodies that contain identifiable organelles (such as mitochondria or granular endoplasmic reticulum) are known as *autophagic vacuoles* or cytolysosomes; these bodies are thought to arise by engulfment of organelles by a cisterna of membrane (5). More work is needed to know whether the enzymes are furnished by the cisternae or by fusion with primary lysosomes. The structure resulting from the formation of all of these *digestion vacuoles* is the *residual body*, which looks like a dense body filled with dense particles and whorls of membrane-like structures termed "myelin figures." In some cases, residual body contents may be released from the cell by fusion of the limiting membrane with the cell surface membrane (6). Or the residual body may be retained, participating over and over in digestive activity, growing larger and more heterogeneous in content, and becoming in time a *lipofuscin granule* (7). It is believed that the lysosomal enzymes are produced on ribosomes, after which they are channeled into the granular endoplasmic reticulum and packaged in the Golgi region into primary lysosomes (the small vesicle or the larger dense body type). (Diagram based upon papers by Novikoff and coworkers and Farquhar and collaborators.)

somewhat limited range of specifities in the battery of contained enzymes, and the variable amount of phagocytized material on which they are acting. These factors affect the efficiency of degradation. Since lipase activity is weak in lysosomes, there is frequently an accumulation of partially degraded lipidic material, some of which has been converted to pigments that are completely resistant to lysosomal digestion. Thus, many cells contain *residual bodies*, the remnants of undigestible components. *Lipofuscin granules* (*aging pigment*) that accumulate in neurons (Fig. 1.42) and in cardiac muscle cells are residual bodies, and in some of the cells lipofuscin granules may become so numerous as to impair normal function.

Peroxisomes

In the middle 1950s studies of liver and kidney cells by electron microscopy led to

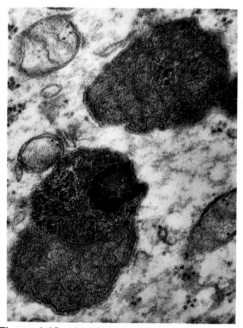

Figure 1.42. Lipofuscin pigment bodies. In untreated but aging animals, dense bodies may become markedly enlarged, very irregular in contour, and highly heterogeneous in appearance, at which point they are known as lipofuscin bodies or granules. They often contain a wealth of thin, curving, dense bands, as in this figure. Mature rabbit neuron (×58,000). (Courtesy of Dr. Virginia Tennyson.)

the discovery of a distinct category of small cytoplasmic dense bodies. These bodies were referred to by the descriptive term *microbodies*. They were of similar size to what were later recognized as lysosomes, were bounded by a single membrane, and frequently contained a distinct crystalline core (Fig. 1.43). A decade later these bodies were successfully isolated by cellular fractionation techniques and found to contain variable quantities of a few oxidative enzymes, the most constant being catalase. The biochemical studies showed that these organelles produce and consume hydrogen peroxide; hence the current name *peroxisomes* was introduced.

Peroxisomes are now known to occur in many different (most) cell types. They are identified positively by utilizing the diaminobenzidine reaction to localize peroxidase activity (catalase), but their morphology is also characteristic. There are two size populations described and the numbers vary under conditions of altered lipid metabolism. Nevertheless, the origin and function of peroxisomes remain equivocal. The proposal that they arise as outpouchings from the endoplasmic reticulum has not been fully substantiated. The morphological evidence remains controversial and there is strong biochemical evidence that the marker enzyme catalase is synthesized by free polysomes, and is not sequestered into cisternae of the endoplasmic reticulum. The mechanism by which this large heme-containing molecule gains access to the interior of the peroxisome is still unexplained. The function of the organelle in living cells is equally obscure. The later is not surprising in view of the recence of their discovery.

Vesicles

The cytoplasm of most cells contains a number of membrane-bounded vesicles of different sizes, some appearing devoid of content, some containing variable amounts of flocculent material, and some having a dense coating material on the cytosol side of the enclosing membrane. Tracer studies have shown that these vesicles have a va-

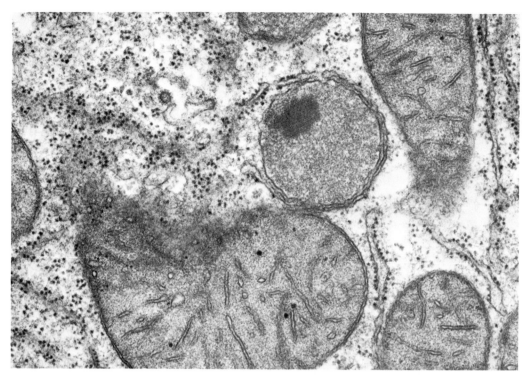

Figure 1.43.   Peroxisome (*right center*) in a rat liver cell. Note the close association with endoplasmic reticulum membranes and the dense crystalline core (×38,800).

riety of sources, but generally are involved in the intracellular transport of materials between several of the membrane-bounded compartments, the redisposition of specific areas of the membranes themselves, the secretion of products that are not stored within the cell (e.g., γ-globulin or collagen), and the uptake of materials at the cell surface. In other words, they are involved with the traffic of both membranes and sequestered products (Figs. 1.41 and 1.44). One category of the *coated vesicles* functions in the incorporation of materials that are selectively bound to the cell surface by receptor molecules located in the membrane. This phenomenon is referred to as *receptor-mediated endocytosis.* The coating material on the cytosol side of these vesicle membranes is a specific protein called *clathrin.* Its role in receptor-mediated endocytosis is not well understood, but it is known that clathrin is shed from the vesicle surface after the vesicle pinches off into the cytoplasm. Limited quantities of clathrin,

then, can be available continuously through recycling. Coated vesicles are also involved in membrane retrieval at neuronal synapses, in the transport of some components between the endoplasmic reticulum and Golgi saccules (Fig. 1.32), and the transport of some components from the Golgi apparatus to other membranous organelles or the cell surface. (Fig. 1.44). It is not clear yet whether clathrin is responsible for the coating of vesicles in all of these situations. It is clear, however, that some shuttle activity among elements of these membranous organelles also occurs by means of uncoated vesicles.

An understanding of the regulation of vesicle traffic in cells is only in its infancy. For example, the sorting of lysosomal enzymes by the Golgi apparatus (*green arrows,* Fig. 1.44) is known to involve the addition of mannose-6-phosphate, but the signal that directs the primary lysosome to fuse with a phagocytic vacuole remains a mystery. In fact, no other signal molecules

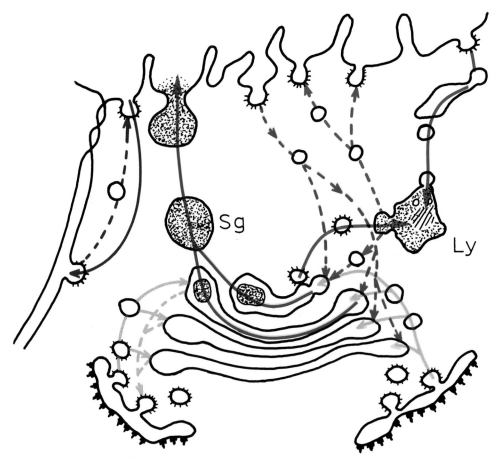

Figure 1.44. Summary diagram illustrating routes in the traffic of secretory products, endocytosed material, and lysosomal enzymes. Also shown are pathways for membrane recycling accompanying these activities. Some of the routes are documented, whereas others are proposed, but not fully documented. The Golgi apparatus plays a central role in the regulation of this traffic. Solid yellow, pathway of protein synthesis from rough endoplasmic reticulum (RER) to the Golgi apparatus. Dashed yellow, pathway for recovery of membrane from Golgi to RER. Solid red, pathway of secretory and membrane protein from Golgi to plasma membrane. Dashed red, pathway for recovery of membrane from plasma membrane to Golgi. Solid green, pathway of lysosomal enzymes from packaging in Golgi to lysosomes, and from plasma membrane (endocytosis) to lysosomes. Dashed green, recovery of membrane from lysosomes to Golgi, and from lysosomes to plasma membrane. Solid blue, pathway of endocytosed material from apical plasma membrane to lateral cell surface. Dashed blue, recovery of membrane from lateral cell surface to apical cell surface. (Courtesy of Dr. Marilyn Farquhar; figure modified.)

involved in vesicle traffic routing are known as yet. It is assumed that many may be comparable simple molecules, making difficult their identification as signal molecules.

Centrosome, Centrioles

The *centrosome* is a specialized, rather homogeneous zone of cytoplasm that con-tains *centrioles*. It usually lies close to or indents the nucleus (Figs. 1.36 and 1.37), although its position varies somewhat in different cell types (Fig. 1.45). In glandular epithelial cells it is situated between the nucleus and the luminal surface. The centrosome can be observed in living cells, and stained by iron hematoxylin in fixed prep-arations. Although it is most distinct during cell division, it can be demonstrated during the intermitotic stage. Its most constant feature is the presence of two centrioles, together called the *diplosome*. This organelle is self-replicating, as is discussed in Chapter 2. The two centrioles of a diplosome are oriented perpendicular to each other. Each centriole is a cylindrical organelle, 0.3 to 0.5 μm in length and about 0.15 μm in diameter, apparently closed at one end. The wall of the cylinder is composed of nine evenly spaced, longitudinally oriented, parallel units embedded in a dense material. Each unit consists of three microtubules (discussed in detail below) joined together. When the centriole is sectioned perpendicular to its long axis, the tubular units are seen as circles (Fig. 1.46). When sectioned parallel to its long axis, the tubules may be visualized as linear elements (Fig. 1.37). Other microtubules radiate into the cytoplasm from the area around the centriole or from closely associated dense clumps of material, which are called *pericentriolar satellites* (Figs. 1.37 and 1.46).

As is indicated later, the centrosome is associated with the process of cell division, particularly in the organization of microtubules within the spindle apparatus. In the nondividing cell, it serves as a center about which other cytoplasmic organelles such as the Golgi apparatus may be polarized and,

as such, it is termed *cell center, centrosphere,* or *cytocentrum* (Figs. 1.12, 1.36, and 1.37). In addition, a centriole may migrate near the cell surface, where it becomes a *basal body* (kinetosome), which gives rise to a motile *cilium* or *flagellum* (discussed in detail in Chapter 5). The mechanisms by which the centrioles exert their important

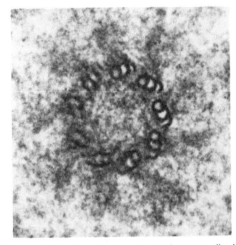

Figure 1.46. Centriole sectioned perpendicular to its length. The "wall" of the centriole is seen here as a circle of nine units, each composed of three united microtubules. Radiating from these units (resembling a pinwheel) are nine densities called pericentriolar satellites. Electron micrograph of rat ovarian follicle cell (×140,000). (Courtesy of Dr. Daniel Szollosi.)

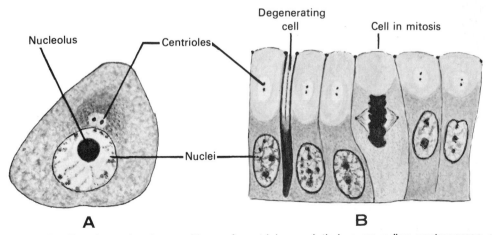

Figure 1.45. Drawings showing positions of centrioles and their surrounding centrosomes as visualized in early light microscopic studies. *A*, an interstitial cell of human testis. *B*, columnar epithelial cells of human stomach. (*A* redrawn after Petersen; *B* redrawn after Zimmerman.)

organizational capabilities are not understood.

Mitochondria

In the 1890s, Altmann and, subsequently, Benda devised histological techniques which preserved and stained a population of small cytoplasmic bodies which came to be known as *mitochondria* (from the Greek *mitos*, a thread, + *chondros*, a grain). These are visible in the light microscope as granules, rods, or filaments in both living (by phase microscopy) and fixed (after special staining) cells. Mitochondria also may be identified in the living cell by applying *supravital dyes*, (nonlethal), particularly Janus green B. The ability of these organelles to utilize O_2 and transport electrons maintains the Janus green in its oxidized or colored form, whereas in the surrounding cytoplasm the dye is reduced to a colorless compound. Under these conditions mitochondria may measure 0.2 to 1 μm or more in diameter, and may be 2 to 12 μm in length. Mitochondria are present in almost all cell types. Any given cell type as a rule contains a characteristic number of these organelles; a rat liver cell is purported to contain 800 to 1000. The number of mitochondria per cell may be as low as 20 (in sperm) and as high as 500,000 (in giant amebas).

In living cells grown in tissue culture, the mitochondria are seen to be in constant agitation—expanding and contracting, fusing, dividing, and changing location. They often react more rapidly than any other cell organelle to temperature, metabolic, pH, or osmotic changes. Studies of mitochondrial fractions indicate that mitochondria undergo swelling and contraction phases related to their physiological activity. Despite these known perturbations, mitochondria appear remarkably consistent in form and in position and orientation in some cell types. In epithelial cells, mitochondria are often polarized such that their long axes are oriented in the direction of the secretory or transport process (Fig. 1.11 *A*).

Electron microscopic studies indicate that each mitochondrion is bounded by *two* membranes. The inner membrane lies closely apposed to the outer one and, in addition, is thrown into folds (*cristae*) which protrude inward (Figs. 1.47 and 1.48). Depending upon the cell type, and correlating with physiological activity, the cristae vary in number and form (usually folds or tubules). They may or may not extend all of the way across the mitochondrion interior, and they are oriented either perpendicular (in most cases) or parallel to the long axis. The basic plan of the mitochondrion is nonetheless strikingly similar in all animal forms, ranging from protozoa to mammals. The cristae provide an increase in membrane surface area. An approximate calculation made for liver cells suggests that the surface area of all of the mitochondrial membrane in one cell is 10 times greater than the surface area of the cell. This vast surface area houses the enzymes associated with electron transport and phosphorylation. Studies by Fernandez-Moran and co-workers in the early 1960s demonstrated the presence on crista membranes of an array of particles which were termed "elementary particles" in the belief that each particle represented a fundamental grouping of oxidative enzymes. Later investigations showed that the particles apparently do not contain the oxidative enzymes but do contain mitochondrial ATPase activity.

The interior not occupied by cristae is filled with a finely granular *mitochondrial matrix*. Highly dense matrix granules (30–50 nm) may be found as well (Fig. 1.48). Their presence and size depend upon the metabolic state and type of cell. These are now known to be, in part, binding sites for ions, particularly cations such as Ca^{2+}. Cytologists puzzled for years over the autonomous behavior of mitochondria and finally were able to demonstrate the presence of a circular form of DNA and of RNA in the mitochondrial matrix. These discoveries provided a plausible explanation for the ability of mitochondria to divide as separate genetic units and to synthesize proteins independently of nuclear control. Mitochondria are not fully autonomous, however, as most of their enzymatic proteins are synthesized in the cell cytoplasm under nuclear control and transferred to mitochondria secondarily. The manner by which this occurs is only partially understood; it appears to involve signal sequences on the proteins and special receptors in the mitochondrial membrane. The self-replicating ability of mitochondria enables the cell to maintain a relatively constant number of these organelles within each daughter cell after division.

Like some of the other cytoplasmic organelles, mitochondria perform diversified functions. Most important, they are the chief source of energy in the cell. During cell respiration, enzymatic breakdown (mostly of carbohydrates but also of fats and amino acids), yields CO_2, water, and energy as end products. The energy freed in this oxidation is converted into phosphate bond energy. This energy, bound in *adenosine triphosphate* (ATP), is required for innumerable vital cellular processes, including transport of ions across the cell membrane, protein synthesis, and muscle contraction.

The formation of ATP by the breakdown of glucose involves three different mitochondrial systems. The initial degradation of glucose occurs in the cytoplasm outside the mitochondria. The resulting product, a 3-carbon compound (pyruvate), enters the mitochondrion, where it is processed by a sequence of enzymes known as the *Krebs citric acid cycle*. Liberated electrons are fed into a complex chain of flavoproteins and cytochromes called the *electron transport system* or *respiratory chain*. Eventually two electrons plus two hydrogen ions combine with oxygen, which is thereby reduced to water. At three points along this respiratory chain, sufficient energy becomes available from the transfer of electrons to form ATP by the addition of phosphate to adenosine *di*phosphate (*phosphorylation*). Because oxygen is the oxidizing agent at the terminus of the respiratory chain and the

phosphorylation apparatus is intimately *coupled* to this chain, the process is termed *oxidative phosphorylation.*

The respiratory and phosphorylation systems are found in highly ordered recurring assemblies in or bound to the mitochondrial crista membrane. That the membranes hold these essential enzyme systems is reflected in the fact that freeze-fracture replicas show high numbers of intramembrane particles in the inner mitochondrial membrane (including cristae). Also, in cells requiring more energy, such as insect flight or mammalian cardiac muscle, the cristae are much more densely packed. In such cells, mitochondria also are more numerous and are situated close to the energy-requiring structures.

Contractile protein has been found in mitochondria, suggesting a basis for the contraction observed earlier by light microscopists. Mitochondrial contraction, known to be related to respiratory activity, is thought to aid in mitochondrial movement and in the exchange of substances such as ATP and ions with the cytoplasm. Additional functions of mitochondria now include the accumulation of calcium as well as the synthesis of nucleic acids and proteins and the oxidation of fatty acids. Much of this activity and the Krebs cycle reactions probably take place in the matrix.

Filaments

Slender threads of *filaments* occur in the cytoplasm of virtually all cells. As a rule, they range from less than 3 nm up to 12 nm in diameter and are of indeterminant length. Whether the filaments are randomly scattered throughout the cytoplasm, clustered into wisplike bundles, or aggregated into a meshwork depends upon the cell type. They make up a large proportion of any cell's *cytoskeleton*. When the filaments occur in bundles, they are visible in the light microscope as *fibrils*, (as in Fig. 1.2*A*), but visualization of individual filaments requires the resolution of the electron microscope (Fig. 1.49).

Recently it has become possible to rec-

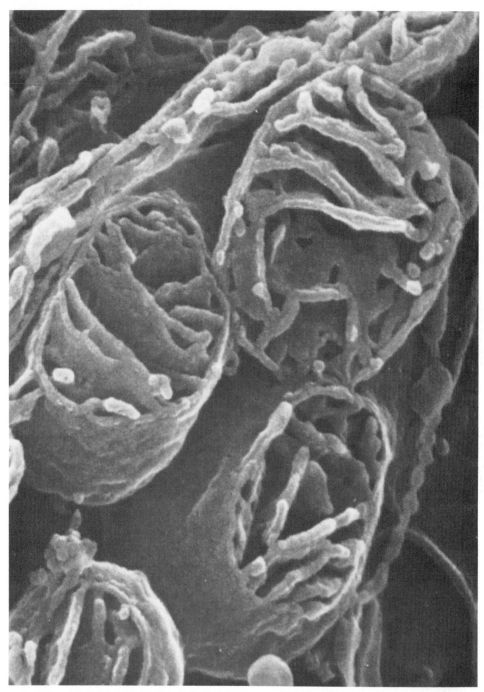

Figure 1.47. High resolution scanning electron micrograph showing four mitochondria which have been sliced to reveal their internal structure. Shelf-like cristae are visible in each; these represent inward foldings of the inner mitochondrial membrane. The space between cristae would be occupied by mitochondrial matrix in the living state. Although present, the outer mitochondrial membrane is not separately resolvable from the inner membrane in this preparation (×128,000). (Reprinted with permission from Tanaka K: In Tanaka K, Fujita T (eds): *Proceedings of the International Symposium on SEM in Biology and Medicine* (Kyoto, Japan, May 11–15, 1980). Excerpta Medica, The Netherlands, Elsevier, 1980.)

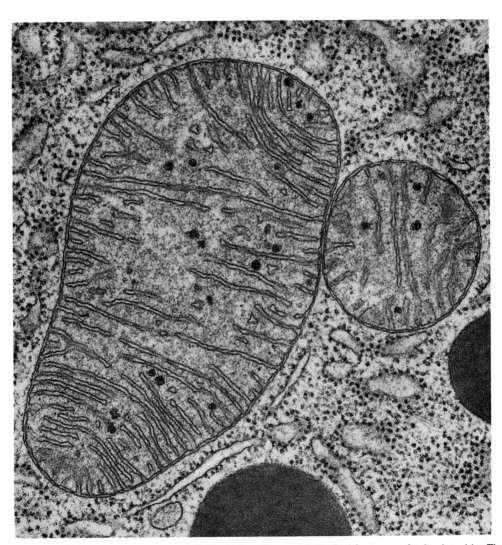

Figure 1.48. This electron micrograph illustrates the morphological features of mitochondria. The inner membrane, unlike the outer one, is thrown into folds (cristae) which may span the interior. Within the mitochondrial matrix, which fills the area not occupied by cristae, are scattered dense granules. Bat pancreas (×64,000). (Reprinted with permission from K. R. Porter and M. A. Bonneville: *Fine Structure of Cells and Tissues*, ed 3. Philadelphia, Lea & Febiger, 1968.)

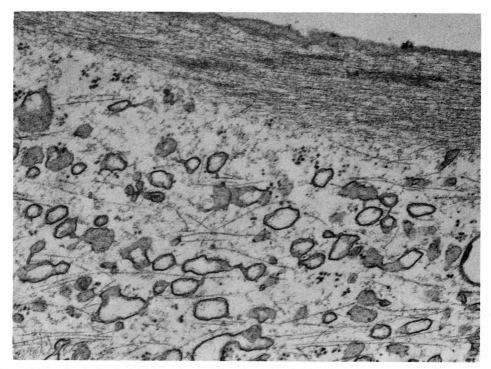

Figure 1.49. Immediately beneath the cell border (which is shown at *upper right*) is a band of closely packed microfilaments. Somewhat thicker intermediate filaments are scattered throughout other areas of the cytoplasm of this cell grown in culture (×42,500). (Courtesy of Drs. M. Bunge and D. Bray.)

ognize two basic categories of filaments; the *microfilaments*, whose diameters measure less than about 8 nm, and the *intermediate filaments* (or *tonofilaments*), whose diameters range from 8 to 12 nm. Substantial evidence now suggests that most microfilaments are contractile, acting to promote cell shape changes or motility in a wide variety of cells. These are mostly varieties of *actin filaments*, so abundantly deployed in the cytoplasm of all types of muscle. Study of highly motile cells in the living state shows relatively clear pseudopods or a clear, thin, peripheral rim of cytoplasm. This is referred to as *ectoplasm*, known for years to be more viscous or gelled than the rest of the cytoplasm. It is now known that these areas are full of microfilaments and that the apparent clarity is due to the exclusion of other organelles from these regions. A narrow band of microfilaments just beneath the cell membrane is a prominent feature of the cleavage furrow of dividing cells. Microfilaments are also found appropriately aligned in various embryonic epithelia which are undergoing rapid morphogenetic cell shape changes.

In muscle, the contractile function of actin filaments requires the interaction with another filamentous protein, *myosin*. In the nonmuscle contractile systems, it is still unclear whether myosin-like molecules always accompany the actin-like filaments. Some good evidence suggests that they do, at least in some cells.

Because recent investigations have revealed that these and other actin-like systems are widespread in nature, it is reasonable to presume that microfilament-induced contractility is a common property of most or perhaps all cells. It is a property which is greatly emphasized in muscle cells, traditionally regarded as the only contractile tissues. But it is a property which is also exerted in subtle fashion in providing localized changes in cellular form or in establishing the shapes of cells and tissues during their development. In addition, actin filaments contribute to the general cytoskeletal support system of most cells. In fact, in some highly specialized cells, the supportive function of actin filaments may be of primary importance.

Intermediate filaments, on the other hand, are not known to be contractile and appear to serve exclusively in a supportive role. They function generally to maintain cellular shape and provide resiliency to forces that might tend to alter that shape. Intermediate filaments are frequently grouped into delicate bundles (fibrils) which course through the cell in an architectural array clearly suited to meet stress and provide an overall girderlike supportive system. Such networks are exceedingly prominent in the cytoplasm of "wear and tear" epithelia, such as the lining surfaces of the skin and the esophagus. Here they are generally referred to as *tonofilaments*. In nerve cells, intermediate-sized filaments are a regular component (along with microtubules; see below) of the axons and, to a lesser extent, of dendrites, where they lie parallel to the long axis. In the cell bodies of nerve cells, they are loosely aggregated into slender bundles. Intermediate filaments are frequently found associated with the firmest sites of adhesion between adjacent cells of epithelial systems, further attesting to their role as a supportive intracellular network important in individual cells and also in transmission of forces among adherent cell populations.

Intermediate filaments display remarkably similar images when observed in all the various cell types where they occur. Hence, it was often assumed that they possess chemical constancy also. However, since 1975 some 20 different intermediate filament proteins have been identified using sensitive electrophoretic and immunocytochemical techniques. Many of the varieties are relatively tissue specific. *Keratan, dermatan, desmin,* and *vimentin* are a few of the many biochemical names used to identify the new protein species.

It can be appreciated from the above discussion that the rich filamentous population which most cells display is finely proportioned to serve the cytoskeletal and contractile requirements of both individual cells and tissues. The mechanisms by which filaments interact with each other, with other cytoplasmic molecules, with membranes, and with microtubules (see below) to perform these roles are current highly active areas of research.

Microtubules

Another of the most active areas of research in recent years has concerned itself with widely occurring, slender, cylindrical structures, the *microtubules*. Their discovery depended not only upon the resolution of the electron microscope but also upon improved preservation with glutaraldehyde fixation. Microtubules vary somewhat in diameter from 18 to 30 nm, but they usually measure about 24 nm, and they have been followed for several microns in thin sections. They are straight or slightly curving, suggesting a rigid structure (Figs. 1.2B, 1.36 and 1.37). When sectioned at right angles to its long axis, the microtubule appears as a circle composed, on the average, of 13 globular subunits, each about 4 to 5 nm in diameter.

Microtubule proteins from diversified sources have been found to be quite similar in their sequences of amino acids, and they closely resemble the muscle protein, actin. These proteins are referred to as *tubulins*, and they are known to circulate between a free monomeric or dimeric form and an aggregated microtubular configuration. Like actin, tubulin has binding sites for nucleotides. Tubulins also contain specific binding sites for *colchicine* and when combined with this drug, tubulins display an inability to aggregate and maintain microtubular structure. Since microtubules are an important functional element of the spindle apparatus in dividing cells, it can readily be appreciated why colchicine is a mitosis-blocking agent frequently used to arrest tumor growth. Microtubules from different locations vary in sensitivity to colchicine, pointing to at least subtle differences in the constituent tubulins.

During cell division, microtubules increase greatly in number, to as many as 3000 per cell, to form the mitotic spindle (which is described in Chapter 2). In nondividing cells, microtubules are scattered throughout the cytoplasm (Fig. 1.2B). They may converge on centrosomes (Figs. 1.36 and 1.37) and are found in units of three (triplets), forming the framework of the basal body and the centriole (Fig. 1.46). Microtubules form the cores of cilia, flagella, and sperm tails, where they are typically organized into nine doublets encircling two centrally situated microtubules (Figs. 4.18 and 4.19). During sperm maturation, hundreds of microtubules are clusted in an orderly fashion around the nucleus at a time when the nucleus begins to elongate. During the development of chick lens epithelium, when cells may undergo a four-fold increase in length, microtubules become prominent in the cortical cytoplasm, lying parallel to the axis of elongation. Microtubules are a regular component of the slender processes of nerve cells. One of the most striking examples of microtubule arrays was discovered in a spherical protozoan, *Actinosphaerium.* Radiating from the cell body, which is about 100 μm in diameter, are numerous long, needle-like extensions or axopodia, often more than 400 μm long and only 5 to 10 μm in diameter. Each axopodium contains as many as 500 microtubules in a highly ordered arrangement. When these microtubules are disrupted, the axopodia collapse.

Findings like those just mentioned have led to the conclusion that microtubules play a role in maintaining diverse cell shape. Their prominence and orientation during periods of changing cell shape have also suggested that they are active in changing cell form, although no exact mechanism for this postulated role has been established.

However, if microtubules are treated with colchicine and thereby prevented from assembly during such a period, normal development may be arrested. As components of the spindle, cilia, and flagella, they not only provide a cytoskeletal framework but also may contribute to the mechanisms by which movement is accomplished. In cilia and flagella, evidence suggests that pairs of microtubules interact directly to cause differential positioning, thereby generating the whiplike motion characteristic of these organelles. Microtubules are also closely associated with microfilaments. It is believed that interactions between microtubules and microfilaments are responsible for at least some kinds of cytoplasmic movement.

Cytoplasmic Inclusions

The cytoplasm of most cells may contain numerous accumulations of *non*-membrane-bounded substances or other materials which are membrane-bounded, but not essential for survival of the cell. These are collectively termed inclusions. Often the non-membrane bounded inclusions are raw food materials or the stored products of the cell's metabolic activity. Thus, deposits of proteins, fats, and carbohydrates are characteristic features in certain cells. The storage of *glycogen* by cells of liver and muscle are outstanding examples of carbohydrate storage (Fig. 1.11D). Glycogen is a polymer formed from glucose. It is stained magenta by the PAS reaction or Best's carmine method. In the electron microscope, glycogen (after lead staining) appears as scattered or clustered small dense particles, 15 to 40 nm in diameter (Fig. 1.50). Although fat cells are the chief sites of *lipid* storage, many other cell types store some lipid in the form of droplets of varying size. If frozen sections are stained with specific fat-soluble dyes or if the tissue is fixed in osmium tetroxide, the lipid droplets are retained and appear black (Fig. 1.1C). In electron micrographs they appear as homogeneous spheres of varying density. Ex-

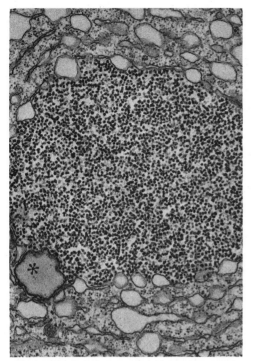

Figure 1.50. An accumulation of glycogen particles in an X-irradiated neuron. These particles may be compared to the smaller ribosomes scattered among the swollen elements of endoplasmic reticulum. A lipid droplet is marked by an *asterisk*. Electron micrograph of rat nervous tissue in culture (×25,000). (Reprinted with permission from E. B. Masurovsky et al.: *J Cell Biol* 32:467, 1967.)

amples of the products of cell activity are *yolk granules*, *secretory granules*, and residual bodies.

Another type of cytoplasmic inclusion is the *pigment granule*. Pigment granules are membrane-bounded and display color without having been stained. The occurrence of aging pigment on *lipofuscin* is considered above in the section describing lysosomes. Certain cells contain dark brown or black granules which are composed of the pigment *melanin*. In the electron microscope, these granules appear as homogeneous dense bodies. In man they are present in the eye, certain areas of the brain, and the skin.

Cell Form and Size

The cells of highly evolved organisms, such as vertebrate animals, have achieved a wide variation in size and form, coincident with their adaptation to perform a diversity of specific functions (Fig. 1.51). Cells of tissues which have acquired a fixed location in the body become polyhedral, columnar, flat (pavement), fusiform, or spindle-shaped, and they may retain a smooth contour or send out numerous processes. The nerve cell, with its processes sometimes several feet in length, is perhaps the most aberrant type. The mechanisms which control or limit cell size as well as body size are not well understood. Some groups of animals have larger cells than do others, but it does not follow that small animals have small cells and large animals have large cells. The size of the individual is in general determined by the number of its cells, not by their size.

Cellular Life and Death

Biologists generally believe that living matter is constructed according to the same basic principles as is the physical world in which it exists. Considering the tenets of physics, particularly thermodynamics, living systems might be expected gradually to decrease in complexity, for energy is always involved in the maintenance of high degrees of organization. Yet the trend in the evolution of living systems is toward greater complexity.

The key to this riddle is, of course, the continual input into living systems of free energy from the sun. This energy was initially used in the synthesis of the simplest of organic substances and is now continuously used to maintain and extend the organization of living things. Many organisms do not, of course, use the energy of the sun directly, but feed on lower forms that do.

The process of cellular growth can occur with remarkable rapidity, for the chemical reactions within the cell are efficiently catalyzed by *enzymes*. The construction of

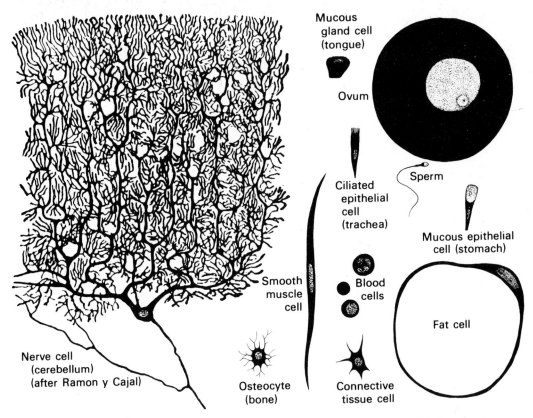

Figure 1.51. Cells vary widely in size and shape and their nuclei occupy differing positions, as depicted diagrammatically here. All of the cells are drawn to scale (100 μm = approximately 1½ inches), with the measurements based on data from humans.

macromolecules, which is the most basic aspect of the process of growth, is called *anabolism*. The cell also uses mechanisms of *catabolism* for the breakdown of its components. These catabolic mechanisms can release stored energy for use by the cell, as in the breakdown of fatty acids, and are a necessary part of the ongoing activities of the cell. Both anabolism and catabolism are important for maintaining the proper functional levels of materials within the cell. Several important diseases, called storage diseases, result not from the lack of anabolic activity within the cell but from the failure of the proper degradation of cellular constituents. In these conditions, specific components accumulate within the cell in abnormal amounts and in time seriously interfere with cellular function.

Cellular death is an integral part of the growth of tissues and organs. During the development of some tissues, large numbers of cells may die. In these cases there is an initial overproduction of certain cell types, and only those required for the functional needs of the tissue survive. Local cell death (*necrosis*) occurs normally in the body, or may be the result of disease or trauma. Morphologically, necrotic tissue can be recognized by the altered structure of the cells and intercellular substance. Coagulation of proteins takes place in the cytoplasm, the latter appearing flocculated or in the nature of a fibrous network. The cells appear fused by the obliteration of cellular boundaries. Or the cell may liquefy, swell, and finally burst (*cytolysis*), the liquefaction often being preceded by the appearance of numerous fat droplets. These degradative processes are in many cases caused by intracellular enzymes liberated after the death of the cell (*autolysis*). The nucleus, likewise, shows various forms of structural disintegration. The chromatin may contract into a dense, deeply staining irregular mass (*pyknosis*), it may fragment into a number of small pieces with obliteration of the nuclear boundary (*karyorrhexis*), or it may gradually disappear, as evidenced by the loss of its staining capacity (*karyolysis*).

References

Afzelius BA, Eliasson R: Flagellar mutants in man: on the heterogeneity of the immotile-cilia syndrome. *J Ultrastruct Res* 69:43–52, 1979.

Alberts B, Bray DM, Lewis J, Raff M, Roberts K, Watson JD: *Molecular Biology of the Cell.* New York, Garland, 1983.

Allen RD: Evidence for firm linkages between microtubules and membrane-bounded vesicles. *J Cell Biol* 64:493–496, 1975.

Andre J, Marinozzi V: Presence, dans les mitochondries, de particules ressemblant aux ribosomes. *J Microsc* 4:615–626, 1965.

Bainton D: The discovery of lysosomes. *J Cell Biol* 91:66s–76s, 1981.

Bainton DF, Farquhar MG: Origin of granules in polymorphonuclear leukocytes. Two types derived from opposite faces of the Golgi complex in developing granulocytes. *J Cell Biol* 28:277–301, 1966.

Bainton DF, Farquhar MG: Differences in enzyme content of azurophil and specific granules of polymorphonuclear leukocytes. II. Cytochemistry and electron microscopy of bone marrow cells. *J Cell Biol* 39:299–317, 1968.

Baker JR: *Cytological Technique; The Principles Underlying Routine Methods,* ed 5. New York, John Wiley & Sons, 1966.

Barr ML. The significance of the sex chromatin. *Int Rev Cytol* 19:35–95, 1966.

Behnke O, Forer A: Evidence for four classes of microtubules in individual cells. *J Cell Sci* 2:169–192, 1967.

Bennett HS. Morphological aspects of extracellular polysaccharides. *J Histochem Cytochem* 11:14–23, 1963.

Bensley RR, Hoerr NL: Studies on cell structure by the freezing-drying method. VI. The preparation and properties of mitochondria. *Anat Rec* 60:449–455, 1934.

Bentler WL, Granett S, Rosenbaum JL: Ultrastructural localization of the high molecular weight proteins associated with in vitro-assembled brain microtubules. *J Cell Biol* 65:237–241, 1975.

Bibb MJ, Van Etten RA, Wright CT, Walberg MW, Clayton DA: Sequence and gene organization of mouse mitochondrial DNA. *Cell* 26:167–180, 1981.

Branton D, Bullivant S, Gilula NB, Karnovsky MJ, Moor H, Muhlethaler K, Northcote DH, Packer L, Satir B, Satir P, Speth V, Staehelin LA, Steere RL, Weinstein RS: Freeze-etching nomenclature. *Science* 190:54–56, 1975.

Bretscher MS, Raff MC: Mammalian plasma membranes. *Nature* 258:43–49, 1975.

Brinkley BR: The cytoskeleton—a perspective. In Wilson L (ed): *Methods in Cell Biology,* vol 24. New York, Academic Press, 1982, pp 1–8.

Caro LG, and Palade GE: Protein synthesis, storage, and discharge in the pancreatic exocrine cell. An autoradiographic study. *J Cell Biol* 20:473–495, 1964.

Cloney RA: Cytoplasmic filaments and morphogenesis: effects of cytochalasin B on contractile epidermal cells. *Z Zellforsch* 132:167–192, 1972.

Coons AH: Histochemistry with labeled antibody. *Int Rev Cytol* 5:1–23, 1956.

Cowdry EV (ed): *General Cytology.* Chicago, The University of Chicago Press, 1924.

Crowther RA, Pearse BMF: Assembly and packing of clathrin into coats. *J Cell Biol* 91:790–797, 1981.

Danielli JF: Experiment, hypothesis and theory in the developing of concepts of cell membrane structure 1930–1970. In Martonosi AN (ed): *Membranes and Transport,* vol I. New York, Plenum Press, 1982, pp: 3–14.

Danielli JF, Davson H: A contribution to the theory of permeability of thin films. *J Cell Comp Physiol* 5:495–508, 1935.

deDuve C, Baudhuin P: Perosixomes (microbodies) and related particles. *Physiol Rev* 46:323–357, 1966.

deDuve C, Wattiaux R: Functions of lysosomes. *Annu Rev Physiol* 28:435–492, 1966.

deHarven E. The centriole and the mitotic spindle. In Dalton AJ, Haguenau F (eds): *The Nucleus* New York, Academic Press, 1968, pp 197–227.

Dingle JT, Fell HB (eds): *Lysosomes in Biology and Pathology.* New York, John Wiley & Sons, 1969.

Drochmans P: Melanin granules: their fine structure, formation, and degradation in normal and pathological tissues. *Int Rev Exp Pathol* 2:357–422, 1963.

Dustin P: *Microtubules.* New York, Springer-Verlag, 1978.

Edelman GM: Surface modulation in cell recognition and cell growth. *Science* 192:218–226, 1976.

Emans JB, Jones AL: Hypertrophy of liver cell smooth surfaced reticulum following progesterone administration. *J Histochem Cytochem* 16:561–570, 1968.

Farquhar M, Palade G: The Golgi apparatus (complex) (1954–1981) from artifact to center stage. *J Cell Biol* 91:77s–103s, 1981.

Fawcett DW: *The Cell,* ed 2. Philadelphia, W.B. Saunders, 1981.

Franke WW, Scheer U, Krohne G, Joresch E-D: The nuclear envelope and the architecture of the nuclear periphery. *J Cell Biol* 91:39s–50s, 1981.

Frye LD and Edidin M: The rapid intermixing of cell surface antigens after formation of mouse-human heterokaryons. *J Cell Sci* 7:319–335, 1970.

Gall JG: Octagonal nuclear pores. *J Cell Biol* 32:391–399, 1967.

Gilula NB: Gap junctions and cell communication. In Brinkley BR, Porter KR (eds): *International Cell Biology.* New York, Rockefeller University Press, 1977, pp 61–69.

Goldfischer S: The internal reticular apparatus of Camillo Golgi. *J Histochem Cytochem* 30:717–733, 1982.

Goldman B, Blobel G: Biogenesis of peroxisomes—intracellular site of synthesis of catalase and uricase.

Proc Natl Acad Sci USA 75:5066–5070, 1978.

Goldman RD, Lazarides E, Pollack R, Weber K: The distribution of actin in non-muscle cells. *Exp Cell Res* 90:333–344, 1975.

Goldstein JL, Anderson RGW, Brown MS: Coated pits, coated vesicles, and receptor-mediated endocytosis. *Nature* 279:679–685, 1979.

Gurdon JB: Transplanted nuclei and cell differentiation. *Sci Am* 219:24–35, 1968.

Gurdon JB: Nuclear transplantation and the control of gene activity in animal development. *Proc R Soc (Lond Biol)* 176:303–314, 1970.

Gurdon JB, Laskey RA, Reeves OR: The developmental capacity of nuclei transplanted from keratinized skin cells of adult frogs. *J Embryol Exp Morphol* 34:93–112, 1975.

Hackenbrock CR, Hochli M, Chau RM: Calorimetric and freeze-fracture analysis of lipid phase transitions and lateral translational motion of intramembrane particles in mitochondrial membranes. *Biochim Biophys Acta* 455:466–484, 1976.

Haguenau F: The ergastoplasm: its history, ultrastructure and biochemistry. *Int Rev Cytol* 7:425–483, 1958.

Harrison R, Lunt GG: *Biological Membranes*. Glasgow, Blackie, 1980.

Hayat MA (ed): *Principles and Techniques of Electron Microscopy: Biological Applications*, vols 1–6; and *Principles and Techniques of Scanning Electron Microscopy*, vols 1–5. New York, Van Nostrand Reinhold, 1970–1976.

Hayat MA: *Fixation for Electron Microscopy*. New York, Academic Press, 1981.

Heuser J: Quick-freeze, deep-etch preparation of samples for 3-D electron microscopy. *Trends Biochem Sci* 6:64–68, 1981.

Hogeboom GH, Schneider WC, Palade GE: Cytochemical studies of mammalian tissues. I. Isolation of intact mitochondria from rat liver; some biochemical properties of mitochondria and submicroscopic particulate material. *J Biol Chem* 172:619–635, 1948.

Hruban Z, Rechigl JR M: Microbodies and related particles; morphology, biochemistry and physiology. *Int Rev Cytol* (Suppl. 1) 1969.

Isenberg G, Rathke PC, Hulsmann N, Franke WW, Wohlfarth-Bottermann KE: Cytoplasmic actomyosin fibrils in tissue culture cells. Direct proof of contractility by visualization of ATP-induced contraction in fibrils isolated by laser microbeam dissection. *Cell Tissue Res* 166:427–444, 1976.

Ishikawa H: Arrowhead complexes in a variety of cell types. Excerpta Medica Congress Series No. 333, 1973, pp 37–50.

Jamieson JD, Palade GE: Intracellular transport of secretory proteins in the pancreatic exocrine cell. I. Role of peripheral elements of the Golgi complex. *J Cell Biol* 34:577–596, 1967.

Jamieson JD, Palade GE: Intracellular transport of secretory proteins in the pancreatic exocrine cell. II. Transport to condensing vacuoles and zymogen granules. *J Cell Biol* 34:597–615, 1967.

Johnson LV, Walsh ML, Bockus BT, Chen LB: Monitoring of relative mitochondrial membrane potential in living cells by fluorescence microscopy. *J Cell Biol* 88:526–535, 1981.

Jones AL, Fawcett DW: Hypertrophy of the agranular

endoplasmic reticulum in hamster liver induced by phenobarbital. *J Histochem Cytochem* 14:215–232, 1966.

Kirkman H, Severinghaus AE: A review of the Golgi apparatus. *Anat Rec* 70:413–431 and 557–573, 1938, 71:79–103, 1938.

Kirschner MW: Microtubule assembly and nucleation. *Int Rev Cytol* 54:1–71, 1978.

Kornberg RD, Klug A: The nucleosome. *Sci Am* 244:52–64, 1981.

Lazarides E: Intermediate filaments as mechanical integrators of cellular space. *Nature* 283:249–255, 1980.

Lazarides E: Antibody production and immunofluorescent characterization of actin and contractile proteins. In Wilson L (ed): *Methods in Cell Biology*, vol 24. New York, Academic Press, 1982, pp 313–332.

Lazarides E, Weber K. Actin antibody; the specific visualization of actin filaments in non-muscle cells. *Proc Natl Acad Sci USA* 71:2268–2272, 1974.

Lewin B. *Gene Expression*, vol 2: *Eucaryotic Chromosomes*, ed 2. New York, John Wiley & Sons, 1980.

Lowenstein WR: On the genesis of cellular communication. *Dev Biol* 15:503–520, 1967.

Lowenstein WR: Junctional intercellular communication: the cell-to-cell membrane channel. *Physiol Rev* 61:829–913, 1981.

Margolis RL, Wilson L: Microtubule treadmills—possible molecular machinery. *Nature* 293:705–711, 1981.

Miller OL: The nucleolus, chromosomes and visualization of genetic activity. *J Cell Biol* 91:15s–27s, 1981.

Miller OL, Beatty BR: Visualization of nucleolar genes. *Science* 164:955–957, 1969.

Neufield EF, Ashwell G. Carbohydrate recognition systems for receptor-mediated pinocytosis. In Lennarz WJ (ed.): *The Biochemistry of Glycoproteins and Proteoglycans*. New York, Plenum Press, 1980, pp 241–266.

Neupert W, Schatz G: How proteins are transported into mitochondria. *Trends Biochem Sci* 6:1–4, 1981.

Novikoff A, Novikoff P, Davis C, Quintana N: Studies on microperoxisomes. V. Are microperoxisomes ubiquitus in mammalian cells? *J Histochem Cytochem* 21:737–755, 1973.

Palade G: Intracellular aspects of the process of protein synthesis. *Science* 189:347–358, 1975.

Pastan IH, Willingham MC: Journey to the center of the cell: role of the receptosome. *Science* 214:504–509, 1981.

Pearse AGE: *Histochemistry, Theoretical and Applied*, ed 3. London, J & A Churchill, 1968 and 1972.

Pearse BMF: Clathrin: a unique protein associated with intracellular transfer of membrane by coated vesicles. *Proc Natl Acad Sci USA* 73:1255–1259, 1976.

Perry RP: RNA processing comes of age. *J Cell Biol* 91:28s–38s, 1981.

Perry RP: The nucleolus and the synthesis of ribosomes. *Prog Nucleic Acid Res Mol Biol* 6:219–257, 1967.

Pinto da Silva P, Branton D: Membrane splitting in freeze-etching. Covalently bound ferritin as a membrane marker. *J Cell Biol* 45:598–605, 1970.

Pollak JK, Sutton R: The differentiation of animal

mitochondria during development. *Trends Biochem Sci* 5:23–27, 1980.

Pollard TD: Cytoplasmic contractile proteins. *J Cell Biol* 91:156s–165s, 1981.

Pollard TD: Myosin purification and characterization. *In* Wilson L (ed): *Methods in Cell Biology*, vol 24. New York, Academic Press, 1982, pp 333–372.

Prescott D. (ed): *Methods in Cell Biology*. New York, Academic Press. (A multivolume series on current techniques).

Rash JE, Hudson CS (eds): *Freeze-fracture: Methods, Artifacts and Interpretations*. New York, Raven Press, 1979.

Revel J-P: Electron microscopy of glycogen. *J Histochem Cytochem* 12:104–114, 1964.

Rogers AW: *Techniques of Autoradiography*, ed 3. New York, American Elsevier, 1979.

Rothman JE, Lenard J: Membrane asymmetry. *Science* 195:743–754, 1977.

Sabatini D, Kreibich G, Morimoto T, Adesnick M: Mechanisms for the incorporation of proteins in membranes and organelles. *J Cell Biol* 92:1–22, 1982.

Sanger JW: Intracellular localization of actin with fluorescently labeled heavy meromyosin. *Cell Tissue Res* 161:431–444, 1975.

Schroeder TE: Cell constriction: contractile role of microfilaments in division and development. *Am Zoologist* 13:949–960, 1973.

Schwartz RM, Dayhoff MO. Origins of prokaryotes, eukaryotes, mitochondria and chloroplasts. *Science* 199:395–403, 1978.

Singer SJ, Nicholson GL: The fluid mosaic model of the structure of cell membranes. *Science* 175:720–731, 1972.

Sjostrand FS: A comparison of plasma membrane cytomembranes, and mitochondrial membrane element with respect to ultrastructural features. *J Ultrastruct Res* 9:561–580, 1963.

Slautterback DB: Cytoplasmic microtubules. I. Hydra *J Cell Biol* 18:367–388, 1963.

Sly WS, Natowicz M, Gonzalez-Noriega A, Grubb JH, Fischer HD: The role of mannose-6-phosphate recognition marker and its receptor in the uptake and intracellular transport of lysosomal enzymes. In Callahan JW, Lowden JA (eds): *Lysosomes and Lysosomal Storage Diseases*. New York, Raven Press, 1981, pp 131–146.

Spencer M: *Fundamentals of Light Microscopy*. Cambridge, Cambridge University Press, 1982.

Steiner DF, Quinn PS, Chan SJ, Marsh J, Tager HS: Processing mechanisms in the biosynthesis of proteins. *Ann NY Acad Sci* 343:1–16, 1980.

Steinert P, Zackroff R, Aynardi-Whitman M, Goldman RD: Isolation and characterization of intermediate filaments. In Wilson L (ed): *Methods in Cell Biology*, vol 24. New York, Academic Press, 1982, pp 399–419.

Steinman RM, Mellman IS, Muller WA, Cahn ZA. Endocytosis and the recycling of plasma membrane. *J Cell Biol* 96:1–27, 1983.

Stephens R, Edds K. Microtubules: Structure, chemistry and function. *Physiol Rev* 56:709, 1976.

Stryer L. *Biochemistry*, ed 2. San Francisco, W. H. Freeman, 1981.

Tanaka K: Scanning electron microscopy of intracellular structures. *Int Rev Cytol* 68:97–125, 1980.

Tanaka K, Iino A, Najuro T: Scanning electron microscopic observation on intracellular structures of ion-etched materials. *Arch Histol Jpn* 39(3):165–175, 1976.

Tandler B, Erlandson RA, Smith AL, Wynder EL. Riboflavin and mouse hepatic cell structure and function. II. Division of mitochondria during recovery from simple deficiency. *J Cell Biol* 41:477–493, 1969.

Tilney LG: Role of actin in nonmuscle cell motility. In Inoue S, Stephens RF (eds): *Molecules and Cell Movement*. New York, Raven Press, 1975, pp 339–388.

Tolbert ME, Essner E: Microbodies: peroxisomes and glyoxysomes. *J Cell Biol* 91:271s–283s, 1981.

Tucker JB: Cytoskeletal coordination and intercellular signalling during metazoan embryogenesis. *J Embryol Exp Morphol* 65:1–25, 1981.

Tzagoloff A: *Mitochondria*. New York, Plenum Press, 1982.

Walter P, Blobel G: Translocation of proteins across the endoplasmic reticulum. III. Signal recognition protein (SRP) causes signal sequence-dependent and site-specific arrest of chain elongation that is released by microsomal membranes. *J Cell Biol* 91:557–561, 1981.

Warner FD, Satir P: The structural basis of ciliary bend formation. *J Cell Biol* 63:35–63, 1974.

Watson JD: *The Double Helix; A Personal Account of the Discovery of the Structure of DNA*. New York, Atheneum Press, 1968.

Watson JD: *Molecular Biology of the Gene*, ed 3. Menlo Park, Calif., Benjamin Cummings, 1976.

Watson JD, Tooze J: *The DNA Story: A Documentary History of Gene Cloning*. San Francisco, W. H. Freeman, 1981.

Weeds A: Actin-binding proteins—regulators of cell architecture and motility. *Nature* 296:811–816, 1982.

Wessells NK, Spooner BS, Ash JF, Bradley MO, Luduena MA, Taylor EL, Wrenn JT, Yamada KM: Microfilaments in cellular and developmental processes. *Science* 171:135–143, 1971.

Whaley WG: *The Golgi Apparatus*. New York, Springer-Verlag, 1975.

Wheatley DM: *The Centriole: A Central Enigma of Cell Biology*. New York, Elsevier/North Holland, 1982.

Wolfe J: Basal body fine structure and chemistry. *Adv Cell Mol Biol* 2:151, 1972.

Wolosewick JJ, Porter KR. Microtrabecular lattice of the cytoplasmic ground substance: artifact or reality. *J Cell Biol* 82:114–139, 1979.

Chapter 2

STUDIES OF LIVING CELLS, CELL CULTURE, CELL DIFFERENTIATION, AND CELL DIVISION

Fixed and stained preparations have the advantage of being more or less permanent and available for repeated microscopic examination. Unfortunately, although significant progress has been made in preserving cells and tissues in life-like condition, even the most modern fixatives, dehydrating agents, and stains may induce significant alterations, or *artifacts*, to the living structure. It is therefore advantageous to study living cells and tissues in action, when many aspects of true structure as well as some functional changes can be observed directly. Studies of living cells also offer the opportunity to control directly the immediate environment of the cell during experimentation.

The living cell is delicate, however, and its study requires great care. The first extensive studies on living tissues were carried out on free-living unicellular organisms and on the eggs and early embryos of lower forms of both plants and animals. Whereas much was learned about the physical properties of cells, the methods used could not be applied directly to most cells from higher animals, particularly man.

The first living human cells studied in detail were blood cells. They could be viewed under the highest powers of the microscope while still surrounded by their natural environment, the plasma. Because of the fluid nature of blood, a thin film could be made between a cover glass and slide. If the coverslip edges were sealed to prevent evaporation and the stage of the microscope was heated to body temperature, the conditions inside the body were approximated. With this preparation, the various types of white blood cells were recognized and their ameboid and phagocytic activity observed.

This simple procedure cannot be used for the more adherent and interdependent living cells from organized tissues. Attempts have been made to study solid tissues by teasing the tissue apart with fine instruments until it is spread thinly enough to be viewed with the light microscope. Subcutaneous connective tissue can be studied effectively this way, as can muscle and nerve fibers. These preparations are short lived, however, and other methods have been evolved for maintaining living cells for extended periods and repeated direct microscopic examinations.

CELL, TISSUE, AND ORGAN CULTURE

New biological methods often arise out of the need to solve a particular question, and the most dramatic early tissue culture experimentation was devised to solve a problem of nerve fiber growth. Early in this century, histologists were debating whether processes of nerve cells, called fibers or axons, grew out from the nerve cell body or formed from the fusion of longitudinally arrayed elements within the peripheral nerve. The available microscopes did not allow a clear resolution of this controversy.

Harrison attacked the problem directly by isolating a part of the developing nervous system of a frog into a clot of sterile lymph and watching nerve fiber formation under the microscope. His experiments provided a clear demonstration that nerve fiber elongation occurs by direct extension and growth of the nerve cell (Fig. 2.1). Soon thereafter many of the tissues of the body found themselves in oddly shaped glass containers surrounded by complex feeding solutions. Such *in vitro* ("in glass") *cultivation* soon became a valuable and commonplace tool of the cytologist.

Three categories of in vitro cultivation are now recognized. *Cell culture* refers to maintenance of nonadherent, usually dividing, cells, which are transferred from vessel to vessel as their numbers continuously increase. *Tissue culture* entails explantation of an immature tissue fragment into culture. The cultured fragment, called the *explant*, generally undergoes some growth and reorganization. Cells growing out from the explant are termed the *outgrowth*. *Organ culture* generally involves explantation and maintenance of mature tissues or organ fragments. This technique is particularly useful for study of the direct effects of drugs or hormones on various tissues of the body.

Successful in vitro studies require that the tissue be obtained in a sterile state (or that it be treated with antibiotics to render it sterile), for the conditions favoring cell growth are similar to those for bacterial multiplication. At all times the tissues must be handled in a fluid environment with salt concentrations and a pH resembling that of the body fluids. Such salt solutions are called *balanced salt solutions* (BSS). Tissues may be dissociated into individual cells, often by mild treatment with a digestive enzyme, such as trypsin, which loosens the adhesions between cells. After being washed in BSS, the cells are provided with a nutrient *medium* and maintained either in suspension culture, where the cells are kept floating by constant agitation, or on a surface to which the cells attach. The surface may be either glass or plastic, sometimes covered with a thin layer of collagen. Sometimes it is advantageous to attach the tissue to this surface (and provide a matrix for growth) by clotting blood plasma around it.

The medium may be completely *defined*,

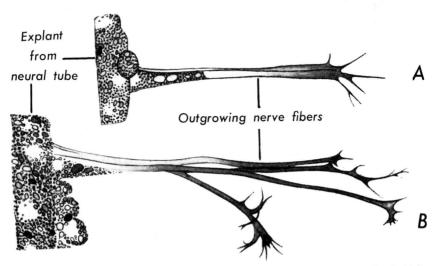

Figure 2.1. Outgrowth of nerve fibers from pieces of embryonic frog neural tube (which contains the nerve cell bodies) grown in tissue culture. *A*, after 25 hr; *B*, after 34 hr. The expanded tips of the elongating nerve fibers, called growth cones, are regions of vigorous motility. (Redrawn from von Möllendorff (ed): *Handbuch der mikroskopische Anatomie des Menschen.* Vienna, Springer-Verlag, after Harrison).

i.e., a mixture of known composition containing vitamins, amino acids, and salts, or *natural*, i.e., a mixture containing one of the complex products of the body, such as blood serum. Certain continuously propagated cell lines can be maintained and continue to grow on completely defined media. The content of one of the simplest of these is given in Table 2.1. For the propagation of certain cells, this medium is often supplemented with 10% serum.

To obtain the fullest possible expression of the organization and functions of certain tissues in culture, it is sometimes necessary to add additional organic ingredients to the medium. The most generally employed aug-

Table 2.1.
Eagle's Minimum Essential Medium[a]

Components	
	mg/l
Amino acids	
L-Arginine HCl	126.4
L-Cystine	24.0
L-Glutamine	292.0
L-Histidine HCl · H_2O	41.9
L-Isoleucine	52.5
L-Leucine	52.4
L-Lysine HCl	73.1
L-Methionine	14.9
L-Phenylalanine	33.0
L-Threonine	47.6
L-Tryptophan	10.2
L-Tyrosine	36.2
L-Valine	46.8
Vitamins	
D-Ca-pantothenate	1.0
Choline chloride	1.0
Folic acid	1.0
i-Inositol	2.0
Nicotinamide	1.0
Pyridoxal HCl	1.0
Riboflavin	0.1
Thiamine HCl	1.0
Inorganic salts and other components	
$CaCl_2$ · $2H_2O$	265.0
KCl	400.0
$MgSO_4$ · $7H_2O$	200.0
NaCl	6800.0
$NaHCO_3$	2200.0
NaH_2PO_4 · H_2O	140.0
Dextrose	1000.0
Phenol red	10.0

[a] From H. Eagle: *Science* 130:432, 1959.

mentations are blood derivatives such as fetal calf serum, bovine serum albumin, or human umbilical cord serum.

Certain specific proteins, called *growth factors*, have also been discovered; these enhance the growth of specific tissues in culture. A dramatic example is the stimulation of the growth of certain types of nerve fibers by a factor present in the salivary gland of the mouse. This protein is termed *nerve growth factor* and this puzzling circumstance—a protein present in a digestive gland exerting a very specific effect on nervous tissue—raises many intriguing questions concerning factors which may control appropriate rates of growth in the various tissues of the body. Other specific growth factors are known such as *epidermal growth factor*. While these promote growth of specific cells in vitro, it is not yet clear how frequently they are used in the body as control mechanisms governing normal growth.

Morphology of the Living Cell

The greatest detail in living animal cells can generally be observed in thinly spread culture preparations. It is necessary to use a phase contrast or differential interference (Nomarski) optical system to enhance contrast because living cells, being composed chiefly of water, are quite transparent. Even under the best light microscopic conditions, however, only a fraction of the great internal complexity of the cell known from electron microscopic work can be seen (see Fig. 2.2 and compare to Fig. 1.12). The nucleus and its contained nucleoli are clearly visible. It is clear that the cell contents are contained within a flexible and often very active covering. The cytoplasm is seen to contain varying numbers of dense granules and somewhat less dense, thread-like elements. The dense, particulate granules are elements of the lysosomal system or lipid inclusions; the less dense linear organelles are mitochondria. Occasionally the Golgi apparatus and endoplasmic reticulum can be visualized.

When the cell contains substantial arrays of molecules in a patterned orienta-

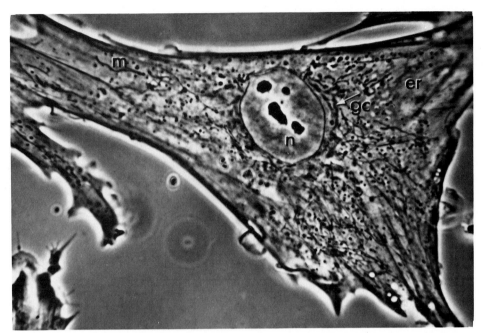

Figure 2.2. Phase contrast photomicrograph of a living rat embryo cell grown in culture. Many cytoplasmic organelles are visible. The Golgi complex (*gc*) may be seen near the nucleus (*n*). Endoplasmic reticulum (*er*) is visible as a shadowy, branching structure. The long sinuous threads are mitochondria (*m*) (×1450). (Reprinted with permission from I. K. Buckley and K. R. Porter: *Protoplasma* 64:349, 1967.)

tion, these alter the path of transmitted light, and the manner in which the light is altered gives some clue regarding the basic molecular organization. Thus, with *polarizing microscopy*, areas containing linear arrays of filamentous material, such as the actin and myosin of muscle cells, can be detected. Similarly, a mass of microtubules such as is found in the mitotic spindle can be visualized (see Fig. 2.18).

EXPERIMENTAL MANIPULATION OF LIVING CELLS

Simple observations of living cells have been usefully supplemented with a host of techniques which can be applied more or less directly to living cells.

Vital and Supravital Staining

In *vital staining*, dyes are injected into the living animal so that the activity of certain cells can be demonstrated by their selective absorption of the coloring matter. An outstanding example has been the dem-

onstration of the distribution of highly phagocytic cells throughout the body. When trypan blue is injected into an experimental animal, accumulations of the dye are found in vacuoles in the macrophages of the loose connective tissue, and in the phagocytic cells of lymphatic organs, bone marrow, and liver.

Supravital staining consists of adding dyes to the medium of cells already removed from the organism. When trypan blue is placed on a tissue culture, the macrophages take it up in abundance. Small phagocytic cells have been marked in this way, and their subsequent development into epithelioid and giant cells has been followed. The use of supravital dyes such as neutral red to mark the lysosomal systems of cells is discussed in Chapter 1, as is the staining of mitochondria by Janus green. Rhodamine is a supravital stain which selectively accumulates in mitochondria of living cells because of its positive charge. It causes the mitochondria to glow brilliantly when viewed by fluorescence microscopy (Fig. 2.3).

The selective staining of organelles with a colored dye combined with the high intensities of light available from laser sources provides the opportunity for a new form of *cellular microsurgery*. Laser light, like other visible light, is not much absorbed by living tissue, unless the cells contain pigment granules. If the mitochondria are colored green, however, and laser light of a wavelength absorbed by the green dye is directed at the cell, the light absorption leads to local heating, as well as other effects, and thus to more or less selective destruction of the mitochondria of the cell. If the cone of laser light is restricted to a part of the cell, only some of the mitochondria are damaged. Similarly, chromosomes which have been supravitally stained with acridine orange can be irradiated during mitosis with a laser microbeam. Using this technique, lesions less than 1 μm can be placed on desired sites of individual chromosomes (Fig. 2.4).

Micromanipulation and Microdissection

Several new techniques have been made possible by the development of an instrument, called a *micromanipulator*, which moves fine glass needles or pipettes with such precision that single cells can be injected, manipulated, or dissected. Experiments with the microneedles have made our concept of the physical nature of cells much clearer. Microdissection provided some of the first direct evidence of the presence of a cell membrane. More recently, micromanipulators have been employed to move or fragment fixed cells while they were being examined under the scanning electron microscope. Thus the value of the technique is being extended to electron microscope levels of resolution.

With these techniques cytoplasm has been shown to be viscous, its viscosity var-

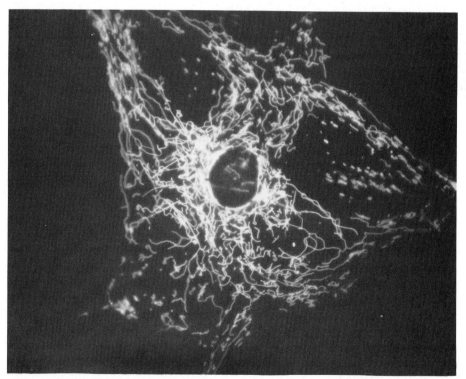

Figure 2.3. Mitochondria of a living fibroblastic cell (gerbil fibroma line) stained with rhodamine 123 and viewed by fluorescence microscopy (×250). (Courtesy of Dr. Lincoln Johnson.)

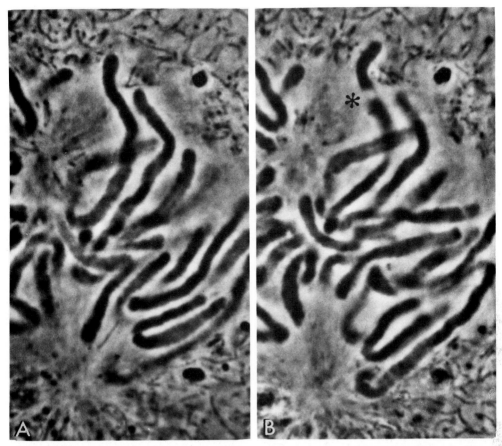

Figure 2.4. Phase contrast photomicrographs of chromosomes in a dividing salamander lung cell before (*A*) and after (*B*) irradiation with laser microbeam. The cells had been previously treated with a nucleic acid stain, acridine orange, to enhance absorption of the microbeam by the chromosomal material. After irradiation, a discrete lesion is seen (at asterisk) in one of the chromosomes (×2500). (Reprinted with permission from M. W. Berns, et al.: *Exp Cell Res* 56:292, 1969.)

ing in different cells. The granules, vacuoles, and mitochondria can be moved about within the cell. The nucleus can be indented by the pressure of the needle and pushed about from one part of the cell to another or even, in some special cases, transplanted from one cell to another.

Microelectrodes, which are extremely fine pipettes (tips less than 1 μm in diameter) filled with concentrated salt solutions, may also be mounted in micromanipulators. If these are inserted into cells with great care, the cell membrane will seal around them and allow measurements of the differences in electrical potential between the inside of the cell and the external environment (Fig. 2.5). This technique has been especially

useful to the physiologist in the study of nerve and muscle, which employ changes in membrane potentials as a method of signaling. A related method has been used to detect ionic fluxes across specialized junctions linking adjacent epithelial cells.

If a microelectrode is filled with a dye carrying a charge and if current of the appropriate polarity is passed into the cell via the electrode, then dye will pass into the cell with the current flow. There are charged dyes which can be made to fluoresce in the light microscope. When injected into cells, these diffuse widely through the cytoplasm. This technique, which may be termed *microdye injection*, is useful in delineating the contour of individ-

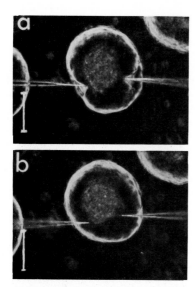

Figure 2.5.   Photomicrographs of frog oocytes being impaled with two extremely fine microelectrodes. The microelectrodes can first be seen to indent the plasma membrane (*a*) and then to penetrate the cell cytoplasm (*b*). This manipulation allows the measurement of intracellular electrical activity. The bar indicates 100 μm. (Reprinted from permission from Y. Kanno and W. R. Loewenstein: *Exp Cell Res* 31:149, 1963.)

ual cells in complexly organized tissues such as the nervous system (Fig. 2.6). Radioactive materials can be similarly employed.

Cinematography

Another technique which has been used with tissue culture cells is cinematography, motion pictures taken through the objectives of a microscope. It is useful not only to obtain permanent records of cell activity but also as an experimental aid in the analysis of movement too slow or too fast to be appreciated by the unaided eye. When the exposures are taken at intervals of several seconds and projected on the screen at the usual speed, the photographed processes are speeded up more than 100 times. The movements of cells and organelles, which are scarcely appreciated by direct observation, become visible. In the division of the cell by mitosis, the shifting of the nucleus during the prophase, the rounding blebs or

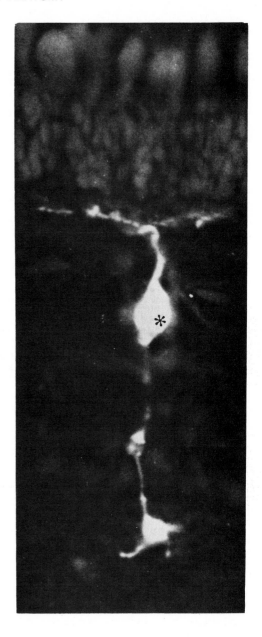

Figure 2.6.   The cell body (asterisk) and cytoplasmic extensions of a neuron in the goldfish retina are here demonstrated after the injection of a fluorescent dye (Procion yellow) directly into the cell soma. After injection the tissue is fixed, embedded, and sectioned for viewing in the fluorescence microscope. At the top of the figure are rod and cone cells, which fluoresce faintly without dye injection (autofluorescence). Scale: 50 μm = 2 inches. (Reprinted with permission from A. Kaneko: *J Physiol* 207:623, 1970.)

pseudopodia which are sent out and withdrawn from every part of the surface of the cell, and the violent agitation just before the chromosomes separate are all aspects which cannot be appreciated by any other means. Within the nondividing cell, the shifting of the granules and mitochondria is beautifully demonstrated by these speeded films.

In order to reverse the process and slow activities too quick for the eye, the exposures are taken three or four times as rapidly as they are to be shown on the screen. The movement of cilia has been studied by this method. The contraction of cardiac muscle in tissue cultures, slowed to one-fourth the actual speed, offers an opportunity to study the mechanism of muscle contraction.

ACTIVITIES OF LIVING CELLS

Application of the techniques discussed above, as well as observations on single-cell organisms, has led to the recognition of a variety of types of cellular movements. All cell types exhibit various intracellular movements.

Intracellular Movements

Inside the living cell, both nuclear motion and movement within the cytoplasm can be observed. The simplest form of movement exhibited to some extent by all cells is a shifting about of the elements within the cytoplasm. This is often very slight and so slow that it is frequently overlooked unless cinematography is employed. The granules and mitochondria move slowly for varying distances. In addition, one observes rapid linear movements of cytoplasmic particles; this distinctive activity is termed *saltatory movement*. Saltatory activity must not be confused with the more random motions of *Brownian movement*, which is dampened in healthy cells but which becomes marked in cells after death. Cytoplasmic movement may sometimes involve the transport of materials from the cell body into cell processes and is especially important in cells with long processes such as neurons.

In certain cells, a surprising rotation of the entire nucleus within the relatively immobile cytoplasm has been observed. These periodic rolling motions can be seen when several nucleoli are present to mark the disposition of the nucleus, thus allowing accurate detection of its movements.

Cellular Locomotion

Cellular locomotion means the movement of the whole cell from one place to another. Studies utilizing tissue culture, immunocytochemical and viral tagging techniques, and cinematography have revealed two at first seemingly different mechanisms by which cells move. In fact the two probably share fundamentally similar mechanisms. Amebae locomote by pseudopodial propagated movement. They dispatch long processes in the appropriate direction and then appear to flow into these processes. Among animal cells, leukocytes and macrophages appear to move in a similar fashion, i.e., by *ameboid movement*.

Other types of animal cells (such as the mesodermally derived fibroblast) flatten and adhere to surfaces on which they are placed and then glide along this surface without extensive pseudopodium formation (or gross changes in their overall shape). The membrane along the flattened edges of these cells ruffles, and this ruffling is most active at the edge of the cell marking the direction of movement. The adhesiveness and other properties of the cell surface and of the substrate are important in determining the extent and speed of this locomotion, for movement can be influenced by the shape and properties of the terrain. Changes in the adhesive properties of the cell membrane are especially important during developmental stages of the organism because these properties will influence the migration of cells.

The mechanisms responsible for the actual movements at the cell border are not clearly understood. It is known that in certain fibroblasts, the Golgi apparatus is localized near the leading edge of the migratory cell. Certain integral membrane proteins can be traced in vesicles which leave this organelle for insertion into the leading edge membrane. It is postulated that as new membrane is added at the leading edge of the cell, trailing edge membrane is retrieved by endocytosis. Coordinated adhesions of the cell to its substrate, as well as contractile activity of actin "stress fibers" and other cytoskeletal elements also are important components of the motility mechanism. It is now known that actin- and myosin-like proteins occur widely in many cell types, suggesting that many cells contain at least some representation of a motility system.

The direction of movement of a cell can be influenced by a concentration gradient of some substance in the surrounding solution. The cell is then said to be influenced by *chemotaxis*. Some white blood cells are chemotactically responsive to certain bacteria and move toward any such organism in their vicinity.

An interesting and important aspect of the control of cell movement is the phenomenon of *contact inhibition*. This property is exhibited well by fibroblasts. When, in vitro, a moving fibroblast contacts an adjacent fibroblast its ruffling membrane becomes paralyzed and movement in this region of the cell stops. The cell then reverses its direction, extending an exploring ruffling membrane from its opposite side. When the population of fibroblasts is sufficiently dense, movement of any cell in any direction brings immediate contact. Ruffling then ceases and both movement and proliferation of the cells are suspended. This is called contact inhibition. The cytological significance of contact inhibition is under active investigation, for it has been observed that some cancer (sarcoma) cells, which, like fibroblasts, are derived from mesodermal tissue, are not contact-inhibited when they approach normal inhibited fibroblasts in culture. It is thus possible that the invasiveness of some types

of cancer is related to a failure in this type of inhibition.

In some cases where two cells come together and exhibit contact inhibition, the involved membranes are known to form low resistance junctions in regions where cell membranes come into especially close apposition (see Chapter 4). This type of cell-to-cell junction is known to allow small molecules or ions to pass from one cell to another without diffusing into the extracellular spaces. These junctions therefore provide special regions for cell-to-cell communication. This type of junction is known to form, sometimes transiently, during various phases of development and has been postulated to play an important integrating role, determining developmental patterns.

Phagocytosis and Pinocytosis

The term *phagocytosis* is generally used to describe the ingestion of solid material by the cell, whereas *pinocytosis* refers to the ingestion of fluids. Both mechanisms involve invagination of the surface membrane and the sequestration of the ingested material within a vacuole in the cell cytoplasm and can be considered types of endocytosis.

The process of phagocytosis (from the Greek *phagein*, to eat) is used by certain single cell organisms for feeding, but in higher organisms it is more commonly used as a defense mechanism for the ingestion of particles foreign to the organism. Actively ameboid cells usually have an enhanced capability for phagocytosis. In the case of the more rapidly moving cells, such as neutrophilic leukocytes, engulfment is facilitated by the passage of the cell over the particle, such as a bacterium, to be ingested. Cells with less rapid locomotion, such as macrophages, come in contact with the material to be engulfed by sending out pseudopodia, which adhere to the debris and surround it, either by drawing it toward the cell or by expanding the pseudopodium.

The ingestion of droplets of fluid by cells in tissue culture was described by Lewis in 1931 as pinocytosis (from the Green *pinein*, to drink). A similar process is known to occur in vivo, and the term pinocytosis is now generally used to describe the ingestion of fluids and their contained solutes, whether observed with the light (Fig. 2.7) or the electron microscope. Recent electron microscopic observations indicate that the presence of tiny vacuoles below the resolution of the light microscope is common to most cells. Because of the minute size of these vacuoles (vesicles), their uptake activity at the membrane is sometimes termed *micropinocytosis*. The presence of protein outside the cell generally acts as a stimulus to pinocytosis. Proteins thus ingested are broken down by the lysosomal system of the cell (discussed in Chapter 1). Certain cell types apparently use the process of pinocytosis for the transcellular transport of large molecules (see "Capillaries," Chapter 12).

OBSERVATION OF LIVING CELLS IN SITU

The descriptions up to this point have dealt with cells surviving after their removal from the body, but cells have been observed by various methods within the living organism (that is, *in situ* or *in vivo* contrasted to in vitro). The earliest attempts were made on the vascular system, on the blood cells circulating in the tadpole's tail fin, in the tongue, foot web, and mesentery of the adult frog, and in the mesentery and omentum of mammals. The transparency of the tail fin of the tadpole is particularly advantageous for the observation of many kinds of cells. Tadpole tail fin has been used to study the outgrowth of nerve fibers and the formation of special sensory nerve endings. The growth of blood vessels and lymphatics and the activity of the endothelium, connective tissue cells, and phagocytes have also been extensively studied.

Mammalian material has been made available for similar observation by the perfection of a technique for inserting a transparent window in the rabbit's ear. Through it, the growth of new blood vessels and lymphatics, the activity of capillaries, the opening and closing of vascular anastomoses, the behavior of the phagocytic cells of connective tissue, and the growth and resorption of other tissues have been studied in detail.

CYTOLOGICAL ANALYSIS IN CELL CULTURE

Cell culture techniques permit certain types of cytological analysis that cannot be undertaken in whole tissues. Several of these are discussed below.

Determination of Karyotype

The chromosomal content of cells is best visualized when the chromosomes are fixed and stained while tightly coiled during the process of cell division. This is accomplished by placing cells in a medium fostering cell division. An agent (colchicine) which prevents completion of the mitotic process is added, and the cells arrested during mitosis accumulate in the culture. These cells are made to swell by the addition of hypotonic medium and are then flattened with pressure. After staining the chromosomes may be counted and classified by size and shape. This analysis allows the determination of the *karyotype* of an organism. A normal karyotype for human cells is 46 chromosomes: 22 pairs not associated with sex determination (*autosomes*) and 2 chromosomes that determine sex (Fig. 2.8).

A variety of human congenital abnormalities relate to abnormal karyotypes. For example, the basis for certain types of abnormal sexual development has been traced to abnormalities in sex chromosome number. Thus, if the normal XX sex chromosome pattern of female human cells is altered so that only one X chromosome is present (a condition called *Turner's syndrome*), or if the normal XY composition of the male is supplemented with a second X to give a XXY complement (a condition called Klinefelter's syndrome), then sexual and other traits of the individual are abnormal. *Down's syndrome* is also a condition of abnormal chromosome content; in these cases there is an extra autosome

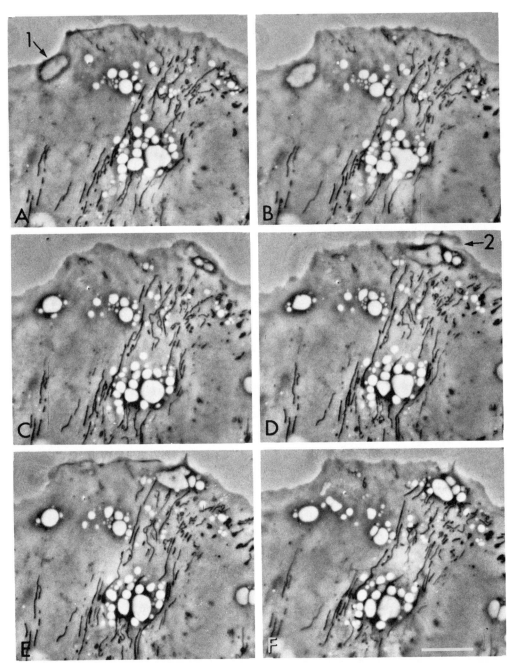

Figure 2.7. Pinocytosis in cultured human sarcoma cells as observed in the phase contrast microscope. The figures shown here are but a few of those obtained every 2 sec for a time lapse film and were obtained over a 12-min period. Pinocytosis occurs in regions of the cell body which are undulating vigorously. Recent intake of fluid appears as an irregular lake just inside the cell (as at 1A and 2D). Secondarily the collected fluid assumes the appearance of more refractile spheroidal droplets which start to migrate interiorly. The bar indicates 5 μm. (Reprinted with permission from A. Gropp: In *Cinemicrography in Cell Biology*, edited by G. G. Rose, p. 279. New York, Academic Press, 1963.)

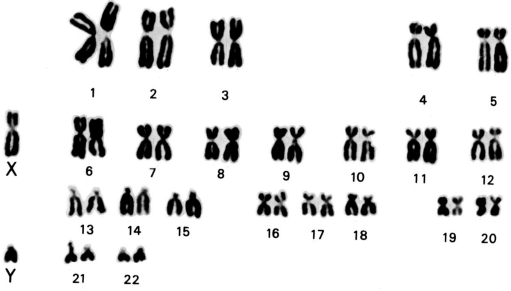

Figure 2.8. A normal karyotype prepared from a human leukocyte dividing in culture. The chromosomes were fixed in acetic alcohol and stained with acetic orcein. When this preparation is viewed in the light microscope the metaphase chromosomes appear in a cluster on the slide. A photograph of these chromosomes is obtained and is then cut up so that the chromosomes may be grouped as shown here (×1500). (Courtesy of Dr. Orlando Miller.)

(chromosome 21), giving a total chromosome number of 47 instead of the normal 46.

Repeated analysis of cultured cell lines has led to the observation that cells carried for long periods in culture often develop abnormal karyotypes. When cells from normal tissues are set out in culture, they have the number of chromosomes characteristic of the species. For human cells this is 46, the *diploid* number of chromosomes. Cells are termed *euploid* if they contain this number of chromosomes or an exact multiple of it; cells with multiples of the diploid number also are referred to as *polyploid*. After long periods in culture, many cell types undergo a transformation and the number of chromosomes per cell changes. The cell line is then said to be *aneuploid* (or *heteroploid*) if the cells contain an odd number of chromosomes. The extensively studied HeLa cell lines, derived from a human cervical cancer in 1952 and whose progeny is still carried in many laboratories, may have from 50 to 350 chromosomes per cell.

Various interpretations have been offered for changes in chromosome number in cultured cells. Some investigators believe that it indicates damage to the replicating mechanism resulting from less than optimal culture conditions. Others have suggested that the change from euploid to aneuploid is the mechanism of adaptation of cells to permanent growth in culture, and that if aneuploidy does not occur, cells will not adapt to permanent culture as cell lines. Hayflick has suggested that if cells remain euploid they have a limited life span in culture and undergo only a limited (preset) number of divisions before losing their capacity to survive in culture. This limited life span of euploid cultured cells has been related to an aging process, and the transformation to the aneuploid state has been related to the origin of malignancy, i.e., cancer. When reintroduced into animal hosts, many transformed cells grow as tumors. It should be noted, however, that not all malignant cells are aneuploid.

Cloning

As the above discussion indicates, cells established in culture may be a diverse group, and it is often desirable to select a single cell and to establish it and its progeny as the only cells present in a cell culture line. This process is called *cloning* (from the Greek for twig). It involves isolation of a single cell, either by dissociating and greatly diluting cell populations before culture or by isolating a single cell in a micropipette. These cells are placed in the most propitious culture environment, and as they multiply, their progeny provide, at least for a time, maximally homogeneous cell populations.

Cloning techniques are utilized in current research to develop sensitive probes for the localization of specific molecules in living systems. Advantage is taken of the specificity of the antigen-antibody reaction and the fact that almost any complex molecule can induce the formation by lymphocytes of one or more highly specified antibodies against that molecule. Since lymphocytes normally do not live for a lengthy time in culture, individual antibody-producing cells are fused with lymphocytic tumor cells that continue to proliferate. Hybrid cells formed in this manner that have the ability to make the desired antibody and retain their ability to divide in culture indefinitely are then selected and propagated as clones. They are referred to as *hybridomas* and the antibodies produced are called *monoclonal antibodies*. By labeling the antibody with fluorescent, radioactive, or electron-dense markers, the specific location of the reacting molecule in cells or tissues can be determined. Antibodies produced by this technique are of high purity because they result from the proliferation of a single lymphocyte and the antibody is specific for a single antigenic determinant on the inducing molecule. Antibodies produced in the regular manner (i.e., injecting an antigen into an animal and collecting serum) are termed *polyclonal antibodies* because the antigenic molecule usually has several antigenic sites, each of which can generate its own specific antibody. A family of related antibodies is produced, since large numbers of lymphocytes in the body can respond to the stimulus simultaneously. The monoclonal antibody technique is especially useful for studies on the appearance of cell surface molecules during development and determining the roles of such molecules in differentiation and normal function. The antibodies can also be used to isolate specific molecules for biochemical characterization.

Cellular Aggregation

Tissue culture techniques have provided an opportunity to study the reaggregation of cells which have been separated and suspended in a fluid medium. Embryonic organs are dissociated into individual cells by loosening intercellular adhesions, with a proteolytic enzyme such as trypsin and/or a reduction in Ca^{2+} concentration of the medium. After dissociation, cells tend to reaggregate, often in structures resembling the tissue of origin. Cells of different organs, and from different species, for example, from kidneys and cartilage from mouse and chick, can be mixed together after dissociation. Under these conditions, kidney cells from both species aggregate in one mass and, similarly, all cartilage cells in another. Cells of a certain organ thus have the ability to recognize cells of similar type and maintain preferential association with them. These observations apply primarily to embryonic organs, for as organs mature the constituent cells lose their capability for cellular reaggregation.

A tissue containing cells from two different sources, for example a mixture of chick and mouse cartilage cells, is called *chimeric*. It is also possible to produce chimeric animals, i.e., animals containing cells from more than one source. Mintz has been able to dissociate the cells of two different mouse embryos at the early cleavage stages and allow them to reaggregate as one blastocyst. This is then reintroduced into a pseudopregnant mother, and subsequently develops and is delivered normally. If dissociated blastomeres from a strain of black and a strain of white mice are mixed together to form a single blastocyst, certain of the newborn mice develop alternating black and white areas of hair pigmentation.

Heterokaryons

In addition to the possibility of deriving tissues composed of cells from a variety of sources, tissue culture provides the opportunity of producing cells with mixtures of genetic material. Human cells can be cultured together with cells of, for example, chick tissues. If certain types of inactivated virus particles are added to these cultures, the two types of cells fuse together to become one cell with two or more nuclei. It is thus possible to observe the reactions of an inactive nucleus when it is introduced into an active cell (Fig. 2.9). As heterokaryons divide, the nuclei sometimes enter mitosis together and are reconstituted as a single larger nucleus. Cells thus formed contain, within a single nucleus, chromosomes derived from different species. With subsequent divisions certain of these chromosomes may be lost. In man-mouse hybrids, for example, the human chromosomes are gradually reduced in number until in some cases only one remains. This circumstance has been used to determine the localization of certain genes to a specific human chromosome.

Other Uses of Cell and Tissue Culture

Tissue culture has been essential in research on viruses. Functioning cells are necessary for virus growth, and tissue cultures offer an opportunity to study virus growth outside the animal host and to prepare large quantities of virus for vaccines. They are also necessary to assay the types and amounts of virus present in any biological preparation.

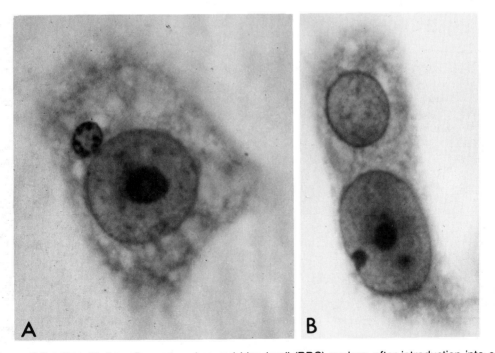

Figure 2.9. Reactivation of a mature hen red blood cell (RBC) nucleus after introduction into an active HeLa cell. The heterokaryon in *A* contains the large, cultured HeLa cell nucleus (about 10 μm in diameter) and a typical small, dotted RBC nucleus. *B* shows the subsequent enlargements and disappearance of heterochromatin in the hen RBC nucleus. By applying radioautographic techniques to this type of preparation, it is possible to demonstrate that DNA and RNA synthesis (which normally does not occur in the mature RBC nucleus) is resumed in RBC nuclei residing in the cytoplasm of a continuously synthesizing HeLa cell. (Reprinted with permission from H. Harris: *J Cell Sci* 2:23, 1967.)

Observations on Organized Tissue in Culture

With the increasing refinement of tissue culture techniques, it has become possible to establish many of the tissues of the body in culture, often with a high degree of organization and function. Three examples are given here to illustrate the degree of organization that can be achieved by cells maintained in vitro.

Skeletal muscle may be established in culture by taking cells from embryonic muscle before the muscle fibers are fully differentiated. A single cell is selected and, if culture conditions are very carefully controlled, it divides repeatedly, producing a prodigious progeny of like cells. After a substantial amount of cell division has occurred, some of these cells fuse together to form long multinucleated muscle fibers. Normally mitosis does not occur in the cells after they have fused. The muscle fibers thus formed develop cross striations, indicating that the muscle proteins actin and myosin are being formed and aligned within the fiber. The fibers are then capable of contraction. A single muscle cell has thus become a group of functioning muscle fibers (Fig. 2.10).

Nervous tissue in culture may similarly attain an impressive degree of histological organization. Young cells may be taken from the developing nervous system of em-

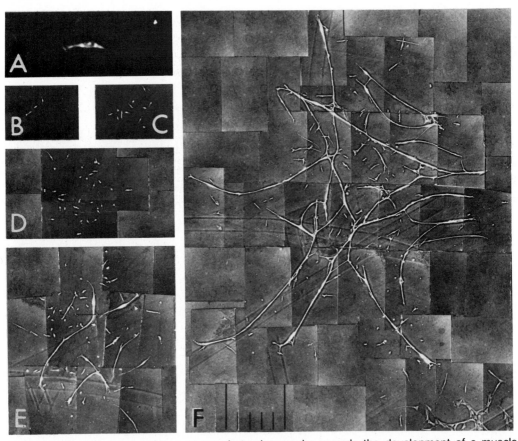

Figure 2.10. This series of low power photomicrographs records the development of a muscle colony from a single cell. The colony produced by the cell in *A* is shown after 1 day (*B*), 2 days (*C*), 3 days (*D*), 5 days (*E*), and 8 days (*F*) of development. After substantial cell division, the cells begin to fuse to form the straplike multinucleate muscle fibers seen in *E* and *F*. The entire muscle mass is a clone because it has arisen from a single cell. In *F*, each division of the scale represents 0.1 mm. (Reprinted with permission from I. R. Konigsberg: *Science* 140:1273, 1963.)

bryos and placed in chambers, where they can be kept for days, weeks, or even months. Development of the tissue continues in vitro much as it would in vivo (Fig. 2.11). The nerve cells send out processes and these form contacts (synapses) with other neurons. The supporting cells around the neuron form a special ensheathment called myelin, just as they do in vivo. In addition, the nervous tissue in vitro demonstrates many of the electrical properties characteristic of its function in the body.

Gland cells, such as those of the pancreas, can also express their activity in culture. Under proper conditions, this tissue forms zymogens, the relatively inactive form of digestive enzymes when they are in secretory granules in the exocrine pancreas in the intact animal.

The list of tissues capable of impressive in vitro performance continues to grow; skin keratinizes, hair and feathers grow, glands secrete, bone is deposited, heart cells beat, blood cells differentiate, collagen forms, and cilia move. The usefulness of tissue culture techniques in the study of the cell is expanding.

CELLULAR DIFFERENTIATION

The central problem in the study of development is the question of how a single cell, the fertilized egg, gives rise to the many cell types of the mature organism. The fertilized egg divides rapidly, forming first a ball of cells called morula; later this mass of cells develops a cavity and is termed a blastula in lower animals and in a slightly modified form, a blastocyst in mammals. In mammals the blastocyst becomes embedded in the uterine wall and is subsequently nourished by the maternal tissues. With time, three classes of cells can be distin-

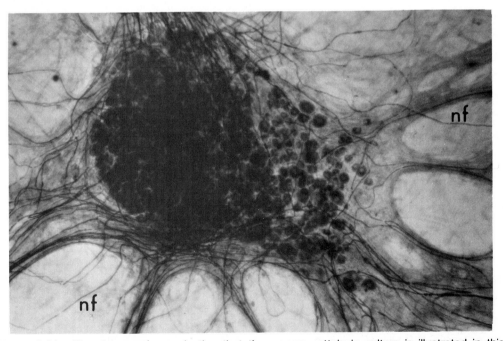

Figure 2.11. The degree of organization that tissues may attain in culture is illustrated in this photomicrograph of a group of nerve cells which have matured in vitro. Clustered in the center are the nerve cell bodies (best seen at the right, where they are less concentrated). Radiating from these nerve cells are nerve fibers, often gathered into fascicles. Some individual nerve fibers are visible because their fatty sheaths (the myelin sheaths) are stained with Sudan black; they are best seen when situated singly, as at *nf*. This fat stain colors the neuron cytoplasm more intensely than the nucleus. Whole mount (unsectioned); dorsal root ganglion taken from a rat fetus and grown in culture for more than 6 months (×100).

guished in the embryonic germ disc of the blastocyst: the ectoderm or outside layer, the endoderm or inside lining, and the mesoderm, the cells between these surface layers. The organization and development of these three fundamental layers of embryonic tissue are discussed in the next chapter. From these layers and from their interaction, ultimately more than a hundred recognizable kinds of cells develop to form the adult mammal. The process of functional and structural specialization of these cells is called *differentiation*. Put another way, differentiation is the process whereby the various cells of a multicellular system acquire, individually or in groups, the structural machinery which allows them to emphasize certain particular functional capabilities. For example, although virtually all cells display some propensity for cytoplasmic contraction only those cells which we term muscle cells have developed the mechanisms which permit the generation of strong and/or lasting contractile force. Such cells display very elaborate cytoplasmic structure for this special function. Other functional capabilities are appropriately reduced, but not necessarily eliminated. Muscle cells also display some ability to conduct impulses (an emphasized property of neurons) and to synthesize some collagen (a principal activity of fibroblasts).

The problem of the mechanism and control of differentiation is broad and beyond the scope of this discussion. It is useful, however, in discussing the principles of cytology, to consider how differentiation might be accomplished by an individual cell. In order to differentiate during embryonic development, cells must make a series of small shifts in their potential, as, for example, when a cell of the blastocyst becomes a cell belonging to the endoderm. These then proliferate to make more cells of their own kind. Then another shift is made, and members of this cell group may become either part of the gut wall or part of the lung. If the former occurs, then a third shift ensues, and the cell becomes

either absorptive or secretory. Once the fate of the cell is set, the cell is said to be *"determined."* It subsequently becomes structurally differentiated to perform and emphasize specialized functions. What a cell is and what it is capable of doing is largely a matter of the structural proteins and enzyme systems which it acquires.

There can be little doubt that this orderly development rests ultimately on the activities of the genetic material in the cell nucleus. It is also generally agreed that the basic codes in the genetic material do not change with development, but that different regions of the genome are "turned on" (and others "turned off") as cells develop. The genome is therefore differentially expressed as the cells are progressively determined.

It is also clear that alterations in the use of genetic material during development are not entirely preprogrammed within the cell but are influenced by interactions with other cells. As soon as an organism becomes multicellular the cells begin to react with one another in ways which trigger (or *"induce"*) the onset of appropriate regional differentiation. As will be seen, the trigger may operate by activation of genetic mechanisms or by alteration of the rate or amount of synthetic activity already underway in responding cells. Cells of different stages of maturity may respond differently to normal or abnormal triggering interactions. The often disastrous effects of the German measles virus and the drug Thalidomide on the embryo, as compared with their mild effect on the older individual, are good examples of interference with normal processes to which cells of a specific stage are highly sensitive.

The Operon

How do the sequential changes that occur in the cell during development take place? In 1961 the French molecular biologists Jacob and Monod suggested a mechanism by which the expression of genetic material in bacteria might be controlled. Their concept is based on the assumption, now generally accepted, that the genetic information of the organism, encoded in the nucleotide sequence of DNA, is transcribed into messenger RNA (mRNA), as has been discussed above. In union with ribosomes, the nucleotide sequences of mRNA are translated into the amino acid sequence of a specific polypeptide. Jacob and Monod suggest that the synthesis of mRNA on the gene is regulated by specific repressors which are products of other genes, called *regulator genes*. The *repressors* are thought to act by becoming engaged with the operator site of a group of genes. The *operator* plus the "structural" genes it controls is termed the *operon*. When the operator site is open, all of the genes of the operon synthesize mRNA, and when it is closed by the repressor, none do. The affinity of the repressor for the operator site is influenced by the concentration of small molecular weight metabolites within the cell. This scheme is summarized in Fig. 2.12.

Considerable evidence supports this concept of gene regulation for procaryotes (e.g., bacteria, viruses) but it is clear that the situation is far more complex for eucaryotic cells. The DNA in eucaryotic cells is much more condensed and is in close association with histones and other DNA-binding proteins. In addition, a nuclear envelope separates the process of RNA synthesis (*transcription*) from protein synthesis (*translation*). Therefore, it is necessary to have mechanisms to loosen the chromatin structure and then to activate selected regions of the decondensed chromatin before the type of regulation outlined for bacteria can occur.

In addition to regulation associated with

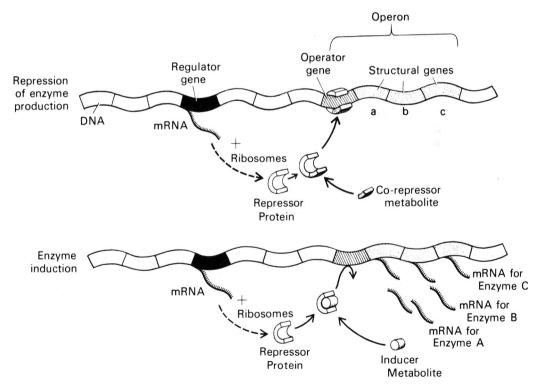

Figure 2.12. Gene control: the operon concept. According to this concept a regulator gene occupying one site on the DNA strand controls the production of a repressor protein which, in combination with a corepressor substance, inhibits the activity of an operator gene on another site of the DNA strand. In the presence of an inducer compound, the repressor protein is unable to block the operator site. This operator gene controls the activity of adjacent structural genes on which there is assembly of messenger RNA (mRNA) molecules involved in enzyme manufacture.

gene activation and RNA synthesis, there is a measure of control that can occur at the level of transport from nucleus to cytoplasm. Additionally, a high degree of control of synthetic mechanisms occurs in the cell cytoplasm. Certain cells of lower forms can live, grow, and in fact differentiate after their nucleus has been removed. This is considered possible because the mRNA codes were made before the nucleus was removed and are stable for periods of several days or even weeks after the removal of the nucleus. Cytoplasmic control mechanisms determine when and to what extent the mRNA is to engage in protein synthesis. Thus it is clear that there are many levels of control of genetic expression, both in the nucleus and in the cytoplasm.

Recent work has led to the recognition that differentiation can be a remarkably reversible process in some cell types. One of the most dramatic examples has been provided by the work of Gurdon utilizing techniques introduced in the pioneering studies of Briggs and King. It is possible to destroy the nucleus of an unfertilized frog egg with ultraviolet light and then, using an extremely fine pipette, to introduce a diploid nucleus into the egg to see whether it will be capable of directing the development of the egg (and subsequently the embryo) as the original nucleus would have done. Gurdon has demonstrated that nuclei from fully differentiated intestinal cells in tadpoles can be obtained in a viable state and injected into anucleate frog eggs. In a small number of cases, these eggs developed into normal frogs (Fig. 2.13).

Experiments relevant to this point have also been undertaken by Harris. He has demonstrated, for example, that the nucleus of the highly differentiated chicken red blood cell is dramatically altered upon introduction into a cell already containing an active nucleus (Fig. 2.9). Normally the red cell nucleus does not synthesize measurable amounts of RNA, but in the heterokaryon it resumes RNA synthesis. Both of these experiments indicate that genes are not lost, nor are they permanently inactivated, in the process of differentiation.

This should not be taken to imply that all differentiation is, in the normal animal, reversible. In fact, the various populations of cells in a mature organism can be demonstrated to display varying levels of differentiation as judged by their structure and their varying capability to reverse a course of differentiation or to respond to injury with appropriate repair. The neurons of the mammalian central nervous system do not reproduce themselves; many have very limited capacities of repair. When nerve cells are lost there is no mechanism for replacement, a point that should not be overlooked in an age which has witnessed an increasing reliance upon adjustment of the activities of the nervous system with drugs of every nature and degree of purity.

Cell–Cell Interactions

It is known that there are critical periods during the development of certain cells when exposure to other cells, or to products of other cells such as hormones, is critical for differentiation. Embryoic *induction* involves the interaction between cells or tissues in which one tissue induces a developmental change in another. A classic example is the formation of the lens of the eye. As the brain develops, that part destined to form the sensory portion of the eye bulges laterally and approaches the overlying ectoderm. As this portion of the nervous system comes in contact with the ectoderm, the ectoderm thickens, and its cells elongate and form a lens placode, the precursor of the lens. If the nervous tissue is prevented from contactng the ectoderm, no lens is formed. The nervous tissue has induced the formation of the lens. Furthermore, if the nervous tissue destined to form the eye is transplanted under the ectoderm on the back of the animal instead of the head, it will often induce lens formation in this region of the overlying ectoderm.

The development of the pancreas provides one of the best studied examples of tisue interaction. Pancreatic cells first develop in an endoderm derivative, the lining of the primitive gut. Wessels and Rutter have discovered that, at a precise time and

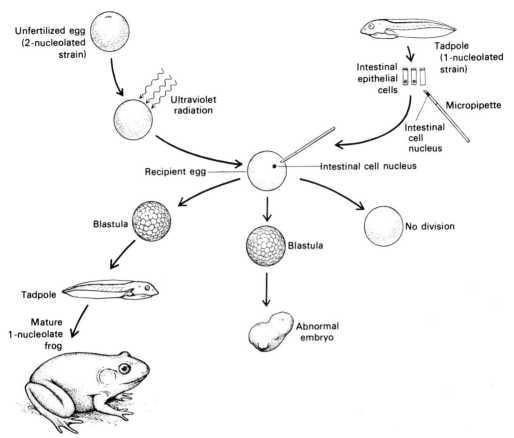

Figure 2.13.   The ability of a nucleus from a differentiated cell to perform all of the basic functions of the unspecialized embryonic nucleus may be demonstrated in the following way. After destruction of the frog egg nucleus by ultraviolet light, a nucleus isolated from an intestinal epithelial cell of a tadpole is substituted by microinjection. In a few cases, development of a normal frog occurs. Because the injected nucleus is the only functional nuclear material it must, in this case, be able to perform all of the functions of the egg nucleus. The use of two different frog strains (one with only one nucleolus in each nucleus and the other with two) allows confirmation of the presence of the intestinal cell nucleus. (After J. B. Gurdon: *Sci Am* 219:24, 1968.)

at a precise site in the gut wall, some of the lining cells begin to make small amounts of digestive enzymes that mark them unmistakably as pancreatic cells. At this point they bear little histological similarity to mature pancreatic cells. But in terms of gene control a critical change has taken place, for some new region of the DNA code is now being used to transcribe mRNA, and the production of the digestive enzymes is thus possible. Then a puzzling dependence develops. The endoderm from which the pancreas cells are forming requires the close proximity of mesodermal tissue to become fully differentiated into pancreatic tissue. Without mesoderm little further de-

velopment takes place, but if mesoderm is present the presumptive pancreatic cells greatly multiply their numbers, form definitive gland tissues, and increase their production of enzymes 50-fold—the tissue is now clearly pancreas. After this critical period the pancreatic cells are no longer dependent upon the mesoderm for normal development.

It is clear from this type of experiment that tissue type may be determined before cell division ceases. Cell multiplication of the determined tissue type goes on until a certain volume of tissue is reached. In some tissues the process of cell division is then permanently halted, as with nerve cells or heart muscle cells. In other tissues, cell division may continue at a slower rate to replace tissue elements lost with time, as in the lining of the gut. In other adult tissues, the ongoing needs of rapid cell turnover are met by the division of multipotential "*stem cells*," cells which themselves do not differentiate but produce progeny that do. An example is the bone marrow stem cell, which gives rise to many different types of blood cells.

CELL DIVISION

Cells arise by the division of preexisting cells. All of the cells of the adult human body, an estimated 10^{14} of them, are derived from just one cell, the fertilized egg. The structure and specificity of cells ultimately depend upon the population of proteins therein, and these proteins are assembled under the direction of mRNA. The mRNA carries the code of the genetic material, the DNA, which is contained within the nucleus. Thus it should be apparent that newly formed cells must be endowed with exact replicas of the parent DNA complement. To accomplish this, the parent cell must exactly duplicate its DNA and then precisely divide it and distribute it to two daughter cells. The process by which the DNA molecules are duplicated is called *rep-*

lication and the mechanism by which the replicated DNA is divided to supply each daughter cell with its complete and exact complement of hereditary material is termed *mitosis*. The division of nuclear material is referred to as *karyokinesis*; the division of the cytoplasm is called *cytokinesis*.

DNA Replication

To achieve replication, the DNA double helix unwinds, and each strand becomes a template for the assembly of a new one, which then becomes incorporated into a new double helix. The end result, therefore, is two double helices, each composed of one parent and one new strand. This mechanism of replication, termed "semiconservative," is the usual one for mammalian somatic (body) cells. In this manner, the linear arrays of genes are copied exactly if conditions are normal. Utilization of radioactive thymidine, incorporated only into duplicating DNA molecules, has been helpful in studying the mechanism of DNA replication, as well as in discovering the time at which it occurs.

Replication is accomplished before the cell visibly enters mitosis. During the nondividing (*interphase* or "resting") period, three different phases have been defined:

Table 2.2
Periods of the Cell Cycle, i.e., From One Cell Division to the Next

Period	Definition	Per Cent Time from One Mitosis to the Next (Generation Time)[a]
	Interphase; period of increasing mass with protein and RNA synthesis	
G_1	Gap$_1$: period between previous mitosis and S	30–40% for regularly dividing cells, but time may vary considerably, even lasting the lifetime of the organism
S	Synthesis: period of DNA and histone synthesis	30–50%; this interval usually constant depending upon cell type or state; may be 7 hr in some species
G_2	Gap$_2$: period between S and beginning of mitosis	10–20%; interval fairly constant, lasting up to 2 hr
	Division	
M	Mitosis: period when chromosomes shorten (and thus become visible), are aligned in the middle of the cell, and are divided equally	5–10%; usually lasts 1–2 hr but depends upon the cell type

[a] The generation time usually ranges from 10 to 30 hr; for certain human cultured cells it is 22 hr, with the S period lasting about 6 hr.

G_1, the gap between the previous mitosis and the start of DNA synthesis (S), and G_2, the gap between the end of S and the beginning of mitosis (M) (Table 2.2). In general, the replication of DNA may occur without cytokinesis, but cell division does not take place without the prefatory replication of DNA. It is known that mitosis is triggered by DNA synthesis, but the stimulus for DNA replication remains a mystery.

Mitosis

The nuclear DNA is contained within *chromosomes* which are not readily visible by light microscopy in the interphase nucleus. The chromosomal material is actually arranged in dispersed networks of delicate submicroscopic strands collectively referred to as *chromatin*. After staining of the interphase nucleus, only scattered condensed areas of chromatin, the *heterochromatin*, are visible. As the cells prepare for division, the entire chromosome becomes visible, as the term mitosis (from the Greek *mitos*, thread) implies. Each chromosome becomes progressively thicker and shorter by a process of coiling. This extreme shortening of the chromosomes allows their disentanglement and precise alignment before their division and distribution into daughter cells.

Although mitosis is a continuous process, it is often divided into four stages: *prophase, metaphase, anaphase,* and *telophase.* During a typical mitotic period, prophase may be the longest stage, perhaps 1.5 hr, whereas metaphase, anaphase, and telophase take approximately 20, 4, and 60 min, respectively. In cultured HeLa cells, mitosis is accomplished in about 80 min, the successive stages requiring about 18, 35, 13, and 14 min, respectively.

Prophase

The onset of prophase is recognizable by an increase in the number and density of stainable chromatin particles, which are gradually replaced by slender threads (Figs. 2.14 and 2.15). With continued coiling they become shorter and thickened in girth; the gyres of the threads (chromosomes) in-

crease in diameter and decrease in number. These chromosomes may be studied in appropriately stained, preserved tissue or examined in the living state by means of phase optics or, better still, the Nomarski (differential interference contrast) system (Fig. 2.16).

Each chromosome now contains twice the normal amount of DNA as a result of the replication before the onset of prophase. This doubling becomes visible for the first time when the chromosome appears to be divided lengthwise into two parallel, closely apposing units called *chromatids.* As long as they remain attached (in one region only, the *centromere*), they are called chromatids (or "sister chromatids";

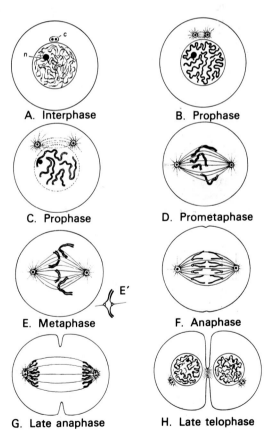

A. Interphase   B. Prophase

C. Prophase   D. Prometaphase

E. Metaphase   F. Anaphase

G. Late anaphase   H. Late telophase

Figure 2.14. Diagram illustrating the successive cellular events in mitosis, which is described in the text. *E'* is an enlargement of the two chromatids of one chromosome, showing completion of separation by detachment at the centromere region. *c*, centrosome; *n*, nucleolus.

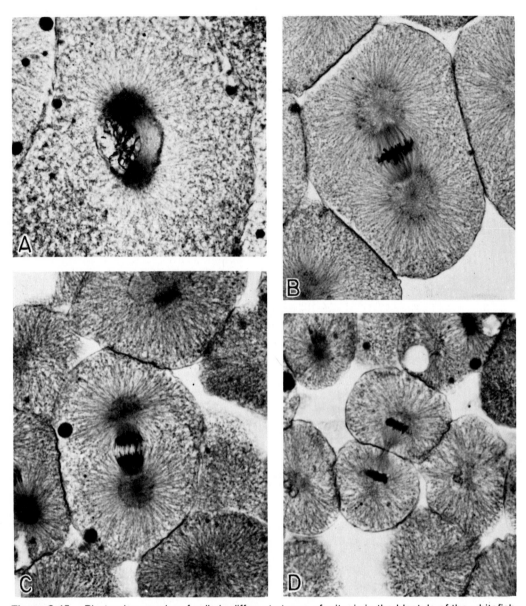

Figure 2.15. Photomicrographs of cells in different stages of mitosis in the blastula of the whitefish. *A*, late prophase, with chromosomes in coiled threads, nuclear membrane still present, and the cell center divided into two new centers which have moved toward opposite poles of the nucleus; *B*, metaphase, in lateral view; *C*, early anaphase; *D*, telophase. (Photographs at ×600, from slides purchased from the General Biological Supply House, Chicago.)

Fig. 2.8); once they become separated (at a later interval) they are called "daughter chromosomes." The chromatids coil on themselves rather than around each other.

During prophase, the nuclear envelope starts to disappear and centrioles begin their migration to opposite poles of the cell.

Before this, the two *centrioles* (a *diplosome*) have been clustered together, lying at right angles to one another. Between the centrioles a *mitotic spindle* of microtubules begins to enlarge into an array roughly the shape of a football. The centrioles thus act as organizing centers for the spindle and

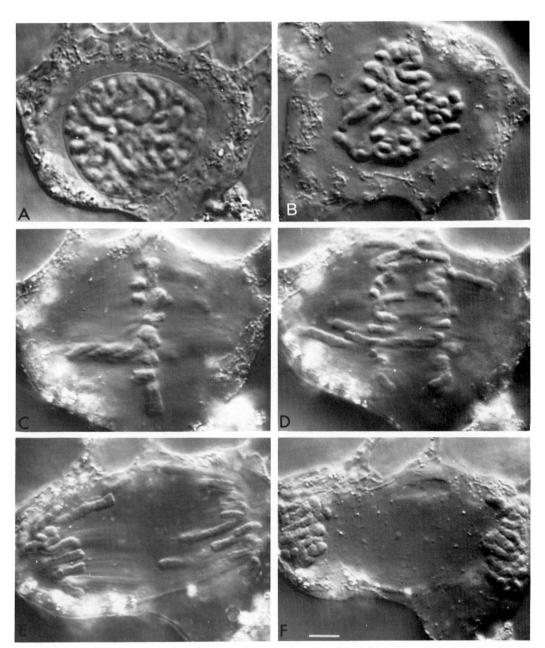

Figure 2.16. Photomicrographs of successive changes in a lily endosperm cell during mitosis, as seen in the Nomarski optical system. This system has the advantage of revealing spindle fibers in living cells. Time after A: B, 14 min; C, 1 hr 4 min; D, 1 hr 14 min; E, 1 hr 33 min; and F, 1 hr 47 min. Compare with Figure 2.14. The bar indicates 10 μm. (Reprinted with permission from A. Bajer: *Chromosoma* 25:249, 1968.)

become its two poles. The spindle microtubules converge on, but are not continuous with, the centrioles. A small disc-like structure, the *kinetochore*, becomes visible (in electron micrographs) at the centromere region of each chromatid. It is in this region that some of the spindle tubules become attached to chromosomes (Fig. 2.17). The kinetochore is considered to participate in microtubule assembly as well. The spindle structure, which according to recent evidence contains actin (but, perhaps not myosin-like molecules) as well as tubulin and microtubules, provides the mechanism for subsequent chromosomal movement. The close of prophase is marked by the disappearance of the nuclear envelope.

Metaphase

During *prometaphase* (Fig. 2.14*D*) the spindle becomes fully developed and the chromosomes, all in a condensed state and thus visible in their entirety, move into it and become situated midway in the spindle. During metaphase the chromatids continue to condense and shift slightly until they are oriented in a precise manner. Actually, it is the centromere portion of the chromatids which becomes aligned in the *equatorial* or *metaphase plate* of the spindle (Fig. 2.15*E*). The kinetochores of each chromatid pair are oriented perpendicular to the spindle axis and face opposing poles, with the attached microtubules extending toward each pole (Fig. 2.17).

In living cells the spindle microtubules are not visible in the phase microscope, although the spindle area is represented by a clear zone around which are clustered organelles, but they can be detected in the Nomarski system (Fig. 2.16) and appear as birefringent structures in the polarizing microscope (Fig. 2.18). The spindle may be demonstrated in fixed and stained preparations (Fig. 2.15) and is beautifully resolved in the electron microscope (Fig. 2.19) as a large array of microtubules which may number in the hundreds or thousands, depending upon the species. A cluster of microtubules is attached to each kinetochore and may extend in bundles, which accounts for their visibility in the Nomarski system. Spindle microtubules are thought to extend from pole to pole ("*continuous*"), from pole to kinetochores ("*chromosomal*"), or to overlap in the equatorial region. The spindle apparatus is highly labile, but it may be isolated from the cell for special study.

When colchicine or vinca alkaloids such as *vinblastine* are administered to dividing cells, mitosis is arrested at the beginning of metaphase. Apparently colchicine blocks the migration of the chromosomes, presumably because some continuous microtubules cannot be assembled to aid in their poleward movement. Because both kinetochores of a chromatid pair do not face opposing centrioles, one of the kinetochores lacks chromosomal microtubules, with the result that the sister chromatids cannot be pulled apart. If the colchicine is washed away, within minutes centriole migration is initiated, the spindle develops, the chromatids are aligned on the metaphase plate, and anaphase movement is visible.

During the paralysis of chromosome separation induced by colchicine, the chromatids nevertheless continue condensing and thus become shorter and thicker than normal, allowing their ready visualization and identification in the light microscope. At this point, each chromosome assumes a characteristic form, depending upon its length and the position of its centromere, or *primary constriction*. This array of chromosomes of varying form is distinctive for a given species and is known as the *karyotype*, explained earlier in the chapter.

Anaphase

After alignment in the metaphase plate, the chromatids are ready to be moved apart. Upon separation of the centromere, the only point of attachment between each chromatid pair, the two daughter chromosomes begin their journey to opposite poles. Each appears to be pulled at the kinetochore, with the remainder of the chromosome trailing behind. They are brought to the polar regions where they become maximally condensed and may appear to fuse with one another. At the same time the entire spindle elongates, and a furrow around the cell (in a plane midway in and perpendicular to the spindle axis) heralds the beginning of cytoplasmic cleavage.

The mechanism by which the separated daughter chromosomes move to opposite poles is not completely understood. It has been proposed by some investigators that

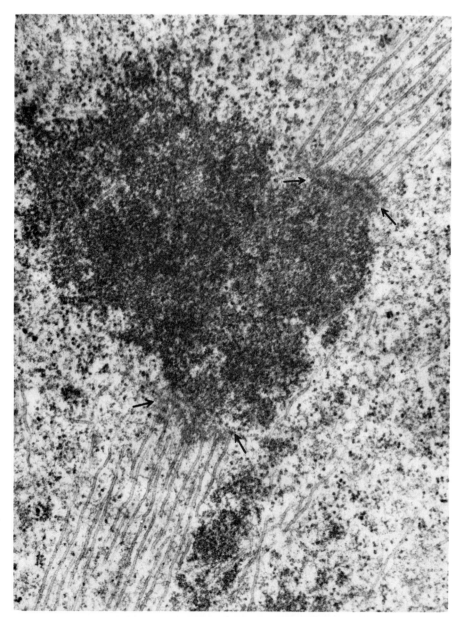

Figure 2.17. Electron micrograph of a portion of a chromosome at metaphase in a dividing fibroblast in tissue culture. The sister chromatids are still joined in the centromere region shown here. On each chromatid, facing the pole to which it will be drawn, is the kinetochore (arrows). The chromosomal spindle microtubules are attached to the chromatid in the kinetochore region (×45,000). (Reprinted with permission from B. R. Brinkley: In *Advances in Cell Biology*, edited by D. Prescott, vol. 1, p. 119. New York, Appleton-Century-Crofts, 1969.)

movement is due to depolymerization of chromosomal microtubules at the centriole region. Tubulin subunits thus freed would then be available for assembly into, and subsequent lengthening of, the continuous tubules, thereby providing the basis for overall extension of the spindle. Since actin is known to be present in the mitotic spindle, the motive force for chromosomal migration might be provided in some manner

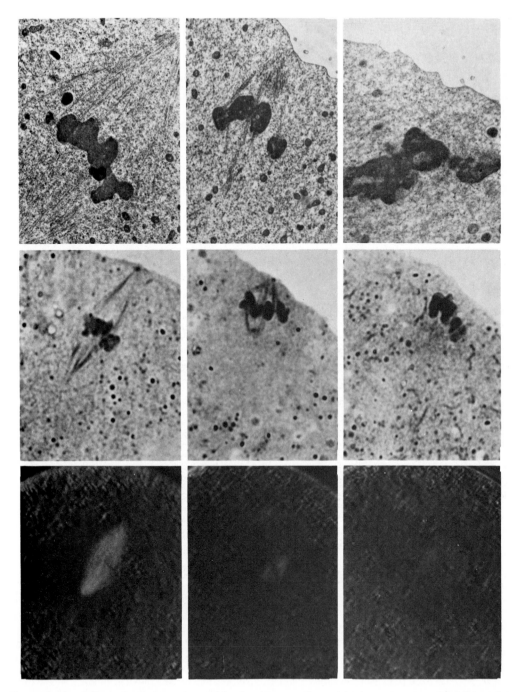

Figure 2.18. Effect of administering vinblastine known, like colchicine, to arrest a dividing cell in metaphase. Division is interrupted because the spindle microtubules disappear, as demonstrated in electron micrographs (*top row*, *left* to *right*), light micrographs (obtained by sectioning at 1 μm the tissue prepared for electron microscopy, staining with toluidine blue, and viewing in the phase microscope; *middle row*), and photographs of living cells taken in the polarizing microscope (*bottom row*). This set of pictures also serves to demonstrate that spindle birefringence depends upon the presence of an array of spindle microtubules. Living marine worm oocyte. (Reprinted with permission from S. E. Malawista et al.: *Science* 160:770, 1968.)

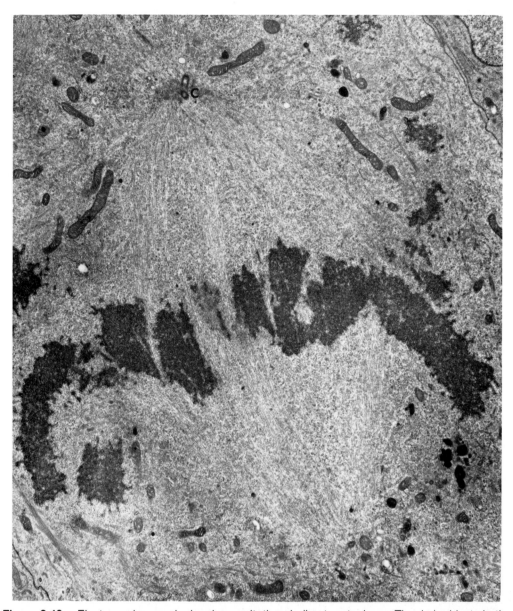

Figure 2.19. Electron micrograph showing a mitotic spindle at metaphase. The dark objects in the center are the chromosomes, oriented in the metaphase plate. The chromosomes are suspended in myriads of linear chromosomal and continuous spindle microtubules. In this plane the centrioles (c) at one pole of the spindle can be seen; the daughter centriole is perpendicular to the parent centriole. Other cytoplasmic organelles such as mitochondria are confined to areas outside the spindle. Kangaroo rat fibroblast in tissue culture (×10,000). (Courtesy of Dr. B. R. Brinkley.)

by this molecule, perhaps also involving the microtubules. The possible roles of contractile proteins and microtubules in chromosomal movement are still under active investigation.

Centrioles usually are duplicated in anaphase or telophase to provide each daughter cell with its interphase complement. Centrioles are self-replicating, apparently not by division but by the action of one as a template for the organization of a new one. Some evidence suggests that RNA is present in the centriole.

Telophase

Once the chromosomes have reached the poles of the spindle, reformation of the nuclear envelope (from cisternae of endoplasmic reticulum) begins. Subsequently the cytoplasm is divided into two new daughter cells. These remain connected for a time by a narrow stalk of cytoplasm into which some of the remaining continuous microtubules and associated dense substance have been gathered. This temporary, dense isthmus is termed the *midbody*. Chromosomal spindle microtubules and the kinetochore structures disappear.

The new daughter nuclei are at first small and very dense. Gradually, these nuclei enlarge and the chromosomes begin to disperse. The reconstruction of the nucleus appears to be the reverse of the changes of prophase: chromosomes become progressively thinner, their presence eventually signified only by the scattered heterochromatin characteristic of the interphase nucleus. One or more nucleoli reappear, in association with the nucleolar-organizer regions of certain chromosomes.

General Considerations of Mitosis

Cell division also has an important function in relation to cell growth because without division cells eventually reach a stage where growth ceases. There is no increase in total cell mass during mitosis, but immediately after division the two daughter cells grow rapidly and continue growing until the mass of cytoplasm reaches a point in relation to nuclear size which is characteristic for a particular cell type. When some of the cytoplasm is removed from an ameba by microsurgery without damage to the nucleus, the cell regenerates the cytoplasm without nuclear division.

The constancy of the number of chromosomes, along with other data, indicates that the chromosomes retain their individuality during the intermitotic stage. Earlier in the chapter evidence was reviewed indicating that the genetic material is not altered during differentiation, but that different sites of this material are expressed at different times. Usually the amount of DNA per given chromosome does not vary, no matter what the metabolic variations may be. The DNA molecule is extremely stable, and this stability is an important aspect in the maintenance of appropriate constancy from generation to generation in the lives of cells—and organisms.

Meiosis

As we have just learned, mitosis is the process by which new daughter cells acquire a complete genetic complement identical to that of the parent cell. In man, the set of 46 chromosomes (the *diploid* number) is thus passed on from generation to generation of daughter cells. If this were the case during the formation of the egg and sperm cells, however, the fusion of nuclei at fertilization would lead to a set of 92 chromosomes. Therefore, a somewhat different division process, *meiosis* (or *reduction division*) is at work in the development of eggs and sperm to provide for the presence of only 23 chromosomes (the *haploid* number). The diploid number of chromosomes is then restored at the time of fertilization. Meiosis is discussed further in Chapter 19.

References

Alberts B, Bray D, Lewis J, Raff M, Roberts K, Watson JD: *Molecular Biology of the Cell.* New York, Garland, 1983.

Allen RD Taylor DL: Molecular basis of amoeboid movement. In Inoue S, Stephens R (eds): *Molecules and Cell Movement.* New York, Raven Press, 1975, pp 239–258.

Amy RL, Storb R, Fauconnier B, Wertz RK: Ruby laser microirradiation of single tissue culture cells vitally stained with Janus green B. *Exp Cell Res* 45:361–373, 1967.

Bajer AA: Interaction of microtubules and the mechanisms of chromosome movement (zipper hypothesis). I. General principle. *Cytobios* 8:139–160, 1973.

Bergmann JE, Kupfer A, Singer SJ: Membrane insertion at the leading edge of motile fibroblasts. *Proc Natl Acad Sci USA* 80:1367–1371, 1983.

Brinkley BR, Stubblefield E, Hsu TC: The effects of colcemid inhibition and reversal on the fine structure of the mitotic apparatus of Chinese hamster cell *in vitro. J Ultrastruct Res* 19:1–18, 1967.

Cande WZ, Lazarides E, McIntosh JR: A comparison of the distribution of actin and tubulin in the mammalian mitotic spindle as seen by indirect immunofluorescence. *J Cell Biol* 72:552–567, 1977.

Carrel A: On the permanent life of tissues outside of the organism. *J Exp Med* 15:516, 1912.

Clarke ER: The transparent chamber technique for the microscopic study of living blood vessels. *Anat Rec* 120:241–252, 1954.

Ebert JD, Sussex IM: *Interacting Systems in Development*, ed 2. New York, Holt, Rinehart and Winston, 1970.

Fitzgerald PH: Chromosomal abnormalities in man. In Bittar EE (ed): *The Biological Basis of Medicine*, vol 4. New York, Academic Press, 1969, pp 133–178.

Furshpan E, Potter D: Low resistance junctions between cells in embryos and tissue culture. In Moscona A (ed): *Current Topics in Developmental Biology*. New York, Academic Press, 1968, pp 95–125.

Furusawa M: Cellular microinjection by cell fusion: technique and application in biology and medicine. *Int Rev Cytol* 62:29–67, 1980.

Gall JG: Chromosome structure and the C-value paradox. *J Cell Biol* 91:15s–27s, 1981.

Gurdon JB: Transplanted nuclei and cell differentiation. *Sci Am* 219:24–35, 1968.

Harrison RG: Observations on the living developing nerve fiber. *Proc Soc Exp Biol Med* 4:140, 1907.

Hayflick L: Human cells and aging. *Sci Am* 218:32–37, 1968.

Hinkley R, Telser A: Heavy meromyosin-binding filaments in the mitotic apparatus of mammalian cells. *Exp Cell Res* 86:161–164, 1974.

Inoue S: Cell division and the mitotic spindle. *J Cell Biol* 91:132s–147s, 1981.

Jacob F, Monod J: Genetic regulatory mechanisms in the synthesis of protein. *J Mol Biol* 3:318–356, 1961.

King TJ, Briggs R: Serial transplantation of embryonic nuclei. In Bell E (ed): *Molecular and Cellular Aspects of Development*. New York, Harper and Row, 1965, pp 171–192.

Kopac MJ: Micrurgical studies on living cells. In Brachet J, Mirsky AE (eds): *The Cell; Biochemistry, Physiology, Morphology*, vol. 1. New York, Academic Press, 1959, pp 161–191.

Leblond CP: The life history of cells in renewing systems. *Am J Anat* 160:113–158, 1981

Lewin B: *Gene Expression*, vol 2: *Eucaryotic Chromosomes*, ed 2. New York, John Wiley & Sons, 1980.

Lewis WH: Pinocytosis. *Bull Johns Hopkins Hosp* 49:17–27, 1931.

Lowenstein WR: On the genesis of cellular communication. *Dev Biol* 15:503–520, 1967.

McGhee JD, Felsenfeld G: Nucleosome structure. *Annu Rev Biochem* 49:1115–1156, 1980.

Metcalf D: Clonal analysis of proliferation and differentiation of paired daughter cells: action of GM-CSF on granulocyte-macrophage precursors. *Proc Natl Acad Sci USA* 77:5327–5330, 1980.

Miller OL: The nucleolus, chromosomes, and visualization of genetic activity. *J Cell Biol* 91:15s–27s, 1981.

Milstein C: Monoclonal antibodies. *Sci Am* 243(4):66–74, 1980.

Mintz B: Genetic mosaicism in adult mice of quadriparental lineage. *Science* 148:1232–1233, 1965.

Mittwoch U: *The Sex Chromosomes*. New York, Academic Press, 1967.

Moscona AA (ed): The cell surface in development. New York, John Wiley & Sons, 1974.

Moscona A, Moscona H: The dissociation and aggregation of cells from organ rudiments of the early chick embryo. *J Anat* 86:287–301, 1952.

Prescott D (ed): *Methods in Cell Biology, New York, Academic Press* (multivolume series of reviews on current techniques).

Puck TT: Marcus PI, Cieciura SJ: Clonal growth of mammalian cells in vitro. Growth characteristics of colonies from single HeLa cells with and without a "feeder" layer. *J Exp Med* 103:273–284, 1956.

Ris H: Ultrastructure of the animal chromosomes. In Konigsberger VV, Bosch L (eds): *Regulation of Nucleic Acid and Protein Biosynthesis*. New York, American Elsevier, 1967, pp 11–21.

Schrader F: *Mitosis*, ed 2. New York, Columbia University Press, 1953.

Schroeder TE: Dynamics of contractile ring. In Inoue S, Stephens R (eds): *Molecules and Cell Movement*. New York, Raven Press, 1975, pp 305–335.

Sheridan JD: Cell coupling and cell communication during embryogenesis. In Poste G, Nicolson GL (eds): *Cell Surface Reviews*, vol 1. Amsterdam, Elsevier/North Holland, 1977, pp 409–448.

Squire J: *The Structural Basis of Muscle Contraction*. New York, Plenum Press, 1981.

Stebbings S, Hyams JS: *Cell Motility*. Harlowe, Longman, 1979.

Stubblefield E, Brinkley BR: Architecture and function of the mammalian centriole. In Warren KB (ed): *Formation and Fate of Cell Organelles* New York, Academic Press, 1967, pp 175–218.

Trinkaus JP: *Cells Into Organs. The Forces that Shape the Embryo*. Englewood Cliffs, N.J., Prentice-Hall, 1969.

Weeds A: Actin-binding proteins—regulators of cell architecture and motility. *Nature* 296:811–816, 1982.

Weisband S. Active chromatin. *Nature* 297:289–295, 1982.

Wessels NT: *Tissue Interactions and Development*. Menlo Park, Calif., Benjamin Cummings, 1977.

Willmer EN (ed): *Cells and Tissues in Culture*, vols 1–3. New York, Academic Press, 1965.

Chapter 3

GENERAL FEATURES OF VERTEBRATE DEVELOPMENT

Adult living organisms are vehicles by means of which the germinative cells (ova or sperm) are produced and their genetic complement is transmitted from generation to generation, thereby perpetuating their respective species. Amid all of the living species, those that we characterize as "high organisms," including man and other vertebrates, display adult body plans that are relatively large and highly complex. They exhibit *sexual reproduction*, a remarkable process which has lent efficiency to the evolution of such complex forms by ensuring variety among the offspring who must contend with new or changing environmental challenges. But sexual reproduction requires that the life of each individual is initiated by the fusion of two tiny cells. From them the new offspring receives the combined set of genetic instructions which dictates all future capabilities. The basic developmental processes of *growth, cellular differentiation, morphogenetic movements* (cellular shape change, migration, and epithelial folding), *inductive interactions*, and *selective cellular death* are coordinated to convert these cells and their instructions sequentially into the complex reproductive unit which is the adult.

John Tyler Bonner has defined development as the inevitable result of the evolution of *sex* on the one hand and *size* on the other. In other words, successful species, more readily able to invade, feed, locomote, and reproduce in demanding environments, have generally evolved increasingly large, complex, and capable adult forms. Development is the sequence whereby each individual begins life in an appropriately small sexually combined package and gradually converts itself into a much more massive, adaptable adult.

Because the evolution of the vertebrates has been one of continual progression and modification, it is not surprising that, at least as embryos, these animals share many common basic properties. They may all be defined as *triploblastic* (having three fundamental tissue layers), *metameric* (segmented), *eucoelomate* (having true body cavities), and *bilaterally symmetrical*. They all possess, at some stage, a *notochord*, a dorsal hollow *central nervous system*, *branchial arches* and *grooves*, and *pharyngeal pouches*.

EARLY MORPHOGENESIS

Early development (or *morphogenesis*; the acquisition of form) commences, by definition, with fertilization, although obviously many events involving maturation of sperm and ovum have occurred in anticipation of this event. In human development, fusion of male and female pronuclei within the new, one-celled individual, the *zygote*, is quickly followed by *cleavage*, a series of mitotic divisions (Fig. 3.1). By the time the zygote is transported from the oviduct into the lumen of the uterus (where it will implant in the endometrium), it is apparent that the newly derived daughter cells, or *blastomeres*, remain together as an adherent aggregate enclosed by a thin, extracellular *zona pellucida*. The total aggregate, now termed a *morula*, has not increased in mass, but will do so rapidly after attachment to and penetration into the uterine wall. By that time its cells have secreted an internal reservoir of extracellular fluid and arranged themselves into a hollow sphere, the *blastocyst*, one side of which is thickened (the *embryoblast* or *inner cell mass*). The rest of the cells, collectively termed the *trophoblast*, form a thin,

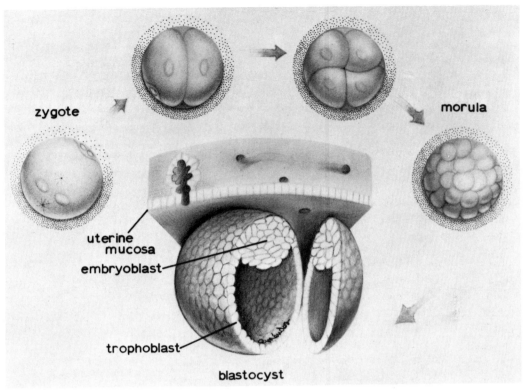

Figure 3.1. Early stages of human development after fertilization (*left*), through cleavage and morula (*right*). The relationship of the blastocyst and its parts just before the commencement of implantation into the uterine mucosa is shown at *bottom*.

surrounding shell. As this occurs, the zona pellucida is lost and the entire blastocyst becomes embedded in the uterine endometrial wall. Within the embryoblast, certain of the cells can be designated as those which will give rise to the embryo proper, and the rest, together with cells of the trophoblast, are destined to proliferate and provide components of four surrounding extraembryonic membranes; *amnion, chorion, allantois,* and *yolk sac* (Fig. 3.2). The detailed structure and fate of these will be covered in a later chapter.

The region of the embryo proper becomes distinct as a *diploblastic* (bilayered) plate of cells (the *embryonic disc*) which, except at its lateral edges, delaminates away from other embryoblastic cells of amnion and yolk sac destiny. Already a head or anterior end of the plate as well as left and right halves can be defined. The two layers of the embryonic disc are termed the *epiblast* (above) and *hypoblast* (below) (Fig. 3.2).

Each layer is *epithelial*, in the sense of displaying a free surface and possessing definite intercellular junctions which secure adjacent cells within each layer. The epiblast is particularly active mitotically.

GASTRULATION

A striking transformation now occurs which is of paramount importance to the modern histologist. It literally sets the stage for all of the organizational features which follow in this book. This is the process of *gastrulation* (Fig. 3.3). Many cells of the epiblast lose attachment with their neighbors and migrate inward to become incorporated as a looser population sandwiched between remaining epiblast and hypoblast. Most of this activity occurs along a midline groove in an elongate region of the posterior epiblast, the *primitive streak*, in such a way that the newly freed cells are crowded into the subepiblastic region along the groove. Mitotically active, these cells commence a

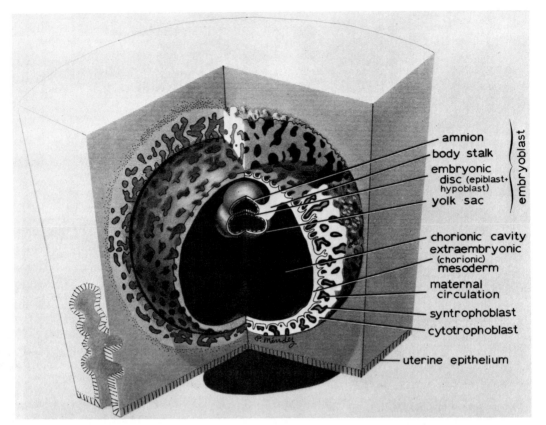

Figure 3.2. The human blastocyst after implantation into the uterine wall is complete. The inner cell mass has delaminated into amnion, embryonic disc, and yolk sac. Collectively these are suspended from the trophoblast (now chorion) by the body stalk.

lateral migration, forming a spreading sheet or network of cells which progressively separates epiblast from hypoblast. The migrating, spreading network, termed the *mesoblast*, proceeds laterally and anteriorly within either side of the embryonic disc, its two "wings" eventually converging to meet medially at the most anterior portion of the embryonic disc (*dotted arrows,* Fig. 3.3). There the fused mesoblast forms the *cardiogenic plate*. In reaching the cardiogenic plate, the mesoblast bypasses a midline region, the *prochordal plate*. Here a small round patch of epiblast remains unseparated from the underlying hypoblast. Along the center line, ahead of the primitive groove, a rodlike core of closely adherent mesoblastic cells is laid down as the embryonic disc elongates and the primitive groove diminishes rapidly in relative dimensions. This core is the future *noto-chord*, and it extends anteriorly nearly to the prochordal plate.

It is essential to note the vastly different behavior assumed by most of the mesoblastic cells as compared with those left to dwell as epithelia in the epiblast or hypoblast. Whereas the latter cells remain relatively stationary and locked tightly to each other, mesoblastic cells (other than those of the notochord) display an opposite tendency, migrating freely, and, for a time, maintaining a remoteness from their neighbors. The adjective "*mesenchymal*" is often applied to these mesoblastic cells, denoting not only this individualistic migratory behavior but also the fact that they are embryonic cells with the potential to proliferate and mature into many diverse types of differentiated cells. Unlike epithelial cells, mesenchymal cells are characterized by the production of large amounts of *extracellular matrix* into

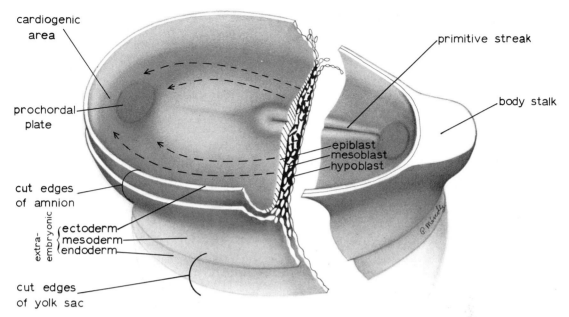

Figure 3.3. The embryonic disc during the process of gastrulation. The amnion has been cut and lifted off to reveal the epiblastic surface. Cells from the epiblast are entering the mesoblast (primarily in the area of the primitive streak) and migrating anteriorly along the paths indicated by *dotted arrows*. The outline of the notochordal proces extending anteriorly from the primitive streak to the prochordal plate delineates the longitudinal axis of the forming embryo.

their immediate environment. Regional variations in the hydration of this matrix may cause expansion of appropriate regions of extracellular space, thus aiding in shaping of the embryo and its organs.

An interesting recently discovered phenomenon reportedly occurs in chick embryos and perhaps also in mammals. There, cell labeling experiments disclose that some of the newly arrived mesoblast cells near the embryonic midline invade the hypoblast, displacing the original hypoblastic cells laterally. It is now thought that all of the hypoblastic cells which eventually remain in the embryo proper are of this mesoblastic origin. Hence one might say that, at least in the chick, all or nearly all of the cells of the embryo originate from the epiblast.

At the close of gastrulation, when mesoblastic development has achieved a complete or nearly complete intermediate middle layer between epi- and hypoblasts, the embryo is said to be *triploblastic*. Its three fundamental layers are often referred to as the "germ layers." They are: the *ectoderm* (formerly the remaining epiblast); the *endoderm* (formerly the remaining hypoblast); and the *mesoderm* (that mesoblast which has become mesenchymal cells and notochord). The ectoderm and endoderm produce a submicroscopic thin extracellular coating, the *basal lamina*, along their interior surfaces, i.e., surfaces facing the mesoblast. This segregates them from the mesoblast. With true deposition of a definitive basal lamina the ecto- and endodermal layers have acquired all the essential features of true *epithelia* (discussed in detail in Chapter 4). Similarly, the adherent cells of the notochord surround that structure with a basal lamina. The remaining mesoblast (now mesoderm) is trapped in a compartment which is enshrouded by the basal lamina of the ectoderm and endoderm and likewise separated from the notochord. This compartment can usefully be termed the *mesenchymal* or *mesoblastic compartment*. Unlike the epithelial layers which now surround it and seal it, the mesenchymal compartment contains much extracellular fluid and matrix. High volumes of those extracellular fluids and materials are retained in some tissues of mesoblastic origin and lost in others where differentiation involves an intimate secondary clumping of mesenchymal cells.

The cells of each of the three germ layers divide, migrate, group, and differentiate in rather precise patterns, ultimately forming organ systems. In general, the early epithelial cells retain firm, close adhesion with their neighbors and achieve final appropriate shapes by processes of *folding, invagination,* and *evagination* of epithelial layers. Mesenchymal components, by contrast, seem at first to clump or spread, often crowding into nooks formed between ecto- or endodermal epithelial folds. There they form mesodermally derived epithelial linings and/or remain mesenchymal to differentiate further. Thus, most organs are formed by a combination of epithelial linings with mesenchymal compartments packed between. Indeed, as careful analysis has shown, the relationship between mesenchyme and epithelium is virtually always of critical importance, for each plays a controlling or *inductive* influence to signal or direct the appropriate developmental pattern for the other. Likewise, the close proximity of one embryonic epithelium to another may exert reciprocal inductive control in the differentiation of each.

DIFFERENTIATION AND HISTOGENESIS

Tissues from different germ layers, while retaining their individuality, frequently associate in the formation of an organ, inducing each other to express new morphological properties collectively characteristic of that organ. With careful cell marking techniques, one can determine (with few exceptions) the original germ layer from which has arisen every cell in each organ of the fully developed body (Table 3.1). The process whereby each constituent cell acquires organelles and other properties necessary to emphasize a particular function is termed *cellular differentiation*. The aggregate, integrated differentiation into the specialized cellular patterns of tissues is termed *histogenesis*.

Table 3.1.
Major Derivatives of the Three Germ Layers and Neural Crest

Origin	Derivatives
Ectoderm	
	Epithelium of skin, hair, nails, sebaceous, mammary, and sweat glands (including myoepithelial cells of some glands)
	Epithelium of mouth, anus, teeth, taste buds
	Epithelium of nose and nasal glands
	Epithelium of penile urethra
	Epithelium of external auditory canal and membranous labyrinth
	Epithelium of anterior cornea, conjunctiva, lacrimal glands, pars ciliaris, and pars retinae (and related muscle), neural retina, and retinal pigment epithelium
	Brain and spinal cord, epithelial cells of all parts of the pituitary gland
Neural crest ("mesectoderm")	
	Cells of spinal, cranial, and autonomic ganglia; ensheathing cells of peripheral nervous system
	Pigment cells of dermis
	Certain muscles, connective tissues, and bone of branchial arch origin
	Adrenal medulla
	Cells of meninges and tunics of the eye
Mesoderm	
	Most connective tissues of body
	Stromal components of all glands
	Lymphatic organs (except Hassall's corpuscles and thymic reticulum)
	All endothelia and mesothelia
	Skeletal, cardiac, and most smooth muscle
	Urogenital epithelia, except urethra and large areas of bladder
	Blood cells and bone marrow
	Adrenal cortex
Endoderm	
	Epithelium of digestive tract except mouth and anus
	Epithelium of glands of digestive tract including liver, gallbladder, pancreas
	Epithelium of thyroid and parathyroid glands and thymic reticulum and Hassall's corpuscles
	Epithelium linning middle ear cavity, inner tympanic membrane, and auditory tube
	Epithelial lining of respiratory tract and its glands (except nostril)
	Epithelium of most of bladder, female urethra, vaginal vestibule, prostatic portion of male urethra, and its glands

In terms of principal tissue components, the outer epithelia and, as will be seen, the central nervous system develop from ectoderm. The epithelial linings of respiratory passages and gut and the glandular cells of appended organs such as liver and pancreas are of endodermal origin. The smooth muscular coats, connective tissues, and vessels supplying these organs are of mesodermal origin. Mesoderm also differentiates into blood, skeleton, skeletal muscles, and organs of excretion and reproduction. An interesting and important exception is in the case of the gonads, testis or ovary, in which the precursor cells of sperm and ova, the so-called *primordial germ cells*, are now believed to be of yolk sac, and possibly endodermal, derivation.

NEURULATION

The pattern by which such organ systems emerge commences with the process of *neurulation*, so named because it involves the establishment of a primitive *central nervous system* (brain and spinal cord).

As the developing notochord and adjacent mesoblastic cells are mobilized into a central layer beneath the midline ectoderm, an induction occurs which governs a highly coordinated growth and movement of the overlying ectodermal cells, collectively termed the *neural plate*. In response to the underlying notochord and adjacent mesoderm, there is initiated within these ectodermal cells the activation of specific genes and a resultant synthesis of specific supportive and contractile proteins. These become arranged as *intracellular filaments* and *microtubules* (discussed in detail in Chapters 1 and 4) which are positioned so as to exert and maintain rather precise changes in the shapes of the induced ectodermal cells. Coupled with regionally specific rates of mitotic activity, directionality in this proliferation, perhaps some mechanical influence by growth of surrounding tissues, and probably also precise patterns of cell-to-cell attachment, the shape-changing mechanisms of all of the cells act in harmony to fold the lateral edges of the neural plate upward, between them forming a *neural groove* (Fig. 3.4). This type of re-

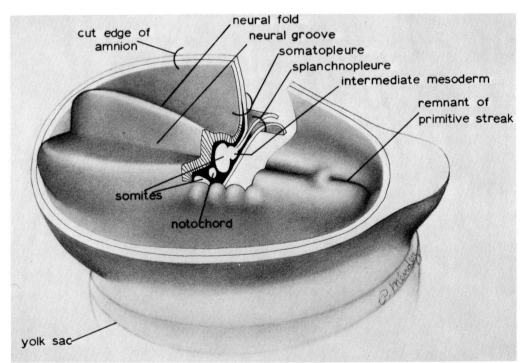

Figure 3.4. The embryonic disc during the process of neurulation. The mesoblast has begun differentiating into notochord, somites, and intermediate and lateral plate mesoderm. Ectoderm above the somites and notochord has been induced to fold upward. Eventually the lateral margins of the folds will fuse progressively to form the neural tube, the future brain and spinal cord. By this stage of development, the embryonic disc is about twice the length of that depicted in Figure 3.3.

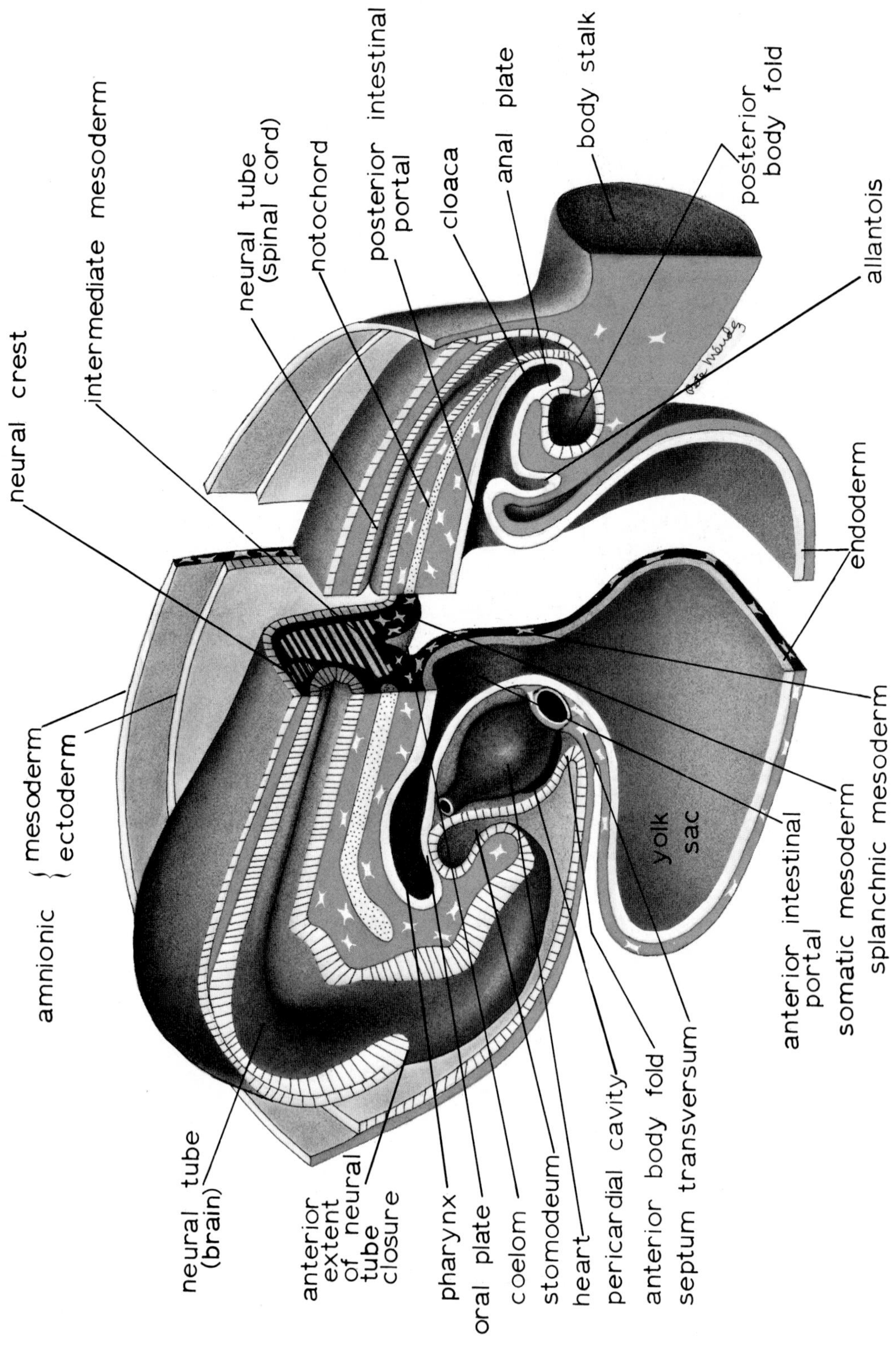
neural crest
intermediate mesoderm
neural tube (spinal cord)
notochord
posterior intestinal portal
cloaca
anal plate
body stalk
posterior body fold
allantois
endoderm
amnionic { mesoderm ectoderm
neural tube (brain)
anterior extent of neural tube closure
pharynx
oral plate
coelom
stomodeum
heart
pericardial cavity
anterior body fold
septum transversum
yolk sac
anterior intestinal portal
somatic mesoderm
splanchnic mesoderm

sponse to an inductive stimulus, resulting in individual and collective cell shape changes, can be detected as a basis for shaping of most tissues, organs, and regions. This is particularly true where the newly forming part is largely of epithelial composition. During neurulation, the process begins earliest in the anterior regions, where the mitotic activity is highest; thus the anterior folds are highest and thickest and, with their correspondingly deep groove, they herald the development of the brain. Gradually, the two elevating folds converge toward each other and fuse. First contact occurs in the posterior brain region, and fusion spreads from that point, zipper-like, anteriorly over the brain and posteriorly down the future spinal cord (Fig. 3.5). Fusion of the folds results also in the detachment from overlying ectoderm of the hollow inner epithelial tube, the *neural tube*, the walls of which will differentiate into the substance of the brain and spinal cord. Note that the spinal cord and posterior brain are immediately underlain by the notochord (Figs. 3.5 and 3.6).

NEURAL CREST

At the time of neural fold fusion and neural tube detachment, an unusual phenomenon occurs which adds still more cells to the mesenchymal compartment. Certain previously ectodermal epithelial cells residing along the crest of each neural fold suddenly lose their epithelial affinities, disengage, and migrate inward to invade the mesoblast along either side of the developing neural tube (Figs. 3.6 and 3.7). These cells rapidly disperse, making their identification immediately obscure, but special tracer techniques disclose that their numbers are considerable and their derivatives quite important. They are referred to collectively as the *neural crest* and they contribute, among other things, to developing spinal and autonomic ganglia, pigment cells, adrenal medulla, meningeal coverings of the brain and spinal cord, and many skeletal and muscular components of the head.

In a sense, neural crest development is a belated finish to the gastrulation process; the new mesoblastic neural crest cells have arrived in the mesenchymal compartment via a detachment process not dissimilar from that displayed some time earlier by gastrulating mesoblastic cells of epiblastic origin. As they detach from the ectoderm, the neural crest cells penetrate the basal lamina of that layer and become typically mesenchymal in their behavior; they are mitotically active and display a high degree of ameboid migratory capability. Having lost their epithelial attachments, they tend to migrate quite independently, displaying negative affinities toward other mesenchymal cells. Later in their various differentiative patterns, many of them will reverse this property and clump into appropriately shaped groups, such as those giving rise to spinal and autonomic ganglia, or sheets, like the enveloping meninges which eventually surround the neural tube. Many examples of specific neural crest development are portrayed in subsequent chapters of this text.

SOMITES AND THE EMBRYONIC AXIS

The notochord and neural tube are formed as single midline (or axial) structures which separate right and left halves of the embryo. Each is segregated from the surrounding mesoblastic compartment by the acquisition of basal laminae. Concomitant with establishment of the notochord, the mesenchymal cells immediately lateral

Figure 3.5. The process of neural tube fusion is nearly complete. The anterior body fold has inverted the cardiogenic region into a position beneath the pharynx. Lateral plate mesoderm has divided to form splanchnic and somatic layers with the interval between indentifiable as coelom. Neural crest migration is active. The posterior body fold has rolled anterior to the cloacal membrane so that allantois and body stalk are included in the forming umbilical cord. Communication between the elongating gut and the diminishing yolk sac is still very wide.

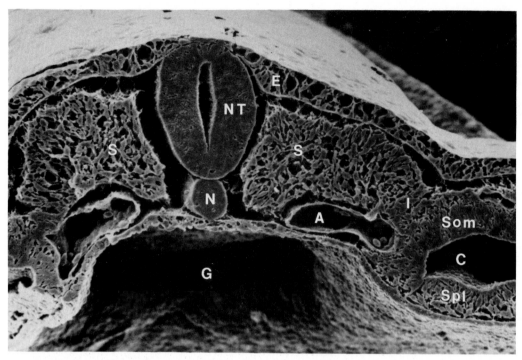

Figure 3.6. Scanning electron micrograph showing a cross-cut trunk region of an embryo following closure of the neural tube (*NT*) and establishment of structures of the embryonic axis. The neural tube is underlain by the notochord (*N*) and flanked by somites (*S*). The overlying ectoderm (*E*) has closed over and separated from the neural tube. Splanchnic (*Spl*) and somatic (*Som*) mesoderm is visible surrounding the embryonic coelom (*C*). *I*, intermediate mesoderm; *A*, dorsal aorta; *G*, developing gut cavity (×60). (Courtesy of Dr. Gary Schoenwolf.)

to it commence a highly regular pattern of clumping that results in development of sequentially arranged *somites* on either side of the midaxial neural tube (figs. 3.4 and 3.6). Some 31 pairs of somites are eventually formed, each representing a first visible representation of the repeating body segment, or *metamere*, which is characteristic of all vertebrate organisms and many invertebrates as well. Somites are compact aggregates of mesenchymal cells whose integrity seems temporarily ensured by a brief encasement in basal lamina material. The encasement is retained only long enough for the somites to achieve their metameric organization; shortly it will disperse as somitic mesodermal cells migrate once again into definite locations and commence differentiation into such serially repeated units of the body as bony vertebrae, axial musculature, ribs, etc. By that time certain neural crest cells have clustered between

adjacent somites to give rise to the equally segmentally ordered spinal ganglia.

Somites, spinal ganglia, neural tube, and notochord are regarded as the *embryonic axis*, around which all other elements of the embryo are assembled. From their beginning all components of the axis are mutually interdependent. Each exerts inductive influence upon the others so that spatial and temporal precision is maintained in the shaping of each unit and the axis as a whole. Somites appear first in the thoracocervical levels, where neural tube fusion has just occurred, newer ones arising progressively anteriorly and posteriorly until the entire miniature segmented individual has been laid out. By 4 weeks, enlargement of the brain and lateral expansion of its walls into ectodermal rudiments of the eyes are apparent. The embryo begins to assume the characteristic shape of a tetrapod vertebrate.

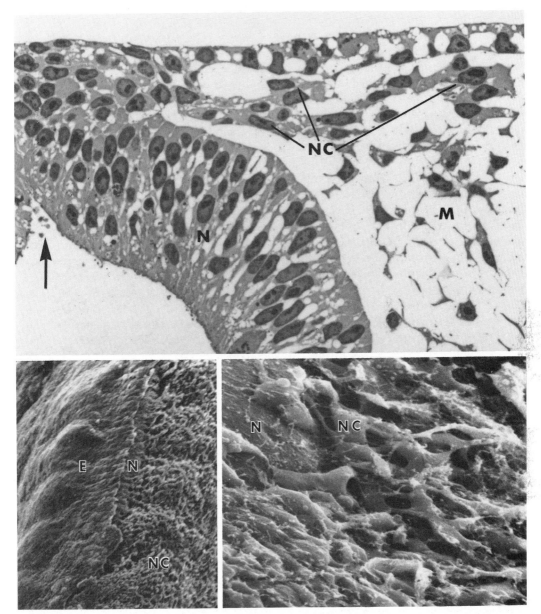

Figure 3.7. Formation of neural crest. *Top,* light micrograph showing a cross section through the neural tube (*N*) of an embryo at the time of neural tube closure (at *arrow*) and release of neural crest cells (*NC*) into the mesenchymal compartment (*M*) (×600). (Courtesy of Dr. Stephen Meier.) *Bottom,* low (*left*) and higher (*right*) magnification scanning electron micrographs showing migrating neural crest cells (*NC*) in an embryo viewed from a dorsal aspect after the ectoderm (*E*) from one side of the body has been removed. Flow of neural crest cells from the neural tube (*N*) region and over the developing somites is apparent (left, ×130; right, ×879). (Courtesy of Dr. Cheryl Anderson.)

SOMATIC AND SPLANCHNIC MESODERM

Lateral to the row of somites on each side of the embryonic axis, cells of the mesoblast group into a recognizable, but not distinctly segregated, mesodermal rod. Eventually these two rods elongate to run the full length of the embryonic trunk region. They constitute the *intermediate mesoderm* (Fig. 3.6), an important precursor to the developing excretory system, the gonads, and the inferior vena cava. Lateral to the intermediate mesoderm, the mesoblast extends as a sheet, the *lateral plate mesoderm*, reaching well beyond the boundaries of the embryonic disc, where it continues as the mesoderm of the amnion above, yolk sac below, and the body stalk behind. Within the embryonic disc, this lateral plate mesoderm exists only briefly as a single mesoblastic stratum; small cavitations appearing in its midst eventually fuse, to split the mesoderm into two layers. That layer above, immediately underlying the ectoderm, is termed *somatic mesoderm* (the two together constituting *somatopleure*), and the lower mesodermal layer, lying adjacent to endoderm, is termed *splanchnic mesoderm*. (Combined with the nearby endoderm, it constitutes *splanchnopleure*) (Figs. 3.5 and 3.6). The large mesoderm-coated cavity thus formed between the two layers within the embryo is the first representation of a true *coelom* or body cavity. For a time, the embryonic coelom will remain continuous with the extraembryonic *chorionic cavity*, or *extraembryonic coelom*. The mesodermal cells which line the coelom rapidly form attachments and acquire a basal lamina to separate themselves as an epithelial lining layer from the underlying splanchnic or somatic mesenchyme. This special mesodermal epithelial lining of the coelom and its derivative body cavities is referred to as *mesothelium*. Students of histology should note that the term mesothelium refers specifically to the lining epithelium of the true body cavities and *not* to other epithelial linings of mesodermal origin (such as the linings of vessels).

Definition of the above splanchnic and somatic components is important in terms of the patterns of differentiation which occur in each. For example, *splanchnic mesoderm* will eventually develop into a high proportion of smooth or cardiac nonvoluntary musculature and will be served largely by the autonomic nervous system. *Somatic* and somite-derived (*somitic*) mesoderm, on the other hand, will be the source of most skeletal musculature under the voluntary control of somatic neural components.

BODY FOLDS AND FORMATION OF THE PRIMITIVE GUT

As the embryonic disc, with its contained mesodermal and neural tube components, grows in length and width, it becomes elevated into the amnionic cavity. The movement is rather like when a low table, with its enshrouding tablecloth, is lifted above a floor just enough that the cloth drapes down from the table and spreads over the floor. If the table has but a single central pedestal, the tablecloth can next be gathered gradually toward the pedestal. This might conveniently be done by a noose or purse string. The portion of the tablecloth left surrounding the table corresponds to embryonic ectoderm, that spread over the floor is equated with extraembryonic ectoderm lining the inside of the amnionic cavity, and that part of the tablecloth cinched around the pedestal eventually represents ectoderm of the growing *umbilical cord*.

The movement is important to understand, for in the early embryo it gradually delineates embryonic from extraembryonic components, determines the position of the mouth, anus, and heart, and forms the gut and umbilical cord. The ectodermal folds, termed *head, tail,* and *lateral body folds*, are really parts of a single fold, a continuous inpocketing around and beneath the elevated embryo (Fig. 3.5). Eventually this ringlike fold constricts sufficiently in relation to the growing embryo that it constitutes the surface of a narrow neck, the rapidly lengthening *umbilical cord*. This latter is covered by ectoderm, contains the *yolk stalk, allantois*, and a mesodermal core, and continues to connect the embryo or fetus with extraembryonic components throughout prenatal life.

One important consequence of the development of the head fold and anterior lateral body folds relates to heart and mouth development. Originally the *cardiogenic plate* of mesoderm was situated well anterior on the midline of the embryonic disc, so far forward, in fact, that a mesoderm-free *prochordal plate* region separated it from the anterior tip of the notochord and overlying neural plate (Fig. 3.3). During head fold development, the cardiogenic plate, with its overlying ectoderm and underlying endoderm, is inverted and tucked under in such a way that it comes to lie beneath the neural plate and notochord and posterior to the prochordal plate, which has also been inverted. The endoderm is also folded and at the same time evaginated, forming an anterior midline diverticulation above the cardiogenic plate (Fig. 3.5). This diverticulation is the primordium of the *foregut*; its anterior extent is the former prochordal plate (now properly called the *oral plate* or *buccopharyngeal membrane*). This latter will ultimately perforate to complete the opening of the mouth. Note that the mouth itself is largely lined by ectoderm, a result of its development as an invagination in the oral plate region. This invagination is the *stomodeum*, (Figs. 3.5 and 3.8) and is the site of origin of several important ectodermal components such as the enamelforming cells of *teeth*, some *salivary gland*, epithelia, and the anterior and intermediate portions of the *pituitary gland* parenchyma.

The endodermally lined foregut remains continuous for a time with a yolk stalk via an *anterior intestinal portal*, and it begins a number of tubular evaginations which will eventually form the secretory or lining epithelia of a number of glands and organs. Prominent among these are *lungs* and *thyroid glands*, and more posteriorly the *liver*,

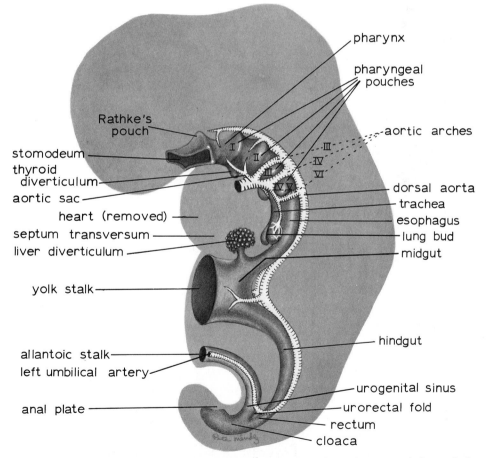

Figure 3.8. Three-week human embryo showing the extent of development of the endodermal epithelium and major arterial vessels associated with it. Pharyngeal pouches are starting expansion into various epithelial derivatives. Lung primordia are expanding. The cloaca is being divided into urogenital sinus and rectum by development of the urorectal fold. The yolk stalk is still relatively wide.

gallbladder, and *pancreas*. The *pharynx* is the most anterior (or superior) part of the foregut, and it develops paired bilateral endodermally lined outpouchings, the *pharyngeal pouches* (Fig. 3.8). Each pouch is met by an inpocketing of ectoderm or *branchial groove*, and occasionally a perforation, a *branchial cleft*, will form at the site of fusion between pharyngeal pouch endoderm and branchial groove ectoderm. Such clefts are usually transitory in mammalian development, but they recall their evolutionary homologues, the gill clefts so prominently retained in present day fishes and other adult lower vertebrates.

On each side of the embryo's developing head, the branchial grooves become apparent in a series of parallel vertical slits. Adjacent grooves bound prominent mesoderm-filled pillars, the *branchial arches*, and these have definite derivates such as the components of the upper and lower *jaws*, the *external ear*, parts of the *larynx*, etc. Their embryonic serial arrangement typifies further the segmented organization now apparent in the head as well as in the trunk of the embryo.

Inside, each pharyngeal pouch displays differentiation of its endodermal lining, which, after extensive invagination, proliferation, and morphogenetic shaping, becomes secretory, supporting, or lining epithelium of such important organs as *parathyroid glands*, *thymus*, *tonsils*, and the *middle ear* and *auditory tube*.

While the pharyngeal components take form, the cardiogenic region just beneath undergoes extensive change. Coelom formation extends anteriorly to separate splanchnic from somatic mesoderm; the anterior coelomic pocket thereby formed will ultimately be separated as the *pericardial cavity* (Fig. 3.5). Splanchnic mesoderm of this region forms a single midline tube lined by mesothelium on its outer surface (the *visceral pericardial mesothelium*) and, eventually, an *endothelium** on its inside aspect;

cardiac muscle will develop in between the two. This tube is attached to and supplied by important venous channels which join it posteriorly. Anteriorly it leads to and feeds paired arterial channels, the *aortic arches*, which course within several of the branchial arches. Quickly this tube initiates a series of contortions and septations which eventually lead to the typical morphology of the four-chambered mammalian heart.

Development of the embryo in the tail fold area has many similarities to that just described in head fold, pharyngeal, and stomodeal regions. A *hindgut* and *posterior intestinal* portal are entrapped within the embryo as the tail fold advances anteriorly, and an *anal plate* is formed by fusion of hindgut endoderm with overlying ectoderm (Figs. 3.5 and 3.8). This particular ectoderm lies at the bottom of an exterior invagination, the *proctodeum*. The proctodeum is the future *anus* of the developing embryo, and will become continuous with the hindgut when the anal plate is ruptured during later fetal stages.

The *allantoic stalk*, which took its origin just before tail fold development as a midventral outpouching of hindgut endoderm, is swung ahead of the tail fold, retaining its connection to the hindgut. It opens into an enlarged part of the hindgut, the *cloaca*, in the region of the anal plate (Figs. 3.5 and 3.8). As tail fold development continues, the allantoic stalk is drawn along so that its distal tip finally resides in the umbilical cord. Later yet, the cloaca will be divided by septation into a *urogenital sinus* (to which the allantoic stalk communicates) and a *rectum* (which drains the hindgut). Before anal plate perforation, the cloacal septation will be completed so that the urogenital sinus (the future *urethra* and *urinary bladder*) and rectum will have separate external openings. The urogenital sinus also receives paired *mesonephric* and *ureteric* ducts, which drain the embryonic excretory system developing within the nearby intermediate mesoderm.

---

*The term *endothelium* is specifically used to denote the interior epithelial lining of the heart, blood vessels, and lymphatic channels. All endothelium is of mesodermal origin. The term endothelium should not be confused with either mesothelium or endoderm.

As head, tail, and lateral body folds tighten around the belly of the enlarging embryo, the gut is elongated. Suspended within the coelom from the dorsal body wall by a splanchnic mesodermal *mesentery*, the emerging *midgut* elongates even more rapidly than the embryonic tissues around it. For a time during late embryonic and early fetal stages the midgut herniates into a rather wide umbilical cord, where it still communicates with a rapidly narrowing yolk stalk. As the umbilical cord becomes more constricted, the yolk stalk obliterates to a tiny ligamentous remnant, and the midgut is pulled back into the fetus, a process which by necessity involves rotation of the previously herniated midgut limbs. As the midgut continues to elongate and differentiate, it assumes the typical form and position of the small intestine and the proximal part of the large intestine.

RELATIONSHIP OF MICROSCOPIC ANATOMY AND EMBRYOLOGY

The foregoing synopsis of early human development is but a glimpse of an obviously complex and highly coordinated series of harmonious events. The histologist or cytologist must at least be aware of these basic patterns for they describe the origins of the four *basic adult tissue types*: *epithelia*, *contractile tissue* (muscle), *neural tissue*, and *connective* and *supportive tissue* (of which blood is a unique close relative).

The art of microscopic anatomy is greatly enhanced by the ability to appreciate that these four classes of tissues are not completely distinct and exclusive, but rather represent portions of a spectrum of morphological and functional intergradations in cellular differentiation. The *differences* among and within these types are emphasized in the study of adult tissues; their *similarities* and common origins are perceived by a consideration of their embryology.

The adult tissues are not composed of cells only. At very early stages, many cells (especially the nonepithelial cells) become separated from each other by their elaboration of important *intercellular substances*.

These substances also display a spectrum of variation and are just as much a part of the differentiation (and definition) of the emerging tissues as are the cells. Thus, each tissue is an aggregate of cells with its own characteristic amount and variety of intercellular substances (or *matrix*). In some tissues, the intercellular material is scanty (epithelia, muscle) and the cells are closely approximated. In such cases, differentiation relates more to the functional machinery developed *within* the cells' cytoplasm. In other tissues, the intercellular substances may become the major bulk of the tissue and assume physiological roles of massive proportions (bone, cartilage, connective tissue, blood, lymph). Here differentiation is really defined more by what the cells have constructed *outside* of themselves. Their cytoplasm may even be relatively nondescript.

Organs of the body are aggregates of the shades and varieties of the basic tissues, blended by appropriate shaping, quantity, and proportion to assume the specialized functions for which organs have evolved. Their construction and synergistic activities can best be appreciated by consideration of embryonic stages when the tissues' relationships are simple and just emerging.

In the chapters ahead, first the basic tissues and then the organs of the body will be examined, not only in terms of final adult microscopic anatomy but also in relation to the embryonic processes and relationships which led to that eventual form. It will be found that adult cells still contain certain organelles which controlled their individual and collective shaping during the embryonic life of their tissue or organ. Likewise it will be seen how both intracellular and extracellular components have gradually been mobilized, first to ensure the inductive tissue interactions controlling development and second, to stabilize and retain the emerging parts of the new individual into its complex, definitive adult form.

References

Bonner JT: *The Evolution of Development*. London, Cambridge University Press, 1958.

Bronner-Fraser ME, Cohen AM: The neural crest: what can it tell us about cell migration and determination? In *Current Topics in Cell Biology*, vol 15. New York, Academic Press, 1980, pp 1–25.

Gasser RF: *Atlas of Human Embryos*. Hagerstown, Md., Harper & Row, 1975.

Hamilton WJ, Boyd JD, Mossman HW: *Human Embryology*, ed 4. Baltimore, Williams & Wilkins, 1972.

Hay ED (ed): *Cell Biology of the Extracellular Matrix*. New York, Plenum Press, 1981.

Hay ED: Organization and fine structure of epithelium and mesenchyme in the developing chick embryo. In Fleischmajer R, Billingham RE (eds): *Epithelial Mesenchymal Interactions*. Baltimore, Williams & Wilkins, 1968, pp 31–55.

Johnson KE: Gastrulation and cell interactions. In Lash J, Whittaker JR (eds): *Concepts of Development*. Stamford, Conn., Sinauer Associates, 1974, pp 128–148.

Langman J: *Medical Embryology*, ed 4. Baltimore, Williams & Wilkins, 1982.

Lash J: Tissue interactions and related subjects. In Lash J, Whittaker JR (eds): *Concepts of Development*. Stamford, Conn., Sinauer Associates, 1974, pp 197–212.

Ledouarin N: Migration and differentiation of neural crest cells. In Moscona AA, Monroy A, Hunt RK (eds): *Current Topics in Developmental Biology*, vol 16. New York, Academic Press, 1980, pp 32–85.

Moore KL: *The Developing Human*, ed 3. Philadelphia, W. B. Saunders, 1982.

Noden D: The control of avian cephalic neural crest differentiation. I. Skeletal and connective tissues. *Dev Biol* 67:296–312, 1978.

Noden D: The control of avian cephalic neural crest differentiation. II. Neural tissues. *Dev Biol* 67:313–329, 1978.

Noden D: Interactions directing the migration and cytodifferentiation of avian neural crest cells. In Garrod D (ed): *The Specificity of Embryological Interactions*. London, Chapman and Hall, 1978, pp. 4–49.

Saxén L: Neural induction: past, present and future. In *Current Topics in Developmental Biology*, vol 15. New York, Academic Press, 1980, pp 409–418.

Spooner BS: Morphogenesis of vertebrate organs. In Lash J, Whittaker JR (eds): *Concepts of Development*. Stamford, Conn., Sinauer Associates, 1974, pp 213–240.

Tosney KW: The segregation and early migration of cranial neural crest cells in the avian embryo. *Dev Biol* 89:13–24, 1982.

Willier BH, Weiss PA, Hamburger V: *Analysis of Development*. Philadelphia, W.B. Saunders, 1955.

Chapter 4

EPITHELIUM

Chapter 2 dealt primarily with *cells* as structural and functional units. Basic information on the constituents commonly found in all cells as well as some of the specializations have been discussed. Through the process of *cellular differentiation*, maturing cells also come to exhibit different and often unique degrees in the development of specific organelles and other cytoplasmic components, and differences in the quantity and quality of extracellular products which they produce. A *tissue* may be defined as a collection of cells and associated intercellular materials specialized for a particular function or functions. It follows, then, that a tissue is the product of the sum total of the properties of its constituent cells. Usually the cells of a given tissue in a given region are relatively uniform in their properties, but from region to region the cellular properties vary, and likewise a given tissue shows gradations in its properties from region to region. Tissues are combined in appropriate patterns and proportions to form *organs*. The organs and organ systems are the subjects of later chapters.

The fundamental properties and patterns of tissues are the subjects of this and the next six chapters. For convenience, tissues are broadly classified into *four basic categories*: (a) *epithelia*, (b) *connective and supportive tissues*, including *blood and lymph*, (c) *contractile tissues* (*muscle*), and (d) *nervous tissue*. This categorization is traditional and useful, but there are important overlaps. As examples, the nervous tissue of the brain and spinal cord can itself be considered an epithelium, a number of epithelial cells are known to display at least subtle degrees of contractility, and in the thymus a major supportive function is carried out by the epithelial component.

In Chapter 3 the earliest multicellular stages of an embryo were seen to consist of closely adherent cells. These are shortly segregated into definable layers. Hence, the earliest beginnings of a new individual can be said to be epithelial, because *an epithelium may be defined as a layered collection of adherent cells, with very little intercellular material, usually covering internal and external surfaces of the body*. It was seen that ectodermal and endodermal epithelial layers cover the external surface of the embryo and its earliest manifestations of a gut. Moreover, and very importantly, these same layers serve as boundaries and seals for the mesenchymal compartment expanding between them. Hence, *adhesion* in an epithelial system is important not only for the maintenance of topographic integrity but also for the provision of relatively leakproof seals for the compartments surrounded by those epithelia.

As the organism matures, epithelium covers the outer surfaces of the body as *epidermis*. Other epithelia line all passages leading to the exterior (the linings of the digestive, respiratory, and urogenital systems, and numerous glands). Epithelia also line most of the closed cavities of the body. Most of these are derived by cavitation of mesenchymal tissues. Their lining epithelial cells are of mesodermal origin. More specifically, the epithelial linings of the *pleural, pericardial*, and *peritoneal cavities* are known as *mesothelia*, in view of their mesodermal origin. Likewise the lining of blood and lymphatic vessels is also an epithelium of mesodermal origin. Curiously, this lining has come to be known as *endothelium*.

During development, many embryonic epithelia send invaginating growths into the underlying connective tissues. Many such epithelial invaginations form the *parenchymal* (functional epithelial) components of glands. These usually contain cavities or passages leading to the surface from which they grew. They are termed *exocrine glands* (discussed below), because the passageway (duct) provides an exit for the products of the epithelial glandular cells. In some of the ingrowths, however, the connection is lost, and deeply lying epithelial cords, follicles, or aggregates of cells are produced and maintained, in spite of the loss of their passages or ducts. Because they must release their secreted products into surrounding connective tissue and thence into the nearby vascular passageways, these are termed *endocrine* glands (discussed below and in Chapter 21).

Epithelia serve widely differing functional demands in different locations. On the surface of the body or along the alimentary canal they are subjected to abrasion, attrition, and drying, and provide protection against these physical demands. In less exposed locations, as in the closed body cavities, the epithelium (mesothelium) is subjected to but little attrition and is covered with a fluid film; in these locations it forms smooth surfaces which glide over each other. In still other locations, epithelia serve not only for protection but also for secretion and absorption. An epithelium may be adapted to great changes in surface area, as in the distensible urinary bladder. Most epithelia are active mitotically throughout the life of the individual, constantly replacing cells which are lost in the normal course of function. In correlation with the differences in all of these functional demands, there are marked differences in epithelial structure. The epithelia vary in cellular shape, in number of cell layers, in physical and structural characteristics, in their mode of attachment to each other, in their relative mitotic activity, and in their secretory or absorptive potential. In some rather localized circumstances epithelial cells display highly specialized morphology related to sensory reception. It is remarkable that with all of these special-

ized activities and structural variations, the cells of epithelia maintain themselves as a closely adherent population serving as partially or tightly sealed barrier to fluids and other substances which might otherwise leak between the cells and cross the epithelium without being selectively recognized and transported by the cells themselves. More remarkable still is the recently emerging evidence that neighboring cells of many epithelia are in ionic or metabolic communication, i.e., able to signal each other by intercytoplasmic transfer of specific ions or molecules. Hence the cells of epithelia appear to be both physically and functionally adherent and interdependent.

CLASSIFICATION

Because epithelia line surfaces and cavities, they commonly have a free margin which faces the outside environment or the lumen of a particular organ, and a surface which faces underlying or surrounding connective tissue. The free margin is termed the *apical* surface or pole of the epithelium, and the connective tissue-facing pole is termed the *basal* surface. The surfaces of cells which face neighboring epithelial cells within an epithelium are sometimes referred to as the *lateral* cell surfaces. In nearly all epithelia (with some outstanding exceptions), the cells bordering the basal surface secrete a submicroscopically thin and complex extracellular coat, the *basal lamina* (discussed in detail below) along that surface. It serves to separate the epithelium from underlying connective tissue. When the basal lamina is itself very thick or sufficiently reinforced by layers of connective tissue collagen to be discerned by light microscopy, the whole structure is referred to as a *basement membrane*.

For convenience, epithelia are classified into different types on the basis of the number of cell layers and the shape of the cells at the apical surface; thus, epithelia of only one layer are termed *simple*, and they are subdivided according to the height of the cells when viewed in cross section, into *simple squamous, simple cuboidal,* and *sim-*

ple columnar (Table 4.1 and Fig. 4.1). One often notes cell heights which fall intermediate to those defined strictly by the above terms. The lateral margins of cells also outline specific shapes in many epithelia, although this characteristic is not frequently used in classification. For example, mesothelial cells which line all body cavities, display fairly regular lateral surfaces, whereas the equally simple epithelial cells of kidney tubules have lateral surfaces that are tortuously interdigitated with those of their neighbors.

An epithelium composed of two or more layers is said to be *stratified*, and is categorized according to the shape of the cells at the apical surface into *stratified squamous*, *stratified cuboidal*, and *stratified columnar*. Stratified squamous epithelium is the most commonly found stratified type. In it, only the upper layers are squamous; those along the basal lamina and for a considerable distance above it are columnar and polyhedral (Fig. 4.1). The cells of the basal areas are frequently mitotically active, serving to replenish the layers above. Moreover, the functions served by the cells of various layers may be quite different. This is particularly true in the epidermis of the skin (Chapter 15).

The epithelium of some parts of the body consists of a single layer of cells of variable height and arrangement, with all cells resting on the basement membrane, but with only some of the cells reaching the apical surface. The nuclei of these cells are seen at different levels above the basement membrane and, on first inspection, one might conclude that the epithelium is stratified. Careful study discloses that this epithelium is really composed of only one layer of cells. It has been traditionally classified as *pseudostratified* (Fig. 4.1).

A special modification of stratified, epithelium is found in the urinary system, where the shapes of cells and the number of layers vary with distention and contraction of the organ. This type of epithelium is classified as *transitional* (Fig. 4.1).

In addition to the above criteria, epithelia are often described in terms of products they accummulate or release, or in terms of cellular appendages that may characterize the apical surface. Hence, an epithelium which has a high population of specialized cells which synthesize and release mucus onto the apical surface (goblet cells) can be termed a *mucous* epithelium. Likewise, because the cells of the apical epidermis accumulate high concentrations of a tough

Table 4.1.
Types of Epithelium

No. of Cell Layers	Shape of Surface Cell	Examples of Location in the Body
Simple (one layer of cells)	Squamous	Endothelium of blood vessels, mesothelium of body cavities, thin segment of Henle's loop in kidney
	Cuboidal	Some kidney tubules
	Columnar	Gastrointestinal tract
Pseudostratified (modification of simple; not all cells reach the surface)	Columnar	Trachea, parts of male reproductive system
Stratified (more than one layer of cells)	Squamous	Epidermis, lining of esophagus, vagina
	Cuboidal	Infrequent; found in duct of sweat gland
	Columnar	Infrequent; found in parts of epiglottis and in the male urethra
Transitional (variety of stratified; varies with distention)	Surface cell varies from dome shape in contracted organ to flat in distended state	Lining of renal pelvis, ureter, urinary bladder, and parts of urethra

EPITHELIUM

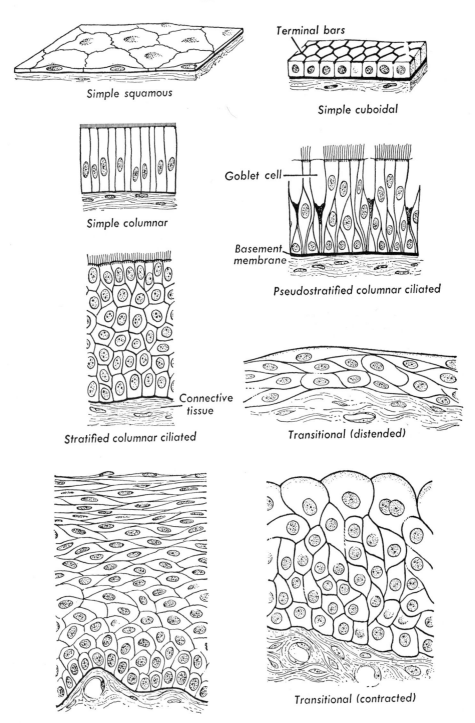

Simple squamous

Terminal bars

Simple cuboidal

Simple columnar

Goblet cell

Basement membrane

Pseudostratified columnar ciliated

Connective tissue

Stratified columnar ciliated

Transitional (distended)

Transitional (contracted)

Stratified squamous

Figure 4.1. Schematic representation of the various morphological types of epithelium. In each case, the epithelium is shown with some of the underlying connective tissue.

proteinaceous material called *keratin,* this epithelium can be said to be *keratinized.* When the apical surface of an epithelium bears cilia, particularly if they are numerous, the epithelium is said to be *ciliated.* If the same surface possesses large numbers of more minute projections, the *microvilli,* the epithelium is said to have a "striated," "brush," or *microvillous* border.

Combining these various schemes, it is common to describe an epithelium in rather complex fashion. For example, the epidermis of the skin is termed *stratified squamous keratinized epithelium* and the lining of the trachea is a *pseudostratified ciliated columnar epithelium.* The lining epithelium of the intestine is a *simple columnar epithelium* displaying a stiated *microvillous* border.

SPECIAL CYTOLOGICAL CHARACTERISTICS

Virtually all substances which enter or leave the body or its components must cross one or several epithelia. Often, materials are sequestered within epithelia to be converted by the cells into specific products. These are subsequently released either apically or basally (see *exocytosis,* Chapter 1). The organelles of epithelial cells are appropriately arranged in a polarized fashion to promote these directional processes; i.e., the cells contain a polarized cytoplasmic content. For example, the Golgi apparatus and accumulated secretion droplets are polarized between the nucleus and the apical border in the parenchymal cells of many epithelial glands. Similarly, rows of mitochondria are arranged between the nucleus and a highly infolded basal surface of the simple epithelial linings in kidney tubules, as part of a polarized mechanism for the pumping of ions across the epithelium. The apical surfaces of many simple epithelia are adorned with cilia and microvilli, whereas such structures are rarely found basally. In stratified epithelia, the progression of young cells from a mitotically active basal region to replace older cells toward the apex, finally to be cast off at that surface,

is also a reflection of epithelial polarization. Collectively, the polarizations inherent in the many epithelia of an organism underscore the directionality of fluxes necessary to the homeostasis of the many compartments comprising that organism.

The above discussion implies also that the cells of epithelia attain and maintain rather specific shapes. Maintenance of a specific cell shape is requisite not only to the functional polarity of an epithelial cell but also to the mechanical integrity of the epithelium as a whole. Subtle or elaborate *cytoskeletal networks* of filaments provide an internal scaffolding for this function, and it may be especially well developed in those epithelia that resist wear and tear (for example, the stratified squamous epithelia). This cytoskeleton is composed of 8- to 12-nm cytoplasmic filaments (often termed *intermediate filaments* or *tonofilaments*) which are woven in specific patterns to resist, again on a polarized basis, the forces most frequently applied to the cells. As will be seen, the cytoskeleton is intimately connected to the points of intercellular adhesion within an epithelium.

Other networks of finer cytoplasmic filaments, the so-called "*microfilaments,*" are also found in epithelial cells. They are well developed components of the more pliable epithelia in which absorption or secretion seems emphasized. Many of these microfilamentous populations are contractile and exert changes in the shapes of the epithelial cells as a part of normal day-to-day function. Microfilaments are particularly prominent just beneath the microvillous apices of many epithelial cells involved in absorption. It is now believed that they not only control the apical diameter of a given cell but may also be involved with subtle movements of the microvilli themselves. During embryonic stages, the shapes of epithelial invaginations and evaginations are probably promoted by microfilaments within the constituent epithelial cells acting in harmony to provide a very specific result. Again, the shapes achieved and maintained within individual cells through this type of

SPECTRUM OF JUNCTIONAL FINE STRUCTURE

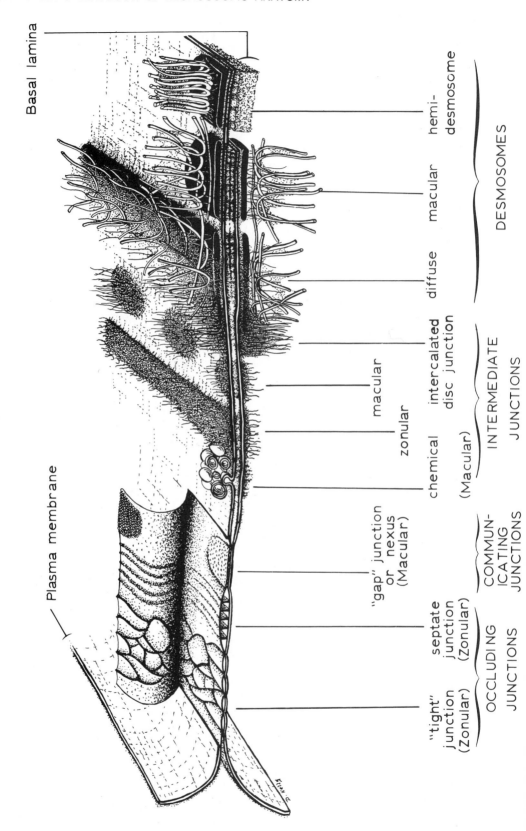

Basal lamina

Plasma membrane

"tight" junction (Zonular)

OCCLUDING JUNCTIONS

septate junction (Zonular)

"gap" junction or nexus (Macular)

COMMUN- ICATING JUNCTIONS

chemical (Macular)

zonular

macular

intercalated disc junction

INTERMEDIATE JUNCTIONS

diffuse

macular

hemi- desmosome

DESMOSOMES

"cytomuscular" activity reflects further the propensity for polarization shown by epithelial cells.

Intercellular Attachment

Most cells invest their plasma membranes to some degree with a *glycoprotein* or *glycosaminoglycan* surface coat (sometimes referred to as "*glycocalyx*"). In epithelia the deposition of this coat may be highly polarized, as seen in the formation of basal lamina. When deposited on the lateral surfaces of epithelial cells, these coatings are much thinner, but they may promote some degree of cell-to-cell adhesion. This type of adhesion seems especially important during initial embryonic stages when the first few cells of an embryo are prevented from dispersing. However, the early epithelial cells of an embryonic system quickly become attached by firmer sites of intercellular adhesion (often termed *junctions*). These not only serve the function of cell-to-cell mechanical anchorage but also provide the mechanism to seal the epithelial system against the escape of fluids between adjacent cells (so-called *paracellular flux*). Some of them also provide channels for ionic communication and flux between the cytoplasms of adjacent cells. The details of these junctional mechanisms have had to await study by electron microscopy. We know now that a spectrum of junctional morphology exists in nature, but for convenience we have classified junctious into several prominent groups (Fig. 4.2).

One of the earliest known types of epithelial attachments is referred to either as a *desmosome* (from the Greek *desmos*, bond, + *soma*, body) or as a *macula adherens* (from the Latin *macula*, spot, + *adhaereo*, to stick). Desmosomes are particularly abundant in stratified epithelium, where they are large and numerous enough to be described by light microscopy. Their distinctness is often accentuated by preparative techniques which cause the cells to shrink and pull apart except in these regions of adhesion. Electron micrographs show that these are not true bridges, and, in fact, a space of about 20 to 25 nm separates the apposing cell membranes in the desmosomal junction (Fig. 4.3). The cell membrane itself is no thicker in this region than elsewhere, but it may appear so because in each of the adjacent cells there is a dense proteinaceous plaque of cytoplasmic material subjacent to the cell membrane (Figs. 4.4 and 4.5). Desmosomes are visible by light microscopy because numerous intermediate filaments (tonofilaments) converge in the region of these plaques and are apparently attached to the plaques and the cell membranes at that point. It was once thought that the intermediate filaments terminate at that point or perhaps proceed into the adjacent cell, but high resolution electron micrographs indicate that these filaments form shallow or hairpin loops that turn back into the cytoplasm (Fig. 4.4). In some desmosomes, the filaments course nearly parallel to the plaque, apparently attached to it en route (Fig. 4.5). The eventual terminus for individual tonofilaments is not known.

The extracellular space of desmosomes is filled with an abundance of sialic acid-rich glycoprotein which apparently serves as a strong adhesive, anchoring the membranes of adjacent cells. It typically displays a dense intermediate line in electron micrographs. This is interpreted by some workers as representing an overlap of the adhesive contribution of the adjacent cells.

Desmosomes represent focalized sites of

Figure 4.2. Schematic diagram of the range of junctional variation known to exist in cells, based on electron microscopic evidence. The plasma membranes of two apposed cells are depicted, one of which has been split over a short segment at left. There, one leaflet is folded back to display intramembranous components revealed by freeze-fracture techniques. The intercalated disc type of junction is a complex intermediate junction characteristic of cardiac muscle, and the chemical synapse is an asymetric, quasi-intermediate junction found between neurons; these are discussed in detail in the chapters on muscle and nervous tissue. Septate junctions are found primarily in epithelia of invertebrates. See text for descriptions of each junctional variation.

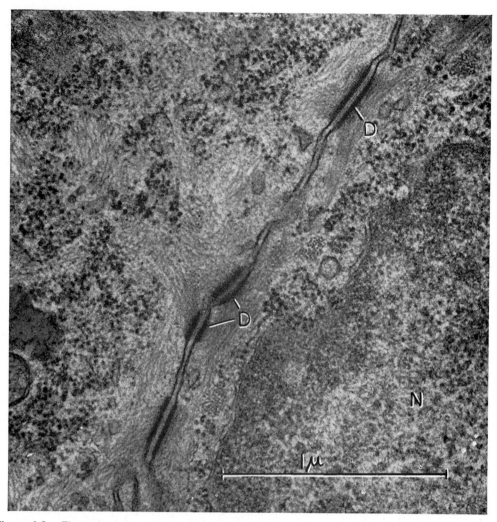

Figure 4.3. Electron micrograph showing attachments between epithelial cells of stratified epithelium of esophagus of bat. *D*, desmosome or macula adherens; *N*, nucleus. Networks of intermediate filaments (tonofilaments) can be seen in the cytoplasm and converging into the desmosomes (×64,000). (Courtesy of Dr. Keith Porter.)

relatively firm adhesion between adjacent cells, but they are also the focalized sites for anchorage, to cell membranes, of the cytoskeletal filaments within adjacent cells. When viewed over the extent of a given epithelium, it can be seen that the desmosomal-cytoskeletal network within an epithelium forms a girder-like supportive system for the epithelium.

In the basal cells of an epithelium, this network extends to the basal cell membrane also, although that membrane is not lying adjacent to a neighboring cell, but rather to the basal lamina and underlying connective tissue substrata. Along that surface there may be *hemidesmosomes*, which resemble one-half of the desmosome described above (Fig. 4.6). There are, in fact, notable differences in the morphology of hemidesmosomes as compared to desmosomes, but the main relationships among tonofilaments, plaques, cell membranes, and extracellular adhesive material follow similar principles. Hemidesmosomes are believed to be basal anchorage sites for cytoskeletal filaments and adhesion points for the basal cell membrane to the basal lamina and connective tissue.

Looping
tonofilaments

Plasma membrane

dense plaque

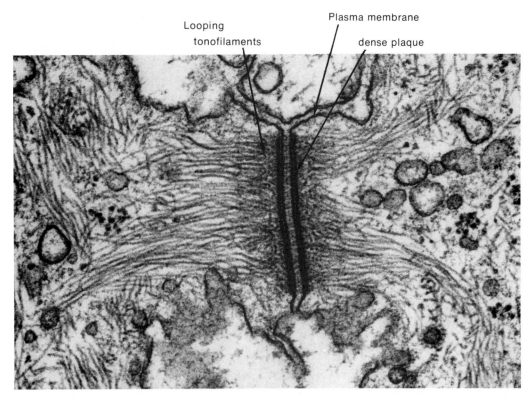

Figure 4.4.   Electron micrograph of a desmosome from stratified squamous epithelium. Note the cell membrane and the presence of an electron-dense plaque in each cell subjacent to the plasmalemma. Tonofilaments of the cytoplasm form loops at or in the dense plaque of the desmosome. Note that a discontinuous midline is present in the material within the intercellular space at the desmosome. From the epidermis of a newt (×81,000).

Pigment granule

Plasma membrane

Plasma membrane

Dense plaque

Tonofilaments

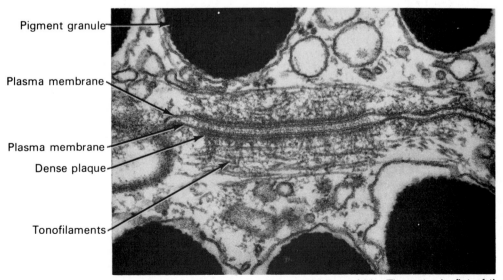

Figure 4.5.   Electron micrograph of a desmosome from epithelium of iris. The outer leaflet of the plasma membrane is more distinct than that depicted in Fig. 4.4 as a result of staining *en bloc* with uranyl acetate. Note that the tonofilaments approach the desmosome in a horizontal direction, in contrast with the pattern seen in Figure 4.4. Iris of newt (×90,000). (Courtesy of Dr. A. Tonosaki.)

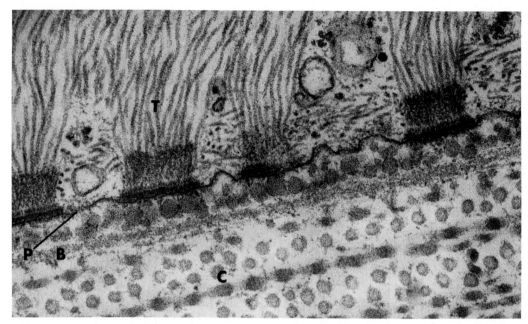

Figure 4.6. High magnification electron micrograph depicting a portion of the most basal cytoplasm of a basal epidermal cell from a larval salamander. The cytoplasm occupying the upper one-half of the micrograph is separated by a plasmalemma (*P*) from the underlying dermis (lower half of the micrograph). The lamina densa of the basal lamina (*B*) and collagenous lamellae (*C*), both parts of the basement membrane, support the epidermis. Four hemidesmosomes are recognizable as densities along the plasmalemma. Bundles of tonofilaments (*T*) converge toward each hemidesmosomal plaque. Presumably, each hemidesmosome is a point of attachment of tonofilaments to the basal plasmalemma and attachment of the plasmalemma to the underlying basal lamina and collagenous substrata. A peculiar, globular lipid-rich layer lies within the lamina rara externa of the basal lamina at this stage of development in this animal (×74,500).

Freeze-fracture studies disclose aggregates of intramembranous particles within the leaflets of desmosomal cell membranes (Figs. 4.7, 4.9, and 4.10). Evidence now suggests that the looping tonofilaments are attached to the cell membrane by a population of smaller diameter filaments (termed "*linker*" or "*traversing*" *filaments*) which course through the dense plaque. These smaller filaments are thought to be related to the desmosomal intramembranous particles. Hemidesmosomes have also been shown in some species to display intramembranous particles, often of larger individual diameters clustered at the hemidesmosomal site (Fig.4.7).

Desmosomes are most frequent in those epithelia that resist wear and tear and, as would be expected, in those epithelia that contain the most complex and highly evolved intermediate filament-dominated cytoskeletal networks.

In nearly all epithelia a prominent circle of close apposition can be detected around the apical neck of each cell. This ring of adhesion firmly attaches each epithelial cell to its neighbors. The adjective *zonular* is used to describe this collar-like ring of attachment in contrast to the *macular* or "*spot weld*" *configuration* described above for desmosomes. This attachment collar could be revealed in some of the earlier light microscopic preparations of mesothelia viewed from the apical aspect, particularly when impregnated with silver. In transverse sections the collars appear as distinct spots at the apical margins of each individual cell (Fig. 4.1). The early light microscopists termed this attachment collar the *terminal bar*, a designation which is

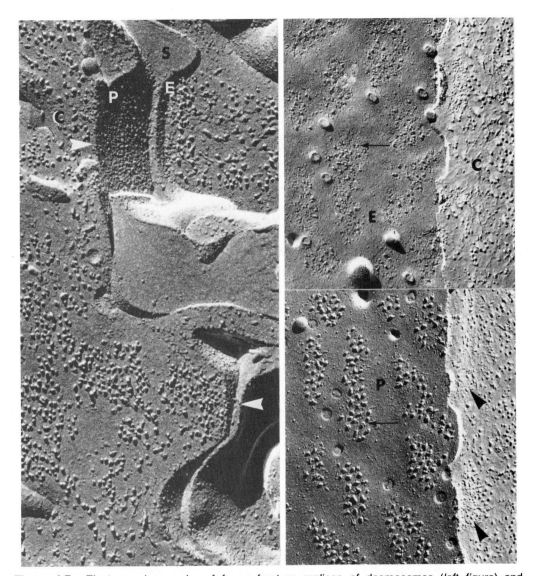

Figure 4.7. Electron micrographs of freeze-fracture replicas of desmosomes (*left figure*) and hemidesmosomes (*right figure*). In the figure at *left*, the fracture plane has passed through the cytoplasm (C) of the first of two adjacent epithelial cells. The same fracture next exposes the P-face (P) of the plasmalemma of that cell before passing through extracellular space (S) and the E-face (E) of the plasmalemma of the adjacent cell. The cytoplasm of that cell is exposed in the *upper right corner*. The fracture plane has passed through two desmosomes (*white arrows*). At these desmosomal sites, it can be seen that closely packed granules occupy the P-faces. Hemidesmosomes are similarly revealed in two complementary, "mirror-image" freeze fracture images to the *right*. The fracture plane has passed through the tonofilament-rich basal cytoplasm (C) of an epithelial cell before splitting the basal membrane of that cell to reveal its E-face (E) in the top image and its exactly complementary P-face in the bottom replica. Clusters of densely packed filamentous material can be seen in the cytoplasm adjacent to the cell membrane in the regions of the hemidesmosomes (*large arrows*). Clusters of granules (*small arrow*) are seen on the P-face, and tiny pits are visible at corresponding points on the E-face. Each cluster corresponds to the cell surface area occupied by one hemidesmosome. The openings of caveolae are also visible on both faces. Both figures prepared using dark shadow imaging. (*Left figure*, ×73,200; *right figure*, ×53,000.) (Micrographs in collaboration with Aileen Kuda.)

now frequently replaced by *"junctional complex"* in view of detailed knowledge of the components found in this region by means of electron microscopy.

In most instances the terminal bar region contains two to four distinct types of attachments (Fig. 4.8). The most universal is the *occluding junction* (often termed *tight junction* or *zonula occludens*). This junction constitutes the principal seal against paracellular passage of extracellular materials which might otherwise cross the epithelium. It may be extensively developed along the lateral surfaces of cells within epithelia that are highly impermeable to such passage or it may be sparse and discontinuous in the case of certain epithelia which are relatively and appropriately "leaky." In electron micrographs of transversely sectioned tight junctions (Figs. 4.8 and 4.17), the essential component of the junction is a series of punctate appositious where the outer dense leaflet of the cell membrane of one cell comes into confluency with that of its neighbor. There may be only one or two such points apparent between the cells of leaky epithelia (e.g., kidney proximal tubule), but in relatively impermeable epithelia (e.g., urinary bladder) many such points of apposition are usually found. Freeze-fracture images of the membranes in the region of tight junctions disclose that the points of membrane apposition are really anastomosing linear contacts. Inside the membranes the areas of contact appear as grooves or ridges forming networks of variable extent (Fig. 4.9). In the leaky epithelia there are but a few of these profiles and they may be discontinuous, whereas in the impermeable epithelia there may be an extensive series of interconnecting, linear strands (Figs. 4.9 and 4.10). Because freeze-fracture splits the cell membrane it will be appreciated that the profile of a tight junction consists of ridges on the P-face and corresponding grooves on the E-face of each membrane. If one were able to look at the true external surfaces of separated cells one would also see ridges.

Since this junction is so crucial to the functional characteristics as well as the structural integrity of a given epithelium, there has been considerable interest in deducing its molecular structure. Prior freeze-fracture evidence suggested that the ridges represent a common fibrous strand shared between the cell membranes of the two adherent cells. More recently, however, it seems clearer that each membrane contributes an equal component to the ridge. One interpretation suggests that the two components are cylindrical elevations of each membrane which became juxtaposed in parallel fashion, but slightly overlapping, to form the ridge. While the ridges have traditionally been considered to be proteinaceous, some newer evidence suggests that the cylindrical components are of micellar lipid composition.

Interestingly, the epithelia of most invertebrate species display a strikingly different junction in this location. It is termed the *septate junction* because of the presence of multiple parallel ridges of intercellular structure between the adjacent cells. It too is believed to provide a seal against the flux of extracellular materials across the epithelium (Fig. 4.2).

Closely associated with the tight junction region of epithelia is the *intermediate junction* (or *zonula adherens*). This junctional area also encircles the apical-lateral margin of the cells; hence its designation as *zonular* (Figs. 4.8 and 4.17). It is also a site of relatively firm adhesion between the adjacent cells, and it displays an extracellular space of about 15nm. The space contains a glycoprotein adhesive material, although not in the apparent abundance seen in desmosomes. The cytoplasms of the apposed cells at intermediate junctions display a density, but this density is not so distinct as the plaques of desmosomes. It appears to be the anchorage point for another system of cytoplasmic filaments often concentrated within the apical cytoplasm of these cells, the so-called *terminal web*. Unlike the larger 10-nm tonofilaments associated with desmosomes, the terminal web filaments are of the *microfilament* variety (less than

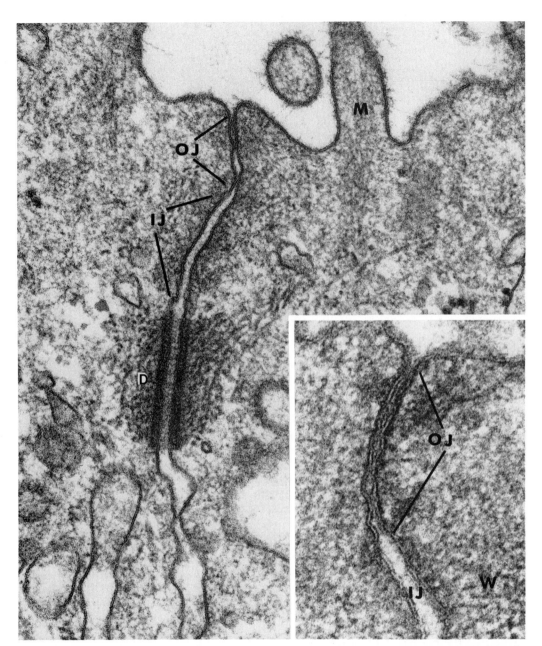

Figure 4.8. Electron micrographs showing the apical junctional region between two epithelial cells. Microvilli (*M*) of the adjacent cells are visible at the top. They are covered by plasmalemma which is continuous over the opposed junctional surfaces in left center. The section plane has passed through an occluding junction (*OJ*), an intermediate junction (*IJ*), and a desmosome (*D*). Microfilaments of the terminal web (*W*) are seemingly attached to the cell membranes at the intermediate junction. The occluding junction displays intermittent points of fusion between the outer leaflets of the plasmalemmas of the two adjacent cells (×124,000). (Courtesy of Dr. Barry King.) Details of an occluding junction (*OJ*) and an intermediate junction (*IJ*) are shown at higher magnification in the *inset* at lower right (×225,000). (Courtesy of Dr. David Chase.)

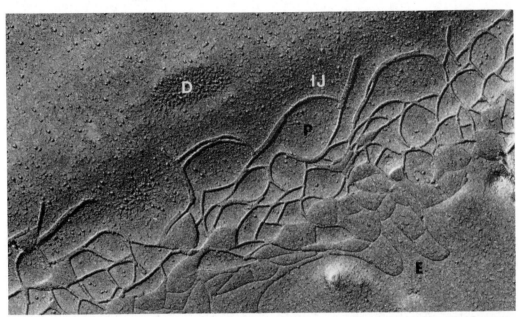

Figure 4.9. Electron micrograph of a freeze-fracture replica taken through the membranes of the apical junctional region of two adjacent epithelial cells like those depicted in Figure 4.8. In the *lower right* of the micrograph the fracture plane has split the plasmalemma of one cell, exposing its E-face (*E*). In a line coursing diagonally from the *upper right* to the *lower left* corner of the micrograph, the fracture plane has deviated into the plasmalemma of the adjacent cell, revealing its P-face (*P*) over the *upper left half* of the micrograph. The region of the occluding junction is revealed as a series of entangled grooves on the E-face and corresponding ridges on the P-face of the neighboring cell membranes. The area along the plasmalemma occupied by the intermediate junction (*IJ*) appears somewhat lighter but not otherwise distinctive. An aggregation of granules demarks the location of a desmosome (*D*). Note also widely scattered membrane particles over the exposed P-face. Figure prepared using dark shadow imaging (×69,500).

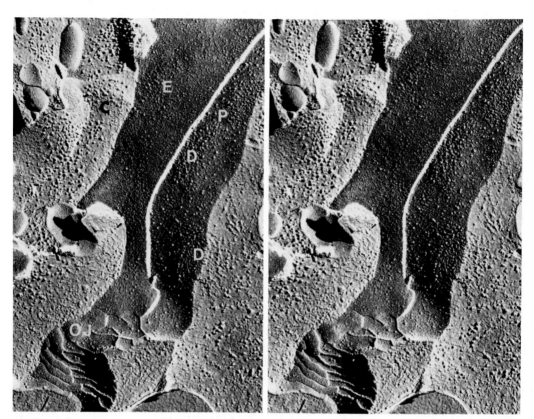

Figure 4.10. Stereo electron micrograph pair depicting a freeze-fracture replica of the apical junctional region of two adjacent epithelial cells similar to those shown in Fig. 4.8. The apical surface is at the bottom of this figure. The figure plane has cleaved the cytoplasm (C) of one cell on the left of the picture, then split the membrane of that cell to expose its E-face (E). A narrow, white intercellular space is next encountered, after which the P-face (P) of the neighboring cell's membrane is revealed. The fracture then courses through the neighboring cell cytoplasm at *lower right*. Elements of an apical occluding junction (OJ) and several desmosomes (D) are visible. This figure may be studied in stereo by utilizing cross-eyed viewing of the two pictures to form a third, middle, combined image. Figure prepared using dark shadow imaging (×55,300). (Micrographs in collaboration with Aileen Kuda.)

8 nm in diameter). The terminal web is particularly well developed in cells that display a *microvillous apical border* (discussed below); it contains the contractile proteins *actin* and *myosin* and may be involved in minute shape changes at the apex of these cells or within the microvilli themselves. Microfilaments, either continuous or associated with the terminal web, extend as cores into microvilli, where they terminate at the apical tips of those structures. In developing epithelia that are undergoing *morphogenetic cell shape changes*, similar areas of microfilamentous attachments are found along apical and other surfaces of the cells. Their positioning appears to relate to the specific shapes that will be assumed by the cells as the result of the contractile activity of those microfilaments.

Intermediate junctions of epithelia have not, as yet, revealed any specialized intramembranous structure in freeze-fracture replicas, although their location can be ascertained from the general contours of the membranes and the positions of other junctions (Figs. 4.9 and 4.10).

The fourth type of intercellular junction frequently found in epithelia is the "*communicating junction*" (also designated *gap junction, nexus,* or *close junction*). Like desmosomes, these junctions may or may not appear within the terminal bar region. For many years after the introduction of electron microscopy "gap junctions" went unrecognized because of close similarity to tight junctions (compare Fig. 4.8 with Fig. 4.11). When epithelia are treated with small molecular weight, electron-dense tracer particles such as *lanthanum hydroxide* or *horseradish peroxidase*, these materials do not penetrate an intercellular space guarded by a tight junction. However, such tracer materials do percolate between the two apposed membranes of nearby regions which previously appeared very similar to the tight junction. By this means, it is recognized that in these latter regions there is a narrow extracellular gap of about 2 to

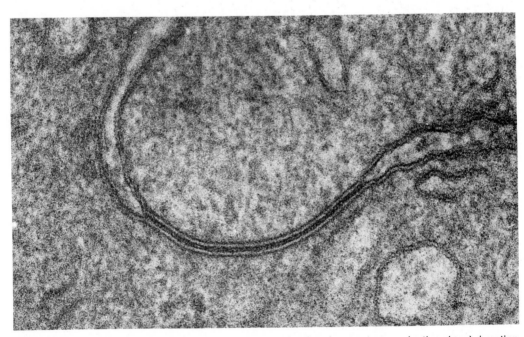

Figure 4.11. High magnification electron micrograph showing a communicating (gap) junction between two adjacent liver cells of a rat. The cell membranes of neighboring hepatocytes come into very close proximity in a region shown in the center of the micrograph. Close inspection discloses a 2- to 4-nm gap between the membranes in this region (×220,000). (Courtesy of Dr. Norton B. Gilula.)

4 nm. between the adjacent cells. (Fig. 4.12).

Face-on views of such "gap junctions" after treatment with tracer materials reveal the junctional area to be macular in form and also disclose that the tracer percolates through the gap following a minute hexagonal pattern (Fig. 4.12). Close inspection of the array suggests that the junction contains hexagonally arranged subunits with a center-to-center spacing of about 9 nm. The tracer particles seem to percolate

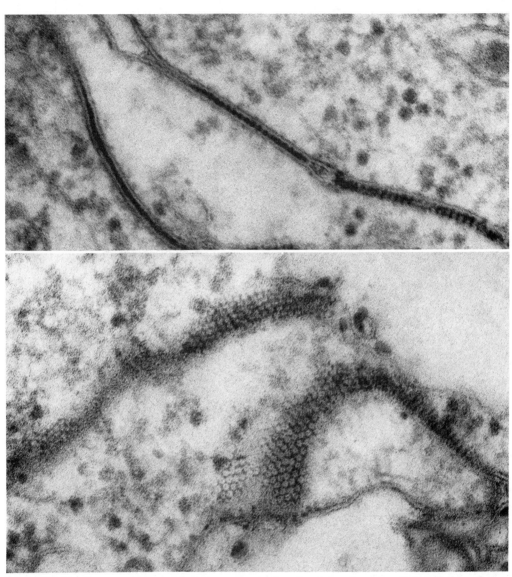

Figure 4.12. Electron micrographs of communicating (gap) junctions treated with a lanthanum impregnation technique. In the *upper figure*, a colloidal form of the heavy metal lanthanum has been deposited between the adjacent cell membranes of the junctions and appears dense in this cross section micrograph. Lanthanum thereby delineates the intercellular gap, which in this animal is about 4 nm wide. It also reveals in negative image regularly arranged bridging components between the adjacent cell membranes. The bridging components are seen to better effect in the *lower figure*, where the plane of section is parallel to the plane of junction. The bridging components appear as doughnut-shaped profiles arranged in a regular hexagonal array. Lanthanum has percolated into the intercellular space remaining between the bridging components. Both figures ×189,000.

through narrow passages between the sub-units.

Freeze-fracture study of these junctions confirms such interpretations. When split and replicated, the membranes of gap junctions reveal arrays of intramembranous particles termed *connexons* (Fig. 4.13). These usually remain with the P-face and may not be preserved in a precise hexagonal or close packed pattern. There remains uncertainty as to functional implications of this variability. The E-face usually displays a complementary array of pits for these particles. There have been a number of interpretations offered as to the molecular arrangement of the proteins, presumably comprising the particles and their relationship to the cell membranes. One model Fig. 4.14 depicts the possibility that the particles, or connexons, are protein complexes which span the width of each apposed cell membrane and extend extracellularly far enough to join an equivalent member from the adjacent cell. The narrow extracellular space is continuous between the tiny pillars provided by the apposition of these protein complexes. The authors of this model have also portrayed hydrophilic channels coursing through the center of the protein complexes. The presence of such channels is occasionally suggested by the presence of a small dimple or dot in the center of the particles seen in freeze-fracture preparations, or a linear density across the membrane in certain special thin sections viewed by transmission electron microscopy. Such images suggest the presence of a communicating pore of approximately 2 nm diameter.

It had been known for some years before the discovery of gap junctions that the cytoplasms of cells within a number of epithelia must be *ionically coupled*. This property can be detected by the insertion of microelectrodes into adjacent epithelial cells or even epithelial cells several cells apart. In either case, an ionic flux can often be detected between the cells under test. This suggests that there are channels interconnecting the cytoplasm of one cell to

that of its neighbor and that these channels are of such minute proportions as to allow only the passage of materials of ionic or small molecular dimensions. Impedance studies indicate the pore diameter to be about 1 nm (10 Å). Since high calcium concentrations in the cell block ionic flux, this ion may regulate the activity of the pores. The passage of certain low molecular weight (up to approximately 500 to 1100 daltons) fluorescent tracers, fluorescein and procion yellow, has subsequently also been demonstrated, and these theoretically require a channel of between 3.5 and 16 Å. Hence, all of the various measurements point toward pore diameters of nearly equivalent ranges.

A number of authors have postulated that such ionic exchanges among cells might serve as mechanisms for coordination of epithelial activities or as signals to promote specified changes or new directions during developmental processes. Theoretically, certain ions or other small molecules, such as nucleotides, exchanged between coupled cells should be small enough to be moved very rapidly and yet large enough to carry some reasonably specific code. It has been calculated that a molecular weight of from 300 to 500 falls into the ideal range.

Whereas ionic coupling between epithelial cells has been known from physiological evidence for some time, the exact site of the exchange could not be immediately ascertained. Junctions other than gap junctions have been suspected in the past, but mounting circumstantial evidence has lessened the likelihood that any of them are involved in this activity—at least in vertebrate tissues. Hence, the term "*communicating junction*" has become a common replacement for *gap junction*. Investigations utilizing mechanical or chemical dissociation of epithelial cells show that, like tight junctions and desmosomes, communicating junctions are also relatively firm sites of adhesion between adjacent cells. We can infer therefore that in communicating junctions a strong anchorage is

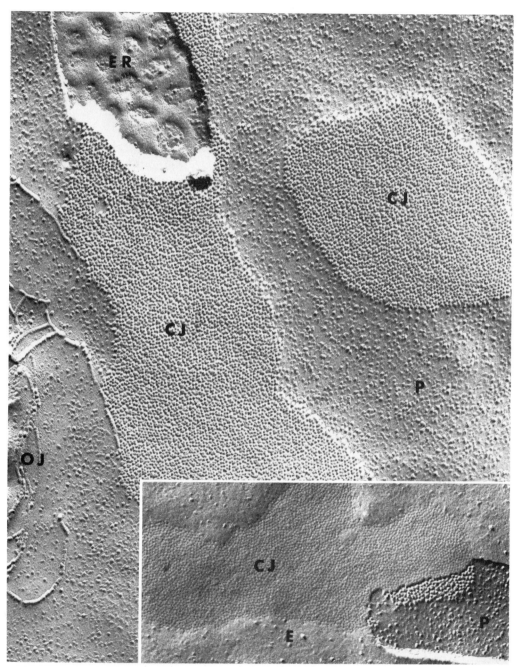

Figure 4.13. Regions of communicating junctions between adjacent rat liver cells as revealed by freeze fracture and electron microscopy. In the *upper figure* the P-face (*P*) has been exposed to reveal closely packed particles in the region of two communicating junctions (*CJ*). A nearby region of occluding junction (*OJ*) is seen at left. In the *upper part* of the figure, the fracture plane has diverted into the cytoplasm of the liver cell to expose the split membrane surfaces of the endoplasmic reticulum (*ER*). In the *lower figure* the fracture plane has exposed the E-face (*E*) over most of the field of view. An area of communicating junction (*CJ*) is identified by the presence of closely aggregated pits. These pits can be shown to correspond in position to the particles exposed on the P-face (*P*) within the cell membrane of the adjacent liver cell. Both figures ×48,000.

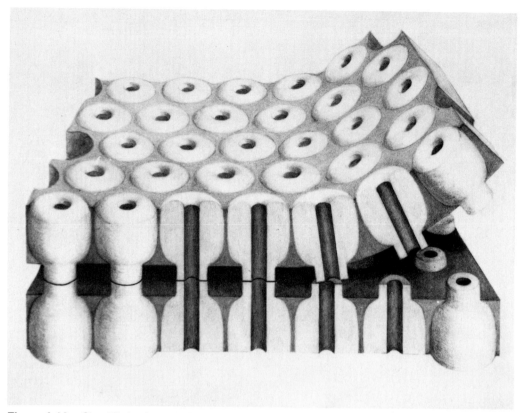

Figure 4.14. Simplified schematic illustration demonstrating the postulated components witin adjacent cell membranes of a communicating junction. Intramembrane particles are seen within each of the two membranes arranged in regular hexagonal pattern. These are the particles revealed as P-face particles when either of the membranes are split by freeze-fracture techniques. Each particle (or connexon) represents a molecular aggregate which theoretically contains a pore. The pore provides a communicating channel of approximately 1 to 2 nm between the cytoplasms of the two adjacent cells. This communication is by virtue of the registration across the intercellular gap of extensions of connexons from the adjacent membranes. (Courtesy of Dr. Norton B. Gilula.)

maintained between adjacent cells to insure an appropriate level of ionic flux.

Strong morphological and physiological evidence points to the existence of communicating junctions or nexuses in tissues other than epithelium. They are well developed between adjacent smooth and cardiac muscle cells (Chapter 8), where they promote the transfer of contraction-producing excitation from one cell to the next. Nexuses are also common between neuronal cells of lower vertebrate nervous tissue, and occasionally similar junctional morphology has been recorded in the brains of mammals. These junctions are often called "*electrotonic synapses*," and again presumably serve a funtion of excitatory transfer (Chapter 10).

Our understanding of both the morphology and function of junctions between epithelial and other cells has advanced very rapidly in the past 15 years and promises to continue to do so in the future. It is not presently certain that all of the basic junctional configurations or their subvarieties are known. Certainly, the finest components of junctional architecture require much further elucidation. At this point in our understanding, however, it is possible to realize that a *spectrum of junctional morphology* exists in nature and that the various basic types we have described, as well as a number of less common subvarieties, fit into that scheme (Fig. 4.2). Potentially all of the junctional configurations can be *macular* (focalized), *diffuse*, or *zonular*. Some of the junctions seem to involve only components of adjacent cellular membranes, whereas others show increasing degrees of involvement of both extracellular and cytoplasmic components. Indeed, the junctions that display the most complex cytoplasmic organization (filaments, plaques, etc.) seem also to display the greatest quantity and complexity of extracellular adhesive materials. Junctions found in other nonepithelial situations can easily be located within the spectrum (for example, intercalated disc junctions of cardiac muscle, chemical synapses of neural tissue), as can the very common septate junction of invertebrate epithelia.

Within epithelia it is typical for many of the junctions to occur together; for example, the type of *junctional complex* shown in Figure 4.8 is particularly characteristic within the *terminal bar* region of intestinal, respiratory, and a number of other epithelia. However, tight junctions, intermediate junctions, desmosomes, and gap junctions may also occur independently. In some epithelia the arrangement of the junction permits relatively large *intercellular clefts* and gaps to be maintained. Good examples are found in the endothelial linings of lymphatic capillaries and vascular sinusoids. These passages become sufficiently large to allow the intercellular passage across the endothelium of large molecules such as plasma proteins or even entire cells (cancer cells, or white blood cells).

Modifications at the Free Surface

Microvilli, microscopic projections of the free surface, are found in most epithelia. They are usually numerous, often regularly arranged and uniform in length, and particularly well developed in the lining epithelium of the small intestine and other absorptive epithelia. Because the microvilli of the intestine collectively appear vertically striated under the light microscope, the apical surface has been termed a *striated border*. Electron micrographs reveal that the microvilli composing the border are cell membrane-covered cytoplasmic extensions about 2 μm long (Figs. 4.15, 4.17, 16.38, 16.39, 16.40 and 16.41). Each microvillus has a core of fine filaments apparently anchored at the tip and extending into the terminal web. These are believed to provide structural support and, because they are composed of a form of the contractile protein actin, also may interact with myosin molecules of the terminal web area to provide subtle degrees of microvillar movement. The actin "core" filaments of microvilli are also attached to the cell membrane along the sides of each microvillus in a complicated fashion—apparently involving an array of the calcium-regulating protein *calmodulin* and also an actin attachment protein known as α-*actinin*. The protein attaching the actin filaments to the tip of each microvillus is apparently yet another protein. Hence, the cytoskeletal structure of microvilli and its mode of action are not simple. Microvilli greatly increase the surface area of the cells in correlation with absorptive functions. Vesicles involved in pinocytotic uptake are frequently found in the basal notches between such microvilli. Microvilli are also numerous on the free surfaces of the proximal convoluted tubules of the kidney. In this location they are somewhat higher and less uniform than in the small intestine, and they appear as a so-called *brush border* under the light microscope (Figs. 18.13 and 18.14). Epithelia of many other locations, where no border modification is visible by light microscopy, are often seen by electron microscopy to possess short, irregular microvilli.

As indicated above, *glycoprotein surface coats* (or *glycocalyx*) are present over the surfaces of epithelial cells, and these extend over the microvilli. These surface coats give a positive periodic acid-Schiff reaction. In the striated border of the small intestine the coat is so well developed that in electron micrographs it gives a decidedly fuzzy appearance to the microvilli (Fig. 4.15). Indi-

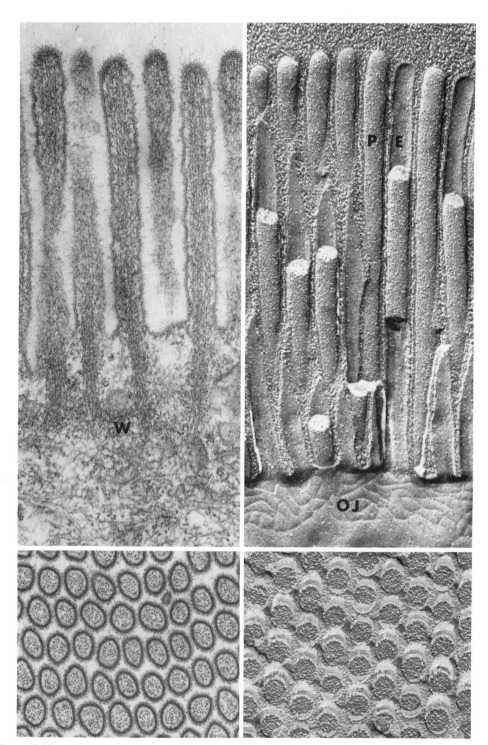

Figure 4.15. Microvilli from the apical surface of intestinal absorptive cells. In the *left hand figures,* several microvilli are seen by transmission electron microscopy in longitudinal (*upper figure*) and cross section (*lower figure*). Note the continuity of the plasmalemma which covers the surface of each microvillus. The membrane in turn is covered with a fuzzy glycosaminoglycan material. The interior of each microvillus contains microfilaments which are anchored to the plasmalemma at the tip and extend to the apical cytoplasm of the cell, where they engage the microfilamentous terminal web (*W*). In the *right figures,* the same views are shown in freeze-fracture preparations. Note that the plasmalemma of each microvillus is split to reveal particle-covered P-faces (*P*) and relatively bare E-faces (*E*). Microfilaments in the core of each microvillus are seen in the cross fracture (*lower figure*). A region of occluding junction (*OJ*) is seen along an E-face in the *upper figure.* All figures approximately ×62,000. (*Upper figures* courtesy of Dr. David Chase, *lower figures* courtesy of Dr. Michael J. Cavey.)

vidual filaments of the "fuzz" are about 2 to 3 nm thick, and they form a radiating and branching network for as much as 0.1 to 0.5 μm above the surface. They are attached to the plasmalemma and probably represent an extension from an integral protein of the cell membrane. They are thought to serve a protective role for the free surface of the cell, act as a selective barrier allowing colloidal particles and dissolved substances to penetrate, while preventing the approach of large particles, and function as an ion trap, serving to concentrate various small molecular weight charged particles that are to be absorbed by the cells.

Stereocilia are unusually long microvilli found in parts of the male reproductive system (Fig. 4.22) and in sensory regions of the inner ear. They do not have the structural characteristics of the true cilia or flagellae (see below). They increase the surface area of the apical cell membrane and may aid in secretion and absorption in the former instance and the reception and transduction of vibratory stimuli in the latter.

Cilia are relatively large, often motile appendages usually formed on the apex of cells. They may be present singly or in massive numbers. Cilia are usually 5 to 10 μm in length and about 0.2 μm in diameter. They are readily seen with the light microscope (Fig. 4.21), but their internal structure cannot be resolved. Electron microscopy discloses that the shaft or free part of each cilium is enclosed by a plasmalemma continuous with that of the cell and that each contains longitudinal microtubules typically arranged in a constant and orderly manner (Figs. 4.16 and 4.17). Most cilia have two single central microtubules and nine peripheral pairs of fused double microtubules, or *doublets*. These microtubules extend from near the tip of the cilium to its base. A *basal body* is located in the cytoplasm just inside the free surface of the cell. Each basal body is a modified centriole constituted of a "wall" of nine *triplet* microtubules. It is quite similar to the centrioles

seen in the cell center of many cells and known to play an important role in cell division. In the course of differentiation of a ciliated cell, the centrioles apparently replicate many times to provide a basal body for each cilium. Where the ciliary shaft joins the basal body, the two central microtubules terminate and each of the nine doublets joins a triplet, each doublet continuing as the two central subunits of a triplet. In many instances striated "*rootlets*" extend from the basal body well into the cytoplasm of the cell. Other footlike connections may extend onto the nearby cell membrane from the basal body. Both of these modifications are believed to be reinforcing anchorage mechanisms for the cilia. It is interesting that the same fundamental plan of ultrastructural characteristics is found in the cilia of all animals.

Cilia are numerous on the surface cells of the epithelium lining the respiratory tract and on some of the cells of the female reproductive system, for example. In these locations they beat in a coordinated rhythmical wavelike manner, promoting movement of materials over the cell surfaces. The beating of the cilia in the trachea produces an upward movement of mucus with its entrapped dust particles, thus preventing foreign materials from blocking the lower respiratory regions, which must remain unobstructed for proper exchange of O_2 and CO_2.

The mechanism which underlies the movement of cilia is currently being elucidated. High resolution electron microscopy and special techniques disclose two arms extending from the central microtubule of each doublet toward the next adjacent doublet (Fig. 4.17). Other less prominent elements extend toward the central pair and the surface membrane. The arms are believed to contain an ATPase (*dynein*) whose action promotes bending of the ciliary shaft in a plane oriented to the substructure within the ciliary shaft. Recent evidence suggests that this is accomplished by an ATP-dependent mechanism which causes sliding of the doublets on one side

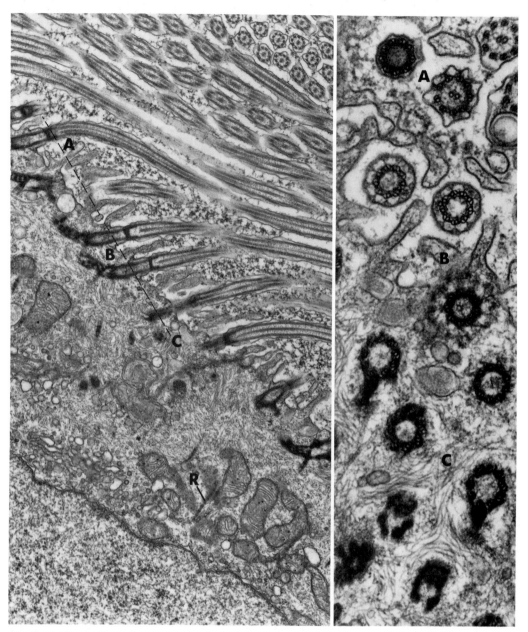

Figure 4.16. *Left*, electron micrograph showing numerous cilia characteristic of the apical surface of the esophagus in a salamander. The shaft of each cilium extends from the surface of the cell, carrying the plasmalemma of the cell with it. At the base of each ciliary shaft a dense basal body can be seen in various planes of section. The basal body contains a centriole capped by a dense plate. Beyond the plate a regular array of microtubules extends into the ciliary shaft. These are seen in various planes of section in the *upper portions* of the figure. Striated rootlets (*R*) radiate from the base of each centriole and extend for some distance into the cytoplasm. Dotted line *ABC* represents the plane of section seen in the inset (×19,000). (Micrograph in collaboration with Mary Ann Cahill.)

Inset (right), higher magnification electron micrograph cut in the plane labeled *ABC* on micrograph at *left*. The section plane courses from just outside the cell membrane (*A*) to just inside the apical cytoplasm (*C*). At level *B* the plane passes through the apical plasmalemma. Details of internal ciliary structure are seen at the various levels. At *A*, the dense plate and the typical 9 + 2 arrangement of microtubular doublets, as well as the surrounding plasmalemma, are seen in cross sections of the cilia. At level *B*, the plane passes through the centriolar region of each cilium and discloses a 9 + 0 arrangement of triplets, each displaying an attachment to the cell membrane. Deeper into the centriole (at *C*), the microtubular triplets transition into the basal body and rootlet (×50,000). (Micrograph in collaboration with Mary Ann Cahill.)

136

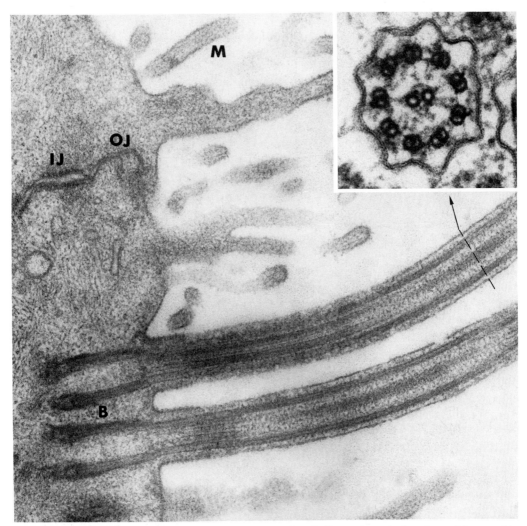

Figure 4.17. Higher magnification electron micrographs of cilia on the apical surface of the monkey trachea. Centriolar components of two basal bodies (*B*) are seen to be in continuity with the microtubules extending into ciliary shafts. A cross section in the plane indicated at the *arrow* is shown at higher magnification in the *inset*. Here the nine peripheral doublet microtubules and the central pair are well defined, as is the surrounding plasmalemma. Arms can be seen extending from the central member of doublet pairs toward their neighbors. Additional connecting structures extend toward the central pair and the surrounding plasmalemma. Other components of the tracheal epithelial apical surface include occasional microvilli (*M*), occluding junctions (*OJ*), and intermediate junctions (*IJ*) (×50,000; inset ×130,000).

of the cilium with respect to those of the other.

Flagella also have the same axial structure as cilia but are much longer and are usually present as but one or two per cell. The best example of flagella to be seen in the mammalian organism is in the tail of the spermatozoon (Chapter 19, Fig. 19.11). Although possessing similar microtubular patterns within their interior, flagellae usually beat in a seemingly more random whip- or wavelike motion.

In certain locations of the body, ciliary projections are highly modified to serve sensory receptor functions. This is strikingly exhibited in the outer segments of the rods and cones of the retina and in some of the hair cells of sensory portions of the inner ear. Such ciliary processes are usually not motile and lack the central pair of microtubules. The nine doublets, however, are retained. In rods and cones, the plasmalemma of the ciliary shaft has been thrown into a highly regular and constantly replaced series of membranous discs. These membranous discs are the site of deposition and action of photosensitive pigments (Chapter 22).

Basal Modifications and Developmental Stabilization

A fundamental characteristic of epithelia is the secretion of a complex cell coat along their basal surfaces. This extracellular layer separates each epithelium from underlying connective tissues. It consists of a *proteoglycan* matrix within which very fine (20 Å) filaments of predominantly *type IV collagen* (discussed in the next chapter) are embedded. This coat is termed the *basal lamina* (or *basement lamina*). It averages 100 to 200 nm in thickness and is usually seen in high resolution micrographs to consist of two layers, a lucent *lamina rara* adjacent to the cell membrane and a more opaque *lamina densa*. The lamina densa is usually about twice the thickness of the lamina rara. Occasionally the lamina densa is much thicker, but seldom enough to allow the entire basal lamina to be resolved by light microscopy.

The basal lamina is mostly a secreted product of the epithelial cells themselves. Both the collagen components and a glycoprotein, *laminin*, have been demonstrated to originate from the epithelial cells, but a third constituent, the glycoprotein *fibronectin*, may be at least partly provided from cells of the underlying connective tissue. Laminin appears to play a role of attachment between the cell surface and the lamina densa, while fibronectin appears to be involved in attachment of other collagen fibrils to the lamina densa or to the cell membrane (see also Chapter 5).

Frequently the basal lamina is reinforced by an underlying and much thicker layered meshwork of *reticular* and other collage-

nous fibers embedded in a similar matrix. This layer is termed the *reticular lamina.* The combination of the basal lamina and the reticular lamina constitutes the *basement membrane* which *is* visible by light microscopy and which has been described for many years. The basement membrane appears deeply black in silver preparations because of the presence of reticular fibers, and it stains red after periodic acid-Schiff because of its polysaccharides. It is easily seen in hematoxylin- and eosin-stained sections of the trachea, where the reticular lamina is exceedingly thick. A similarly disposed layer around the basal surfaces of kidney tubules is almost entirely composed of basal lamina. In that instance it is occasionally thick enough to be discerned by light microscopy. In other locations, such as beneath transitional epithelium, the basement membrane is so thin as to be unresolvable by light microscopy.

The basal lamina appears as a thin deposit very early in the development of most epithelial rudiments of the embryo. It seems to serve an important function in the segregation of tissues within the embryo. As will be outlined in the next chapter, it becomes the peripheral boundary of a broad and complex connective tissue compartment. However, it should not be considered an impenetrable boundary; it is more analogous to a mesh fence. Many molecules easily diffuse across basal laminae to interact with epithelial cells on the one side and connective tissue components on the other. As noted above, the ultimate seals for preventing fluid loss from these extracellular compartments lie in the tight junctions of the epithelial cells. Figure 4.18 illustrates a vascular channel, the adjacent connective tissue compartment, two basal laminae, and an epithelial region which have been perfused with the tracer colloidal thorium dioxide, previously introduced into the bloodstream. It can be seen that after an appropriate period of time this molecule has penetrated in clumped aggregates through the endothelium of the blood vessel and its basal lamina to occupy the connec-

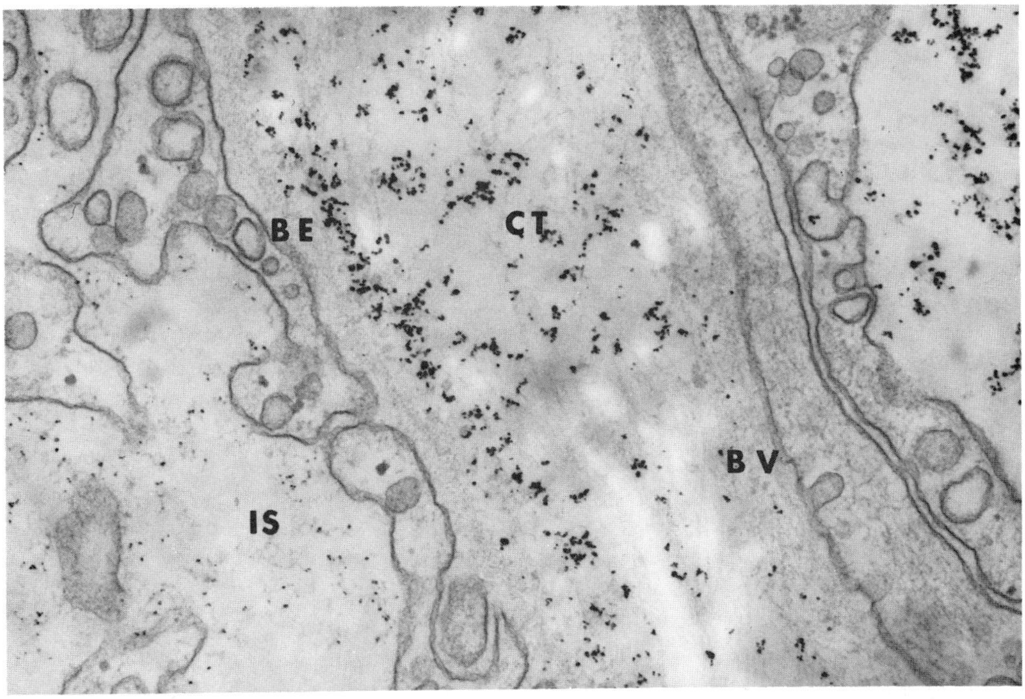

Figure 4.18.   Medium magnification electron micrograph of the connective tissue compartment (*CT*) between a thin-walled blood sinusoid at the *right* of the figure and the basal region of an epithelium at the *left*. There are large intercellular spaces (*IS*) in this epithelium. A heavy metal tracer (colloidal thorium dioxide) has been injected into the blood stream of the animal and allowed to circulate for several minutes. Tracer particles are visible in the sinusoidal lumen at the *right*. They have also leaked through the vessel wall and crossed the vascular basal lamina (*BV*) to occupy the connective tissue. Note that large clusters of the tracer are piled up against the epithelial basal lamina (*BE*) and only fine particles of the tracer have managed to penetrate that basal lamina to gain access to the epithelial intercellular space. The experiment demonstrates that basal lamina material is not impervious to the passage of materials but can serve as a sieve to select the size of molecules that are allowed to pass (×48,500).

tive tissue compartment. The basal lamina of the epithelium, on the other hand, is more selective and has permitted the diffusion of only the smallest aggregates of thorium dioxide into epithelial extracellular compartments. The larger aggregates are seen clumped along the basal lamina. Hence, in addition to their segregative potential, basal laminae may serve to regulate selective movement of colloidal-sized aggregates or macromolecules among the compartments of an embryo or an adult.

As embryonic epithelial rudiments develop, they assume particular shapes. The initiation of *rudiment shaping* is probably a function of contractile microfilaments and their associated attachments within the epithelial cells themselves. However, it seems that as the rudiments enlarge, additional reinforcement and stabilization are required to maintain the emergent shapes. The acquisition of basal laminae around these rudiments may be the first step in such an extracellular stabilization construction. Collagenous and reticular fibers may also be laid down, most frequently through the action of connective tissue cells, eventually reaching reticular lamina proportions. Thus, an extracellular collagen-glycoprotein encasement for such rudiments serves as a reinforcing framework. It should be realized, then, that the shapes that cells and epithelial rudiments attain and maintain are dependent upon the harmonious interaction of cytoplasmic cytoskeletal (filamentous) networks and their attachments on the one hand and extracellular collagenous stabilizing frameworks on the other.

Epithelia are not the only tissues which deposit basal lamina material. During embryonic development, certain other cells segregate themselves from surrounding connective tissues by the acquisition of similar coats. When the coat completely or nearly completely surrounds such cells, as smooth, skeletal, and cardiac muscle as well as fat cells, the encasement is more properly termed an *external lamina*. Reticular lamina is seldom well developed in association with such external lamina. Otherwise, the appearance of basal and external laminae is essentially similar. There is emerging evidence, however, to suggest that there are chemical differences in both the collagen and the glycoproteins found in various basal laminae and external laminae.

The basal cell membranes of various epithelia may acquire a wide range of modifications which increase the basal surface area exposed to the connective tissues and their interstitial fluids. Deep infoldings of the basal surface of individual cells (*basal infoldings*) are prominent in epithelia which are differentiated to promote transport of fluids and salts between the lumen and the connective tissue (Figs. 18.13 and 18.15). There may also be numerous *caveolae* or *pinocytic vesicles* along the basal cell membrane, ostensibly engaged in uptake or release of metabolic constituents. In all these cases, the basal lamina generally does not accompany the diverted membrane, but rather runs a relatively straight course as seen in section. If, however, the basal surface of an epithelium is more grossly undulated into folds which each involve several cells, the basal lamina also undulates accordingly.

Vascular Supply to Epithelia

Epithelium is avascular. Nutritive materials and oxygen enter it by diffusion through the cells and across basal laminae

and basement membranes. Capillaries are present in the epithelium of the stria vascularis of the internal ear, an apparent exception to this rule, and the tissues of the spinal cord and brain might also be considered exceptions on first glance. In these cases, however, blood vessels make only apparent entrance into the epithelia. Close examination by electron microscopy shows that their excursions into the epithelium are looping ones; they carry with them both the basal lamina of the epithelium itself and a basal lamina of the vascular endothelium. Therefore, these vessels do not actually invade the epithelium, but rather remain separated by at least some basal lamina material. This point will be discussed in greater detail in Chapters 10 and 11.

SIMPLE EPITHELIA
Simple Squamous Epithelium

Simple squamous epithelium (*pavement epithelium*) consists of flat scalelike or platelike cells arranged in a layer only one cell thick. On surface view the cells appear as a delicate mosaic, as demonstrated well by precipitation of silver at the boundaries of the cells (Fig. 4.1). The edges of the cells are usually slightly interdigitated with those of their neighbors, but may be smooth. The nucleus, situated in the center of the cell, is spherical or ovoid, causing a bulge.

Simple squamous epithelium is widely distributed. It lines the peritoneal, pleural, and pericardial cavities (*mesothelium*), the heart and all blood and lymph vessels (*endothelium*), the membranous labyrinth of the internal ear, portions of the uriniferous tubule, and portions of the rete testis.

Pinocytotic vesicles are particularly numerous in the cytoplasm of endothelial cells, and they apparently play a role in the transport of some substances (e.g., large molecules such as proteins) across the cell. The significance of this in relation to other mechanisms for transport is discussed under the circulatory system (Chapter 12). It appears that regeneration of endothelium, like that of most other types of epithelium, involves multiplication and rearrangement of cells of its own type. Mesothelium apparently can be regenerated from cells of the underlying connective tissue. Mesothelial cells can also change into fibroblasts. They seem to be less specialized than other types of epithelial cells and appear to retain some of the multipotency of mesenchyme. However, in the embryo at least one instance is known (development of the endocardial cushions of the heart) wherein endothelial cells convert and contribute to formation of fibroblasts.

Mesenchymal epithelium is a name sometimes given to the simple squamous cells which line certain other connective tissue-enclosed cavities: the subarachnoid and subdural cavities, the chambers of the eye, and the perilymphatic spaces of the ear. The structure of this epithelium is generally similar to that of mesothelium, although in some sites (e.g., the anterior surface of the iris) its cells are very loosely joined to each other.

The cells lining bursae and synovial membranes of joint cavities are associated with an underlying mat of collagenous fibers and are more loosely joined to each other than are typical mesothelial cells. While often described as fibroblasts, electron microscopy discloses that these cells really represent an intermediate state between typical mesothelial and fibroblastic cells.

Simple Columnar Epithelium

Simple columnar epithelium (Fig. 4.19) in its various modifications represents the chief secretory and absorptive tissue of the body. It consists of a single layer of tall cells resting on a continuous basal lamina. The height varies considerably and the term *cuboidal* epithelium is applied when height and thickness of the cells are about equal (isodiametric). All transitions from low cuboidal to high columnar types of cells are encountered (Fig. 4.20). The secretory units or *acini* of most glands are lined by

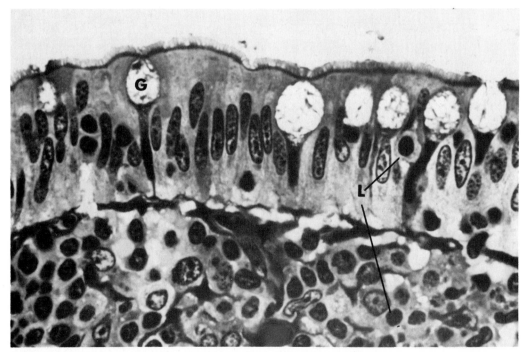

Figure 4.19. Light micrograph of simple columnar epithelium. All epithelial cells reach both apical and basal surfaces of the epithelium, although some (*G*) are differentiated as mucus secreting goblet cells. Lymphocytes (*L*) occasionally invade the epithelium from underlying connective tissue. Monkey intestine (×1,420).

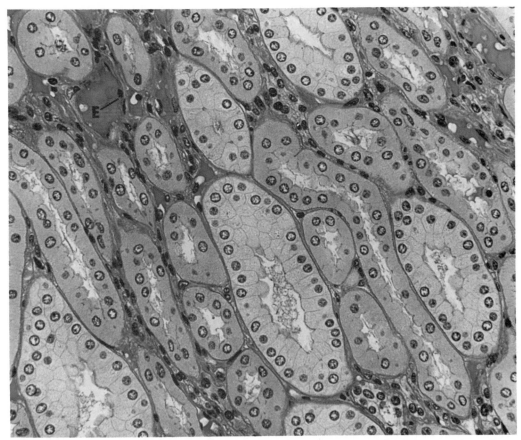

Figure 4.20. Simple cuboidal epithelium lining tubules in monkey kidney. Some regions appear stratified owing to the plane of section, which courses tangentially through the wall of a tubule. Connective tissue and blood vessels occupy the space between tubules. Close inspection reveals simple squamous endothelium (*E*) lining blood vessels which are filled with darkly stained blood plasma (×430).

cuboidal or columnar epithelial cells whose broad bases rest on the basal lamina and whose apices face the narrow lumen. This is termed *pyramidal* or *glandular* epithelium. In simple columnar epithelial cells, the nucleus is oval and usually placed basally; in cuboidal cells, it is spherical and central. In the basal perinuclear portion of the cytoplasm, there are numerous mitochondria and abundant rough endoplasmic reticulum, particularly in cells that are secretory. The apical portion may contain granules or vesicles of stored products of the cell (zymogen, mucin, etc.). The cytoplasmic constitution varies greatly under different conditions of cellular activity. A striated border may be absent, as in most glandular epithelium, or very prominent, as in the high columnar absorptive epithelium of the small intestine (Figs. 1.9C and 4.19).

An important cellular variation found in many columnar epithelia is the *goblet cell* (Figs. 4.19 and 4.29; discussed in detail later in this chapter). This cell is characterized by a long narrow base and apical region swollen by the accumulation of membrane-bounded *mucigen vesicles*. There is a relative paucity of microvilli. Most mucins are not preserved and stained in the routine preparations for light microscopy. Contents of the vesicles may wash out of the cell, leaving a clear space, or they may partially dissolve and then fuse into a faintly staining meshwork composed of remnants of mucin and remaining cytoplasm.

PSEUDOSTRATIFIED EPITHELIUM

In this type of epithelium (Figs. 4.1, 4.21, and 4.22), the nuclei lie at different levels, giving it a stratified appearance. All of the cells reach the basal lamina, but not all of them extend to the free surface. The processes which extend to the basal lamina may be multiple and difficult to see in routine histological preparations as they extend between basal-lying ovoid or spindle-shaped cells. This type of epithelium usually has either cilia or stereocilia. It occurs mainly as the lining of the passages of the respiratory and the male reproductive systems.

STRATIFIED EPITHELIA

Stratified Squamous Epithelium

Stratified squamous epithelium (Figs. 4.1 and 4.23) is the main protective epithelium of the body and consists of many cell layers. The number of layers varies considerably in different places, but the shape and arrangement of the cells are quite characteristic. The deepest layer, which rests on a basal lamina, is formed by columnar or prismatic cells which in sections of the tissue appear as a distinct row. Hemidesmosomes are seen along the basal surface

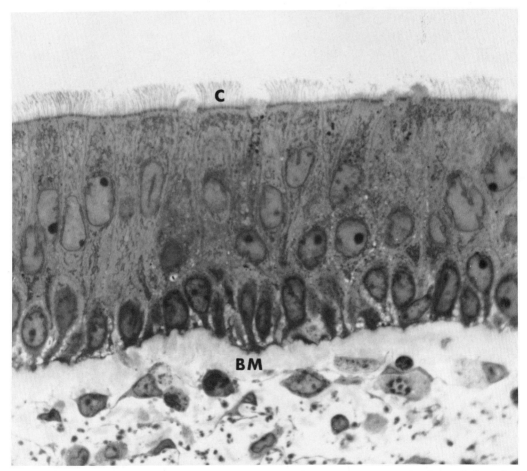

Figure 4.21. Pseudostratified epithelium from the trachea of a monkey. Not all cells reach the apical surface, giving the epithelium a stratified appearance. Note that this epithelium is richly ciliated (*C*) and is characterized by a very thick basement membrane (*BM*) (×1,168).

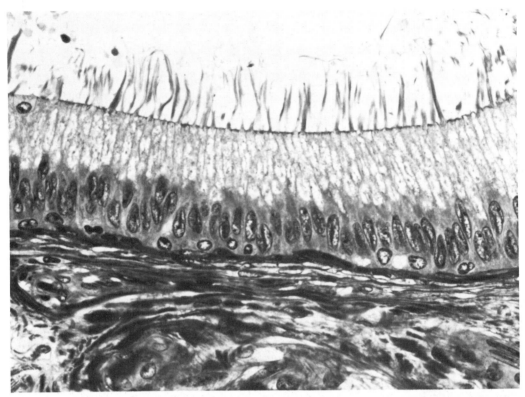

Figure 4.22. Pseudostratified epithelium lining the epididymis of the male reproductive tract. The cells which do not reach the apical surface are relatively few in number. Their nuclei appear small and located basally. This epithelium bears stereocilia (×570).

of each cell adjacent to the basal lamina. Further apically, the cells are cubical or polyhedral in shape and larger than the cells of the basal layers. Just beneath the free surface, the cells are flattened and, at the surface, squamous. It is the flattened character of the surface cells which identifies the entire epithelium as stratified squamous. The deeper cells of the basal and polyhedral layers have relatively large nuclei rich in chromatin. The cytoplasm is finely granular and somewhat basophilic because of its content of RNA. The desmosomal tonofilament bundles are prominent, giving the cell a prickly appearance (*"prickle cells,"* Figs. 15.3 and 15.5).

The extent of change in the superficial cells varies with the location and environment of the stratified squamous epithelium. The epidermis, for instance, is subjected to more attrition and drying than is the epithelium of the mouth, pharynx, and esoph-agus. Its surface cells are non-nucleated, scalelike, and *keratinized.* On the other hand, the epithelium of moist surfaces such as that of mouth, pharynx, and esophagus is usually not keratinized. The surface cells are flattened, but usually remain nucleated.

The mitotic activity of the cells in the lower layer and the lack of mitosis in the upper layers may reflect the fact that the deeper cells are in closer relation to the underlying capillaries which supply nutritive substances. As new basal cells are formed, their neighbors are pressed upward. Surface cells are constantly cast off, to be replaced by cells from the deeper strata. In man this is a slow and continuous process; in some of the lower vertebrates (e.g., snakes) there is a periodic shedding of the whole superficial layer of the epidermis.

Stratified squamous epithelium covers the entire surface of the body and the ori-

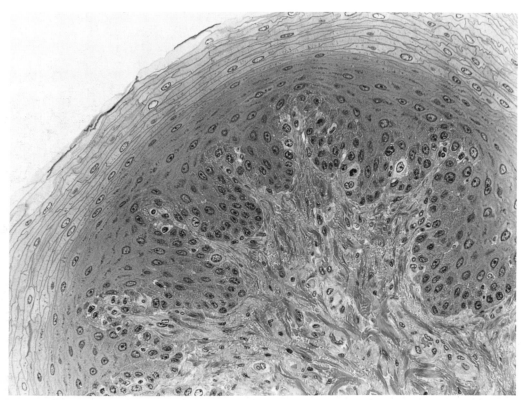

Figure 4.23.   Nonkeratinized stratified squamous epithelium from the esophagus. The basal surface of the epithelium is thrown into folds and contains cells which are distinctly rounded in comparison to flattened cells of the apical surface from which the epithelium gains its name (×465).

fices of cavities opening upon it. It lines the mucous membranes of the mouth, pharynx, esophagus, portions of the larynx, external auditory canal and conjunctiva, vagina, vestibule, labia majora, and portions of the urethra.

Stratified Columnar and Stratified Cuboidal Epithelium

A *stratified columnar epithelium* is comparatively rare. It consists of columnar surface cells which rest on several layers of irregular cubical cells. Stratified columnar epithelium is found chiefly where a stratified squamous adjoins a pseudostratified columnar type, as for instance at the juncture of the oropharynx with the nasopharynx and with the larynx (Fig. 17.5). It is said to occur also in part of the penile portion of the male urethra.

In a few locations, a stratified epithelium has surface cells which are definitely cu-

boidal, thus forming a *stratified cuboidal epithelium*. Examples are the ducts of salivary and sweat glands (Figs. 4.24 and 15.11) and the lining of the antra of ovarian follicles (Fig. 20.3). The sebaceous glands possess epithelial cells which are polyhedral in shape and several layers in thickness (Fig. 15.20).

The epithelium of seminiferous tubules of the testis is a highly specialized type (Fig. 19.6). Functionally, it is cytogenic; structurally, it probably approximates a stratified cuboidal type more closely than any other, although certain of its cells (cells of Sertoli) are elongated and extend from the basal lamina to the lumen. The shape of the surface cells varies greatly with stages of growth and differentiation.

Transitional Epithelium

All epithelial cells are pliable to some degree, but these properties are especially

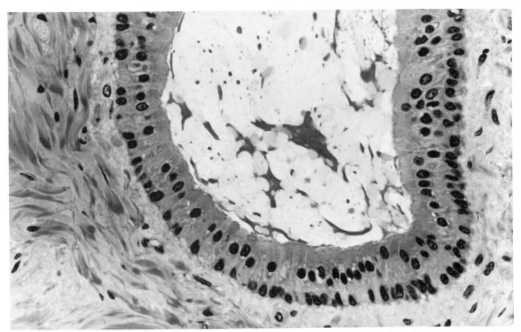

Figure 4.24. Stratified columnar epithelium. This example of a relatively rare epithelial type is from the duct of a salivary gland. The epithelial cells are cuboidal to columnar in shape and stratified to the extent of two layers (×475).

striking in the transitional epithelium (Figs. 4.1 and 4.25 to 4.27) of the urinary passages and bladder. In the dilated bladder, the epithelium consists of two or three layers of cells. The superficial cells are large, low, cuboidal plates; the lower ones are smaller and irregularly cubical. In the contracted bladder, the epithelium becomes five- or six-layered. The surface cells are large and cuboidal, with a condensed, darkly staining superficial layer of cytoplasm reflective of the abundant microfilaments there. These cells have characteristic convex free surfaces and facet-like indentations in their undersurfaces (Figs. 4.1 and 4.27). The lower cells have rearranged themselves, owing to a reduction of the surface area. They overlap each other and have assumed a flask- or pear-shaped form. The luminal surface of transitional epithelial cells is not smooth in electron micrographs, but rather displays alternating crests and hollows. The apical cytoplasm contains numerous membrane-bounded fusiform vesicles which derive from the surface membrane. When the bladder contracts, the tips of the surface crests rise and join, perhaps under control of the closely related web of subapical microfilaments, and pinch off the intervening troughs into the underlying cytoplasm, thereby forming the vesicles. The process thus serves to reduce the area of the surface membrane. The excess membrane which accumulates as vesicles may either be returned to the surface during distention or be digested by lysosomes. The synthesis of new membrane for replacement would presumably occur in the rough endoplasmic reticulum as is true for plasma membranes of other cell types (see Chapter 1).

The surface membrane of the bladder has an important function as a barrier to prevent undue water loss from underlying tissues into the hypertonic urine in the lumen. The plasmalemma of the luminal surface is unusual in that its outer leaflet is definitely thicker than its inner leaflet. In freeze-fracture preparations it displays plaques with a highly structured particulate array, reflective of an unusually high protein content. While the exact significance of these features remains obscure, it is thought that since about 70% of the surface is structured in this way, it is likely an adaptation promoting a high degree of membrane impermeability. Diffusion via intercellular routes is prevented by extensive tight junctions between the surface cells. Desmosomes are scarce in the deeper cells; this seems to be correlated with the ability of the cells to adapt during contraction and distention of the organ. Another structural adaptation for contraction and expansion is the presence of numerous interfoldings and interdigitations of the membranes of the deeper cells. The folds tend to disappear when the bladder is distended. A basement membrane is usually indistinct by light microscopy. Electron microscopy shows it to be limited to a basal lamina and a thin mat of reticular collagen fibers.

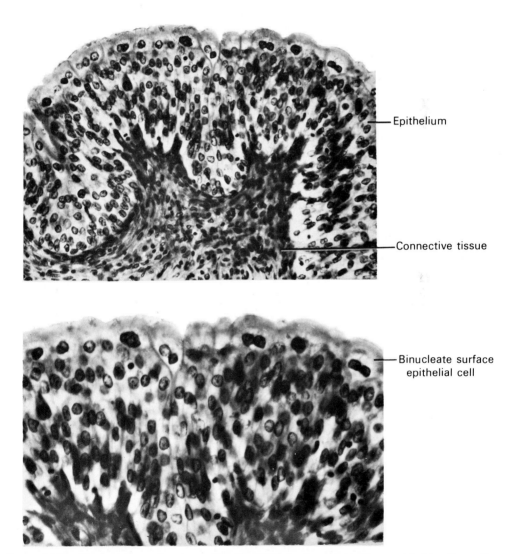

— Epithelium

— Connective tissue

— Binucleate surface epithelial cell

Figure 4.25. Photomicrographs of transitional epithelium of contracted human bladder. *Upper figure*, ×250; *lower figure*, a portion of the same region, ×390. Note that some of the surface cells have two nuclei and most of the surface cells are umbrella-shaped at their upper border in the contracted bladder. Hematoxylin and eosin stain.

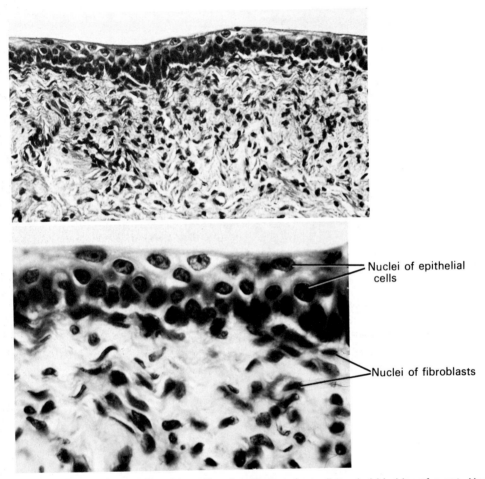

Figure 4.26. Photomicrographs of transitional epithelium from distended bladder of a cat. *Upper figure*, ×250; *lower figure*, a region of the same field ×390. Note that the cells are arranged in only a few layers and that each stretched surface cell usually covers several of the underlying cells. Transitional epithelium, as indicated by its name, varies in different functional states, and there are numerous gradations between the appearance seen in Figure 4.25 and that seen here.

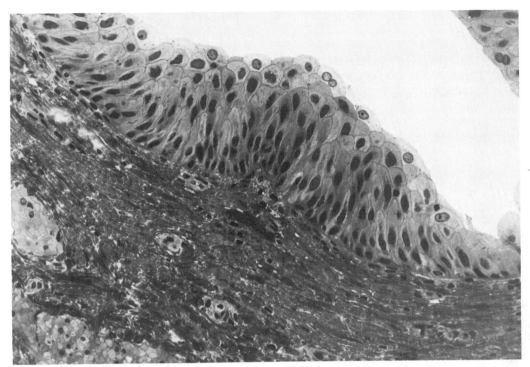

Figure 4.27. Higher magnification light micrograph of transitional epithelium in a plastic-embedded specimen. This epithelium lines the ureter. Note the rounded free surface of apical cells and the distinct curved boundaries between adjacent epithelial cells. Bundles of smooth muscle are visible at *lower left* amid the connective tissue (×420).

Transitional epithelium is found only in the urinary system—pelvis of kidney, ureter, bladder, and a portion of the urethra.

GLANDULAR EPITHELIA

All cells of the body take up oxygen and nutritive substances from the blood, via intercellular fluid, and give off waste products. In this sense, all cells secrete and excrete. Certain cells of the body, in addition to carrying on these metabolic processes necessary for their own existence, also manufacture specific substances not for their own use but to be extruded from the cells and used elsewhere in the body (secretions, e.g., gastric juice) or discarded (excretions, e.g., urine). Such cells are known as *gland cells* or *glandular epithelium*, and an aggregation of these cells into a definite structure for the purpose of carrying on secretion or excretion is known as a *gland.*

A gland may consist of a single cell, as,

for example, the goblet cell or the *unicellular glands* of invertebrates. Such a cell produces within itself a substance which is to be used outside the cell. The appearance of any glandular cell depends upon the stage of secretion. It is thus possible to differentiate between a "resting" and an "active" cell or between an "empty" and a "loaded" cell.

Most glands are composed of more than one cell (*multicellular glands*). Usually there is a large number of cells, and these line more or less extensive epithelial invaginations into which they pour their secretions (*exocrine glands*), or from which they release normal products to the perivascular connective tissue and thence to the blood stream (*endocrine* glands).

General Structure and Function of Secretory Cells

The goblet cell of the intestine is one of the simple columnar cells that constitute the surface epithelium of the mucous membrane. It is distinguishable as a mucous cell in ordinary histological preparations only after the formation of secretion has begun. When filled with secretion, the apical portion of the cell becomes dilated and the basal portion remains slender, giving the cell a goblet shape. The swollen apical portion in the living cell contains vesicles of *premucin* or *mucigen.* The mucigen vesicles are not generally visible in sections prepared by routine methods because the commonly used fixatives dissolve the mucigen, leaving a loose filamentous network in the cytoplasm. However, the mucigen can be seen readily under the light microscope in sections prepared by appropriate technical procedure (Fig. 4.28).

At the height of the "active" phase of secretion, the mucigen vesicles are released at the apical end of the cell (Figs. 4.28 and 4.29) and are dissolved and immediately converted into *mucin.* In some cases, the vesicles are released gradually while new vesicles are formed, and the goblet shape of the cell is retained for a considerable length of time. In other cases, the vesicles are released rapidly and the cell quickly loses the goblet shape and reverts to a more slender form. After a period of rest, the same cell may become active again and pass through the same stages of secretion.

The process of protein synthesis and secretion is explained in Chapter 1. Goblet cells have been utilized for studies of the coupling of protein and carbohydrate synthetic pathways because these cells contain appreciable quantities of carbohydrate in the mucigen they secrete.

Classification of Glands

As has been mentioned, a gland may consist of a single secretory cell (unicellular gland), or it may be composed of many cells (multicellular gland); the secretory cells (often termed the *parenchyma* of a gland) usually line an epithelial invagination from the free surface. In the simplest form of a glandular invagination, all of the cells lining the lumen are secreting cells. In more highly developed glands, secretion is primarily by the deeper cells and the remainder of the gland serves to carry the secretion to the surface. This latter part is then

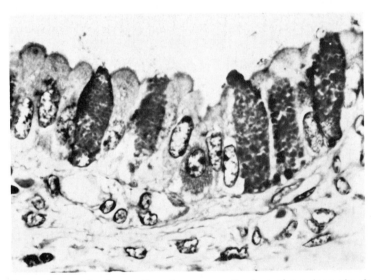

Figure 4.28. Photomicrograph of a portion of a pancreatic duct of a guinea pig showing several goblet cells interspersed among the columnar lining cells. The mucigen is preserved in droplet form but the resolution of the light microscope is not sufficient to show whether the plasmalemma is complete at the apical end of the cell. Compare with electron micrograph in Figure 4.29. Chrome hematoxylin and phloxine stain (×1125).

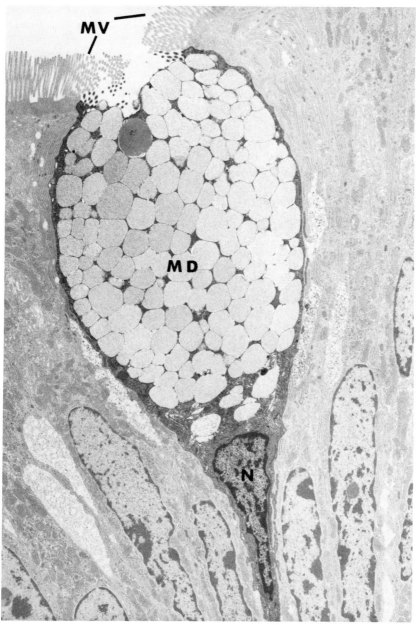

Figure 4.29. Electron micrograph of a section of the small intestine showing a goblet cell between columnar absorbing cells. Mucigen droplets (*MD*) fill most of the cell above the nucleus (*N*). An intact plasmalemma, with a few microvilli, is seen at the adluminal surface of the goblet cell. Numerous microvilli (*MV*) are present on the adluminal surface of the absorbing cells (×8,000). (Courtesy of Dr. Barry King.)

known as the *duct*, in contradistinction to the deeper *secreting portion*. In both the duct portion and the secreting portion of a gland, the epithelium rests upon a more or less definite *basement membrane*. Beneath the basement membrane, separating and supporting the glandular elements, is a fine vascular connective tissue which constitutes the *stroma* of the gland.

Glands are sometimes classified, according to the nature of their secretion, into *mucous* (producing a viscous, slimy secretion), *serous* (producing a thin, watery secretion), and *mixed glands* (producing both types of secretion). Although this classification is particularly useful for some of the glands, such as those of the oral cavity, it cannot be satisfactorily used for all glands of the body.

The cells of mucous and serous glands differ in structure. The structure of the unicellular mucous gland or goblet cell has already been described. In the multicellular mucous glands or *mucous alveoli* (e.g., of the palatine glands) the cells are usually more or less pyramidal in shape as a result of their arrangement around the lumen of the terminal tubule. When the cell is filled with secretion, the nucleus is flattened against the basal part of the cell. As already described for the goblet cell, the mucigen of these cells is not well preserved with ordinary techniques and is dissolved, leaving a loose network that, with hematoxylin and eosin, remains unstained or stains very faintly with hematoxylin.

The cells of *serous alveoli* secrete a clear, watery, proteinaceous product. The secretion of many serous glands (e.g., pancreas and parotid gland) contains digestive enzymes. In these cells, the secretory granules are the enzyme precursors or *zymogen granules*. Serous cells are usually pyramidal, with rounded nuclei lying in the basal one-half of the cells. The cells pass through active and resting phases of secretion, like mucous cells. During the resting phase, the secretory granules may become so numerous as to almost fill the cell, but the nucleus does not become flattened as in the mucous cell. The secretory granules, if they are preserved, are acidophilic. Basophilic rough endoplasmic reticulum is found in high concentration in the basal portion of serozymogenic cells, giving that part of the cell a strongly basophilic, striated appearance.

The alveoli of mixed glands (e.g., submandibular and sublingual) contain both mucous and serous cells.

According to whether the secretion is merely a product of the cell or whether it consists of gland cells, the glands may be classified as *eccrine* (*merocrine*), *apocrine*, or *holocrine*. The majority of the glands are eccrine. The secretion is a product of the cell, extruded without loss of other cellular components. In the sebaceous glands, entire cells laden with secretory material are extruded as the secretion. This is the holocrine type of secretion. Because they secrete living cells (ova and sperm), the ovary and testis are sometimes called *cytogenic* glands. An intermediate type of secretion is apocrine, found in axillary and circumanal modified sweat glands. In these glands, a microscopic portion of the cell apex may be released along with the secretory material.

The exocrine glands may further be subdivided and classified in accordance with the type of duct system contained. When a gland consists of a single secretory passage or a single system of secretory passages opening into an unbranched duct it is called a *simple gland* (Fig. 4.30, *A* to *G*). When a gland contains a duct system that is elaborate and branched, it is called a *compound gland* (Fig. 4.30, *H* to *J*). Both the simple and compound glands may be subdivided in accordance with the form of the terminal secretory portions. When the secreting portion is a tubule, the lumen of which is of fairly uniform diameter, the gland is known as a *tubular gland* (Fig. 4.30, *A* to *C*). When the secreting portion is dilated in the form of a sac (termed an *acinus* or an *alveolus*), the gland is known as a *saccular, alveolar,* or *acinar gland* (Fig. 4.30, *E, F, G, J*). In many glands, the secretory passages are neither typically tubular nor alveolar but intermediate in type, combining certain characteristics of both; such glands are called *tubuloalveolar* or *tubuloacinar* (Fig. 4.30, *D, I*). The serous salivary glands and pancreas are typical examples of this type; they have acinar enlargements which are produced by an increase in the height of the secretory epithelium while the lumen remains undilated and tubular (Fig. 4.30, *I, a, e, f,* and *g*). In some of the glands usually

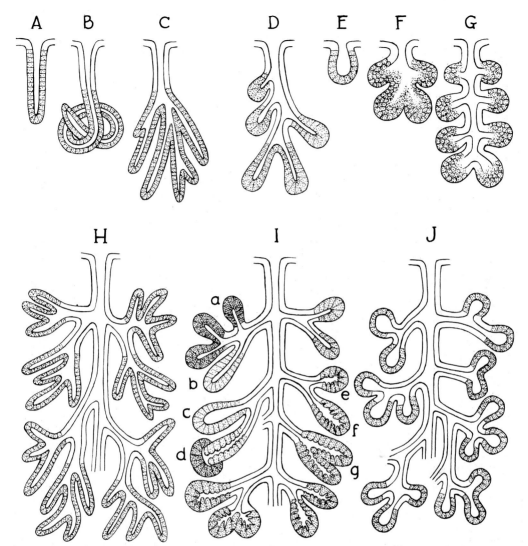

Figure 4.30. Schema of various types of exocrine glands. *A* to *G*, simple glands; *H* to *J*, compound glands. *A*, simple nonbranched tubular; *B*, simple coiled tubular; *C*, branched tubular; *D*, branched tubuloacinar (tubuloalveolar); *E*, simple nonbranched alveolar; *F* and *G*, branched alveolar as in sebaceous glands; *H*, compound tubular; *I*, compound tubuloacinar, showing some of the various types of terminations. *a*, serous acinus with simple nonbranched canal; *b* and *c*, variations in size of lumen of mucous terminations, as in sublingual, etc.; *d*, tubuloalveolus of mucous tubule and serous demilune; *e*, *f*, and *g*, serous terminations with branched canals, or intercellular secretory canaliculi as in parotid, etc.; *J*, compound alveolar gland.

included in this group, such as the mucous salivary glands, mucous portions of the mixed salivary glands, and Brunner's glands of the duodenum, the secretory passages vary in type of lumen from tubular forms to dilations resembling elongated alveoli (Fig. 4.30, *I*, *b*, *c*).

Glands may thus be classified as follows:

A. Exocrine glands (or glands with ducts)
　1. Simple glands
　　(a) Tubular $\begin{cases} \text{straight} \\ \text{coiled} \\ \text{branched} \end{cases}$
　　(b) Tubuloalveolar (tubuloacinar)
　　(c) Alveolar (acinar, saccular)

2. Compound Glands
  (a) Tubular
  (b) Tubuloalveolar (tubuloacinar)
  (c) Alveolar
B. Endocrine glands (or glands without ducts)

EXOCRINE GLANDS

Simple Tubular Glands

These glands consist of simple, epithelia-lined tubules which open to the surface. All of the cells may be secretory, or only the more deeply situated ones may be. In the more highly developed of the simple tubular glands, we distinguish a mouth opening upon the surface, a neck which is usually somewhat constricted, and a fundus, or deep secreting portion of the gland.

Simple tubular glands are divided according to the appearance of the fundus into (a) straight, (b) coiled, or (c) branched.

Straight Tubular Gland. This is one in which the entire tubule runs a straight unbranched course, e.g., the crypts of the large intestine (Fig. 4.30A).

Coiled Tubular Gland. This is one in which the deeper portion of the tubule is coiled or convoluted (Fig. 4.30B). The sweat glands of the skin are the most typical examples.

Branched Tubular Gland. This is a simple tubular gland in which the deeper portion of the tubule divides into branches that are lined with secreting cells and that open into a superficial portion which serves as a duct (Fig. 4.30C). Examples of branched tubular glands are the glands of the stomach and the glands of the endometrium of the uterus. Many of the pyloric glands of the stomach are also slightly enlarged and coiled at their terminations, so that they resemble to some extent both the convoluted tubular and the tubuloalveolar glands.

Simple Tubuloalveolar Glands

Simple tubuloalveolar or tubuloacinar glands are found only in the branched form (Fig. 4.30D). Included in this group are the smaller glands of the following types: salivary glands of the oral cavity, seromucous glands of the respiratory tract, mucous glands of the esophagus, and submucosal glands of the duodenum. Many of these, such as the esophageal and the duodenal submucosal glands, are classified by some authors as branched tubular, but, because they are frequently enlarged at their terminations, they may be included in the branched tubuloalveolar group.

Simple Alveolar Glands

The simplest form of alveolar gland, consisting of a single sac with a dilated lumen and connected with the surface by a constricted portion, the neck, is shown in Figure 4.30E. This simple form of alveolar gland is found in the skin of certain amphibians but does not occur in man. Simple alveolar glands in which there are several saccules are represented by the smaller sebaeous glands (Fig. 4.30F). In the sebaceous glands, the secreting cells are extruded as the secretion. Consequently, there are a number of layers of cells filling the space that would otherwise represent the lumen of the alveolus. Simple branched alveolar glands (Fig. 4.30G), in which a common duct gives rise to a number of saccules, are seen in the larger sebaceous glands and in the Meibomian glands.

Compound Tubular Glands

The compound tubular glands consist of a number of distinct duct systems, which open into a common or main excretory duct (Fig. 4.30H). The kidney and testis are examples of compound tubular glands. Some authors, as already stated, classify the smaller mucous glands of the esophagus, etc., as branched tubular glands; accordingly, the larger of the mucous glands of the esophagus, mucous terminations of the salivary glands, and submucosal glands of the duodenum are then classified as compound tubular, but because these glands frequently terminate in enlargements they are usually classified as compound tubuloalveolar.

Compound Tubuloalveolar Glands

The glands of this type (Fig. 4.30I) are numerous and widely distributed; they include the parotid, pancreas, mandibular, sublingual, the larger of the mucous glands of the esophagus and seromucous glands of the respiratory tract, many of the duodenal submucosal glands, etc. The structure of the terminal tubules and duct systems varies somewhat in the different glands (see later chapters).

Compound Alveolar Glands

The compound alveolar glands resemble the compound tubular and compound tubuloalveolar glands in having a large number of duct systems, but the terminal ducts, instead of ending in tubular and tubuloacinar secreting passages, end in alveoli with dilated, saclike lumina (Fig. 4.30*J*). The mammary gland is the best example of a compound alveolar gland.

Architecture of Compound Glands

All compound glands are surrounded by connective tissue which forms a more or less definite *capsule*. From the capsule, connective tissue *septa* or *trabeculae* extend into the gland. The broadest septa usually divide the gland into a number of compartments or *lobes*. Smaller septa from the capsule and from the interlobar septa divide the lobes into smaller compartments, usually microscopic in size, the *lobules*. A lobule not only is a definite portion of the gland separated from the rest of the gland by connective tissue but also represents a definite grouping of tubules or alveoli with reference to one or more terminal ducts.

During the development of gland tubules, the connective tissue is also developing but proportionately less than the more rapidly growing tubules (see discussion of patterns below). The gland tubules do not develop irregularly but in definite groups, each group being dependent upon the tubule (duct) from which it originates. Thus the main excretory duct gives rise to a few large branches which may lie either between or within the developing *lobes* (*interlobar* and *intralobar ducts,* respectively); a lobe is formed by all of the subdivisions of one of the lobar branches. From each intralobar duct there arise within the lobe a large

number of smaller branches, each of which gives rise to subdivisions which make up a lobule of the gland. These branches lie first between *lobules* (*interlobular ducts*) and finally within the lobules to which they give rise (*intralobular ducts*). As groups of tubules develop into lobes and lobules, the largest strands of connective tissue are left between adjacent lobes (interlobar connective tissue), smaller strands between lobules (interlobular connective tissue), and the finest connective tissue between the tubules or alveoli within the lobule (intralobular connective tissue). The liver and kidney are notable exceptions to this developmental pattern.

ENDOCRINE GLANDS

Certain glands, as already stated, are lacking in ducts; they are called *endocrine glands* or glands of internal secretion, in contrast to those glands with ducts, the exocrine or external secreting glands. Some glands, such as the pancreas and testis, secrete both externally, by way of ducts, and internally, by way of the bloodstream. The endocrine glands secrete specific substances called *hormones* which have specific effects on the other tissues or organs of the body. The endocrine glands include the thyroid, parathyroid, adrenal, hypophysis, islands of Langerhans of the pancreas, and parts of the ovary and testis. The pineal gland is also usually included in this group. Detailed histology of each of these glands will be discussed in Chapter 21. However, it is necessary at this point to outline several other patterns of epithelial organizaton to gain an understanding of the origin of most endocrine glands as contrasted to exocrine gland development.

OTHER PATTERNS OF EPITHELIAL ORGANIZATION

In addition to the commonly described epithelial types and configurations noted above, certain other epithelia progress through patterns of development which alter them considerably. In past years they have been largely ignored because they are hardly discernible as epithelia and because they constitute relatively isolated instances. Recently, however, the importance of their recognition and understanding has become more obvious. A glance at their development aids comprehension.

The derivation of various glands as epithelial invaginations into mesenchymal or connective tissue beds has been discussed above. Retention of the original invagination stalk, or in some cases the development of a new one, leads to the formation of exocrine glands (Fig. 4.31A). On the other hand, detachment or loss of that stalk gives rise to isolated islands or follicles of epithelial cells which develop into endocrine glands. These must release their secretory products from their basal surface into the surrounding connective tissue and nearby

vascular pathways. In this endocrine pattern, the original apical surface of the invaginating cells may either be retained or obscured. The basal surface of the cells in all cases will be retained as that portion of the epithelial mass facing the surrounding connective tissues. When a lumen is retained or emerges secondarily, as is the case in the development of thyroid follicles (Fig. 4.31B), a cavity is created which is bounded on all sides by the apical surfaces of lining epithelial cells. In the case of thyroid follicles, the cavity serves as a temporary storage site for secretions first released from the apices of the cells, later to be reabsorbed back through the cells and released basally in the usual endocrine fashion. In this instance it can be seen that both apical and basal surfaces of the epithelium are present

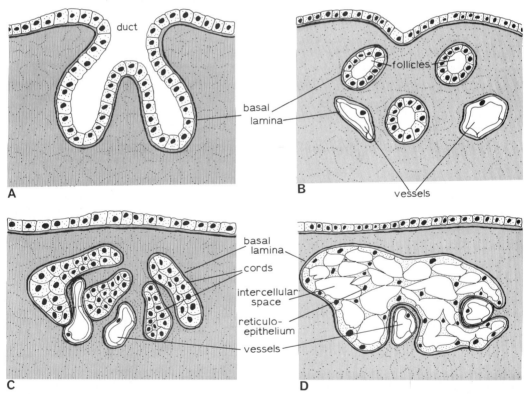

Figure 4.31. Schematic diagram illustrating examples of progressive degrees of specialization in the development of glandular epithelium: *A*, retention of developmental stalk as the *duct of a gland*; *B*, loss of stalk leading to *follicular pattern*; *C*, loss of stalk and lumen leading to *cord pattern*; and *D*, loss of stalk and lumen but expansion of intercellular spaces resulting in a *reticular epithelial pattern*. Note that in each example a basal lamina is retained, marking the basal surface of the epithelial mass. Blood vessels may indent but not penetrate that basal lamina.

in the final adult configuration. In other instances the epithelial cells may become so closely compacted that a lumen is lost and apical surfaces are pressed against each other and thereby obscured (Fig. 4.31C). This is the typical configuration that one sees in the development of cords of parathyroid epithelia and the cords of liver parenchyma, and to a somewhat lesser extent in the pars distalis (anterior lobe) of the pituitary gland (hypophysis). The secretory cells of these organs are all epithelial by derivation and retain some of their epithelial characteristics including an apparent basal surface and typical epithelial cell-to-cell attachment mechanisms.

A further elaboration on this theme is found in the development of thymus (Fig. 4.31D). The epithelial precursor of this gland is from endodermal epithelium of one, or perhaps two, pair of pharyngeal pouches. These epithelial masses are relocated over considerable distances, proliferating as they go, to form the eventual epithelial component of the thymus during fetal stages. During this development the epithelial masses lose their apical surfaces and lumina in a manner similar to that described above, but in addition the central cells of the epithelial masses become separated from their neighbors so that large intercellular spaces intervene between them. A basal surface around the whole mass is retained and can be identified by the presence of a typical basal lamina.

The internal morphology of such a mass is now sufficiently obscured that its epithelial identity is difficult to appreciate. Electron microscopy, however, discloses that the cells remain attached by desmosomes. By light microscopy the internal parts of such masses bear a distinct resemblance to reticular connective tissue and cells, and have in the past often been described as such. In the thymus, vascular channels invaginate the mass, particularly in the cortex of that organ, carrying with them a basal lamina of the endothelial cells as well as the basal lamina of the thymic epithelium (or *thymic reticulum*) itself. In subse-

quent development the intercellular spaces of the reticular epithelium are invaded by lymphocytes, which there proliferate and complete the typical histological characteristics of that organ (see Chapter 14).

An example similar to the epithelial reticular development outlined for the thymus can be found in the development of tooth buds, wherein the enamel organs proliferating from an epithelial *dental lamina* also form an enclosed epithelial bag, the central regions of which assume a reticular appearance. Along one basal surface of each of these masses the epithelial cells differentiate as enamel-forming *ameloblasts*. The other cells of the epithelial mass are retained during development of the crown of the tooth as the so-called *stellate reticulum* (see Chapter 16).

EPITHELIAL REPAIR

Epithelia in certain locations are in a constant state of cellular loss and renewal. The continuous loss of epidermal surface cells with replacement from the deeper layers of stratified epithelium is a case in point. Less obvious, but perhaps just as active, is the loss of columnar cells from the simple epithelium covering the villi, crypts, and other surfaces along the digestive tract. These cells are regularly replaced by mitosis somewhat distant along the epithelium and continual movement of new, maturing cells toward the site of loss. These are normal renewal processes involving little or no trauma. But many epithelia are also able to respond to injury by a timely increase of mitotic activity and motility in areas adjacent to a wound. The response of epithelium in the healing of wounds in mammals has been more extensively studied in the epidermis than in other types of epithelium.

Both epithelium and the underlying connective tissue are injured in abrasions and most other wounds, and both have a capacity for cell division and for repair, in contrast with more highly differentiated tissue such as nerve cells and skeletal muscle fibers. The response of the epidermis depends somewhat on the size of the injured surface, but there is generally an enlargement and migration of the deeper cells near the wound. These exhibit a sort of ameboid movement, with the formation of tongue-like processes which grow over the denuded area or, if there is a scab, grow under it and help to absorb it. Mitoses are decreased for the first few (four to five) days but soon thereafter exceed the normal rate. In wound repair, as in tissue culture, epithelium exhibits the propensity of forming a cellular layer on a surface.

MEMBRANES

Epithelium assumes its full significance only when considered in conjunction with the underlying connective tissue. In that combination, it forms so-called membranes (in the grosser sense) of varying toughness and thickness, as exemplified by the skin and peritoneum. In conjunction with a stratum of connective tissue, it forms the *mucosa* of the gastrointestinal, respiratory, and genitourinary systems. In general, the connective tissue lying beneath the epithelium is extremely fine but closely woven. This passes gradually into a stratum of coarser, closely woven fibers. The membrane thus formed permits a variable amount of stretching, depending on the location, but prevents an excessive expansion which might separate the epithelial cells. The denseness of the connective tissue varies with the membranes formed; thus, in the mucosa it is not nearly as dense as it is in the skin.

The denser connective tissue of a membrane ultimately grades with no abrupt transition into a looser stratum, which attaches the membrane to the underlying structures and usually permits a movement over them. This underlying zone of looser tissue is well exemplified by the *subcutaneous fascia* of the skin and the *submucosa* of the gastrointestinal tract.

Serous Membranes

Serous membranes line the *peritoneal*, *pleural*, and *pericardial* cavities as the *peritoneum*, *pleura*, and *pericardium*, respectively. A serous membrane consists of mesothelium and an underlying layer of delicate fibroelastic connective tissue. It should be noted that serous membranes line closed cavities and do not contain glands. They are moistened by a thin fluid similar to lymph.

Mucous Membranes

Mucous membranes (*mucosae*) line all of those cavities and canals of the body which connect with the exterior; that is, they line the alimentary tract, the respiratory passages, and the genitourinary tract. Although differing in details, the mucous membranes of these various locations all have a similarity in the general plan of their structure. The essential parts are (*a*) surface epithelium, (*b*) basement membrane, with all its constituents and (*c*) a stratum of connective tissue, the *lamina propria*.

Although the name mucous membrane suggests that mucous glands are present, this is not always the case. Both mucous and serous glands are present in the mucous membrane of the alimentary and respiratory tracts, but no glands are present in the mucous membrane of most of the genitourinary tract.

References

Bernfield M, Banerjee SD: The turnover of basal lamina glycosaminoglycan correlates with epithelial morphogenesis. *Dev Biol* 90:291–305, 1982.

Bennett HS: Morphological aspects of extracellular polysaccharides. *J Histochem Cytochem* 11:2–13, 1963.

Bonneville MA, Weinstock M: Brush border development in the intestinal absorptive cells of *Xenopus* during metamorphosis. *J Cell Biol* 49:151–171, 1970.

Brandt PW: A consideration of the extraneous coats of the plasma membrane. *Circulation* (suppl.) 26:1075–1091, 1962.

Briggaman RA, Wheeler CE: The epidermal-dermal junction. *J Invest Dermatol* 65:7–84, 1975.

Chambers R, de Renyi, GS: The structure of the cells in tissues as revealed by micro-dissection. *Am J Anat* 35:385–402, 1925.

Claude P, Goodenough DA: Fracture faces of zonulae occludentes from "tight" and "leaky" epithelia. *J Cell Biol* 58:390–400, 1973.

DiBona DR, Civan MM, Leaf A: The anatomic site of the transepithelial permeability barriers of toad bladder. *J Cell Biol* 40:1–7, 1969.

Farquhar MG, Palade GE: Junctional complexes in various epithelia. *J Cell Biol* 17:375–412, 1963.

Farquhar MG, Palade GE: Cell junctions in amphibian skin. *J Cell Biol* 26:263–291, 1965.

Fawcett D: Cilia and flagella. In Brachet J, Mirsky AE (eds): *The Cell; Biochemistry, Physiology, Morphology,* vol 2. New York, Academic Press, 1961, pp 217–297.

Fawcett DW: Surface specializations of absorbing cells. *J Histochem Cytochem* 13:75–91, 1965.

Fawcett DW: *The Cell,* ed 2. Philadelphia, W. B. Saunders, 1981.

Gabe M, Arvy L: Gland cells. In Brachet J, Mirsky AE (eds): *The Cell; Biochemistry, Physiology, Morphology,* vol 5. New York, Academic Press, 1961, pp 1–88.

Gibbons IR: Molecular basis of flagellar motility in sea urchin spermatozoa. In Inoue S, Stephens RE (eds) *Molecules and Cell Movement.* New York, Raven Press, 1975, pp 207–232.

Gibbons IR: Cilia and flagellae of eukaryotes. *J Cell Biol* 91:107s–124s, 1981.

Goodenough DA: The structure and permeability of isolated hepatocyte gap junctions. *Cold Spring Harbor Symp* 40:37–44, 1975.

Goodenough DA: *In vitro* formation of gap junction vesicles. *J Cell Biol* 68:220–231, 1976.

Haimo LT, Rosenbaum JL: Cilia, flagella, and microtubules. *J Cell Biol* 91:125s–130s, 1981.

Hay ED, Extracellular matrix. *J Cell Biol* 91:205s–223s, 1981.

Hicks RM: The fine structure of the transitional epithelium of rat ureter. *J Cell Biol* 26:25–48, 1965.

Ito S: The surface coat of enteric microvilli. *J Cell Biol* 27:475–491, 1965.

Kefalides NA, Alper R, Clark CC: Biochemistry and metabolism of basement membranes. *Int Rev Cytol* 61:167–228, 1979.

Kelly DE: Fine structure of desmosomes, hemidesmosomes, and an adepidermal globular layer in developing newt epidermis. *J Cell Biol* 28:51–72, 1966.

Kelly DE, Kuda AM: Traversing filaments in desmosomal and hemidesmosomal attachments: freeze-fracture approaches toward their characterization. *Anat Rec* 199:1–14, 1981.

Lazarides E: Intermediate filaments: a chemically heterogenous, developmentally regulated class of proteins. *Annu Rev Biochem* 51:219–250, 1982.

Leblond CP, Walker BE: Renewal of cell populations. *Physiol Rev* 36:255–276, 1956.

Loewenstein WR, Junctional intercellular communications: the cell-to-cell membrane channel. *Physiol Rev* 61:829–913, 1981.

Matoltsy AG: Desmosomes, filaments, and keratohyaline granules: their role in the stabilization and keratinization of the epidermis. *J Invest Dermatol* 65:127–142, 1975.

Mooseker MS, Howe CL: The brush border of intestinal epithelium—a model system for analysis of cell-surface architecture and motility. In Wilson L (ed): *Methods in Cell Biology,* vol 25, part B. New York, Academic Press, 1982, pp 143–174.

Mooseker MS, Tilney LG: Organization of an actin filament-membrane complex. Filament polarity and membrane attachment in the microvilli of intestinal epithelial cells. *J Cell Biol* 67:725–743, 1975.

Mooseker MS: Brush border motility. Microvillar contraction in Triton-treated brush borders isolated from intestinal epithelium. *J Cell Biol* 71:417–432, 1976.

Odland GF, Ross R: Human wound repair. I. Epidermal regeneration. *J Cell Biol* 39:135–151, 1968.

Overton J: Cell junctions and their development. *Progr Surf Membr Sci* 8:161–208, 1974.

Petersen M, Leblond CP: Synthesis of complex carbohydrates in the Golgi region as shown by radioautography after injection of labeled glucose. *J Cell Biol* 21:143–148, 1964.

Pollard TD: Cytoplasmic contractile proteins. *J Cell Biol* 91:156s–165s, 1981.

Porter KR, Bonneville MA: *Fine Structure of Cells and Tissues,* ed 4. Philadelphia, Lea & Febiger, 1973.

Revel J-P, Ito S: The surface components of cells. In Davis B, Warren L (eds): *The Specificity of Cell Surfaces.* Englewood Cliffs, N.J., Prentice-Hall, 1967, p 211.

Ross R, Odland GF: Human wound repair. II. Inflammatory cells, epithelial-mesenchymal interrelations, and fibrogenesis. *J Cell Biol* 39:152–168, 1968.

Satir P: Studies on cilia. III. Further studies on the cilium tip and a "sliding filament" model of ciliary motility. *J Cell Biol* 39:77–94, 1968.

Schaffer J: Das Epithelgewebe. In von Möllendorff (ed): Die Drusen. *Handbuch der Mikroskopische Anatomie des Menschen,* vol 2, part 1. Berlin, Springer-Verlag, 1927, pp 132–231.

Staehelin LA: Structure and function of intercellular junctions. *Int Rev Cytol* 39:191–283, 1974.

Stanley JR, Woodley DT, Katz SI, Martin GR: Structure and function of basement membrane. *J Invest Dermatol* 79:69s–72s, 1982.

Tucker JB: Cytoskeletal coordination and intercellular signalling during metazoan embryogenesis. *J Embryol Exp Morphol* 65:1–25, 1981.

Turner CD: *General Endocrinology.* Philadelphia, W. B. Saunders, 1966.

Weiss P: The biological foundations of wound repair. *Harvey Lect* 55:13–42, 1961.

Zimmerman KW: Die Speicheldrusen der Mundhole und die Bauchspeicheldruse. In von Möllendorff (ed): *Handbuch der Mikroskopische Anatomie des Menschen,* vol 5, part 1. Berlin, Springer-Verlag, 1927, pp 61–244.

Chapter 5

THE CONNECTIVE TISSUES

The connective and supporting tissues are characterized by cells which function to elaborate and maintain a variety of extracellular materials (matrix) about themselves. These extracellular materials are of such volume that in most cases the cells of connective tissues are rather widely separated, in contrast to epithelia, where cells are closely associated. The character of the extracellular matrix is determined from region to region by the abundance and proportion of fluid, fibers, ground substance molecules, and mineral aggregates. The cells have either synthesized and released these products or promoted their establishment by delicate control of the immediate environment. In connective tissue proper, the extracellular substance is soft; in cartilage, it is firm yet flexible and may be readily cut; in bone, it is rigid because of the deposition of inorganic salts in the matrix.

The cells of one type of connective tissue are often not easily distinguished from those of another on the basis of cytoplasmic structure. Rather, the histologist relies primarily on the appearance and physical properties of the extracellular matrix in assigning a given area of connective or supportive tissue to an appropriate subcategory such as *loose connective tissue, dense connective tissue, regular or irregular connective tissue, cartilage, bone,* etc. (Scheme 5.1). Even with appropriate criteria, however, such assignments are often difficult. This is so because in the organism the character of the extracellular matrix may grade imperceptibly from that characteristic of one tissue to that of another. *Hence, one is really dealing with a spectrum of connective and supportive tissues rather than a series of easily defined categories.*

EMBRYONAL CONNECTIVE TISSUES

The spectral nature of connective tissues is more easily appreciated when one considers their common embryology. All connective and supportive tissues of the body have originated from the mesenchyme of the embryo. It will be recalled that, except for the notochord, the original cells of the mesoblast were mesenchymal in their morphology and behavior, dispersing widely and migrating freely as they produced a loose tissue network emphasizing a fluid extracellular matrix interspersed with a network of fine collagenous fibers (Figs. 5.1 and 5.2). The embryonal connective tissue of this stage has classically been referred to as *mucous connective tissue.* Very early in development the mesoblast became a compartment, separated physically from its surrounding epithelial neighbors by the deposition of a basal lamina. This early mesoblastic compartment can be termed the *mesenchymal compartment.* It is a principal staging area within or around which much further development will occur. The development of many glands and other organs involves extensive invaginations of one or another epithelium into the territory of the mesenchymal compartment. These are sites of intensive epithelial-mesenchymal inductive interaction through which the epithelium is transformed into a functionally differentiated epithelium appropriate to a particular organ (the *parenchyma* of the organ) and the mesenchymal component differentiates into the appropriate vascular and connective tissue parts (the *stroma* of the organ). Throughout these processes, separation of the mesenchymal compartment from the epithelial components is maintained by the interposed basal

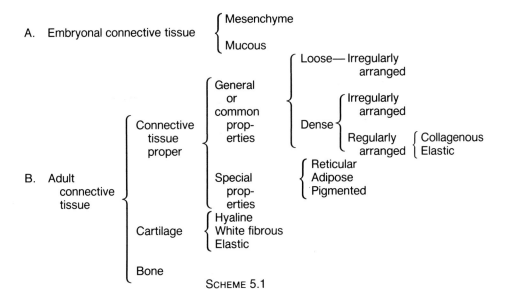

A. Embryonal connective tissue { Mesenchyme / Mucous

B. Adult connective tissue {

Connective tissue proper {

General or common properties {

Loose— Irregularly arranged

Dense {

Irregularly arranged

Regularly arranged { Collagenous / Elastic

Special properties { Reticular / Adipose / Pigmented

Cartilage { Hyaline / White fibrous / Elastic

Bone

SCHEME 5.1

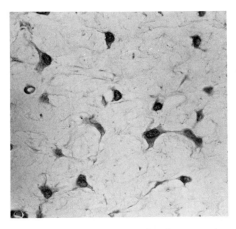

Figure 5.1. Light micrograph of mesenchyme cells from the embryonal connective tissue of the human umbilical cord. The cells are separate although they may contact neighboring cells at the tips of extenuated processes (×370).

lamina, but it can be seen that the mesenchymal compartment becomes much more restricted and tortuous. A number of cavities also appear within the mesenchymal compartment (coelomic cavities, vascular channels, etc.) which, to a high degree, are also separated from the parent compartment by development of intervening basal laminae. In other areas of the body (for example, in areas of muscle differentiation) mesenchymal cells clump together and de-

velop into highly differentiated cells which soon segregate themselves from the mesenchymal compartment by acquiring a basal or external lamina.

THE CONNECTIVE TISSUE COMPARTMENT

The net result of these types of development is that during later embryonic and early fetal stages, the once simple mesenchymal compartment of the gastrulating embryo is transformed into a tortuous array of narrow mesenchyme-filled passages interdigitated among the various other epithelial (including endothelial and mesothelial), muscular, and neural components. With very few exceptions, the mesenchymal compartment is separated from those components by a basal or an external lamina which can be visualized as the outer boundary of the compartment. Within this compartment, then, the differentiation of the connective and supportive tissues takes place. The result is the emergence of the connective tissue compartment, an even more complicated compartment whose perimeter remains defined by basal and external laminae. The contents of this compartment are not segregated from each other by basal or external laminae. This is

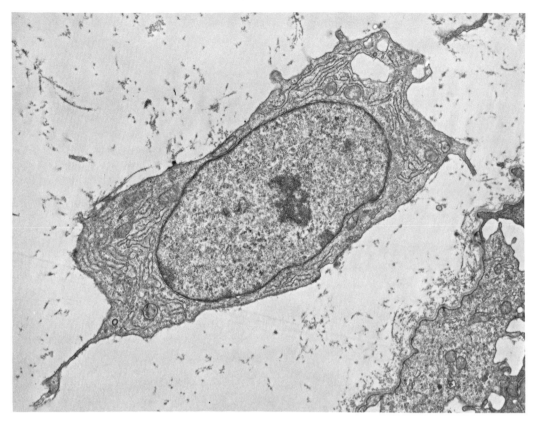

Figure 5.2. Electron micrograph of a mesenchymal cell (×8100).

to say that basal and external laminae are not found within connective and supportive tissues. A possible exception to this rule, the case of fat cells, is discussed later.

It is important to recognize the various connective and supportive tissues as intrinsic territories of this single, vast compartment for several reasons. The compartment is one of the body's largest circulating systems. Interstitial body fluids find their way through its most minute passages to bathe all of its cells. Integrity against leakage is maintained by tight junctions between the epithelial cells which guard the perimeter of the compartment. Turnover of the fluid is provided by leakage of blood fluids into the compartment and drainage via venous and lymphatic capillaries. The compartment is the main arena within which the immune mechanisms of the body operate and most storage is achieved. It is literally a channel which must be crossed by most

metabolites entering or leaving the cells and tissues of the body. All of these functions, and more, are in addition to the usually emphasized aspects serving skeletal support and structural integrity among tissues and organs.

ADULT CONNECTIVE TISSUE
Loose Connective Tissue

Loose, irregularly arranged, or areolar connective tissue is widely distributed in the human body. It forms the superficial and most of the deep fascia; it forms a part of the framework (stroma) of most of the organs; it surrounds blood vessels and nerves and fills otherwise unoccupied spaces. It generally contains a varying number of fat cells, or *adipocytes*. When the latter are abundant the tissue is designated as *adipose* or *fat tissue*. Subcutaneous tissue (*superficial fascia*) which is heavily laden with fat cells in many parts of the body is often given a special name, *panniculus adiposus*.

Loose connective tissue, like all of the other connective tissues, is composed of *cells* and extracellular *matrix*. The latter consists of *fibers*, and *ground substance*. The composition of fibers and ground substance is described later under separate headings, but it should be noted immediately that the matrix of loose connective tissue is much more fluid in nature than that of cartilage and bone.

The loose connective tissue derives its name from the fact that its intercellular fibers are loosely arranged, in contrast with the closely packed fibers of dense connective tissue. The name *areolar* is descriptive of the general appearance produced by small spaces which contain only an amorphous ground substance.

Loose connective tissue contains most of the types of cells, all of the kinds of fibers and many of the ground substance components found in the other varieties of connective tissue. Hence, a thorough knowledge of its structure serves not only for understanding its own important functions but also as a basis for understanding the other types of connective tissue.

Connective Tissue Cells

By means of various methods, the following cell types have been distinguished and found to be more or less constant inhabitants of loose connective tissue: *fibroblasts*, (fixed connective tissue cells), *histiocytes* or *macrophages, mast cells, plasma cells, fat cells*, and *wandering cells from the blood*.

Fibroblasts

The *fibroblasts* (Fig. 5.3) are one of the two most numerous cell types of loose connective tissue, the other being macrophages. Fibroblasts are little different morphologically compared to the mesenchymal cells from which they originated. As their name suggests, they are the principal cells responsible for fiber formation. There is evidence that they also form the ground substance.

They are large, somewhat flattened, frequently ovoid cells, with branching proc-

esses. Their nuclei are oval and somewhat flattened, resembling the shape of the cell. They usually stain lightly in fresh connective tissue spreads. In sections prepared by ordinary methods, the fibroblast nuclei are usually shrunken and stain deeply with basic dyes. The chromatin is distributed through the nucleus, with a tendency to become aggregated at intervals along the inner surface of the nuclear envelope. Because the cytoplasm takes little or no stain in its outer (ectoplasmic) region and because the cell membrane is too thin to be resolved under the light microscope, it is difficult to identify the cell boundary.

The appearance of the fibroblast varies in relation to its functional activity. When the cell is actively producing intercellular materials, as in normal development and in tissue regeneration after injury, the cell assumes a more mesenchymal appearance and is enlarged in correlation with an increase in its organelles. The nucleus is larger, the nucleoli are more prominent, the cytoplasm stains more deeply and is basophilic in contrast with the lightly staining, slightly acidophilic cytoplasm of the relatively inactive cell. Scanning electron micrographs of cultured fibroblasts show characteristic surface processes (Fig. 5.4). In thin section there is prominent rough-surfaced endoplasmic reticulum, numerous free ribosomes and an enlarged Golgi complex (Fig. 5.5). The cell membrane may be difficult to resolve in places where aggregates of filamentous material in the peripheral portion of the cytoplasm face aggregates of extracellular dense material. The significance of these structural changes in relation to fiber formation is discussed further in the section on the origin of fibers. Some investigators prefer to confine the term fibroblast to the active stage of the cell and to use the term *fibrocyte* for the relatively inactive cell. This seems unnecessary, because they are only different functional states of the same cell.

Macrophages

Macrophages or *histiocytes* (Figs. 5.3 and 5.6) are found in all loose connective tis-

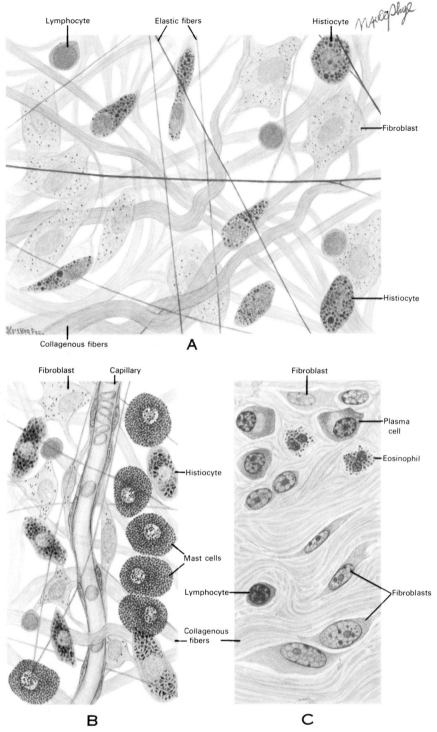

Figure 5.3. *A*, spread of subcutaneous areolar connective tissue from a rat which had received several intraperitoneal injections of trypan blue over a period of two weeks. The animal was autopsied one week after the last injection and the spread was made immediately. After fixation in Bouin's fluid, it was stained with resorcin-fuchsin for elastic fibers and with azocarmine to show cells and collagenous fibers. All of the blue color shown in histiocytes and fibroblasts represents the trypan blue which was phagocytosed by the cells preceding autopsy. No trypan blue is present in the nuclei, although a few vacuoles may appear to be within the nuclei when they are in the overlying cytoplasm (×650). *B*, subcutaneous spread from the same trypan blue rat, stained with neutral red for mast cells (×650). *C*, a section through the loose connective tissue of the submucosa of the colon. The field shown is directly beneath the muscularis mucosae. Rhesus monkey. Hematoxylin and eosin-azure (×1250).

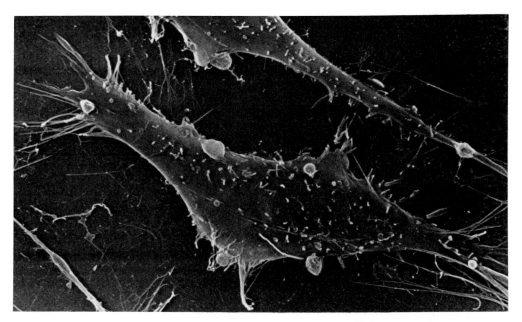

Figure 5.4. Scanning electron micrograph of cultured mouse fibroblastic cells (×2250).

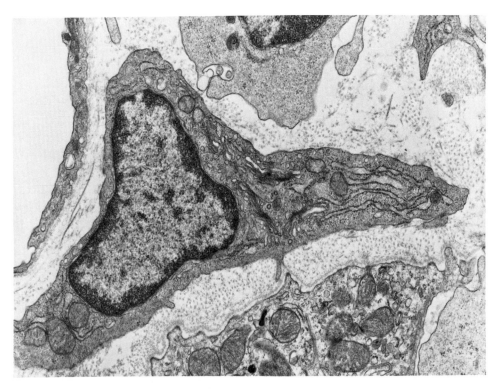

Figure 5.5. Electron micrograph of a fibroblast in the lamina propria of rat intestine. A venule lies at the *left*, a lymphocyte at the *top* and the intestinal epithelium at the *bottom* in this field (×17,000) (Courtesy of Dr. David Chase.)

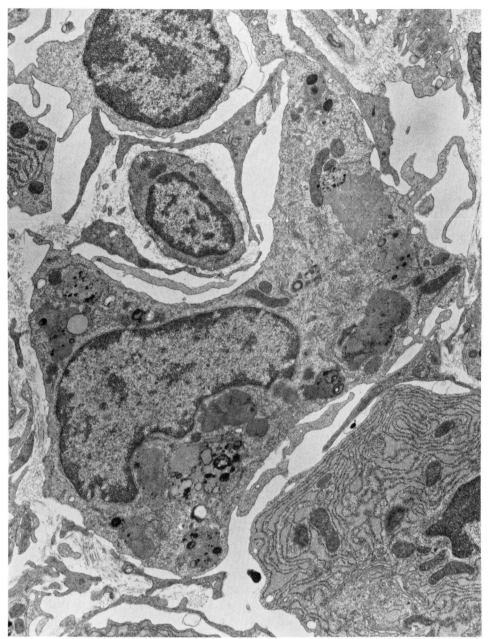

Figure 5.6. Macrophage in lamina propria of rat intestine. Part of a plasma cell is at *lower right* and two lymphocytes are at *upper left* (×9900). (Courtesy of Dr. David Chase.)

sues. They are irregularly shaped cells with processes which usually are short and blunt but occasionally long and slender. The nucleus is more rounded and somewhat smaller and darker-staining than that of the fibroblast. In the quiescent cell, the cytoplasm, like that of the fibroblast, stains lightly but may contain a few granules and vacuoles. It should be noted that the diagnostic features just listed are minor. The characteristics of the relatively inactive macrophages do not differ sufficiently from those of the fibroblasts to enable one to distinguish the two cell types readily in most light microscope preparations. However, macrophages become clearly distinguishable from fibroblasts when they are activated. The entire cell becomes larger, with a more prominent nucleolus, and a cytoplasm more or less filled with granules and vacuoles of ingested material.

Light microscopic studies of macrophages in tissue culture preparations show that foreign material is surrounded by protoplasmic processes and taken into the cell by ameboid activity. Electron micrographs show that the ingested materials are membrane-bounded in vesicles called *phagosomes*. These vesicles combine with primary lysosomes to form secondary lysosomes, as shown schematically in Figure 1.41. Most of the ingested materials are digested by the proteolytic enzymes acquired from the primary lysosomes, but some materials, e.g., carbon particles in the connective tissue macrophages of the lung, are not digestible and may remain in the cytoplasm for a long period.

Objects too large to be engulfed by a single cell are attacked en masse and become surrounded by macrophages, which eventually fuse to form a *multinucleated foreign body giant cell.* These are not to be confused with blood platelet-producing *megakaryocytes* of bone marrow (Fig. 13.2).

A common experimental method for identifying macrophages is to study their physiological reaction to dyes or inert particulate material applied to living preparations (supravital preparations). Sections of tissue from animals which have had one or more injections of trypan blue show extensive ingestion and segregation of the dye in vacuoles in the cytoplasm of macrophages and relatively little ingested material in fibroblasts (Fig. 5.3). Active macrophages are readily distinguished in transmission electron micrographs (Fig. 5.6).

Macrophages are widely distributed in the body. They are in loose connective tissue and in all fascia. They also occur in the connective tissue which is present in organs, although the proportion of them to fibroblasts may vary considerably in differ-

ent regions of an organ. The phagocytic cells are also found in specific locations in some organs, e.g., in association with the lining cells of the sinusoids of the liver, lymphatic organs, and bone marrow. In these locations macrophages were once thought to be modified endothelial cells, but studies of tissues after labeling with tritiated thymidine indicate that these cells are derived from promonocytes. Together with the macrophages of loose connective tissue they form the *macrophage system*, which is discussed in more detail at the end of this chapter.

It has been noted that macrophages become *active* and more numerous in regions of inflammation. The increase in numbers results from (*a*) migration of macrophages from neighboring areas, and (*b*) transformations of monocytes which migrate into the area from the blood vessels. These reactions occur in response to chemotactic factors released at the inflammatory site.

Plasma Cells

The *plasma cells* (Figs. 5.3 and 5.7) are relatively rare in most connective tissues under normal conditions, although they are fairly numerous in the connective tissue of the alimentary mucous membrane and greater omentum. They are also fairly numerous in the reticular connective tissues of blood-forming organs. Their number is greatly increased in areas of chronic inflammation. They are ovoid, irregularly shaped cells, smaller than macrophages but larger than lymphocytes from which they are derived (Fig. 5.3). The nucleus is relatively small and eccentrically placed. The chromatin appears in deep-staining, coarse granules, many of which are clumped in a regular manner against the nuclear membrane. This imparts a typical "cartwheel" appearance to the nucleus.

The cytoplasm of the plasma cell is highly basophilic, but there is a characteristic unstained or lightly stained area at the side of the nucleus (Fig. 5.3). The unstained area represents the region of the Golgi complex (Fig. 5.7). In comparison with a lym-

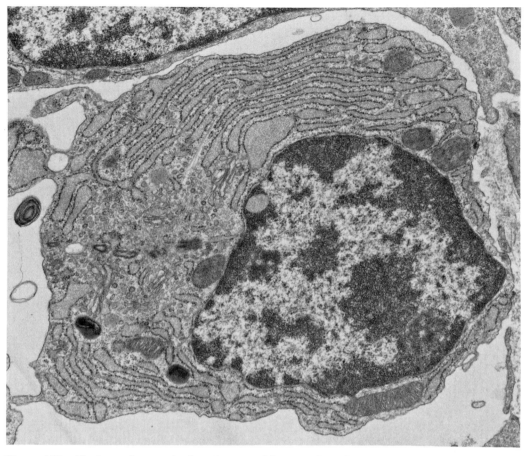

Figure 5.7. Electron micrograph of a plasma cell from rat intestine. Note the eccentrically placed nucleus with peripheral clumps of chromatin, the prominent rough endoplasmic reticulum and the Golgi zone containing a centriole (×16,000). (Courtesy of Dr. David Chase.)

phocyte, the plasma cell has more cytoplasm in proportion to the size of the nucleus; i.e., the cytoplasmic-nuclear ratio is greater. The cytoplasm of the two types of cells also shows significant differences in electron micrographs. The plasma cell has an extensive endoplasmic reticulum with associated ribosomes, whereas the lymphocyte contains mostly free ribosomes with little reticulum (Figs. 5.7 and 7.2). The Golgi complex is large (Fig. 5.7) and is associated with secretory vesicles that migrate to the surface where they liberate the secretory material by exocytosis in a manner similar to that described for exocrine glands (Fig. 1.12). Some unusually large masses of electron-dense material are seen

occasionally within the cisternae of the rough-surfaced endoplasmic reticulum; these apparently correspond to the *Russell bodies* first described by light microscopists. They probably represent an aberrant secretory pathway and may forecast degenerative changes in the cell.

The plasma cell precursor is an activated B-type lymphocyte. It is known from fluorescent antibody techniques and from other lines of evidence that the plasma cell is the major producer of *circulating antibodies*. The mature plasma cell is an end stage, that is, it does not continue to divide. The different roles of the lymphocytes and the macrophages of lymphatic organs in the immune mechanism are discussed in the

The secretory
bounded and, i
of the granules
characteristic p

The granules
coagulant, and
vasodilation and
of capillaries ar
cells of a few sp
contain seroton

The earliest
contain heparin
tions which sh
and mast cells
was shown later
mast cells also
those with only
it was found th
have a very hig

The evidence
tamine is based
resembling thos
rin. For exampl
containing an a
tain more hista
tively few mast
by chemical stu
duce and secret

The importar
agulant in clini
role in the no
mains obscure.
ing effect of his
of venules pro
functional rela
and connective
cumstances.

Mast cells ar
phylactic sensit
ver, extrinsic a
etc.) characteri
of smooth mus
laries. The mas
surface for a spe
When a sensiti
the appropriate
mast cells and
ulation. In add
of histamine ar
mediators are re

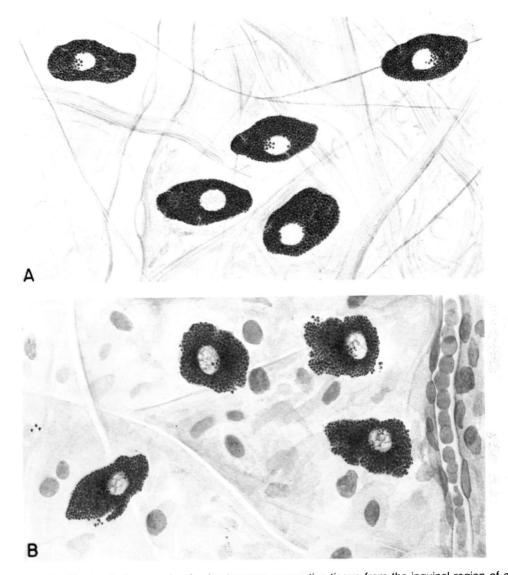

Figure 5.8. Mast cells in spreads of subcutaneous connective tissue from the inguinal region of a rat. *A*, basophilia of mast cell granules seen after staining with an alcoholic solution of toluidine blue. The pH of the stain was lowered by the addition of HCl and the nuclei of cells remained unstained. Nuclei, connective tissue fibers, and the wall of a capillary are visible in the background by their refraction (×730). *B*, metachromasia of mast cell granules seen after staining in a dilute aqueous solution of toluidine blue. The mast cell granules give a reddish color with the blue dye. Nuclei of fibroblasts, of histiocytes, and of capillary endothelial cells (*right side of field*) stain blue. Erythrocytes are bluish green. The pH of the stain in this case was relatively high (×730).

sections on lymphocytes (Chapter 7) and lymphatic organs (Chapter 14).

Mast Cells

These cells (Figs. 5.3, 5.8 to 5.10) occur in varying numbers in most loose connec-tive tissue, being especially numerous along the blood vessels. They are large cells with relatively small ovoid nuclei and numerous cytoplasmic granules that are usually ba-sophilic. These cells resemble the baso-philic leukocytes of the blood in some re-

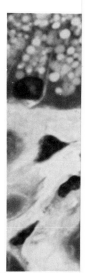

Figure 5.9. Li*(ter*) from monke

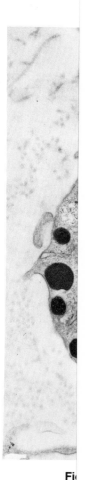

Fi

Wandering Cells from the Blood

Besides the cells enumerated, migratory cells from the blood and lymph stream are seen in varying numbers. These may include lymphocytes and eosinophilic and neutrophilic leukocytes. Although individuals of these cells are mostly short-lived and cannot be regarded as permanent members of the loose connective tissue cell population, their important biological functions are carried out predominantly in this location. This aspect will be pursued in detail in the context of the functions of blood cells (Chapters 7, 13, and 14).

Connective Tissue Fibers

Three types of fibers occur in adult connective tissue. Each of these types is present in loose connective tissue, and thus a study of the fibers in this type of tissue gives an understanding of the fibrillar elements of all adult connective tissue.

White or Collagenous Fibers

The *white* or *collagenous* fibers generally course together in bundles of indefinite length and variable thickness ranging from 10 to 100 μm or more. The individual fibers seen in routine preparations vary in diameter from 1 to 12 μm (Fig. 5.3). When these are studied under the higher magnifications of oil immersion objectives, and particularly after special treatment, it is found that they are composed of smaller fibers, the so-called *fibrils of light microscopy*, only 0.2 to 0.5 μm in diameter. These are held together by an amorphous material which can be dissolved by weak alkalis or by trypsin. They are aligned in a parallel direction, giving the appearance of longitudinal striation. In loose connective tissue, these fibers follow an irregular and undulating course; this allows for movement and flexibility of the other tissues with which they are associated. The collagenous fibers themselves are flexible but so slightly elastic as to be practically nonextensible.

Collagen is a protein which stains with most acid dyes. Hence, the fibers are red in hematoxylin-eosin-stained sections, blue from the aniline blue of Mallory's triple

stain, and green or blue in Masson's trichrome, depending on the modification used. The fibers are rapidly digested by gastric secretions but resist digestion by trypsin in alkaline solution. They swell in dilute acids and are dissolved by strong acids and alkalis. They yield gelatin on boiling; thus, meat with a high content of collagen is made more tender by boiling. Collagen is also a source of glue; animal hides which are composed largely of dense collagenous fibers can be made into leather by tanning.

Electron micrographs show that each of the collagenous fibrils of light microscopy is composed of still smaller *fibrils*. The latter are relatively uniform in diameter in any given connective tissue region but vary in different locations and in different stages of development, ranging from about 20 to 200 nm. In adult human dermis, they are about 100 nm in diameter. In regions where collagen is being formed, there are slender collagenous fibrils only about 20 nm in diameter. In these regions, one may also find very thin *microfibrils* (3 to 15 nm) which are collagen-like but lack the characteristic periodicity of collagen.

The electron microscope fibrils of mature collagen have periodic cross bandings at intervals of about 64 nm (Fig. 5.11). Information on the periodicity and the structure of collagen has evolved from the discovery that collagen can be disassembled in vitro and that its constituent molecules can be reassembled either into their previous native form or into other forms. Analysis of the morphology and chemistry of in vitro preparations of collagen established by the early 1960s that the extracellular collagen macromolecule is approximately 280 nm long and 1.5 nm in width. Each macromolecule is composed of three helically intertwined polypeptide chains and is structurally polarized. Alignment of these macromolecules end to end, but not touching, and with the molecules in adjacent rows arranged in parallel but staggered by about one-fourth of their length, gives rise to the 64-nm periodicity of collagen commonly seen by electron microscopy (Fig. 5.11).

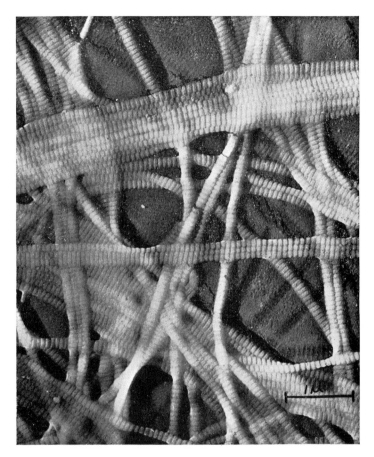

Figure 5.11. Electron micrograph of collagen fibrils from the adult human dermis. Chromium-shadowed (×19,300). (Courtesy of Drs. Gross and Schmitt.)

More recent studies using autoradiography and sophisticated biochemical techniques have clarified the sequence of collagen synthesis. The polypeptide chains (α-chains) are synthesized independently and are sequestered into the lumen of rough endoplasmic reticulum cisternae. Here, signal peptide sequences are removed and the chains commence post translational processing involving hydroxylation of proline and lysine, glycosylation, the formation of interchain disulfide bonds, and helix formation. Most of the processing occurs in the endoplasmic reticulum, but it is not certain whether helix formation is accomplished in the endoplasmic reticulum or in the Golgi apparatus. In any event, the fully formed tripeptide complex, now termed *procollagen*, passes through the Golgi where it is packaged within Golgi vesicles and transported to the cell surface for release by exocytosis (Fig. 5.12). The procollagen molecule is larger than the collagen molecule found outside the cell by virtue of extra amino acid sequences at both the amino and carboxyl ends of the molecule. These sequences are removed concurrent with or shortly after secretion, and the definitive collagen molecules (*tropocollagen*) spontaneously assemble into fibrils. The final stabilization of collagen macromolecular aggregates is dependent on cross-linking by a series of interactions involving lysine and hydroxylysine residues that produce covalent bonds.

Collagen consists of about 30% glycine and 25% proline and hydroxyproline, with the remainder consisting of other amino

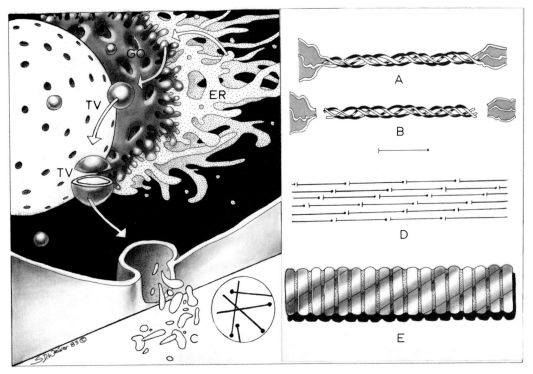

Figure 5.12. Diagram of the formation and structure of collagen. *A*, procollagen molecule showing three polypeptide chains and extra amino acid sequences at each end. *B*, tropocollagen molecule, formed by removal of extra amino acid sequences. The asymmetric bar represents this molecule schematically. The intracellular pathway for synthesis of procollagen is depicted at *left*; *ER* → Golgi (*GO*) → transport vesicles (*TV*) → cell surface. Tropocollagen is formed at the time of or immediately following exocytosis (*C*). Polymerization of tropocollagen molecules in quarter-stagger array (*D*) is postulated as the mechanism of formation of the 64-nm banding pattern of the type I collagen fiber, shown at *E*.

acids, including hydroxylysine. Glycine recurs at a constant position and frequency along the alpha chain, whereas the other amino acids recur at variable positions. Because hydroxyproline is not found in any significant amount in any other tissue, a determination of its amount in any organ indicates the amount of collagen in that organ. Proline and hydroxyproline prevent easy rotation of the strand where they are located, and thus they add stability to the macromolecule.

Collagen macromolecules are not identical throughout the body. This is because the three helically intertwined polypeptide chains can differ individually in their amino acid sequences. The α-chains have now been separated into two basic classes,

a_1 and a_2, and, in addition, the a_1 class appears to consist of several *types*. For example, the collagen macromolecules made by fibroblasts in skin and tendon contain two a_1, type I polypeptides linked to an a_2 polypeptide, whereas those made by chondroblasts have three a_1, type II polypeptide chains. The five different types of collagen now identified and their distribution in the body are summarized in Table 5.1. Types IV and V are currently attracting considerable attention because they are associated with the epithelial basal lamina and appear to be synthesized primarily by epithelial cells. The polymerized form of types IV and V collagen do not exhibit the characteristic 64-nm periodicity at the electron microscopic level of resolution originally

Table 5.1.
Types of Collagen and Their Distribution

Collagen Type	Polypeptide Chains	Location in Body
I	$[\alpha_1 (I)][\alpha_2]_2$	Skin, tendon, bone, cornea
II	$[\alpha_1 (II)]_3$	Cartilage, intervertebral disc, vitreous body
III	$[\alpha_1 (III)]_3$	Fetal skin, cardiovascular system, basal lamina
IV	$[\alpha_1 (IV)]_3$	Basal lamina, external lamina
V	$\alpha_A (\alpha_B)_2$ or $(\alpha_A)_3 + (\alpha_B)_3$	Basal lamina, external lamina

thought to be diagnostic for all collagen. It is now recognized that the final appearance of collagen morphologically is dependent on its polypeptide composition, the degree of cross-linking and the types and quantities of associated sugar moieties.

Reticular Fibers

These are small, branching fibers which frequently form a netlike supporting framework or reticulum. Their caliber is so small that they are masked by surrounding structures in ordinary preparations, but they blacken intensely after silver impregnation (Bielchowsky's method), whereas collagenous fibers are colored yellow or brown. Because they impregnate with silver, reticular fibers are frequently designated as *argyrophilic* fibers.

Reticular fibers are often continuous with collagenous fibers, and it is difficult to obtain any quantity of their substance, for chemical analysis. In most respects, they appear to be chemically similar to collagenous fibers, although they are more resistant to peptic digestion. They also have relatively more carbohydrate, which is apparently associated with each fibril in the form of a surface coat. This explains the fact that reticular fibers give a strongly positive reaction with the periodic acid-Schiff (PAS) technique, whereas collagenous fibers give only a slight reaction. The

associated carbohydrate is also responsible for the more intense reaction with silver. The reticular fibers have the same 64-nm cross banding as skin-type collagenous fibers and are morphologically similar to them except for diameter. Because collagenous fibers pass through a developmental stage in which they are argyrophilic and appear identical with reticular fibers, the latter have been regarded by some investigators as merely immature stages of the former. The fact that reticular fibers remain small in diameter and have a somewhat restricted distribution seem valid reasons for considering them a separate fiber type, even though the protein core is collagen. Recent evidence suggests that the collagen of reticular fibers is type III.

Reticular fibers are relatively sparse in adult loose connective tissues, except for regions around muscle fibers and around blood vessels, nerves, and epithelial structures. They are numerous in glandular organs (Fig. 16.86).

In lymphatic organs and in red bone marrow, the fibers are associated with a special type of cell known as the *reticular cell*; the two elements (reticular fibers and reticular cells) form a type of tissue, the *reticular tissue*. In other locations, reticular fibers, have the same relationship to fibroblasts as do collagenous fibers.

Elastic Fibers

The *elastic* fibers (Fig. 5.3) are highly refractile and are as a rule thinner than the white fibers but may reach a diameter of 10 to 12 μm in some *elastic ligaments* (e.g., ligamentum nuchae of an ox). They branch and anastomose freely, forming networks. The smaller fibers are round in cross section; the larger are flat or polygonal. They are highly elastic. When seen in large masses (elastic ligaments) in the fresh state, they have a distinctly yellow appearance. In arteries, the elastic tissue often occurs in the form of fenestrated membranes or lamellae.

Elastic fibers are best demonstrated in the fresh condition by immersing the tissue in dilute acid solutions. The collagenous fibers swell and become transparent. The elastic fibers are then seen as highly refractive, shining threads. The elastic fibers react poorly to most stains, but they are colored selectively by certain dyes such as orcein and resorcinfuchsin (Fig. 5.3).

Electron micrographs show that elastic fibers are not made up of cross-banded fibrils as is collagen. In fact, most electron micrographs give the impression that elastic tissue is composed only of an amorphous substance of varying electron density. However, high resolution electron micrographs show that the elastic fiber has two components: homogeneous ("amorphous") material, *elastin*, and slender *elastic fiber microfibrils* about 120 Å in diameter (Fig. 5.13).

The formation of elastic fibers is not as well understood as that of collagen, but the synthetic pathway appears to be similar. Whether the two components are produced simultaneously or sequentially is not known, but morphologically the microfibrils appear in the extracellular matrix prior to the amorphous elastin. Consequently the microfibrils are more obvious in young elastic tissue. On the other hand, elastin is the most obvious component in mature elastic fibers, and the microfibrils are limited chiefly to the periphery of the fiber, with only a few scattered through the elastin. Whether the elastin appears light or dark in electron micrographs depends on the method of fixation. Furthermore, the appearance of the microfibrils may vary with the functional state of the fiber: it has been postulated that the fibrils are randomly oriented in relaxed fibers and more parallel in stretched fibers.

Chemically, the elastic fiber contains proline, glycine, valine, and a number of other amino acids. It differs from collagen in the fact that there is little hydroxypro-

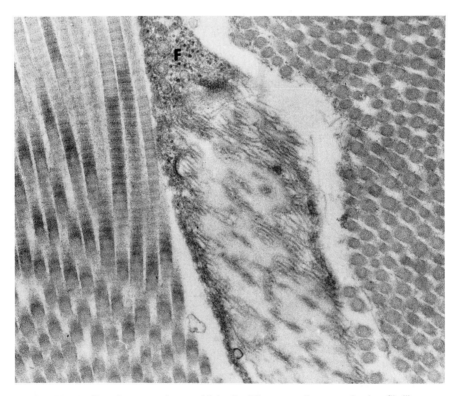

Figure 5.13. Elastic fiber from monkey epididymis. The amorphous and microfibrillar components of elastin are evident. A fibroblast process (*F*) and collagen fibrils in cross and longitudinal section are also shown (×102,000).

line, a much higher concentration of valine, and it contains desmosine and isodesmosine, two amino acids not found in collagen. These specialized amino acids are now known to be involved in the cross-linking of elastin. Elastin and the elastic tissue microfibrils differ from each other in the proportions of their amino acids. Elastin has a higher content of valine than the microfibrils, whereas the latter have a much greater content of cystine and completely lack hydroxyproline and desmosine. The microfibrils also contain sugar moieties such as hexose and hexosamine, thus suggesting that they contain glycoproteins.

Elastic fibers are usually formed by fibroblasts, but in certain locations, such as the media of the aorta, they are produced by smooth muscle cells.

The surface of an elastic fiber seems to be continually undergoing changes which involve a turnover of material. In the aging of arteries, small regions of degenerating elastic tissue form seeding sites for mineralization. In elastic fibers of the skin, age changes occur in the associated glycosaminoglycans. There is an increase in chondroitin sulfate and keratosulfate in proportion to the other glycosaminoglycans, and this gives a loss of resiliency.

Origin of the Connective Tissue Fibers

The development of connective tissue fibers has been studied extensively, both by light microscopy and by electron microscopy. In locations where connective tissue fibers first appear in embryos, one can see with the light microscope that the accompanying cells differ little from the more primitive mesenchymal cells from which they are derived. They have prominent nucleoli and basophilic cytoplasm and the name fibroblast, given by early histologists, was based on the belief that the cells participate in some manner in the formation of fibers. However, it has been long recognized that a number of other mesenchymally derived cells also are capable of producing collagen and elastin. Chondroblasts (cartilage-producing cells), osteoblasts (bone-forming cells), reticular cells, and smooth muscle cells all secrete collagen. In addition, it is now clear that most epithelial cells, regardless of embryonic origin, also produce collagen as a component of their basal lamina. Therefore, we must modify categorical definitions of cells and recognize the spectrum of functional activities in which most cells are involved. Nevertheless, we still acknowlege fibroblasts as being especially active in the production of connective tissue fibers, as well as ground substance, and that they have an important role in the maintenance of the connective tissue matrix in much of the body.

Ground Substance

The cells and fibers of connective tissue are embedded in an amorphous background material known as *ground substance*. It is a colloidal substance in the form of a gel of variable viscosity, which binds varying amounts of water. The bound water serves as a medium for diffusion of gases and metabolic substances from the blood vessels to the cells of the tissues, and vice versa. Thus the amorphous matrix and the tissue fluids are intimately associated. Most of the extravascular fluid is bound within the matrix and is not present in any appreciable amount as free water in the connective tissues under normal conditions. Whereas the matrix is normally fluid, it rapidly becomes much more so in areas of injury and inflammation.

In fresh spreads of connective tissue, the ground substance has the same refractive index as water and isotonic saline solutions, and therefore it is invisible in spreads mounted in these media. The ground substance is quite soluble in the reagents generally used in preparing tissues for sectioning, and it is not seen in the areolar connective tissue of routinely prepared sections. It is preserved best by fresh freezing and freeze-drying techniques, provided that the tissues are fixed subsequently in vapors of ether-formol. In these preparations, the ground substance stains metachromatically, indicating the presence of acidic glycosominoglycans. In some connective tissues, such as cartilage and bone, it can be preserved by appropriate fixatives in sufficient quantities for histochemical studies. In fact, the proteoglycan content of cartilage and bone is sufficient to affect the tinctorial results in sections routinely prepared and stained with hematoxylin and eosin (Chapter 6).

The *proteoglycans* of the ground substance consist of about 95% carbohydrate and 5% protein. The carbohydrate is a polymer of disaccharide units referred to as *glycosaminoglycan*, which may be *sulfated* or *nonsulfated*. The nonsulfated group includes *hyaluronic acid* and *chondroitin.* The sulfated group includes: *chondroitin 4-sulfate* (chondroitin sulfate A), *chondroitin 6-sulfate* (chondroitin sulfate C), *dermatan sulfate* (chondroitin sulfate B), *keratan sulfate* (keratosulfate) and *heparan sulfate. Heparin,* produced by mast cells, is also a glycosominoglycan, and it has a relatively high content of sulfate. Most of the sulfated glycosaminoglycans are gel-like, and when they are abundant, as in cartilage, they provide support.

Hyaluronic acid is a viscous glycosaminoglycan isolated by Meyer and Palmer in 1934. It is found in synovial fluid, loose connective tissue, etc. (Table 5.2). Because of its capacity to bind water, it has a major responsibility for changes in the viscosity and permeability of ground substance. It probably also plays a role in preventing the spread of noxious agents in localized infections. An enzyme, *hyaluronidase,* hydrolyzes it, reducing its viscosity with a consequent increase in the permeability of the tissue. For example, subcutaneous injections of India ink to which hyaluronidase has been added spread much more rapidly than injections of ink alone. This enzyme (known as "spreading factor") was first isolated from testicles and snake venom. An enzyme with similar effects on hyaluronic acid is produced by some bacteria.

The sulfated glycosaminoglycans are generally much more metachromatic than the nonsulfated ones. The sulfated form also stains with hematoxylin when it is sufficiently abundant, as in cartilage, to overshadow the associated acidophilic collagenous fibers.

The ground substance also contains *glycoproteins.* Some of these have been characterized biochemically and they are known to have a variety of important functions. Probably the best known of these com-

Table 5.2.
Main Types of Connective Tissue Glycosaminoglycans*

Name	Some Locations Where Found	Sulfate/Disaccharide Unit	Hyaluronidase Susceptibility	
			Testicular	Bacterial
Hyaluronic acid	Synovial fluid, umbilical cord, vitreous humor, loose connective tissue, group A streptococci capsules	0	+	+
Chondroitin	Cornea	0		
Chondroitin 4-sulfate (chondroitin sulfate A)	Aorta, bone, cartilage, cornea	1	+	−
Chondroitin 6-sulfate (chondroitin sulfate C)	Cartilage, nucleus pulposus, sclera, tendon, umbilical cord	1	+	−
Dermatan sulfate (chondroitin sulfate B)	Aorta, heart valve, ligamentum nuchae, sclera, skin, tendon	1	−	−
Keratan sulfate (keratosulfate)	Bone, cartilage, cornea, nucleus pulposus, kidney glomerulus	1	−	−
Heparin	Mast cells	2	−	−
Heparan sulfate	Lung, arterial wall, cell surfaces	1–2	−	−

* Modified from Spicer et al., 1967.

pounds is *fibronectin.* It is elaborated by many different cell types but is produced in particularly large amounts by fibroblasts. Fibronectin and its counterparts in cartilage and bone, *chondronectin* and *osteonectin,* appear to have a major role in the attachment of cells and other components to collagen fibers. Both free and cellular bound forms of the molecule exist and, despite minor chemical differences, the two forms appear to function identically. Fibronectin is of considerable interest to developmental and cancer biologists because it is implicated in the regulation of a variety of cellular interactions, including adhesion and migration. Cells rendered cancer-like by viral or other inducing agents (transformed cells) have reduced quantities of membrane-bound fibronectin and this is correlated with their altered behavior. Fibronectin is a characteristic glycoprotein of the connective tissue but it is also produced by epithelial cells.

The PAS Reaction in Connective Tissues

The PAS (periodic acid-Schiff) technique is based on the fact that free aldehydes restore the reddish color to basic fuchsin which has been bleached previously with sulfurous acid. In Chapter 1 it is noted that the Schiff reagent (i.e., bleached basic fuchsin) is specific for DNA in the Feulgen reaction because the sections are treated to only a mild hydrolysis which liberates aldehydes from DNA but not from RNA. When a stronger oxidizing agent, such as periodic acid, is used, aldehydes are liberated from polysaccharides in general. Cartilage matrix gives a positive PAS reaction, and the ground substances of other connective tissues also give PAS reactions of varying degrees in different locations. However, *pure* hyaluronic acid is PAS-negative, and the same is apparently true for *pure* chondroitin sulfate. The PAS-positive reaction given by reticular fibers is apparently due to a higher quantity of carbohydrates in the surface coat of this fiber as compared to ordinary collagen fibers.

Functions of Loose Connective Tissue

Nutrient substances in their passage from the blood vessels to the cells of the body traverse connective tissue, as must also those products of metabolism which reach the blood and lymph capillaries (see Fig. 12.28.) Loose connective tissue loosely binds structures together and holds them in position. It acts as a padding and serves as a pathway for nerves and blood vessels.

The loose connective tissue plays an extremely important role in limiting the spread of localized infections and in the healing process. The localization invokes all elements of the connective tissue. The ground substance, although permeable, tends to inhibit the passage of the noxious agent. In addition to the phagocytic cells (neutrophilic leukocytes and monocytes) which migrate to the area from the blood, the tissue phagocytes (macrophages) mobilize. The fibroblasts also become active and, after a considerable time, deposit a surrounding barrier of fibers.

In repair of wounds, the fibroblasts increase in number and form fibers. Sprouts from the blood vessels penetrate into the delicate regenerating tissue, which is known as *granulation tissue.* Some of the fibroblasts in wound areas assume morphological characteristics resembling smooth muscle. These cells are called *myofibroblasts* and they are thought to play an important role in drawing together tissues at the wound edge to promote the healing process.

Changes in connective tissues occur in a number of disease states. For example, in a condition known as *scurvy,* collagen is not formed in normal amounts because there is a deficiency of vitamin C which is necessary in order for fibroblasts to hydroxylate normal amounts of proline to hydroxyproline and lysine to hydroxylysine. Many aging changes are closely related to changes in collagen and ground substance. In *rheumatoid arthritis,* there is an excessive production and abnormal organization of collagen. In fact, the various rheumatic conditions are so intimately related to abnormalities in the formation and repair of connective tissue that they are often spoken of as collagen diseases. Some diseases are clearly related to abnormal function of genes. *Hurler's syndrome*, a condition involving stunted skeletal growth and abnormal fat metabolism, is an hereditary disorder involving an excessive accumulation of dermatan sulfate and heparan sulfate.

Dense Connective Tissue

Dense connective tissue is chiefly characterized by the close packing of its fibers. It occurs in the form of sheets, bands, and cordlike structures. Examples are the dermis, capsules of certain organs, aponeuroses, ligaments, and tendons. Some of the deep fascia is intermediate between dense and loose connective tissue. In most locations, the main component is collagenous fibers, but in a few of the ligaments, elastic fibers predominate.

Dense, irregularly arranged connective tissue is composed chiefly of coarse collagenous fibers, but elastic and reticular fibers are also present. The fibers interlace and form a coarse tough feltwork, and some of them continue into adjacent tissue. Fibroblasts and some macrophages are present but show no special modifications. Examples of dense irregularly arranged connective tissue are dermis (Figs. 5.14), periosteum and perichondrium, and the capsules of some organs. The capsule of the testis (tunica albuginea) is extremely dense.

Dense, regularly arranged connective tissue occurs as cordlike structures and as bands, some of which, as in aponeuroses, may be very broad. The fibers are densely packed and lie parallel to each other, forming structures of great tensile strength. This type of tissue comprises the tendons, ligaments, and aponeuroses.

Tendons are composed almost entirely of white fibrous tissue. The collagen fibers are parallel and are closely packed in bundles which are so dense that they appear almost homogeneous. Fibroblasts are the only cell type present, and they are relatively few in number. In longitudinal sections of tendon, the fibroblasts are elongated and aligned in rows between the bundles of collagenous fibers (Fig. 5.15). In cross sections, the cells appear stellate in shape, with platelike extensions between the collagenous bundles (Fig. 5.15).

Around each bundle of fibers is a small amount of loose tissue, and the whole tendon is surrounded by interlacing fibers.

Aponeuroses have the same composition as tendons but are broad and relatively thin. The fibers may be arranged in several superimposed layers, those of one layer running at an angle to those of adjacent layers. The layers may interweave.

Ligaments in most cases are structurally similar to tendons, being formed predominantly of collagenous fibers, but a few are composed almost entirely of elastic fibers.

The *yellow elastic ligaments* are formed of parallel-coursing yellow elastic fibers which are bound together by a small amount of loose tissue. The elastic fibers may be very large, as in the ligamentum nuchae. The series of ligaments (ligamenta flava) coursing between the arches of the vertebrae are also of the elastic type.

RETICULAR CONNECTIVE TISSUE

The special tissue forming the supporting framework of bone marrow and most lymphoid tissues (except thymus) is characterized by the presence of a mesenchymally derived cellular reticulum and fine extracellular fibrils. Because of their morphology, these cells and fibrils have been called "reticular cells" and "reticular fibers" and the tissue so formed has been referred to as "reticular tissue." The reticular cells are frequently stellate in shape and are in contact with each other along extended cellular processes (Fig. 5.16). Cells with this morphology in the thymus were long assumed to be identical in structure and origin, but thymic reticular cells are now known to be modified epithelial cells derived from pharyngeal endoderm (see Chapter 3, Chapter 4, and Chapter 14). True connective tissue reticular cells of the bone marrow and lymphoid tissues are associated with reticular fibers which are argyrophilic, contain col-

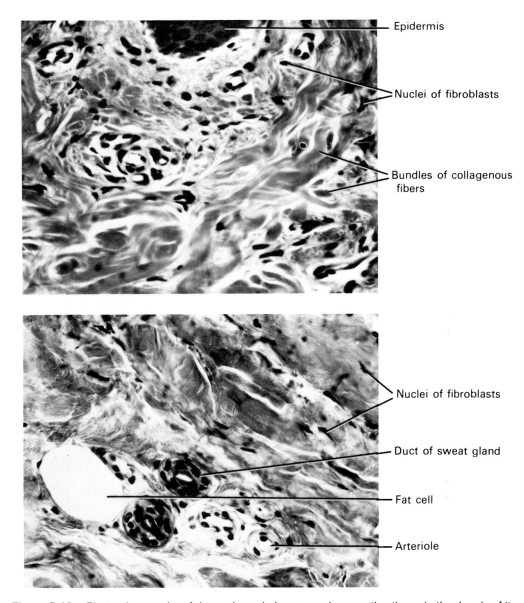

Epidermis

Nuclei of fibroblasts

Bundles of collagenous fibers

Nuclei of fibroblasts

Duct of sweat gland

Fat cell

Arteriole

Figure 5.14. Photomicrographs of dense, irregularly arranged connective tissue in the dermis of the dorsum of the thumb. *Upper figure*, a field just below the epidermis; *lower figure*, a deep region of the dermis just above the subcutaneous tissue. Note variations in the diameter and course of the bundles of fibers in different fields. For example, the bundles of fibers are coarse in the deep portions of the dermis and more slender in the subepidermal region. Even greater variations are found in other parts of the body, and there are many gradations between the loose and dense varieties of irregularly arranged connective tissue. Hematoxylin and eosin-stained section (×390).

lagen and are apparently identical to reticular fibers formed by fibroblasts in loose connective tissue. Reticular fibers are scarce in the thymus and those present are not formed by the epithelial reticular cells (see Chapter 14).

Several different functional and developmental potencies have been attributed to connective tissue reticular cells, i.e., the formation of reticular fibers, phagocytosis, the formation of blood cells, the formation of fat cells, and the presentation of antigens

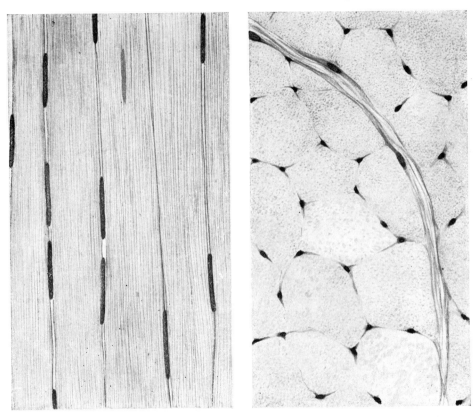

Figure 5.15. Sections of human achilles tendon. At left is a longitudinal section which shows rows of dense-staining nuclei of fibroblasts (tendon cells) between bundles of regularly arranged fibrils. At *right* is a cross section. Note that the nuclei and the pale-staining cytoplasm of the tendon cells appears stellate in shape. A band of irregularly arranged connective tissue separating tendon bundles is seen in the *right side* of the drawing. Both figures ×575.

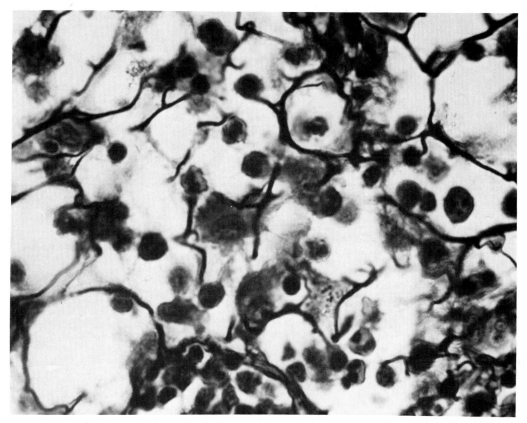

Figure 5.16. Light micrograph of reticular tissue from lymph node of monkey. The two large cells in the center are reticular cells. The reticular fibers are stained with silver in this preparation (×1360).

to B lymphocytes in the immune response. Recent evidence seriously challenges the role of reticular cells in phagocytosis and the formation of blood cells or true fat cells, and even raises some question about their ability to form reticular fibers. It is generally accepted, however, that reticular cells in lymphoid tissues adsorb antigens to their surfaces and present them to B lymphocytes. In view of the wealth of evidence challenging many of the traditional views of the significance of reticular cells, it seems wise to deemphasize the concept of a specialized reticular tissue.

ADIPOSE TISSUE (FAT)

Fat cells are found isolated or in groups in all loose connective tissue, but in certain places they are present in such large numbers and have such an organization as to justify the designation of adipose tissue. The largest deposits of fat are found in the subcutaneous connective tissue (panniculus adiposus), in the kidney region, in the mesenteries and mediastinum, and in the cervical, axillary, and inguinal regions.

Fat is different from the other connective tissues in that the cells, and not the intercellular substance, make up the bulk and determine the nature of the tissue. The cells are large and have an ovoid or spherical shape. The cytoplasm is displaced to the peripheral region of the cell by the presence of a single large fat droplet (Fig. 5.17). The nucleus, flattened and surrounded by a small amount of cytoplasm, is usually found pressed against the periphery. In sections of fixed preparations in which the fat has been dissolved out, the cells appear as empty rings or ovals, or they have a "signet ring" shape if the plane of section passes

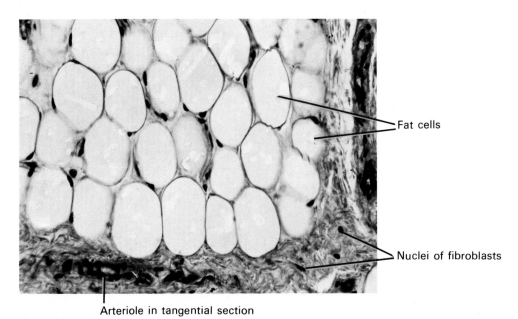

Arteriole in tangential section

Figure 5.17. Photomicrograph of fat from human subcutaneous tissue. Because the fat dissolves and escapes from the cell during the dehydration and clearing of the tissue for preparing paraffin sections, the cells appear empty. The cells are large and only a few are sectioned, by chance, in the plane of the nucleus. Hematoxylin and eosin stain (×250).

through the nucleus. When occurring singly or in small groups the cells retain their spherical or ovoid form; in denser masses they become polyhedral as a result of the pressure of adjacent cells. Fat cells are usually arranged in groups or lobules, each lobule being separated from its neighbor by loose connective tissue. Delicate strands of irregularly arranged connective tissue consisting of reticular, collagenous, and elastic fibers surround the fat cells and serve as a bed for the numerous capillaries.

The appearance of the adult fat cell can be best understood by a reference to its histogenesis. In places where fat is to be formed, certain cells of the embryonal connective tissue become grouped in the meshes of a rich capillary network which marks the end of a small artery. Such groups, each of which is destined to become an adult fat lobule, can be distinguished in man in the fourth month of embryonic life. The changes in morphology accompanying maturation can be most readily studied by electron microscopy. The preadipocytes enlarge, become rich in endoplasmic reticu-

lum and begin to accumulate small lipid droplets (Figs. 5.18 and 5.19). The latter fuse into a single large droplet which occupies more and more of the cytoplasmic volume (Fig. 5.20). The nucleus is pushed to one side and the cytoplasm is eventually reduced to the thin peripheral layer of the adult adipocyte. Each fat cell is surrounded by an external lamina, differing in this respect from all other types of connective tissue cells.

The blood supply of fat is rich, and the adult lobule retains its embryonal vascular relations, the vascular supply of each lobule being complete and independent. One artery runs to each lobule, where it breaks up into an intralobular capillary network which in turn gives rise to the intralobular veins, usually two in number.

Chemically, fat consists of the esters of glycerol and certain fatty acids (palmitic, stearic, and oleic). It is not soluble in water or cold alcohol but dissolves readily in ether, chloroform, benzol, and xylol. Because the latter reagents are commonly used in histological technique, the fat is

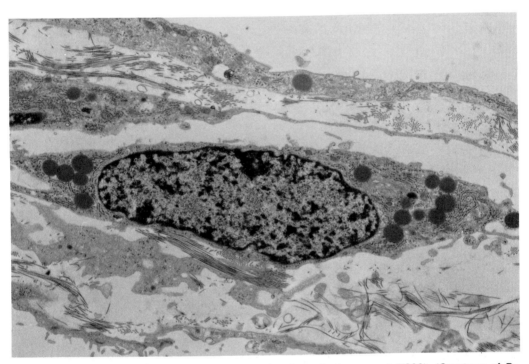

Figure 5.18. Electron micrograph of a developing fat cell of mouse (×7200). (Courtesy of Dr. Bernard Slavin.)

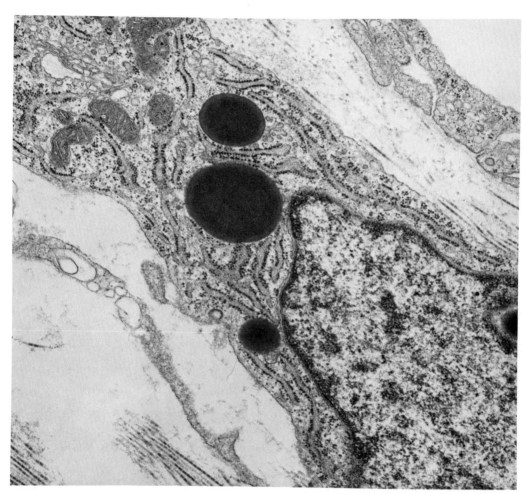

Figure 5.19. Higher magnification electron micrograph of a developing fat cell. Note the well developed rough endoplasmic reticulum, the dense fat droplets and the prominent Golgi apparatus (*lower right*). The external lamina is not yet formed on this cell (×26,000). (Courtesy of Dr. Bernard Slavin.)

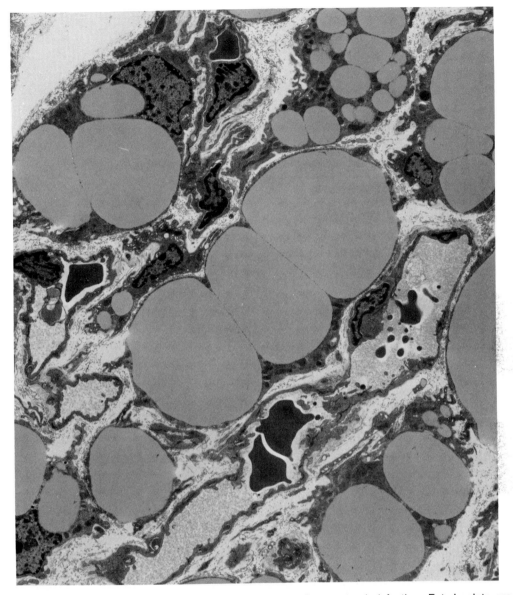

Figure 5.20. Developing fat cell of rat during recovery from extended fasting. Fat droplets are increasing in size as a result of fusion of smaller droplets. Handling procedures have caused some tissue shrinkage and distortion (×3600). (Courtesy of Dr. Bernard Slavin.)

usually dissolved, leaving an empty space or vacuole. Fat and fatlike substances stain black with osmic acid (osmium tetroxide) or with certain coal tar dyes such as Sudan III and Scharlach R.

The so-called fat deposits of the body are not inactive storehouses. Labeled or "tagged" molecules of carbohydrates, are incorporated into fats and are rapidly re-

placed; the turnover in mice requires only about six days.

Besides its nutritive value, fat has important mechanical functions. It forms plastic, shock-absorbing pads in the subcutaneous tissue of parts exposed to pressure, such as the gluteal region and the soles of the feet. It packs the orbital cavity and the angles of joints, acting as a guard against exaggerated movements. Such fatty pads are especially prominent in the hip, knee, shoulder, and elbow joints, where they may be retained even in states of extreme emaciation.

As a nonconductor, fat is also an important agent in the conservation of the body heat.

Brown fat, in addition to the above described white fat, is present in numerous species of animals, being particularly prominent in hibernating animals such as the hedgehog and bat. The brown fat of insectivores, bats, and true rodents retains its characteristic appearance throughout life, whereas that of other mammals begins to show variable degrees of regression soon after birth.

Brown fat is well developed in particular regions of the body, e.g., the interscapular region, inguinal area, etc., and it is not distributed widely in the body, as is white fat.

The histological appearance of brown fat is quite different from that of white fat. The nuclei of brown fat cells are round rather than flattened and are often located in the central portions of the cells. The cytoplasm contains numerous lipid droplets which are generally seen as vacuoles after routine histological techniques; thus brown fat is described as *multilocular* in contrast to *unilocular* white fat.

The mitochondria are larger and more numerous in brown fat than in the white variety and the mitochondrial cristae are more closely packed and commonly extend completely across the organelle. Histochemical studies show that these mitochondria are rich in succinic dehydrogenase and cytochrome oxidase. Rough endoplasmic reticulum is scarce in brown fat cells and smooth-surfaced membranes are less numerous than in white fat. The Golgi complex is also quite small.

Both types of fat are richly vascularized and innervated, but in each case the supply to brown fat exceeds that for the white variety. The postganglionic sympathetic endings have synaptic vesicles of the type that is characteristic for norepinephrine-containing nerves. Recent correlated physiological and electron microscopic studies show that brown fat cells are electrically coupled and are attached to each other by communicating (gap) junctions. White fat cells do not seem to be functionally interconnected in the same way, at least in mature cells.

Whereas white fat cells function as storehouses for triglycerides which can be mobilized for fuel by other parts of the body, the masses of brown fat are specialized for transducing the energy stored in fatty acids into heat which warms the blood passing through their capillaries and venules and subsequently increases body temperature. This process is particularly important in newborn and young animals exposed to cold and in the arousal of hibernating animals. In this process, there is evidence that the transduction of energy into heat results from a failure of the usual oxidative phosphorylation in the mitochondria of brown fat cells.

Brown fat does not respond to nutritional changes as readily as ordinary fat. On the other hand, hypophysectomy brings about a more rapid lipid depletion in brown than in white fat.

PIGMENTED CONNECTIVE TISSUE

Pigmented connective tissue cells (melanocytes) occur in the choroid and iris of the eye (Figs. 5.21 and 5.22). The cytoplasm is filled to a varying degree with brown or black pigment, which is usually *melanin.* Experiments with tissue culture indicate that pigmented connective tissue cells are a specialized type. The cells form true pigment in the cultures only if they are explanted from a tissue which would have grown pigment in the body. There is considerable evidence that melanocytes are of neural crest origin.

BLOOD AND NERVE SUPPLY OF CONNECTIVE TISSUE

Blood vessels and lymphatics are numerous in loose connective tissue. The rich

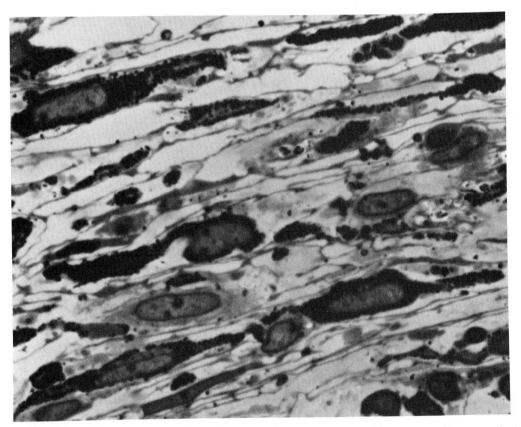

Figure 5.21.   Light micrograph of pigment cells in the choroid layer of human eye. From a patient with choroidal melanoma (×1120). (Tissue supplied by Dr. Ann Bunt-Milam. Micrograph courtesy of Dr. Gregory Hageman.)

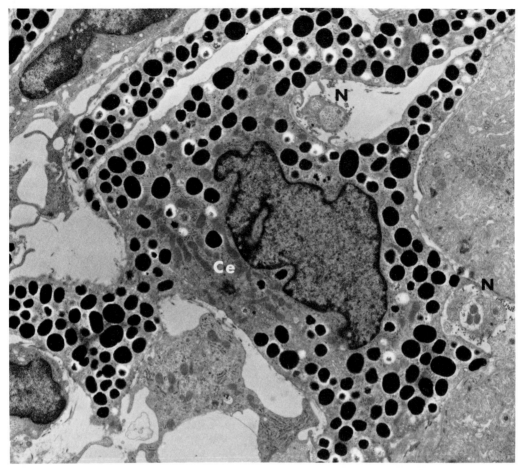

Figure 5.22. Electron micrograph of a pigment cell from the choroid layer of hamster eye. Note the centriole in the pigment cell (*Ce*) and small unmyelinated nerve (*N*) (× 7800). (Courtesy of Dr. Gregory Hageman.)

capillary plexuses are not, however, in the main destined for the tissue itself but for the more active cells of epithelium and muscle. The connective tissue forms the supporting bed for all blood vessels and incidentally receives its own nutrition from them. In the dense connective tissues and tendons, the blood supply is less abundant. In tendons, the blood vessels follow a straight course between the large collagen bundles and communicate with each other by short branches which run across the bundles, forming a scanty capillary network with oblong meshes. The fibrous membranes of the periosteum and dura mater are more vascular, but here too the blood vessels are mainly destined for bone.

Lymphatics are numerous and form extensive networks, especially in the submucous, subserous, and subcutaneous connective tissue. They are also present in fibrous membranes and tendons, where they form both superficial and deep lymphatic plexuses.

Connective tissue is richly supplied with nerves which end in the tissue itself or go to epithelium and muscle. Special nerve endings are found in the tendons, in fibrous membranes, and in the periarticular connective tissue.

THE MACROPHAGE SYSTEM

It was found by Metchnikoff in the latter part of the 19th century that certain connective tissue cells are markedly phagocytic; he named them *macrophages*, in contrast with the relatively small neutrophilic leukocytes which become *microphages* in the connective tissues during localized inflammations. In the early part of this century, it was found that phagocytic cells are also present along the lumina of liver sinusoids (Kupffer cells) and along the lumina of the venous sinuses of the spleen and the lymphatic sinusoids of lymph nodes. Aschoff proposed the name *reticuloendothelial system* for the macrophages of the body based on the phagocytic *reticular cells* in the framework of lymphatic organs and the so-called *endothelial cells* of the sinusoids of the liver and lymphatic organs. This term was criticized by Maximow and others on the grounds that reticular refers to only one type of connective tissue macrophage, thus omitting the connective tissue macrophage ("histiocyte"). Furthermore, the term endothelial might give the incorrect impression that the endothelial cells of ordinary blood vessels are included. Nevertheless, the term *reticuloendothelial system* was generally adopted.

The simplest method for identifying the cells of this system is to give living animals injections of certain nontoxic dyes such as trypan blue or of some inert particulate matter such as carbon particles of India ink. The macrophages avidly take up the dye (or particles) and are easily identified in light microscope preparations (Fig. 5.3). Although the cells containing the dye are found in widely separated organs, the reaction is quite specific. Epithelium, nerve cells, and muscle cells take up the dye very slightly, if at all. Fibroblasts take up the dye more slowly and in smaller amounts than do the histiocytes (Fig. 5.3). True endothelial cells of blood and lymphatic vessels either fail to react or react so slightly that when a macrophage is near an endothelial cell a quantitative difference is readily seen (Fig. 16.83). The microglia of the nervous system ingest the dye, and therefore they are included in the system. In fact, all highly phagocytic cells except the neutrophils are included.

Electron micrographs show that macrophages have a well developed Golgi complex and a more or less well developed rough endoplasmic reticulum, dependent on the species (prominent in rodents but present in relatively small amounts in humans). There are, as would be expected in phagocytic cells, numerous cytoplasmic vacuoles, lysosomes, and residual bodies.

Electron micrographs have helped to resolve the relationship between endothelial cells and Kupffer cells of the liver. Although these cells are intimately associated with each other along the lumina of the sinusoids, there is no indication of cells with transitional characteristics even after prolonged stimulation of the macrophage system. Furthermore, the Kupffer cells differ from endothelial cells in that they give a strongly positive reaction for endogenous peroxidase. High resolution electron micrographs of lymphatic organs and bone marrow also cast doubt on the presence of any markedly phagocytic endothelial cells in these organs.

The use of tritiated thymidine, incorporated into DNA only during replication, has been useful in tracing the lineage of Kupffer cells and other macrophages. In testing the role of monocytes, promonocytes from bone marrow were used because the mature monocytes do not usually divide and thus do not usually incorporate DNA. Tissues from various regions of the animals which had received transfusions of labeled promonocytes from compatible strains were fixed and processed for studies by the combined use of radioautography and electron microscopy. Studies of the liver showed the label in a number of Kupffer cells but not in any endothelial cells. It is evident that the new Kupffer cells observed in these studies developed from the labeled promonocytes and not from endothelial cells. The combined evidence from different studies indicates that there is no *endothelial* component of the so-called reticuloendothelial system. The promonocytes from bone marrow used in these studies apparently develop from "stem cells" with morphological characteristics that have not been defined.

As already noted, there is also a question concerning the *reticular* component of the so-called reticuloendothelial system. Are the highly phagocytic cells of lymphatic organs a functional stage of the reticular cells or are they derived from precursor mononuclear cells brought in by the vascular system? It has not been shown that the phagocytic cells of lymphatic organs participate in the formation of reticular fibers or that the fiber-producing cells change to macrophages. There is increasing evidence in favor of the view that the macrophages of the lymphatic organs, Kupffer cells of the liver, and "dust cells" of the lung develop from mononuclear cells of bone marrow origin. Hence, a more appropriate name for the reticuloendothelial system is *mononuclear phagocyte system* or simply *macrophage system*.

During embryonic development the mesenchyme differentiates into numerous types of cells, including the connective tissue fibroblasts and cells described by Maximow as wandering cells. The latter were considered as relatively undifferentiated and as capable of taking one of several lines of differentiation according to the stimulus of body needs. It was thought at that time that many of the wandering cells become histiocytes of the loose connective tissues and that some remain as *undifferentiated mesenchymal cells*. Cells of a relatively undifferentiated type are identifiable along the blood vessels, where they are known as *pericytes*. These may be able to develop into mast cells, as noted in the preceding section. There is evidence that pericytes can also develop into smooth muscle on regenerating blood vessels, and also into fibroblasts. Although the possibility that some macrophages can develop from the undifferentiated perivascular cells cannot be ruled out, it seems unlikely. Furthermore, there is no evidence that any macrophages develop from lymphocytes or that the monocytes develop from lymphocytes.

References

Bensley SH: On the presence, properties and distribution of the intercellular ground substance of loose connective tissue. *Anat Rec* 60:93–109, 1934.

Bienkowski RS, Baum BJ, Crystal RG: Fibroblasts degrade newly synthesized collagen within the cell before secretion. *Nature* 276:413–416, 1978.

Bornstein P, Sage H: Structurally distinct collagen types. *Annu Rev Biochem* 49:957–1003, 1980.

Brissie RM, Spicer SS, Thompson NT: The variable fine structure of elastin visualized with Verhoeff's iron hematoxylin. *Anat Rec* 181:83–94, 1975.

Carpenter JC, Perrelet A, Orci L: Morphological changes of the adipose cell membrane during lipolysis. *J Cell Biol* 72:104–117, 1977.

Castro CW, Prince RK, Dorstewitz EL: Characteristics of human fibroblasts cultivated in vitro from different anatomical sites. *Lab Invest* 11:703–713, 1962.

Evans HM, Scott KJ: On the differential reaction to vital dyes exhibited by the two great groups of connective-tissue cells. *Carnegie Inst Contrib Embryol* 10:1–55, 1921.

Fahimi HD: The fine structural localization of endogenous and exogenous peroxidase activity in Kupffer cells of rat liver. *J Cell Biol* 47:247–262, 1970.

Fawcett DW: A comparison of the histological organization and cytochemical reactions of brown and white adipose tissue. *J Morphol* 70:363, 1952.

Fawcett DW, Jones IC: The effects of hypophysectomy, adrenalectomy and of thiouracil feeding on the cytology of brown adipose tissue. *Endocrinology* 45:609–621, 1949.

Furth R, van Cohn ZA, Hirsch JG, Humphrey JH, Spector WG, Langevoort HL: The mononuclear phagocyte system: a new classification of macrophages, monocytes and their precursor cells. *Bull WHO* 46:845–852, 1972.

Godleski JJ, Brain JD: The origin of alveolar macrophages in mouse radiation chimeras. *J Exp Med* 136:630, 1972.

Grant RA, Horne RW, Cox RW: New model for the tropocollagen macromolecule and its mode of aggregation. *Nature* 207:822–826, 1965.

Hymes, RO: Fibronectin and its relation to cellular structure and behavior. *In* Hay ED (ed): *Cell Biology of Extracellular Matrix.* New York, Plenum Press, 1981, pp 295–334.

Kazayama M, Douglas WW: Electron microscope evidence of calcium-activated exocytosis in mast cells treated with 48/80 or the ionophores A-23187 and X-537 A. *J Cell Biol* 62:519–526, 1974.

Leduc EH, Scott GB, Avrameas S: Ultrastructural localization of intracellular immune globulins in plasma cells and lymphoblasts by enzyme-labeled antibodies. *J Histochem Cytochem* 17:211–224, 1969.

Maximow AA: Bindegewebe und blutbildende Gewebe. In von Möllendorff (ed): *Handbuch der mikroskopische Anatomie des Menschen*, vol 2, part 1. Berlin, Springer-Verlag, 1930, pp 232–583.

Maximow AA: The macrophages or histiocytes. In Cowdry EV (ed): *Special Cytology*, vol 2. New York, P.B. Hoeber, 1932, pp 709–770.

Meyer K: 1946 The biological significance of hyaluronic acid and hyaluronidase. *Physiol Rev* 27:335–359, 1946.

Murata F, Spicer SS: Ultrastructural comparison of basophilic leukocytes and mast cells in the guinea pig. *Am J Anat* 139:335–351, 1974.

Napolitano L: The differentiation of white adipose cells. An electron microscope study. *J Cell Biol* 18:663–679, 1963.

Nopajaroosi C, Simon GT: Phagocytosis of colloidal-carbon in a lymph node. *Am J Pathol* 65:25–42, 1971.

Papadimitriou JM, Archer M: The morphology of foreign body multinucleate giant cells. *J Ultrastruct Res* 49:372–386, 1974.

Perlstein E, Gord LI, Garcia-Pardo A: Fibronectin: a review of its structure and biological activity. *Mol Cell Biochem* 29:103–128, 1980.

Prockop KJ, Kivirikko KR, Tuderman L, Guzman NA: The biosynthesis of collagen and its disorders. *New Engl J Med* 301:13–23, 77–85, 1979.

Riott IA: *Essential Immunology*, ed 4. Oxford, Blackwell Scientific Publications, 1980.

Romchetti IP, Fornieri E, Baccaroni-Contri M, Volpim D: The ultrastructure of elastin revealed by freeze-fracture electron microscopy. *Micron* 10:89–100, 1979.

Ross R, Bornstein P: The elastic fiber. I. The separation and partial characterization of its macromolecular components. *J Cell Biol* 40:366–381, 1969.

Ross R, Everett NB, Tyler R: Wound healing and fiber formation. V. The origin of the wound fibroblast studied in parabiosis. *J Cell Biol* 44:645–654, 1970.

Schmitt FO, Gross J, Highberger HJ: Tropocollagen and the properties of fibrous collagen. *Exp Cell Res* 3 (suppl.):326–334, 1955.

Slavin BG: The cytophysiology of mammalian adipose cells. *Int Rev Cytol* 33:279–334, 1972.

Smith RE, Horwitz BA: Brown fat and thermogenesis. *Physiol Rev* 49:330, 1969.

Spicer SS, Horn RG, Leppi TJ: Histochemistry of connective tissue mucopolysaccharides. In Wagner BM, Smith DE (ed): *The Connective Tissue*. Baltimore, Williams & Wilkins, 1967, pp 251–303.

Squier CA, Kremerak CR: Myofibroblasts in healing palatal wounds of the beagle dog. *J Anat* 130:585–594, 1980.

Stryer L: Biochemistry, ed 2. San Francisco, W.H. Freeman 1981.

Termine JD, Kleinman HK, Whitsong SW, Conn KM, McGarvesy ML, Martin GR: Osteonectin, a bone-specific protein linking mineral to collagen. *Cell* 26:99–105, 1981.

Weinstock M, Leblond CP: Synthesis, migration, and release of precursor collagen by odontoblasts as visualized by radioautography after [^{3}H] proline administration. *J Cell Biol* 60:92–127, 1974.

Wislocki GB, Bunting H, Dempsey EW: Metachromasia in mammalian tissues and its relationship to mucopolysaccharides. *Am J Anat* 81:1–38, 1947.

Wisse E: Kupffer cell reactions in rat liver under various conditions as observed in the electron microscope. *J Ultrastruct Res* 46:499–520, 1974.

Chapter 6

THE CONNECTIVE TISSUES: CARTILAGE AND BONE

While the adult human connective tissue compartment is differentiated for the most part into the pliable, fluid-rich tissues described in the previous chapter, a nearly equal volume is committed in the embryo and fetus for the differentiation of much more firm supportive structures. The elaboration of the skeletal framework, cartilage and bone, occurs by the patterned and properly proportioned deposition of specific matrix molecules and inorganic salts in specified regions of the compartment. In simplest terms, the various configurations of cartilage and bone can be understood conceptually as extensions of the connective tissue spectrum in those regions where relatively or extremely rigid, yet adaptable, support is required. Obviously, this specialization is best evolved in the larger, most mobile and complex vertebrates.

CARTILAGE

Cartilage, like other regions of the connective tissue compartment, consists of cells, fibers, and ground substance. The last named, however, has physical properties which give to the tissue an elastic firmness, rendering it capable of withstanding a considerable degree of pressure and shear. In some of the lower vertebrates (e.g., elasmobranchs) the whole adult skeleton consists of cartilage, and in the mammals much of the skeleton is first laid down in cartilage. In the adult body, cartilage covers the articular surfaces of bones, and it forms the sole skeletal support of the larynx, trachea, bronchi, and certain other structures.

According to the nature and visibility of the fibrillar elements, cartilage is subdivided into three varieties: (a) *hyaline*, (b) *elastic*, and (c) *fibrous*. Of these, hyaline cartilage is the most widely distributed type.

Hyaline Cartilage

Hyaline cartilage (Figs. 6.1 and 6.2) appears as a bluish white, translucent mass in the fresh condition. It forms the costal cartilages and the cartilages of the nose, larynx, trachea, and bronchi. It is also a major component of the epiphyseal cartilages of growing long bones. In the fetus, nearly all of the skeleton is first laid down as hyaline cartilage and is replaced later by osseous tissue in the formation of the bones.

With the exception of the free surfaces of articular cartilages, hyaline cartilage is always invested by a layer of dense fibrous connective tissue, the *perichondrium* (Fig. 6.1). Hyaline cartilage is composed of cells and an *extracellular matrix* of ground substance and connective tissue fibers.

Cartilage is usually devoid of blood vessels except in areas where vessels may be passing through it to other tissues and in particular zones which are forming ossification centers in intracartilaginous bone development. Exchange of substances between cartilage cells and blood vessels of the perichondrium is mediated by the tissue fluid of the cartilage, i.e., by the bound water which is the dispersion medium of the glycosaminoglycans of the intercellular matrix.

The Cells

The cartilage cells, *chondrocytes*, occupy chambers known as lacunae (Figs. 6.1 to 6.3). The cells appear irregularly shaped and shrunken away from the walls of their

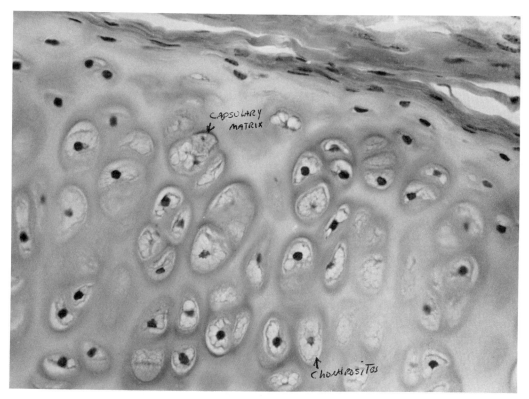

Figure 6.1. Light micrograph of hyaline cartilage from monkey trachea. Perichondrium is seen at the top of the figure (×575).

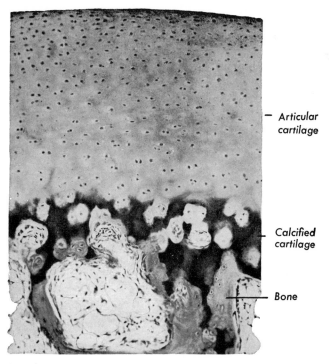

Figure 6.2. Articular cartilage from a metatarsal bone of a rhesus monkey two months old. Photomicrograph (×165).

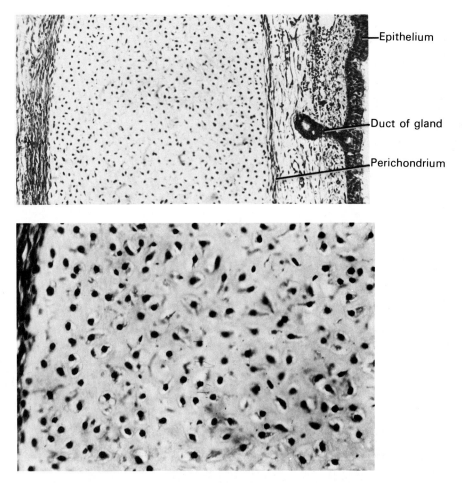

— Epithelium

— Duct of gland

— Perichondrium

Figure 6.3. Light micrographs of hyaline cartilage from the trachea of a five-month-old human fetus. *Upper figure* is at low magnification to cover a relatively large field. Note that the cartilage cells are distributed singly throughout the fetal cartilage, instead of being in groups as they are in later periods (Fig. 6.1). *Lower figure*, a higher magnification of a portion of the field above. Note that the cartilage matrix appears homogeneous and stains uniformly. The irregular shape of the cells is accentuated by the usual shrinkage that occurs during fixation and dehydration for preparing sections. *Upper*, ×146; *lower*, ×390.

lacunae in most light microscope preparations. However, the cells fill the lacunae in fresh preparations, as verified by electron microscopic studies of well-fixed material (Fig. 6.4). Although the cell surface is irregular and has short processes extending into depressions in the matrix, there is no obvious space between the cell and its surrounding matrix. Chondrocyte cytoplasm contains, in addition to glycogen and lipid, the usual characteristics of a secretory cell (see below).

Chondrocytes and their lacunae vary in shape in relation to their position within the cartilage. For example, the subperichondrial cartilage grades almost imperceptibly into the perichondrium (Fig. 6.1) and hence the cells, like nearby fibroblasts, are flat. Deeper within the cartilage, the cells and their lacunae are usually rounded (Figs. 6.1 and 6.2).

Chondrocytes are often arranged in groups which represent the offspring of a parent cartilage cell (Fig. 6.1). Such groups,

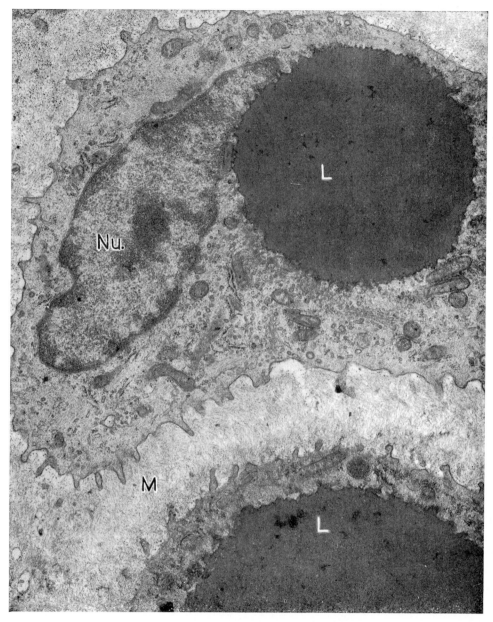

Figure 6.4. Electron micrograph of hyaline cartilage from the trachea of a bat. Portions of two chondrocytes are seen, one with a nucleus (*Nu*). Large lipid droplets (*L*) are often found in the cytoplasm of mature cartilage cells. Note that the cartilage cells have numerous processes extending into the matrix and that the cells fill the lacunae. A fine feltwork of collagen is seen in the matrix (*M*) (×17,000). (Reprinted with permission from Dr. Keith Porter: *Biophys J* 4:1964.)

termed *isogenous groups*, are found particularly in costal and tracheal cartilages. A special arrangement with the isogenous groups aligned in longitudinal rows is seen in intracartilaginous bone formation (Fig. 6.25).

In embryonal cartilage (Fig. 6.3), the cells are randomly distributed and variable in shape. Some have processes and resemble the mesenchymal cells from which they are derived. Intercellular matrix is relatively scant.

The Intercellular Substance

The intercellular substance, or matrix, appears homogeneous in the fresh condition and in most routine histological preparations. However, some areas are more basophilic than others and also more metachromatic after toluidine blue staining. For example, each lacuna is surrounded by a thin layer of substance which is strongly metachromatic and presumably composed chiefly of chondroitin sulfate. Such thin metachromatic *lacunar linings* are sometimes described as *capsules*, although this term is ambiguous because the broad zones of basophilic substance around groups of isogenous cells are more frequently described as capsules.

The apparently homogeneous intercellular substance contains fine collagenous fibrils which are masked by a ground substance of similar refractive index. Although these fibrils can be detected by light microscopy after treatment of the cartilage with trypsin or dilute acids, our knowledge of their structure is based on biochemistry and electron microscopy. They are mostly slender fibrils of only about 10 to 25 nm in width and they usually lack the 64 nm cross banding characteristic of collagen. The fibrils are arranged in a feltwork in most of the matrix, but they become parallel with the surface in the subperichondrial region and gradually blend with the perichondrial fibrils, which are wider and cross-banded (Fig. 6.5). As noted in Chapter 5, the collagen of cartilage differs in chemical nature from that of skin in that it has three α_1-type II polypeptide chains.

The intercellular substance contains proteoglycan complexes containing *chondroitin 4-sulfate* and *chondroitin 6-sulfate*, some *hyaluronic acid*, and some *keratan-sulfate*. The latter is insignificant in amount at birth but increases with age and may reach relatively high levels in senile, degenerate cartilage.

The basophilia of the cartilage matrix in routine hematoxylin and eosin preparations is due to the basophilia of the sulfate dominating the eosinophilia of the collagen. The matrix just outside the lacunar lining is generally quite basophilic and is known as *pericellular matrix*. The region around a cell group is also often more basophilic than the general matrix, and is then named the *capsular* or *territorial* matrix (Fig. 6.1). Intervening regions with less sulfate and more collagen are less basophilic and are known as *interterritorial matrices*.

The ground substance also gives a positive reaction with the periodic acid-Schiff (PAS) technique. Because *pure* chrondroitin sulfate is apparently not PAS-positive, it is assumed that the reaction by the cartilage ground substance is due to an undetermined carbohydrate component. The proteoglycans of the ground substance appear in electron micrographs as electron-dense granules about 10 to 40 nm in diameter. *Membrane-bounded vesicles (matrix vesicles)* of high electron density are present in the matrix of epiphyseal cartilages in regions where calcification is occurring. These vesicles apparently arise from chondroblasts by exocytosis, and they range from about 30 nm to 1 μm in diameter. They contain alkaline phosphatase and are often seen in close association with hydroxyapatite. They apparently indicate sites where initial calcification is occurring (see below).

Development and Growth

As mentioned before, cartilage is a part of the connective tissue spectrum. Like all other connective tissues, it originates within the mesenchymal compartment of the embryo. The blastema of a future intracartilaginous mass is first recognized as an area of mesenchymal cell concentration resulting from cell proliferation and enlargement. The cells in the interior of the precartilage blastema show a marked cytoplasmic basophilia resulting from an increase in rough-surfaced endoplasmic reticulum, and they are known as *chondroblasts*. They form the collagenous fibrils and the ground

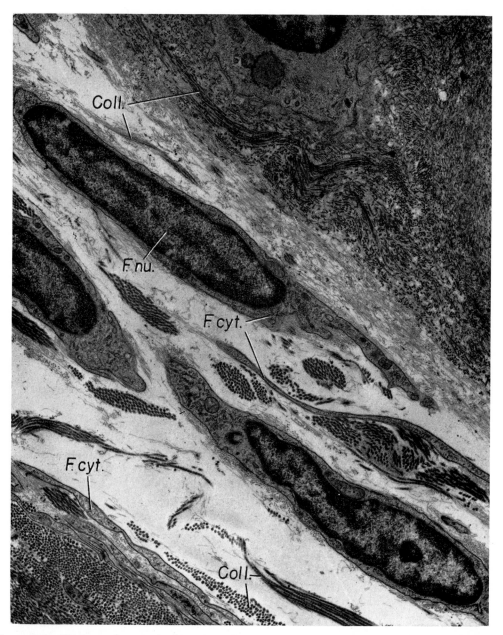

Figure 6.5. Electron micrograph of junction of hyaline cartilage and perichondrium from the trachea of a bat. A portion of a cartilage cell is seen in the *upper part* of the photograph, and portions of several fibroblasts with their nuclei (*F. nu.*) and cytoplasm (*F. cyt.*) are seen in the *lower part* of the figure. Collagen fibers (*Coll.*) are seen in cross and longitudinal sections. Note that the fibrils adjacent to the surfaces of the fibroblasts are generally smaller than the bundles of fibrils found at some distance from the cells (×12,250). (Courtesy of Dr. Keith Porter.)

substance of the matrix. As the cells of the central region continue to form more matrix, they become separated from each other and become the chondrocytes, whereas those of the periphery continue as chondroblasts. The matrix components of cartilage are formed in the usual manner, the proteins being synthesized in rough endoplasmic reticulum and most of the carboyhydrates being added at the Golgi complex prior to secretion. Studies of the pathways for synthesis of glycosaminoglycans indicate that these compounds are formed predominantly in the Golgi complex.

Growth of cartilage takes place in two ways: (*a*) formation of new cartilage by chondroblasts at the surface, known as *appositional growth*, and (*b*) expansion of the internal mass of cartilage by division of chondrocytes and deposition of surrounding matrix, known as *interstitial growth.*

In appositional growth, chondroblasts of the perichondrium multiply, and some form cartilage matrix as described above, whereas others remain as a part of the chondroblast population. In interstitial growth, cartilage cells divide, and the daughter cells may divide again, each isogenous group representing the progeny of a single parent cell. The cells become separated, each surrounded by its own capsule and matrix. The old capsules and the territorial matrices merge into the newly formed territorial matrix. Interstitial growth occurs mainly in young cartilage and gradually ceases, further growth being chiefly appositional (subperichondrial).

Nutrition of Cartilage

Cartilage is devoid of vascular and lymphatic channels; hence, nutrition is entirely by diffusion and imbibition.

Age Changes

The poor nutrition is probably responsible for certain degenerative changes found in old cartilage, especially in cartilages of considerable thickness. The deeper portions of the cartilage show areas, extending through many cell territories, where the homogeneous matrix is replaced by closely packed coarse fibers. Cavity formation resulting from the softening and liquefaction of these areas may ultimately result.

With old age, cartilage loses its translucency and bluish white color and appears yellowish and cloudy. This change is due to a decrease of glycosaminoglycans and an increase in noncollagenous proteins.

Calcification is likewise of common occurrence in old cartilage and is usually associated with degenerative changes of the cartilage cells. Calcification of cartilage is a normal process during bone formation and is described below.

Regeneration and Transplantation

Regeneration of cartilage is a slow process and occurs primarily by activity of the perichondrium. When cartilage is broken or injured, the wound is invaded by the perichondrial connective tissue, which gradually develops into cartilage. This type of regeneration depends on the presence of a perichondrium. Regeneration in part by interstitial growth has been observed, but is doubtless comparatively rare. In many instances of cartilage fracture, the pieces become united by dense fibrous tissue which may partly be replaced by a bony clasp.

A high percentage of cartilage *autografts* survive provided that they contain living cells and receive sufficient nutrition. *Homografts* also survive in a fairly high percentage of cases provided that they contain living cells and receive good nutrition. Grafts of cartilage apparently do not stimulate host antibody production to the extent that other tissue grafts do. The factors responsible for this are not completely understood, but lack of a direct blood supply and the relatively poor permeability of the cartilage matrix to large molecules are undoubtedly involved.

Elastic Cartilage

Elastic cartilage appears more yellow and opaque than hyaline cartilage in the fresh condition because of the large number of elastic fibers in its matrix (Fig. 6.6). These branch and course in all directions to form a dense network of anastomosing and interlacing fibers. In the peripheral layers, the fibers are thin and the network is widemeshed; in the deeper portions, they are thicker and more closely packed. The ground substance also contains collagenous fibrils, particularly in the subperichondrial region.

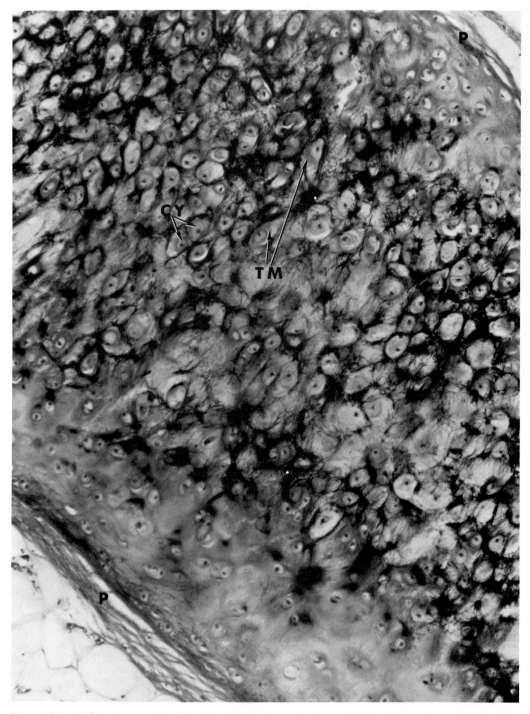

Figure 6.6. Light micrograph of elastic cartilage from human epiglottis. The mature chondrocytes have condensed nuclei and a vesicular cytoplasm (*CY*). They are surrounded by a territorial matrix (*TM*) that is free from prominent elastic fibers. *P*, perichondrium. Verhoeff's elastic stain (×195).

Elastic cartilage develops from a hyaline-like blastema. Elastic fibrils are assembled just peripheral to the cells and traverse the matrix as an elastic network. Growth of the cartilage takes place interstitially and subperichondrially. Calcification of elastic cartilage occurs rarely, if at all.

Elastic cartilage occurs in the external ear, the Eustachian tube, the epiglottis, and some of the laryngeal cartilages.

Fibrous Cartilage

Fibrous cartilage (Fig. 6.7) is a combination of dense collagenous fibers with cartilage cells and a scant cartilage matrix. It is generally not circumscribed by a perichondrium. The relative proportions of cells, fibers, and matrix vary greatly. The cells are frequently in rows, with intervening bundles of type I collagenous fibers that have the characteristic 64 nm cross banding.

Fibrous cartilage is found in considerable amounts in the intervetrebral discs, pubic symphysis, ligamentum teres of the femur, glenoid and cotyloid ligaments, and interarticular cartilages. Because the articular cartilages have numerous fibrils with the 64 nm cross banding, they are classified by some authors as fibrocartilage, even though they have a hyaline-like matrix and other hyaline cartilage characteristics.

The *intervertebral discs* consist largely of fibrocartilage which is continuous above and below with the articular cartilage of the adjacent vertebrae and peripherally with the spinal ligaments. In the center of each disc is a gelatinous ellipsoid mass of variable extent known as the *nucleus pulposus*, a remnant of the embryonic notochord. Its center may contain fluid and cellular debris. Rupture of the disc and herniation of the nucleus pulposus into the spinal canal may be the cause of severe pain and other neurological symptoms.

BONE (OSSEOUS TISSUE)

Osseous tissue is a rigid form of connective tissue and is normally organized into

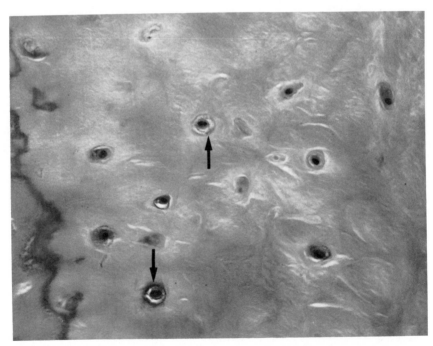

Figure 6.7. Light micrograph of fibrocartilage (*center*) at the attachment site of ligament (*right*) to bone (*left*). The isolated cartilage cells are surrounded by basophilic territorial matrix (*arrows*) (×320).

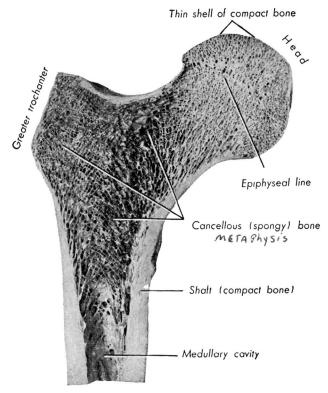

Thin shell of compact bone

Head

Greater trochanter

Epiphyseal line

Cancellous (spongy) bone
META physis

Shaft (compact bone)

Medullary cavity

Figure 6.8. A longitudinal section through the upper end of the femur of an adult male. The epiphyseal line of the great trochanter is not evident. Photograph.

definite structures, the bones. These form the skeleton, serve for the attachment and protection of the soft parts, and, by their attachment to the muscles, act as levers which bring about body motion. Bone is also a storage place for calcium which can be withdrawn when needed to maintain a normal level of calcium in the blood.

Gross Organization of Bone Tissue

Grossly, two types of bone may be distinguished: the *spongy* or *cancellous*, and the *dense* or *compact*. When a long bone is cut longitudinally (Fig. 6.8), it will be seen that the head, or *epiphysis*, has a spongy appearance and consists of slender irregular bone trabeculae, or bars, which anastomose to form a latticework, the interstices of which contain the marrow. The thin outer shell, however, appears dense. As the shaft, or *diaphysis*, is approached, the irregular marrow spaces of the epiphysis become

continuous with the central medullary cavity of the shaft, whose wall is formed by a thick plate of compact bone (Fig. 6.9).

The spongy and compact varieties of bone have the same types of cells and intercellular substance, but they differ from each other in the arrangement of their components and in the ratio of marrow space to bone substance. In spongy bone, the marrow spaces are relatively large and irregularly arranged, and the bone substance is in the form of slender anastomosing trabeculae and pointed spicules. In compact bone, the spaces or channels are narrow and the bone substance is densely packed.

With very few exceptions, the compact and spongy forms are both present in every bone, but the amount and distribution of each type vary considerably. The diaphyses of the long bones consist mainly of compact tissue; only the innermost layer immediately surrounding the medullary cavity is

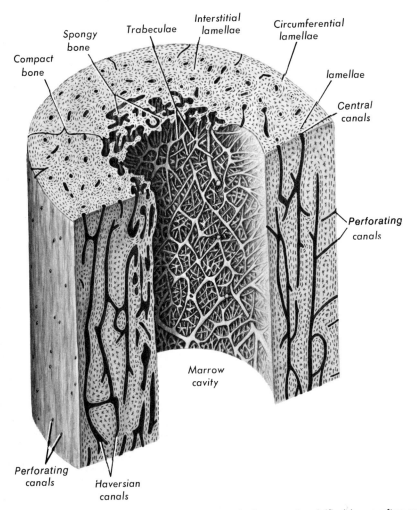

Figure 6.9. Shaft of human humerus. Drawing is made from undecalcified bone after removal of marrow and other organic components by maceration techniques. (From a chart by H. Poll.)

spongy. The tabular bones of the head are composed of two plates of compact bone enclosing marrow space bridged by irregular bars of spongy bone (*diploë*). The epiphyses of the long bones and most of the short bones consist of spongy bone covered by a thin outer shell of compact bone.

Each bone, except at its articular end, is surrounded by a vascular fibroelastic coat, the *periosteum*. The so-called *endosteum*, or inner periosteum of the marrow cavity and marrow spaces, is not a well-demarcated layer. It consists of a variable concentration of medullary reticular connective tissue which contains osteogenic cells that are in immediate contact with the bone tissue.

Organic and Inorganic Components of Bone

Bone is composed of cells and an intercellular matrix of organic and inorganic substances. The organic fraction consists of collagen, glycosaminoglycans, proteoglycans, and glycoproteins. The matrix is acidophilic in stained sections, in contrast to the basophilic reaction of cartilage matrix. This is due to the high content of collagen and the relatively low content of sulfated glycosaminoglycans in bone. The collagen of bone is generally type I.

The inorganic component of bone is responsible for its rigidity and may constitute up to two-thirds of the fat-free dry weight. It is composed chiefly of calcium phosphate and calcium carbonate, with small amounts of magnesium, hydroxide, fluoride, and sulfate. The composition varies with age and with a number of dietary factors. X-ray diffraction studies show that the minerals are present as crystals having an *apatite* pattern or structure. More specifically, they are *hydroxyapatites*.

Microscopic Structure

The microscopic structure of bone can be studied either using slices of dried bone ground sufficiently thin to transmit light (ground bone) or using sections made after decalcification by treatment with dilute acids or chelating agents. Although the slices of dried bone contain only the inorganic material, they show considerable detail (Fig. 6.10). The inorganic substance is also retained after the organic constituents are destroyed by burning with free access of air (calcination), but the inorganic material is then very brittle and useless for the preparation of sections.

A characteristic feature of adult bone tissue is its layered structure, with the cells and fibers organized in *lamellae*. The osseous tissue of long bones, especially in the compact regions, is also chracterized by longitudinal passages or *central canals* (*Haversian canals*) which anastomose with each other by oblique and transverse communications (Fig. 6.9). From the periosteal and endosteal surfaces, somewhat narrower *perforating canals* (*nutrient canals, Volkmann's canals*) pierce the bone obliquely or at right angles to its long axis and communicate with the central canals, thus establishing a continuous and elaborate system which houses the blood vessels and nerves of the bone.

In a cross section of the bone, the central canals are seen to be surrounded by a varying number (8 to 15) of concentric lamellae and accompanying bone cells. The concentric lamellae of intercellular substance, the cells, and the central canal constitute an *osteon* or *Haversian system* (Figs. 6.10 and 6.11). The whole bone does not, however, consist of such concentric systems. In the periphery, the lamellae run parallel with the surface and form a relatively thin outer layer of the bone. These are the outer *circumferential* lamellae (Fig. 6.9). A few similarly arranged inner circumferential lamellae separate the osteons from the marow cavity. Finally, the intervals between the osteons are occupied by more irregular layers of bone, which constitute the *interstitial* lamellae (Fig. 6.10). Adjacent lamellar systems are as a rule delimited from each other by a darkly staining thin layer

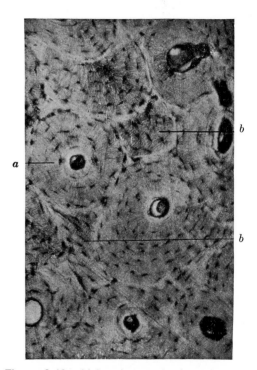

Figure 6.10. Light micrograph of a transverse section from the shaft of an undecalcified, dried long bone. A slab of the dried bone was ground very thin and then mounted in thick balsam. In the spaces within the bone (lacunae, canaliculi, and some of the central canals), air was imprisoned, so that they appear dark. *a*, osteon; *b*, interstitial lamellae.

Haversian system   Partly destroyed
                          Haversian system

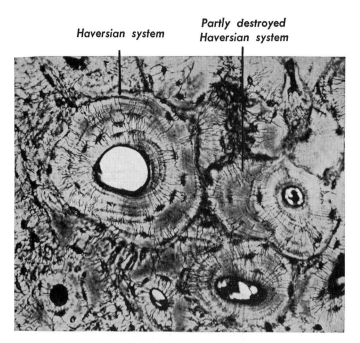

Figure 6.11. Light micrograph of a transverse section through the shaft of the femur of a young adult rhesus monkey. Decalcified 6-μm section. The walls of the lacunae, canaliculi, and central canals are stained with Schmorl's thionin phosphomolybdic acid method (×270).

of modified matrix (cement line, cement "membrane").

Compact bone thus consists of branching and anastomosing concentric tubular lamellae, with intervals filled in by interstitial lamellae, which are covered externally and internally by the more parallel circumferential lamellae. The perforating canals which pierce the bone from its outer and inner surface and become continuous with the central canals are not lined by concentric lamellae.

The bone cells (*osteocytes*) fill the flattened, almond-shaped spaces or lacunae situated between or within the lamellae (Fig. 6.12). Tiny *canaliculi* course across the lamellae and interconnect neighboring lacunae. Cytoplasmic processes of the osteocytes are found within these canaliculi, but neither the cell processes nor their canaliculi can be traced far in routine hematoxylin and eosin-stained sections. However, the canaliculi are readily seen after special stains (Fig. 6.12), and the cell processes can be seen in well-fixed and well-stained sec-

tions of fetal bone. The full extent of the cell processes is more readily appreciated by electron microscopy, which has revealed that the processes of neighboring cells are in contact within the canaliculi by communicating (gap) junctions (Figs. 6.13 and 6.14). Electron micrographs show that the osteocytes and their processes do not rest directly on the mineralized matrix but are separated from the walls of their lacunae and canaliculi by a thin layer. Histochemical studies demonstrate that material in this layer is PAS-positive. It probably serves as an extra medium by which substances can be transported and exchanged between the cells and the blood vessels present in the Haversian canals.

The osteocytes are matured bone-forming cells (*osteoblasts*) which have become imprisoned in the bone as it was deposited. *Osteoprogenitor cells* also persist as an incomplete lining of the central and perforating canals and are present in the endosteum and inner layer of the periosteum. With a stimulus such as is supplied by a fracture

Canaliculi   Haversian canal   Lacuna   Interstitial lamellae

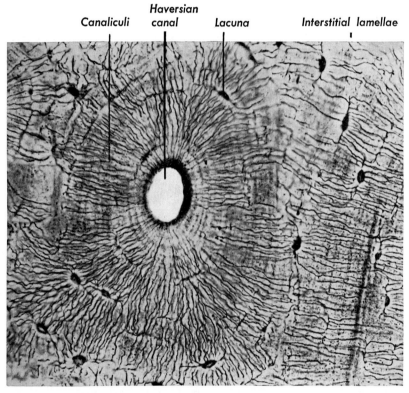

Figure 6.12. Light micrograph of a transverse section through an osteon and adjacent interstitial lamellae. Decalcified bone from the shaft of the femur of a young adult rhesus monkey, 6-μm section. Schmorl's thionin phosphomolybdic acid method ($\times$420).

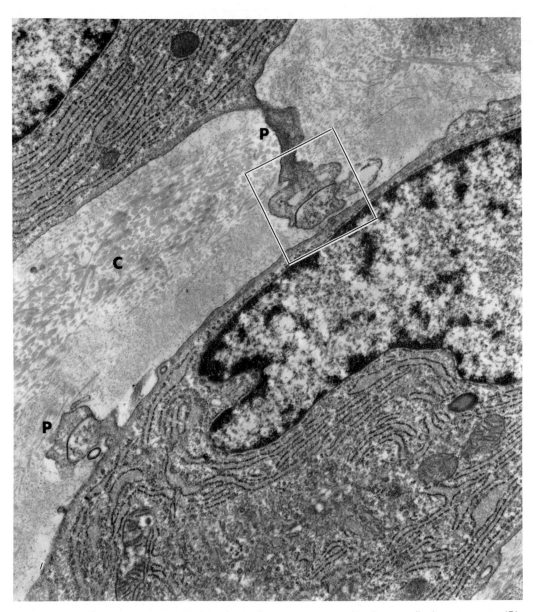

Figure 6.13. Electron micrograph of portions of two osteocytes showing canalicular processes (*P*). The decalcified matrix shows collagenous fibers (*C*) and a more finely textured halo adjacent to the osteocyte surfaces. The rough ER and Golgi zone are prominent in these cells, indicating continued synthetic activity (×23,000). The region in the box is shown at higher magnification in Figure 6.14. (Courtesy of Dr. Carol Itatani.)

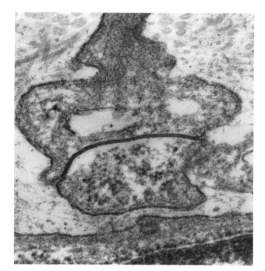

Figure 6.14. Higher magnification of the gap junction joining osteocyte processes included in the outlined square in Figure 6.13 (×54,000). (Courtesy of Dr. Carol Itatani.)

or physiological stress, they differentiate into osteoblasts, the active bone-forming cells.

When the collagenous fibrils are studied in preparations in which precautions have been taken to prevent collagenous swelling, the fibrils are found in delicate fascicles coursing parallel with one another within a single lamella. They follow a helical course in each lamella, with differences in slope and direction in alternate lamellae. This is apparently the reason why transverse sections of osteons show the concentric lamellae alternately striated and punctuated. In the former, the fibrils are coursing circularly at the level of the section and are cut lengthwise. In the punctuated lamellae, the fibrils are parallel to the long axis of the Haversian system at the level of the section and are cut across.

Besides the lamellar fibrils, there are found within the outer layers of the bone the coarser, *perforating fibers* of Sharpey (Fig. 6.15). These are continuations of the periosteal fibers that pierce the bone obliquely or at right angles to its long axis. They consist of collagenous or fibroelastic bundles with uncalcified or only partly calcified matrix. Purely elastic perforating fibers are also found. Perforating fibers extend into the outer circumferential and interstitial lamellae but do not penetrate the osteons. They are especially numerous in places where ligaments and tendons are inserted, and they serve for firmer anchorage of these structures.

Spongy bone shows the same lamellar structure but differs from compact bone in the more irregular arrangement of the lamellae in trabeculae and spicules, and in the presence of relatively few osteons.

Nonlamellar (Woven) Bone

Although the bone of all vertebrates consists of collagen, ground substance, calcium salts, and a permeating system of spaces occupied by cells and their processes, different samples of bone differ in the manner in which their constituents are combined. Thus, the skeletons of fish, amphibians, and birds differ from each other and from those of mammals, and the bone of man shows marked structural changes during ontogenesis. The human embryonic skeleton consists of coarsely bundled *woven*

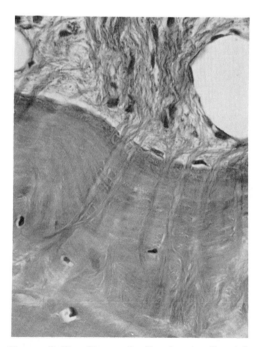

Figure 6.15. Sharpey's fibers extending into decalcified bone (*bottom*) from the periosteum. Note the continuity of the collagenous fibers with those of the periosteum (*top*) (×540).

bone; i.e., the collagenous fibers are in coarse bundles and are irregularly woven or plaited, and the lacunae are irregularly dispersed. Stratified or *lamellar bone,* i.e., with fibrils oriented similarly in any given stratum and in different directions in alternating lamellae, gradually replaces woven bone, beginning before birth and continuing until only traces of woven bone persist in the adult (for example, in tooth sockets, bony sutures, osseous labyrinth, and regions of tendon-bone attachment). The first bone formed during repair of fractures is of the woven type.

Development and Growth of Bone

According to the embryological origin, there are two types of bone development, *intramembranous* and *intracartilaginous* or *endochondral.* In intramembranous bone formation, the bone develops within a layer of connective tissue. It does not involve the removal and replacement of cartilage. In endochondral bone formation, cartilage forms a framework for bone deposition, and the cartilage is eventually totally replaced

by bone. The development of the flat bones of the skull involves only the intramembranous type of bone formation (Figs. 6.16 to 6.19). The development of the bones of the base of the skull, of the face, and of the axial skeleton involves both types of bone formation: the bone around a cartilage precursor (subperiosteal bone) is formed by the intramembranous type, and the bone which directly replaces the cartilage is formed by the endochondral method. It should be kept in mind, however, that *the fundamental process of bone deposition is the same in both types.* In intracartilaginous bone formation, there is simply the additional feature of the presence of a cartilage model and its partial removal preparatory to the deposition of the bone.

Cell Types in Osteogenesis

One can identify different types of cells in sites of bone formation as follows: (*a*) *osteogenic* or *osteoprogenitor cells,* (*b*) *osteoblasts,* (*c*) *osteocytes,* and (*d*) *osteoclasts.* Because the cells of a given type have similar characteristics regardless of whether

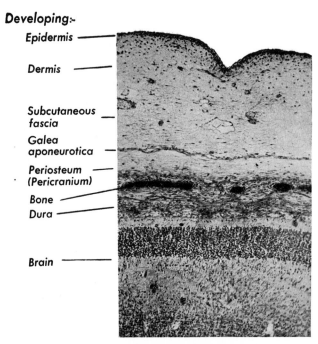

Developing:-
Epidermis ———
Dermis ———
Subcutaneous fascia ——
Galea aponeurotica ——
Periosteum (Pericranium) ——
Bone ——
Dura ——
Brain ———

Figure 6.16. Light micrograph showing the first appearance of bone in the parietal region of the developing skull. Human embryo of about 2½ months (×60).

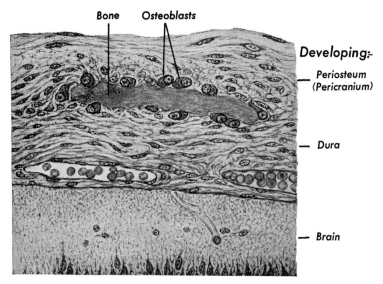

Figure 6.17. One of the spicules of developing bone. Parietal region of the skull of a human embryo of about 2½ months. Camera lucida drawing (×420).

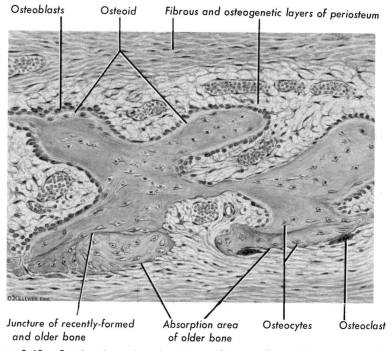

Figure 6.18. Section through parietal bone of human fetus of three months (×115).

they are found in intramembranous or intracartilaginous bone-forming regions, the cytological features of the cell types are described before the topographical aspects of bone formation.

Osteogenic or Osteoprogenitor Cells

In regions of the embryonic mesenchymal compartment where bone formation is beginning and in areas near the surfaces of

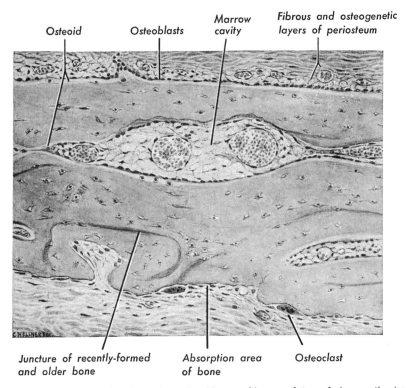

Osteoid   Osteoblasts   Marrow cavity   Fibrous and osteogenetic layers of periosteum

Juncture of recently-formed and older bone   Absorption area of bone   Osteoclast

Figure 6.19.   Vertical section through parietal bone of human fetus of six months (×115).

growing bones, one finds irregularly shaped and somewhat elongated cells which have pale-staining cytoplasm and pale-staining nuclei. They differ structurally only slightly from the mesenchymal cells from which they have arisen. They are identified chiefly by their location and by their association with osteoblasts. They multiply by mitosis, and some of them change into osteoblasts, which change later into osteocytes. Although it was once thought that mature osteocytes were capable of reverting to osteogenic cells under appropriate conditions, current evidence does not support that claim. It now seems established that osteoblasts and osteocytes are no longer mitotic and that a population of osteogenic cells persists throughout life. The osteogenic cells occur in the inner portion of the periosteum and in the endosteum of mature bone.

Osteoblasts

These cells are generally larger than the osteoprogenitor cells, and they have a more rounded nucleus, a more prominent nucleolus, and cytoplasm which is much more basophilic (Fig. 6.17). The nucleus is often toward one side of the cell, and close to it, one can frequently see a clear zone which is the negative image of the enlarged Golgi complex. Electron micrographs disclose numerous mitochondria, a well developed rough endoplasmic reticulum (Fig. 6.20), an active Golgi complex with numerous vesicles, and microtubules. The cells have microvillous processes during early development, and some of these elongate and remain as protoplasmic processes within the canaliculi as the matrix increases in amount. The processes of both osteoblasts and osteocytes contain 5- to 6-nm diameter microfilaments which course parallel with the long axes of the processes (Fig. 6.14).

The basophilia of the osteoblasts is due to the abundance of rough endoplasmic reticulum. It has been shown by studies in which labeled precursors are used, that the osteoblasts secrete the organic components of the matrix, i.e., the collagen fibers and

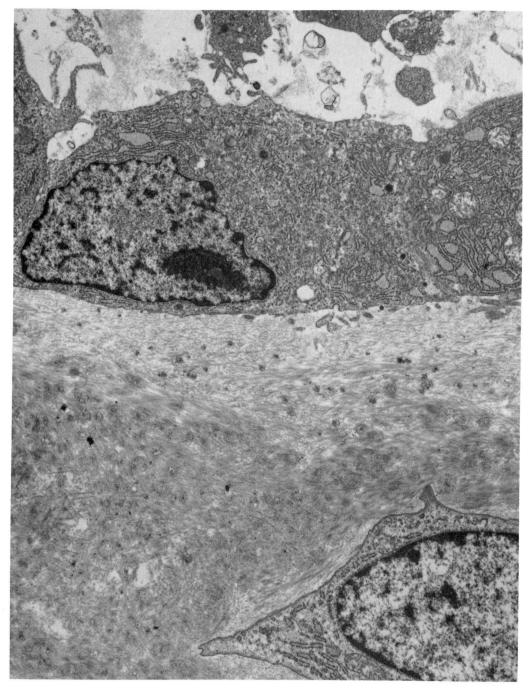

Figure 6.20. Electron micrograph of decalcified developing bone showing osteoblasts at the surface (*top*) and part of an osteocyte embedded in the matrix (*bottom*). Note the layer of less dense matrix near the osteoblasts. This is presumed to be osteoid (×8800). (Courtesy of Dr. Carol Itatani.)

the glycosaminoglycans. From histochemical studies it is known that the cytoplasm of osteoblasts also contains considerable alkaline phosphatase. Although the exact role of this enzyme in calcification is not understood, there is evidence that it is important in controlling the deposition of calcium. It is known, for example, that calcification continues in growing long bones of animals after the cells have been killed, provided that alkaline phosphatase is added to the solutions in which the bone is kept.

The formation of bone in unusual regions of the adult body (*ectopic* bone formation), as in the walls of sclerotic arteries, calcified foci in the lungs, and connective tissue adjoining transplants of transitional epithelium in experimental animals, is difficult to harmonize with the view that bone formation can only be accomplished by differentiated osteogenic (osteoprogenitor) cells. The most commonly accepted explanation for metaplastic bone formation is that either fibroblasts or persisting primitive mesenchymal cells lying in close association with blood vessels (*pericytes*) can differentiate into osteoprogenitor cells under altered environmental conditions.

Osteocytes

These cells are described above under "Microscopic Structure." It has been pointed out that they arise from osteoblasts by differentiation. Their synthetic activity is less than that of osteoblasts but they are by no means inactive cells. The presence of living osteocytes is essential for the maintenance of the organic matrix of bone and they may also play an important role in control of normal levels of blood calcium. Bone calcium is resorbed under the stimulation of elevated *parathyroid* hormone (PTH) and some investigators believe that osteocytes are involved in this activity through *osteolysis.* The preponderance of current evidence does not support this view, however, as osteocytes do not appear to secrete products that could be responsible for degradation of matrix components.

Osteoclasts

On the surfaces of bones where resorption is occurring, one frequently finds large, multinucleated giant cells known as osteoclasts (Figs. 6.18, and 6.21). They are often found in depressions in the bone referred to as *Howship's lacunae.*

The number of nuclei in osteoclasts varies greatly. The cytoplasm has a foamlike or vacuolated appearance and gives a variable staining reaction. It is less basophilic than the osteoblast cytoplasm and, in some cells, particularly in the older ones, it becomes slightly acidophilic. Electron micrographs show a paucity of granular endoplasmic reticulum, but reveal clusters of free ribosomes. The mitochondria are relatively short and they are most numerous in the cytoplasm facing the bone. There are multiple paired centrioles corresponding to the number of nuclei and also numerous Golgi complexes. Vacuoles of various sizes are abundant, as are lysosomes. The surface of the osteoclast facing toward the bone being resorbed has numerous cytoplasmic processes and microvilli, described as a *ruffled border* (Fig. 6.21).

The fact that osteoclasts are often present in depressions where bone is being resorbed supports the view that they have an important role in the process. There is an increase in number and activity of osteoclasts when *calcium resorption* is stimulated by intravascular injection of *PTH.* Conversely, osteoclastic activity is suppressed by injection of *calcitonin,* a hormone produced by *parafollicular* cells of the thyroid gland. These hormones also affect urinary excretion of electrolytes, including phosphates, which in turn affect the level of blood calcium. Bone represents the primary storage site for calcium in the body, so fluctuations in blood calcium are smoothed out by alternate deposition and resorption of calcium in bone. The maintenance of a constant level of calcium ions in the blood and interstitial fluids of the body is crucial for normal cellular function and is kown as *calcium homeostasis.*

The origin of osteoclasts has been controversial, but recent experiments have shown conclusively that these cells arise from blood-borne monocytic cells. When an irradiated animal incapable of forming osteoclasts was parabiosed with a normal littermate, the irradiated animal regained the ability to form osteoclasts. If the donor animal had been injected with tritiated thy-

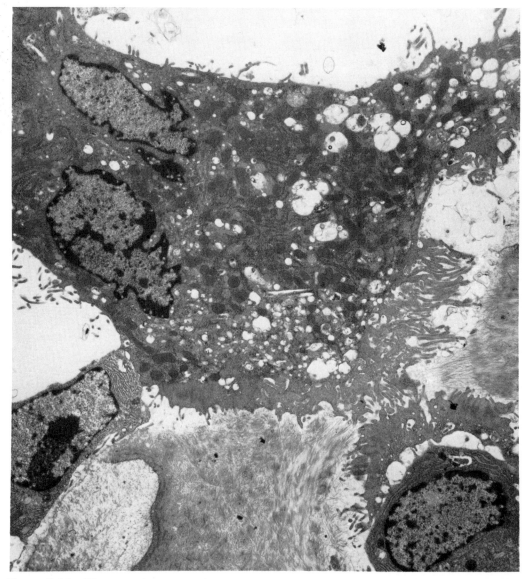

Figure 6.21. Electron micrograph of an osteoclast at the surface of decalcified bone (×6000). (Courtesy of Dr. Carol Itatani.)

midine to label monocytes, the nuclei of the rejuvenated osteoclasts contained the label.

Studies with labeled thymidine also show that there is a turnover of nuclei in osteoclasts. Some of the older nuclei become pyknotic and are extruded from the cell, whereas new nuclei are added by fusion of new monocytic cells with the osteoclasts.

In the clinical condition known as *osteopetrosis*, bone is not resorbed normally. The defect involves abnormal osteoclasts. This condition can now be alleviated by providing a source of normal monocytes through bone marrow grafting or injection of histocompatible normal monocytes.

In regions of cartilage resorption, as in stages of endochondral bone development, there are multinucleated cells with the same characteristics as osteoclasts. They appear to be formed in the same manner as osteoclasts but because they are associated with cartilage, they are known as *chondroclasts*.

Intramembranous Bone Formation

Because the development of the flat bones of the skull involves only intramembranous bone formation, it is an excellent place to study the structural features of the deposition of osseous tissue uncomplicated by changes in cartilage. In the locations where bone is to be laid down, the mesenchyme becomes richly vascularized, and active proliferation of the mesenchymal cells takes place. Within the primitive connective tissue bed, some of the cells show structural changes which enable one to identify them as osteoprogenitor cells and osteoblasts.

Between the enlarged osteoblasts, an acidophilic ground substance appears. It masks the fibrils which were already present in the embryonal connective tissue, as well as those that are subsequently formed by the osteoblasts. The intercellular substance, or matrix, which thus is composed of a clear ground substance and collagenous fibrils, is usually not calcified at first and is soft and easily cut. It is given the name *osteoid* (resembling bone) and it is the organic part of bone matrix without appreciable inorganic constituent. As the deposition of the matrix progresses, the osteoblasts, with their processes, are imprisoned by matrix being deposited around them; lacunae and canaliculi are thus formed. Because processes of adjoining cells make contact with each other, the canaliculi of adjoining lacunae connect with each other. New osteoblasts, arising by differentiation of osteoprogenitor cells, maintain a layer of bone-forming cells at the surface of the newly formed bone. The osteoprogenitor cells multiply by mitosis, and they probably continue to increase for a certain embryonic period by differentiation of undifferentiated neighboring mesenchymal cells.

Calcification of bone is dependent upon (*a*) the availability of adequate amounts of minerals, particularly phosphorous and calcium, at the region to be calcified and (*b*) requisite chemical and physical conditions within the calcification site. The minerals are present in the blood and are carried to the calcification site, where calcium and phosphate ions are present in metastable solution under normal conditions.

In the process of calcification, minerals are deposited as minute crystals of hydroxyapatite. This process is initiated by a "seeding" phenomenon. Two forms of seeding have been described. In one it is accomplished by the fibrils of type I collagen. Electron micrographs show that the microcrystals of hydroxyapatite appear first on the surface of the collagen in association with the visible 64-nm periodicity. In the second mode of seeding, matrix vesicles similar to those described for calcifying cartilage are involved. The vesicles arise from osteoblasts and are membrane-bounded. The matrix of these vesicles contains calcium and phosphate which precipitates as a minute crystal of hydroxyapatite. This in turn serves as a nidus for continued mineral deposition. The matrix vesicle mode of mineral seeding appears to be limited primarily to embryonic and ectopic bone formation and is not prevalent in the remodeling of adult bone.

In some disease states, such as *rickets*, the body lacks an adequate amount of vitamin D, which is essential for absorption and maintenance of the minerals at an appropriate level in the blood. In this condition, collagen and glycosaminoglycans continue to form and the increase of uncalcified osteoid at the growing ends of long bones give abnormal shapes. The lack of sufficient minerals leads to decreased rigidity.

The local factors responsible for calcification are controlled by the cells in the ossification center. Although many of the details remain obscure, there is evidence on some of the requisites. It is noted in Chapter 5 that collagen can be dissolved and reconstituted in vitro, either in its native form or in other types. When different types of reconstituted collagen are exposed in vitro to metastable solutions of calcium phosphate, calcification occurs only in the 64 nm periodicity type. In other words, a "precise stereochemical configuration" is necessary for the initiation of calcification. This raises the question why calcification does not occur in all 64 nm periodicity collagen in the body. Further studies have shown that reconstituted collagen from tendon, which does not calcify in the body, does calcify in metastable solutions of calcium phosphate in vitro, provided that components of the associated ground substance are removed. Apparently, certain glycosaminoglycans and glycoproteins associated with collagen have a role in inhibiting and regulating calcification.

Scurvy is a disease state related to local changes in the calcification site. In this condition, the diet is deficient in vitamin C, which is essential for osteoblasts to form collagen capable of normal cross-linkage. The collagen which is formed can become mineralized, but its abnormality affects skeletal growth and maintenance and retards healing of fractures.

Further Growth and Resorption of Intramembranous Bone

Osteogenic cells around the foci of newly formed intramembranous bone continue to multiply and change into osteoblasts and osteocytes. By this process, irregular plates and trabeculae are formed. These enclose spaces (primary marrow spaces) which contain blood vessels, reticular cells, and primitive marrow cells (Fig. 6.19).

During early development of intramembranous bone, osseous tissue is deposited in both the inner and outer surfaces of the flat bones of the skull and also on their peripheral margins. Deposition in the latter area increases the surface area of the bone and also accompanies an enlargement of the cranial cavity to accommodate the growth of the brain. A further increase in the cranial cavity is achieved by resorption along the inner surface, a process which begins relatively early. Continued growth involves new bone deposition, primarily on the outer and marginal surfaces, and resorption, chiefly along the inner surface. However, new bone formation is not entirely absent from the inner surfaces; *the processes of formation and resorption accompany each other in the constant remodeling of bone.*

Intracartilaginous (Endochondral) Bone Formation

In this form of ossification, an embryonal type of hyaline cartilage precedes the formation of bone, and the shape of the bone corresponds more or less closely to that of the prior cartilage. However, it must be realized that the initial cartilaginous model of the bone-to-be is minute in comparison to the eventual mass of the bone. During development, the cartilage is replaced by bone, except at the joint surfaces. This replacement is not completely accomplished, however, until the bone has achieved its full size and growth has ceased.

During the replacement of the cartilage by bone, not only does the supporting function have to be maintained but there is a continual increase in length and diameter as well.

Stages in Intracartilaginous Bone Formation

The first indication of beginning ossification in the cartilaginous model of a long bone is seen near the center of the future shaft, the diaphyseal or *primary ossification center* (Fig. 6.22). The cartilage cells proliferate and hypertrophy, and their lacunae correspondingly increase in number and size. The matrix between the lacunae becomes reduced in amount and forms but thin partitions. These, except for the cartilage capsules, then become calcified. Such calcified cartilage is not to be confused with mineralized bone. The inorganic salts are similar but the organic matrix is quite different. The calcified cartilage is much more basophilic than the normal cartilage at either end of the ossification center.

At about the time that these intracartilaginous changes are clearly evident, the perichondrium assumes an osteogenic func-

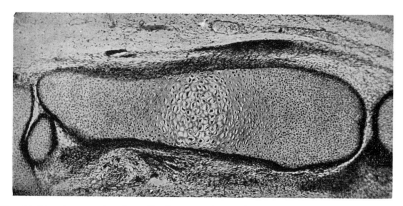

Figure 6.22. Light micrograph of cartilaginous anlage of metacarpal bone of 4-cm human fetus, showing changes in the central portion preparatory to ossification. The bone collar is beginning to form (×90).

tion. Some of the cells of the inner part of the perichondrium change into *osteogenic cells* and, in turn, into *osteoblasts*, which deposit a perforated *bony ring* or *collar* around the cartilage of the ossification center. This bone collar is thin-walled and short at first but becomes progressively thicker-walled and longer as the ossification progresses. It is closely adherent to the cartilage and forms a splint that assists in maintaining the strength of the shaft, which has been weakened by the dissolution of part of the cartilage. It is formed by an intramembranous type of bone development. The perichondrium which surrounded the cartilage has, in this region of ossification, become a periosteum.

Vascular connective tissue from the periosteum, known as *periosteal buds*, grows through apertures in the bone collar and enters the periphery of the changed cartilage matrix (Fig. 6.23). It contains blood vessels and osteogenic cells from the periosteum. These penetrate the thin-walled partitions between the hypertrophied cartilage lacunae and thus form cavities, the *primary marrow spaces*. The osteogenic cells multiply by mitosis, and some of them transform into osteoblasts around the periphery of the calcified cartilage remnants.

The hypertrophied cartilage cells of endochondral bone-forming centers become increasingly abnormal and eventually degenerate. Early experiments with isotope labeling suggested that some of the cartilage cells survive and become chondroclasts and osteoblasts. This has not been confirmed in more recent studies. The degree to which partially differentiated cartilage and bone cells may be capable of interconversion is not fully known. It is reported that cartilage cells derived from neonatal mesenchymal cells grown in vitro in association with bone matrix transform into bone cells after subsequent transplantation into isogenic host animals. This type of dedifferentiation and transition into a new type of tissue cell is known as *metaplasia*.

The primitive marrow cavity of developing endochondral bone regularly contains remnants of calcified cartilage matrix on which osteogenic cells align themselves and differentiate into osteoblasts. Thus, the calcified cartilage becomes enclosed first by osteoid and then by mineralized bone. The initial trabeculae of cartilage and bone thus formed is subsequently resorbed as the marrow cavity enlarges during bone growth. Hence, the initial trabeculae of cartilage and bone serve only as a temporary framework (Figs. 6.24 to 6.26).

The extension of the zone of ossification toward the ends of the cartilage model is accomplished by an orderly sequence of changes in the cartilage similar to those which took place in the formation of the primary ossification center. However, the changes show a more distinct zonal ar-

Periosteal bud   Primitive
marrow cavity   Bone collar

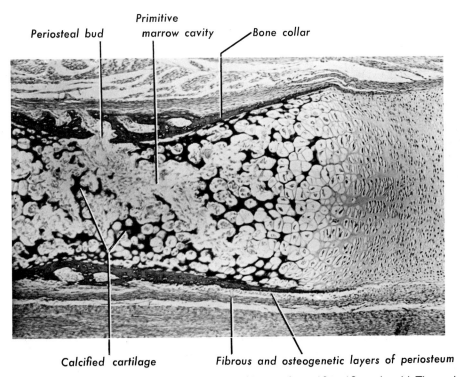

Calcified cartilage   Fibrous and osteogenetic layers of periosteum

Figure 6.23. Light micrograph of metacarpal bone of human fetus 10 to 12 weeks old. The periosteal bud is only one of several, as shown by an examination of serial sections. The primary marrow cavity is quite extensive. The zones of cell and lacunar enlargement and of cell multiplication are evident. Only a small amount of reserve cartilage has been included in the figure (×120).

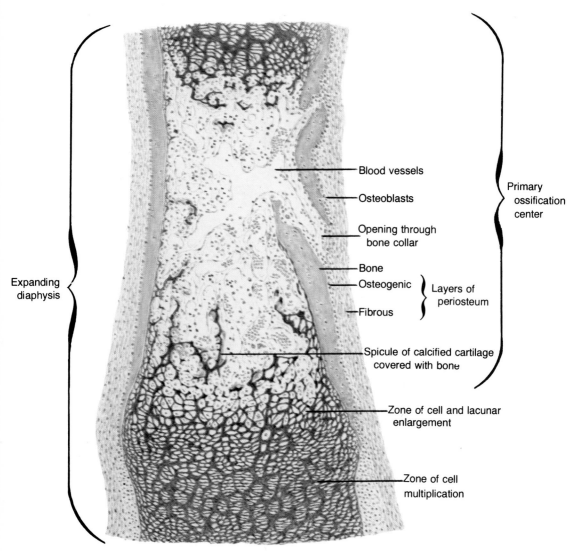

Figure 6.24.   Longitudinal section of middle phalanx of finger of a human embryo of about four months. Hematoxylin and eosin-azure II (×80).

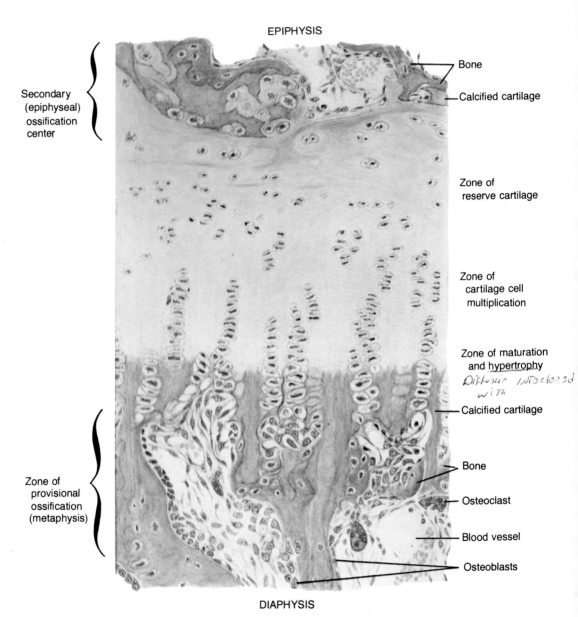

EPIPHYSIS

Secondary (epiphyseal) ossification center

Bone

Calcified cartilage

Zone of reserve cartilage

Zone of cartilage cell multiplication

Zone of maturation and hypertrophy

Calcified cartilage

Zone of provisional ossification (metaphysis)

Bone

Osteoclast

Blood vessel

Osteoblasts

DIAPHYSIS

Figure 6.25. Longitudinal section through the distal end of a metatarsal of a rhesus monkey two months of age. The epiphyseal (secondary) ossification center is well formed. Bone formation is taking place both at the epiphyseal and the diaphyseal surfaces of the epiphyseal plate and is particularly pronounced on the diaphyseal side. Delafield's hematoxylin and eosin (×280).

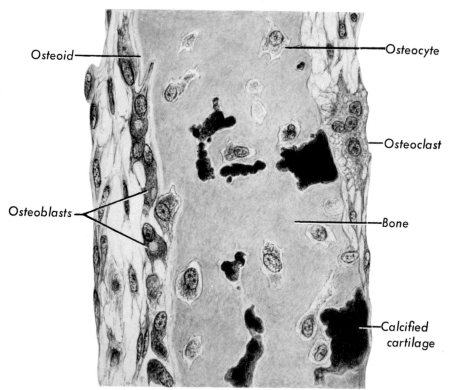

Figure 6.26. Section of a trabecula in developing endochondral bone. Tibia of human fetus about 3½ months old. Azure II-eosin stain (×950).

rangement (Fig. 6.25), and the whole process of bony replacement proceeds as a wave of osteogenic activity toward the extremities of the eventual bone.

Several zones can be distinguished in the cartilage. Beginning at the ends of the cartilage and passing toward the ossification center, these zones, which overlap each other somewhat, are as follows:

Zone of Reserve Cartilage

This zone is relatively long prior to the formation of the secondary (epiphyseal) centers of ossification which develop in some parts of the skeleton at about the time of birth. After the secondary centers form, the zone of reserve (or resting) cartilage becomes relatively short (Fig. 6.25).The cells are randomly arranged and the growth of the zone is relatively slow.

Zone of Cell Proliferation or
Multiplication

In this zone the cells are more or less aligned in rows which course parallel with the long axis of the growing bone. The lacunae containing the daughter cells are broad but flattened, as are the cells, their long axes being perpendicular to the longitudinal axis of the cartilage. By divisions of cartilage cells and their distribution in rows, the length of the cartilage is increased more than is its diameter as new matrix is formed.

Zone of Cell Maturation and Hypertrophy

In this zone there is no further multiplication of the cells, but they mature and enlarge. This increases still further the length of the cartilage of this region. The cytoplasm of the cells contains considerable amounts of glycogen and alkaline phosphatase at this stage. Poor preservation of glycogen in routine preparations for light microscopy is partly responsible for the vacuolated and lightly stained appearance of the cytoplasm seen in the hypertrophied cartilage cells. The cartilage between adjacent cells within a row, previously small in amount, becomes even thinner.

Zone of Cartilage Calcification

This is a zone of variable length, but is always narrow. The matrix between adjacent lacunae within a row has practically disappeared and the matrix between the rows begins to calcify. The mechanism of calcification in the cartilage matrix has been the subject of much investigation and debate. Recent evidence suggests that prior to their degeneration, hypertrophied chondrocytes release membrane-enclosed vesicles (*matrix vesicles*) containing calcium ions into the surrounding cartilage matrix. These tiny vesicles and their contained calcium are thought to serve as nucleation sites for the calcification process. The mechanism by which the large amounts of additional calcium necessary to complete the calcification are made available selectively to the nucleation sites remains unclear.

Zone of Cartilage Removal and Bone Deposition (Zone of Provisional Ossification)

In the outer part of this zone, the thin partitions between the lacunae within a row undergo dissolution. This is accompanied by death of the cartilage cells and is apparently aided by an erosive action that is associated with the blood vessels that grow in from the marrow cavity. Longitudinal canals, filled with vessels and marrow, are thus formed in tunnels surrounded by calcified cartilage matrix. There are considerable numbers of chondroclasts in this area. Farther toward the marrow cavity, the calcified cartilage matrix between the newly formed tunnels becomes reduced in amount by resorption, but remnants of calcified cartilage matrix persist; upon these, osteoblasts deposit lamellae of bone (Figs. 6.24 to 6.26). All of the cartilage remnants and their bony coverings are subsequently resorbed as the marrow cavity enlarges. Osteoclasts and chondroclasts remain prominent and are involved with the resorption.

The region where the diaphysis joins the epiphysis, i.e., where the calcified cartilage is being first reinforced and then replaced by bone, is known as the *metaphysis*. This includes the region described above as the zone of cartilage removal and bone deposition.

The overall region of newly formed bone is known as the *spongiosa* on the basis of its spongy appearance. This is subdivided into *primary spongiosa* (equivalent to the zone of provisional ossification) and *secondary spongiosa*. The former is a relatively short region beginning just below the level where the hypertrophic cartilage cells disappear; it is characterized by marrow spaces of fairly uniform width. The secondary spongiosa is a relatively long region with wide and irregularly contoured marrow spaces extending toward the center of the diaphysis.

While these changes within the cartilage are taking place, the bone collar is increasing in length and in diameter by the deposition of new bone by the osteoblasts of the periosteum. The marrow cavity also increases in size, not only by its longitudinal extension as a result of cartilage removal, but also in diameter, owing to resorption of the inner part of the bone collar or splint. These processes continue as development proceeds. The zone of reserve cartilage is maintained by continued cell division, as outlined above.

At about the time of birth, additional ossification centers (epiphyseal or *secondary ossification centers*) appear in each end of the long bones. The cartilage in these centers passes through the same changes as seen in the diaphysis. The proliferation of the cartilage cells leads to nearly equal growth in all directions, however. The cartilage cells, each of which is enclosed in a lacuna, are arranged in irregularly shaped nests and not in rows, and the partitions between the nests run in various directions. As in the diaphysis, the center is invaded by osteogenic buds, and cartilage removal and bone deposition take place. Bone trabeculae, however, remain in the epiphyseal cavity, giving it grossly a spongy appearance, and the cartilage forming the articular surface persists, anchored to and supported by the underlying bone (Fig. 6.27).

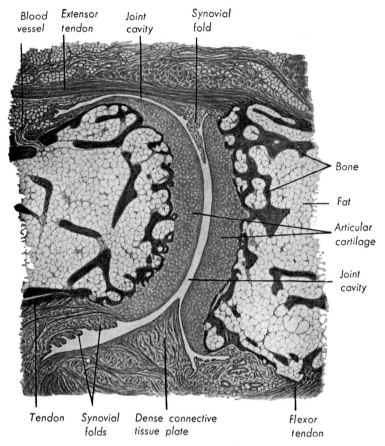

Blood vessel   Extensor tendon   Joint cavity   Synovial fold

Bone

Fat

Articular cartilage

Joint cavity

Tendon   Synovial folds   Dense connective tissue plate   Flexor tendon

Figure 6.27.   Median sagittal section through the joint between the middle and terminal phalanges of middle toe. Human, 10 years of age. The terminal phalanx is at the *right* (×14).

The diaphysis continues its growth in length long after the epiphyseal centers appear. The cartilage plate which separates the primary and secondary ossification centers is called the *epiphyseal plate* (Fig. 6.25).

Eventually, the epiphyseal plate is replaced by bone development on both of its faces (epiphyseal and diaphyseal). At this time, growth of a bone ceases and the diaphysis is bound to the epiphysis by a bony union. The zone of this union is visible in the adult. It is called the *epiphyseal line.*

Osteons

During the growth of the skeleton, some of the spongy bone becomes transformed into compact bone. In this process, lamellae of bone are deposited progressively inward on the surface of the cavities in the spongy bone until they are reduced to narrow canals. Each canal is traversed by blood vessels which originally were in the large cavity. The system of concentric lamellae with its canal and blood vessels forms an osteon (Haversian system).

The osteons of the shafts of long bones are formed by a more complicated process than that described above for transformation in areas of cancellous bone. The first step in the formation of osteons in compact bone is the erosion of tunnels in it by vascular sprouts and osteoclasts from the medullary and periosteal surfaces. The tunnels thus formed (Howship's lacunae) have irregular, roughened surfaces but are of a fairly uniform diameter. When the absorption phase leading to the formation of the tunnel has been completed, osteoblasts arise from the osteogenic cells in the vascular sprouts. They come to lie next to the walls of the tunnel and deposit concentric lamellae of bone characteristic of an osteon. The lamellae are laid down progressively inward until only a narrow canal containing blood vessels is left, the central canal. Parts of the original circumferential lamellae remain between the osteons. However, new generations of osteons keep forming throughout life, although at a reduced rate in later years. In this process, parts of osteons formed earlier, as well as additional parts of the original circumferential lamellae, are sequentially destroyed. Stages in the destruction of bone and its replacement by newer osteons are illustrated in Figure 6.28. The osteons have an important function in providing channels for blood vessels through compact bone. They also provide better structural support and presumably make the bone less brittle.

Because bone serves as a storehouse for calcium and phosphate, the rate of bone resorption increases whenever either of these essential elements tends to fall below a normal blood level. This leads to changes in osteons and in the trabeculae at the ends of the long bones. The minerals are not withdrawn independently; both minerals and matrix are withdrawn simultaneously. Destruction of bone can be produced by the experimental administration of parathyroid extract or by a tumor of the parathyroid gland. The latter usually causes pronounced resorption of bone and its replacement by connective tissue (von Recklinghausen's disease).

It has been pointed out that perforating fibers of Sharpey do not enter the osteons. An understanding of the developmental process will make the reason for this clear. Perforating fibers of Sharpey do not grow into bone. Rather they are radially or obliquely directed fibers which have been imprisoned by the advancing deposition of subperiosteal bone in much the same way that a branch of a tree becomes more and more enclosed in the expanding trunk. When a vascular sprout forms a tunnel

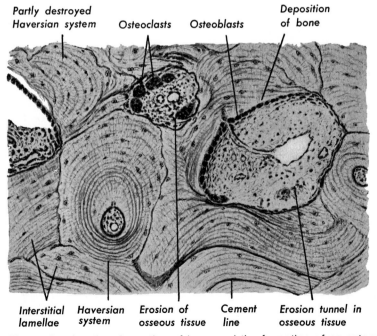

Figure 6.28. Figure showing the absorption of bone and the formation of an osteon in compact osseous tissue. Proximal phalanx of the thumb of a child 6 years old (×150). (After Petersen.)

preceding the deposition of an osteon, the perforating fibers of Sharpey as well as the bone substance are resorbed, and because of their method of formation the perforating fibers are not replaced.

Development of Short Bones

The development of the short bones is similar to that of the epiphyses of long bones. Ossification begins in the center of the cartilage and extends in all directions in the wake of the growing cartilage. Near the end of growth, the endochondral bone is invested with a thin compact layer of subperiosteal bone, except at the articular surfaces which remain cartilaginous.

Remodeling of Bone

Although bone is dense, hard, and rigid, it is able to change somewhat in shape and amount in response to environmental conditions. These changes are not brought about by a remodeling, such as might be done with a plastic wax, but involve the formation of new bone and the removal of bone already formed or the combination of both processes. This capacity to change in shape is well illustrated by the moving of improperly aligned teeth by the orthodontist and by the spontaneous movement of neighboring teeth after a tooth is extracted. The bony socket is resorbed ahead of the tooth undergoing movement, and the shape and size of the socket maintained by the formation of new bone in back of the tooth. In other situations, as, for instance, in increased muscular development, bone may be remodeled to meet the additional stresses imposed upon it. In old age, resorption of the surfaces of some bones occurs. The changes in bone are slower and less pronounced in the adult than during the period of growth, but they occur to some degree throughout life.

Healing of Fractures

A fracture, like any traumatic injury, causes hemorrhage and tissue destruction. The first reparative changes thus are characteristic of those occurring in any injury of soft tissue. Proliferating fibroblasts and capillary sprouts grow into the blood clot and injured area, thus forming granulation tissue. The area also is invaded by polymorphonuclear leukocytes and later by macrophages which phagocytize the tissue debris. The granulation tissue gradually becomes denser, and in parts of it, cartilage is formed. This newly formed connective tissue and cartilage is designated as a *callus*. It serves temporarily in stabilizing and binding together the fractured bone.

As this process is taking place, the dormant osteogenic cells of the periosteum enlarge and become active osteoblasts. On the outside of the fractured bone, at first at some distance from the fracture, osseous tissue is deposited. This formation of new bone continues toward the fractured ends of the bone and finally forms a sheathlike layer of bone over the fibrocartilaginous callus. As the bone increases in amount, osteogenic buds invade the fibrous and cartilaginous callus and replace it with a bony one. In the replacement of the fibrocartilaginous callus, the cartilage undergoes calcification and absorption, as described in "Intracartilaginous Bone Formation." Typical intramembranous bone formation also takes place. The newly formed bone is at first a spongy and not a compact type. It becomes transformed into a compact type, and the callus becomes reduced in diameter. At the time when this subperiosteal bone formation is taking palce, bone also forms in the marrow cavity. The medullary bone growing centripetally from each side of the fracture unites, thus aiding the bony union. The process of repair is, in general, an orderly process, but it varies greatly with the displacement of the fractured ends of the bone and the degree of trauma inflicted. Uneven or protruding surfaces are gradually removed, and the healed bone, especially in young individuals, assumes its original contour.

The Periosteum and Endosteum

The *periosteum* is a fibrous connective tissue investment of the bones, except at their articular surfaces. Its adherence to the bone varies in different places and at different ages. In the young bone, it is easily stripped off. In the adult bone, it is more firmly adherent and especially so at the insertion of tendons and ligaments, where more periosteal fibers penetrate into the bone as the perforating fibers of Sharpey.

The periosteum consists of two layers, the outer of which is composed of coarse, fibrous connective tissue containing few cells but numerous blood vessels and nerves. The inner layer is less vascular but more cellular and contains many elastic fibers. During growth, an osteogenic layer of primitive connective tissue forms the inner layer of the periosteum. In the adult, this is represented only by a row of scattered, flattened cells closely applied to the bone.

The periosteum serves as a supporting bed for the blood vessels and nerves going to the bone and for the anchorage of tendons and ligaments. Its importance for bone regeneration has been a much disputed topic. If the osteogenic layer is considered a part of the periosteum, the latter undoubtedly furnishes osteoblasts for growth and repair. However, the fibrous periosteum of the adult is itself a differentiated end product of the osteogenic layer, and it probably plays no direct part in bone repair but acts as an important limiting layer controlling and restricting the extent of bone formation.

Because both the periosteum and its contained bone are regions of the connective tissue compartment, they are not separated from each other or from other connective tissues by basal laminar material or basement membranes.

The *endosteum* lines the surface of cavities within a bone (marrow cavity and central canals) and also the surfaces of trabeculae in the marrow cavity. In growing bone, it consists of a delicate stratum of myelogenous reticular connective tissue, beneath which is a layer of osteoblasts. In the adult, the osteogenic cells become flattened and are indistinguishable as a separate layer. They are capable of transforming into os-

teogenic cells when there is a stimulus to bone formation, as after a fracture.

Marrow

Marrow is a soft connective tissue which occupies the medullary cavity of the long bones, the larger central canals, and all of the spaces between the trabeculae of spongy bone. It consists of a delicate reticular connective tissue, in the meshes of which lie various kinds of cells.

Two varieties of marrow are recognized: *red* and *yellow*.

Red marrow (Figs. 6.29, 6.30, and 13.2) is the only type found in fetal and young bones, but in the adult it is restricted to the vertebrae, sternum, ribs, cranial bones, and epiphyses of long bones. It is the chief site for the genesis of blood cells in the adult body. The architecture of red marrow is discussed below under "Blood Vessels and Nerves," and the cells of marrow are described under "Blood Development," Chapter 13.

Yellow marrow consists in the main of fat cells (Fig. 6.27) which have gradually replaced the other marrow elements. Under certain conditions, the yellow marrow of old or emaciated persons loses most of its fat and assumes a reddish color and gelatinous consistency. It is then known as *gelatinous marrow*. With an adequate stimulus, yellow marrow may resume the character of red marrow and play an active part in the process of blood development.

Blood Vessels and Nerves

Bone is richly supplied with blood vessels which pass into it from the periosteum. Near the center of the shaft of a long bone, a canal passes obliquely through the compact bone. This is known as the *medullary* or *nutrient* canal, and its external opening is known as the *nutrient foramen*. A medullary artery courses through this canal to the marrow cavity. In its passage through the compact bone, it communicates by branches with the blood vessels of the osteons. On reaching the marrow cavity, the artery divides into ascending and descending branches which supply all portions of

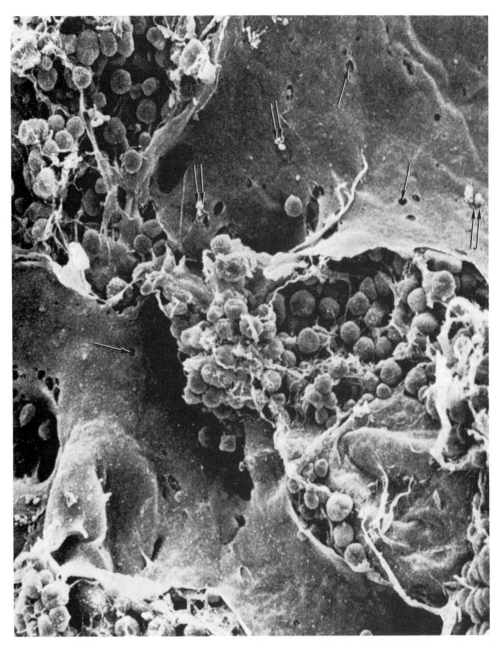

Figure 6.29. Scanning electron micrograph of rabbit bone marrow showing sinusoids and interstitial tissue. The walls of the sinusoids have fenestrations (*single arrows*). Some of the fenestrations have processes of underlying phagocytic cells extending through them (*double arrows*) (×1000). (Courtesy of Dr. Masayuki Miyoshi.)

the marrow. The terminal branches of the arterioles connect with *sinusoids*, which differ from capillaries by their larger diameter and by their close association with phagocytic cells. There are fenestrations in the walls of the sinuoids (Figs. 6.29 and 6.30), and the basal lamina is thin and incomplete. Consequently, the sinusoids are more permeable than are ordinary capillaries.

The sinusoids are drained by narrow and thin-walled veins which have no valves.

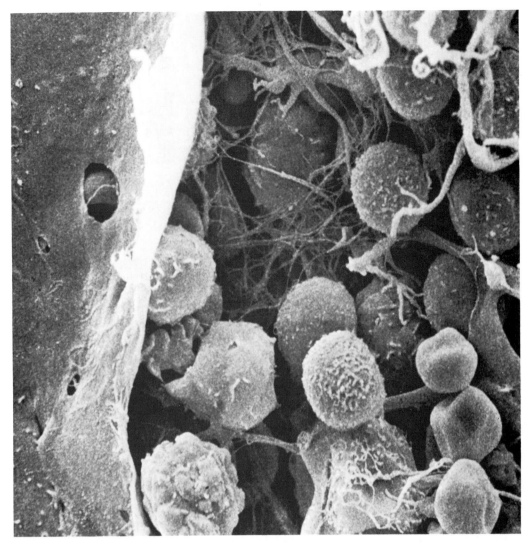

Figure 6.30. Scanning electron micrograph of rabbit bone marrow showing part of a sinusoid (*left*) and some of the reticular tissue framework filled with hemopoietic, migratory, and phagocytic elements (×4200). (Courtesy of Dr. Masayuki Miyoshi.)

The larger medullary veins pass through the medullary canal accompanying the medullary artery and, like the latter, communicate by branches with the veins of the osteons.

Besides the medullary canals, the bone is everywhere pierced by the perforating canals, which serve for transmission of the numerous smaller vessels. In compact bone, these vessels give rise to a network of branches which run in the osteons. In spongy bone, the network lies in the marrow spaces. Branches from these vessels pass to the marrow cavity and there break up into a sinusoidal network which anastomoses freely with that formed by the branches of the medullary artery.

Lymphatics with distinct walls are present in the outer layer of the periosteum. Cleftlike lymph capillaries lined with endothelium accompany the blood vessels in the perforating canals and osteons. The amorphous material which surrounds the osteocytes and cytoplasmic processes in the lacunae and canaliculi serves for the exchange of substances between the cells and blood vessels and as a pathway for lymph.

Both myelinated and nonmyelinated nerves accompany the vessels from the periosteum through the perforating canals into the osteons and marrow cavities. Periosteum is highly sensitive to painful stimuli, whereas osseous tissue is relatively insensitive.

Joints (Articulations)

Two main types of connections between bones are distinguished: (*a*) union without an articular cleft (*synarthrosis*), the joint being immovable or only slightly movable; (*b*) connection of bones with an articular cleft (*diarthrosis*, movable joint, Fig. 6.27).

Synarthrosis

In *synarthrosis*, union may be by ligaments or dense fibrous tissue (*syndesmosis*) or by means of cartilage (*synchrondrosis*).

In *syndesmosis*, the connecting ligaments may be fibrous or elastic. Of the latter type are the ligamenta subflava which unite the vertebral arches. In the immovable articulations of the cranial bones (*sutures*), short fibers (which are, in the main, continuations of the fibers of Sharpey) unite the serrated edges of adjacent bones.

In *synchondrosis*, the cartilage is usually of the fibrous form, except nearest the bone, where it is hyaline (see under "Cartilage"). The intervertebral discs are examples of synchondrosis and consist of a fibrocartilaginous ring surrounding a central gelatinoid mass, the nucleus pulposus.

Diarthrosis

In *diarthrosis*, the bones are separated by an articular cleft (synovial cavity) and are more or less freely movable. The following structures must be considered: (*a*) the articular cartilage, (*b*) the interarticular cartilages, or *menisci*, and glenoid ligaments, and (*c*) the joint capsule.

The *articular cartilage* (Figs. 6.2 and 6.27) covers the ends of the bones and is usually of the hyaline variety, being the remains of the original cartilage in which the bones

were formed. No perichondrium is present. The most superficial cartilage cells are flattened and arranged in rows parallel with the surface. In the deeper portion, the cells are rounded and arranged in typical groups. The deepest layer, firmly apposed to the bone, is calcified.

In the acromioclavicular, sternoclavicular, and costovertebral articulations, the cartilage is of the fibrous form. The same is true of the cartilage covering the head of the ulna, whereas the surface of the radius which enters into the wrist joints is covered not by cartilage but by dense fibrous tissue.

Articular cartilage, like cartilage elsewhere, is devoid of blood vessels. Metabolic exchange is made by diffusion through the ground substance of the cartilage to and from (*a*) synovial fluid, (*b*) capillaries in the periosteum around the periphery, and (*c*) vessels in the underlying bone. Exchange is chiefly with the synovial fluid.

The *interarticular cartilages* and labra glenoidea serve to deepen the sockets for the articular ends; they usually consist of fibrous cartilage.

The *joint capsule* consists of two strata: an outer dense *fibrous layer*, which blends with the ligaments and periosteum of the articulating bones, and an inner layer, the *synovial membrane*, which lines the joint cavity, with the exception of the surfaces of the articular cartilages. Prominent infoldings of the synovial membranes are known as *synovial folds* (Fig. 6.27) and more slender projections are known as *synovial villi.*

The synovial membrane consists of an inner layer composed chiefly of cells and an outer layer of variable types of irregularly arranged connective tissue. On the basis of structural variations, the synovial membranes have been classified as fibrous, areolar, and adipose types. In the fibrous type (e.g., over tendons), a thin cellular layer rests on connective tissue fibers that are intimately blended with the fibrous capsule. The adipose type is found over intraarticular fat pads. The areolar type allows mobility of the synovial membrane over the fibrous capsule. Its outer layer contains irregularly arranged collagenous and elastic fibers plus the usual connective tissue cells, including mast cells and macrophages. Its inner cellular layer is thicker than that of the other types and consists of two to four layers of irregularly arranged cells that are usually described as fibroblasts. Electron micrographs show that the cells have numerous cytoplasmic processes, particularly at the adluminal cell surfaces. No basal lamina is seen between the surface cells and the underlying tissue.

The *synovial fluid, synovia,* is apparently secreted by the synovial cells. It is a viscid, mucoalbuminous fluid, rich in hyaluronic acid. It acts as a lubricating fluid, facilitating the smooth gliding of the articular surfaces.

The larger blood vessels of the joint capsule lie in the outer layer of the stratum synoviale, from which smaller vessels and capillaries pass to the inner layer and to some of the villi. The inner layer is richly and the outer layer more poorly supplied with lymph capillaries. Nonmyelinated nerve fibers are found in the connective tissue, some of them ending in end bulbs and Pacinian corpuscles.

References

Anderson HC: Vesicles associated with calcification in the matrix of epiphyseal cartilage. *J Cell Biol* 41:59–72, 1969.

Brighton CT, Sugioka Y, Hunt RM: Cytoplasmic structures of epiphyseal plate chondrocyte. *J Bone Joint Surg* 55A:771–784, 1973.

Cameron DA, Paschall HA, Robinson RA: Changes in the fine structure of bone cells after the administration of parathyroid extract. *J Cell Biol* 33:1–14, 1967.

Clark SM, Iball J: The x-ray crystal analysis of bone. *Progr Biophys* 7:226–252, 1957.

Clarke IC: Articular cartilage: a review and scanning electron microscope study. II. The territorial fibrillar architecture. *J Anat* 118:261–280, 1974.

Eyre DR: Collagen: molecular diversity in the body's protein scaffold. *Science* 207:1315–1322, 1980.

Glimcher MJ: The role of the macromolecular aggregation state and reactivity of collagen in calcification. In Edds MV, Jr (ed): *Macromolecular Complexes*. New York, Ronald Press, 1961, pp 53–84.

Godman GC, Lane N: On the site of sulfation in the chondrocyte. *J Cell Biol* 21:353–366, 1964.

Gomori G: Calcification and phosphatase. *Am J Pathol* 19:197–210, 1943.

Ham AW, Harris WR: Repair and transplantation of bone. In Bourne GH (ed): *The Biochemistry and Physiology of Bone*, vol 3. New York, Academic Press, 1972, pp 338–397.

Holtrop ME: The ultrastructure of the epiphyseal plate. II. The hypertrophic chondrocyte. *Calcified Tissue Res* 9:140–151, 1972.

Jotenau FV, Le Dourin NM: The developmental relationship between osteocytes and osteoclasts: a study using quail-chick nuclear marker in endochondral ossification. *Dev Biol* 63:253–265, 1978.

Leblond CP, Weinstock M: Radioautographic studies of bone formation. In Bourne GH (ed): *The Biochemistry and Physiology of Bone*, vol 3. New York, Academic Press, 1972, pp 181–198.

Matukas VJ, Panner BG, and Orbison JL: Studies of ultrastructural identification and distribution of protein-polysaccharide in cartilage matrix. *J Cell Biol* 32:365–375, 1967.

McLean FC, Urist MR: *Bone: Fundamentals of the Physiology of Skeletal Tissue*, ed 3. Chicago, University of Chicago Press, 1968.

Nogami H, Urist MR: Substrata prepared from bone matrix for chondrogenesis in tissue culture. *J Cell Biol* 62:510–519, 1974.

Petersen H: Die Organe des Skelet-systems. In von Möllendorff (ed): *Handbuch der Mikroskopische Anatomie des Menschen*, vol 2, part 2. Berlin, Springer-Verlag, 1930, pp 521–676.

Ramagen W: The bone cell system; form and function. (a review). *Beit Pathol* 150:1–10, 1973.

Rasmussen H, Bordier P: *The Physiological and Cellular Basis of Metabolic Bone Disease*. Baltimore, Williams & Wilkins, 1974.

Revel JP, Hay ED: An autoradiographic and electron microscopic study of collagen synthesis in differentiating cartilage. *Z Zellforsch* 61:110–144, 1963.

Salomon CD: A fine structural study on the extracellular activity of alkaline phosphatase and its role in calcification. *Calcified Tissue Res* 15:201–212, 1974.

Sognnaes RF (ed): Calcification in Biological Systems. A. A. A. S. Publication No. 64, Washington, D.C., 1960.

Termine JD, Kleinman HK, Whitson SW, Conn KM, McGarvey ML, Martin GR: Osteonectin, a bone-specific protein linking mineral to collagen. *Cell* 26:99–105, 1981.

Vaughn J: *The Physiology of Bone*, ed 3. Oxford, Clarendon Press, 1981.

Walker DG: Bone resorption restored in osteopetrosic mice by transplanting normal bone marrow and spleen cells. *Science* 190:784–785, 1979.

Weniger JM, Holtrop ME: An ultrastructural study of bone cells: the occurrence of microtubules, microfilaments and tight junctions. *Calcified Tissue Res* 14:15–29, 1974.

Chapter 7

BLOOD AND LYMPH

During embryonic development, certain areas of the mesenchymal tissues form irregular enclosed spaces and become lined by endothelial cells (see Chapter 3). These initial vessels coalesce, eventually forming a complex tubular network of vascular passageways—the blood and lymph circulatory systems. The endothelial lining of this network is a continuous one, serving not only the venous and arterial vessels but also the lymphatic channels and the chambers of the heart. Within the network the blood and lymph circulate, but it should be realized that the fluids of both blood and lymph also percolate through the connective tissues as interstitial fluid. Basically, fluid components of the blood leak out of certain vascular passages (the capillaries and venules) to supply the interstitial fluid. It is recirculated to the blood via uptake into venules and lymphatic channels. The detailed structure of vascular and lymphatic channels is discussed in Chapter 12.

Blood may be considered as a specialized connective tissue consisting of free cells and a fluid intercellular *plasma*. Both genetically and structurally, blood is related to the connective tissues. The blood cells develop in the reticular connective tissues of blood-forming organs and enter the bloodstream in a fully formed condition. Although functioning erythrocytes are limited to the bloodstream, the white or colorless corpuscles function in the loose connective tissues and use the bloodstream merely as a vehicle of transportation.

Because the structural components of mammalian blood are not all true cells, they are sometimes designated as the *formed elements*. They include the red cells (*erythrocytes*), the white cells (*leukocytes*), and the *platelets*. The total quantity of blood (formed elements and plasma) constitutes about 8% of the body weight. There are 5 to 6 liters of blood in a person weighing 150 pounds.

Blood may be studied under the microscope in the living animal by placing a mesentery or web of a frog's foot under a microscope. In small vessels, the blood flow is sufficiently slow that the individual corpuscles can be distinguished floating in clear plasma. More detailed observations on living blood cells can be made by placing a fresh drop of blood on a slide beneath a coverslip for studies with the oil immersion objective. By adding relatively nontoxic dyes such as neutral red to a drop of blood, i.e., by the use of *supravital staining*, one can readily study the reactions of the living cells.

In most of the methods commonly used in clinical work, the blood cells are observed in the nonliving state because they are exposed to special techniques for providing particular kinds of information. To determine what percentage of total blood consists of formed elements, the blood is centrifuged in a graduated tube—the percentage of formed elements is known as the *hematocrit*.

To determine the number of erythrocytes per cubic millimeter of blood, a special pipette is used to dilute a known quantity of blood by a known amount of isotonic fluid, and a drop of the mixture is placed in the chamber of a *hemocytometer* slide. The bottom of the counting chamber is ruled in fine squares and is at a known depth beneath the cover slip. Because the cubic dimension of the space over each square is known, one can readily calculate the total number of erythrocytes per cubic millimeter from a count of the erythrocytes lying over a given number of ruled squares. This is known as the *total erythrocyte count*, and is of particular importance in studies of different types of anemia. The *total leukocyte count* is done by a similar method, although less dilution is needed for making the observations in the counting chamber because the leukocytes are not as concentrated in whole blood as are erythrocytes. In hospital hematology laboratories where large numbers of blood counts are being performed routinely, electronic counting devices are used to speed the process.

To determine the relative proportions of leukocytes, dried blood smears are stained with particular types of compound dyes (e.g., Wright's stain) to differentiate neutrophilic, eosinophilic, and basophilic components of the cells. Details on this technique are given in the discussion of the morphology of the formed elements. The determination of different leukocyte percentages by this method is known as the *differential count*. Since differential counts require recognition of each cell individually, automatic counting is not possible.

The stains which are commonly used for blood cells consist of mixtures of acidic and basic dyes. The development of this procedure stems from the works of Ehrlich published over the period from 1879 to 1898. He noted that the cytoplasmic granules of some leukocytes bind the acidic component of a mixed dye, whereas those of other leukocytes bind the basic component, and those of a third group bind both components of the dye. Hence, he described the leukocytes as acidophilic, basophilic, and neutrophilic.

Romanovsky (1891) used a mixture of methylene blue and eosin to demonstrate the nucleus of the malarial parasite, which had not been seen before. It soon became evident that this combination gave superior results for blood cells, and most of the stains currently used for blood smears are modifications of the Romanovsky stain. The best known modifications are those of Giemsa and Wright.

The basic dyes used in the preparation of Wright's stain are methylene blue and polychromed (oxidized) methylene blue consisting of methylene azure and methylene violet. When solutions of the basic dyes are added to a solution of the acidic dye eosin, a precipitate is formed. The precipitate is dissolved in acetone-free methyl alcohol and, in usage, the alcoholic solution is placed on the slide and water is added during the staining. The alcoholic solution fixes, or preserves, the cells, and the dilution by water permits dissociation of the dye for differential staining. The dye will eventually precipitate in water, but staining should be completed before this occurs.

In Wright's stained blood smears, the erythrocytes are usually colored buff or orange-pink with eosin, the nuclei of leukocytes are stained metachromatically with methylene azure, and the cytoplasm of lymphocytes and monocytes is stained blue with methylene blue. The cytoplasmic granules of basophils have an affinity for methylene blue and are metachromatic also, whereas the granules of eosinophils have an affinity for the acidic dye. The explanation for the staining of the neutrophilic granules is not understood as clearly. The cells originally received their name because it was thought that their granules stained with the neutral dye. In the case of Wright's stain, the neutral dye is an eosinate of methylene azure. It is likely that most of this is rapidly dissociated when the dye is diluted with water. The larger granules of the neutrophils in man usually show a lavender color after Wright's stain, probably from methylene azure and methylene violet.

BLOOD PLASMA

The plasma is a histologically homogeneous, slightly alkaline fluid. Chemically, it contains globulins, albumins, and inorganic salts, chiefly the chloride, bicarbonate, and phosphate of sodium. Calcium is present in a remarkably constant quantity (1 mg/10 cc of blood). The plasma constitutes 55% of the total quantity of blood and the formed elements constitute 45%; i.e., 45 is the hematocrit value for normal blood. The proportions are altered in a number of pathological conditions: e.g., in microcytic anemia there is a reduction in size and number of erythrocytes, which lowers the hematocrit value.

When blood is exposed to the air or when blood vessels are injured, *fibrinogen*, one of the plasma proteins is converted to *fibrin* which forms a network of delicate filaments, leaving a clear yellowish fluid, the *serum*. The blood cells become entangled in the fibrin network and a clot is formed. The clot acts as a plug, preventing further hemorrhage. A clot may, however, become of great danger to the individual if it is torn off by the bloodstream and circulates in the blood vessels (embolus), in which case it may block the blood supply of vital organs.

The plasma mediates the transport of nutritive substances derived from the alimentary canal, the waste substances from the tissues, and the secretions of the various endocrine glands. Even the oxygen which is bound by the red blood cells is first dissolved in the plasma before reaching the cells. The plasma differs from the tissue fluids by the greater constancy of its protein constitutents.

RED BLOOD CELLS (ERYTHROCYTES)

The red blood corpuscles, or erythrocytes, are highly differentiated and specialized for the function of transporting oxygen. In the lower vertebrates, the erythrocyte is a nucleated cell, but in man and all other mammals it is unique in that it normally loses its nucleus, Golgi apparatus, centrioles, endoplasmic reticulum, and most of its mitochondria during the process of maturation before entering the bloodstream as a functional element. When fresh preparations of blood are examined under the microscope, it is seen that the individual red corpuscles have a greenish yellow color (Fig. 7.1*C*); en masse they give the red color characteristic of blood. In dried smears they are acidophilic and stain orange or pink in Wright's stain.

The erythrocytes are biconcave discs. When observed on its flat surface, the cell has a circular outline and the central depression appears as a lighter or darker area, depending on the focus.

Erythrocytes average about 7.7 μm in diameter and 1.9 μm in greatest thickness in dried smears. They are slightly smaller in the living state (about 7.2 μm) and smaller in sections (about 6.5 to 7.0 μm). Although slight variations in size are not uncommon, forms showing marked variations (1 to 2 μm above or below the normal diameter) are relatively rare in normal blood. Large erythrocytes are commonly found in some types of anemia (e.g., pernicious anemia) and are known as macrocytes or megalocytes. Small forms are characteristically present in some other types of anemia (e.g., iron deficiency anemia) and are known as microcytes.

The erythrocytes readily change their shape, as may be seen when they squeeze through the narrowest capillaries or pass around the bend of a branching vessel. They also tend to adhere to each other along their concave surfaces, forming rows or *rouleaux* like stacked coins. Although the cause of this phenomenon is not entirely clear, it is usually explained as the result of surface tension. Rouleaux formation is a transient phenomenon which is not to be confused with "sludging" of erythrocytes. Sludging refers to a clumping of red corpuscles after severe trauma. As a result of burns of the skin and other types of trauma, there is a leakage of fluid from the blood vessels into the surrounding tissue. The trauma may also produce a generalized reaction, in that sludges may circulate and block small vessels in other parts of the body.

The most important component of the erythrocyte cytoplasm is *hemoglobin*. Hemoglobin has the remarkable property of binding oxygen in a very loose combination (*oxyhemoglobin*). The hemoglobin becomes saturated with oxygen in the capillaries of the lung, and the circulating blood distributes this oxygen to the cells of the body in

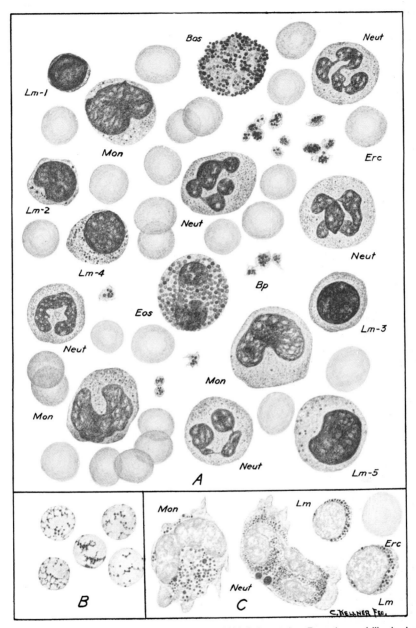

Figure 7.1. *A*, cells from normal human blood. Wright's stain. *Bas*, basophilic leukocyte; *Bp*, aggregations of blood platelets; *Eos*, eosinophilic leukocyte; *Erc*, erythrocytes; *Lm-1* to *5*, lymphocytes: *1* to *3* are small and medium sizes and *4* and *5* are the less numerous larger forms; *Mon*, monocytes; *Neut*, neutrophilic leukocytes. *B*, reticulocytes from normal human blood stained with dilute cresyl blue. *C*, blood cells as seen after about 20 min of staining with neutral red and Janus green B in a supravital preparation. *Erc*, erythrocyte; *Lm*, small lymphocytes with bluish green mitochondria and a few neutral red granules; *Mon*, monocyte with mitochondria and numerous neutral red granules and vacuoles of varying size; *Neut*, neutrophilic leukocytes with staining of the neutrophilic granules and the formation of a few large vacuoles, which frequently appear after 15 to 20 min of staining. All figures ×1550.

exchange for carbonic acid which constantly accumulates as a waste product of metabolism in the tissues. Oxygen is not yielded directly by the corpuscle to the cells, but is first dissolved in the plasma at a level held constant by the erythrocytes.

The contents of the corpuscle are in osmotic equilibrium with the plasma. Normal plasma is said to be *isosmotic* or *isotonic*. Isotonic solutions may be prepared for study of the corpuscles outside the body; a 0.85% solution of sodium chloride is approximately isotonic for mammalian blood. When *hypertonic* solutions are added to blood, the erythrocytes become shrunken and irregular in surface contour. In this configuration they are referred to as *crenated*. The membranes of the corpuscles are permeable to water and impermeable to sodium and potassium ions, and therefore water passes from the corpuscles to restore partially osmotic equilibrium between the corpuscles and the surrounding medium whenever the latter is hypertonic. A few crenated corpuscles are usually found in fresh preparations of blood studied without the addition of hypertonic solutions; this results from evaporation, which produces a slightly hypertonic solution and an altered pH. It should be added that crenation has also been produced experimentally in isotonic media and may not be entirely dependent on osmotic phenomena.

When blood is placed in distilled water or any *hypotonic* solution, water enters the corpuscles and they assume a spheroidal shape. The corpuscles lose their color by the escape of hemoglobin into the diluted plasma, and the colorless part which remains is known as the *stroma*, "blood shadow," or "ghost." Eventually, the ghosts may also undergo solution. The process of extraction of hemoglobin is called *hemolysis*, and the substances which effect it are known as hemolysins or hemolytic agents. Hypotonic solutions are not the only substances which produce hemolysis. Of particular interest is the fact that the plasma of one species may hemolyze the erythro-

cytes of another and that, in man, the serum of certain individuals may produce hemolysis in others. Hemolysis is of interest in clinical work, because one of the types of anemia, *hemolytic anemia*, occurs when the erythrocytes within the body are hemolyzed at a rate which exceeds that of their formation.

Certain substances also bring about an *agglutination* or clumping of corpuscles. Agglutination may occur within the blood stream during certain pathological and experimental conditions and may thus produce a multiple thrombosis of the smaller vessels. Agglutinating factors occur normally on the surfaces of erythrocytes. These are genetically determined and are dependent on specific sugar moieties. They are responsible for "typing" into several "blood groups" and have obvious importance clinically in selecting compatible blood groups for blood transfusions. The agglutination of erythrocytes from mismatched blood groups is an immunological reaction and has severe consequences.

The cytoplasm of the mature erythrocyte appears homogenous in the fresh condition and is seen as an amorphous, moderately dense material in electron micrographs. The plasmalemma is basically similar in structure and composition to that of other cells, although differing in detail. The red cell membrane continues to provide important insight into the structure of membranes because of the ease in obtaining material for biochemical analysis.

A few of the erythrocytes of peripheral blood have a reticulated appearance when supravitally stained with cresyl blue (Fig. 7.1B). They are known as *reticulocytes* or *reticulated erythrocytes*. They are the youngest erythrocytes in the circulating blood, and their reticulated appearance is apparently produced by a clumping of ribosomes by the supravital dye. Electron micrographs of reticulocytes show scattered groups of ribosomes (polysomes) and occasional mitochondria. These cells apparently correspond to the slightly polychromatophilic erythrocytes seen in Wright's stained smears.

The erythrocytes are much more numerous than any of the other formed elements. The average is about 5,000,000/mm^3 of blood in normal adult males (4,500,000 in females), with normal variations ranging from 4,000,000 to 6,000,000. Normal variations occur within the same individual in association with physiological changes, e.g., they increase after exercise. Many of these variations apparently represent a redistribution to the peripheral vessels rather than an actual change in total numbers. Life in high altitudes is accompanied by an increase to about 8,000,000. Whereas the initial change in this case may be a redistribution (Chapter 13), there is also a real increase in total numbers in response to the lower oxygen tension. More pronounced variations occur under pathological conditions.

The surface area of a red corpuscle has been given at 128 μm^2. From this, one may calculate that the total surface area of 5,000,000 corpuscles in 1 mm^3 of blood is 640 mm^2 and that in 6 liters of blood the total area available for respiratory function is 3840 m^2. This enormous area suggests the importance and the rapidity of the exchange phenomena between the corpuscles on the one hand and the plasma and air on the other.

Under pathological conditions, not only the number but the size, shape, and hemoglobin content of the corpuscles may vary strikingly. The normal number may be present, but the amount of hemoglobin is reduced, as in some of the *secondary* (chlorotic) anemias. In the *macrocytic anemias*, e.g., pernicious anemia, which results from a deficiency of an erythrocyte maturation factor, vitamin B$_{12}$, the red cells are reduced in number but are abnormally large, and some cells have an increased content of hemoglobin. In *microcytic anemia*, e.g., iron deficiency anemia, there is a decrease both in the number and in the size of the cells. Under most of these conditions, the cells may show a multiplicity of distortions in shape (poikilocytosis).

WHITE BLOOD CELLS (LEUKOCYTES)

The white blood cells contain no hemoglobin and differ from the red corpuscles in many other important respects. They have a nucleus and hence are true cells, and they have the power of active ameboid movement, which aids in their passage through the walls of blood vessels and enables them to travel within the connective tissues. They are much less numerous than the red cells, the proportion being about one white cell to 600 red cells, or about 8000/mm^3 of blood, with a normal variation from 6,000 to 10,000. Under pathological conditions, the number may be greatly increased (*leukocytosis*); more rarely there is a reduction in number (*leukopenia*). At birth the leukocytes are more numerous (15,000 to 18,000/mm^3).

The leukocytes, unlike the erythrocytes, perform their functions in the connective tissues. They arise, function, and die outside the bloodstream, which is to them merely a means of transportation from their place of origin to their destination in the connective tissues.

The white blood cells are more or less rounded in shape in fresh preparations and in sections of routinely fixed material. The diameters of the leukocytes in sections of fixed tissue are less than those seen in fresh preparations as a result of shrinkage produced by the technique. On the other hand, the diameters of cells in Wright's stained dried smears are even greater than those seen in fresh preparations because the flattening of the cells more than compensates for the shrinkage caused by the fixation and dehydration. Thus, comparing the diameter of one cell type with that of another is only meaningful when both types are studied by the same method. The diameters given in the following descriptions refer to cells seen in dried smears unless stated otherwise.

The white blood cells may be subdivided into nongranular forms (*agranulocytes*) and granular leukocytes (*granulocytes*). The cytoplasm of the granulocytes is characterized by numerous granules which may be seen in living cells and in fixed and stained preparations. The cytoplasm of some of the agranulocytes contains a few granules which are azurophilic in Wright's stained dry smears, but these are not specific for a particular type of cell, as are the neutrophilic, eosinophilic, and basophilic granules of the cells that are classified as granular leukocytes. Electron microscopic cytochemistry shows that the *azurophilic granules* are primary lysosomes.

Nongranular Leukocytes (Agranulocytes)

The nongranular leukocytes include the *lymphocytes*, which are mostly small cells about the size of erythrocytes, and a group of larger cells, *monocytes*, which have more cytoplasm and a more indented nucleus. The nongranular leukocytes are comparatively undifferentiated and can reproduce by mitosis. Such division does not usually occur in the bloodstream but rather in the connective tissues and blood-forming organs.

Lymphocytes

The lymphocytes of the normal circulation measure from 6 to 10 μm, with the majority being about 7 to 8 μm. They normally constitute about 20 to 25% of the white blood cells (Table 7.1). There is a considerable range for normal individuals, and it is not uncommon to find lymphocyte counts as high as 35 or even 45%. They have a relatively large, spherical nucleus

Table 7.1.
Leukocytes

Type	Size (μm)	% of Leuko-cytes
Lymphocytes	6–10	20–45
Monocytes	12–20	3–8
Granulocytes		
Neutrophils	9–12	50–75
Eosinophils	10–14	2–4
Basophils	8–10	0.5–1

which may have a slight indentation on one side. The densely packed chromatin stains intensely. The nuclei have a purplish blue color in many Wright's stained preparations (Fig. 7.1). Lymphocyte nuclei have a "smudgy" appearance due to a lack of distinct separation between chromatin and nonchromatin regions. It is important to realize that the nuclear color varies with different batches of Wright's stain and with variations in technical procedures. The nucleus is regularly more on the reddish side in immature lymphocytes.

The cytoplasm of lymphocytes is basophilic and is a pale blue in Wright's stain. It varies in amount according to variations in cell size (Fig. 7.1A). It is usually homogeneous but may be slightly more basophilic at the border of the cell and paler adjacent to the nucleus. Electron micrographs demonstrate an abundance of free ribosomes (Fig. 7.2), relatively few mitochondria, and a rather small Golgi complex. The endoplasmic reticulum is sparse in the lymphocyte of the circulating blood (Fig. 7.2). Purplish azurophilic granules are occasionally seen in lymphocytes in Wright's stained dry smears, but they are not specific because they are also found in monocytes and in granular leukocytes. The number of lymphocytes containing these granules varies at different times and in different individuals. A few cells resembling lymphocytes found in blood smears may be as large as 10 to 12 μm in diameter. Some of these cells may be partially differentiated precursors of plasma cells and some may belong to special categories of recirculating cells described below. They are not to be confused with the large lymphoblasts found in blood and blood-forming organs during certain pathological states, e.g., lymphatic leukemia (Fig. 13.4B). The latter differ from the normal cells in appearance and function.

When lymphocytes are studied in supravital preparations kept at body temperatures, they are generally stationary for a short time, but after 15 or 20 min they occasionally move in a manner which differs from that of the other leukocytes. They

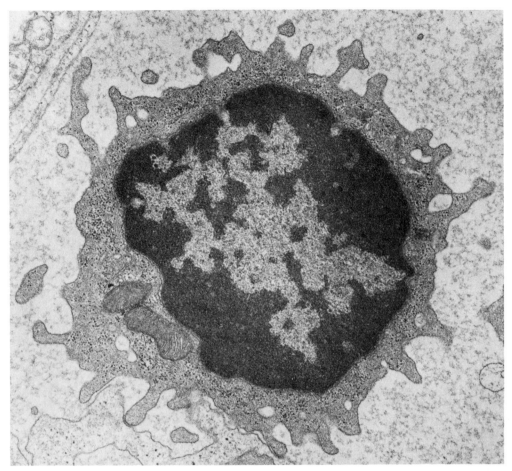

Figure 7.2. Electron micrograph of a section of a human lymphocyte. Note the numerous free ribosomes, the lack of endoplasmic reticulum, and the condensed nuclear chromatin (×25,500). (Courtesy of Dr. June Marshall.)

elongate by sending out a blunt pseudopod and advance by a sort of wormlike motion with the nucleus usually in front (Fig. 7.3). In supravital preparations stained with dilute solutions of neutral red and Janus green B, the mitochondria (stained bluish green by the Janus green B) are in the form of granules and rods (Fig. 7.1*C*). Most of the lymphocytes also show a few neutral red granules (probably the azurophilic granules of Wright's stained preparations).

In the description of connective tissue cells (Chapter 5), it is noted that plasma cells, the principal producers of circulating antibodies, are derived from lymphocytes. The substances which stimulate the formation of antibodies (*immunoglobulins*) by plasma cells are high molecular weight proteins and carbohydrates known as *antigens.* Although the body accepts new proteins formed during embryonic and fetal life as a part of itself, it develops the ability soon after birth to distinguish new proteins as nonself, or antigens. Some lymphocytes acquire the ability to react against extracellular antigens (*exotoxins*) produced by bacterial infection. They migrate into lymphatic organs and into the loose connective tissues of particular regions, where they differentiate into plasma cells which in turn secrete antibodies that enter the bloodstream to counteract the toxins; this is known as a *humoral antibody response.* Other lymphocytes reject foreign grafts and

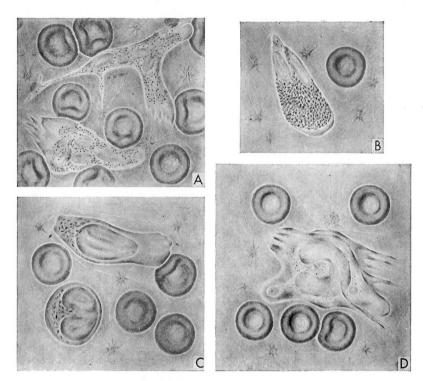

Figure 7.3. Drawings of living human blood cells from a thin film preparation. *A,* polymorphonuclear neutrophils pushing their way between the red blood cells and the delicate fibrin network extending out from the small platelet masses; *B,* polymorphonuclear eosinophil; *C,* lymphocytes, the round resting stage and the elongated motile stage; *D,* monocyte with pseudopodia in the form of delicate undulating membranes. (Courtesy of Dr. C. M. Goss.)

react against numerous viral and fungal infections; this is done by a localized cytotoxic response by lymphocytes that have emigrated from the blood vessels, which is known as *cell-mediated immunity.* The lymphocytes which perform these different functions appear to be a homogenous population in light micrographs, but they can be divided into at least two categories by the study of transfused cells identifiable from isotope labeling, from chromosomal characteristics or from specific surface receptors and immunoglobulins.

The lymphocytes which function in graft rejection and other types of cell-mediated immunity probably arise embryonically from the yolk sac and seed the thymus by way of the liver and the bone marrow. In the thymus, these lymphocytes multiply and differentiate into *T* (thymus-depend-

ent) *lymphocytes.* In mice, the T lymphocytes have a surface marker known as theta antigen, identifiable by special techniques, but as yet such a marker has not been identified in humans. However, human T lymphocytes have the peculiar property of attaching to sheep erythrocytes in a rosette arrangement. Although the reason for this attachment is unknown, it serves as a useful method for distinguishing them from B lymphocytes. There is evidence that in the adult there is a continual reseeding of the thymus with stem cells of bone marrow origin.

The lymphocytes which function as precursors for plasma cells are termed *B lymphocytes* because it was found that, in birds, they develop from a derivative of the cloaca known as the bursa of Fabricius. The bursa apparently provides a special environment for the development for this class of lymphocytes, which is endowed with the ability to differentiate into plasma cells. Mammals lack a bursa of Fabricius, and the exact site of formation of B lymphocytes is controversial. However, there is mounting evidence that, in the adult, a stem cell continues to produce B lymphocytes within the bone marrow. These cells are programmed for response to all conceivable antigens, and on stimulation they proliferate clones of identical cells that differentiate into plasma cells and elaborate humoral antibodies. The latter proliferation occurs in germinal center areas of peripheral lymphatic tissues. The important point is that the B lymphocyte is not proliferated in the thymus. The T and B lymphocytes cannot be distinguished reliably by their morphological characteristics. Early studies reporting characteristic surface features visible in scanning electron micrographs have not been confirmed.

Other cells of the lymphocyte morphology that do not display specific surface markers of either T or B lymphocytes have been termed *null cells*. Some authorities believe that null cells may be developing stages of T or B lymphocytes. There is experimental evidence that a small percentage of such cells represent a multipotent cell of bone marrow origin, the CFU stem cell. (See Chapter 13).

The recognition of an antigen by a lymphocyte is dependent on the arrangement of the amino acids in its surface membrane. Very slight differences in amino acid sequences are sufficient for recognition or nonrecognition of any given antigen. There are so many different combinations in the gene sequence that at least a few lymphocytes are coded with receptors for every conceivable antigen to which an individual could be exposed in a lifetime. When an individual is exposed to a new antigen, the lymphocytes with the specific receptor respond by multiplication and differentiation. At the first response, there are relatively few cells coded for the particular antigen. Only a few cells at a time leave the vessels to differentiate into antibody-forming plasma cells, and the response is relatively slow; this is known as the *primary response*. Some of the newly formed B cells remain in the circulation as *memory cells*. When the individual is reexposed to the same antigen, there are more cells available and a more rapid response occurs; this is known as the *secondary response*. Repeated injections of small amounts of a toxin are sometimes given to induce an *acquired immunity*. Injections of toxoids, i.e., toxins treated in a manner which destroys their toxic properties while retaining antigenicity, are used to provide *active immunity*.

A reaction against an antigen that stimulates the formation of antibodies by plasma cells involves the collaboration of several types of cells. Bacteria that gain entrance to the body are phagocytized by neutrophilic leukocytes that die in the process. The dead neutrophils are phagocytized in turn by macrophages which ingest foreign materials indiscriminately. When a T lymphocyte (termed a *"helper" T lymphocyte*) makes contact with a macrophage it aids in transferring the antigen from the macrophage to a B cell specifically coded for the particular antigen. T cells also survive for a long period as memory cells. The B cells generally depend on the collaboration of T cells for differentiation into plasma cells.

T lymphocytes have a prime function in generating cell-mediated immune responses. That is, these cells are able to recognize and destroy cells infested with organisms capable of living and multiplying in their cytoplasm, or cells of different genetic origin (grafted cells). This is accomplished by two mechanisms: (*a*) the production of cytotoxic T cells (*killer cells*), and (*b*) the elaboration of pharmacologically active agents known as *lymphokines*. The cytotoxic function is important in graft rejection since T lymphocytes will recognize antigenic substances on the surface of genetically dissimilar donor cells and form specific cytotoxic cells to destroy the donor cells. The cytotoxic reaction is highly specific and requires cell contact. Target cells subsequently lyse as a result of an induced focal leakiness in their plasma membranes. The lymphokines produced by T cells include a variety of factors affecting macrophage activity, leucocytic chemotactic factors, mitogenic factors, and many others.

T lymphocytes differentiate into several other recognizable subtypes in addition to helper and killer cells. Some of these are *memory cells, suppressor cells,* and *amplifier cells.* The precise functions of many of the subtypes of T lymphocytes are still under active investigation and are not fully understood.

Antibodies are plasma proteins which belong to a family known as *immunoglobulins* (Ig). Each molecule is composed of four polypeptide chains. The two pairs are joined by several disulfide bridges. The amino acid sequence is constant in the major portion of each chain but variable in the terminal fragment (*Fab*), which functions in antigen binding. On the basis of differences in the variable portion of the heavy chain, the immunoglobulins are divided into five classes, namely, mu, gamma, alpha, delta, and epsilon (*IgM, IgG, IgA, IgD,* and *IgE*). Experimental studies on mice and other mammals have shown that some of the lymphocytes begin to synthesize IgM during the latter part of fetal life. IgG appears at about the time of birth and can apparently form in the same cells that were previously synthesizing IgM. The IgG-producing cell can apparently also switch to IgA production. The function of IgD is not fully understood, but it is commonly believed that this immunoglobulin serves as an antigenic receptor. IgE is a reaginic antibody, that is, it binds to the surface of blood basophils and tissue mast cells and induces them to release their granule contents when subsequently exposed to antigen in allergic reactions.

A high percentage of the lymphocytes present in the bloodstream are recirculating cells. Lymphocytes leave the blood vascular system at the lymph nodes by adhering to the endothelial cells of high endothelial venules, then passing between these cells into the underlying reticular tissue, commonly referred to as parenchyma.* Although some of the cells proliferate in the lymphatic organs and some differentiate into plasma cells, the majority return to the systemic circulation by way of the efferent lymphatic channels and the thoracic duct.

Because the total number of lymphocytes entering and leaving the bloodstream every 24 hr is several times the number present in the circulation, lymphocytes must enter and leave at an equivalent rate to maintain their approximately constant percentage in normal blood. Studies of transfused labeled cells in mice indicate that approximately 85% of the recirculating cells belong to the T type and that only about 15% are of the B type. A high percentage of the recirculating lymphocytes are long-lived and survive for many months in rodents and for many years in humans. It is thought that the long-lived lymphocytes (both B and T) are the memory cells.

Because lymphocytes have a major role in immunity, it is not surprising that they are abundant in connective tissues beneath the epithelial lining of the digestive and respiratory systems. For example, they are aggregated in the Waldeyer's ring of faucial, lingual, and pharyngeal tonsils, in the Peyer's patches of the ileum, and in solitary nodules of other segments of the digestive and respiratory systems. They add to the total body pool of lymphocytes by multipli-

---

*The term *parenchyma* as applied to animal tissues carries two definitions. The traditional histological definition denotes prenchyma as the functional, cellular component of an organ. Embryologically, the "parenchyma" of most organs is that functional part derived from epithelium. In this context, *parenchyma* is in contrast to *stroma,* which is the mesenchymally derived component of an organ. Both definitions apply well to such organs as glands. The embryological definition, however, is not applicable to such organs as lymph nodes, spleen, and bone marrow, which are totally of mesenchymal origin. In this text, the term parenchyma is avoided in discussing such organs.

cation in these locations, and they are also strategically situated for their functions.

Monocytes, or Large Mononuclear Leukocytes

Monocytes are large cells which constitute from 3 to 8% of the leukocytes. In dry smears, they usually vary from 12 to 15 μm in diameter, but when extremely flattened and stretched they may reach 20 μm. In supravital preparations, their diameter varies with the activity of the cell. The active monocytes send out numerous pseudopodia and naturally appear larger than the more rounded, inactive forms. The active cells are especially large when flattened in thin film preparations.

The monocyte nucleus is ovoid, kidney- or horseshoe-shaped, very rarely spherical, and usually eccentrically placed (Fig. 7.1). Its chromatin network is finer and stains less densely than that of the lymphocytes. Nucleoli are not obvious within the monocytes in blood smears but are shown in electron micrographs. The cytoplasm is abundant and has a somewhat reticulated or vacuolated appearance; it is slightly less basophilic than the lymphocyte cytoplasm and is more of a grayish blue after Wright's stain. A Golgi apparatus in the cytoplasm near the indentation of the nucleus can be seen by light microscopy after special techniques. There are also some fine azurophilic cytoplasmic granules that are near the limits of resolution of the light microscope.

Electron micrographs (Fig. 7.4) reveal more rough-surfaced endoplasmic reticulum in monocytes than in lymphocytes but fewer free ribosomes. There are also numerous microfilaments that are associated with cell motility. By a combination of electron microscopy and cytochemistry, it is found that there are membrane-bounded granules that give a positive peroxidase reaction; they are the azurophilic granules of light microscopy and they function as primary lysosomes after the monocytes migrate into the connective tissue. The monocytes do not form any new azurophilic granules after migrating into the connective tissue. However, some additional granules that are peroxidase-negative have been demonstrated by cytochemistry and electron microscopy.

In supravital preparations treated with neutral red and Janus green B, the azurophilic granules are colored by neutral red, and vacuoles of neutral red form by phagocytosis. The vacuoles are often arranged as a rosette around the region containing the cell center, and they increase in size as the supravital staining is continued. Mitochondria are stained bluish green and are usually more numerous around the rim of the rosette than in other parts of the cytoplasm (Fig. 7.1C). Large monocytes are more active than small ones, but none of them travel about rapidly like the neutrophils and eosinophils. The monocytes also exhibit a different type of activity. They continually extend and withdraw pseudopodia and assume an appearance somewhat like an octopus (Fig. 7.3D). The pseudopodia are of different shapes, ranging from threadlike filopodia to broad lamellipodia, and are transparent.

In tissue cultures, the monocytes, or promonocytes, can enlarge and take on all of the characteristics of typical *macrophages*. In the body, they migrate readily through the capillary walls into the connective tissues where they display their phagocytic characteristics. They provide the mobilized macrophages found in areas of focal infection.

Granular Leukocytes (Granulocytes)

The granular leukocytes are characterized by the presence of specific types of granules in their cytoplasm, and according to the nature of this granulation, they have been subdivided into three groups: the *neutrophilic*, *eosinophilic*, and *basophilic* leukocytes. They are further characterized by the presence of a many-lobed (polymorphous) nucleus; hence they are called *polymorphonuclear* leukocytes. The lobes of chromatin are connected by very delicate

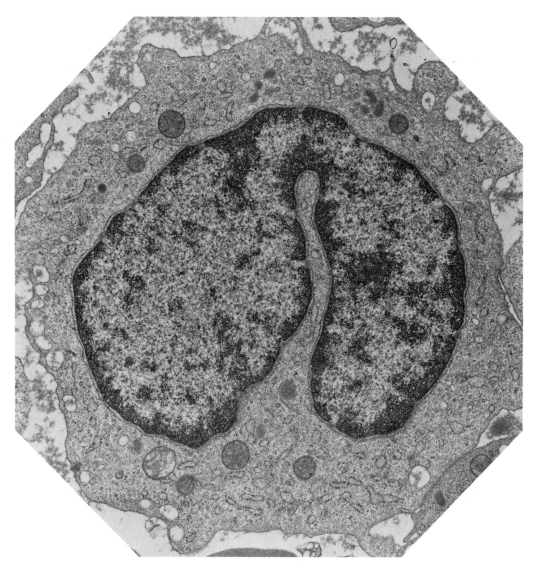

Figure 7.4. Electron micrograph of a section of a human monocyte. The nucleus is deeply indented and the cytoplasm contains endoplasmic reticulum, vacuoles, and a few small membrane-bounded granules (azurophilic granules) (×18,000). (Courtesy of Dr. June Marshall.)

chromatic strands. Occasionally, some of these strands are broken in dry smear preparations, so a few cells may appear to be polynuclear. The granulocytes also differ from the nongranular leukocytes in that they are more highly differentiated and can no longer undergo mitosis.

Neutrophils

The neutrophilic polymorphonuclear leukocytes (Fig. 7.1) vary in size from 9 to 12 μm in blood smears and are the most

numerous of white blood cells. Although they usually constitute about 60 to 70% of the total white blood cells, they have been found to range from 50 to 75% in normal individuals. Under pathological conditions, the range is much greater. The polymorphic nucleus shows a variety of forms, usually consisting of three to five sausage-shaped masses of chromatin connected by fine threads and arranged in the form of an S or a horseshoe. In blood smears from human females, one can see a small appendage attached to the remainder of the nucleus by a narrow filament, giving a drumstick appearance in almost 3% of the neutrophils (Fig. 7.5). The drumstick is the heterochromatin of one of the two X chromosomes of the female. It is presumably present in all of the cells in females, but it is closely packed with one of the lobes of the nucleus in most cells and is obscured. Some of the neutrophils of males have hook-shaped and nodule-like appendages, but they generally do not have the drumstick forms.

The cytoplasm is filled with fine granules which are neutrophilic. In some animals, e.g., rabbit and guinea pig, the granules bind the acid stain and may be called *pseudoeosinophils*. Because these cells vary in their staining reactions in different species, they are sometimes called *heterophils* rather than neutrophils.

In addition to the neutrophilic granules, there are other granules that have a reddish

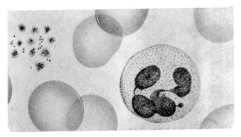

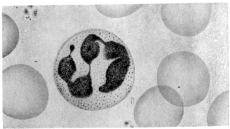

Figure 7.5. Portions of two oil immersion fields of a Wright's stained blood smear from a human female. Fields have been selected to show the drumstick appearance of the sex chromatin which is seen in a number of the neutrophilic leukocytes in the female. It is seen as a hanging drop of chromatin attached by a thin strand to one of the lobes of the nucleus. A relatively large cluster of blood platelets is seen in the *upper left corner* of the figure (×1335). (From a preparation made by Miss Karen Fu.)

purple or azure color in Wright's stained smears. The existence of two types of granules has been confirmed by electron microscopy and by biochemical assays of particles separated by differential centrifugation. In many animals there are relatively large electron-dense granules (Figs. 7.6 and 7.7) that correspond to the azurophilic granules of light microscopy and that develop only during the promyelocyte stage of cell differentiation; they are classified as *azurophilic* or *primary granules*. They contain myeloperoxidase and many acid hydrolases that are characteristic of lysosomes. Another group of granules that are smaller and less electron-dense have a pink color in Wright's stained smears and develop only in the myelocyte stage of leukocyte development; they are known as *neutrophilic* (secondary or specific) granules. They comprise about 80% of the granules of the mature neutrophil and contain alkaline phosphatase and other hydrolases that function at a neutral or alkaline pH and some antibacterial constituents (lysozyme, lactoferrin). Both types of granules are membrane-bounded and both have intracellular functions described below. The mature human neutrophil contains both types of granules, but they cannot be readily distinguished by morphological criteria alone.

In differential counts, the neutrophils are sometimes subdivided on the basis of nuclear differentiation. A commonly used classification proposed by Schilling divides the neutrophils into segmented nuclears, about 57% of the total leukocytes, and nonsegmented nuclears, about 4%. The latter group is subdivided into cells with the nuclei either shaped like bands or shaped like stab wounds, about 3%; juveniles or metamyelocytes with indented or kidney-shaped nuclei, 0 to 1%; and myelocytes, approaching 0%. An increase in relative numbers of nonsegmented nuclears is known as a "shift to the left," whereas an increase in segmented types is known as a "shift to the right." The latter is considered a good sign because it usually indicates that there is no

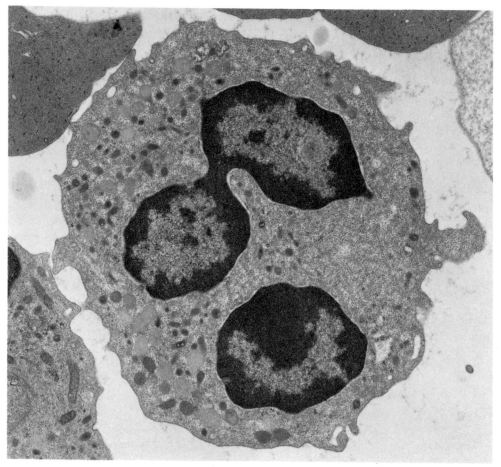

Figure 7.6. Electron micrograph of a section of a human neutrophil. Three nuclear lobes are obvious. The cytoplasm contains granules of different sizes and densities, mitochondria, free ribosomes, and some strands of endoplasmic reticulum. Some of the granules are probably azurophilic granules, but their positive identification would require histochemical procedures (see text). (×15,400). (Courtesy of Dr. June Marshall.)

longer any unusual demand on the bone marrow for younger cells.

In supravital preparations the neutrophilic leukocyte is more active than any other blood cell. It advances by an ameboid movement, usually with the nucleus in the rear. At times, it is difficult to see the strands connecting the nuclear lobes, and the cells may appear to be polynuclear instead of polymorphonuclear. In supravital preparations, the cytoplasmic granules become colored by the neutral red within a few minutes (Fig. 7.1*C*). After 15 or 20 min, some of the neutrophils form phagocytic vacuoles of neutral red that occasionally become as large as one of the nuclear lobes.

A few small mitochondria stain with Janus green B.

Neutrophils circulate in the blood for a relatively brief time (6–12 hr) and then migrate into the connective tissue where they phagocytize bacteria and other small particles. They have been called the *microphages*, in contrast with the macrophages, which are larger cells that characteristically engulf larger particles. They are chemotactically attracted by devitalized tissue, bacteria, other foreign bodies and factors produced by antigen-antibody interactions with certain blood proteins (*complement*), and they migrate to the site of an infection. They engulf bacteria by endocytosis and

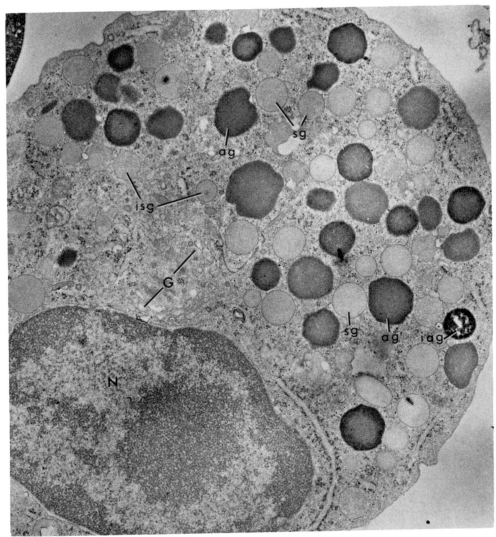

Figure 7.7. Electron micrograph of a section of a neutrophilic myelocyte from rabbit bone marrow. The tissue was reacted for the enzyme peroxidase during the technical procedure. Note that the reaction product is present in the azurophilic granules (*ag*) but not in the specific granules (*sg*). The reaction product is distributed uniformly throughout most of the mature azurophilic granules, but it is present in flocculent form in an immature azurophilic granule (*iag*) seen at the *right*. Several small and immature specific granules (*isg*) are seen in the vicinity of the Golgi complex (*G*). The nucleus (*N*) is not lobed at this stage (×18,000). (Reprinted with permission from D. F. Bainton and M. G. Farquhar: *J Cell Biol* 39: 1968.)

form phagosomes. Then the membranes of first the azurophilic and then the neutrophilic granules fuse with the membranes of the phagosomes, thus forming secondary lysosomes. The neutrophilc granules contribute their alkaline phosphatase and antibacterial lysozyme and lactoferrin about 3 to 4 min before the azurophilic granules empty. This sequential discharge correlates with the development of a lower pH in the phagosomes by the time the azurophilic granules contribute their peroxidase and lysosomal enzymes which function at a lower pH. These enzymes completely destroy the bacteria, and eventually the neutrophils die to become the pus corpuscles of an abscess. Although the neutrophils serve as the shock troops or as the first line of defense against invading organisms, they are not equally effective against all types of bacteria. For example, they cannot successfully combat tubercle bacilli; in this case, the macrophages are the efficient agents. Neutrophils have a life span of a few days at most and do not normally recirculate.

Eosinophils

The eosinophilic leukocytes (Fig. 7.1) normally constitute from 2 to 4% of the white blood cells. They are somewhat larger than the neutrophils (about 10 to 14 μm), and are characterized by an abundance of coarse, refractile granules of a uniform size which stain intensely with eosin or other acid dyes.

In electron micrographs the granules are membrane-bounded and have a matrix of fine particles surrounding an irregularly shaped dense bar or crystalloid (Fig. 7.8). The granules are larger than either the specific or azurophilic granules of the neutrophils. The specific granules of the eosin-

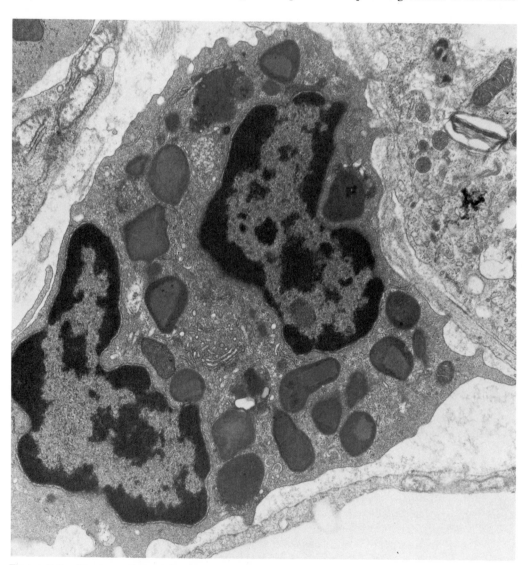

Figure 7.8. Electron micrograph of a section of a human eosinophil. The two nuclear lobes and the large specific granules containing irregular crystalloid inclusions are characteristic. In this preparation the crystalloids are less dense than the granule matrix. A Golgi region appears between the nuclear lobes ($\times$16,400). (Courtesy of Dr. June Marshall.)

ophils resemble the azurophilic granules of the neutrophils in the sense that they give a positive peroxidase reaction and function as lysosomes.

In supravital preparations, the eosinophils occasionally travel as rapidly as the neutrophils but not for as long a period. Their granules stain intensely and uniformly with neutral red, and a few mitochondria can be demonstrated with Janus green B.

The eosinophils are more common in the connective tissue of certain areas (e.g., intestinal mucosa) than in the bloodstream. They increase greatly in allergic conditions such as hay fever and asthma, in skin diseases, and in parasitic infestations. Their functional role in these conditions is not entirely clear, but it has been shown that they produce a histaminase, and moderate the response to allergenic stimulus. They contain arylsulfatase and a specific basic protein in addition to peroxidase and histaminase.

Basophils

The basophilic leukocytes (Fig. 7.1) are present in blood in an almost negligible quantity, forming 0.5 to 1% or even less of the total number of leukocytes. In size they vary from 8 to 10 μm. The nucleus of a basophil is relatively large and irregularly polymorphous. The lobed nature is not as clearly defined as in other granulocytes, and the chromatin network, which is less compact, stains more lightly. The cytoplasm contains a variable number of coarse granules which are basophilic and metachromatic. These granules also vary in size; a few may be as large as or larger than the eosinophilic granules, but the majority are intermediate between the neutrophilic and eosinophilic types. The granules are membrane-bounded structures containing fine particles (Fig. 7.9). Some granules which are more electron dense than others are presumably immature. Because the granules are soluble in water, they are usually not found in sections prepared by the ordinary methods.

In supravital preparations, the basophils are relatively inactive. The basophilic granules are not as refractile as eosinophilic granules, are more variable in size and do not stain as uniformly. Most of the granules give a deeper red reaction with neutral red than do the eosinophilic granules.

Although the blood basophils resemble the connective tissue mast cells in many respects, they have some differential characteristics. For example, they have a more polymorphous nucleus and their cytoplasmic granules have a different ultrastructure. Their main function is to form heparin and histamine, which are stored in their granules before release by exocytosis. They increase in relatively few pathological conditions, e.g., in smallpox, chicken pox, and chronic sinus inflammations. They increase, along with all other leukocytes, in leukemia. Although they normally constitute only about 0.5% of the leukocytes, their total number in an average individual having 6 liters of blood is approximately 200 million. In some of the lower vertebrates (hellbender, mudpuppy, and certain turtles), they are more numerous than the other types of leukocytes.

BLOOD PLATELETS

Blood platelets (*thromboplastids*, Fig. 7.1) are biconvex disc-shaped bodies 2 to 4 μm in diameter. They arise as fragments of cytoplasm of megakaryocytes of bone marrow, and they are colorless in the fresh state. Because they are small and readily clump when blood is drawn, it is difficult to obtain a precise count, but their number in normal blood is given as 150,000 to 300,000/mm^3. They are found only in mammals. The *thrombocytes* of lower vertebrates are nucleated cells that are wholly unlike those of man and other mammals.

In Wright's stained blood smears, the platelets are frequently aggregated, but it can be seen that each platelet is composed of a central area (granulomere, chromomere) that stains purple and a peripheral zone which is light blue (the so-called hyalomere). The platelets have numerous granules, a few mitochondria, considerable glycogen, vacuoles, microtubules, and micro-

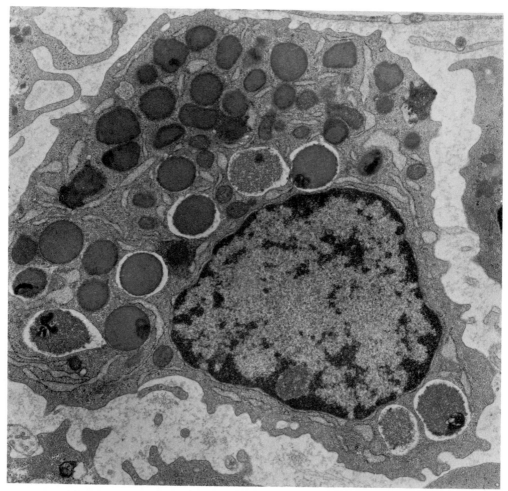

Figure 7.9. Electron micrograph of a section of a human basophil. Note the large granules containing relatively homogeneous material. Some granules show a separation between the contents and the membrane and a partial dispersion of the contents. Basophilic granules are frequently lost entirely during processing. Note the relatively prominent cisternae of endoplasmic reticulum (×14,000). (Courtesy of Dr. June Marshall.)

filaments. Although the granules are widely dispersed in the cytoplasm, the majority are in the granulomere region. Most of the granules (alpha granules) range from 0.15 to 0.2 μm in diameter. A particularly prominent bundle of microtubules courses circumferentially just beneath the membrane that encloses the platelet. It is thought that the microtubules aid in maintaining the shape of the platelet and that the filaments have a role in contraction. The plasma membrane of each platelet is covered externally by a glycoprotein-rich fuzzy coat. It

is thought that this plays a role in the adherence of the platelets to each other.

The platelets presumably liberate an enzyme, *thromboplastin*, which affects the coagulation of the blood. Thromboplastin transforms *prothrombin* into *thrombin*, and the latter, in turn, transforms fibrinogen into fibrin. Thromboplastin is present in the plasma, as well as in the platelets. Blood free of platelets coagulates, although much more slowly, and lymph, which has no platelets, likewise coagulates.

The platelets are most commonly known

for their role in blood clotting, but they also have an important role in maintenance of endothelial cells. Moreover, they contain serotonin and other vasoreactive substances which can cause vascular contractions upon their release. Other platelet factors elicit a proliferative response by vascular smooth muscle cells and, thus, contribute to the pathology of atherosclerosis. The platelets also may by agglutination give rise to colorless intravascular clots or thombi. Deficiencies of circulating platelets are encountered clinically in various forms of the condition known as thrombocytopenia.

LYMPH

Lymph, like blood, consists of a fluid plasma in which are suspended various cells. Red blood cells and platelets are entirely missing and granulocytes are few in number, the chief cellular elements being lymphocytes.

The plasma of lymph is similar to that of blood but of less fixed constitution. It carries carbonic acid but very little oxygen.

During digestion, the lymphatics of the intestine become filled with a large number of lipid containing *chylomicrons*. The lymph assumes a white color and is known as *chyle*. Many of the chylomicrons are removed and stored temporarily by the lymphatic organs before the lymph reaches the blood stream.

Lymph coagulates, although much more slowly than blood, the fibrin forming a colorless clot in which the cells are entangled.

DISPOSAL OF BLOOD CELLS

In contrast with many other cells of the body, the red and white cells of the blood survive for only a relatively short period of time. The life span of the human erythrocyte as determined by tracer doses of radioactive isotopes is about 127 days. From these data, it is obvious that billions of corpuscles are destroyed daily. The destruction is balanced so well by new blood for-mation that the characteristic number of corpuscles is constantly maintained under normal conditions.

Destruction of erythrocytes frequently begins within the bloodstream itself by a disintegration of corpuscles into small hemoglobin-retaining fragments and is completed by the macrophages of the blood-destroying organs, chiefly by the spleen (see Chapter 14). These cells remove the fragmented forms and also engulf many senile erythrocytes in toto. The macrophages break up the hemoglobin into an iron-free portion (*globin*) and an iron-retaining part (*hematin*). Hematin is further separated into *bilirubin* and *iron*. The bilirubin is transported to the liver to be excreted in the bile, and the iron (in protein complexes as ferritin and hemosiderin) is conserved by the macrophages to be used again in new erythrocytes developing in the bone marrow.

The life span of the different types of leukocytes is quite variable. The time spent in circulation is also quite variable. The neutrophils spend 8 hr or less in the circulation before migrating into the connective tissue, where they survive for a few days and function as microphages. The lymphocytes generally remain in the bloodstream for only a short period, about 8 hr, at any one time, but some of them (long-lived lymphocytes) recirculate and survive for many years. Monocytes circulate in the blood for only 1 or 2 days and then migrate into the connective tissues, where they become macrophages which may survive for many months.

Senile and dead cells are removed by phagocytosis in the spleen and liver. The migration of neutrophils, especially pronounced during infection, and their disintegration in the connective tissues have already been pointed out. They also escape by penetration through the lining epithelia of mucous membranes, as illustrated by their presence in saliva. Eosinophils show a particular tendency for migration into the connective tissues of the respiratory and gastrointestinal tracts, where they eventually disintegrate. Some of the lympho-cytes may undergo dissolution in the cir-culatory system, some may be destroyed while the blood courses through organs where cells of the macrophage system are particularly numerous, and large numbers migrate into the connective tissues where they apparently disintegrate. Some are lost by migration into the lumen of the intes-tinal tract.

References

Ackerman G: Cytochemical properties of the blood basophilic granulocyte. *Ann NY Acad Sci* 103:376–393, 1963.

Bainton DF: Sequential degranulation of the two types of polymorphonuclear leukocyte granules during phagocytosis of microorganisms. *J Cell Biol* 58:249–264, 1973.

Bainton DF, Farquhar MG: Differences in enzyme content of azurophil and specific granules of poly-morphonuclear leukocytes. II. Cytochemistry and electron microscopy of bone marrow cells. *J Cell Biol* 39:299–317, 1968.

Bainton DF, and Farquhar MG: Segregation and pack-aging of granule enzymes in eosinophilic leukocytes. *J Cell Biol* 45:54–73, 1970.

Bentfield ME, Nichols BA, and Bainton DF: Ultra-structural localization of peroxidases in leukocytes of rat bone marrow and blood. *Anat Rec* 187:219–240, 1977.

Davidson WM and Smith DR: A morphological sex difference in the polymorphonuclear leucocytes. *Br Med J* 2:6–7, 1954.

DeBruyn PPH: Locomotion of blood cells in tissue culture. *Anat Rec* 89:43–63, 1944.

Everett NB, Caffrey RW, and Rieke WD: Recircula-tion of lymphocytes. *Ann NY Acad Sci* 113:887–897, 1964.

Gowans JL: The recirculation of lymphocytes from blood to lymph in the rat. *J Physiol* 143:84–85, 1958.

Nichols BA, Bainton DF, and Farquhar MG: Differ-entiation of monocytes. Origin, nature, and fate of their azurophil granules. *J Cell Biol* 50:498–515, 1971.

Nichols, BA and Bainton DF: Differentiation of hu-man monocytes in bone marrow and blood: sequen-tial formation of two granule populations. *Lab In-vest* 29:27–40, 1973.

Rifkind RA, Bank A, Marks PA, Nossel HL, Ellison RR, and Lindenbaum J: *Fundamentals of Hematol-ogy*, ed 2. Chicago, Year Book Medical Publishers, 1980.

Roitt I. *Essential Immunology*, ed 4. London, Black-well Scientific Publications, 1980.

Sabin FR: Studies of living human blood cells. *Bull Johns Hopkins Hosp* 34:277–288, 1923.

Shemin D and Rittenberg D: The life span of the human red blood cell. *J Biol Chem* 166:627–636, 1946.

Vietta ES and Uhr JW: Immunoglobulin-receptors revisited. A model for the differentiation of bone marrow-derived lymphocytes. *Science* 189:964–969, 1975.

Wintrobe M, Lee G, Boggs D, Bithell T, Foerster J, Athens J, and Lukens J: *Clinical Hematology*, ed 8. Philadelphia, Lea & Febiger, 1981.

Zucker-Franklin D: The ultrastructure of mega-karyocytes and platelets. In Gordon AS (ed): *Regu-lation of Hematopoiesis*, vol 2, New York, Appleton-Century-Crofts, 1970, pp 1533–1586.

Chapter 8

MUSCLE

Virtually all cells in animal tissues are, at some time in their life cycle, contractile. The degree of contractility may be very subtle or quite obvious, but mobility and cellular shape change are fundamental properties. The tissues which we classify as *muscle* are those which in their differentiation have come to emphasize the property of contractility to a remarkable extent. These tissues are composed of cells whose cytoplasm is predominantly structured with the machinery necessary to bring about extreme, force-generating, and sometimes quite rapid changes in cell shape. Collectively the cells of muscular tissue are able to provide the motile force for activities as subtle as the constriction of an arteriole, as quick as the beat of a fly's wing, or as massive as the effort of a weight lifter. Indeed, even the morphogenetic cell shape changes and tissue movements associated with molding the proper shape of embryos (Chapter 3) involve delicate mechanisms of contractility not unlike the mechanisms found in mature muscle cells.

In nature, there is a wide spectrum of forms and varieties of muscular cells. It ranges from cells which show only small portions of the cytoplasm specialized for contractility to others in which a massive and highly ordered array of organelles performs highly specified degrees and patterns of movement. In mammals, it has been traditional to recognize three major classes of muscular tissue; *smooth* (or nonstriated), *skeletal*, and *cardiac* (the latter two classed together as *striated*). All are derived embryonically from mesenchyme, with a very few interesting exceptions. Most smooth muscle is involuntary in action and takes its origin in splanchnic mesenchyme or somatic mesenchyme associated with blood vessels and glands in the periphery of the body. All skeletal muscle is of somatic mesenchymal origin and most of it is controllable voluntarily. The cardiac muscle of the heart is derived from a rather specialized splanchnic portion of the mesenchymal compartment, and of course it is involuntary.

SMOOTH MUSCLE

The most prominent masses of smooth muscle originate from mesenchymal cells of the splanchnic mesoderm surrounding the embryonic endodermal gut epithelium and its appendages. However, when the collective amount of smooth musculature contained in the walls of peripheral blood vessels and glands is considered, it will be realized that considerable smooth muscle also arises from somatic mesoderm. Exceptions to mesodermal origin are found in the iridic muscle of the eye and in modified muscle cells in the walls of sweat glands which are derived from ectodermal epithelial cells.

As smooth muscle differentiation proceeds, some of the mesenchymal cells become recognizable as *myoblasts* by their elongated nuclei and spindle shape. New myoblasts continue to differentiate from mesenchymal cells during the early stages of development. Later, the division of existing myoblasts gradually takes the place of this differentiation in the production of new muscular elements.

As the young muscle cells differentiate, their cytoplasms become crowded with filamentous contractile elements, and the exterior surface of each acquires a surrounding *external lamina*. They are thus individually segregated from the surrounding connective tissue compartment. In many regions, neighboring smooth muscle cells develop interconnecting *nexuses (communicating* or *gap junctions)*; these occupy macular interruptions of the external lamina and provide an intimate anatomical and functional attachment between the cells involved.

Scattered oval nuclei around and among groups of elongating myoblasts mark the presence of connective tissue fibroblasts. As the muscle cells develop into sheets or bundles, the fibroblasts and/or the muscle cells themselves synthesize and lay down extracellular networks of collagenous, elastic, and reticular fibers.

Mature smooth muscle consists of fusiform or spindle-shaped cells with abundant cytoplasm, in whose central thickest portion the nucleus lies. As a rule, the cells are concentrated into dense sheets or bands, but they may also occur as isolated units scattered among connective tissue.

When concentrated, smooth muscle cells are roughly parallel to each other but irregularly and densely packed, so that the narrow portion of one cell lies against the wide portions of its neighbors. The shape varies according to the organ containing the muscle: for example, very long and slender in the walls of the intestine, short and relatively thick in walls of small arteries, or thrown into irregular folds and twists by the surrounding elastic fibers in the walls of large arteries. The greatest diameter varies from 3 to 8 μm and the length from 15 to 200 μm, except in the pregnant uterus, where it may exceed ½ mm (500 μm). Outlines of the cells are indistinct in longitudinal views of either fresh material or prepared sections because of overlapping, but are easily seen in cross sections. Here outlines are round, oval, or flattened and vary in size because the fusiform cells may be cut through thick central portions or at narrow ends (Figs. 8.1 and 8.2).

The *nucleus* conforms to the outline of the cell, and its shape may therefore be oval, elongated, or flattened (Fig. 8.1). The nuclei of contracted cells usually have a folded or pleated outline, which can be seen in longitudinal sections.

The *cytoplasm* is dominated by longitudinally aligned contractile filaments, but in addition it contains mitochondria, a Golgi complex, centrioles, endoplasmic reticulum, ribosomes, some glycogen, and occasional fat droplets. The filaments are not clearly visible in routine sections, but they can be detected as "fibrils" in fresh preparations after maceration in nitric or trichloracetic acid. These represent aggregates of *myofilaments* which can be seen in electron micrographs (Fig. 8.3). The filaments of smooth muscle cells differ from those in striated muscle in that they are not arranged in registered order (see under "Skeletal Muscle") and are not as readily preserved. From a variety of biochemical and immunocytochemical studies it is well known that the two major contractile proteins, *actin* and *myosin*, are both contained in the filament systems of smooth muscle. However, in routine electron micrographs, the most readily seen filaments are *thin* and composed of *actin*. Coarse filaments, identified as *thick (myosin)* filaments, can be seen in vertebrate smooth muscle, contracted or relaxed, after special fixation procedures (Fig. 8.4). Some workers have postulated that most of the myosin of vertebrate smooth muscles is present in an unaggregated form, and furthermore that aggregation into visibly thick filaments occurs during tension production, a state requiring special fixation procedures for preservation. Thick and thin filaments are seen more readily in invertebrate than in vertebrate smooth muscle cells. The actin filaments of smooth muscles (vertebrate and invertebrate) often course obliquely in the cell and generally attach in characteristic condensations along the inner surface of the plasmalemma (Figs. 8.2 through 8.4). Because the filaments are responsible for contraction of the muscle cell, the force generated by such an arrangement must also have an oblique component. The resultant tension is transmitted to dense regions seen at intervals along the bundles of thin filaments and where the filaments attach to the plasmalemma. These dense areas form sites for interconnection be-

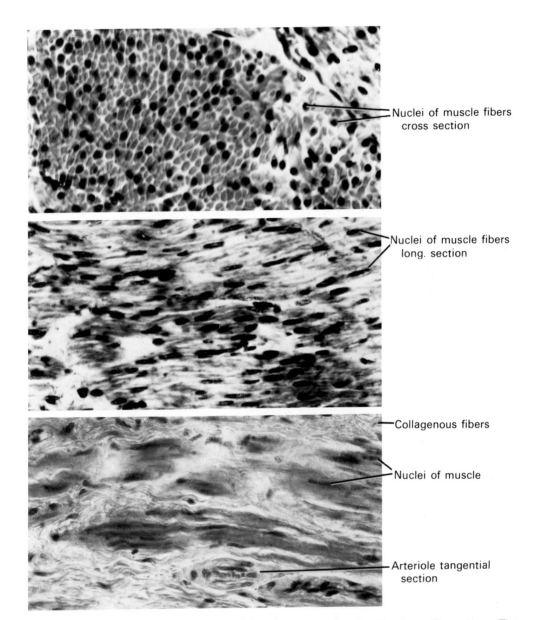

Nuclei of muscle fibers
cross section

Nuclei of muscle fibers
long. section

Collagenous fibers

Nuclei of muscle

Arteriole tangential
section

Figure 8.1. Smooth muscle as viewed by light microscopy of conventional paraffin sections. The *upper figure* shows the muscle fibers cut transversely; the *central* and *lower figures* show the fibers cut longitudinally. In the *central figure*, the fibers are seen in compact arrangement, with a minimum of associated connective tissue, whereas in the *lower figure* the fibers are interspersed with considerable connective tissue. *Upper* and *central* micrograhs are from human urinary bladder, *lower* micrograph is from human rectum. All figures ×390.

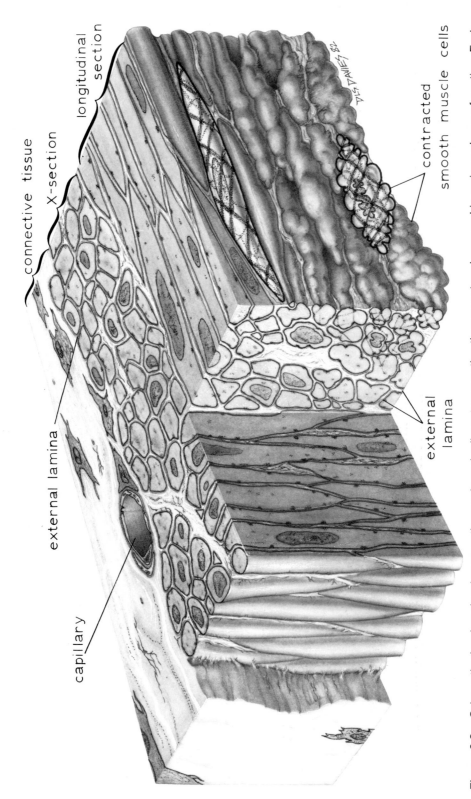

Figure 8.2. Schematic drawing showing smooth muscle and adjacent connective tissues cut and exposed in various planes of section. Each muscle cell is surrounded by an external lamina. Two muscle cells (at *right*) are depicted as translucent in order to show the arrangement of myofilaments during relaxed and contracted states.

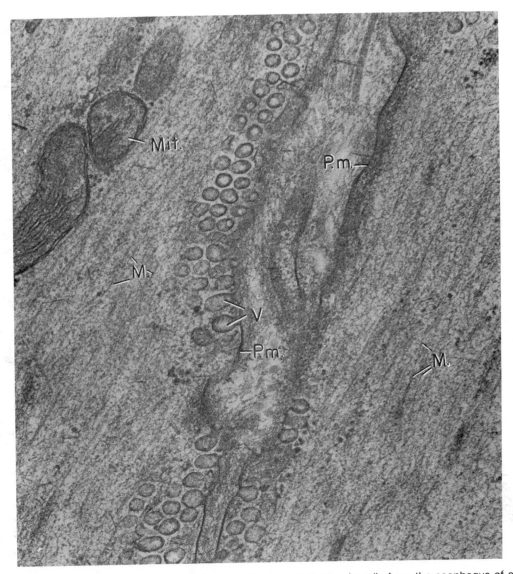

Figure 8.3.   Electron micrograph of portions of two smooth muscle cells from the esophagus of a bat. Note fine myofilaments (*M*.), mitochondria (*Mit.*), caveolae and vesicles (*V*.), and plasma membranes (*P.m.*) (×57,750). (Courtesy of Dr. Keith Porter.)

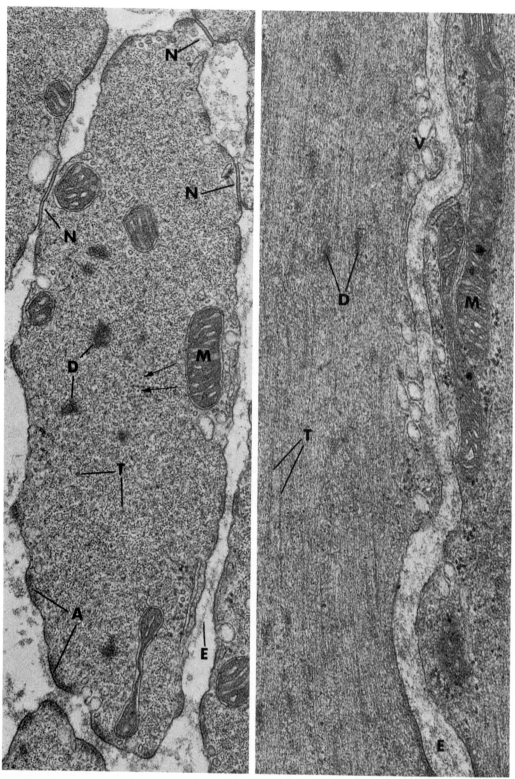

Figure 8.4. Electron micrographs of smooth muscle from rat small intestine. The cells in the *left figure* are cut transversely. Thick (14-nm) filaments (*T*), perhaps consisting of myosin, are seen distributed among numerous thin (5-nm) actin filaments. Near the center of the *left micrograph*, a

tween actin filaments and also with transversely oriented intermediate filaments. They have been likened to the Z discs of striated muscle that appear to hold actin filaments in register (see below).

In routine hematoxylin and eosin-stained sections, the cytoplasm of smooth muscle usually appears more or less homogeneous. The color tone differs slightly from that of nearby collagen fibers because ribosomes in the eosinophilic muscle cytoplasm bind hematoxylin, giving the muscle a slight purplish tint, in contrast with a more pure eosin color in collagen. These reactions are variable and the identification of the tissues should be based more on morphological characteristics than on tinctorial reactions. Classically, Masson's trichrome stain simplifes the differentiation of smooth muscle from collagen because muscle is usually stained red in this technique, whereas collagen is colored blue or green. Identification of smooth muscle in routine preparations stained with hematoxylin and eosin is further complicated when some of the cytoplasmic constituents are not preserved. Consequently the cytoplasm of smooth muscle cells often appears vacuoloated and pale and is easily confused with bundles of nerve fibers.

The *plasma membrane* of the smooth muscle cell in high resolution electron micrographs is characterized by numerous membranous *caveolae* which protrude into the cytoplasm (Fig. 8.3). Together with the densities along its internal aspect plus the prominent external lamina over its outer surface these impart a notably thickened appearance. Where adjacent muscle cells form *nexuses*, or *communicating (gap) junctions*, an external lamina is lacking and intimate membrane-to-membrane contact is achieved by special junctional polypeptide structures which, like the *connexons* of

epithelial cells, (Chapter 4, Figs. 4.12 through 4.15) probably facilitate transmission of impulses from one cell to another. In smooth muscle, these signals probably relate to coordination of contractile waves across the muscle mass. Apparently, nexus formation among certain populations of smooth muscle cells can occur profusely and rapidly. In at least some mammals, there is an enormous increase in numbers of these junctions among smooth muscle cells of the pregnant uterus just prior to parturition, apparently as a response to hormonal signals and as a means to coordinate uterine contracture.

The external lamina of each smooth muscle cell forms a complete covering, except for the regions of nexuses, and appears to aid in holding the cells together. It is composed of specialized filamentous *linkage proteins* and *glycosaminoglycans* which blend into the surrounding reticular and other collagenous fibrils and transmit muscular tension to these connective tissue elements. The reticular fibers can be demonstrated for light microscopy either by Bielchowsky's silver method or by the periodic acid-Schiff (PAS) technique. With resorcin-fuchsin, neighboring elastic fibers can be demonstrated. These are occasionally seen in macerated preparations as tiny coils around the cells. Between the larger bundles of smooth muscle cells, coarser collagenous and elastic fibers are found (Figs. 8.1 and 8.2). Because smooth muscle in mammals either ends in soft parts or forms more or less continuous circular or spiral bands within various organs, there is no specialized connective tissue attachment such as the tendon of skeletal muscle.

Although the filaments are not arranged in orderly register, as they are in striated muscle (discussed below), the *contraction* of smooth muscle is apparently dependent

---

cluster of a third class of filaments, the noncontractile 10-nm intermediate filaments, can be identified (*arrows*). Note the nexuses (*N*) between adjacent smooth muscle cells and attachment placques (*A*) which may anchor filaments to the cell membrane. In the *right figure* the smooth muscle cells are cut longitudinally. Thick filaments (*T*) are seen paralleling the numerous thin filaments. Cytoplasmic dense bodies (*D*), which may function as anchoring devices among the thin filaments, are observed in both figures. Note also pinocytotic vesicles (*V*), external lamina (*E*), and mitochondria (*M*) (×67,200). (Courtesy of Dr. Richard M. Bois.)

upon interaction of thick and thin myofilaments. However, details of the contractile mechanism are not as well understood as they are for skeletal muscle. The thick filaments are considerably longer (~2.2 μm) than those of skeletal muscle and are disposed in a ratio of about 1 thick filament per 15 thin filaments.

As will be seen in the discussion of striated muscle contraction, interaction of thick (*myosin*) and thin (*actin*) filaments requires activation on the part of calcium ions released into the cytoplasm. The calcium reservoir is known in striated muscle, but not in smooth muscle. However, some evidence points toward the possibility that calcium ions are sequestered into smooth muscle cells through the action of the numerous caveolae and vesicles which line the plasmalemma (Fig. 8.3). The specialized endoplasmic reticulum which serves calcium storage and release in skeletal muscle is only sparsely present in smooth muscle.

As will be better appreciated after discussion of the dynamics of skeletal muscle contraction (see below), the regulation of interaction between actin and myosin filaments is different in smooth muscle. Here phosphorylation of a component of the myosin (termed *light chain myosin*) is required to regulate the energetics of contraction, whereas a protein complex associated with actin (called *troponin*) serves this regulatory function in skeletal muscles.

The contraction of smooth muscle is slow and sustained; it contrasts with the range of skeletal muscle activity, which is generally rapid and fatiguing. Each smooth muscle cell may contract in its entirety, or the contraction may pass over the cell in a wave, only part of each cell being in a state of contraction at a given instant. The oblique direction of the filaments and their attachment at the side of the cell, rather than a longitudinal end to end arrangement, seems to correlate with this ability for localized contraction. When the cells have been caught in a completely contracted state by the fixative, they appear shortened and stain more intensely. If a wave has been caught passing over the cell by the fixing reagent, the contracted portion is bulged and shortened and is more heavily stained than the rest of the cell, so that it looks like a swollen dark segment of the cell. These *contraction bands* have a tendency to extend in lines across the whole sheet of muscle so that the contracted swelling involves the center of one cell and the narrower extremities of its neighbors at the same time. Electron micrographs sometimes disclose the contraction bands more clearly (Fig. 8.5).

There are *nerve endings* about smooth muscle cells, but motor terminations for every cell have not been demonstrated. It seems, therefore, that a supplemental type of transmission must be utilized to activate the cells distant from nerve endings. This might involve: (*a*) communicating junctions or nexuses as described above; (*b*) mechanical pull of a contracting cell on its neighbors by their connective tissue investments; and (*c*) action of diffusely spreading chemical agents.

Smooth muscle is not as richly supplied with blood vessels as is skeletal or cardiac muscle. The arteries and veins are carried in the coarser septa of connective tissue. The capillaries lie in connective tissue between thin layers or small groups of cells rather than about individual cells. Connective tissue cells are rare or absent among the reticular fibrils between the muscle cells, unless associated with the blood vessels or larger connective tissue laminae. Evidence from several directions suggests strongly that smooth muscle cells are capable of synthesizing considerable amounts of elastin and collagen, at least early in their differentiation.

Smooth muscle is found in the wall of the alimentary canal from the middle of the esophagus to the anus; gallbladder and hepatic ducts; dorsal wall of trachea and whole bronchial tree; ureter, bladder, urethra, corpora cavernosa, testes and ducts, prostate and Cowper's glands; broad ligament, ovary, oviduct, uterus, and vagina; blood vessels; and larger lymphatics and

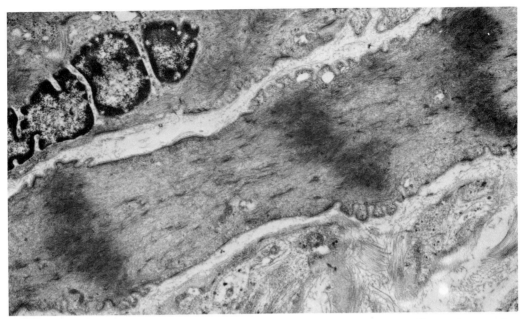

Figure 8.5. Electron micrograph of a smooth muscle cell which displays several dense "contraction bands" across its cytoplasm. The plasma membrane is ruffled at the level of the bands. The nucleus of a neighboring smooth muscle cell (*upper left*) is wrinkled, a characteristic of the contracted state (×23,600). (Courtesy of Dr. David Chase.)

spleen. It also is found in the skin in connection with hairs (*arrectores pilorum*) and occasionally in other places (e.g., corrugator cutis ani), and in the iris and ciliary body of the eye.

Proliferation of smooth muscle cells by mitotic division has been found in the uteri of virgin rabbits treated with female sex hormone, and formation of new muscle cells from undifferentiated cells during pregnancy has been described. Regenerative capabilities of the muscle coats of the alimentary tract are limited, however, and healing of wounds takes place principally by scar formation. The muscle cells of the walls of new blood vessels associated with healing processes have been described as originating from primitive types of perivascular connective tissue cells.

Smooth muscle is often regarded as the most primitive of the body's musculature because of the seemingly diffuse arrangement of its contractile and supportive filaments. In this regard the similarity between smooth muscle filamentous systems and the less obvious or concentrated contractile filaments of epithelial or mesenchymal cells is notable. However, one might also regard smooth muscle as rather highly specialized to provide the necessary slow and sustained contractility that underlies many visceral and vascular activities. By either interpretation it is in distinct morphological contrast to skeletal muscle.

SKELETAL MUSCLE

Of all the cells of the body, those in skeletal muscle present perhaps the most concentrated and highly ordered array of cytoplasmic filaments and membranous compartments. Skeletal muscle has evolved its complexity coincident with the evolution of efficient mobility of organisms. It generally serves relatively quick, voluntary movement and displays morphological variation which reflects gradations in the speed of contractility.

The smallest independent cellular units of mature skeletal muscle are called *fibers*, although they are frequently referred to as cells. They are more complicated than the cells of smooth muscle; they have many nuclei and are larger. The fibers are grouped together into bundles called *fasciculi*. In some muscles (gluteus maximus, deltoideus), the bundles become larger than in others, giving the muscle a coarse-grained appearance when seen with the naked eye. The larger muscles are composed of many fasciculi.

The skeletal muscles of the trunk are derived from myotomal mesoderm of the embryonic somites. Their eventual innervation and action reflects this segmental (*metameric*) origin. The limb muscles are formed from the mesenchyme of the limb buds. Muscles of the tongue are formed from head mesenchyme, and many muscles of the face, jaws, neck, and shoulders derive

from mesenchyme of the branchial arches (the *branchiomeric* musculature). Much of the head and branchial mesenchyme is of neural crest origin.

As in the case of smooth muscle, the first evidence of differentiation is the elongation of mesenchymal cells to form myoblasts (Fig. 8.6). Then an unusual step occurs. Fusion of *myoblasts* gives rise to multinucleated *myotubes*. Growth occurs by continued fusion of myoblasts and myotubes. There is no evidence of nuclear division either by amitosis or mitosis in the new multinucleated muscle cells (fibers). The specialized *myofilaments* make their appearance in the cytoplasm during or shortly after the fusion of myoblasts. Actin and myosin filaments appear separately and seem, at first, to be randomly arranged.

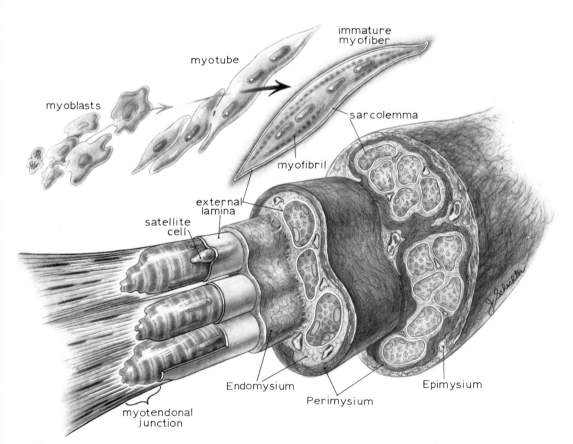

Figure 8.6. Schematic representation of the stages in skeletal muscle fiber development (*top*) and the eventual organization of adjacent muscle fibers and their connective tissue ensheathments and attachments.

They generally arise amid polyribosomal clusters in scattered regions of the cytoplasm and gradually become aligned into *myofibrils* as they accumulate, first as irregular bundles of filaments, and later with filaments aligned in lateral register at Z discs of the fibrils (see below). It has been shown that the cytogenesis of skeletal muscle in vitro is similar to that in vivo and that the organelles essential for contraction can differentiate in the absence of any nerve supply to the muscle.

The number of muscle fibers apparently does not increase significantly during the last month of fetal life or after birth. Increase in the overall size of a muscle is then brought about by the increase in diameter of the fibers through the formation of more myofilaments. As myotubes differentiate into uniform muscle fibers, they invest themselves, individually or in groups, with *external lamina*, thus segregating themselves from surrounding connective tissue.

Not all of the primitive muscle fibers survive. Many of them fail to establish themselves as necessary units of the muscle and degenerate.

Fibers

The *fibers* are cylindrical, multinucleate, cellular structures which vary greatly in length. A common average length for a fiber in man is 3 cm, but lengths of 4 cm or more are not uncommon, and the shortest fibers in small muscles (e.g., stapedius) are less than 1 mm in length. Within a given muscle, the fibers conform to one of three modes of attachment: (a) those extending from one end of the fasciculus to the other; (b) those beginning at one or the other end of the fasciculus and terminating within the substance of the bundle; and (c) those having both ends within the muscular substance. Actually, each muscle is composed of many fasciculi, and the connections from the different fasciculi to the main tendon are via interfascicular, dense, regularly arranged connective tissue (i.e., by subdivisions of the main tendon).

The diameters of fibers vary from 10 to 100 μm, so that, in many cases, the fibers are visible to the naked eye. Although fibers of different thickness are intermingled in the same muscle, there is a more or less typical size for each muscle, and some correlation has been found between the heaviness of the work a muscle performs and the thickness of its fibers. Fibers in the delicate ocular muscles are much smaller than those of a bulky muscle like the gastrocnemius (Fig. 8.7). The fibers of a well nourished individual are thicker than those of one who is emaciated. Moreover, the increase in size of a muscle which takes

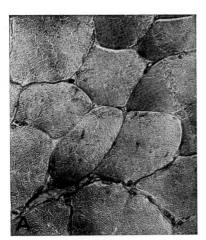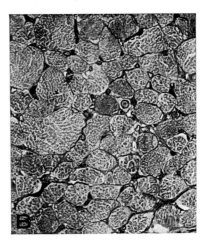

Figure 8.7. Relative diameters of human muscle fibers. *A*, gastrocnemius; *B*, ocular muscle. The muscles were taken from the same subject, a middle-aged adult, and were photographed at the same magnification (×335).

place during the growth of an individual or which is brought about by exercise is due to an increase in the size of its fibers rather than an increase in their number.

Skeletal muscle fibers also vary in diameter in different classes of vertebrates. For example, the fibers of amphibians and fishes are generally thicker, whereas those of birds are thinner, than those of mammals.

When a fresh muscle fiber is teased and broken, a thin, transparent covering membrane known as the *sarcolemma* (from the Greek *sarx*, flesh, + *lemma*, husk) is visible under the light microscope. Electron micrographs reveal that it is composed of a plasmalemma plus an external lamina and occasional reticular fibers. Nevertheless, it has become common to use the term *sarcolemma* for the plasmalemma of muscle cells. As differentiation of a fiber proceeds in the skeletal muscles of mammals, the numerous myonuclei become ovoid and flattened. They assume a position just inside the sarcolemma and usually vaguely aligned in rows or spirals (see Figs. 8.8, 8.9, and 8.11). The vast majority of the volume of each fiber is occupied by the massive cross-striated contractile organelles, the *myofibrils.* Surrounding the fibrils and accumulated near the nuclei are the remaining cytoplasmic components of the fiber, collectively called the *sarcoplasm.*

Each average-sized skeletal muscle fiber comes to possess several hundred *myonuclei,* and each is approximately the same size as the nuclei of neighboring connective tissue cells. In fresh muscle, they are difficult to see by light microscopy, faintly outlined against the background of striated fibrils. In fixed preparations, they show a loose network of chromatin threads and granules. Interior nuclei are common in the lower vertebrates, and in skeletal muscles of insects it is usual for the nuclei to form an axial column in the center of the fiber.

Myofibrils and Sarcomeres

Skeletal muscle examined by light microscopy at low magnification displays striking regular light and dark stripes arranged *across* each fiber (Figs. 8.9 and 8.10). These *cross striations* are visible whether the muscle is fresh, or fixed and stained,

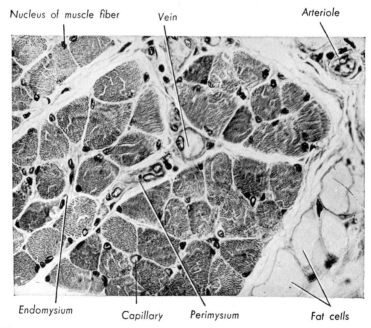

Nucleus of muscle fiber   *Vein*   *Arteriole*

Endomysium   *Capillary*   *Perimysium*   *Fat cells*

Figure 8.8. Cross section of skeletal muscle. Human tongue. Hematoxylin and eosin. Photomicrograph (×510).

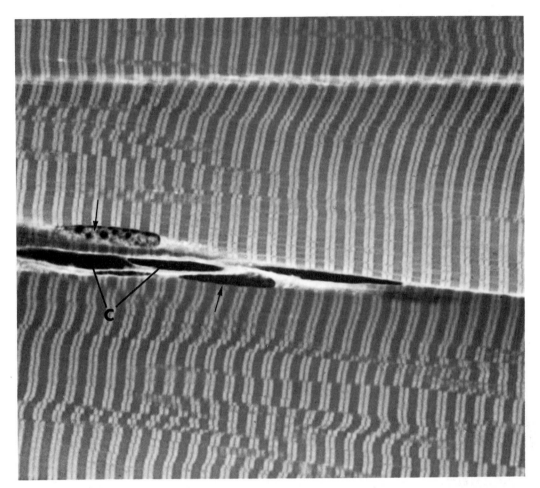

Figure 8.9. HIgh magnification light micrograph of plastic-embedded longitudinally sectioned skeletal muscle. Portions of three fibers are visible. Flattened myonuclei (*arrows*) lie beneath the cell membranes of two of the fibers. Equally flattened connective tissues cells (*C*) lie nearby. Although it is difficult to discern individual myofibrils, the registered banding patterns which form the cross striations of each fiber are obvious. A bands are dark and wide and I bands are light and of about equal width. Each I band is bisected by a narrow dark line, the Z disc. Close inspection reveals a slightly lighter midportion of each A band, the H zone. In a few regions a faint dark line, the M disc, can be discerned midway within H zones (×2,000).

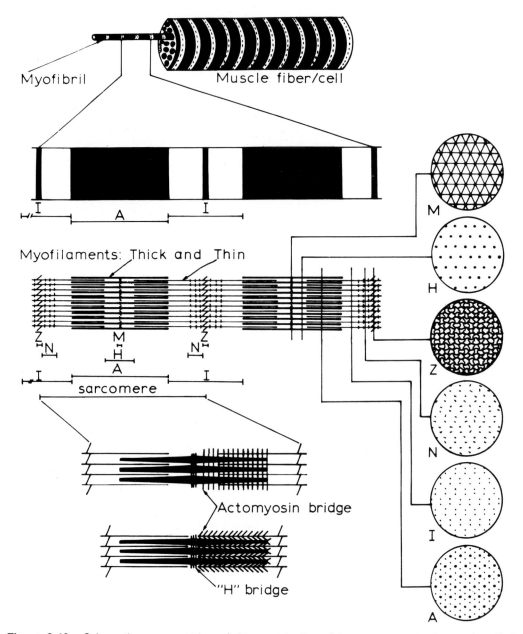

Figure 8.10. Schematic representation of the organization of two sarcomeres along a myofibril removed from a muscle fiber. Details of the sarcomeres and their bands as revealed by electron microscopic techniques are shown in the *lower portion* of the diagram. The *circled images* to the *right* represent thin cross sections through various regions of a sarcomere. At *bottom left*, component filamentous parts of a single sarcomere are shown in relaxed and contracted states. (Diagram courtesy of Dr. Michael J. Cavey.)

and in either transmitted or polarized light. They are the result of regular side-by-side alignment of repeating dense and less-dense components arrayed along longitudinal cables, termed *myofibrils*, which pack

the interior of each muscle fiber. Myofibrils range from 1 to 2 μm in diameter, but may be as small as 0.2 μm. In a cross section of a fiber, the myofibrils are usually visible as punctate densities with individual size and shape separated from each other by narrow clear sarcoplasmic regions (Fig. 8.8). Sometimes the fibrils seem segregated into groups, known as Cohnheim's fields.

Electron microscopy has confirmed that the cross striations result from internal structure of repeating subunits, the *sarcomeres*, which are arranged in series along each myofibril. A sarcomere is the fundamental structural and functional unit of contraction in skeletal muscle. Each sarcomere is composed of smaller segments or "bands" recognized by distinct refractive differences. The more refractive segments color readily with a variety of dyes, the less refractive are broadest, and alternate with less refractive ones. Because the broad, darkly staining band is doubly refractive or *anisotropic* when studied under polarized light, it is known as the *A band*. The light-staining band is relatively monorefringent or *isotropic* when studied under the polarizing microscope, and therefore it is known as the *I band*. Each of these bands is bisected by a narrow zone. It is dense in the I bands and designated *Z line* or disc (from the German *Zwishenscheibe*, between disc). The zone bisecting the A band is pale and is designated *H* (both from the German *Hell*, light, and from the name of the discoverer, Hensen) (compare Figs. 8.9 and 8.12).

The portion of fibril between two successive Z discs is a sarcomere. Its length in relaxed mammalian muscle is 2 to 3 μm. It may be stretched to a greater length, and in greatly contracted fibers it may be reduced to about 1 μm. Insect muscles with sarcomeres 14 μm long have been described.

With the electron microscope all of the cross bands or discs observed with the light microscope are revealed, plus some additional zones (Fig. 8.10). Moreover, the sarcomeres of each myofibril can be seen to be an orderly three-dimensional assembly of much finer filaments. Two filament types predominate; these are known collectively as *myofilaments* because their interaction results in the generation of contractile force. One of the myofilament types has a diameter of about 10 nm, whereas the other type is only 5 nm in diameter. The *thick* (*myosin*) *filaments* have a length of approximately 1.5 μm and occupy the A bands. The *thin* (*actin*) *filaments* extend from either side of the Z disc, across the adjacent I band, and into the A band as far as the H zone (Figs. 8.10 through 8.13). Thus, the electron microscope reveals that the cross bands seen with the light microscope are related to the distribution and overlap of interdigitating myofilaments.

The distribution of the myofilaments can be seen to advantage in electron micrographs when the myofibrils are sectioned transversely (Figs. 8.14 and 8.15). Sections across the I band show only thin filaments, those through the extremities of the A band have both thick and thin filaments, and those through the H zone have only thick filaments. The two types of filaments have a precise relationship to each other in the A band regions where they interdigitate. As seen in cross sections, they have a constant arrangement, with one thick filament in the center of a hexagon of six thin filaments (see also Fig. 8.16). The thick filaments are arranged as triangles with one thin filament at the center of each triangle. Close inspection reveals thin cross bridges extending from each myosin filament to link it with its neighboring actin filaments.

The Z disc is a filamentous network which serves to link the actin filaments of one sarcomere to those of the next. Z disc filaments appear reinforced with a dense sarcoplasmic matrix material in many striated muscles. These reinforcing matrices may impart different patterns and consistencies to Z discs of different muscles, and to muscles fixed by different methods. *Tonic* skeletal muscle, for example, displays very broad, dense, and irregular Z discs compared to those of fast muscle (Figs. 8.14 and 8.15). Although the pattern of filamentous arrangement within the Z disc can be deduced from high resolution electron micrographs (Fig. 8.17), the precise molecular mechanism for actin-to-actin linkage there is not well understood. Various models have

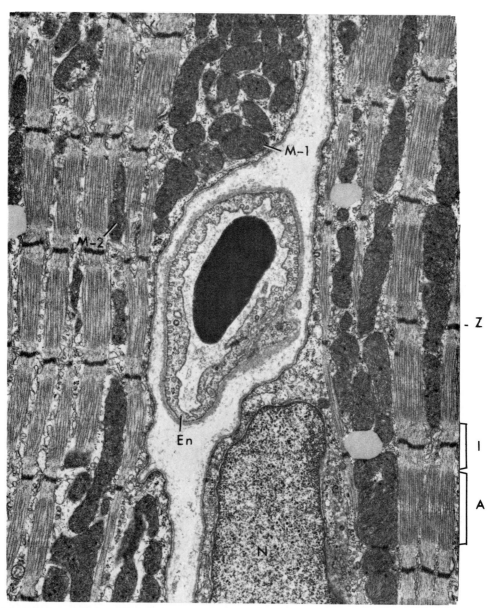

Figure 8.11. Electron micrograph showing portions of two skeletal muscle fibers. The plane of the section cuts only one of the muscle fiber nuclei (*N*). Numerous mitochondria (*M-1*) are seen in the sarcoplasm of the subsarcolemmal region of each fiber and additional mitochondria (*M-2*) are present in the sarcoplasm between myofibrils. The anisotropic or A bands (*A*) of each myofibril are dark and the isotropic or I bands (*I*) are relatively light. Each of the latter is bisected by a dense Z disc (*Z*). Caveolae and vesicles can be seen in the cytoplasm of the endothelium (*En*) of a capillary located in the connective tissue between the muscle fibers. Extrinsic eye muscle of slow loris (×14,000). (Micrograph in collaboration with Mary Ann Cahill.)

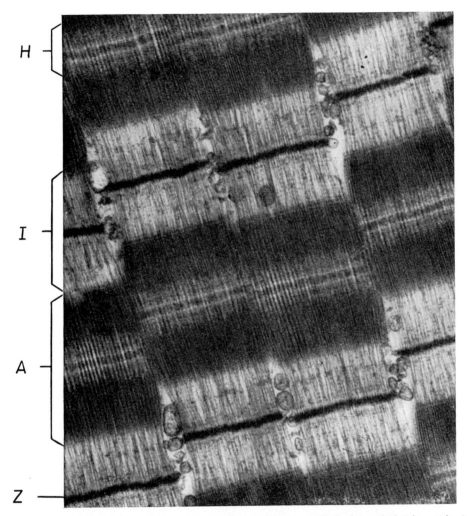

Figure 8.12.   Electron micrograph showing portions of four myofibrils from skeletal muscle, taken from rabbit psoas muscle. The anisotropic bands (*A*) are dense for most of their extent; they are bisected by lighter zones (*H*), within which there is a thin dense M disc (unlabeled). The isotropic bands (*I*) are light regions, each bisected by a relatively dense, narrow disc (*Z*) (×26,000). (Courtesy of Dr. H. E. Huxley.)

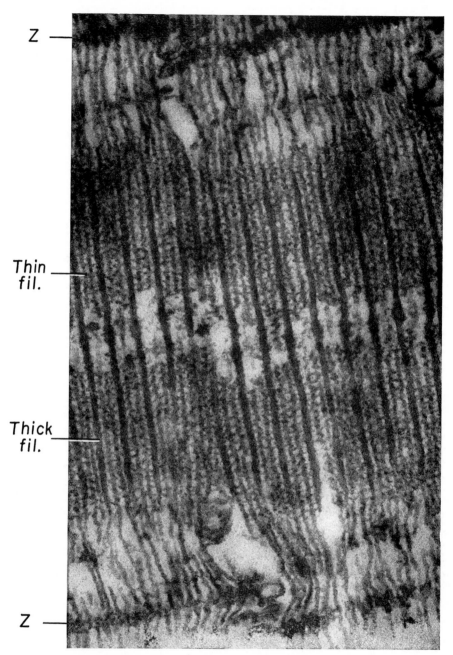

Figure 8.13. High magnification electron micrograph of longitudinal section of relaxed skeletal muscle, taken from rabbit psoas muscle. The thick myosin filaments (*Thick fil.*) extend throughout the length of the A band and the thin actin filaments (*Thin fil.*) are found in the I band and in a part of A; they do not continue through the H zone, although there is some indication of a connecting protein of undetermined nature linking thickened portions of the thick filaments in the center of the H zone (M disc). The actin filaments are twice as numerous as the myosin ones, but they are seen in this manner only when the section passes through the fibers in a plane, as indicated in Fig. 8.16D. Heavy meromyosin cross linkages from myosin to actin are visible (×148,000). (Courtesy of Dr. H. E. Huxley.)

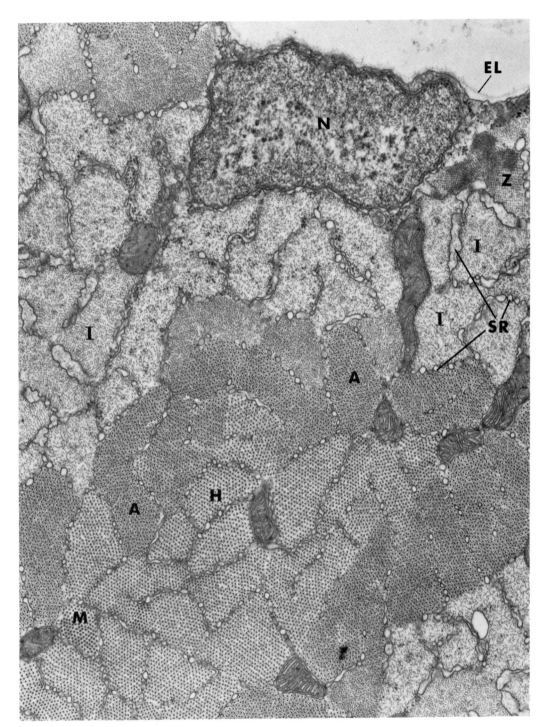

Figure 8.14. Electron micrograph of a cross section of a small portion of a "fast" skeletal muscle fiber. The nucleus (*N*) lies just inside the sarcolemma and the external lamina (*EL*). *Z*, *I*, *A*, *H*, and *M* refer to planes of section through corresponding bands of sarcomeres (compare to diagram in Fig. 8.10). The sarcoplasmic reticulum (*SR*) is abundant and forms an ensheathment around individual myofibrils. Note that the tubular sarcoplasmic reticulum expands into terminal cisternae in regions where it approaches the Z disc. This sample is from amphibian skeletal muscle (×32,500). (Micrograph in collaboration with Mary Ann Cahill.)

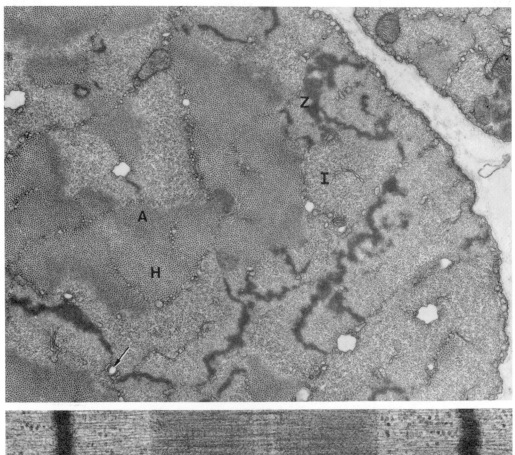

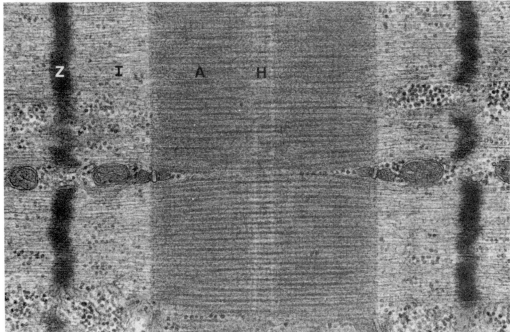

Figure 8.15. Electron micrographs of tonic ("slow") skeletal muscle. *Top,* cross section from amphibian muscle showing similarity of A, H, and I bands to those of "fast" muscle (compare to Fig. 8.14). However, the Z disc (*Z*) is much more dense in its matrix component and irregular in profile. The sarcoplasmic reticulum is also more sparse. A T tubule (*arrow*) is visible between two terminal cisterns. Other T tubules are probably artifactually dilated. *Bottom,* longitudinal section of guinea pig tonic muscle. Note thick Z discs and scanty sarcoplasmic reticulum. Triads are located at junction of A and I bands in this relaxed specimen (*top* ×22,000, *bottom* ×40,000). (Micrographs in collaboration with Mary Ann Cahill and Aileen Kuda).

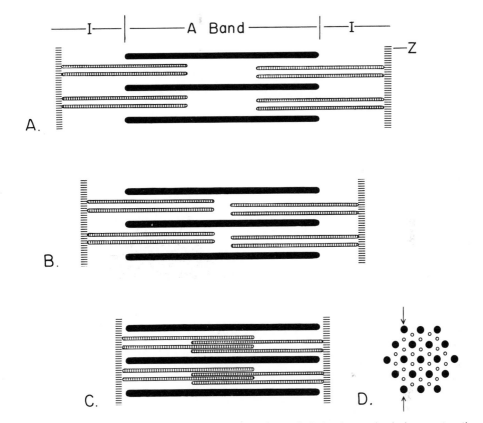

Figure 8.16. Diagram showing changes in fine structure of skeletal muscle during contraction. *A*, resting muscle; *B*, partially contracted; *C*, contracted; and *D*, arrangement of myofilaments as seen in a cross section through the anisotropic band. Note that longitudinal sections (*A*, *B*, *C*) show the thick (myosin) filaments separated by two thin (actin) filaments when the plane of the section corresponds with that shown by the *arrows*; in sections perpendicular to the one indicated, two actin filaments usually are superimposed and appear as one thin filament for each thick one. Note that the isotropic (*I*) band shortens and disappears during contraction, whereas the anisotropic (*A*) band maintains its length over a wide range of muscle lengths. In extreme contractions, beyond that illustrated, the ends of the myosin filaments of one sarcomere meet with those of adjacent sarcomeres and crumple along the *Z* disc, giving rise to new band patterns. Not illustrated is the fact that sarcomeric girth is increased concurrently with contracture. (Diagrams based on illustrations and descriptions by H. E. Huxley.)

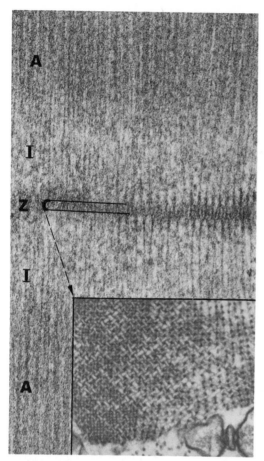

Figure 8.17. High magnification electron micrograph showing a portion of a Z disc (Z) as seen in a longitudinal section of skeletal muscle. The Z disc is flanked by its adjacent I band (I) and nearby A bands (A) of two adjacent sarcomeres. The *inset* depicts details of the Z disc when seen in a cross section, the plane and thickness of which is indicated by *brackets* and *arrow*. A nearby T tubule and two terminal cisterns are seen in the *lower right* of the *inset*. Amphibian skeletal muscle (×90,000). (Micrograph in collaboration with Mary Ann Cahill.)

been proposed; some anticipate direct actin-to-actin interaction, whereas others rely upon looping filament patterns and/or the presence of intermediary linking proteins such as *tropomyosin* or *α-actinin*. According to the most widely accepted model, four Z disc filaments radiate diagonally from the tip of each actin filament at the edge of a Z disc. These each cross the Z disc to attach (with three like members) to an

actin tip in the adjacent sarcomere. In certain muscular diseases, and in muscle which has been detached from its tendinous anchorage, the Z discs become greatly thickened as a result of multiple layering of the linkage mechanism.

Myosin filaments seem held in register by virtue of some form of attachment in the center of the H zone, the so-called *M line* or *disc* (Figs. 8.10 and 8.12). Here each myosin filament is connected with its neighboring myosin filaments by slender, transversely oriented filaments about 4 nm in diameter, and these latter filaments may be interconnected and supported by other slender filaments that course parallel to the myosin filaments. Again, the appearance of an H zone is highly variable among different muscles.

In addition to the above well-recognized banding patterns, some muscle preparations disclose a faint cross striation in the I band, usually near the Z disc. The significance of these so-called *N bands* is as yet unclear. Like smooth muscle cells, striated muscle is known to contain 10 nm supportive filaments (*intermediate filaments*). The exact architecture of this non-contractile cytoskeleton and its relation to the contractile system has not been resolved completely. It is clear from recent immunocytochemical evidence that intermediate filaments containing two special proteins, *desmin* and *vimentin*, form a series of supportive ring-like frameworks around the Z discs, linking each to Z discs at the same level of adjacent myofibrils and possibly to the sarcolemma (Fig. 8.18). The proteins of this peri-Z disc lattice are different from those of the Z disc proper. Microtubules may also play an important supportive role, particularly in myoblasts and myotubes. None of these filaments and microtubules are to be confused with cross bridges between myosin and actin filaments, which have an important role in the mechanisms of contraction.

Further details on actin and myosin filaments have been obtained by electron microscope studies of negatively stained, iso-

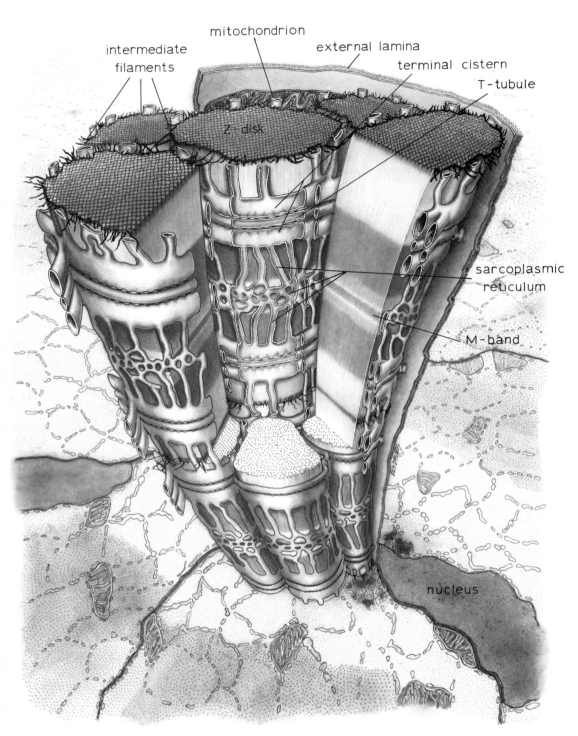

Figure 8.18. Schematic representation of the components in and associated with several mammalian skeletal myofibrils. Note the three-dimensional arrangement of the sarcoplasmic reticulum and T tubular system. Triadic junctions are seen between T tubules and terminal cisterns. A portion of the sarcolemma and its external lamina is included to illustrate the continuity of T tubules and the myofiber's surface membrane. Intermediate filaments interconnect Z discs of adjacent fibrils.

lated filaments and from X-ray diffraction studies (Fig. 8.19). Each actin filament is composed of two strands of *F actin* (fibrous actin) coiled in a helix. Each F actin filament is a polymer of about 200 small globular units, *G actin* monomers. *Tropomyosin* and *troponin*, newly described regulatory proteins, are associated with the actin filaments. Tropomyosin is believed to be helically wound along the grooves of the F actin double helix and troponin is thought to occupy specific active sites as tripartite complexes of globular molecules inserted at each half-turn of the same helix.

Myosin filaments are made up of a number of myosin molecules. Each molecule is composed of two long, 200,000-dalton polypeptides plus four smaller polypeptides of about 20,000 daltons each. The two longer polypeptides are helically intertwined over about half their length, forming a rod-like structure. A number of these packed longitudinally form the rigid backbone of the myosin filament. The remaining free ends of the long polypeptide chains plus the 20,000-dalton polypeptides (*light chain myosins*) are folded into two globular regions which retain connections to the backbone through short, flexible neck regions.

Isolated myosin molecules can be fragmented by proteolytic enzymes. The two major fragments thus formed are called *light meromyosin* and *heavy meromyosin*. The former constitutes the backbone of the myosin filament and the latter includes the globular ends of the long polypeptide chains, the flexible connecting necks, and the associated light chain myosins. Additional proteolysis of heavy meromyosin frees the globular portion, or S_1 fraction, from the connecting neck, or S_2 fraction. The light chain myosins remain associated with the S_1 fraction.

The flexible neck lies parallel to the backbone myosin filament in relaxed muscle, and the globular heads extend laterally towards the actin filaments (Figs. 8.13 and 8.19). The myosin molecules are polarized in the sense that the heavy meromysin subunits are always aligned with their globular heads directed away from the midpoint along the length of the backbone filament. Thus they face in opposite directions on opposite sides of the M discs. The cross bridges are absent from a central region extending 75 nm on either side of the M line of each myosin filament (the so-called "bare" region). *Adenosine triphosphatase* and *actin-binding sites* are apparently located in or on the globular (S_1) region of the heavy meromyosin.

The globular heads of the heavy meromyosin protrude on their flexible necks from the backbone filament, forming the *cross bridges*, at intervals of about 14.3 nm (143 Å, Fig. 8.19). Moreover, successive cross bridges along the filament protrude at an angle of approximately 60° relative to each other, forming 60° steps in a spiral. Actually a double spiral of heavy meromyosin cross bridges is achieved by the myosin molecular organization, and the 60° steps of these correspond closely, but not exactly, with the placement of troponin complexes and binding sites along the six actin filaments that come to surround each myosin filament. The implications of this arrangement will be apparent from a discussion of changes during contraction (see below).

In a given muscle there is established during development an appropriate proportion of skeletal muscle fibers which contract rapidly (*phasic* fibers) and ones which contract in a slower and more prolonged fashion (*tonic* fibers). Although these have been occasionally rigidly classified as "*fast*" (*red* or *dark*) and "*slow*" (*white* or *light*) respectively, it now appears that there is a fairly continuous range in speed of contraction, and the extremes of the range display corresponding fine structural differences. With respect to filamentous components, the most obvious difference is in Z disc structure which is more dense and irregular in "slower" fibers (compare Figs. 8.14 and 8.15). In fact, over the breadth of muscle that we commonly describe as skeletal there are far more variations than are usually implied in histology textbooks. Recent

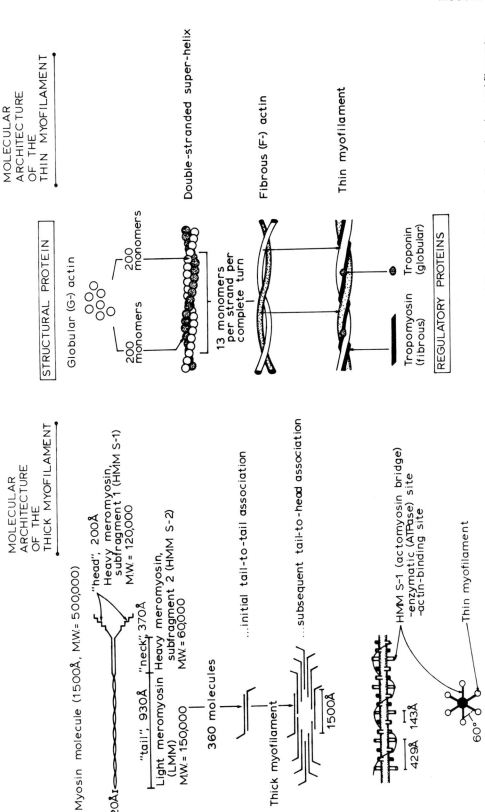

Figure 8.19. Diagrammatic representations of the molecular components of myosin molecules and filaments (*left*) and actin molecules and filaments (*right*). The probable location of tropomyosin and troponin complexes in relation to actin helices is also shown. Dimensions are given in Ångstrom units (Å); Å = 1/10 nm. See text for further explanation. (Diagrams courtesy of Dr. Michael J. Cavey.)

evidence has emerged from experiments in which the innervation to groups of predominantly tonic muscle fibers has been exchanged for that which normally supplies predominantly phasic fibers. The results suggest strongly that the character of the muscle fibers can be converted to match the innervation provided. However, the mechanism of conversion remains to be elucidated.

The Sarcoplasm

The sarcoplasm should *not* be thought of as a structureless fluid phase in which the above contractile mechanism is suspended. Rather, it is a complex assemblage of organelles which provides special structural and energetic support for the contractile apparatus, while serving also the general metabolic requirements of this living cellular system. It includes an elaborate endoplasmic reticulum (the *sarcoplasmic reticulum*), a supportive framework of intermediate and finer filaments, microtubules, a Golgi complex, variable amounts of mitochondria, few ribosomes, glycogen, and occasional lipid droplets.

Fibers which are rich in mitochondria and display less extensive sarcoplasmic membranes tend to be slower. Due to an abundance of a special oxygen transporting pigment, *myoglobin*, they also have a dark appearance in the fresh state, whereas faster fibers have less sarcoplasm and are lighter in color. In some species, e.g., turkey, the *dark fibers* are characteristically predominant in particular muscles and the *light fibers* predominate in other muscles. The two types of fibers as well as intermediate varieties are appropriately intermingled in human and most other mammalian muscles.

The *sarcoplasmic reticulum* is seen in electron micrographs as a network of cisterns or membranous tubules which course between and around the myofibrils (Figs. 8.14, 8.18, and 8.20 through 8.22). It is an agranular reticulum because the relatively few ribosomes present are scattered through the cytoplasm and not aligned on the membranes. The cisterns course chiefly parallel with the myofibrils. Lateral anastomoses between the parallel or longitudinal cisterns form a perforated collar around the myofibrils at the level of the H zone. In the vicinity of the I band or Z disc, the sarcoplasmic reticulum is expanded into *terminal cisterns*. These tend to be arranged into pairs which flank another, single membranous passage, the *transverse tubule* (often called a *T tubule*). (Figs. 8.21 and 8.22). Each transverse tubule and its closely apposed two terminal cisterns constitute a *triad*. Studies of mammalian skeletal muscle show a triadic organization typically with transverse tubules and accompanying terminal cisterns at the level of each A-I junction, rather than at the Z disc (which is the pattern common in lower vertebrate skeletal muscle; Fig. 8.22). This provides two sets of tubules and terminal cisterns per sarcomere.

The transverse tubules are narrow, regularly arranged invaginations of the plasmalemma. Hence, their walls provide narrow tubular extensions of the cell membrane into the depths of the muscle fiber where, within each triad, they form complex membrane-to-membrane junctions (but not actual confluency) with the membranes of the terminal cisterns. These are termed the *triadic junctions* or *triadic couplings*. It now seems clear that an action potential traveling along the transverse tubule membrane is able to signal the terminal cisterns across the junctions. Transverse tubules, therefore, serve for rapid transmission of impulses from the exterior to the deepest regions of the cell, thus giving coordinated activity of all myofibrils. Several models have been proposed for the finest architecture of the *triadic junctions*. The most recent arise from freeze-fracture evidence that discloses that the junctional terminal cistern membranes contain integral subunits which correspond, in their spatial arrangement, with pillars or densities spanning the narrow gaps between each T tubule and its adjacent terminal cisterns (Fig. 8.23). Since similar subunits have not

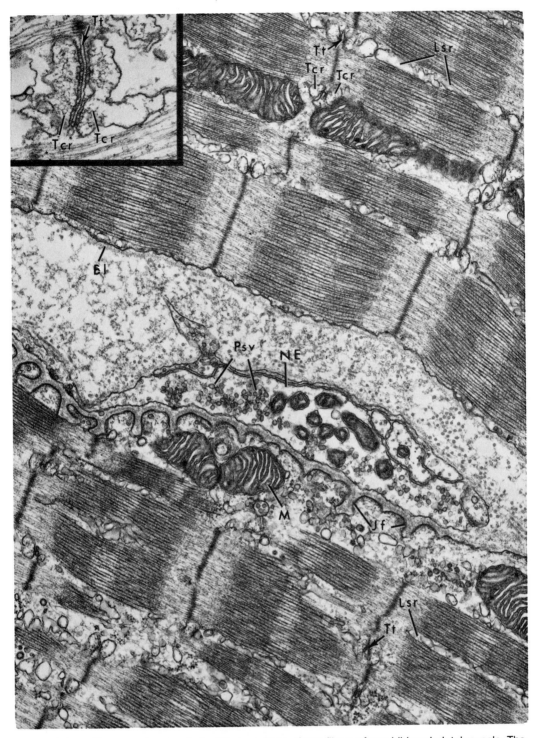

Figure 8.20. Electron micrograph depicting portions of two fibers of amphibian skeletal muscle. The picture shows the interfibrillar components of the muscle fiber in addition to the fine structure of the myofibrils. Note the external lamina (*El*), the mitochondria (*M*), the longitudinally oriented elements of the sarcoplasmic reticulum (*Lsr*), and the dilated terminal cisterns (*Tcr*) of the reticulum. The transverse tubules (*Tt*), invaginations of the sarcolemma, are also seen. The *inset, upper left*, shows, at higher magnification and in a plane perpendicular to the rest of the plate, the relationship of a transverse tubule to the terminal cisterns of the reticulum. The transverse tubule with a dilated cistern on each side constitutes a triad. A nerve ending (*Ne*) on a muscle fiber is seen in the *lower half* of the picture. Note the presynaptic vesicles (*Psv*) in the nerve terminal and the junctional folds (*Jf*) of the sarcolemma (×27,300; *inset*, ×61,870). (Micrograph in collaboration with Mary Ann Cahill.)

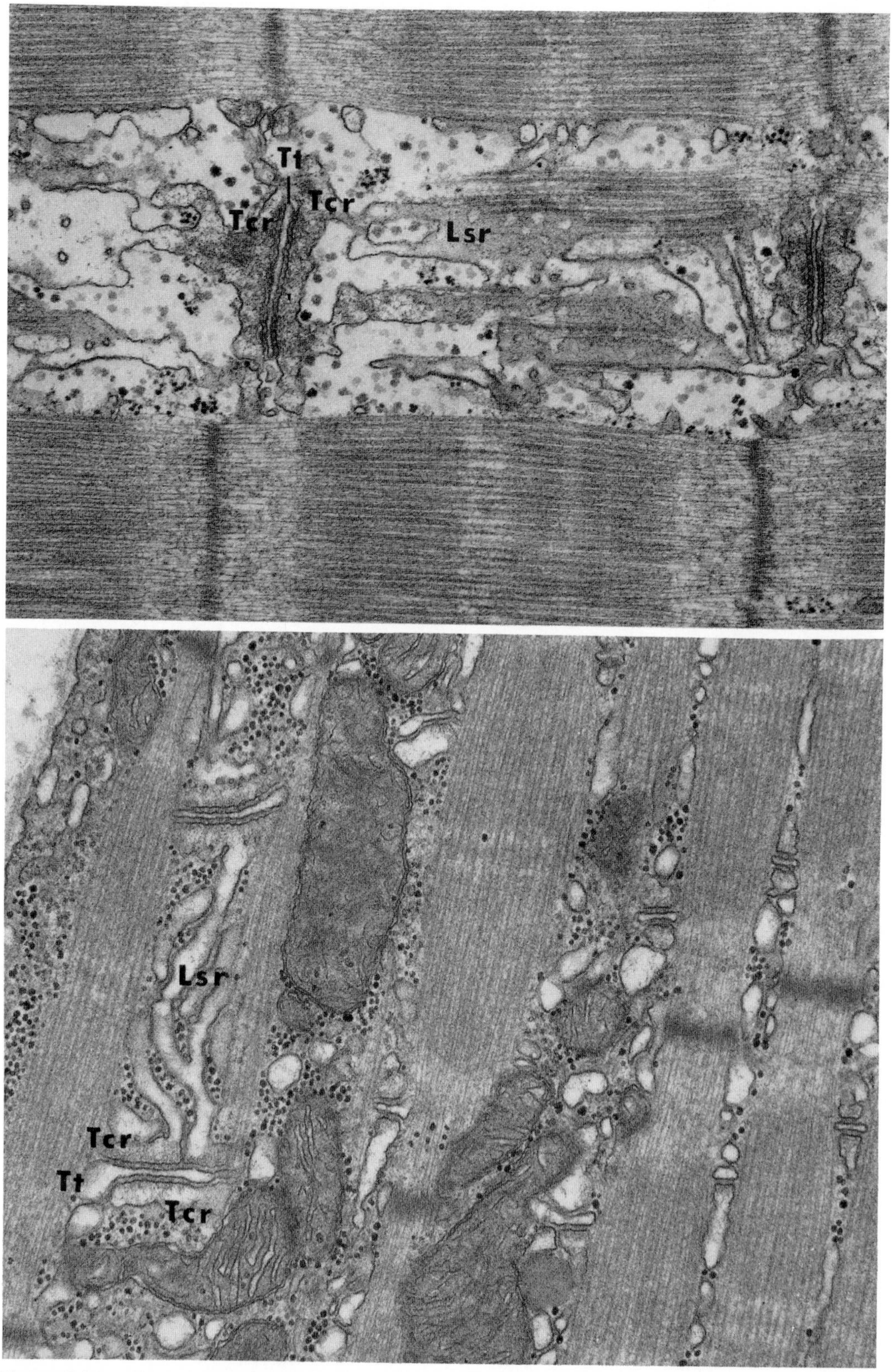

Figure 8.21. Electron micrographs showing components of sarcoplasmic reticulum and T tubular system of fast amphibian (top) and mammalian (bottom) skeletal muscle. In the labeled portions of

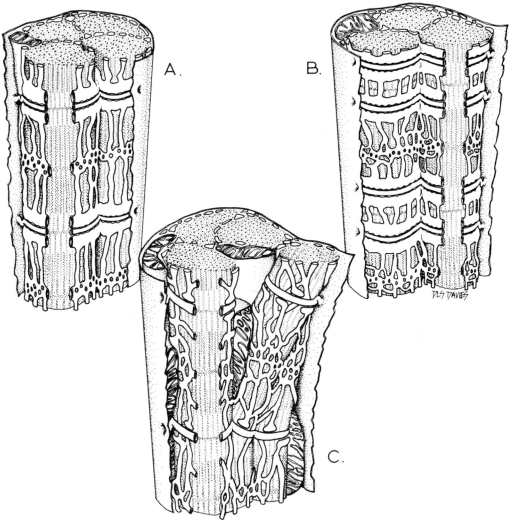

Figure 8.22. Schematic diagrams to compare internal membranous components of lower vertebrate (*A*) and mammalian (*B*) fast skeletal muscle fibers with similar elements in cardiac muscle (*C*). Note narrow sarcoplasmic reticulum network in cardiac muscle. T tubules are wide and irregularly distributed in cardiac muscle and make contact with the sarcoplasmic reticulum in more focal diadic junctions. Compare *A* and *B* with Figures 8.18 and 8.21, and *C* with Fig. 8.30.

been found in T tubule membranes, the junction appears asymmetrical. It is reasonable to suspect that some of the complex structure of triadic junctions relates to maintenance of adhesion, and some relates to the mechanism of signal transfer, but the identity of these as functional units is still obscure.

Freeze-fracture studies also disclose that the *non*-junctional regions of the entire sarcoplasmic reticulum membrane contain closely packed P face particles (Fig. 8.23).

these micrographs, the section plane has passed just to one side of a myofibril, thus intersecting the nearby sarcoplasmic reticulum network (compare to Fig. 8.18). Longitudinal elements of the sarcoplasmic reticulum (*Lsr*) communicate with terminal cisterns (*Tcr*) which, in turn, are attached to T tubules (*Tt*) within triadic junctions. These lie at the level of Z discs in amphibian muscle, but over the A-I junction in mammalian muscle. Note flocculent (calcium-storing?) material in terminal cisterns (*top* ×35,000; *bottom* ×40,000). (*Top figure* in collaboration with Mary Ann Cahill.)

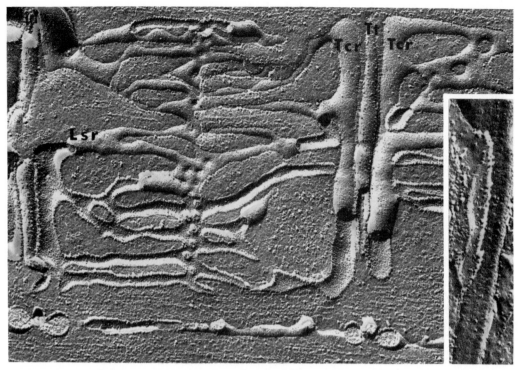

Figure 8.23. Freeze-fracture replica of the sarcoplasmic reticulum and T tubule system from amphibian fast skeletal muscle. The plane of fracture corresponds to that seen in section in Figure 8.21 (*top*). Regions of triadic junction between terminal cisterns of sarcoplasmic reticulum (*Tcr*) and T tubules (*Tt*) are seen at *left* and *right*. Longitudinal elements of the sarcoplasmic reticulum (*Lsr*) extend between the triadic junctional regions. Note richly granulated P faces of the sarcoplasmic reticulum. *Inset (right)* shows a higher magnification view of the triadic junction in which the fracture plane has exposed the E face of the junctional part of the terminal cistern. Note regularly spaced subunits which are characteristic of this membrane (×46,500; *inset* ×72,700). Figures prepared using dark shadow imaging. (Micrographs in collaboration with Aileen Kuda).

These are presumably proteins involved in the transfer of calcium ions into the sarcoplasmic reticulum. A network of dense material is seen in the terminal cisterns in electron micrographs of sectioned muscle cells (Figs. 8.20 and 8.21). This is thought to be involved with calcium, storage within the cistern, prior to its release upon signaling from the T tubule, a point to be elaborated below.

In the study of longitudinal sections, it appears that Z discs, sarcomeres, and triads are aligned in perfect lateral register—from myofibril to myofibril—across the breadth of a muscle fiber. However, recent evidence gained from high voltage stereo electron microscopy of thick sections and serial re-constructions discloses that there is actually a slight displacement of register from one myofibril to the next such that the alignment of Z discs and triads courses spirally along the fiber, rather like the alignment of steps down a shallow spiral staircase. The slight variation is thought to function in integrating and smoothing the contractions of sarcomeres throughout a given muscle cell.

The *mitochondria* of the muscle cell or are found beneath the sarcolemma, around the nuclei, and in the sarcoplasm between the myofibrils (Figs. 8.11 and 8.20). In the last location, they are generally aligned with their long axis parallel to the direction of the myofibril, although they may be found encircling the myofibril transversely, particularly in the region overlying the Z disc.

Changes During Contraction

Morphological changes associated with contraction have been studied both in living and in fixed muscle. In both cases, the fiber as a whole becomes shorter and broader when it contracts. Each sarcomere also becomes shorter and broader. The isotropic or I band becomes shorter as the sarcomere becomes shorter, and it disappears when the fibers are stimulated to contract to about 50% of their resting length. The H zone of the A band gradually disappears concurrently. The total length of the A band, on the other hand, remains constant during normal cycles of contraction and relaxation. The A band seems to shorten only when contraction is so extreme that it produces a concentration of dense material along the Z disc, forming a darkly staining *contraction band*. It is postulated that this is due to overlap of the ends of the thick (myosin) filaments against the Z disc.

Electron micrographs of contracted muscle show an interdigitation of the thick and thin filaments throughout the length of the sarcomere, in contrast with the arrangement seen in resting muscle. Based on these findings, Hanson and Huxley first proposed a *sliding filament mechanism* of contraction (Fig. 8.16). In resting muscle, the thick and thin (myosin and actin) filaments are presumably not firmly attached to each other because a relaxed muscle can be stretched mechanically beyond its normal rest length. During muscle contraction, the heavy meromyosin heads of the cross bridges attach to and interact sequentially with active sites along the actin filament helix as the latter is pulled into the A band.

It has been calculated that the distances between actin binding sites on the heavy meromyosin heads and the active sites along the actin double helix are such to promote a smooth and progressive, wave-like chain of attachment and release as any given actin filament is moved to interdigitate more deeply with the surrounding myosin filaments of the A band. This "stroking" of the actin toward the center of the sarcomere may require flexibility on the part of the neck-like portion of the heavy meromyosin. Some workers postulate that a spiraling of either actin or myosin occurs as contraction and relaxation proceed.

When a nerve to a muscle is stimulated, a *depolarization wave* (*action potential*) spreads rapidly over the muscle cell membrane and over the membranes lining the T tubules to the deepest regions of the cell. Presumably a change in the membrane potential of the T tubules induces, in some manner, a reaction in the adjacent terminal cisterns. The result is that calcium is released from its storage place in the sarcoplasmic reticulum to enter the sarcoplasm immediately bathing the myofibrils. Such freed calcium is necessary for the actin-myosin interaction to occur. According to one of several current theories, calcium operates by invoking a steric conformational change on the regulatory protein complex of *troponins* which, in concert with *tropomyosin*, otherwise acts as a safety catch, preventing activation of myosin *adenosine triphosphatase* by actin (when calcium is absent). The activation occurs as soon as calcium can be bound by one part of the troponin complex and the troponin-tropomyosin assembly is warped so as to expose actin active sites to nearby adenosine triphosphatase-laden globular heavy meromyosin heads. The latter then readily swing to join with active actin sites, an action which in an as yet obscure way promotes movement of the actin helix relative to myosin. In the process, adenosine triphosphate (ATP) is changed by action of the adenosine triphosphatase to *adenosine diphosphate* (ADP), with the release of energy. This energy is believed to provide the motive force for contraction, perhaps by promoting bending of the flexible "neck" of heavy meromyosin. Apparently a phosphate group is split from ATP each time a cross bridge goes through a cycle of attachment and release at each successive actin binding site. When removal of phosphate groups from ATP stops, there is no further action of cross bridges, and the muscle returns to its resting state. At the same time, calcium is withdrawn from the sarcoplasm back into the sarcoplasmic reticulum. ADP is rephosphorylated into ATP before the muscle is ready for contraction again.

While the above postulated mechanism seems to fit well with morphological and physiological data from vertebrate skeletal muscle, it can by no means be precisely universal. Many invertebrate striated muscles, for example, possess much thicker myosin filaments which, unlike those described above, appear to contract *within themselves*. This contraction is in addition to that achieved by interaction with actin, and helps to account for the extreme sarcomeric shortening which those muscles can achieve. Clearly, there is great diversity in patterns of myosin-actin relationships in nature beyond that typically described in medical histology textbooks.

Phosphorylation of ADP back to ATP can be provided by aerobic glycolysis within nearby mitochondria, or under anaerobic conditions from a storage compound, *phosphocreatine*. The latter is regenerated during periods of relaxation. In tonic muscles, abundant mitochondria provide ATP rather directly, but somewhat slowly. By contrast, the "faster" muscles rely heavily and immediately on phosphocreatinine stores and are adapted for prolonged anaerobic operation.

ATP is also required to break the bonding between actin and heavy meromyosin heads. Death results in the loss of available ATP from any source, with the result that bonding persists for some hours—a state referred to as *rigor mortis*.

Connective Tissue

Surrounding each muscle fiber is an external lamina and then a sheath of very delicate, irregularly woven reticular fibrils plus their surrounding ground substance fluids and other molecules (Fig. 8.6 and *center*, Fig. 8.20). It is called the *endomysium*. At many points, the delicate fibrils combine into stronger strands, which merge with collagenous connective tissue fibers. The collagenous fibers, mingled with elastic fibers, form a more or less complete connective tissue sheath about groups of a dozen or more muscle fibers to make up a *fasciculus*. The fasciculi are in turn bound into larger and larger orders of bundles, and the entire muscle has as its outer investment the deep fascia seen upon gross dissection. The outermost sheath of connective tissue is called the *epimysium*, and the tissue surrounding the fasciculi and dividing the muscle by septa is called the *perimysium*.

Muscle-Tendon Attachment

At the ends of a muscle, its fibers are attached securely either to tendon, to periosteum, or to some fibrous connective tissue structure. In light microscopic sections, the fibrils of the muscle fiber often appear to be "continuous" with those of the tendon. The striations of the muscle fiber decrease in distinctness, so that the exact point at which they disappear and the tendon fibers begin is uncertain. Sections stained by the Bielschowsky silver method show that reticular fibers associated with the sarcolemma become aggregated into strands as they converge around the end of the muscle fiber, and that the strands become continuous with fiber bundles of the tendon (Fig. 8.24). Connective tissue fibers do not penetrate the sarcolemma but merely extend into indentations. Electron micrographs confirm these conclusions and show in detail how the connective tissue fibers are inserted into invaginations of the sarcolemma (Fig. 8.24). There they are apparently attached firmly to the external lamina, which in turn is adherent to the sarcolemma. Within the muscle fiber, the actin (thin) filaments distal to the last sarcomere are drawn out and anchored by an as yet obscure mechanism to the cell membrane. Hence, tension generated by the series of sarcomeres aligned in a fibril is

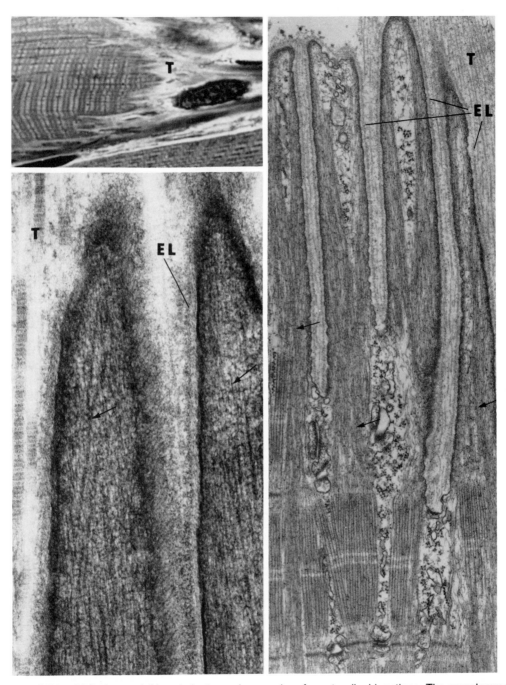

Figure 8.24.   Light (*upper left*) and electron micrographs of myotendinal junctions. The sarcolemma and its surrounding external lamina (*EL*) are folded into long finger-like extensions which interdigitate with collagen and ground substance of a tendon (*T*). Thin filaments (*arrows*) extending from actin filaments of the last sarcomeres are drawn out into the extensions where they attach the sarcolemma along the lateral axes of the interdigitations. Transmission of contractile force involves all of the labeled structures as well as the sarcolemma (*upper left* ×640, *lower left* ×60,000, *right* ×24,600). (Figures at *left* courtesy of Dr. John Trotter; figure at *right* in collaboration with Mary Ann Cahill.)

transmitted successively to the cell membrane, to the external lamina, and then to collagen fibers of the tendon.

Blood Vessels

The larger branches of the arteries penetrate the muscle by following the septa of the perimysium. The arterioles which penetrate the fasciculi give off capillaries at abrupt angles. The capillary supply is rich, several capillaries having proximity with each muscle fiber. The veins follow the arteries; even their smallest branches have valves.

Lymphatic capillaries are not found between individual muscle fibers. They are present, however, in the connective tissue septa and along the blood vessels.

Nerves

Every skeletal muscle fiber receives at least one motor nerve ending from the central nervous system. The minute anatomy of the *motor end plates* is described in chapter 10. The sensory or afferent fibers are principally associated with specialized end organs known as *neuromuscular spindles*, also described in chapter 10.

Regeneration

In adult mammals, *skeletal muscle regeneration* seems quite limited. However, regeneration of vertebrate skeletal muscle can occur after certain chemical, mechanical, or disease-mediated injuries. In most cases, shortly after injury, mononucleated myoblasts appear between the external lamina and the underlying degenerating muscle fiber. Subsequent stages of regeneration closely parallel embryonic myogenesis in that myoblasts proliferate and then undergo fusion to form multinucleated myotubes. Myotube differentiation is characterized principally by synthesis of contractile proteins leading to the maturation of a myofiber. Although motor end plates typically develop in association with the regenerating muscle fibers, complete return of functional activity is usually limited by the amount of scar tissue, which also develops within the regenerating muscle. The major source of regenerating myoblasts, at least

in young mammals, appears to be *satellite cells* (Fig. 8.25), a small population of morphologically undifferentiated cells located between the external lamina and sarcolemma of uninjured muscle fibers. Satellite cells are probably derived from embryonic myoblasts. During postnatal muscle growth they fuse with their adjacent growing myofiber, resulting in an increase in the number of myonuclei. However, not all satellite cells fuse during muscle growth, and those that remain in adult skeletal muscle may have an important role in the repair and regeneration that does occur in mature skeletal muscle.

CARDIAC MUSCLE

The heart muscle, or *myocardium*, is derived from splanchnic mesoderm and, as noted in Chapter 3, is recognizable at a very early age in mammals. The mesenchymal primordium of the heart is at first sequestered well anterior to the neural plate in the early embryo, but with development of the head fold, it is swung into a position just beneath the developing foregut. Here it is formed into a two- and then three-layered tube which will ultimately be contorted and partitioned into the definitive four-chambered heart. The early two layers are an internal endothelium and an outer *epimyocardium*. These are separated by an increasingly thick layer of "*cardiac jelly*," a mesenchymal mass relatively devoid of cells and rich in hyaluronic acid and other hydrated ground substance. In areas of the heart wall which will become muscular, a separate *myocardium* emerges from the epimyocardium at the relative expense of cardiac jelly. Some endothelial cells are known also to contribute fibroblasts to the interior of the heart wall. The resultant adult layers are: an internal endothelial lining, which together with underlying connective tissue constitutes the *endocardium*; an external mesothelium, which together with its adjacent connective tissue comprises the *visceral pericardium*; and between those two layers, the *myocardium*, a distinct layer surrounding all of the chambers of the heart

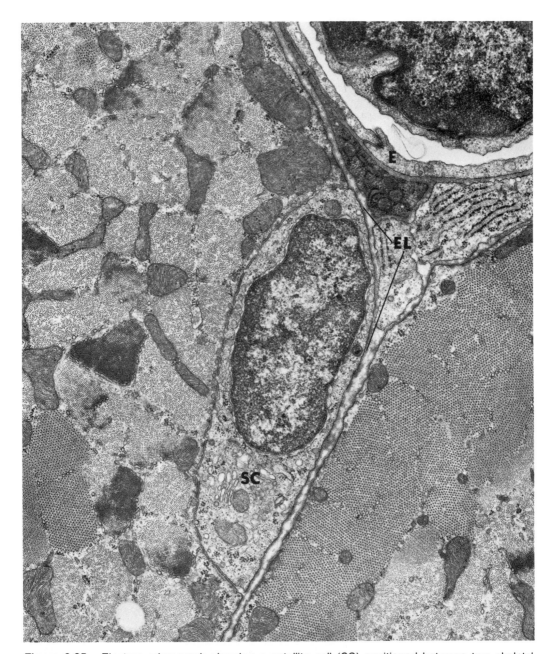

Figure 8.25. Electron micrograph showing a satellite cell (*SC*) positioned between two skeletal muscle fibers, shown here in cross section. Note that the satellite cell lies entirely within the external lamina (*EL*) of the muscle fiber to the *left*. The endothelium (*E*) of a capillary and several processes of connective tissue cells are seen in the *upper right corner* (×11,500). (Courtesy of Dr. Mikel H. Snow.)

but much thicker around the ventricles than around the atria. Cardiac muscle fibers arise by differentiation and growth of single myocardial myoblasts, not by a fusion of cells, as is the case for skeletal muscle fibers. Growth of the fibers occurs by formation of new myofilaments, particularly in the peripheral portion of the cytoplasm.

The myocardium of vertebrate hearts is

therefore composed of *non-syncytial* muscle fibers (cells) which adjoin in an irregular manner to form a branching network. In mammals, the network of cells is partially subdivided by connective tissue into bundles and laminae that wind about the heart in long spirals, particularly in the ventricular walls. The fibers within a bundle are roughly parallel, but the bundles themselves course in different directions in the deeper and more superficial layers, so that any section through the myocardium presents groups of fibers cut longitudinally, transversely, and with varying degrees of obliquity.

Fibers

The cells or fibers of adult cardiac muscle fit together so tightly that under the light microscope they give the false impression of comprising a syncytium (Figs. 8.26 and 8.28). Electron micrographs show, however, that cardiac muscle is definitely composed of elongated, branching cells with irregular contours at their junctions. The fibers are usually about 14 μm in diameter in a normal adult heart, but they vary during normal growth and under pathological conditions. In a newborn, the fibers are only 6 to 8 μm, or approximately one-half the diameter of those of an adult. In hearts showing hypertrophy, the fibers may be 20 μm or more in diameter.

Each fiber is enclosed by a *sarcolemma* which is similar to that of skeletal muscle. The structure seen with the light microscope includes a cell membrane, an external lamina outside the plasmalemma, and associated reticular fibers.

The nuclei, unlike those of skeletal muscle, are generally located in the central portion of the fiber, and number one per cell, or occasionally two, in contrast with the multinucleated condition in skeletal muscle. They are oval in shape and quite large, sometimes one-half of the diameter of the fibers (Figs. 8.26 and 8.28).

The fibers contain *myofibrils* with constituent *actin* and *myosin myofilaments* organized into *sarcomeres* similar to those

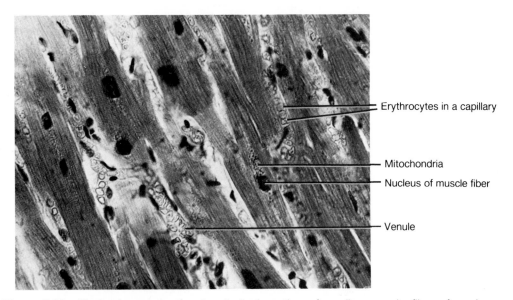

Erythrocytes in a capillary

Mitochondria
Nucleus of muscle fiber

Venule

Figure 8.26. Photomicrograph of a longitudinal section of cardiac muscle fibers from human ventricle. Note that the fibers branch and become apposed to each other in a complicated pattern. The intercalated discs at the sites of intercellular attachment are not obvious in this section, and they are frequently obscured in hematoxylin and eosin-stained preparations of human cardiac muscle. Cardiac muscle has a rich blood supply and the capillaries and venules are seen clearly in this preparation. The 10-μm section is sufficiently thick to show some of the vessels winding around and over the muscle fibers (×390).

Venule   Nuclei of capillary endothelial cells

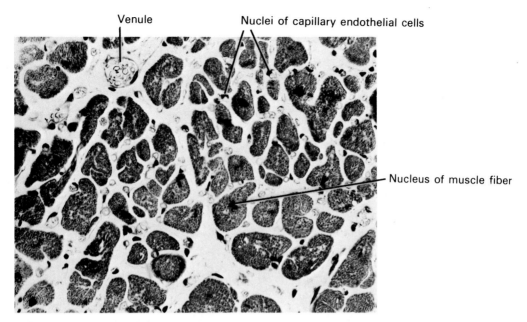

Nucleus of muscle fiber

Figure 8.27. Photomicrograph of a transverse section of cardiac muscle from human ventricle. Note the central portion of the nuclei and the irregular contour of branching fibers cut in cross section. The myofibrils are also cut in cross section, giving the cytoplasm of each fiber a stippled or punctate appearance. Hematoxylin and eosin (×390).

in skeletal muscle. However, the myofibrils course more irregularly than in skeletal muscle, and they frequently branch. Sarcomeres and bundles of myofilaments of one myofibril often become confluent with those of an adjacent myofibril. Consequently, the myofibrils are not as well demarcated as they are in skeletal muscle. In cross sections, the arrangement of the cut ends of the myofibrils often gives the appearance of bands or spokes of a wheel (Fig. 8.27). In longitudinal sections they diverge around the nucleus, leaving a paler-staining zone of *sarcoplasm* at each pole of the nucleus (Fig. 8.28). This zone contains the usual organelles plus some bundles of specialized myofilaments. It has a *sarcoplasmic reticulum* (endoplasmic reticulum), fat droplets, and glycogen. Lipochrome pigment granules may be present in older hearts. As would be expected in this rhythmic and continuously contracting organ, mitochondria are much more abundant than in skeletal muscle and are characterized by their numerous cristae. They

are clustered around the nucleus, beneath the sarcolemma, and between the bundles of myofilaments. In the latter region, there are usually one or two per sarcomere.

The Golgi complex is also located near the nucleus. Curiously, in atrial fibers this region is often rich in dense, membrane-bounded granules, whereas ventricular fibers seldom display this organelle. The functional significance of these "*atrial granules*" is unknown (Fig. 8.29).

The *sarcoplasmic reticulum* consists mainly of smooth-surfaced membranes, but small segments occasionally have polyribosomes attached. The cisterns are narrow and tend to course longitudinally, but they anastomose so frequently that they give a plexiform pattern (Figs. 8.22 and 8.30). The reticulum is continuous from one sarcomere level to another, and there are no dilated terminal cisterns around the Z disc or at any other level. The membranes of the cisterns come into close association at various points with the membranes of wide and less regularly arranged *transverse tu-*

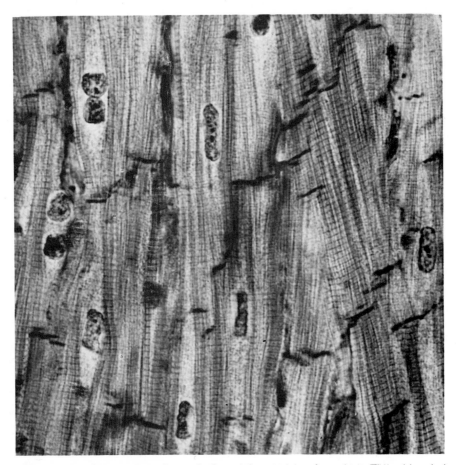

Figure 8.28. Longitudinal section of muscle from left ventricle of monkey. The wider dark cross lines are intercalated discs. Mitochondria occupy the clearer areas adjacent to the nuclei. Photomicrograph ×920.

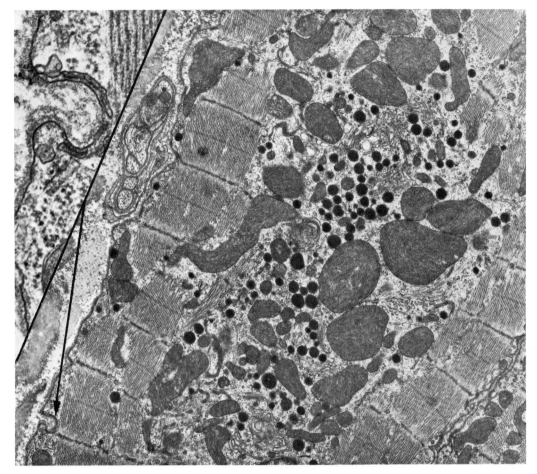

Figure 8.29.   Electron micrograph of cardiac muscle from the wall of the atrium. Large mitochondria plus smaller, dense "atrial granules" are prominent cytoplasmic features. A small nerve bundle courses within surrounding connective tissue at *left.* The *inset* and *arrow* display at higher magnifications the details of a diadic peripheral coupling round the opening of a wide T tubule onto the surface of the myocardial cell (×11,200; *inset* × 50,400). (Courtesy of Dr. David Chase.)

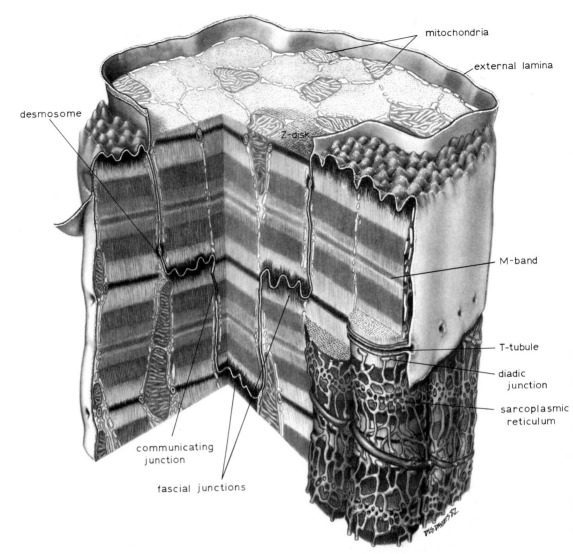

Figure 8.30. Schematic diagram illustrating the major features of the intercalcated disc region between the cardiac muscle cells. Note the presence of desmosomes and communicating (gap) junctions as well as the contractile force-transmitting fascial junctions. The arrangement of components of the sarcoplasmic reticulum and the T tubular system are also portrayed.

bules (T tubules) and with the sarcolemma at the cell surface (Figs. 8.29 and 8.30, discussed below).

In those mammals studied thus far, it appears that cardiac T tubules are formed during neonatal stages as invaginations of the sarcolemma which extend into the deepest regions of the fiber. The tubules course mainly in a transverse direction but are often interconnected by longitudinally oriented branches. T tubules are generally seen at the level of the Z disc in all vertebrates studied; this location is similar to that in lower vertebrate skeletal muscle and different from that in mammalian skeletal muscle (Fig. 8.22). The transverse tubules of cardiac muscle have a much wider lumen than those of skeletal muscle, and unlike skeletal muscle T tubules, they contain external lamina-like material. Their openings at the surface of the fiber are quite large and obvious in electron micrographs of glutaraldehyde-fixed material (Fig. 8.29). The tubules do not open into the cisterns of the sarcoplasmic reticulum, but their membranes become closely associated with the cisternal membranes along various junctional regions and in various patterns. The membranes are separated by a space of about 15 nm, in which poorly defined densities are observed. Because most transverse tubules are associated with only one cistern at any point, the association is called a *diad*, in distinction from *triads* of skeletal muscle. The membranes of the transverse tubule transmit the stimulus for contraction from the surface of the fiber to all depths of the fiber, and the *junctional couplings* at the diads presumably effect a response within or along the sarcoplasmic cisterns that results in the release of stored calcium to the sarcoplasm around the bundles of myofilaments. The presence of calcium is necessary for the actin-myosin reaction in contraction, as described for skeletal muscle.

Cisterns of the sarcoplasmic reticulum lying just beneath the sarcolemma often have couplings with the sarcolemma. These are also diads, and are termed *peripheral couplings*. Because the membrane of the transverse tubule is invaginated sarcolemma, the sarcoplasmic cisterns associated with the T tubules, as well as those associated with the surface of the fiber, are actually all *subsarcolemmal cisterns*.

The cytological changes during contraction of cardiac muscle are similar to those in skeletal muscle. The movement of actin filaments farther into the A band during contraction appears to involve the same sequence of events. However, there are a number of differences in the functional reactions of these two types of muscle, such as differences in speed and strength of contraction, in factors affecting contraction, and in autorhythmicity. For example, heart muscle is more dependent upon calcium in the surrounding medium than is skeletal muscle. This may be correlated with the fact that heart muscle lacks the dilated terminal cisterns of skeletal muscle and has less space for internal storage of calcium. The contraction of cardiac muscle is relatively prolonged, somewhat like that of tonic skeletal fibers. In this respect, it is interesting that the myofilaments of both tonic skeletal and cardiac muscle are arranged in less distinctly defined myofibrils. Skeletal muscle usually contracts only after an external stimulus that is provided under normal conditions by the motor nerve endings. By contrast, cardiac muscle cells possess the ability to contract rhythmically at an intrinsic basic rate in the absence of a nerve supply or other external stimulus. The mechanism underlying this capability remains largely unexplained. Interestingly, when myocardial cells are grown in vitro, they display rhythmic contractions individually until the colony is crowded enough that intercellular contacts are established. At this time contraction is coordinated among the cells, apparently mediated by nexuses (gap junctions).

Intercalated Discs

Intercalated discs are peculiar to cardiac muscle. They are seen by light microscopy as cross bands 0.5 to 1 μm thick (i.e., less than a cross striation or sarcomere) and are strongly refractive in fresh muscle and deeply stained in fixed material (Fig. 8.28). They often follow an irregular or stepwise course. Electron micrographs show that the intercalated discs represent a complex pattern of specialized cell junctions (Figs. 8.30 through 8.32). In some regions, particularly at the tips of interdigitations between adjacent muscle fibers, the cytoplasm along the inner surfaces of the membranes of the firmly adherent cells is densely filamentous. Here also the cells are separated by a uniform 15- to 20-nm space. This portion is termed the *fascial junction* of the intercalated disc and relates to the attachment of actin filaments to the sarcolemma and the transmission of contractile force from cell to cell. The structure of this region resembles that encountered on the cyto-

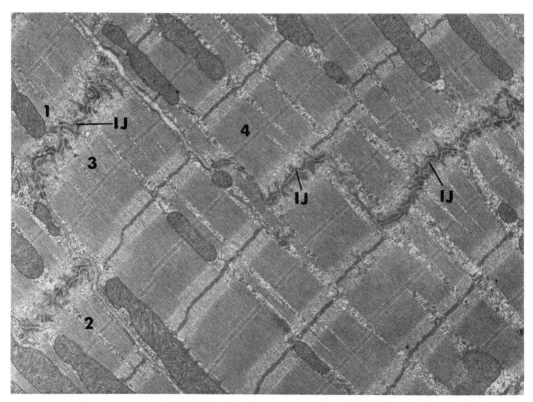

Figure 8.31. Low magnification electron micrograph showing a longitudinal section in the region of intercalated disc joining four myocardial cells (*1*, *2*, *3*, and *4*). Note the stepwise arrangement of the junctional faces, in register with Z discs, as well as shallow interdigitations in each junctional area (*IJ*) (×12,600). (Courtesy of Dr. N. Scott McNutt.)

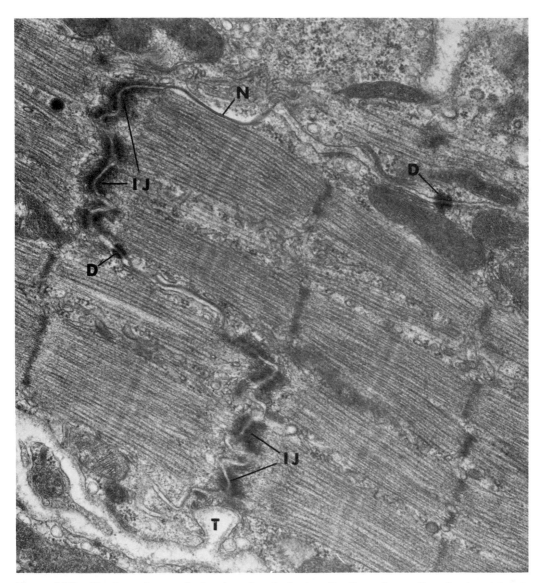

Figure 8.32. Electron micrograph showing a longitudinal section through a portion of an intercalated disc. Intercalated disc junctions (*IJ*) anchor the actin filaments of abutting myocardial cells at areas of firm intercellular adhesion. True desmosomes (*D*) and nexuses (*N*) (gap junctions) are also found, mainly along the lateral surfaces of the intercalated disc interdigitations. The opening of a T tubule (*T*) is visible on the surface of one myocardial cell (×33,000). (Courtesy of Dr. David Chase.)

plasmic side of myotendonal junctions (Fig. 8.24). Such fascial junctions are focal, but otherwise not greatly dissimilar from intermediate junctions; hence their occasional classification as *fasciae adhaerentes*. Desmosomal portions of the intercalated disc regions apparently function chiefly for additional firm cell adhesion and the anchorage of noncontractile cytoskeletal *interme-*

diate filaments. In still other regions, in or near the intercalated disc, particularly where the cells meet laterally, there are focal *nexuses* or *communicating (gap) junctions* (Figs. 8.30 and 8.32). These junctions are currently believed to provide electrotonic coupling among the cardiac muscle cells and thus contribute to a network of communicative pathways over which the overall rhythmic activity of the heart may be coordinated.

The regions identified by light microscopy as intercalated discs are really the aggregate image of all the above junctional elements, many of which stain darkly and/or are electron dense.

Connective Tissue of Cardiac Muscle

In the mammalian heart, a net of reticular fibrils and fine collagenous fibrils surrounds each muscle fiber and its external lamina. This net corresponds to the endomysium of skeletal muscle, but it is more irregular in its arrangement because the cardiac muscle cells are apposed to each other in a complicated pattern. Between bundles of muscle fibers, there are coarser collagenous and elastic fibers. These regions correspond to the perimysium of skeletal muscle. The connective tissue is particularly dense at the atrioventricular junction. The topographical arrangement of the connective tissues in the heart is described in Chapter 12.

Blood Vessels and Nerves of Cardiac Muscle

Branches of the coronary arteries and cardiac veins penetrate the myocardium by coursing among the larger bundles of connective tissue. An extensive plexus of blood and lymph capillaries is found in the connective tissue network surrounding each muscle fiber. The blood supply of cardiac muscle surpasses that of skeletal muscle.

Branches of sympathetic and parasympathetic nerves follow the connective tissue pathways and terminate in fine endings scattered among the muscle fibers. Here *norepinephrine* (sympathetic) and *acetylcholine* (parasympathetic), and other neurotransmitter substances are released to diffuse to the nearby myocardial cell surfaces. The frequency of muscle contraction is accelerated by stimulation of the sympathetics and retarded by the parasympathetics.

Conduction System

Cardiac muscle fibers, because of their intimate network of junctional contacts

and their inherent capacity to conduct, are capable of transmitting a contractile impulse over the entire heart. However, some of the fibers are modified in structure and conduct at a rate surpassing that of the typical cardiac fibers. These special conduction elements are known as *Purkinje fibers*; a description of their structure and distribution is given in Chapter 12.

Regeneration of Cardiac Muscle

There is little or no regenerative capacity of cardiac muscle fibers after injury or destruction. Healing is accomplished by scar formation.

Hypertrophy of the heart after any condition which places an excessive functional demand on the organ is accomplished by an increase in the size of the fibers rather than by an increase in their numbers. Likewise, growth of the heart during childhood is accomplished by an increase in the size of the fibers.

References

Allbrook D: Skeletal muscle regeneration. *Muscle Nerve* 4:234–245, 1981.
Ashton FT, Somlyo AV, Somlyo AP: The contractile apparatus of vascular smooth muscle: intermediate high voltage stereo electron microscopy. *J Mol Biol* 98:17–29, 1975.
Berenger T: A freeze-fracture study of sarcoplasmic reticulum from fast and slow muscle of the mouse. *Anat Rec* 184:647–664, 1975.
Bois RM, Pease DC: Electron microscopic studies of the state of myosin aggregation in the vertebrate smooth muscle cell. *Anat Rec* 180:465–480, 1974.
Bourne GH (ed): *The Structure and Function of Muscle.* Three volumes. New York, Academic Press, 1960.
Bozler E, Cottrell CL: The birefringence of muscle and its variation during contraction. *J Cell Comp Physiol* 10:165–182, 1937.
Brandt PW, Lopez E, Reuben JP, Grundfest H: The relationship between myofilament packing density and sarcomere length in frog striated muscle. *J Cell Biol* 33:255–263, 1967.
Chowrashi PK, Pepe F: The Z-band: 85,000-dalton amorphin and alpha-actinin and their relation to structure. *J Cell Biol* 94:565–573, 1982.
Cooke P: A filamentous cytoskeleton in vertebrate smooth muscle fibers. *J Cell Biol* 68:539–556, 1976.
Daniel EE, Daniel VP, Duchon G, Garfield RE, Nichols M, Malhotra SK, Oki M: Is the nexus necessary for cell-to-cell coupling of smooth muscle? *J Memb Biol* 28:207–240, 1976.
Dewey MM, Barr L: Intercellular connection between smooth muscle cells: the nexus. *Science* 137:670–672, 1962.

Eisenberg BR: Quantitative ultrastructure of mammalian skeletal muscle. In Peachey LD, Adrian R (eds): *Handbook of Physiology*. Bethesda, American Physiology Society, 1982 (in press).

Eisenberg BR, Eisenberg RS: The T-SR junction in contracting single skeletal muscle fibers. *J Gen Physiol* 79:1–20, 1982.

Eisenberg BR, Kuda AM: Discrimination between fiber populations in mammalian skeletal muscle by using ultrastructural parameters. *J Ultrastruct Res* 54:76–88, 1976.

Fawcett, DW: The sarcoplasmic reticulum of skeletal and cardiac muscle. *Circulation* 24:336–348, 1960.

Fawcett DW, McNutt NS: The ultrastructure of the cat myocardium. I. Ventricular papillary muscle. *J Cell Biol* 42:1–45, 1969.

Fischman DA, Shimada Y: Cardiac cell aggregation by scanning electron microscopy. Lieberman M, Sano T (eds): *Development and Physiological Corelates of Cardiac Muscle*. New York, Raven Press, 1976, pp 81–102.

Fishman AP (ed): The myocardium; its biochemistry and biophysics. *Circulation* 24(2) and American Heart Association, New York, 1960.

Forbes MS, Sperelakis N: Myocardial couplings: their structural variations in the mouse. *J Ultrastruct Res* 58:50–65, 1977.

Forer A: Electron microscopy of actin. In Hayat MA (ed): *Principles and Techniques of Electron Microscopy*; vol 9: *Biological Applications*. New York, Van Nostrand Rheinhold, 1978.

Franzini-Armstrong C: The comparative structure of intracellular junctions in striated muscle fibers. In Rowland LP (ed): *Pathogenesis of Human Muscular Dystrophies* Amsterdam, Excerpta Medica, 1977, pp 612–625.

Franzini-Armstrong C: Structure of sarcoplasmic reticulum. *Fed Proc* 39:2403–2409, 1980.

Franzini-Armstrong C, Peachey LD: Striated muscle—contractile and control mechanisms. *J Cell Biol* 91:166S–188S, 1981.

Gabella G: Smooth muscle junctions and structural aspects of contraction. *Br Med Bull* 35:213–218, 1979.

Gauthier GF: The structural and cytochemical heterogeneity of mammalian skeletal muscles. In Podolsky RJ (ed): *The Contractility of Muscle Cells and Related Processes*. Englewood Cliffs, N.J., Prentice-Hall, 1971.

Gauthier GF: Ultrastructural identification of muscle types by immunocytochemistry. *J Cell Biol* 82:391–400, 1979.

Goldstein MA, Schroeter JP, Sass RL: The Z lattice in canine cardiac muscle. *J Cell Biol* 83:187–204, 1979.

Goldstein MA, Stromer MH, Schroeter JP, Sass RL: Optical diffraction and reconstruction of Z bands in skeletal muscle. *J Cell Biol* 87:261a, 1980.

Granger BL, Lazarides E: Desmin and vimentin coexist at the periphery of the myofibril Z-disc. *Cell* 18:1053–1064, 1979.

Hanson J, Huxley HE: The structural basis of contraction in skeletal muscle. *Symp Soc Exp Biol* 9:228–264, 1955.

Huxley HE: The fine structure of striated muscle and its functional significance. *Harvey Lect* 60:85–117, 1964.

Huxley HE: The mechanism of muscular contraction. *Science* 164:1356–1366, 1969.

Ishikawa H: Formation of elaborate networks of T-system tubules in cultured skeletal muscle, with special reference to the T-system formation. *J Cell Biol* 38:51–66, 1968.

Ishikawa H, Bischoff R, Holtzer H: Formation of arrowhead complexes with heavy meromyosin in a variety of cell types. *J Cell Biol* 43:312–328, 1969.

Ishikawa H, Yamada E: Differentiation of the sarcoplasmic reticulum and T-system in developing mouse cardiac muscle. In Lieberman M, Sano T (eds): *Developmental and Physiological Correlates of Cardiac Muscle*. New York, Raven Press, 1975, pp 21–35.

Kannan MS, Daniel EE: Formation of gap junctions by treatment *in vitro* with potassium conductance blockers. *J Cell Biol* 78:338–348, 1978.

Kelly DE: Models of muscle Z-band fine structure based on a looping filament configuration. *J Cell Biol* 34:827–839, 1967.

Kelly DE: Myofibrillogenesis and Z-band differentiation. *Anat Rec* 163:403–425, 1969.

Kelly DE, Cahill MA: Filamentous and matrix components of skeletal muscle Z-disks. *Anat Rec* 172:623–642, 1972.

Kelly DE, Kuda AM: Subunits of the triadic junction in fast skeletal muscle as revealed by freeze-fracture. *J Ultrastruct Res* 68: 220–233, 1979.

Kelly RE, Rice RV: Ultrastructural studies on the contractile mechanism of smooth muscle. *J Cell Biol* 42:683–694, 1969.

Knappeis GG, Carlsen F: The ultrastructure of the Z disc in skeletal muscle. *J Cell Biol* 13:323–336, 1962.

Knappeis GG, Carlsen F: The ultrastructure of the M-line in skeletal muscle. *J Cell Biol* 38:202–211, 1968.

Landon DN: The influence of fixation upon the fine structure of the Z-disk of rat striated muscle. *J Cell Sci* 6:257–276, 1970.

Lazarides E, Granger BL, Gard DL, O'Connor CM, Breckler J, Price M, Danto SI: Desmin and vimentin-containing filaments and their role in the assembly of the Z-disk in muscle cells. *Cold Spring Harbor Symp Quant Biol* 46:351–378, 1981.

Manasek FJ: The extracellular matrix of the early embryonic heart. In Lieberman M, Sano T (eds): *Developmental and Physiological Correlates of Cardiac Muscle*. New York, Raven Press, 1976, pp 1–21.

Mauro A: *Muscle Regeneration*. New York, Raven Press, 1979.

McNutt NS, Weinstein RS: The ultrastructure of the nexus. *J Cell Biol* 47:666–688, 1970.

Murphy RA: Filament organization and contractile function in vertebrate smooth muscle. *Annu Rev Physiol* 41:737–748, 1979.

Neville H: Ultrastructural changes in diseae of human skeletal muscle. In Winter PJ, Broyn GW (eds): *Handbook of Clinical Neurology: Disease of Muscle*. Amsterdam, North Holland Publishing, 1979, pp 63–123.

Nonomura Y: Myofilaments in smooth muscle of guinea pig's taenia coli. *J Cell Biol* 39:741–745, 1968.

Ontel, M: The growth and metabolism of developing muscle. In Jones CT (ed): *Biochemical Development of the Fetus and Neonate*. Amsterdam, Elsevier

Biomedical Press, 1982, pp 213–247.

Padykula HA, Gauthier GF: The ultrastructure of the neuromuscular junction of mammalian red, white, and intermediate skeletal muscle fibers. *J Cell Biol* 46:27–41, 1979.

Panner BJ, Honig CR: Locus and state of aggregation of myosin in tissue sections of vertebrate smooth muscle. *J Cell Biol* 44:52–61, 1970.

Peachey LD: Structure and function of T-system of vertebrate skeletal muscle. In Tower DB, Brady RD (eds): *The Nervous System*, vol 1: *The Basic Neurosciences*. New York, Raven Press, 1975, pp 81–90.

Peachey LD, Eisenberg BR: Helicoids in the T system and striations of frog skeletal muscle seen by high voltage electron microscopy. *Biophys J* 22:145–154, 1978.

Pepe FA: Structure of muscle filaments from immunohistochemical and ultrastuctural studies. *J Histochem Cytochem* 23:543–562, 1975.

Porter KR: The sarcoplasmic reticulum in muscle cells of Amblystoma larvae. *J Biophys Biochem Cytol* 2(Suppl.):163–170, 1956.

Rayns DG, Devine CE, Sutherland CL: Freeze fracture studies of membrane systems in vertebrate muscle. I. Striated muscle. *J Ultrastruct Res* 50:306–321, 1975.

Rayns DG, Simpson FO, Bertaud WS: Surface features of striated muscle. 1. Guinea pig cardiac muscle. *J Cell Sci* 3:467–474, 1968.

Resnick JS, Engel WK, Nelson PG: Changes in the Z disk of skeletal muscle induced by tenotomy. *Neurology (NY)* 18:737–740, 1968.

Rice RV, Moses JA , McManus GM, Brady AC, Blasik LM: The organization of contractile filaments in a mammalian smooth muscle. *J Cell Biol* 47:183–196, 1970.

Robbins N, Karpati G, Engel WK: Histochemical and contractile properties in the cross innervated guinea pig soleus muscle. *Arch Neurol* 20:318–329, 1969.

Sawada H, Ishikawa H, Yamada E: High resolution scanning electron microscopy of frog sartorius muscle. *Tisue Cell* 10:179–190, 1978.

Shibata Y, Yamamoto T: Freeze-fracture studies of gap junctions in vertebrate cardiac muscle cells. *J Ultrastruct Res* 67:79–88, 1979.

Shimada Y, Fischman DA, Moscona AA: The fine structure of embryonic chick skeletal muscle cells differentiated *in vitro. J Cell Biol* 35:445–453, 1967.

Shoenberg CF, Needham DM: A study of the mechanism of contraction in vertebrate smooth muscle. *Biol Rev* 51:53–104, 1976.

Small JV, Sobieszek A: The contractile apparatus of smooth muscle. *Int Rev Cytol* 64: 241–306, 1980.

Snow MH: Myogenic cell formation in regenerating rat skeletal muscle injured by mincing. I. A fine structural study. *Anat Rec* 188:181–200, 1977.

Snow MH: Myogenic cell formation in regenerating rat skeletal muscle injured by mincing. II. An autoradiographic study. *Anat Rec* 188:201–218, 1977.

Somlyo AP, Somlyo AV, Shuman H: Electron probe analysis of vascular smooth muscle. Composition of mitochondria, nuclei, and cytoplasm. *J Cell Biol* 81:316–335, 1979.

Somlyo AV: Bridging structures spanning the junctional gap at the triad of skeletal muscle. *J Cell Biol* 80:743–750, 1979.

Sommer JR, Johnson EA: Ultrastructure of cardiac muscle. In Berne R (ed): *Handbook of Physiology: The Cardiovascular System*. Bethesda, American Physiological Society, 1979, pp 113–186.

Sommer JR, Waugh RA: The ultrastructure of the mammalian cardiac muscle—with special emphasis on the tubular membrane systems. *Am J Pathol* 82:191–232, 1976.

Squire J: Muscle regulation: a decade of the steric blocking model. *Nature* 291:614–616, 1981.

Thornell LE, Edstrom L, Eriksson A, Henriksson KG, Ängovist KA: The distribution of intermediate filament protein (skeletin) in normal and diseased human skeletal muscle. An immunohistochemical and electronmicroscopic study. *J Neurol Sci* 47:153–170, 1980.

Toyota N, Shimada Y: Differentiation of troponin in cardiac and skeletal muscles in chicken embryos as studied by immuno-fluorescence microscopy. *J Cell Biol* 91:497–504, 1981.

Trotter JA, Corbett K, Avner BP: Structure and function of the murine muscle-tendon junction. *Anat Rec* 201:243–302, 1981.

Yamaguchi M, Stromer MH, Robson RM, Anderson B, Anderson WD: Studies on the basic structural unit of muscle Z lines. *J Cell Biol* 87:259a, 1980.

Zampighi G, Vergara J, Ramon F: On the connection between the transverse tubules and the plasma membrane in frog semi-tendinosus skeletal muscle. Are caveolae the mouth of the transverse tubule system? *J Cell Biol* 64:734–740, 1975.

Chapter 9

ORGANIZATION OF NEURAL TISSUE

The evolution of increasingly complex and larger animals has necessitated the parallel emergence of extensive systems of communication. In mammals and other vertebrates, these systems involve highly complex circuitry of specialized cells operating with a high degree of integration and coordination. Collectively this cellular circuitry and related supportive cells are termed neural tissue.

Neural tissue is characterized functionally by its ability to transmit impulses from one part of the body to another, often over long distances. The cellular unit immediately responsible for this functional capability is a cell type known as the *neuron*. Neurons, however, cannot function without the support and protection of other neighboring cells of the neural tissue known as *glia* (or *neuroglia*). Together neurons and glia provide for the capability of the generation and conveyance of a nerve impulse along the length of a neuron. These impulses are waves of membrane depolarization (often termed *action potentials*) and they provide a means of rapid signaling between the various regions of the body. Combining many neurons into the intricate circuitry of the nervous system, the organism is able to receive information about its environment and its internal state, analyze this information, and respond in an appropriate manner.

As noted in Chapter 3, neurons and their supporting glial companions take their origin embryonically from two sources, later to be combined into development of the total nervous system. The first and most massive source of neural tissue appears on the dorsal surface of the embryonic disc shortly after gastrulation. Here an oval plate of surface ectoderm (the *neural plate*) thickens along the embryonic axis and soon folds along its lateral margins to form a deep median longitudinal groove. Eventually, this groove closes over and becomes a long hollow tube (the *neural tube*) extending over the entire length of the developing embryo (Figs. 9.1 and 3.4). This tube is epithelial at its origin, is epithelial during its development, and, although highly modified, will always retain basic epithelial characteristics. Eventually it becomes the substance of the brain and spinal cord, i.e., the *central nervous system* (CNS). Differential proliferation along the internal aspect of this tube leads to a rapid increase in the number of its epithelial cells. More massive proliferation anteriorly heralds the formation of the brain (Fig. 3.5); posteriorly the thickening of the neural tube is less apparent (Fig. 9.3), but a rather precise developmental pattern is established and persists in the spinal cord (Figs. 9.2 and 9.4). Some of the newly proliferating cells (*neuroblasts*) of the epithelial neural tube are destined to become neurons, and others (the *glioblasts*) will differentiate into various glial elements.

As cellular proliferation proceeds, three concentric regions become apparent within the wall of the tube (Fig. 9.2). The most internal region is termed the *ependymal* or *ventricular layer* and contains actively dividing cells. After division, the nuclei of daughter cells take up positions in the intermediate (or *mantle*) layer. Those which differentiate as neuroblasts send out processes called *neurites*. Some neurites become *axons* which may grow out of the neural

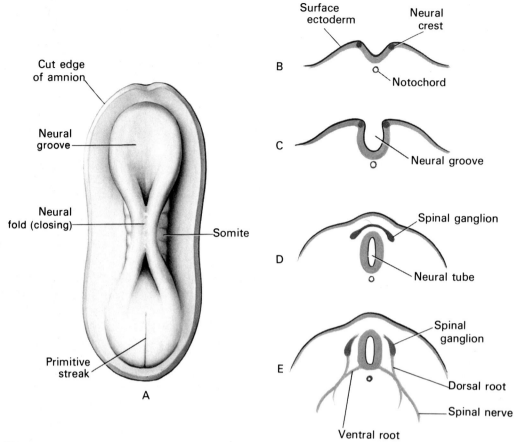

Figure 9.1. Surface and cross sectional views of the development of the neural tube on the dorsal surface of the embryo. The lips of the neural fold fuse to enclose a hollow tube, the neural tube. This fusion progresses anteriorly and posteriorly until the neural tube is completely shut off from the amnionic fluid. Parts *B, C, D,* and *E* show cross sections through the neural tube at various stages of development. The derivation of the spinal ganglion from the neural crest and the joining together of the dorsal and ventral nerve root to form the spinal nerve are shown.

tube (e.g., to form *ventral root motor fibers*), or they may course up or down the neural tube to form the relatively anuclear outermost *marginal* layer. In the differentiated CNS, the derivatives of these three layers (marginal, mantle, and ventricular) have matured to become, respectively, (*a*) the *white matter,* (*b*) the *gray matter,* and (*c*) the *ependyma* and an immediately subjacent layer in which proliferation of glial cell precursors continues into adulthood. Within these layers, the neurons generally develop first, with two glial derivative cell types, the *astrocytes* and then the *oligodendrocytes* appearing somewhat later.

The enlarged upper (or anterior) end of the neural tube develops three dilations which form the *forebrain,* the *midbrain,* and the *hindbrain* of the CNS. In these regions, additional cell proliferation and cell migration lead to the development of superficial *cortical regions* containing large numbers of neurons.

Concurrent with the development of the neural tube, a second source of neural tissue arises in a peculiar fashion. Along the lips of the neural groove some of the ectodermal cells which originally lay just lateral to presumptive neural tube separate from the ectodermal epithelium to invade the underlying mesenchymal compartment. Their release from the ectoderm coincides closely

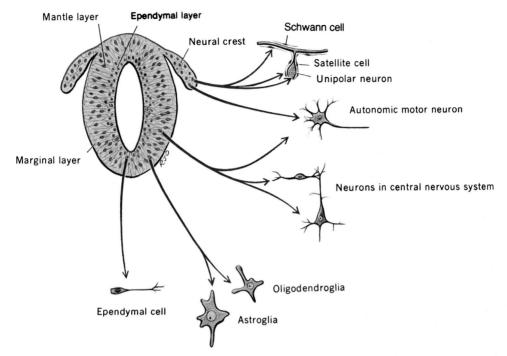

Figure 9.2. This schemtic diagram indicates the cells which derive from the neural tube and the neural crest. Note that mitotic activity in the neural tube is restricted to cells near the ependymal layer. (Reprinted with permission from C. Noback: *The Human Nervous System.* New York, McGraw-Hill, 1967.)

with the time of closure of the neural tube. These cells are termed *neural crest* and can be found migrating lateral to the neural tube along its entire length (Fig. 9.1).

Neural crest cells are at first quite mesenchymal in their behavior and unrecognizable from other mesenchymal cells around them. Eventually, they can be shown to give rise to a number of specific derivatives, not all of which are neural tissue. A very large number of them will, however, contribute to the *peripheral nervous system* (PNS).

The first indication of this differentiation is the clumping of some neural crest cells in a repeating serial fashion along either side of the neural tube between adjacent somites. These are rudiments of spinal *ganglia*. A *ganglion* (singular) is a clumped group of neurons lying outside the CNS, i.e., within the peripheral nervous system. Similar clustering will occur later in a more ventral position, giving rise to ganglia of the *sympathetic* portion of the

autonomic nervous system (ANS). Other *parasympathetic ganglia* will arise from neural crest clumping in various regions to be discussed later. Within each ganglion, growth will occur by proliferation, and some of the new cells will differentiate into neurons, whereas others will differentiate into supportive components not dissimilar from the glia emerging within the neural tube. Hence, populations of neuroblasts and glioblasts can be found in both neural tube and neural crest derivatives. That is to say, *both* neural tube epithelium and neural crest cells give rise to neurons and glia.

Other cells of the mesenchymal compartment, at least some of which are of neural crest origin, surround and ensheath the neural tube. These are the protective and nourishing meningeal layers (*meninges*) of the CNS. As will be seen, these are continuous with similar protective coverings of elements of the peripheral nervous system.

The CNS (at this stage, the neural tube)

is brought into contact with other parts of the body through development of the peripheral nervous system. Extensions of neurons (the longest of which are termed *axons* or *fibers*) grow out from certain regions of the brain and spinal cord to make functional contact with the *effectors* of the body—the muscles or glands. These outgrowing fibers constitute one portion of the PNS and will carry output impulses from the CNS to peripheral structures. They are called *efferent* or *motor* because they control the activities of the outlying tissues. Neuroblasts within spinal ganglia develop fibers which course in two directions—to the periphery and toward the neural tube. The latter penetrate the neural tube and establish connections with neurons of the CNS. These fibers are thus able to provide an input of signals from the periphery to the CNS. They are therefore termed *afferent* or *sensory*. It can be seen that motor and sensory neurons and their fibers become intermixed to form *cranial* and *spinal nerves* of the *peripheral nervous system* (Figs. 9.3 and 9.4). It is clear also that fibers of some CNS neurons extend into the peripheral nervous system and fibers from some ganglionic neurons extend into the CNS. In this way the basic integration of the two components is established.

Although neurons exhibit a great variety of shapes and forms, each is characterized by having one or more cytoplasmic processes. Some of these are specialized to receive signals from other neurons. These processes are called *dendrites*, or the *dendritic zone* of a neuron; this part of the neuron constitutes most of the receptive portion. Neurons also develop a main trunk or principal process which generates the *action potential* and conducts this impulse along the length of the neuron to its most distant regions. This main trunk is the *axon* (or *neuronal fiber*). The termination of an axon most frequently forms a special contact, a *synapse*, with the dendritic portion, axon, or the cell body of another neuron, or it may form a similar contact (*neuro-*

muscular junction) with a muscle cell. Many neurons receive a great number of signals from a variety of sources on their dendritic, or receptive, surface. Those incoming signals may be either *inhibitory* or *excitatory*. The summation of these influences will determine whether the neuron will fire (i.e., generate its own action potential) and thus influence the dendritic portion of the next nerve cell in the pathway.

BASIC ORGANIZATION

An arrangement whereby a motor and a sensory neuron are linked together synaptically as a receptor-effector mechanism constitutes the simplest type of *reflex arc*. An example of this type of combination is illustrated in Fig. 9.4*A*, which represents a cross section through the spinal cord and a spinal nerve. The cell body of the sensory neuron is located outside the spinal cord, where, together with other similar cell bodies, it forms a spinal ganglion. The sensory neuron is *unipolar*; that is, it has only one process. A short distance from the cell body, this single process, which is structurally an axon, divides into a peripheral process with a receptor ending in the skin and a central process which enters the spinal cord by way of the *dorsal root* of the spinal nerve. The central process may terminate in contact with either the dendrites or the cell body of a *multipolar* motor neuron located in the ventral part of the cord. The axon of this second neuron leaves the cord by way of the *ventral root*, runs along side the sensory fibers to form the *spinal nerve*, and courses peripherally to terminate on an effector (skeletal muscle, in the example illustrated in Fig. 9.4*A*).

The two-neuron reflex, described above, although theoretically possible, is a much more simple arrangement than that which is usually found in mammals. More commonly, a series of neurons is interposed between the sensory and motor neurons of the basic reflex arc. These are commonly called *interneurons* (or *internuncial neurons*). Simpler nervous systems, as in some

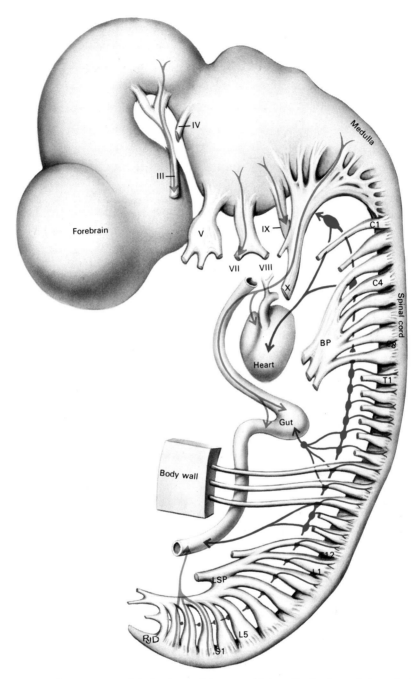

Figure 9.3. Simplified diagram of derivatives of the neural tube after brain parts have begun to form and after the cranial and spinal nerves have developed. Cranial nerves are given *Roman numerals*, and spinal nerves of the cervical (*C*), thoracic (*T*), lumbar (*L*), and sacral (*S*) regions are indicated by *numbers*. The craniosacral (*blue*) and thoracolumbar (*red*) parts of the autonomic nervous outflow are derived from the "head and tail" and the "middle" part of the neuraxis and provide dual innervation to visceral structures. The dominance of the vagus nerve (*X*) in the innervation of the trunk viscera is apparent. The fact that autonomic outflow is always a two-neuron system is not shown.

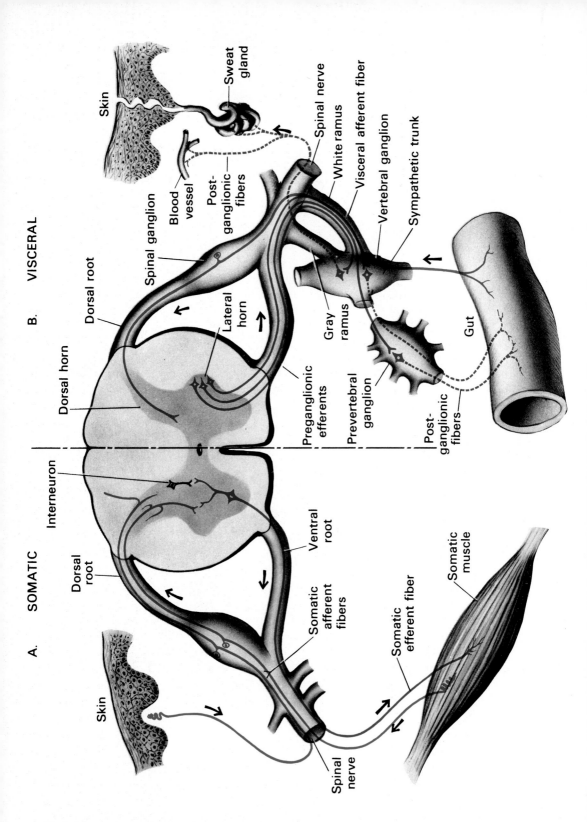

Figure 9.4. *A*, somatic nerves. *B*, visceral nerves. A cross section of spinal cord is shown connected via dorsal and ventral roots to the spinal nerve and to one of the ganglia of the autonomic system. The patterns of afferent (*blue*) and efferent (*red*) nerve fibers in both the somatic and visceral system may be directly compared. For details see text.

invertebrates, often have relatively few interneurons interposed between receptors and effectors, and the reactions of the organism are quite stereotyped and predictable. In higher animals, the pathways provided by interneurons can be very complex; nerve impulses generated in receptors in the periphery are carried to many levels of the nervous system, including the highest centers of the brain. In the various parts of the brain, incoming information is sorted, stored, and used in determining the appropriate motor responses. Complex interneuronal pathways lead from the brain back to the cranial or spinal motor neurons and are influential in determining whether these neurons will generate nerve impulses (and thus cause a muscle to contract or a gland to secrete). In the vertebrate nervous system, the cranial or spinal motor neurons constantly receive "advice" in the form of hundreds or thousands of inhibitory and excitatory synapses applied to their dendritic portion or to their cell bodies. These motor neurons provide the *final common pathway* from the CNS to its effector organs. Once they fire, there is no mechanism of recall; the muscle contracts or the gland secretes.

The basic reflex arc is not controlled by local sensory influences alone but by information converging on the motor neurons from many levels of the CNS, including the cerebral cortex, the midbrain, and the hindbrain. How these complex synaptic networks become organized is one of the most challenging questions in neurobiology. There is no doubt that some synaptic contacts are genetically determined, for certain synapses form in nerve tissue completely isolated from the other tissues of the body and from sensory influences. There is strong evidence to suggest that, after having been guided to the correct region by mechanical forces and chemical gradients, young axons make appropriate contact with other neurons or muscle cells through the intermediary action of specific *receptor macromolecules* on the surfaces of those cells. Certain synapses appear to require

some degree of use to be retained, others do not. Are most synapses permanent? Are new synapses formed with learning? Are some synapses superfluous? Are more synapses formed in animals exposed to an "enriched" environment? These are some of the questions that present neurobiological experimentation is attempting to answer.

THE SPINAL CORD AND ITS NERVES

The arrangement of the nerve cells and fibers within the spinal cord makes it possible to differentiate two distinct areas of tissue: a thick peripheral layer of *white matter* and a central column of *gray matter* (Fig. 9.4). The white matter is composed primarily of longitudinally directed nerve fibers, many of which are covered by white lipid-rich sheaths provided by the membranes of certain glial cells. Such membranous sheaths are termed *myelin*. The gray matter is composed principally of nerve cells and their fibers and glial cells. Many of the fibers of the gray matter are *unmyelinated*, but a considerable number of myelinated ones are present also. In transverse section, the gray matter is shaped like the letter H. Its dorsal wings constitute the *dorsal horns* and its ventral ones the *ventral horns* (in which lie the cell bodies of the motor neurons). The two lateral gray areas are connected across the midline by a transverse bar, the *gray commissure*, in which lies the small central canal, the remnant of the previously wide neural tube lumen. It is, of course, evident that the dorsal and ventral horns seen in cross section actually are continuous columns of gray matter extending the length of the cord.

The *dorsal roots* are composed of the *afferent* or *sensory fibers*; these fibers have their cell bodies grouped into an enlargement of the dorsal root called the *dorsal root ganglion* (Fig. 9.4). The *ventral roots* contain the *efferent* or *motor fibers*, and these join the dorsal root forming a common trunk called a *spinal nerve*. Those afferent fibers which are distributed to sensory endings in the body, exclusive of the viscera, are termed *somatic afferent* fibers;

those providing the sensory innervation of the viscera are the *visceral afferent* fibers. Both functional types have their cell bodies in the spinal ganglia (Fig. 9.4).

A great many of the efferent fibers are distributed to the voluntary skeletal muscle of the body and are therefore termed *somatic efferent* fibers. Other efferent fibers terminate on smooth or cardiac muscle and glandular epithelium of visceral structures; these are the *visceral efferent* fibers.

THE AUTONOMIC NERVOUS SYSTEM

The visceral efferent components of both the cranial and the spinal nerves pursue a different course than do the somatic efferent fibers, for two neurons are always involved in the conduction of a visceral impulse from the CNS to the effector organ. They also differ physiologically in that the essentially visceral reflexes which they mediate are often not subject to direct voluntary control and are also more or less diffuse, rather than localized, in their effects. Because of these and certain other differences, it has been found convenient to consider the visceral efferent neurons of the body as a separate physiological system, the *autonomic nervous system*. According to the original definition, the autonomic system included only the visceral efferent (motor) innervation and did not include either the visceral afferent (sensory) fibers or those higher centers in the CNS which influence the visceral activities. In recent years, however, the use of the term "autonomic" increasingly has included all of the neural apparatus concerned with visceral function.

It must be emphasized that the autonomic nervous system is purely a functional grouping of efferent neurons and is in no sense an anatomical division. Some neuron cell bodies lie within the CNS; others are located in visceral ganglia in distant regions of the body. Autonomic nerve fibers are present in all spinal nerves and in most of the cranial nerves. The reflexes which they govern may be initiated by sensory impulses flowing over somatic afferent or visceral afferent fibers or coming from any

receptor organ. The stimuli may be in the external environment or they may arise within the body.

The efferent fibers to visceral structures leave the CNS at three levels, making it possible to recognize three divisions of the autonomic nervous system (Fig. 9.5). In the *cranial division*, autonomic fibers leave by way of cranial nerves III, VII, IX, and X. Other visceral efferent fibers emerge through the thoracic and the upper lumbar spinal nerves; these constitute the *thoracolumbar division*. The *sacral division* includes visceral efferent fibers that generally leave by way of the sacral spinal nerves, mostly S2 to S4.

Whatever their level of origin, all visceral efferent pathways involve two successive neurons (Figs. 9.4 and 9.5). The first of these has its cell body within the central nervous system and its axon terminating in a peripheral autonomic ganglion; it is therefore termed a *preganglionic neuron*. In the ganglion, it makes synaptic connection with a second neuron, the *postganglionic neuron*, whose axon terminates on an effector organ (muscle or epithelium).

In the cranial and sacral divisions, the preganglionic fibers generally end in *terminal ganglia* which lie near or within the walls of the structures that they innervate. In this and other respects, as well as in their response to certain drugs, the cranial and sacral divisions resemble each other and differ from the thoracolumbar components. They are therefore grouped together as the craniosacral or *parasympathetic division* of the autonomic nervous system.

The thoracolumbar visceral efferent outflow is the *sympathetic division* of the autonomic nervous system. Its preganglionic fibers terminate in either *vertebral* or *prevertebral ganglia*. The vertebral ganglia are a series of ganglia, connected linearly by nerve fibers, that lie along the ventrolateral aspects of the vertebral column and thus form two *sympathetic trunks* extending on either side the length of the vertebral column. The prevertebral, or *collateral*, ganglia are aggregations of postganglionic neurons

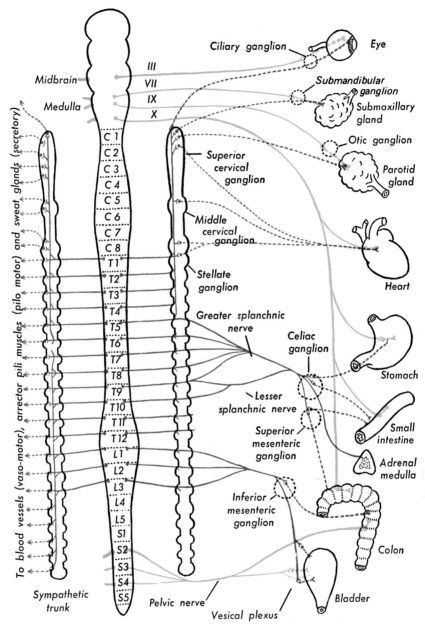

Figure 9.5. Diagrammatic representation of some of the chief conduction pathways of the autonomic nervous system. For clearness, the nerves to blood vessels, arrector pili muscles, and sweat glands are shown only on the *left* side of the figure and the pathways to other visceral structures are shown only on the *right* side. The sympathetic division is shown in *red*, the parasympathetic division in *blue*. *Solid lines* represent preganglionic fibers; *broken lines* represent postganglionic fibers.

associated with visceral nerve plexuses in the abdomen (Figs. 9.4 and 9.5).

In general, most visceral organs are innervated by both the parasympathetic and sympathetic divisions, the effects of which are usually, but by no means always, antagonistic. For example, the parasympathetic fibers to the heart transmit impulses which tend to slow the heart rate; impulses from the sympathetic fibers, on the other hand, accelerate it. In the stomach, parasympathetic impulses excite muscular contraction, and sympathetic impulses inhibit it. Parasympathetic stimulation contributes to the conservation of bodily energy; sympathetic stimulation assists the body in meeting emergencies.

Sympathetic Division

The sympathetic trunks are composed of a series of vertebral ganglia containing the cell bodies of postganglionic neurons and connected in linear order by ascending or descending nerve fibers (Figs. 9.3 to 9.5). In the cervical region there are three ganglia: the *superior cervical ganglion*, which is the largest; the *middle cervical*, sometimes absent; and the *inferior cervical*, which may be fused with the first thoracic to form the *stellate ganglion*. In the thoracic region, the ganglia, 10 or 11 in number, are segmentally arranged. Three or four ganglia are associated with the lumbar level and four or five with the sacral region.

Each sympathetic trunk is connected with the spinal nerves of its side by a series of communicating rami composed of nerve fibers. These are of two types. One type, the *gray communicating rami*, consists of fibers mostly devoid of myelin; these are found connecting the trunk to every spinal nerve. The other type, the *white communicating rami*, is limited to the thoracic and first three or four lumbar nerves and is not present at cervical or sacral levels (Fig. 9.5). *Preganglionic fibers* of the sympathetic division have their cell bodies located in the *intermediolateral cell column* (*lateral horn*) of the thoracic and upper lumbar levels of the spinal cord (Fig. 9.4). The myelinated fibers emerge through the ventral roots and reach the nearby sympathetic trunk by way of the white communicating rami. Within the sympathetic trunk the preganglionic fiber may take one of three courses:

1. It may terminate in this level of the trunk in synaptic relation to a *postganglionic neuron* whose nonmyelinated axon joins the corresponding spinal nerve by way of the gray communicating ramus. The postganglionic fiber courses peripherally to terminate in the smooth muscle of a blood vessel (*vasomotor*), in the arrector pili muscle of a hair (*pilomotor*), or among the epithelial cells of a sweat gland (secretory) (Fig. 9.4).

2. Many of the preganglionic fibers from the white rami pass directly through the sympathetic trunk without interruption and continue to the prevertebral (collateral) ganglia, from which postganglionic fibers course to the visceral organs. Preganglionic fibers such as these emerge as branches from the sympathetic trunks. Those from the 5th to 10th thoracic ganglia form the *splanchnic nerves* and terminate in the *celiac ganglia*, which are prevertebral. The postganglionic fibers contribute to the formation of the *celiac plexus* and pass directly to their terminations in the viscera.

3. A great many of the preganglionic fibers, upon reaching the sympathetic trunk, course either caudally or cranially in this trunk before they have a synaptic juncture with postganglionic neurons. These fibers form the pathways for the visceral efferent outflow to regions of the trunk which do not possess white rami. For example, preganglionic fibers originating at levels as low as the seventh thoracic terminate in the superior cervical ganglion. From this ganglion, nonmyelinated postganglionic nerve fibers run to various visceral structures. Some accompany the internal carotid artery as the *internal carotid plexus* and furnish the pathway by which impulses reach the dilator pupillae muscle of the eye. Other fibers form the *superior cervical cardiac nerve* to the *cardiac plexus* and conduct impulses which accelerate the rhythm of the heart.

Other pathways of the sympathetic division are shown diagrammatically in Figure 9.5.

Parasympathetic Division

The cranial parasympathetic preganglionic neurons lie in the midbrain and medulla, sending their axons out over the *oculomotor, facial, glossopharyngeal, vagus,* and *spinal accessory cranial nerves* (Fig. 9.3). These preganglionic fibers are myelinated and course in their respective nerves to terminal ganglia located near or within visceral structures.

In the case of the oculomotor nerve, the preganglionic fibers reach the *ciliary ganglion,* which lies against the lateral surface of the optic nerve and contains the postganglionic neurons whose axons course to the eye. In the eye, they are distributed to the *ciliary muscle* of accommodation and the sphincter muscle of the iris. The antagonistic action of parasympathetic and sympathetic nerves is here evident, for the parasympathetic fibers bring about contraction of the pupil; sympathetic postganglionic fibers from the superior cervical ganglion cause dilation of the pupil.

The vagus nerve contains many preganglionic fibers. The cell bodies lie in the medulla, and many of the fibers pass to the cardiac plexus and terminate in synaptic relation to ganglion cells located within the cardiac atrial walls and roots of the great vessels. The axons of these cardiac ganglion cells are short postganglionic fibers which end in the heart muscle. They are inhibitory in function.

The parasympathetic innervation of the gastrointestinal tract and other abdominal viscera is through efferent fibers of the vagus nerve and also the pelvic nerve, which arises from nerve cells in the lateral horn of the second, third, and fourth sacral segments of the spinal cord. These are preganglionic fibers. Those which innervate the gastrointestinal tract course without interruption to terminate in its wall. Here they are synaptically related to postganglionic neurons, which, with associated plexuses of nerve fibers, form two extensive *enteric ganglionated plexuses.* One of these, the *myenteric plexus* or *plexus of Auerbach,* is situated between the longitudinal and circular layers of muscle. The other, the *submucosal plexus* or *plexus of Meissner,* lies in the submucosa.

Preganglionic fibers which pass to pelvic reproductive and urinary organs terminate in synaptic relation to the cell bodies of postganglionic neurons located in or near the walls of these viscera.

The nerve fibers of the enteric plexuses fall into the following classes.

Postganglionic Sympathetic Fibers

These are derived from postganglionic neurons located chiefly in prevertebral ganglia. They end on the smooth muscle of the gut and among epithelial cells. Their impulses usually inhibit gastrointestinal activity.

Preganglionic Parasympathetic Fibers

These are fibers of the vagus or, in the descending colon and rectum, the visceral branches of sacral nerves. They end in synapses with the ganglion cells of the myenteric or submucosal plexuses.

Postganglionic Parasympathetic Fibers

These are axons of the above mentioned ganglion cells. They innervate smooth muscle and epithelium of the gut, and their impulses usually excite gastrointestinal activity.

Visceral Afferent Fibers

These fibers are sensory and intermingle with the visceral efferent fibers. They play an important part in gastrointestinal reflexes. Some of the sensory fibers from the gut course in the vagus to the sensory ganglia of this nerve and from there to the medulla. Other sensory fibers course in the visceral nerves, then through the vertebral sympathetic ganglia and the white rami communicantes to their cell bodies in the spinal ganglia and then to the spinal cord (Fig. 9.4).

References

Ariëns Kappers CU, Huber GC, Crosby EC: *The Comparative Anatomy of the Nervous System of Vertebrates, Including Man.* 3 vols. New York, Hafner Publishing Company, 1960.

Bourne GH (ed): *The Structure and Function of Nervous Tissue,* 3 vols. New York, Academic Press, 1968–1969.

Bullock TH, Horridge GA: *Structure and Function in*

the Nervous Systems of Invertebrates, 2 vols. San Francisco, W. H. Freeman, 1968.

Bullock TH, Orklund R, Grinnell A: *Introduction to Nervous Systems*. San Francisco, W. H. Freeman, 1977.

Carpenter MB, Sutin, J: *Human Neuroanatomy*, ed 8. Baltimore, Williams & Wilkins, 1983.

Crosby EC, Humphrey T, Lauer EW: *Correlative Anatomy of the Nervous System*, New York, Macmillan, 1962.

Ebbesson SOE: The parcellular theory and its relation to interspecific variability in brain organization, evolutionary and ontogenetic development, and neuronal plasticity. *Cell Tissue Res* 213: 179–212, 1980.

Jacobson M: *Developmental Neurobiology*. New York, Plenum Press, 1978.

Patton HD, Sundsten JW, Crill WE, Swanson PD: *Introduction to Basic Neurology*. Philadelphia, W. B. Saunders, 1976.

Ramon y Cajal S: *Histologie due Système Nerveux de l'Homme et des Vertébrés*, 2 vols. Paris, A. Maloine, 1909–1911.

Chapter 10

NEURAL TISSUE

In vertebrate animals, the great majority of neurons are within the central nervous system (CNS). The microscopic anatomy of this tissue reflects its origin. Like other epithelia, its cells are closely packed, with little extracellular space or substance, and are connected by frequent cell-to-cell junctions. Unlike most epithelia, however, central nervous tissue is characterized by enormous diversity among its cells, many of which display great complexity. The tissue of the peripheral nervous system (PNS) is also complex, but less diverse, and it shares with the CNS a number of fundamental properties. Foremost among these is a special type of intercellular junction: the *chemical synapse* (see Fig. 4.3). All neurons, whether CNS or PNS, participate in synaptic contact, and must be so connected to survive. The human brain contains billions of neurons, and certain of these receive thousands of synapses. The enormous number of neurons in the human body and the complexity and specificity of their circuitry provide for the functional capabilities of the nervous system and give man his rich variety of reaction and behavior.

In the central nervous system, the neuronal cell bodies are the most conspicuous elements. They tend to occur in groups called *nuclei* (not to be confused with the nucleus of a single cell) if they occur as a cluster, *layers* if they occur in a laminar array, and *columns* if they occur in a linear configuration. Related to the nerve cell bodies are great entanglements of nerve cell processes (*axonal* and *dendritic*) along with processes of supportive cells, collectively called *neuropil*, where many of the synaptic contacts occur. Nerve fibers (generally axons) grouped into bundles that travel to other parts of the nervous system are called *tracts*.

Special techniques are required to work out the circuitry of nervous tissue, delineate the whole of the neuronal contour, demonstrate synapses, or detect certain types of neurotransmitters; other procedures demonstrate degenerating cell processes. Only at the electron microscope level of resolution do these various techniques begin to reveal the full complexity of the nervous system.

The CNS epithelium is marked by compactness, in contrast with the peripheral nervous tissues, in which nerve cell bodies and nerve fibers are interspersed with distinctive connective tissue investments. Supportive cells—the *neuroglia*—are the helper cells of all neurons. These cells, often referred to simply as *glial* cells, include the various supportive cells of the central nervous system, the *Schwann cells* of the peripheral nerve fibers, and the *satellite cells* of the craniospinal and autonomic ganglia. Connective tissue forms part of the membranous *meninges* surrounding the entire CNS and provides tubular investments around peripheral nerves. It also contributes to the capsules of the ganglia and is associated with the sensory nerve fiber endings in the formation of certain sense organs.

THE NEURON

The *neuron* may be defined as the nerve cell body with all of its extensions. Neurons are generally elongated—some over 100 cm—to provide communication between various regions of the body (Fig. 10.1). Despite their elongation, neurons seldom are multinucleated. The portion of the nerve cell that surrounds the nucleus, the *perikaryon*, is vital for the survival of the entire cell. The processes extending from the perikaryon are specialized for three primary

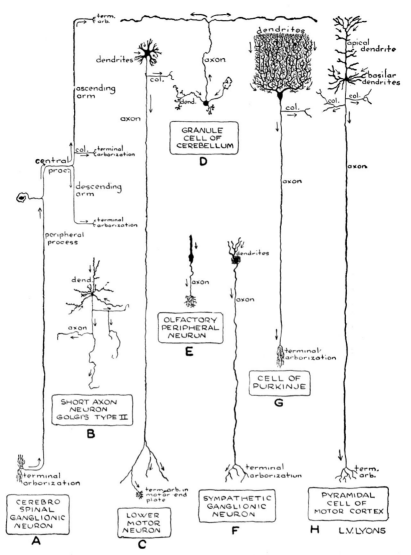

Figure 10.1. Some of the principal forms of neurons as depicted from silver impregnation light microscope studies. Myelin sheaths or other investments are not shown. The axons, except in *B*, are shown much shorter in proportion to the size of body and dendrites than they actually are. The direction of conduction is shown by the arrows. *Col*, collateral branch; *proc*, process; *term. arb*, terminal arborization.

functions (Fig. 10.2): (*a*) *reception* of various stimuli—this is generally the function of the *dendritic zone* (receptor portion) of the neuron, including those areas of the cell body or the axon that receive signals from other cells; (*b*) *conduction* of the nerve impulse (action potentials) to regions distant from the receptive area—this is generally the function of the axon, but dendrite regions and cell bodies may also propagate impulses; and (*c*) *synaptic transmission* of

the signal to subsequent neurons in the neural pathways or to muscle or gland. This *effector* function generally occurs in the nerve terminals, where minute amounts of chemical compounds called *neurotransmitters* are released. Each neuron is thus equipped to receive information, to act on the basis of this information to signal its distant portions, and then to influence other neurons or other tissues.

In addition to interactions served by

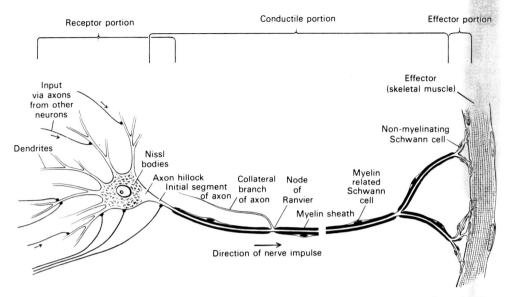

Figure 10.2. This diagram illustrates the receptor, conductile, and effector portions of a typical large neuron. The effector endings on skeletal muscle identify this as a somatic motor neuron; in many neurons the effector endings are applied to the receptor portions of other neurons. The presence of the myelin sheath on the conductile portion of the neuron (the axon) increases conduction velocity. The axon is shown to be interrupted, for it is much longer than can be illustrated here.

chemical synapses, neurons may also be coupled by *gap* or *communicating junctions*, although these are rare in mammals. Such couplings are sometimes referred to as *electrotonic synapses.*

Classification of Neurons by Shape

The general form of the neuron is best studied after staining thick sections of nervous tissue with heavy metals such as silver or gold (Fig. 10.3). Adaptation to different functional needs in various parts of the body leads to a great spectrum of neuronal shapes and sizes (Fig. 10.1). *Multipolar neurons* (Fig. 10.1B, C, D, F, G, and H) frequently have a number of dendritic processes arising directly from the cell body. The axon may also arise from the cell body or from the proximal part of one of the dendrites. The axon sometimes branches soon after its formation to provide recurrent collateral branches which return to the region of the cell body (Fig. 10.2). Except for these collaterals, there is often no further branching until the axon reaches the region of terminal arborization and transmitter release (Figs. 10.1 and 10.2). In *bi-*

polar neurons, one process emerges from each pole of an elongated cell body (Fig. 10.1E). The receptor and effector portions of these cells are often limited to the extreme ends; the entire intermediate portion, including the cell body, is conductile in function. In *unipolar neurons* (as found in most sensory ganglia), the nerve cell body possesses a single process which divides not far from the cell body into two branches, one proceeding to some peripheral structure and the other entering the CNS (Fig. 10.1A). Both arms of the single process have the structural and functional characteristics of an axon; together they form the conductile portion of the cell. The receptor part is located in some peripheral sense organ and the central part arborizes within the CNS to provide effector influence upon the dendrites of various CNS cells. It should also be noted that in some specialized areas of the CNS there appear to be cells which do not possess axons. These are small cells, called *anaxonic neurons*, which have both receptor and effector regions on their dendritic portions. They thus require no conductile portion to con-

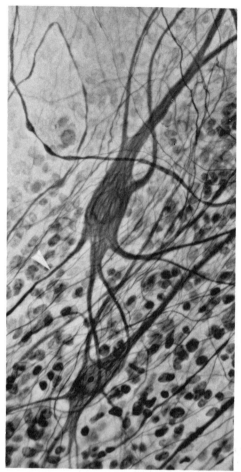

Figure 10.3. This photomicrograph shows two large neurons that have matured in tissue culture. The culture has been fixed and then stained with silver. In the *lower neuron* the nucleolus is stained deeply, as are many of the nuclei of the surrounding glial cells. Within the neurons neurofibrils are seen interlacing in the nerve cell body and extending into the numerous dendrites. The axon of the *upper neuron* is indicated by a *white arrowhead* (×310). (Courtesy of Dr. C. D. Allerand.)

vey receptor influences to distant regions. One example, the *amacrine cell* of the retina, is discussed in Chapter 22.

The Nerve Cell Body

The nerve cell body consists of a mass of cytoplasm, the perikaryon, surrounding a nucleus. The usual cell organelles are present, but it is primarily the quantities and dispositions of many of these components that underlie the special functional capacities of the neuron. The generally accepted *neuron doctrine* recognizes the individuality of neurons and that the cell body is the trophic (nutritional) and genetic center of these complex cells. The various cell processes depend on the cell body for survival and if severed will degenerate.

Nerve cell bodies vary considerably in size. The small *granule cells* of the cerebellum are about 4 μm in diameter, whereas large motor cells in the ventral horn of the human spinal cord may attain diameters of 135 μm (certain invertebrate neurons may be 4 times this size). The size of the neuron cell body generally reflects the amount of cytoplasm being supported in the cell processes. Thus, some of the largest neuronal cell bodies are those with the longest and thickest axons.

Nucleus of the Nerve Cell

The *nucleus* of the nerve cell is spherical in form, proportional to the size of cell it occupies, and characterized by widely dispersed chromatin, suggesting a high volume of transcriptional activity. Certain large neurons are known to contain a tetraploid amount (i.e., twice the normal amount) of DNA. Usually the nucleus is situated approximately in the center of the cell body in large nerve cells, the most striking exceptions being its eccentric position in the cells of Clarke's column in the spinal cord, in cells of sympathetic ganglia, in various pathological conditions, and when the axon of the cell is injured. Although most neurons have a single nucleus, some binucleate neurons are generally present in sympathetic ganglia and a few are occasionally present in sensory ganglia.

The *nucleolus* is relatively large and prominent. In tissues from females, the sex chromatin (or *Barr body*) is often clearly visualized. In some animals (such as the cat, in which it was first observed), this body is seen as a satellite of the nucleolus about 1 μm in diameter; in human females it is adjacent to the nuclear envelope. The appearance of this body is described in Chapters 1 and 7.

Cytoplasm of the Nerve Cell Body

The cytoplasm surrounding a neuron's nucleus is termed the *perikaryon*. It contains ribosomes and endoplasmic reticulum, Golgi apparatus, mitochondria, filaments, microtubules, lysosomes, and cytoplasmic inclusions such as fat, glycogen, lipofuscin, and sometimes the pigment melanin.

When neurons are grown in tissue culture and visualized in the living state by phase microscopy, extensive homogeneous regions in the cytoplasm may be observed (Fig. 10.4). These are distinct from the granular lysosomes and mitochondria or the clear linear aggregates of filaments and microtubules. These regions absorb the same wavelengths of ultraviolet light as do nucleic acids, and stain strongly with basophilic dyes except after prior treatment with ribonuclease (Fig. 10.5). The German histologist Nissl first noted that these distinctive areas in fixed neurons stain with basic aniline dyes. Hence, light microscopists have long referred to them as *Nissl bodies*, usually seen as small granules clumped together in a variety of shapes (Fig. 10.5), larger in motor than in sensory neurons. The *Nissl substance*, as these areas are now commonly called, is one of the hallmarks in identifying neurons. Nissl substance is found in the perikarya and in the proximal parts of the dendrites of all large and many small neurons but *not* in the axon and the axon hillock (Figs. 10.2 and 10.5*A*).

Electron micrographs show that the Nissl substance is composed of clusters of endoplasmic reticulum plus ribosomes bound to the outer surfaces of cisternae or free in the cytoplasm between (Fig. 10.6). Free ribosomes frequently are arranged in rosettes or linear arrays of five or more

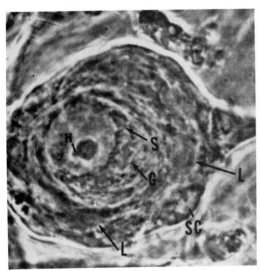 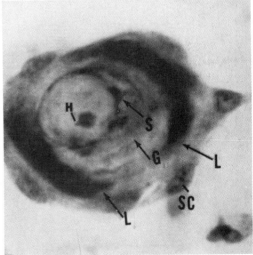

Figure 10.4. Photomicrographs of the same neuron before (*left*) and after (*right*) fixation and staining of Nissl substance. The picture on the *left* is of a living chick neuron in tissue culture photographed with a phase microscope. The large, relatively homogeneous masses (*L*) apparent in the phase microscope are seen to be heavily stained by the basic dye employed to stain Nissl substance (*right*). *S* marks a patch of Nissl material often found near the nuclear envelope and commonly called the nuclear cap. *H* calls attention to heterochromatin adjacent to the nucleolus. *G* points to some granular material seen in the living state that proved not to be Nissl material after staining. *SC* marks a satellite cell nucleus. *Left*, ×1800; *right*, ×2000. (Reprinted with permission from A. D. Deitch, and M. R. Murray: *J Biophys Biochem Cytol* 2:433, 1956.)

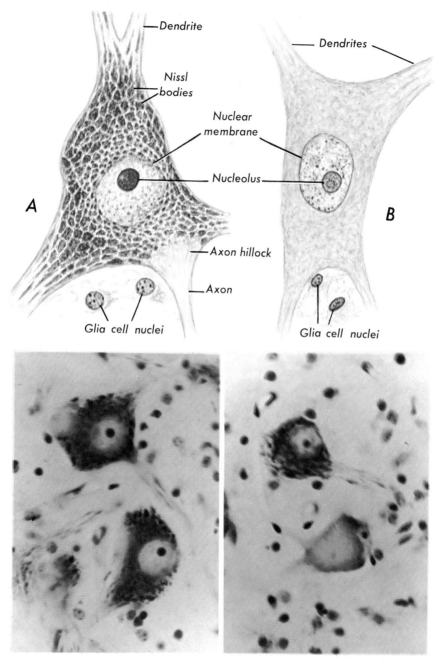

Figure 10.5. These neurons from the ventral horn of the spinal cord are stained for Nissl substance by the toluidine blue method. *A* is a drawing of a normal neuron illustrating the absence of Nissl substance in the axon hillock region; *B* is a drawing of a neuron similarly stained after treatment with the enzyme ribonuclease to remove RNA. This preparation is counterstained with erythrosin. The pictures *below* are photomicrographs showing three normal neurons and one neuron showing chromatolysis in response to axon section several days earlier (*lower right*). The comma-shaped nucleus is at the cell body periphery, and the center of the perikaryon stains very lightly. *Above*, ×1,000; *below*, ×750.

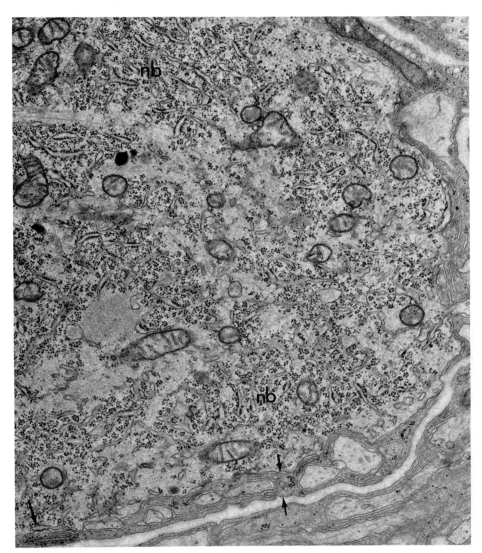

Figure 10.6. This electron micrograph shows a portion of a neuron perikaryon ensheathed by satellite cell processes. The Nissl substance seen in Figure 10.5 is shown here to be aggregates of ribosomes and endoplasmic reticulum cisterns (as at *nb*). Light, often linear areas (sometimes called roads) separate the Nissl material. Cisterns of endoplasmic reticulum lying very near the surface of the neuron are referred to as subsurface cisterns (*single arrow*). The width of the satellite cell investment is indicated by the *paired arrows*. Rat sensory ganglion neuron (×21,500).

granules (Fig. 10.7). The basophilia depends upon the presence of RNA in the ribosomes, not upon components in the endoplasmic reticulum. Certain cisternae of endoplasmic reticulum come to lie unusually close to the plasma membrane of the perikarya. These *subsurface cisternae* are a distinctive characteristic of neurons visible only in electron micrographs (Fig. 10.6).

The fact that neurons exhibit a large nucleolus and abundant granular endoplasmic reticulum indicates that they are actively synthesizing proteins. This may seem surprising, because mature neurons are not increasing in size or number. However, most protein synthesis for the nerve cell body and its vast extensions is accomplished in the region of the cell body (and

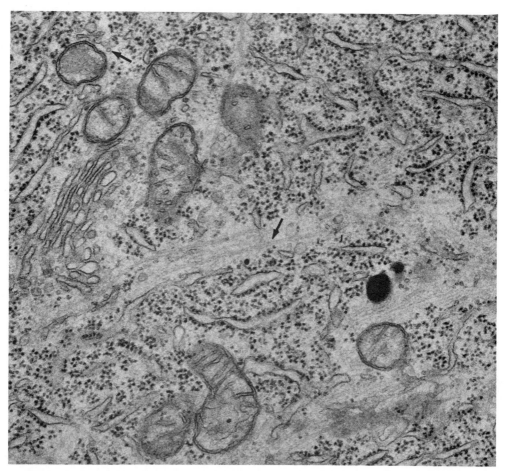

Figure 10.7. A typical region of neuronal cytoplasm is shown in this electron micrograph. Within Nissl substance, many of the ribosomes are in polysomal aggregates that either lie free in the cytoplasm or are arrayed on cisternal membrane. Also illustrated are a Golgi region (*left*), microtubules in cross and longitudinal section (*arrows*), and two small, dense lysosomes. Rat sensory ganglion neuron (×43,000).

the proximal dendrites). Material constantly moves from these areas of production to the farthest reaches of the axon and dendrites.

After repeated electrical stimulation or after amputation of a substantial part of the axon the disposition of the Nissl substance in the nerve cell body is altered. In this condition, known as *chromatolysis*, the nucleus becomes eccentrically located and the basophilic material in the cytoplasm is concentrated in the cell periphery (Fig. 10.5). Certain types of neurons undergo this change as a prelude to degeneration, but others are able to reverse the chromatolytic

pattern, regenerate amputated parts, and return to their former organization. Chromatolysis may be observed as early as the 1st day after an axon is cut and is most marked at about two weeks. There is little change in the total quantity of RNA in the perikaryon during the early stages of regeneration, although its concentration decreases, because the cell imbibes water and increases in volume by more than 200%. In neurons capable of axonal regeneration, the amount of RNA and protein in the neuron increases after several days, and the amputated part is slowly regenerated. The neuronal cytoplasm then returns to normal.

The extent and rapidity of the changes depend upon the type of neuron and the nature and location of the injury: an injury near the cell body causes more effect than one at a distance. Injury near the cell body is more likely to lead to cell death.

Clear areas of neuronal cytoplasm between Nissl substance (Fig. 10.6), as well as in both axons and dendrites, contain numerous *filaments* and *microtubules*. The microtubules are 20 to 30 nm in diameter and are similar to those found in other cell types. Typically, the filaments are linear elements about 7 to 10 nm in diameter, occurring in groups interspersed with microtubules (Fig. 10.7). They are often called *neurofilaments*, and while morphologically similar to intermediate filaments of other cell types, they are chemically distinct. The filament content of neurons varies between species and between regions of the nervous system. The success of microscopic *silver staining* is sometimes related to these variations. Successful silver preparations characteristically show dark, slender elements called *neurofibrils*. The neurofibrils visible in the light microscope are aggregates of filaments on which silver has been deposited. These neurofibrils course parallel with one another in the axon and dendrite but cross and interlace in the cell body (Fig. 10.3). The frequent association between filaments and microtubules and their location among Nissl substance and in axons and dendrites suggest a possible role in intercellular transport (described below under "Axoplasmic Transport").

The *Golgi apparatus* is limited to the perikaryon. Its prominence in neurons probably relates to the fact that much of the protein manufactured by the neuron is channeled through the Golgi region, as it is in secretory cells. *Mitochondria* are plentiful in the perikaryon, as well as in the dendrites and axons. Neither the mitochondria nor the lysosomal elements of nerve cells are morphologically distinctive. *Lipofuscin pigment granules* begin to appear at an early age and increase in number with advancing age; hence they are known as "wear and tear pigment." This pigment is yellow or brown and stains with lipid dyes. These granules are apparently secondary lysosomes (Chapter 1) which represent the end product of incessant lysosomal activity during the long life of the nerve cell. Their accumulation has been postulated to inhibit eventually the normal function of some neurons—a normal part of the aging process.

Some nerve cells contain granules of dark brown pigment, *melanin*. This occurs in certains cells of the olfactory bulb, the locus ceruleus in the floor of the fourth ventricle, the substantia nigra of the midbrain, and certain cells of the reticular formation. Melanin is also present in some spinal and sympathetic ganglion cells.

Dendrites

Like a tree spreading its limbs to allow each leaf exposure to the sun, the highly branched dendrites (from the Greek *dendron*, tree) allow an expansion of the neuron surface for the reception of many axon terminals. Dendrites are generally shorter than axons, but they branch repeatedly and their surface is often studded with fine spiny or knobbed excrescences (*spines* or *gemmules*, Fig. 10.8); this elaboration of surface area allows large neurons to receive as many as 100,000 separate axon terminals on their dendritic surfaces. These axonal inputs are not randomly arranged; axons from one source occupy a specific region of the dendritic tree, whereas axons from another source terminate elsewhere. The contents of the dendrites resemble those of the cell body except that Nissl substance is generally restricted to the more proximal regions. Microtubules and mitochondria are conspicuous, and there are a few microfilaments (Fig. 10.9). The dendrites, like the axons, also contain a few channels of smooth membranes.

Axons

Axons (sometimes termed axis cylinders) arise either from the nerve cell body (Fig. 10.3) or from the proximal part of a dendrite. They are slender extensions with a

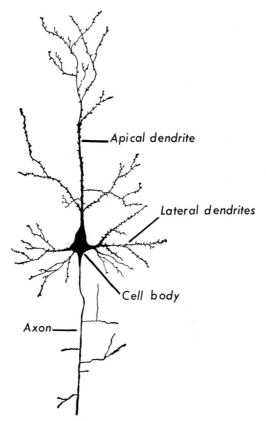

Figure 10.8. This drawing shows part of a pyramidal cell from human cerebral cortex, including the dendritic portion, the cell body, and the proximal part of the axon. The tiny protuberances on the dendrites are called spines or gemmules. Gold chloride method.

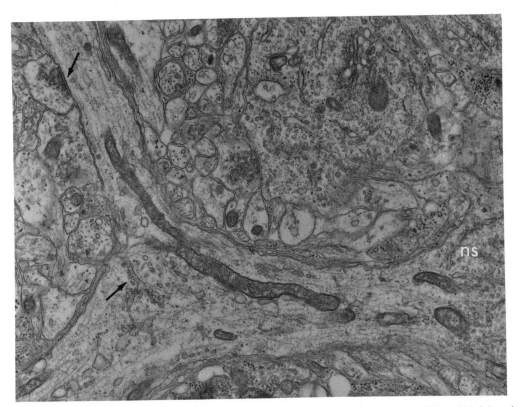

Figure 10.9. This electron micrograph shows a primary dendrite arising from a cell body (*right*) and branching into two secondary dendrites (*left*). Nissl substance in the periphery of the parent neuron is marked *ns*. The *upper arrow* indicates an axodendritic synapse. The *lower arrow* points to endoplasmic reticulum related to ribosomes within the dendrite. Note that the dendritic shaft is covered in many places by flattened processes of astrocytes. The compactness and complexity of the cellular elements is characteristic of central nervous tissue. Rat spinal cord (×17,000). (Reprinted with permission from R. P. Bunge, et al.: *J Cell Biol* 24:163, 1965.)

smoother contour and a more uniform diameter than dendrites. The axon may have side or *collateral* branches along its length, but its most prominent branching generally occurs shortly before its termination. These terminal branches are termed *telodendria*, and the actual point of ending, where the axon is frequently enlarged, is called the *terminal*. The plasma membrane of the axon is often termed the *axolemma*; morphological specializations of this membrane have been observed in the region of the *initial segment* of the axon, at *nodes of Ranvier* (see below) and at the terminals. The axonal contents are termed the *axoplasm*; this cytoplasm differs from that of the cell body in that the only formed organelles normally observed are mitochondria,

filaments, microtubules, and channels of smooth membrane. Nissl substance and Golgi elements are lacking. At the point of egress of the axon from the nerve cell body (or dendrite), there is generally a region of cytoplasm from which Nissl substance is conspicuously absent (Fig. 10.2). This region marks the emerging process as the axon (rather than a dendrite) and is called the *axon hillock*.

That portion of the axon between the cell body and the point at which there is some form of axonal ensheathment (such as myelin, see below) is termed the *initial segment* (Figs. 10.2 and 10.10). In many neurons, this region is known to have a much lower threshold of electrical excitability than does the dendrite or the perikaryon (see

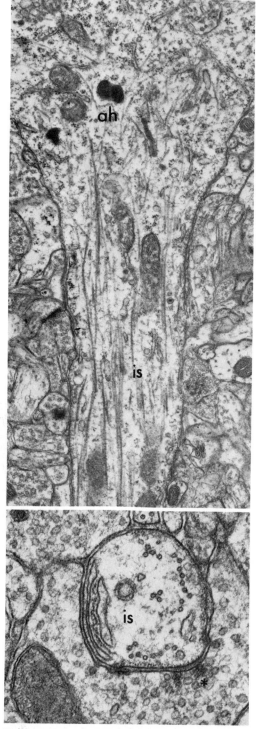

below). Morphologically, it is characterized by three special features: (a) a dense layer of finely granular material undercoating the axolemma, (b) scattered clusters of ribosomes but no discrete Nissl substance and (c) microtubules gathered into slender fascicles (Fig. 10.10).

Axoplasmic Transport

Although there is evidence that some axons contain minute amounts of nonmitochondrial RNA and that they undertake a small amount of protein synthesis, the acknowledged protein assembly center of the neuron is the cell body. The transport of manufactured material into the processes of the cell, especially the long axon, presents special problems. From observations on constricted axons, and from radioautographic studies after labeling of the proteins formed in the cell body, it is known that materials constantly travel from the cell body into the axon and are transported peripherally to the extremities of these processes. The microtubules (and perhaps the filaments) are believed to be involved in this process. A small amount of material travels rapidly (at rates of 40–400 mm/day), but the bulk moves slowly, at a rate of about 1 mm/day in mammals. The material transported at the faster rate is utilized for membrane renewal, neurotransmitter synthesis and recycling, and perhaps also exerts trophic effects on innervated tissues. Molecules comprising cytoskeletal elements (microtubules, neurofilaments) are transported at a rate of about 1 to 3 mm/day, and this is also the approximate rate of regrowth for a cut axon. Material is

Figure 10.10. Electron micrographs of the initial segment of an axon of the cerebral cortex of a rat. The *upper figure* shows a longitudinal section through the initial segment (*is*) arising from the axon hillock (*ah*). Note the absence of Nissl substance and only occasional free ribosomes, the presence of dense material undercoating the axolemma, and fascicles of microtubules. The *lower figure* shows a cross section of the initial segment beyond the level of the axon hillock. In the field shown, the initial segment is partially surrounded by a large axonal terminal that forms a synaptic complex in the region marked by a *, *lower right*. Two flattened cisterns surrounded by dense material are seen on the *left side* of the segment; similar structures are sometimes found in dendritic spines. *Upper figure*, ×23,000; *lower figure*, ×49,000. (Reprinted with permission from A. Peters, et al.: *J Cell Biol* 39:604, 1968.)

also transported from nerve terminals back along an axon to the perikaryon. This *retrograde transport* facilitates recycling of certain molecules that require reprocessing in the perikaryon, and it may also be a means by which the peripheral extremities of a neuron signal its trophic center and effect appropriate control. Endocytosis at nerve terminals, coupled with retrograde transport, may also provide the means by which certain pathogens, such as polio virus or tetanus toxin, gain access to the neuron cell bodies of the CNS.

AXON TERMINALS, SYNAPSES, RECEPTORS, AND NEUROTRANSMITTERS

As the action potential of an axon is carried into the region of its terminal, the mechanism of signaling is generally changed from electrical to chemical. In certain special terminals, however, the electrical signal may be carried directly to an adjacent cell via a *communicating junction* (gap junction or nexus). In neural tissues, such junctions are also frequently termed *electrical synapses, electrotonic junctions,* or *ephapses.* These junctions are similar to those observed in other epithelial tissues, in smooth and cardiac muscle and between certain connective tissue cells (Fig. 10.11). This type of cell-to-cell communication has the advantage of great rapidity.

More commonly, the signal entering the axon terminal has no direct electrical effect on the adjacent cell. Instead, it causes the release of a neurotransmitter from the axon terminal. This chemical diffuses across a narrow (20 nm) intercellular space to react with a specialized *receptor* region on the adjacent cell. Interaction of neurotransmitter with receptor leads to electrical activity in the second cell. The site at which this "chemical" form of transmission (as opposed to the "electrical" transmission discussed above) takes place is called a *chemical synapse* (or in common usage, a *synapse*).

A synapse is defined as a region of specialized attachment between nerve cells or between nerve cells and effector organs. Light microscopic observations disclose synapses to be areas of axon enlargement containing mitochondria and neurofibrillar material. Electron microscopy reveals that the axon characteristically contains clusters of *synaptic vesicles* in the region of the synapse and that the plasma membrane of both the axon and the contacted cell is often modified in this area. These modifications consist of dense material applied to the inner surface of one or both of the apposed membranes, in addition to the presence of demonstrable extracellular material between the apposed membranes (Figs. 10.12 and 10.13). Unlike epithelial junctions such as desmosomes, the intracellular dense material is not disposed similarly on both membranes. This difference and the presence of vesicles in the axon correlate with the physiological observation that the synapse transmits the nerve signal in one direction only—from the axon to the cell contacted. The electrotonic junctions discussed above are thought to transmit the impulse with equal efficacy in either direction.

At the *synapse,* the axon terminal is termed the *presynaptic* element, the cell being contacted is called the *postsynaptic* element, and the intervening extracellular space is designated the *synaptic cleft* (Figs. 10.12 and 10.13). At synapses, axonal enlargements are often called *boutons terminaux* (or end feet) if they are terminating, or *boutons en passage* if they continue on to make additional contacts elsewhere (Fig. 10.12). Thus, a single axon may display synapses with many different neurons. The dense material within the synaptic cleft apparently attaches the pre- and postsynaptic elements. This attachment is strong enough to survive tissue homogenization and differential centrifugation, and it is possible to prepare a tissue fraction composed, in large part, of the axon terminals still attached to cleft substance and postsynaptic membrane. Such preparations are termed *synaptosomes* and are now widely used in biochemical studies.

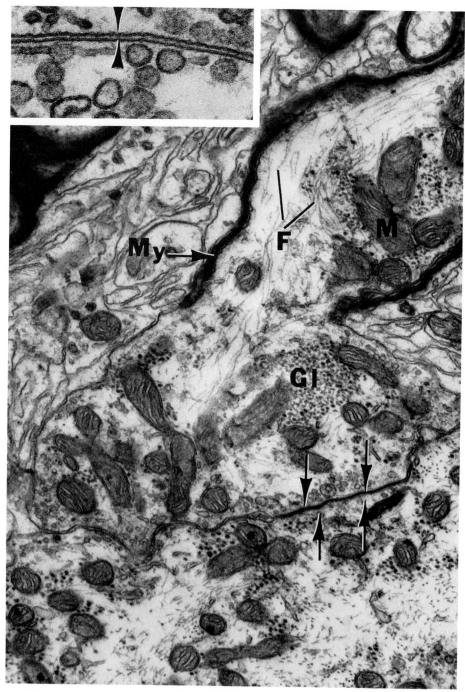

Figure 10.11. These electron micrographs illustrate the type of close apposition of cell membranes that allows direct electrical coupling between nerve cells. This is a section of an axosomatic electrotonic synapse from the medulla of a gymnotid fish, Sternopygus. Filaments (*F*), mitochondria (*M*), and glycogen (*Gl*) are present in the axon. Termination of the myelin sheath (*My*) may be seen. At the *paired arrows* the axonal membrane and the membrane of a neuron cell body are very closely apposed. The *inset* (*upper left*) shows a similar junction at higher magnification to illustrate the closely apposed membranes (at *arrows*). ×27,500; inset, ×110,000. (Courtesy of Dr. George Pappas.)

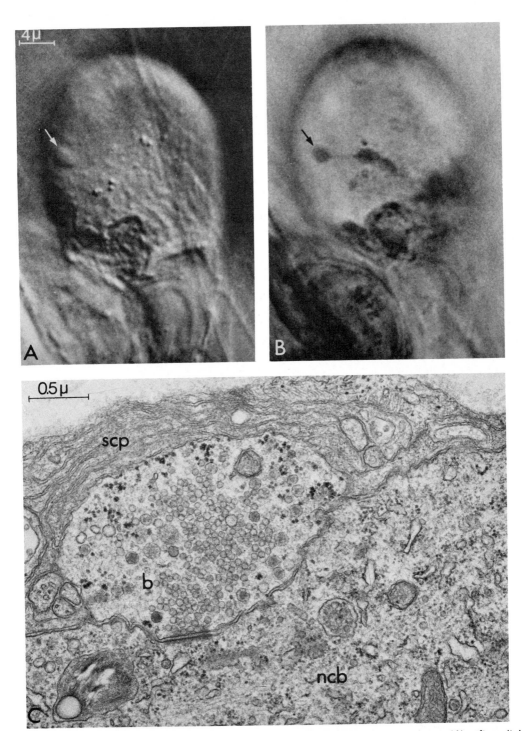

Figure 10.12. These three photographs show a synaptic bouton in living tissue (*A*), after vital staining (*B*), and after preparation for electron microscopy (*C*). *A* shows a bouton (*arrow*) on the cell body of a parasympathetic neuron in the interatrial septum of the frog heart. The septum has been removed from the heart, pinned out in tissue culture medium, and viewed with a Nomarski differential interference contrast optical system. *B* shows the same nerve cell 15 min after adding a dilute solution of methylene blue to the medium. The terminal synaptic bouton (*arrow*) seen in *A* and two others (apparently boutons en passage) not visible in the unstained preparation have taken up the dye. *C* is an electron micrograph of this type of bouton. A bouton (*b*) contains a mitochondrion, glycogen particles, a few granular vesicles, and numerous small agranular vesicles, some of which are clustered next to a region of specialized membrane. Layers of Schwann cell processes (*scp*) cover the bouton, except where it is in contact with the postsynaptic nerve cell body (*ncb*). (Reprinted with permission from U. J. McMahan and S. W. Kuffler: In *Excitatory Synaptic Mechanisms*, edited by P. Andersen and J. K. S. Jansen. p. 57, 1970.)

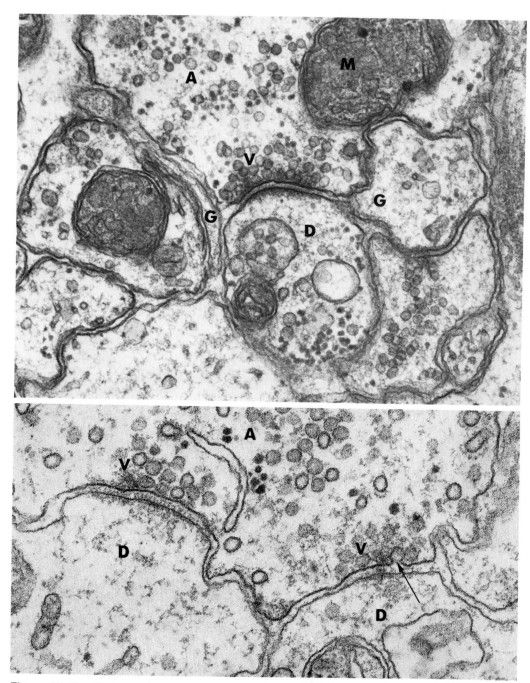

Figure 10.13. Electron micrographs showing synaptic regions from the brain of a salamander. In the *upper figure*, an axonal terminal (*A*) is in synaptic juxtaposition with a dendritic terminal (*D*). The presynaptic cytoplasm of the axon is characterized by clustered synaptic vesicles (*V*). A filamentous web can be seen along the postsynaptic (dendritic) side of the contact zone. A dense intercellular material occupies the synaptic cleft between axonal and dendritic surfaces. Glial cell processes (*G*) appear to encircle and seal the synaptic cleft. Dense glycogen granules are found within both axonal and dendritic cytoplasms, and mitochondria (*M*) are characteristic of axonal terminals. In the *lower figure*, an axonal terminal (*A*) abuts upon portions of two dendrites (*D*). Two synaptic sites are characterized by synaptic vesicles (*V*), one of which appears to have been fixed at the moment of its continuity with the presynaptic plasma membrane (*arrow*). Upper figure, ×71,000; lower figure, ×81,000.

Synapses have been classified on the basis of position, membrane specialization, or organelle content. On the basis of position, they are termed *axodendritic, axosomatic,* or *axoaxonic,* thus indicating whether an axon abuts upon a dendrite, a nerve cell body, or another axon. Axoaxonic synapses are most often found on the initial segment region or near the axon terminal. Some axodendritic synapses are distinguished by an increased amount of dense material coating the cytoplasmic side of the synaptic membranes and a widening of the synaptic cleft (Fig. 10.14).

Variations in the quantity and quality of *synaptic vesicle* content of the axon terminal also aid in the classification of synapses. Although the vesicle population of a given terminal is often not homogeneous, one type generally predominates. At neuromuscular junctions (where nerve contacts skel-

etal muscle) and in many CNS terminals, the majority of synaptic vesicles are 30 to 60 nm in diameter and are spherical with apparently clear centers (Figs. 10.12 and 10.13). In axon terminals of autonomic nerve fibers supplying smooth muscle (e.g., in the intestine), the synaptic vesicles may be slightly larger. They are also round but contain a prominent dense particle or short rod (Fig. 10.15). This allows the distinction between terminals with "*clear*" and those with "*dense-cored*" (or *granular*) *vesicles.* It has been observed that synapses known to release the neurotransmitter *acetylcholine* (i.e., *cholinergic* synapses) contain clear vesicles, whereas terminals known to release *noradrenaline* (i.e., *adrenergic* synapses) contain vesicles with dense cores (see additional discussion below under "Termination of Visceral Efferent Fibers").

Aldehyde fixation of neural tissue pro-

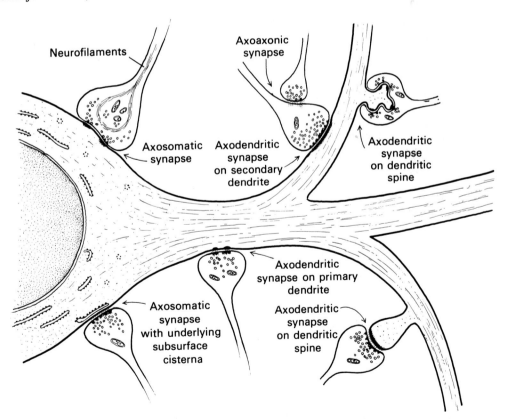

Figure 10.14. The types of synapses occurring on various parts of the neuron are depicted here. Note that the degree of membrane "thickening" varies in different types of synapses, and that the material applied to the cytoplasmic side of the presynaptic membrane is often seen as a regular pattern rather than as a solid plaque. Variations in synaptic vesicle morphology are not shown.

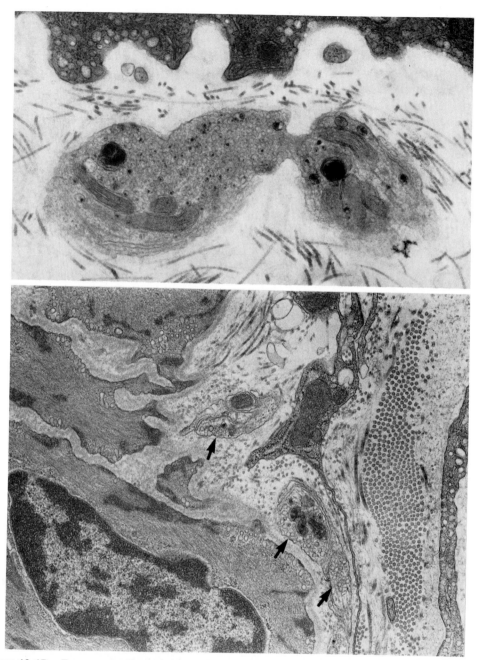

Figure 10.15. *Top*, a sympathetic (adrenergic) postganglionic axonal ending. The nerve terminal lies free within loose connective tissue and contains a vesicle population frequently displaying dense granules (×73,500). *Bottom*, several parasympathetic axonal endings (*arrows*) in the vicinity of smooth muscle (*left side* of figure). These endings lie free in connective tissue rather than in synaptic contact with the muscle cells. They are characterized by clear vesicles. A capillary wall is seen at extreme right (×18,500). (Both figures courtesy of Dr. Bernard G. Slavin.)

duces varying images of endings which contain predominantly clear vesicles. In these preparations, the clear vesicles in certain axonal endings appear smaller and are flat-tened instead of spherical. Clusters of this type of vesicle have been observed after aldehyde fixation of axonal terminals that are known to be *inhibitory* in funtion (Fig.

10.16). This is in contrast to known *excitatory* synapses where the presynaptic vesicles are spherical. However, the correlation is not consistent. Varying degrees of "flattening" among inhibitory synapses are known. When unfixed synapses are prepared for electron microscopy by quick freezing, the vesicles of known inhibitory synapses remain spherical, although smaller than those of neighboring excitatory synapses (Fig. 10.17).

The demonstration of vesicles in axonal endings and the physiological observation that certain transmitters are released in "packets" (i.e., in pulses of several thousand molecules rather than in a continuous stream) have together led to the suggestion that the vesicles contain or bind the neurotransmitter. It was also suggested that vesicles release the neurotransmitter by dumping it into the synaptic cleft after fusing with the presynaptic membrane, i.e., by exocytosis (Fig. 10.13). It seems certain that neurotransmitters are located in synaptic vesicles, but the mechanism of their release is not as clear and may differ in synapses which release different transmitter substances.

The synaptic complex is also known to contain mechanisms for the breakdown and/or uptake of released neurotransmitter. Certain cholinergic synaptic areas contain the enzyme *acetylcholinesterase* in the pre- and postsynaptic elements, in the synaptic cleft, and in the adjacent tissues. This enzyme hydrolyzes acetylcholine with the formation of acetate and choline. Part of the choline is taken up by the presynaptic element and reutilized in subsequent acetylcholine synthesis. In adrenergic endings, the transmitter has not been observed to be similarly broken down; it is simply taken up intact from the surrounding extracellular spaces for reuse.

The past few years have seen a rapid increase in the number of known naturally occurring chemical entities that are suspected of acting as neurotransmitters. These include the familiar *acetylcholine* and *norepinephrine* (*noradrenaline*) as well as *dopamine, serotonin,* some amino acids such as *glycine, taurine, glutamate,* γ-*ami-*

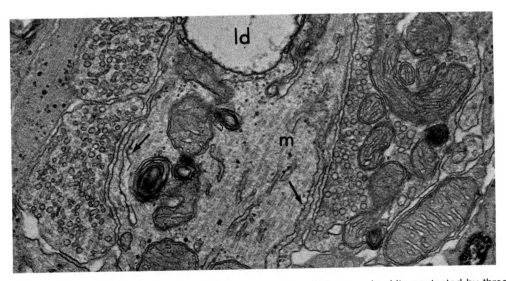

Figure 10.16. This electron micrograph from rat spinal cord shows a dendrite contacted by three axonal boutons. The dendrite contains microtubules (*m*), mitochondria, a large lipid droplet (*ld*) and cisterns of endoplasmic reticulum underlying its surface membrane (*arrows*). Note that the axonal terminal on the *right* contains predominantly round synaptic vesicles, whereas the two terminals on the *left* contain vesicles that are generally somewhat smaller and somewhat flattened. These differences in synaptic vesicle morphology are revealed only after primary fixation in aldehyde. ×46,000. (Reprinted with permission from M. B. Bunge, et al.: *Brain Res* 6:728, 1967.)

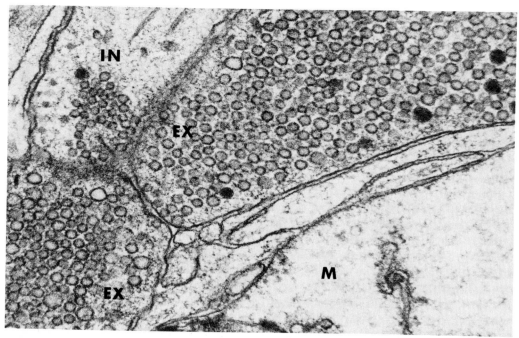

Figure 10.17. One inhibitory (*IN*) and two excitatory (*EX*) axonal terminations along a muscle cell (*M*) in a crayfish stretch receptor organ. This electron micrograph is of a specimen prepared by rapid freezing and freeze-substitution. Note that vesicles of the excitatory endings are larger and round (similar to those that are chemically fixed), but inhibitory ending vesicles are small and round (unlike flattened vesicles in similar endings after aldehyde fixation). (×110,000) (Courtesy of Drs. Yasuko Nakajima and Thomas S. Reese.)

nobutyric acid (*GABA*), and *aspartate*, and a number of recently discovered polypeptides including *enkephalins, endorphins,* and *substance P*. It seems clear that this list will increase as more specific knowledge of synapses and their actions is gathered. In general these are all small molecules which, after release, combine with specific *receptor sites* on the postsynaptic membrane. The receptor sites react with specific neurotransmitters and not with others, and these reactions engender permeability changes to certain ions. If a permeability change leads to a decrease in the electrical polarization of the postsynaptic membrane (*depolarization*), the effect is *excitatory*, making it more likely that the postsynaptic element will generate an action potential. When recording from the postsynaptic cell, the physiologist observes an *excitatory postsynaptic potential* (often abbreviated EPSP). If the effect is to increase electrical

polarization of the membrane (hyperpolarization), making it less likely that the postsynaptic element will "fire," the effect is said to be *inhibitory* and an *inhibitory postsynaptic potential* (IPSP) is recorded. The specificity of synaptic action depends upon the receptor site rather than on the neurotransmitter, for a transmitter may have an excitatory influence at one synapse and an inhibitory effect at another.

It seems certain that molecules other than neurotransmitters must also pass between cells at synaptic junctions, for many synapses also have a *trophic action* on the postsynaptic element. The normal state of skeletal muscle, for example, is dependent upon the continuing presence of neuromuscular junctions; if the nerve is cut, the neuromuscular contact degenerates and the electrical, chemical, and anatomical properties of the muscle fiber are permanently altered unless nerve regeneration occurs.

Certain neurons of the CNS do not survive if a substantial portion of their synaptic input is removed.

The *neuromuscular* (myoneural) *junction* between nerve terminal and skeletal muscle has many of the properties of the basic synaptic apparatus described above. The functional relationship between nerve and cardiac or smooth muscle, on the other hand, presents some basic differences; all these are discussed below under "Nerve Terminations."

Neurons, like many other cells, maintain a negative electrical potential across their plasma membrane, the inside of the cell being about 70 mV more negative than the outside. If this potential is made progressively less negative, a point is reached at which major permeability changes in the surface membrane cause the generation of an action potential; once generated, this action potential tends to be propagated rapidly and with little loss of amplitude over the neuron surface. On many neurons, however, there is a limited number of sites at which action potentials are generated. The dendritic tree and the cell body are often not very excitable. The action of synaptic contacts in these areas leads to transient local shifts, some inhibitory and some excitatory, in the properties of the postsynaptic membrane. Generally, only when several excitatory synaptic inputs act together (and are not canceled by inhibitory influences) does a change in membrane potential reach sufficient strength to be carried down over the dendrite and cell body to excite the initial axonal segment. In most neurons, this region is much more sensitive to membrane potential shifts than is the dendrite or the cell body, and it is here—at the initial segment—where the all or none action potential of the axon is initiated.

NEUROGLIA

Most organs of the body have a connective tissue framework which not only serves as a vascular bed but also provides a supporting skeleton for the particular cellular elements of the organ. Peripheral nerve has such a framework, albeit rather specialized (as discussed below), whereas the CNS does not. This is not difficult to appreciate if one recalls that the CNS is an epithelium and that epithelia are segregated from connective tissues. The brain and spinal cord are suspended in a fluid environment, the *cerebrospinal fluid*. Connective tissue associated with the CNS is limited to the enveloping membranes (the *meninges*) and to a small amount which accompanies blood vessels. The CNS *neuroglia* (from the Greek *neuron*, nerve, + *glia*, glue) or more simply, *glia*, are several varieties of cells which lie among the neurons of the CNS and essentially cover, in various patterns, the surfaces of neurons that are not overlain by synapses. Like the neurons, they arise developmentally within the neural tube (with one possible exception), being the offspring of the embryonic *glioblast* population. The neuroglia provide both structural and metabolic support for the neurons. For example, certain glial cells invest axons with a *myelin sheath*, dramatically increasing the speed of impulse conduction. It has been suggested that they provide neurons with high energy compounds, or aid in chemical control of the neuronal environment.

Glial cells do not generate action potentials, and they have seldom been observed to develop synapse-like junctions. Studies of glial function are presently a fertile frontier in neurobiological research.

Before the era of the electron microscope, neuroglia could be studied only by special and often difficult selective staining procedures. Electron microscopy has provided the means for studying all elements of nervous tissue simultaneously and for delineating the relationships of cell membranes. Hence, many of the features described below are seen only in electron micrographs.

In routine preparations of CNS tissue, (e.g., Fig. 10.5), the majority of cell nuclei seen with the light microscope belong to the glial cells, and careful study of their morphology often permits identification of the following classes: (*a*) *astrocytes*, (*b*) *oli-*

godendrocytes, (*c*) *microglia*, and (*d*) *ependyma* (Fig. 10.18). The *cells of Schwann* of peripheral nerves and the *satellite cells* which surround the cell bodies of the spinal and cranial ganglia are the glial elements of the peripheral nervous system. They are considered to be *glioblast* derivatives, but in this case, of *neural crest* rather than neural tube origin.

Astrocytes

As the name implies, the astrocytes are stellate cells with many cytoplasmic processes (Figs. 10.18 and 10.19). They are often divided into two general types, *protoplasmic* and *fibrous*, which have in common their shape (which provides a large surface area), the presence of characteristic cytoplasmic filaments and glycogen, a generally loosely packed cytoplasm, and a tendency to have one or more processes terminating in the immediate vicinity of a blood vessel (*perivascular feet*). In both astrocytic types, the nucleus is irregularly ovoid and less compact than in other glial cell types.

Protoplasmic Astrocytes

These are found principally in the gray matter of the brain and spinal cord. In addition to their perivascular cellular extensions, these cells also provide flattened processes which cover much of the nonsynaptic neuronal surface, and they circumscribe synaptic zones, suggesting that they may function to separate the activities of synaptic regions from adjacent tissues (Fig. 10.13). In some areas of the brain, protoplasmic astrocytes are connected to one another by low resistance communicating (gap) junctions. There are also isolated reports of similar junctions between the membranes of neurons and astrocytes. The significance of such junctions is not obvious in terms of the present state of knowledge.

Fibrous Astrocytes

Although intergradations between typical protoplasmic and fibrous astrocytes are known, the two are relatively distinct throughout most regions of the CNS. Fibrous astrocytes differ from the protoplasmic type in having fewer processes which are much straighter and longer (Fig. 10.18). They possess many more filaments coursing in bundles through their cytoplasm (Fig. 10.20). When specially stained in light microscopic preparations, these bundles appear as straight, unbranched "astroglial fibers." Fibrous astrocytes are found chiefly in the white matter. They have been observed to be attached to each other by communicating, intermediate, and desmosomal types of junctions. Some of these properties correlate well with the epithelial origins of these cells and suggest also that a primary function is the provision of a semi-rigid, cellular, supportive framework for the CNS. Fibrous astrocyte processes are particularly numerous near the periphery (basal, or meninx-facing surfaces) of the brain and spinal cord. Here their end feet form the continuous outer perimeter of the neural tissue. As such, this *astrocytic border* (or *outer glia limitans*) abuts directly upon the basal lamina surrounding the entire CNS, including those regions (*perivascular space*) where that basal lamina courses deeply into the brain or cord to accompany blood vessels. *Hence, the astrocytic border constitutes the basal, cellular surface of the entire CNS epithelium.*

Fibrous astrocytes are the scarring cells of the nervous system, filling in gaps after tissue is lost in various disease processes. Connective tissue may also participate in CNS scarring. The result is generally a hardened mass of tissue within the normally soft brain tissue. This scarring process is termed *sclerosis* ("hardening").

Oligodendrocytes

These cells are also called oligodendroglia (from the Greek *oligos*, few, + *dendron*, tree, + *glia*, glue). They were given their name because their branches are small, delicate and few as compared with those of astrocytes. By light microscopy their nuclei are generally smaller, rounder, and denser than astrocytic nuclei—this is the chief identifying characteristic in the standard histological preparation. The entire cell body of an oligodendrocyte is smaller and

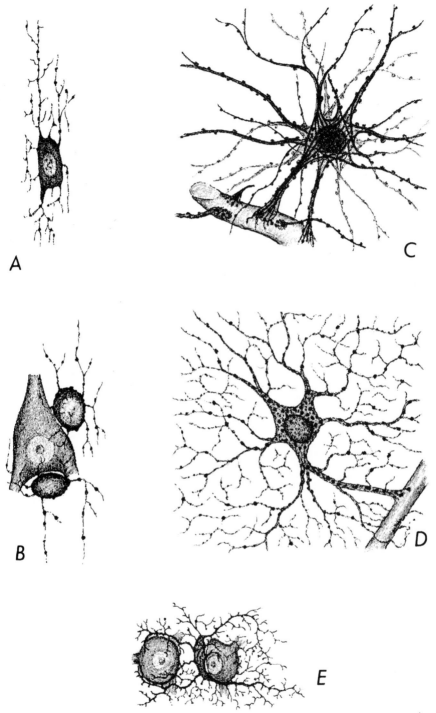

Figure 10.18. CNS neuroglial cell types as described from early, careful light microscopic observations. *A*, oligodendrocyte in white matter (interfascicular form) (see also Fig. 10.35); *B*, two oligodendrocytes lying against a nerve cell (perineuronal form); *C*, astrocyte of fibrous type with processes forming foot plates against a neighboring blood vessel. Astrocytic fibrils (bundles of filaments) are visible in the cell body and the processes. *D*, astrocyte of protoplasmic type with foot plate on blood vessel; *E*, microglial cell in vicinity of two nerve cell bodies. Redrawn from a preparation by Penfield; del Rio-Hortega's modified silver method.

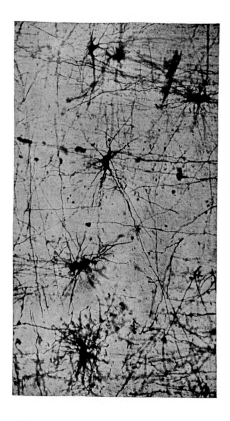

Figure 10.19. This photomicrograph shows several astrocytes in the white matter of spinal cord. The straight unbranched processes are characteristic of the fibrous astrocytes of this region. Golgi's chrome-silver method.

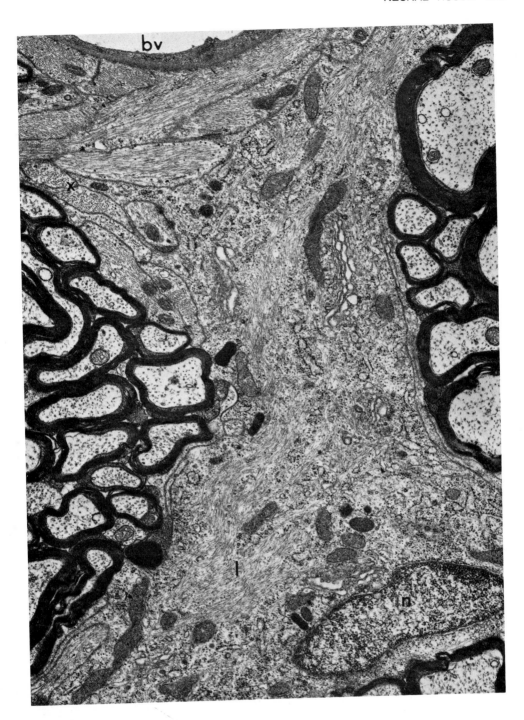

Figure 10.20. This electron micrograph from rat optic nerve shows a fibrous astrocyte interposed between myelinated axons (cut in cross section). Part of the astrocyte nucleus (*n*) is shown, as well as astroglial filaments cut in longitudinal (*l*) and in cross (*x*) section. A series of filament-filled astrocytic processes are applied to the basal lamina surrounding a blood vessel (*bv*) at the *top* of the picture. Some of these processes contain glycogen particles (×15,000). (Reprinted with permission from J. E. Vaughn and A. Peters: *J Comp Neurol* 133:269, 1968.)

its cytoplasm is denser, containing chiefly ribosomes, mitochondria and microtubules. The filaments and glycogen prominent in astrocytic cytoplasm are absent (Figs. 10.21 and 10.22).

Oligodendrocytes found in groups adjacent to blood vessels are termed *perivascular*; their function in this position is unknown. When found directly adjacent to neuron cell bodies (as in gray matter), they are termed *perineuronal* (or *gray matter satellite cells*). This close relationship suggests some type of symbiosis between glia and neuron, but efforts to identify positively what might exchange between them have not yet been successful.

When oligodendrocytes are found in white matter, they are termed *interfascicular*. Many, perhaps most, of these are directly related to myelin formation and maintenance in a manner in many ways similar to that of the peripheral Schwann cell (discussed below). The anatomical connection between the myelin supporting oligodendrocyte cell body and the myelin sheath is narrow and joins one oligodendrocyte with several myelin sheaths—a connection thought to be permanent and to provide a route through which may pass the necessary materials for the maintenance of the myelin sheath. Thus, such myelin sheaths appear to be metabolically related to the oligodendrocyte cell body in much the same way that the axon is related to the neuron cell body (Fig. 10.37).

Certain of the smaller cells in neural tissue (which may be classified as small oligodendrocytes) may be multipotential reserve or "stem" cells capable of reacting to various types of nervous system damage and providing whatever type of glial cell is needed for repair.

Microglia

This glial type has usually been described by light microscopists as a small, densely staining cell with a rounded, deeply staining nucleus. In preparations stained by special silver techniques, the cells identified as microglia have delicate and tortuous cytoplasmic processes with delicate spines (Fig. 10.18*E*). From fine structural and radioautographic tracing studies it seems likely that many of the cells identified as microglia by silver techniques are varieties of oligodendrocytes. The true microglia are generally considered to be macrophages and hence derived from *promonocytes* which have the capability to invade the neuroepithelium of the CNS. Hence these are the only CNS glial component not currently considered to be of neural tube glioblast origin (see "The Macrophage System," Chapter 5). There has been much contro-

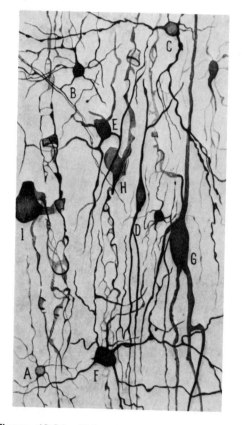

Figure 10.21. This early drawing shows the various types of oligodendrocytes found in white and gray matter. Note that the cells have few processes but that these may be very complex. The elaborate interfascicular forms of oligodendrocytes shown at *H* and *I* are depicted in more detail in Figure 10.35. (Reprinted with permission from P. del Rio-Hortega: *Mem Real Soc Espan Hist Nat* 14:5, 1928.)

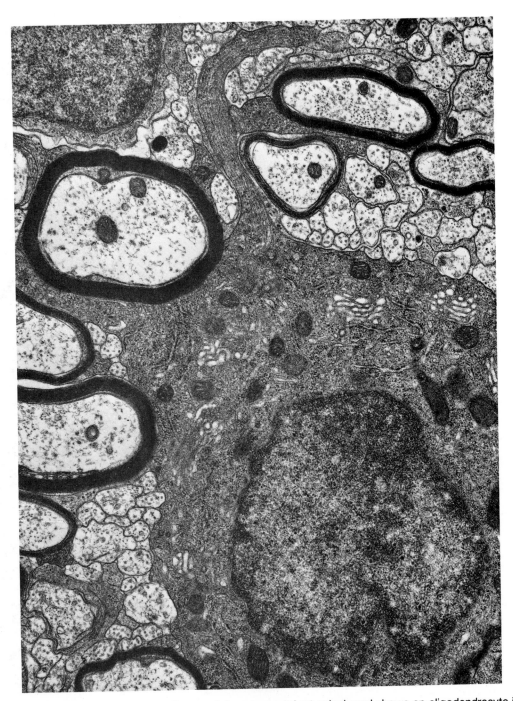

Figure 10.22. This electron micrograph from neonatal rat spinal cord shows an oligodendrocyte in apposition to both myelinated and unmyelinated axons. Oligodendrocytes present this dense appearance after aldehyde fixation. They characteristically contain many ribosomes and microtubules and lack bundles of filaments. The slender processes of this cell are related to myelin segments (as is shown schematically in Fig. 10-37) (×16,000). (Courtesy of Drs. P. L. Hinds and J. E. Vaughn.)

versy concerning the identity and origins of microglia and the question of the role of such CNS macrophage precursors. However, it seems that there are relatively few macrophages present in normal neural tissue, mononuclear precursors of macrophages circulating in the bloodstream rapidly enter the neural tissue after injury, and most of the neuroglial cells can participate to some extent in phagocytic activities required for the removal of cell debris. In cases of minimal injury astrocytes dispose of the debris, and invasion by macrophage precursors is not required.

In extensive injury, the phagocytic cells become greatly enlarged and filled with debris, so that the nucleus appears compressed or indented (Fig. 10.23). These cells are called *compound granular corpuscles* or *gitter cells*. Most are derived from cells that migrate from the bloodstream, and whether some also differentiate from glial cells remains controversial. These cells are capable of taking up impressive amounts of cellular remnants (especially myelin); laden with this material, they appear to accumulate around blood vessels, and the contained material is slowly degraded over several weeks or months.

Ependyma

The ependyma (Figs. 10.24 and 10.25) consists of closely packed cells with elongated nuclei, lining the cavities of the spinal cord and brain (central canal and ventricles). Their long axes are perpendicular to

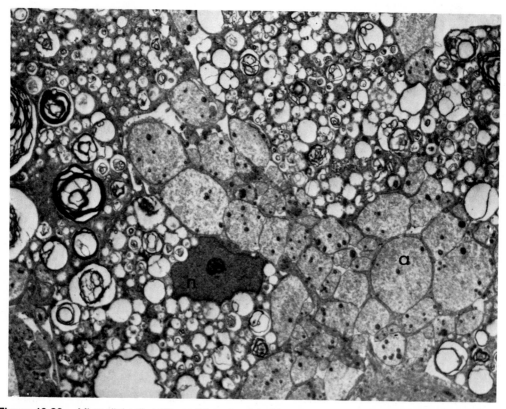

Figure 10.23. Microglial cells (gitter cells) engorged with remnants of degenerating myelin are shown in this electron micrograph from a demyelinating lesion in cat spinal cord. Cross sectioned axons which have lost their myelin sheaths occupy the *lower right* and *central* areas of the picture (e.g., *a*). The remainder of this field is filled with the cytoplasm of four microglial phagocytes. These become so engorged with debris that the nucleus of a macrophage may be indented (as in *n*) (×4500). (Reprinted with permission from R. P. Bunge, et al.: *J Biophys Biochem Cytol* 7:685, 1960.)

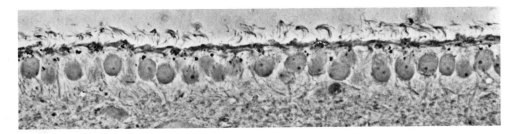

Figure 10.24.   This photomicrograph shows the row of ependymal cells lining the wall of the third ventricle of an adult rabbit brain. Bundles of cilia protrude from the ventricular surfaces of these cells. (Reprinted with permission from V. M. Tennyson and G. D. Pappas: In *Pathology of the Nervous System*, edited by J. Minckler, p. 518. New York, McGraw-Hill, 1968.)

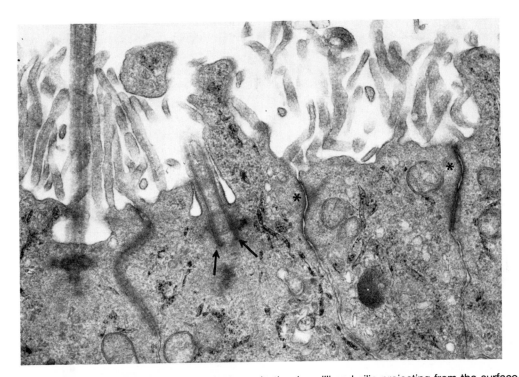

Figure 10.25.   This electron micrograph shows both microvilli and cilia projecting from the surface of ependymal cells lining the spinal cord central canal in a human fetus. The *arrows* indicate a basal body at the base of the cilium. Junctional complexes (∗) occur between lateral cell borders near the free cell surface (×23,500). (Reprinted with permission from V. Tennyson: In *Developmental Neurobiology*, edited by W. A. Himwich, p. 47. Springfield, Ill., Charles C Thomas, 1970.)

the cavity, and although they present the appearance of a columnar or cuboidal epithelium, this is a false impression. Ependymal cells are in reality derived as the most apical cells of the neural tube epithelium. In the adult, therefore, they are closely adherent cell bodies lining the apical (ventricular) surface of the CNS epithelium; the basal surface is the outer perimeter of the brain and cord. These cells have inner processes ramifying more or less deeply into the epithelial walls of the CNS and sometimes providing end feet to the outer glia limitans or to perivascular areas. Ependymal processes are not unlike those of fibrous astrocytes in their fine structure.

They may have, in certain forms and in certain places, cilia which protrude into the neural cavity (Fig. 10.25).

Peripheral Glia

As peripheral axons course among various body tissues, they are found everywhere in association with companion cells which provide various types of ensheathment. When these companion cells are in association with a nerve cell body (as in the peripheral ganglia of the autonomic or sensory system), they are called *satellite cells*; when they provide ensheathment for axons, they are called *cells of Schwann*. During development, these companion cells arise from neural crest and migrate peripherally along the outgrowing axons. They provide sheaths which everywhere enclose each axon, except at certain axon tips, as discussed below. Two basic forms of ensheathment, *myelinated* and *unmyelinated*, are provided by Schwann cells as these become arranged along the axons of a given periph-

eral nerve. Some indication of the structure of each can be gained by light microscopy of osmium-fixed nerves viewed in cross- and longitudinal section (Fig. 10.26). However, the details and modes of formation of these ensheathing patterns were only discovered with the advent of electron microscopy, and these are diagrammed in Fig. 10.27. During the initial phases of the ensheathment process a given Schwann cell embraces one or several axons in a trough formed from its plasma membrane. The axons remain outside the Schwann cell cytoplasm but are surrounded by its plasma membrane. With maturation, each axon comes to occupy its own smaller trough entirely encircled by Schwann cell membrane. The region in which the lips of the encircling Schwann cell approach each other is termed a *mesaxon* (Fig. 10.27). Each Schwann cell extends over a distance of several hundred micrometers along the axon, and the external surface of each Schwann cell becomes encased in basal

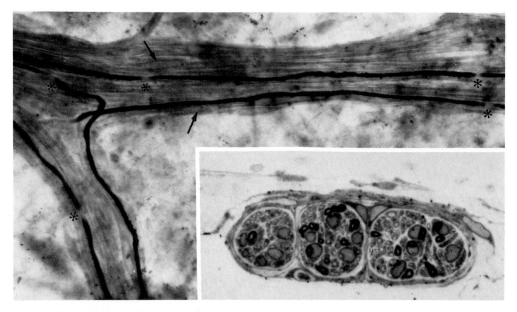

Figure 10.26.   These light micrographs show a small nerve fascicle viewed longitudinally (*above*) and in cross section (*inset*). The tissue has been fixed in OsO₄, which preserves and blackens myelin. In the *upper picture*, individual segments of myelin are delineated by nodes (∗). The remainder of the fascicle is composed of unmyelinated nerve fibers and their associated Schwann cells. Cell nuclei (*arrows*) are not stained but are visible as elliptical structures between the nerve fibers. In the cross section, a perineurial sheath is seen around each of three small nerve fascicles. Myelin sheaths, some with related Schwann cell nuclei, and individual unmyelinated fibers with Schwann cell investments are shown (×500; *inset*, ×1600).

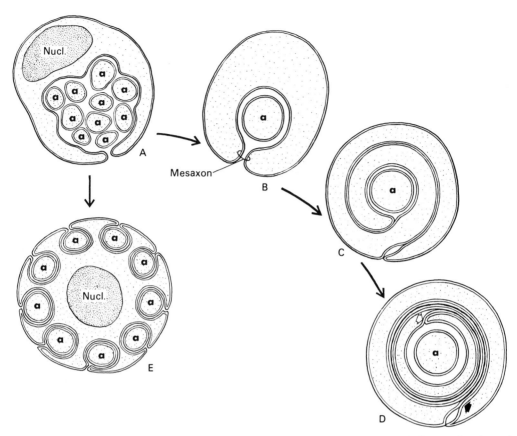

Figure 10.27. Forms of ensheathment in peripheral nerve. During development, the small embryonic nerve fibers are surrounded in groups by Schwann cells (*A*). Those fibers which will become myelinated enlarge and become ensheathed by individual Schwann cells (*B*). The encircling lips of the Schwann cell slide by one another, and the mesaxon is elongated (*C*). As the mesaxon is compacted (*D*), myelin is formed. Note that the apposition of the cytoplasmic surfaces of the plasma membrane forms the major dense line of the myelin sheath; the apposition of the external surfaces of the plasma membrane forms the intraperiod line (*D*). Axons which will not be myelinated remain small and obtain ensheathment within individual troughs in the Schwann cell (*E*). *a*, axon; *nucl.*, nucleus; inner mesaxon marked by *white arrow*; outer mesaxon marked by *black arrow*.

lamina. This basic pattern of ensheathment, with a single Schwann cell embracing from one to a dozen separate axons, is found throughout the peripheral nervous systems of both invertebrates and vertebrates. In many species, this is the most complex form of peripheral nerve ensheathment found.

Nerve fibers (axons) ensheathed in this manner are termed *unmyelinated*; they comprise the majority of the postganglionic axons from the autonomic ganglia and axons from the smaller neurons of the sensory ganglia. These unmyelinated peripheral nerve fibers are sometimes called *C fibers*

or *fibers of Remak*. They conduct nerve impulses at the rate of about 1 m/sec. In light microscopic observations of routine histological preparations, these smaller diameter unmyelinated fibers are often not directly visible, but the presence of a nerve fascicle in the tissue can be distinguished by the elongated nuclei of the ensheathing Schwann cells, as well as by the connective tissue layers, discussed below, which are external to the Schwann cell ensheathment (Fig. 10.26). Beyond obvious physical support and protection, the function of Schwann cell ensheathment of unmyelinated nerve fibers is not known, but it is known that the axolemma, and not the plasmalemma of the Schwann cell, is the membrane responsible for the propagation of the action potential.

PNS Myelination

The majority of the peripheral nerve fibers have a diameter of more than 1 μm; these fibers become ensheathed by *myelin*, which is actually the spirally disposed plasma membrane of the Schwann cell, compacted and modified chemically to provide a highly resistant but regularly interrupted sleeve of insulation around the axon. During development of the sheath, the apposing lips of a single embracing Schwann cell slide by one another, forming a spiral membrane as the original mesaxon elongates (Fig. 10.27B to D).

There is some evidence that this configuration of myelin is accomplished by the repeated circumnavigation of the axon by the outer mass of Schwann cell cytoplasm—that part containing the nucleus. This deposits a great length of spirally wrapped and specialized plasma membrane which becomes compacted together to form the lamellae of the *myelin sheath* (Fig. 10.28). As compaction occurs, the cytoplasm of the sheath is excluded and the cytoplasmic surfaces of its membranes come together. The inner or cytoplasmic leaflets of the membranes are thus fused to form a thickened *major dense* (*major period*) *line* when seen in cross section (Figs. 10.27 and 10.28). The outer surfaces of the membrane of adjacent turns of the spirals become closely apposed, but do not fuse with each other. These outer leaflet images thereby form two thinner *intraperiod lines* which are separated by a small *intraperiod space*. This space is potentially continuous with extracellular space outside the Schwann cell and periaxonal space near the axon surface (Figs. 10.27, 10.28, and 10.32). By this mechanism, one Schwann cell forms one segment or *internode* of the myelin wrapping of one axon, with the Schwann cell nucleus located external to the compacted lamellae and about midway along the myelin segment. The Schwann

cell also invests its external surface with a basal lamina as myelination proceeds toward completion. At each end of the internode, there is a gap of a few micrometers, which is called a *node of Ranvier*, beyond which the next internode of myelin will be found (Fig. 10.26). As nerves elongate during growth, the diameter of the axon is further increased and the segments of myelin are increased in length and in diameter, so that the thickest axons will eventually have the longest internodes, the thickest investments of myelin, and the greatest distance between the interrupting nodes of Ranvier.

One might suspect that a very narrow extracellular space might wind itself between the layers of myelin, thus providing a spiral path for the flux of extracellular material from outside in to reach the axon. However, freeze-fracture evidence discloses a narrow occluding junction that seals the gap at its outer margins, i.e., along outer- and innermost mesaxon and along the edges of the nodes of Ranvier (Figs. 10.29 and 10.33).

Figures 10.30 to 10.32 illustrate that myelin is an integral part of the Schwann cell and that Schwann cell cytoplasm is retained both external and internal to the compact myelin layers and in the *paranodal areas*. The amount of cytoplasm in these regions decreases with development, but substantial amounts remain in the region of the Schwann cell nucleus and near the nodes of Ranvier. The cytoplasm external to the compact myelin is visible in the light microscope and has frequently been termed the *neurilemma sheath*. Unfortunately, this term has also been used in the past to include the compact myelin sheath and various connective tissue elements external to the Schwann cell, including the basal lamina that borders all Schwann cells. It is important to distinguish between the cytoplasm of the myelin-related Schwann cell and the adjacent connective tissue.

At the node of Ranvier, the lamellae of *paranodal myelin* also appear more widely separated because Schwann cell cytoplasm has been retained. Each myelin lamella is

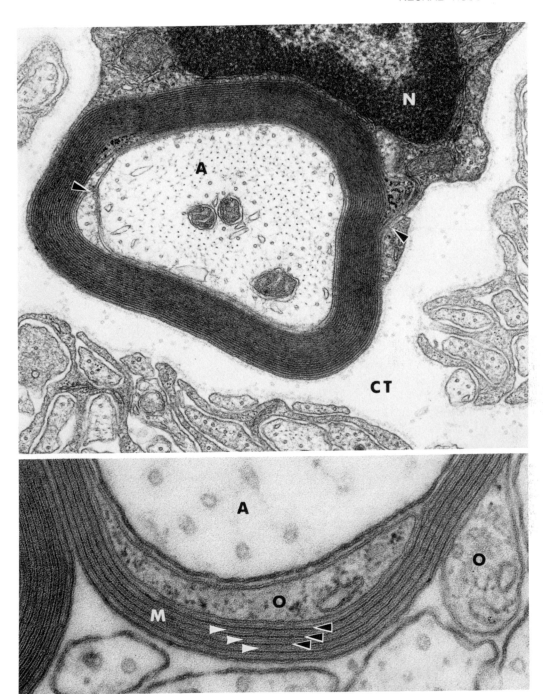

Figure 10.28. *Top*, electron micrograph showing Schwann cell-axon relationships in a tissue culture of rat dorsal root ganglion. A large axon seen in cross section (*A*) has been myelinated by a Schwann cell whose nucleus (*N*) is visible. Internal and external mesaxons are visible (*arrowheads*) as are microtubules and neurofilaments within the axon. Smaller, unmyelinated axons, occupying individual troughs along other Schwann cells are visible at *right* and *lower left*. Note that basal lamina surrounds each Schwann cell, separating them and their contained axons from endoneurial connective tissue (*CT*) (×47,000). (Courtesy of Mr. David S. Copio and Dr. Mary B. Bunge.) *Bottom*, higher magnification view of a cross sectioned CNS axon (*A*) and its thin surrounding myelin sheath (*M*). Internal and external oligodendrocyte cytoplasm is visible (*O*). *Dark arrowheads* indicate major dense lines (see Fig. 10.27), while *white arrowheads* indicate narrow spaces within intraperiod lines. Unmyelinated axons are seen at the *lower edge* of this micrograph (×120,000). (Courtesy of Dr. Michael J. Cullen.)

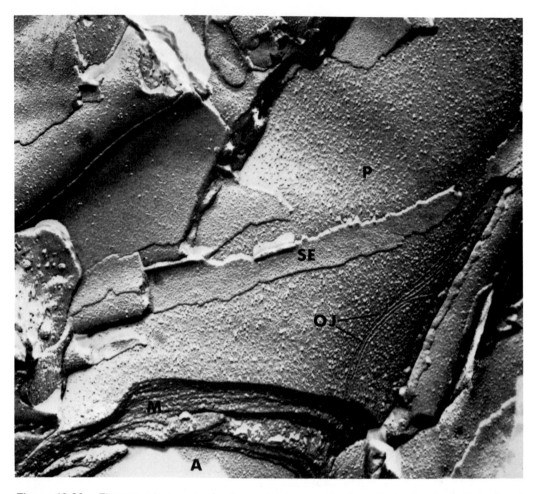

Figure 10.29.   Electron micrograph of a freeze-fracture replica from the brain of a salamander. A myelinated axon (*A*) has been exposed at the *lower edge* of the picture after its myelin investments (*M*) and much of its Schwann cell have been cleaved away. The P-face (*P*) of the outermost myelin lamella is exposed to view, as is a small slip of Schwann cell membrane E-face (*SE*). Ridges of an occluding junction (*OJ*) are seen on the myelin P-face near the area of the outer mesaxon (×60,000).

brought successively into contact with the axon, so that the outermost lamellae of myelin approach the axon nearest the node. At the node itself, loosely interdigitating Schwann cell processes partially fill the nonmyelinated interval (Figs. 10.31 and 10.32). The basal lamina surrounding one internode is directly continuous with that of the next internode, thus bridging the node of Ranvier.

Recent freeze-fracture studies of the nodal region disclose that the axonal membrane is also specialized here (Fig. 10.33). A series of circumferential indentations are apparent along the axonal membrane, and

these correspond positionally with the successive paranodal loops of the Schwann cell. Intramembranous particles of the axonal membranes are arranged in diagonal rows within the paranodal regions, but a much denser population appears randomly within the nodal region itself. These may relate to an abundance of sodium channels known from physiological studies to characterize the nodal region (discussed below).

The finer details of the myelin sheath are not visible in light microscopic preparations. However, after a fixative that preserves lipid (such as osmium tetroxide) has been used, the compacted regions of myelin

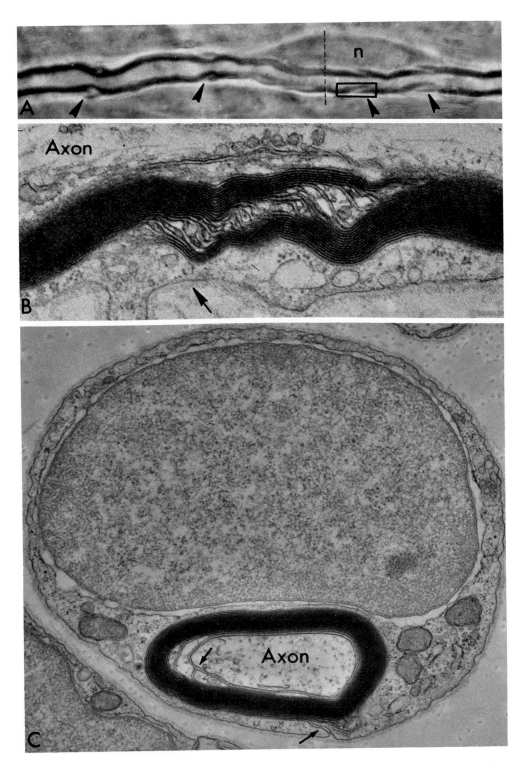

Figure 10.30. The *upper figure* (*A*) is a photomicrograph of part of a living myelin segment (in tissue culture) displaying a series of Schmidt-Lanterman clefts (*arrowheads*) and the nucleus (*n*) of the Schwann cell related to this internode. In an electron micrograph (*B*) a cleft, as in the box in *A*, is seen to be a region where the myelin lamellae are separated by cytoplasm but retain their continuity. The *arrow* in the *middle picture* indicates the basal lamina external to the Schwann cell. *C* is an electron micrograph of a myelin sheath cut in cross section at the level of the *dotted line* in *A*. The *arrows* indicate the inner and outer mesaxons, the points where the membrane spiral which forms the compact myelin begins and ends. Rat peripheral nerve. *A*, ×3,000; *B*, ×60,000; *C*, ×30,000.

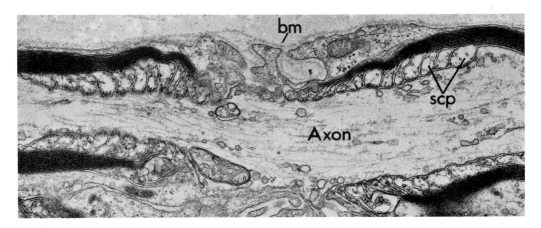

Figure 10.31. This electron micrograph shows a node of Ranvier on a small axon of a rat sensory ganglion cell. The myelin lamellae terminate in loops in which a small amount of Schwann cell cytoplasm is retained. The innermost lamellae terminate farthest from the node. *bm*, basal lamina; *scp*, Schwann cell processes (×27,500).

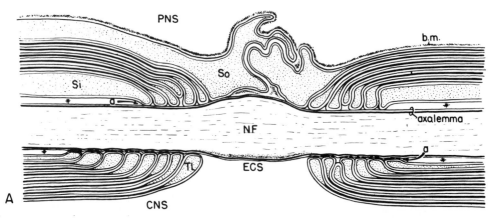

Figure 10.32. This drawing compares nodal regions from the peripheral nervous system (*PNS*), (*above*) and *CNS* (*below*). In the PNS the Schwann cell provides both an inner collar (*Si*) and an outer collar (*So*) of cytoplasm in relation to the compact myelin. The outer collar (*So*) extends into the nodal region as a series of loosely interdigitating processes. Terminating loops of the compact myelin come into close apposition to the axolemma in regions near the node, apparently providing some barrier (*arrow* at *a*) for movement of materials into or out of the periaxonal space (∗). The Schwann cell is covered externally by a basal lamina (*bm*). In the CNS the myelin ends similarly in terminal loops (*tl*) near the node, and there are periodic thickenings of the axolemma where the glial cell membrane is applied in the paranodal region. These thickenings may serve to confine material in the periaxonal space (∗) so that movement in the direction of the *arrow* at *a* would be restrained. At many CNS nodes there may be considerable extracellular space (*ECS*), but usually this region is occupied by processes of astrocytes. (Reprinted with permission from R. Bunge: *Physiol Rev* 48:197, 1970.)

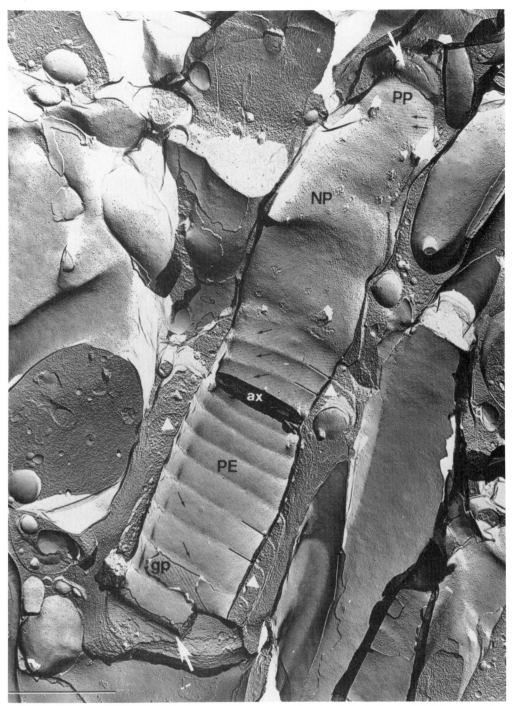

Figure 10.33. Freeze-fracture replica of CNS axons and their myelin sheaths. One axon has been cross-fractured at *ax* and its split membrane faces are exposed in nodal and paranodal regions. Compare with lower half of Figure 10.32 and Figure 10.37. Note the dense population of particles spread randomly over the P-face of the nodal region (*NP*), the diagonal arrays of particles over the paranodal P-face (*PP*), and diagonal arrays of pits over the paranodal E-face (*PE*). Similar diagonal particles are exposed along the P-face of a surrounding oligodendrocyte (*gp*). Cross-fractured paranodal oligodendrocyte membrane loops are seen to either side of the axonal E-face. These lie in register with circumferential furrowing of the axonal surface (*small arrows*). *Large white arrows* point to segments of tight junctions within the myelin lamellae (×29,000). (Reprinted with permission from B. J. Schnapp and E. Mugnaini: Membrane architecture in myelinated nerve fibers. In *Physiology and Pathobiology of Axons*, edited by S. G. Waxman, p. 104. New York, Raven Press, 1978.)

are visualized as a sleeve around the axon. In preparations involving the use of lipid solvents, much of the myelin sheath is dissolved, leaving a residue called "*neurokeratin.*" In silver-stained preparations, the axon appears in cross sections as a central density apparently surrounded by a space because the myelin has been largely extracted. These points are illustrated in Figure 10.34. If not injured, the myelin-Schwann cell unit, like the neuron, is thought to be maintained for the lifetime of the individual. As it ages, myelin develops distortions and redundancies in its basic tubular form. Oblique, funnel-shaped clefts, called *Schmidt-Lanterman* clefts are present along all myelin sheaths, but they may become more common with age and they too interrupt the smooth contour of the internode. These clefts have been observed in the living myelin sheath, and electron microscopic examination has established that they are focal areas along successive layers of myelin where there is incomplete membrane compaction and Schwann cell cytoplasm is retained (Fig. 10.30). Three-dimensionally, each such cleft is a spiral tube of cytoplasm connecting the cytoplasm at the Schwann cell periphery with the small cytoplasmic remnant of the innermost lamella.

Myelin contains about 80% lipid, including cholesterol, phospholipids, glycolipids, and plasmalogens, and about 20% protein, including some proteolipids. The high lipid content gives myelin a whitish appearance in the fresh state. This explains the whiteness of peripheral nerves (e.g., the *white rami* of the autonomic nerves, as compared with the *gray rami* that contain primarily unmyelinated fibers), as well as the distinction between *white* and *gray matter* of the CNS.

The myelinated axon is the superhighway of the nervous system, the periodic interruptions at the nodes of Ranvier providing "limited access" to current flow which allows myelin ensheathment to speed greatly the process of impulse conduction. In the typical myelinated nerve fiber, the action potential is first generated in the initial segment of the axon (Fig. 10.2). This current flows through the axon to depolarize and "fire" the first node of Ranvier. The action potential thus generated forces a pulse of current into the axon interior. Because of the high resistance and low capacitance of the surrounding myelin, the current remains confined to the axon and flows forward, not radially, until the next node is reached. Thus, myelination of an axon functions to force ionic currents to flow great distances before regeneration of the action potential. Both physiological and morphological evidence now suggests that the axonal plasmalemma is far richer in *sodium channels* in the nodal region. Specific proteins termed *ionophores* are accumulated and maintained in the membrane at each node, each such molecule providing an ion pump or pore for ionic influx or outflux associated with excitation of the axonal membrane of each successive node. This leaping of current from node to node has acquired the designation *saltatory conduction*. This process is not only faster than the sequential depolarization of unmyelinated fibers but also more economical of ionic interchange between the inside and outside of the fiber.

Myelinated fibers vary considerably in size, from large (10 to 20 μm in overall diameter) to medium (4 to 10 μm) to small (2 to 4 μm) (Fig. 10.34). In physiological classification, the large and medium fibers are type A, the small myelinated fibers are type B, and unmyelinated fibers are type C. The largest diameter fibers have the longest myelin segments (between 1 and 2 mm); they thus have the greatest spacing between nodes and hence the fastest nerve conduction rates (up to 140 m/sec).

CNS Myelination

The *oligodendrocyte* (a neural tube glioblast derivative) is the cell which is responsible for myelination of axons within the CNS. However, its pattern of myelination is different from that performed by PNS Schwann cells in several important respects. First, there is little cytoplasm associated with the mature CNS myelin sheath.

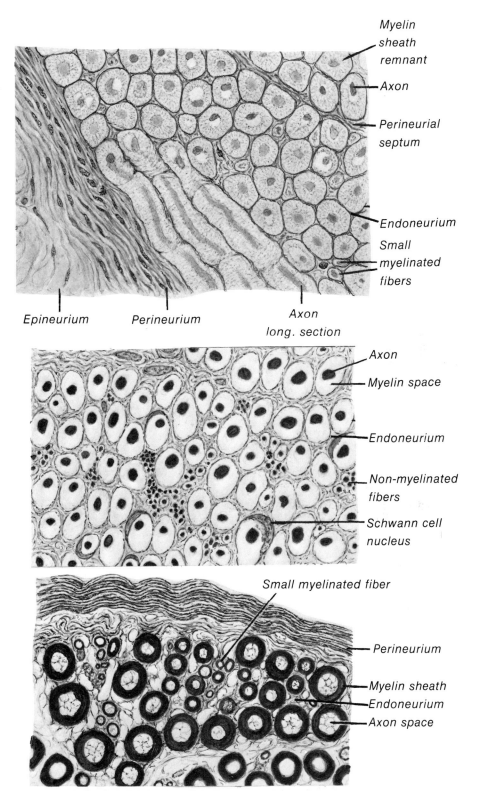

Figure 10.34. These drawings illustrate cross sections of peripheral nerve after standard histological preparation and hematoxylin and eosin staining (*top*), after silver staining to show the axons (*middle*), and after fixation with OsO₄ to preserve the myelin sheaths (*bottom*). The spoke-like remnants of myelin seen in H & E preparations are called neurokeratin.

Second, the oligodendrocyte cell body is not as directly apposed to CNS myelin segments as is the Schwann cell to PNS myelin. Third, each oligodendrocyte may be related, at least during development, to more than one axon and to more than one segment of forming myelin (Figs. 10.35 to 10.37). In addition, there is not basal lamina associated with myelin sheaths in the CNS. This is expected because the CNS is an epithelium and basal lamina material is deposited only outside epithelia. Whereas the basic pattern of myelin deposition is the same, the relation of the oligodendrocyte to more than one axon makes it difficult to think that the myelin membrane spiral can be formed by oligodendrocyte circumnavigation around the axon; the actual mechanism of CNS myelin deposition is unknown.

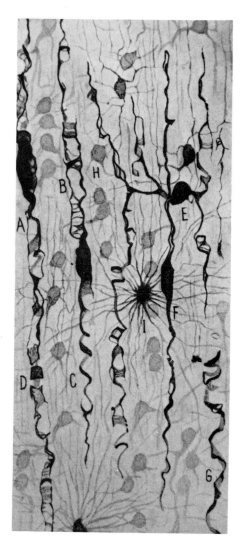

Figure 10.36. An early diagram derived from a special silver impregnation which demonstrates some oligodendrocytes in white matter of cat central nervous tissue. The densely impregnated cells labeled *AD*, *BC*, *E*, *F*, and *G* display multiple processes leading to underlying myelin sheaths, which are not stained in this preparation. Other, unimpregnated oligodendrocytes are labeled *H*, and an astrocyte appears at *I*. (Reprinted with permission from P. del Rio-Hortega: *Mem Real Soc Espan Hist Nat* 14:5, 1928.

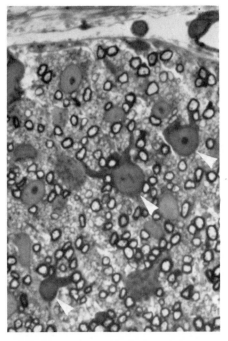

Figure 10.35. Photomicrograph of 5-day old kitten spinal cord with the surface of the cord above. Darkly stained myelin sheaths in varying stages of formation have been cut in cross section. Three myelin-related cells (*white arrowheads*) each display two processes which appear to extend to at least two different myelinated axons. A 1-μm section of OsO_4-fixed material embedded in plastic and stained with toluidine blue (×1200).

The very small amount of cytoplasm external to the CNS myelin sheath has led to the frequent statement that there is no neurilemma cell in the CNS. There is, in fact, some cytoplasm related to CNS myelin both internally and externally and at the

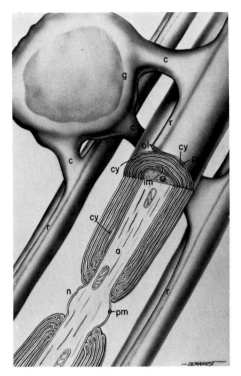

Figure 10.37. This diagram illustrates the relationship of the oligodendrocyte to the central myelin sheath. The trilaminar plasma membrane (*pm*) is here designated as two lines separated by a space, except in the mitochondrion, where it is represented by a single line. The inner mesaxon (*im*), formed as a glial process completes the initial turn around an axon (*a*) and starts a second, is retained after myelin formation is completed. Some cytoplasm of the glial process is present here. Cytoplasm is trapped occasionally at *cy*. On the fully formed sheath exterior, a bit of glial cytoplasm is also retained. In transverse sections, this cytoplasm is confined to a loop (*ol*), but along the internode length, it forms a ridge (*r*) which is continuous with a glial cell body (*g*) at *c*. When viewed transversely, the sheath components are oriented in a spiral, only the innermost and outermost layers ending in loops; in the longitudinal plane, every myelin unit terminates in a separate loop near a node (*n*). Within these loops glial cytoplasm is also retained. (Reprinted with permission from M. Bunge, et al.: *J Biophys Biochem Cytol* 10:67, 1961.)

nodes of Ranvier (Figs. 10.32 and 10.37), but it is too scant to be seen in the light microscope. Myelinated CNS axons also have no connective tissue coats, as do peripheral nerves.

The integrity of myelin depends upon both the axon (as discussed below) and the myelin-supporting cell—the Schwann cell or the oligodendrocyte. If the myelin-supporting cell is damaged, as in certain demyelinating diseases, the myelin will break down even though the axon is preserved. If the axon is preserved, remyelination sometimes occurs in both central and peripheral nervous tissue.

THE PERIPHERAL NERVES

Axons, coursing from neuronal cell bodies to their terminations in some peripheral structure or in the CNS, are grouped together in bundles to form the peripheral nerves. The axons connected with the spinal cord form the *spinal nerves* and those connected with the brain comprise the *cranial nerves*.

When the spinal cord is viewed grossly, it is readily observed that the rootlets of a peripheral nerve are associated with both its dorsal and its ventral regions. The *dorsal root* is distinguished from the *ventral* by an enlargement, the *dorsal root ganglion*, containing nerve cell bodies. The dorsal root contains the sensory or afferent nerve fibers from both somatic and visceral structures; the ventral root contains the motor or efferent fibers to somatic muscles and fibers to the visceral effectors. These are smooth muscle (as in the wall of the gut), cardiac muscle, and glands. The dorsal and ventral roots join together to form the spinal nerves; the spinal nerve is thus a mixed nerve of both sensory and motor fibers. Some of the sensory fibers are myelinated, whereas others are not; the same applies to motor fibers. For this reason, it is generally not possible in the standard histological preparation to distinguish afferent from efferent fibers or visceral from somatic fibers.

Of the cranial nerves, some are purely efferent, others are purely afferent, and still others contain both efferent and afferent fibers. The same fundamental relations hold for the cranial nerves as for the spinal nerves. The afferent fibers arise from cell bodies in ganglia outside the CNS and the efferent fibers arise either from neuron bodies lying within the brain or from cells in autonomic ganglia. The optic "nerve" and parts of certain other cranial nerves form exceptions to this statement. The *optic nerve* actually is a fiber tract connecting the retina—an outlying evaginated part of the neural tube—with the brain.

Epineurium

In all peripheral nerves, the delicate nerve fibers, both myelinated and unmyelinated, are strengthened and protected by substantial connective tissue investments (Figs. 10.34 and 10.38). In histological sections, the connective tissue sleeves in which the nerve fibers course are often the most conspicuous elements. Enclosing the entire nerve is a thick sheath of connective tissue, the *epineurium.* It is composed of irregularly arranged collagenous and elastic fibers, together with fibroblasts and macrophages. When the nerve fibers are arranged in several distinct fascicles, as is often the case, these bundles are separated by extensions of the epineurium.

Perineurium

Inside the heavy epineurial layer is a more delicate sleeve of connective tissue, the *perineurium.* Recent studies indicate that flattened cells on the inner aspect of this layer form continuous epithelioid sheets, neighboring cells being joined by well developed occluding junctions. The perineurium may be several such layers thick, each layer surrounded by basal lamina material. As such, the perineurium provides an effective barrier to the penetration of material into or out of the nerve (Fig. 10.39). Thus, when marker proteins are applied to the nerve externally, they are excluded from the inner regions not by the heavy and coarse connective tissue of the epineurium but by the occluding junctions of the continuous cellular sleeves of the inner part of the perineurium.

Endoneurium

Inside the perineurium are the scattered cells (fibroblasts and macrophages) and the

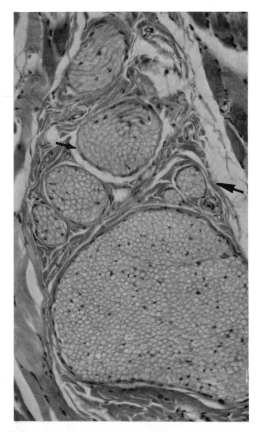

Figure 10.38. This photomicrograph shows seven peripheral nerve fascicles of varying sizes within the muscles of the tongue. At places, the encasing epineurium (*large arrow*) is separated from the underlying perineurium (*small arrow*). The nuclei of Schwann cells and endoneurial cells are visible as darkly stained elements within the fascicles. Individual axons and their myelin sheaths are visible, although preparation extraction gives each sheath a light, ring-like profile surrounding a darker central spot of cross sectioned axon. Hematoxylin and eosin, ×130.

delicate connective tissue fibers of the *endoneurium.* A basal lamina surrounding the Schwann cells separates the latter from the surrounding endoneurial connective tissue (Figs. 10.28 and 10.39). Hence, it can be seen that the relatively loose, fluid connective tissue of the endoneurium constitutes a connective tissue well isolated from the general connective tissues of the body, except at the distal tips of nerves. This *endoneurial space* is of potential importance in the metabolism and conductance of its

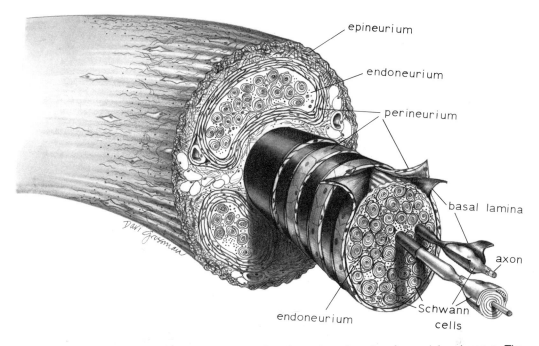

Figure 10.39. Diagram illustrating the connective tissue investments of a peripheral nerve. The perineurium is composed of a variable number of epithelial cell layers which collectively enclose an endoneurial space. Note also the position of basal laminae in relation to Schwann cells and perineurium.

contained axons and may present a pathway for viral or bacterial infection. Further aspects of this compartmentalization are discussed in relation to the meninges.

THE GANGLIA

Cranial and Spinal Ganglia

The cranial and spinal ganglia consist of aggregates of afferent neuron cell bodies situated along the sensory roots of their respective nerves. Each ganglion is surrounded by a connective tissue capsule which is continuous with the epineurium and perineurium of the peripheral nerve. Connective tissue trabeculae extend from the capsule into the ganglion, and the neurons are separated into irregular groups by strands of connective tissue and by bundles of nerve fibers (Figs. 10.40 and 10.41).

Each ganglion cell is invested with both cellular and fibrous connective tissue elements. The inner aspect of this investment consists of flattened cells closely applied to the plasma membrane of the neuron. These

cells are the *satellite cells*; they form a mosaic which completely envelops the neuronal cell body. These cells are akin to the Schwann cells of the nerve fibers; both are peripheral glial cells and both are derived from neural crest tissue. Satellite cells have been reported to myelinate sensory ganglion neuron cell bodies in the guinea pig, further attesting to their similarity to Schwann cells. As with Schwann cells, the outer aspect of the satellite cell investment is made up of a basal lamina reinforced externally by connective tissue fibers intermingled with flattened fibroblasts (sometimes called *capsule cells*; Fig. 10.42). The connective tissue elements outside the satellite cell basal lamina are continuous with the endoneurium of the contiguous nerve fibers.

The nerve cells of cranial and spinal ganglia are unipolar neurons whose cell bodies vary in size from 15 to 100 μm. The smaller neurons, which give rise to unmyelinated fibers, contain closely packed Nissl substance, giving these cells a dark appearance

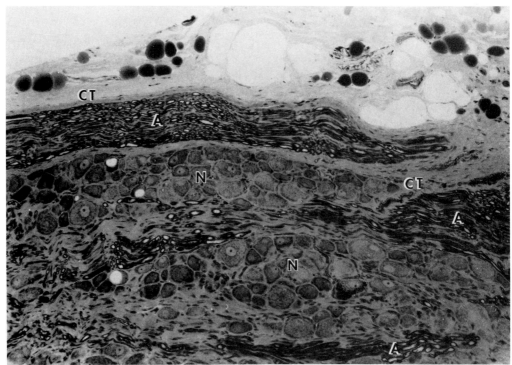

Figure 10.40. Light micrograph showing a longitudinal section through a plastic-embedded spinal ganglion. Large groups of neuron cell bodies (*N*) are visible as well as darkly stained fascicles of axons (*A*) (mostly myelinated) coursing through the ganglion. Connective tissue (*CT*) investments (epi- and perineurial) appear gray in this photomicrograph (×133).

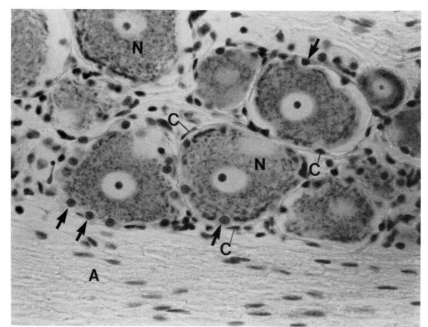

Figure 10.41. Neuron cell bodies (*N*) and nearby axonal fascicles (*A*) within a paraffin-embedded Nissl-stained spinal ganglion. Pale areas within ganglion cell cytoplasm denotes axon hillocks. Myelin has largely been extracted from the fascicles. Satellite cells (*arrows*) are distinct, closely applied to the neuron cell bodies. "Capsule" fibroblasts (*C*) are also visible. Nuclei of Schwann cells within the fascicles appear flattened (×500).

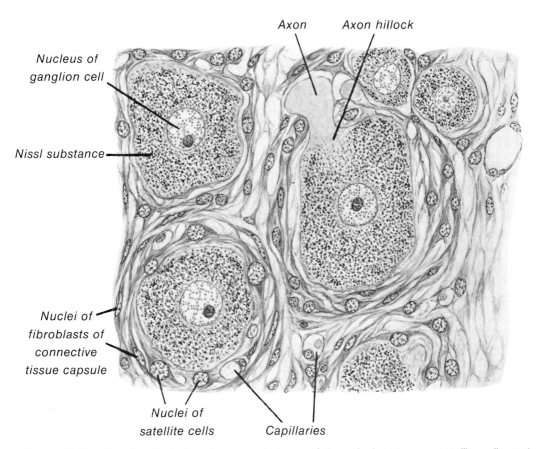

Figure 10.42. Drawing illustrating the major features of the unipolar neurons, satellite cells, and "capsule" fibroblasts from a cranial ganglion. Compare with Figure 10.41. Gasserian ganglion stained by the Nissl method. Human, 19 years of age (×835).

in conventional stains. The large neurons, on the other hand, have Nissl substance separated into groups by microtubules and neurofilaments which course through the cell body and extend into the axonal process. This gives these cells a lighter appearance (Figs. 10.40 and 10.41).

The ganglion cells have one principal myelinated process, which at some distance from the cell body, divides into a peripheral branch which courses in the peripheral nerve and a central branch which enters the CNS. The course of the axon in the neighborhood of the cell body varies for different neurons. In some cases, the axon is coiled and looped around the cell body to form an intracapsular "*glomerulus*"; in other cases, it follows a relatively straight course from its cell body to the point where it divides. The majority of the large gan-

glion cells have axons of the "glomerular" type, whereas most of the small, darkly staining cells have the uncoiled type. *These cell bodies do not receive synapses*; the sensory ganglion is *not* an integrative center.

The Autonomic (Sympathetic and Parasympathetic) Ganglia

The majority of the autonomic ganglia resemble the cranial and spinal ganglia in having a similar connective tissue capsule and framework. *Unlike sensory ganglia, these ganglia contain synapses*, for they are the way stations where certain of the first neurons of the two-neuron efferent system form a synapse with the second neuron of the visceral motor pathway (Fig. 10.12).

The neurons are multipolar cells with numerous branched dendrites and a single axon which forms the unmyelinated postganglionic visceral efferent fiber. The cell bodies vary in size from 15 to 60 μm. The nucleus is relatively large and pale, round or oval in shape, and often eccentrically placed. Binucleate cells are not uncommon. The Nissl substance may be distributed uniformly throughout the cytoplasm or may be confined either to the perinuclear zone or to the peripheral cytoplasm. Lipofuscin granules are somewhat more frequent here than in corresponding sensory ganglia. In the larger ganglia, each cell is surrounded by a layer of satellite cells, as in the spinal ganglia (Fig. 10.43). Often, two ganglion cells may share a single satellite cell-connective tissue investment.

Located in a confusing array throughout these ganglia are frequent axosomatic and axodendritic synapses. The preganglionic elements contain numerous round, clear vesicles, as would be expected in a synapse known to be cholinergic (see above). It has been demonstrated that there are small, densely staining *interneurons* in certain sympathetic ganglia which apparently allow some integrative activity within the ganglion itself.

It will be recalled from the discussion in Chapter 9 that the synaptic contact between the first and second neuron (*pre-* and *postsynaptic neurons*) of the parasympathetic system is frequently not in a discrete ganglion but directly in the wall of the organ innervated (heart, gut, bladder, etc.; see Fig. 10.44). Here presynaptic fibers make contact with neurons in isolated groups. The postsynaptic neurons often have no definitive dendrites. The synapse frequently occurs on the cell body of the second neuron; it is the activity of the axons of this postsynaptic neuron, then, that results in neurotransmitter release in relation to the smooth muscle or glands of the visceral structures of the body.

DEGENERATION AND REGENERATION OF NERVE FIBERS

The individuality of the neuron and the interdependence of its parts are strikingly exemplified by its behavior when injured.

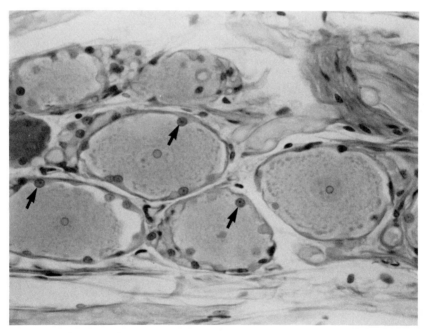

Figure 10.43. Photomicrograph showing neuron cell bodies in a sympathetic ganglion. Satellite cells (*arrows*) are less numerous compared to those of sensory ganglia (compare to Fig. 10.41), but they form a nearly continuous shroud over the perikaryon surface. Nissl substance is not stained; dense material in the perikarya is lipofuscin pigment which is common in autonomic ganglia (×500).

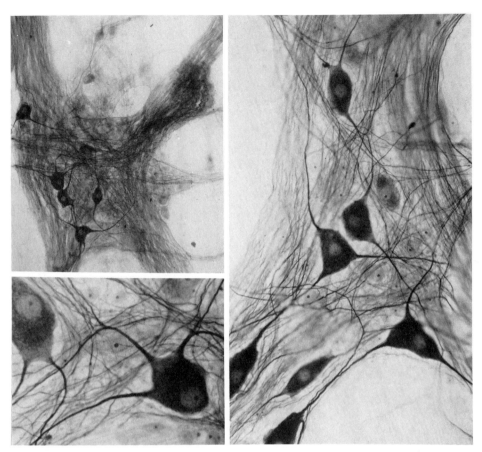

Figure 10.44. Three light micrographs of the fibers and postganglionic neuron cell bodies of the myenteric plexus. Muscle layers of the gut wall were separated to reveal the plexus. Together with the outer muscle layer, the plexus was then whole-mounted and impregnated with silver to reveal neuronal components. Pre- and postganglionic axons course in a rich network within which the neuron cell bodies are interspersed ×100, 260, and 400. (Preparation by Dr. Keith Richardson.)

When a nerve trunk is transected, certain changes taken place for a short distance on either side of the cut. These are degenerative changes of a traumatic nature, involving necrosis of the injured parts. On the proximal side of the injury (toward the cell body), degenerative changes may extend the distance of a few internodes, but very soon regenerative processes are initiated, leading to a new growth from the end of this central stump.

Distal to this site of injury, however, the degenerative changes are progressive and in time lead to the complete breakdown and disappearance of this portion of the nerve fibers, including their terminal arborizations. This process is known as *secondary* or *Wallerian degeneration*. This means that an axon cut off from its cell of origin degenerates and disappears; this behavior of the axon accords with the fact that the cell body is the trophic center of the neuron.

The first changes seen in the distal portion of the cut nerve occur in the axons themselves. They lose their uniform contour and swell intermittently, and the nerve fiber takes on a beaded appearance. Within 3 to 5 days after section of a peripheral nerve, the axons break up into irregular, twisted segments which finally undergo complete disintegration. In the CNS, this axon breakdown is often very much slower, and special stains (e.g., the Nauta stain) which selectively delineate the degenerating axons and their terminals are useful in tracing fiber pathways.

Coincident with these changes in the axon are degenerative changes in the myelin sheath. During the first few days, there is a fragmentation of the myelin, so that it becomes broken into spherical, oval, or elongated segments which surround the fragments of the axon (Fig. 10.45). In the succeeding days, these myelin fragments undergo further breakdown within Schwann cells or invading macrophages. The myelin fragments become smaller and smaller until finally they disappear. The chemical changes taking place as the myelin is digested are the basis of the selectivity of the Marchi stain for degenerating myelin. This stain allows degenerating

tracts (which contain myelin) to be identified, and it is a useful adjunct to the axonal stains mentioned above.

In peripheral nerve tissue, the degeneration of the axon and myelin sheath occurs within the confines of the connective tissue framework. The endoneurial elements which originally surrounded the axon-Schwann cell unit form a tubular envelope within which the reacting Schwann cells are confined (Fig. 10.45). While the breakdown and digestion of axon and myelin are progressing, certain Schwann cells enlarge and undergo mitosis. Confined by the sleeve of connective tissue mentioned above, these cells accumulate in tubular or bandlike arrays ("*band fibers*" or "*protoplasmic bands*") along the length of the

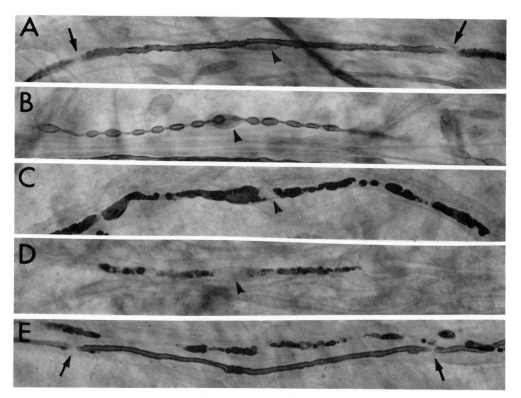

Figure 10.45. *A*, normal short myelin segment delineated by two nodes of Ranvier (*arrows*) and showing the myelin-related Schwann cell nucleus (*arrowhead*). Myelin segments are shown breaking down several hours after the axon has been cut (*B*), several days later (*C*), and about 1 week later (*D*). In each case the Schwann cell involved in disposal of the myelin remnants is marked by an *arrowhead*. *E* is a small nerve fascicle containing one normal myelinated nerve fiber and remnants of a myelinated axon severed about 1 week earlier. If larger amounts of myelin must be digested, macrophages invade the tissue and assist the Schwann cells. Cultured rat sensory ganglia fixed in OsO_4 and stained with Sudan black (×520).

nerve. This tubular framework is very important in supplying pathways for regenerating axons as they grow out of the proximal and into the distal stump of the damaged nerve.

The extensive degenerative processes in the proximal and peripheral stump are not the only changes which follow nerve section. Degenerative changes also occur in the neuron body itself. An apparent *chromatolysis* may be observed as early as the first day after nerve section and is marked at about two weeks. The cytological changes that characterize chromatolysis have been discussed above. It should be noted that this response to axon section is another useful tool in identifying neurons with damaged axons. Thus, if a neuron is observed in chromatolysis after a particular neurological lesion, it is presumed that this neuron supported an axon which coursed through the lesion area.

Regrowth from severed axons is generally considered to be vigorous in the autonomic nervous system and active in the somatic PNS but minimal and generally ineffective in the CNS. If the neuron cell body which supports nerve fibers within the PNS survives, regeneration can be expected in time. The axons of the proximal stump of the severed nerve form bulbous enlargements and axonal sprouts within a few days (Figs. 10.46 and 10.47). Usually it takes about two weeks for the axonal sprouts to cross the scar to enter the endoneurial tubes of the distal stump of the severed nerve. The growing tip of the axonal sprout advances more rapidly after it has entered the endoneurial tube. Axonal growth across the scar is facilitated by bridges formed chiefly by proliferation and migration of the Schwann cells and fibroblasts. The axonal sprouts are unable to cross the gap when it is too long or filled with dense collagenous fibers.

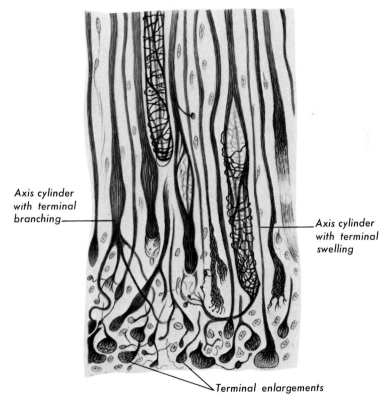

Axis cylinder with terminal branching

Axis cylinder with terminal swelling

Terminal enlargements

Figure 10.46. Diagram taken from an early description of axonal regeneration. Various patterns of axonal regenerative response are shown at the stump of a severed sciatic nerve of a cat 2½ days after section of the nerve. (Redrawn from Ramon y Cajal.)

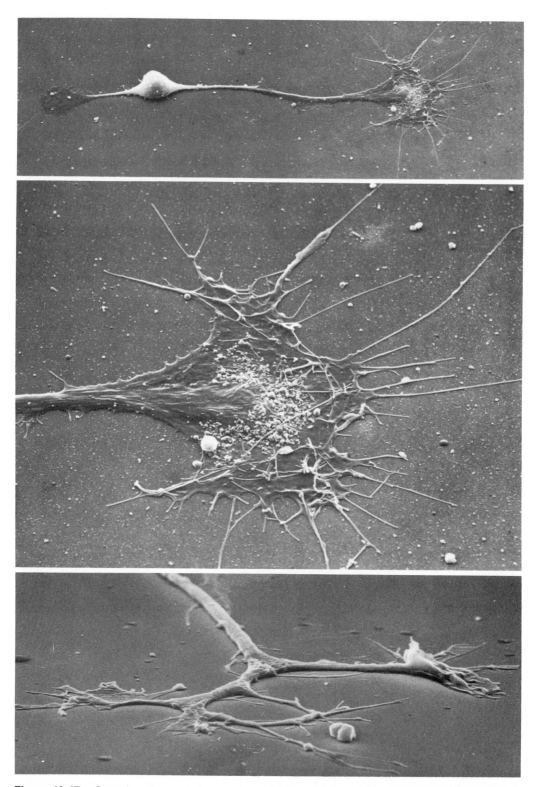

Figure 10.47. Scanning electron micrographs of neurons isolated from an 8-day-old chick embryo and grown in culture. In the *upper* figure, a parasympathetic neuron from the ciliary ganglion displays its cell body toward *left center* and a growth cone at the tip of its axon toward the *right*. The growth

Nerve transplants are made in order to facilitate the growth of axonal sprouts across gaps of any appreciable size (e.g., after gunshot wounds); the transplanted nerve provides the important guiding connective tissue framework and thus may be effective even though it contains no viable cells.

Each sprout from the proximal end of a severed nerve usually splits into a number of branches, sometimes as many as 50. This increases the chance of appropriate connections. A number of branches may enter a single Schwann tube. Some of these branches enlarge; others degenerate. In fibers which will become myelinated, generally only one axon is left per tube.

When only a fraction of the nerve fibers of a peripheral nerve are cut, the remarkable process of *collateral sprouting* appears. If 75 of 100 nerve fibers innervating a region are cut, the 25 remaining fibers sprout numerous collateral branches (at the point of the node of Ranvier in myelinated fibers), and these appear to take up the positions of the 75 lost fibers. This is often partially successful, and the 25 remaining fibers then have expanded regions of nervous influence. In practical terms, this means that the number of muscle fibers supplied by each motor nerve fiber is increased, or that the field of sensation served by a sensory neuron is enlarged. This type of regeneration is common after motor neuron loss in poliomyelitis and helps to explain the partial recovery of motor function that occurs.

In the CNS of mammals, where Schwann cells are lacking and no band fibers are formed, regeneration does not occur as readily as in the peripheral nervous system.

Recent studies have shown, however, that axons bridge the gap between the cut ends of a transected spinal cord in mammals when special efforts are made to prevent connective tissue from growing into the gap. Even under the best conditions, however, effective regeneration accompanied by functional recovery does not occur.

NERVE TERMINATIONS

The axons of peripheral nerves terminate in peripheral structures to which or from which they convey nerve impulses. The *efferent* fibers terminate in tissues in which they excite activity by releasing a neurotransmitter. In the somatic effectors (skeletal muscle), the transmitter released is *acetylcholine*. By reacting with special sites on the muscle membrane, acetylcholine causes the generation of an action potential in the muscle fiber, with subsequent muscle contraction. In many of the visceral effectors, at least two different transmitters are involved: acetylcholine released by the parasympathetic nerve terminals and *norepinephrine* released by sympathetic endings. It should be recalled that in the former case the endings contain small, round, clear vesicles; in the latter case they contain dense-cored vesicles of slightly larger size. The dual autonomic innervation provides for shifts in organ activity; parasympathetic nerves stimulate digestive action in the intestine after eating, whereas sympathetic nerves inhibit intestinal activity during exercise.

In the case of afferent fibers, on the other hand, the receptor portions are located throughout the body, where nerve fibers end freely in the tissues or in specially

cone is shown at higher magnification in the *center* figure. It displays many active microvillus-like microspikes which move about over the free surface of the growth cone, appearing and disappearing as the axonal process is extended. This type of growth cone may move over a substratum at a rate of 50 to 150 μm/hr. The growth cone contains smooth endoplasmic reticulum, but no ribosomes or other granules. Cytoplasmic particles do appear in culture to move up and down the axon to and from the growth cone, presumably reflecting active axonal flow patterns. In the *lower* figure, a growth cone on the axon from a dorsal root ganglion neuron has split during its extension to form two subsidiary growth cones (*right* and *left center*). Upper figure, ×850; center figure, ×2850; lower figure ×4400. (Courtesy of Dr. Norman Wessells.)

organized structures. In either case, they received stimuli which cause them to convey nerve impulses to the CNS.

Terminations of Somatic Efferent Fibers

The cell bodies of these axons lie in the ventral gray matter of the spinal cord or in the motor nuclei of cranial nerves in the brain. The axons are myelinated and form part of the ventral roots and efferent fibers of the peripheral nerves, terminating in the skeletal muscles of the body and head. The nerve fibers enter the *perimysium*, in which they may bifurcate several times, thus permitting one neuron to innervate more than one muscle fiber. A motor neuron and the muscle fibers innervated by it constitute a *motor unit*. The finer muscles that are concerned with precise movement have an abundent nerve supply. For example, muscles which move the eyeball often have a 1:1 ratio of neuron to muscle fiber, whereas the motor units of many regions may include as many as 1600 muscle fibers.

After repeated branchings in the perimysium, the fibers pass to the individual muscle fibers, where they terminate in structures known as *motor end plates* (Fig. 10.48). At the end plate region, the myelin is lost and the endoneurium becomes continuous with a layer of reticular fibers over the sarcolemma. The fiber terminates in a series of bulbous expansions, and in these regions the Schwann cell covering (which has replaced the myelin as an axon sheath) is withdrawn from between the nerve and muscle fiber (Fig. 10.49). At the regions of termination, the nerve indents the plasma membrane of the muscle fiber, forming a "*synaptic gutter.*" Within the nerve terminal are a multitude of small, round, clear vesicles about 45 nm in diameter, and an abundance of mitochondria. Details of this junction, which has many similarities to the synapses of the CNS, are diagrammed in Figures 10.50 and 10.51. It has been suggested that the general configuration of nerve endings on "fast" muscle fibers differs from that of endings on "slow" fibers and that the "tropic" characteristics of the nerve terminal determine whether the muscle fiber contacted is of the slow or fast type.

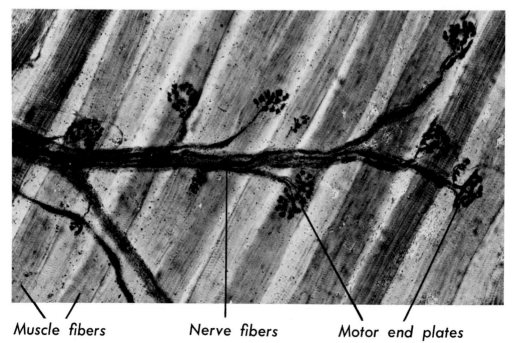

Muscle fibers   *Nerve fibers*   *Motor end plates*

Figure 10.48. Photomicrograph of motor nerve ending in intercostal muscle. Gold chloride method (×315).

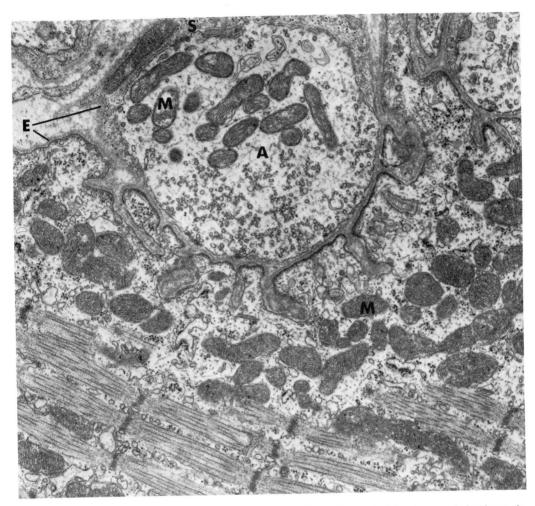

Figure 10.49. Electron micrograph showing a portion of a motor end plate along a skeletal muscle fiber in the extraocular muscle of a mammal. An axonal terminal (*A*) is seen in cross section situated in an indentation of the surface of the muscle cell. A small portion of the terminus of its Schwann cell (*S*) is visible at the *upper edge* of the micrograph. The axonal terminal displays numerous vesicles similar to those seen in other cholinergic synaptic endings. Both the axonal terminal and the nearby muscle cell cytoplasm are richly endowed with mitochondria (*M*). Note that the external (or basal) lamina (*E*) of both the Schwann cell and the muscle cell course into the indentation occupied by the axonal terminal. Several folds are seen along the muscle cell surface within the indentation. These also contain external lamina material (×22,700).

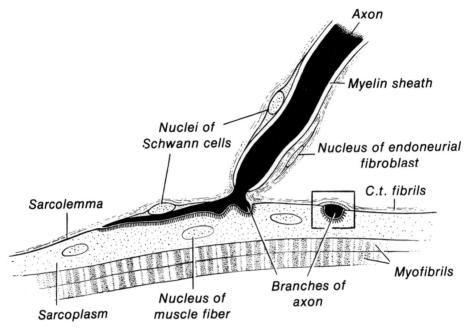

Figure 10.50. Somatic motor nerve ending on a skeletal muscle fiber. The myelin ends just before the axon reaches the muscle fiber. Schwann cells associated with myelin end at the same point. Other Schwann cells continue onto the branches of the axon. Their cytoplasm is so thin that it can be seen under the light microscope only at the level of the nuclei. The branches of the axon lie in invaginations of sarcolemma known as primary synaptic clefts. The subneural sarcolemma and subjacent sarcoplasm, often described as a "subneural apparatus," may appear as a series of myonuclei and mitochondria in special preparations under the light microscope.

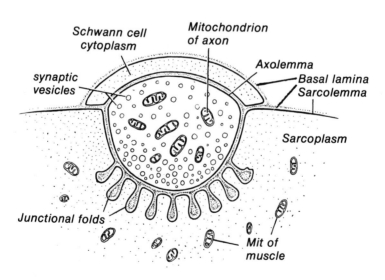

Figure 10.51. Diagram of a portion of the motor end plate (enclosed in the box in Fig. 10.50) showing a branch of an axon in a synaptic indentation as seen in electron micrographs (Fig. 10.49). Secondary clefts or junctional folds extend inward from the primary cleft or gutter. The axon is covered by a thin layer of Schwann cell cytoplasm on the side away from the muscle, but no Schwann cell cytoplasm extends into the indentation. The space between the axolemma and sarcolemma contains an amorphous material, continuous with the basal (external) lamina material around the muscle cell. (Diagram based on descriptions and illustrations by Robertson and Couteaux.)

In the part of the muscle fiber beneath the motor end plate region, there is an increase in number of muscle nuclei. In ordinary sections, the muscle nuclei may appear adjacent to or even between some of the Schwann cell nuclei where nerve fibers course in grooves of the muscle fiber, but electron micrographs have clearly shown that the axon terminals do not penetrate the sarcolemma and therefore do not intermingle with the constituents of the muscle cell (Fig. 10.49).

Terminations of Visceral Efferent Fibers

Postganglionic visceral efferent fibers from the autonomic ganglion cells terminate in the following *effectors*: heart muscle (*cardiomotor*); smooth muscle of viscera (*visceromotor*), of blood vessels (*vasomotor*) and of hairs (*pilomotor*); and glandular epithelia (*secretory*). These axons are unmyelinated.

In heart muscle and in smooth muscle, the fibers form plexuses around the muscle bundles. From these plexuses, fine nerve fibers course in relation to individual muscle fibers. Electron microscopic examination indicates that no special junctions are formed but that bulbous enlargements of the nerve fiber in the vicinity of (and occasionally directly adjacent to) smooth muscle fibers contain aggregates of synaptic vesicles (Fig. 10.15). Some enlargements contain the small, clear vesicles; others contain the larger, dense-cored variety. The former are considered characteristic of postganglionic parasympathetic fibers; the latter are components of postganglionic sympathetic nerve fibers. Apparently, neurotransmitter released from these areas is able to influence responsive cells in the surrounding tissues without establishing discrete neuromuscular junctions.

In glandular epithelium, the visceral efferent fibers form a plexus beneath the basement membrane, through which the fibers pass to terminate in relation to individual gland cells.

Terminations of Afferent Fibers

Those parts of the body which receive stimuli and contain the terminations of peripheral afferent fibers are known as receptors. The receptors have the function of responding to various physical and chemical stimuli, and furthermore, certain receptors have the function of reacting primarily to one particular kind of stimulus. The mechanism of reception must provide for the initiation of a nerve impulse, and in this sense the action of a receptor is considered analogous to the chemical excitability of the dendritic portion of the typical neuron. In some receptors (as in the *taste bud*), special cells receive the stimulus and respond by producing *receptor potentials* which, in turn, activate the afferent nerve ending. In other receptors (as in the *Pacinian corpuscle*), the nerve ending itself receives the stimulus and develops a *generator potential* which triggers the action potential of the nerve fiber. The concept that each type of sensation (touch, heat, etc.) has its own specific receptor has been modified, for it has been observed that different receptors may respond to the same stimulus (e.g., both Pacinian corpuscles and free nerve endings respond to tactile stimuli).

The receptors may be classified in several more or less overlapping ways:

1. Some receptors are found widely distributed over the body. These may be collectively termed receptors of general body or *somatesthetic* sensibility (touch, pressure, pain, temperature, position, movement). Other receptors are found aggregated only in certain places in the head, where they constitute the *organs of special senses* (smell, sight, taste, hearing, and head position and movement).

2. Another distinction may be made between *exteroceptors*, the receptors affected by external stimuli (touch, light pressure, cutaneous pain and temperature, smell, sight, and hearing); the *proprioceptors*, which are affected by stimuli arising within the body wall, especially those of movement and posture; and the *enteroceptors*, which are affected by stimuli arising within the viscera. In receptors, the modes of termination of the peripheral processes of the cranial or spinal ganglion cells are so varied and complicated as to make impracticable

any structural classification except in the broadest sense. The terminal arborizations of the afferent fibers, however, follow one of two structural arrangements. Either they terminate freely among the body tissues or they are surrounded by special connective tissue capsules. The distinction can thus be made between *free* or *nonencapsulated* sensory endings and *encapsulated* ones.

Nonencapsulated Afferent Endings

These endings are found in practically all epithelia of the body, in connective tissue, in muscle, and in serous membranes. They are the most common type of sensory ending in the body.

In the skin and in those mucous membranes which are covered by stratified squamous epithelium, the nerve fibers of a given branch separate as they approach the epithelium, lose their myelin sheaths, and form a subepithelial plexus. From this plexus, axons or their branches enter the epithelial layer and split into minute arborizations, which terminate between the cells in little knoblike swellings. In the skin, the nerve endings do not penetrate beyond the cells of the stratum granulosum.

Essentially similar free nerve endings are seen in other epithelial surfaces, such as the mucosa of the respiratory tract (Fig. 10.52).

Another form of free nerve ending is the *peritrichial* ending, in which sensory fibers encircle the hair follicle and terminate principally in the connective tissue sheath and vitreous membrane of the follicle. Fine nerve fibers may also extend into the outer epithelial root sheath.

In general, these intraepithelial endings terminate among epithelial cells that do not differ from the adjoining epithelial cells. In deeper epithelial layers of the skin, however, are leaflike expansions of a nerve terminal, each of which forms a *meniscus* in contact with an epithelial cell which stains differently from the other cells. This is a *tactile cell*, and the whole apparatus is known as a *tactile corpuscle of Merkel*.

Sensory fibers also terminate diffusely in connective tissue. They all end variously by a branching of the sensory fibers among the fibers and cells of the connective tissue. Such endings are found extensively in the dermis and subcutaneous tissue and in the connective tissue of mucous and serous membranes, the periosteum, and the blood vessels, to name a few instances.

In addition to arborized terminations in the interstitial connective tissue of muscle,

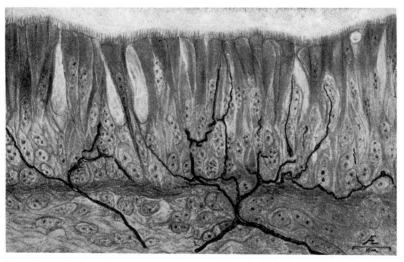

Figure 10.52.   An early drawing illustrating nerve endings in bronchial epithelium (pseudostratified ciliated columnar epithelium). Reduced silver method of Ramon y Cajal. (After A. Elftman.)

nonencapsulated sensory nerve endings are also found around the individual muscle fibers themselves.

Encapsulated Afferent Endings

These include such structures as the *end bulb*, the *tactile corpuscles of Meissner*, the *lamellar* or *Pacinian corpuscles*, the *muscle spindles*, and the *tendon organs* (or *organs of Golgi*).

Of the encapsulated sensory endings, probably the simplest are the so-called end bulbs. These are spherical or oval in shape and consist of a thin, lamellated capsule of flattened connective tissue cells and fibers surrounding a central cavity, the *inner bulb*. Within the inner bulb, the naked axons of one or more myelinated fibers end. In some inner bulbs, the axon may terminate in a number of branches which twist and interlace to form a spherical, skeinlike mass known as a glomerulus. An example of this type is seen in the *end bulbs of Krause* in the conjunctival connective tissue.

End bulbs are found in the lips, in the mucous membranes of the tongue, cheeks, soft palate, epiglottis, nasal cavities, lower end of rectum, peritoneum, serous membranes, tendons, ligaments, connective tissue of nerve trunks, synovial membranes of certain joints, and the external genitals, especially the glans penis and clitoris.

The *tactile corpuscle of Meissner* (Fig. 10.53) is a more complex encapsulated tactile corpuscle. It occurs especially in the hairless portions of the skin and is most

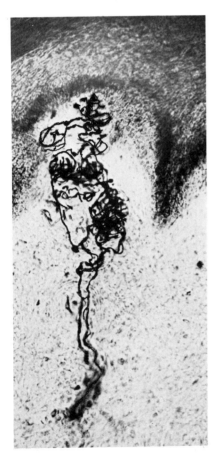
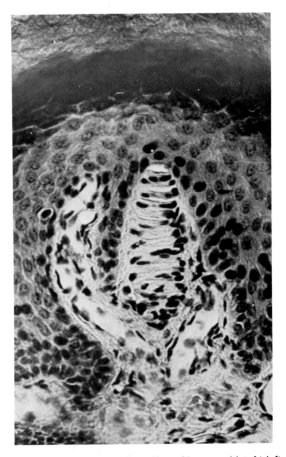

Figure 10.53. Photomicrographs of Meissner's corpuscles in dermal papillae of human skin. At *left*, stained with silver, showing the axon; at *right*, stained with hematoxylin and eosin, showing the connective tissue elements of the nerve ending. Only a portion of the epidermis is included in the field. (Courtesy of Dr. A. Elwyn.)

numerous in the finger tips, the palms of the hands, and the soles of the feet. Lying within the connective tissue of the dermal papillae, these corpuscles are oval bodies which are composed of flattened connective tissue cells in the form of horizontal lamellae surrounded by a connective tissue capsule. Two or more myelinated nerve fibers are distributed to each corpuscle. As the fibers reach the corpuscle, the connective tissue sheath of the nerve joins the connective tissue capsule, the myelin sheaths disappear, and the naked axons pass into the corpuscle, where they branch and pursue a spinal course among the connective tissue elements. In addition to the myelinated fibers, many tactile corpuscles and other encapsulated receptors may also contain the endings of unmyelinated fibers, the significance of which is not clear. The corpuscles of Meissner are known to respond to tactile stimuli.

Ruffini endings are found throughout the subcutaneous connective tissue and in joint capsules. They display branched, spray-like endings emanating from a single myelinated axon. They are surrounded by a very thin capsule and an apparent fluid-filled space. Collagen fibers of the space and capsule interlace with the surrounding connective tissue outside and the axonal endings inside. These tiny but quite common receptors respond to mechanical deformation of surrounding connective tissue.

The *lamellar* or *Pacinian corpuscles* are large laminated elliptical structures which differ from the simpler end bulbs chiefly in the greater development of the connective tissue capsule. They are visible to the naked eye (Fig. 10.54). The capsule is formed by concentric lamellae; each consists of connective tissue fibers and a single layer of flat connective tissue cells. The lamellae are separated from one another by a clear fluid. As in the simpler end bulbs, there is a central cavity within the capsule known as the inner bulb. Each Pacinian corpuscle is supplied by a single myelinated nerve fiber. After losing its myelin sheath, the axon extends through the center of the inner bulb, terminating in a knoblike expansion.

Fine blood vessels enter the base of the corpuscle along with the nerve fiber and break up into capillary networks among the lamellae. They do not enter the inner bulb.

Pacinian corpuscles are found in deeper subcutaneous connective tissue, especially of the hand and foot, in parietal, peritoneum, pancreas, mesentery, penis, clitoris, urethra, nipple, mammary gland, and in connective tissue in the vicinity of tendons, ligaments, and joints. Their form and to some extent their position indicate that they are stimulated by deep or heavy pressure.

In skeletal muscle, sensory nerves terminate in end bulbs and in complicated end organs called *muscle spindles*. The muscle spindle (Figs. 10.55 and 10.56) is an elongated cylindrical structure within which are one or several small muscle fibers of various types, connective tissue, blood vessels, and myelinated nerve fibers. The whole is enclosed in a connective tissue capsule which is pierced at various points by one or more nerve fibers. The thinner axons are generally motor fibers and end on the muscle fibers in typical motor end plates. The thicker myelinated axons are sensory fibers, which lose their myelin as they branch repeatedly within the spindle. The axons then terminate around the enclosed muscle fibers in close apposition to the sarcolemma. Frequently, the ending is in the form of a spiral (*primary annulospiral endings*); it may also form a series of rings or an arborization. The whole structure functions as a unit in reflex regulation of muscle tone.

The muscle fibers of the spindle are thinner than usual, contain a noncontractile filament-poor region in their swollen midsections, and often can be categorized as two types. Usually there are one or two fibers which are long enough to extend well beyond the capsule. These are more slowly contracting muscle fibers which are characterized by an aggregate of nuclei within their sarcoplasm-rich middle regions. They

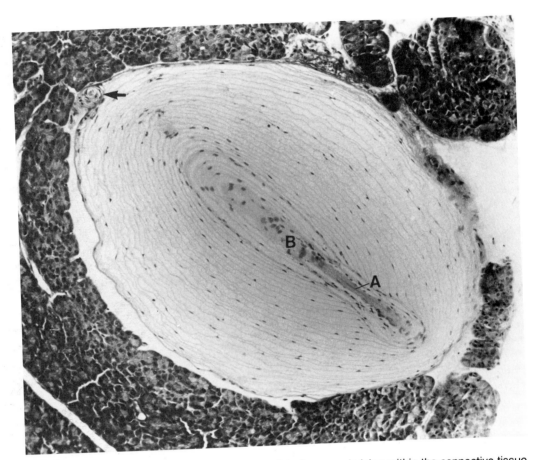

Figure 10.54. Light micrograph of a lamellar (Pacinian) corpuscle lying within the connective tissue of the pancreas. Concentric lamellae occupy most of the volume of this large encapsulated sensory ending. The inner bulb (*B*) is visible and contains a central axon (*A*). The axon has entered the capsule at the *arrow* in another plane of section (×160).

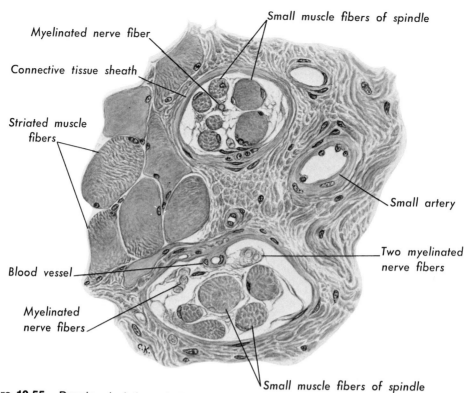

Figure 10.55. Drawing depicting principal features to be found in a cross section of two muscle spindles within a skeletal muscle.

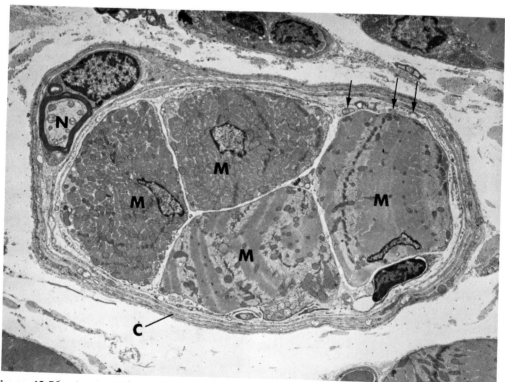

Figure 10.56. Low magnification electron micrograph depicting a muscle spindle in cross section. Four small intrafusal muscle fibers (*M*) are visible within the connective tissue capsule (*C*). A large myelinated primary afferent axon (*N*) and its Schwann cell are seen penetrating the capsule. Small unmyelinated (probably efferent) axons are visible within the capsule (*arrows*) (×3000). (Courtesy of Dr. Mikel Snow and A. Erisman.)

are termed *nuclear bag fibers* as contrasted to more numerous, shorter, intracapsular, rapidly contracting *nuclear chain fibers,* each characterized by a single row of nuclei occupying the central region. Ultrastructurally, nuclear bag fibers resemble tonic skeletal muscle fibers in the arrangement of their filaments and M-lines. Nuclear chain fibers, like other fast (twitch) muscle fibers, display only a faint M-line. Collectively, both populations within the spindle capsule are referred to as *intrafusal fibers,* as opposed to the *extrafusal fibers* of the muscle proper. The motor neurons of the spinal cord that innervate the intrafusal fibes are termed *gamma motor neurons*; the motor neurons supplying the remainder of the muscle fibers are termed *alpha motor neurons*. Details of the structure of the muscle spindle are given schematically in Figure 10.57. Within the capsular region, the connective tissue sheath is separated from the sarcolemma by a space filled with tissue fluid and traversed by connective tissue and nerve fibers. The intrafusal muscle fibers are supplied by three types of nerve fibers: (*a*) small *efferent* fibers (*gamma efferents*) which terminate in motor end plates; (*b*) *primary afferents*, which are large and wind around the muscle fibers to form *annulospiral endings*; and (*c*) *secondary afferents*, which are small and branch to terminate in clusters known as *flower spray endings.*

Because the intrafusal fibers are parallel with the extrafusal fibers, they are stretched and their afferent nerves are stimulated whenever the extrafusal fibers of the muscle as a whole are stretched. Hence, the spindle afferents function as stretch receptors. Contraction of extrafusal fibers reduces tension on the muscle spindle, whereas localized contraction in the poles of the intrafusal fibers under stimulation of gamma efferents increases tension on the nuclear regions and stimulates the stretch receptors.

The afferents have their neuron cell bodies in the spinal ganglion. The central processes from the cells with annulospiral re-

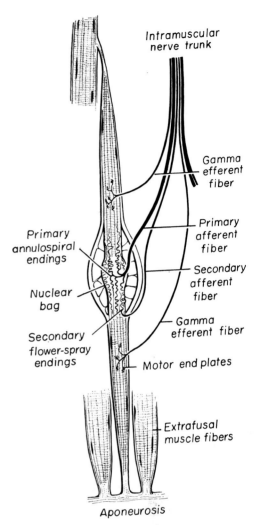

Figure 10.57. Diagram of muscle spindle. Each spindle contains several slender muscle fibers (intrafusal) enclosed by a connective tissue sheath which becomes continuous at its ends with the connective tissue endomysium of regular muscle fibers (extrafusal). For purposes of clarity, only one intrafusal fiber is shown. (Diagram based on illustration from D. Barker: *Q J Microsc Sci* 89:143, 1948.)

ceptors form synapses in the spinal cord with alpha motor neurons which send axons to motor end plates on extrafusal muscle fibers. Thus, a two-neuron (monosynaptic) path is established, functioning as a stretch or *myotactic reflex*. This type of reflex activity maintains muscle tonus and provides a background for voluntary movements after stimulation of the alpha motor

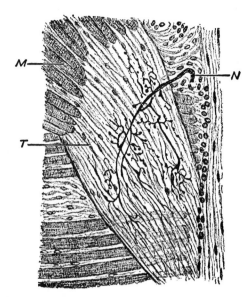

Figure 10.58. An early drawing from a silver impregnated tendon organ with a musculotendinous bundle from a 6-month human fetus. *M*, muscle fibers; *N*, nerve fiber; *T*, tendon fibers. (Redrawn from Tello.)

neurons from higher centers. Stretch receptor reflexes associated with the so-called *flower spray endings* are more complicated and involve polysynaptic pathways.

At the junction of muscle and tendon are found the elaborate sensory structures known as the *tendon organs* or *organs of Golgi* (Fig. 10.58). These are spindle-shaped bodies composed of several tendon bundles covered by a thin capsule. Into this there enter one or several afferent nerve fibers which break up into complicated arborizations upon the tendon bundles.

The proprioceptive stimuli of position and movement resulting from the constant or varying tension of voluntary muscles and their attached tendons are received by muscle spindles and tendon organs. The information gathered in these receptors guides the CNS in governing the attached muscle in the fine degrees of contraction or relaxation necessary for precise motor control.

References

Akert K, Sandri C, Weibel ER, Peper K, Moor H: The fine structure of the perineural endothelium. *Cell Tissue Res* 165:281–295, 1976.

Akert K, Waser PG (eds): Mechanisms of synaptic transmission. *Prog Brain Res* 31, 1969.

Brady ST, Lasek RJ: Axonal transport—a cell biological method for studying proteins that associate with the cytoskeleton. In Wilson L (ed): *Methods in Cell Biology*, vol 25, part B. New York, Academic Press, 1982, pp 365–398.

Bisby MA: Functions of retrograde axonal transport. *Fed Proc* 41:2307–2311, 1982.

Bodian D: The generalized vertebrate neuron. *Science* 137:323–326, 1962.

Bourne G (ed): *Structure and Function of the Nervous System*, vols 1 and 2. New York, Academic Press, 1968, 1969.

Brightman MW, Palay SL: The fine structure of the ependyma in the brain of the rat. *J Cell Biol* 19:415–539, 1963.

Brimijoin S: Microtubules and the capacity of the system for rapid axonal transport. *Fed Proc* 41:2312–2316, 1982.

Bunge, MB: Fine structure of nerve fibers and growth cones of isolated sympathetic neurons in culture. *J Cell Biol* 56:713–735, 1973.

Bunge R: Glial cells and the central myelin sheath. *Physiol Rev* 48:197–251, 1968.

Clemente CD: Regeneration in central nervous system. *Int Rev Neurobiol* 6:257–301, 1964.

Cooper JR, Bloom FE and Roth RM: *The Biochemical Basis of Neuropharmacology*. New York, Oxford University Press, 1974.

Cooper PE and Martin JB. Neuroendocrinology and brain peptides. *Trends Neurosci* 5:186–189, 1982.

Couteaux R: Motor end-plate structure. In Bourne GH (ed): *Structure and Function of Muscle*, vol 1. New York, Academic Press, 1960, pp 337–380.

Droz, B: Protein metabolism in nerve cells. *Int Rev Cytol* 25:363–390, 1969.

Eccles JC: *The Physiology of Nerve Cells*. Baltimore, Johns Hopkins Press, 1957.

Eccles JC. *The Physiology of Synapses*. New York, Academic Press, 1964.

Geren BB: Structural studies of the formation of the myelin sheath in peripheral nerve fibers. In Rudnick D (ed): *Cellular Mechanisms in Differentiation and Growth*. Princeton, Princeton University Press, 1956, pp 213–220.

Gray EG, and Guillery RW: Synaptic morphology in the normal and degenerating nervous system. *Int Rev Cytol* 19:111–182, 1966.

Guth L: Regeneration in the mammalian peripheral nervous system. *Physiol Rev* 36:441–478, 1956.

Haymaker W, Adams RD (eds): *Histology and Histopathology of the Nervous System*, vols 1 and 2. Springfield, Il., Charles C Thomas, 1982.

Heuser JE and Reese TS: Evidence for recycling of synaptic vesicle membrane during transmitter release at the frog neuromuscular junction. *J Cell Biol* 57:315–344, 1982.

Heuser JE, Reese TS, and Landis DMD: Functional changes in frog neuromuscular junctions studied with freeze-fracture. *J Neurocytol* 3:109–131, 1974.

Hild W: Das Neuron. In Möllendorff v, Bargmann W (eds): *Handbuch der mikroskopischen Anatomie des Menschen*, vol 4, part 4. Berlin, Springer-Verlag, 1959, pp 1–184.

Hubel DH: The brain. *Sci Am* 241:44–53, 1979.

Jones DG: Ultrastructural approaches to the organization of central synapses. *Am Sci*, 69:200–210, 1981.

Katz B: *Nerve, Muscle and Synapse.* New York, McGraw-Hill, 1966.

Kiernan JA: Hypotheses concerned with axonal regeneration in the mammalian nervous system. *Biol Rev* 54:155–197, 1979.

Kuffler SW, and Nicholls JG: The physiology of neuroglial cells. *Ergeb Physiol* 57:1–90, 1966.

Lasek RJ. Translocation of the neuronal cytoskeleton and axonal locomotion. *Philos Trans R Soc Lond (Biol)* 299:313–327, 1982.

LeDouarin N: The ontogeny of the neural crest in avian embryo chimeras. *Nature* 286:663–669, 1980.

Lund RD: *Development and Plasticity of the Brain. An Introduction.* New York, Oxford University Press, 1978.

Morales R, and Duncan D: Specialized contacts of astrocytes with astrocytes and other cell types in the spinal cord of the cat. *Anat Rec* 182:255–266, 1975.

Ochs S: Calcium and the mechanism of axoplasmic transport. *Fed Proc* 41:2301–2306, 1982.

Palay SL, and Palade GE: The fine structure of neurons. *J Biophys Biochem Cytol* 1:69–88, 1955.

Payton BW, Bennett MVL, and Pappas GD: Permeability and structure of junctional membranes at an electrotonic synapse. *Science* 166:1641–1643, 1969.

Peters A, Palay S, and Webster H de F: *The Fine Structure of the Nervous System. The Neurons and Supporting Cells.* Philadelphia, WB Saunders, 1976.

Pfenninger KH, Rees RP: Properties of membranes in synapse formation. In Barondes SH (ed): *Neuronal Recognition, Current Topics in Neurobiology.* New York, Plenum Press, 1976.

Purves D and Lichtman JW: Elimination of synapses in the developing nervous system. *Science* 210:153–157, 1980.

Quarton GC, Melnechuk T, and Schmitt FO: *The Neurosciences.* New York, Rockefeller University Press, 1967.

Rambourg A and Droz B: Smooth endoplasmic reticulum and axonal transport. *J Neurochem* 35:16–25, 1980.

Ramón Y Cajal S: *Degeneration and Regeneration of the Nervous System.* London, Oxford University Press, 1928.

Ramón Y Cajal S: *Histologie du Systeme Nerveux de l'Homme et des Vertebres, 1909–1911,* vols I and II. London, Oxford University Press, 1928.

Rosenbluth J: Intramembranous particle distribution at the node of Ranvier and adjacent axolemma in myelinated axons of the frog brain. *J Neurocytol* 5:731–745, 1976.

Schnapp B and Mugnaini E: Membrane architecture of myelinated fibers as seen by freeze-fracture. In Waxman SG (ed): *Physiology and Pathobiology of Axons.* New York, Raven Press, 1978, pp 83–123.

Schnapp B, Peracchia C, and Mugnaini E: The paranodal axo-glial junction in the central nervous system studied with thin sections and freeze-fracture. *Neuroscience* 1:181–190, 1976.

Shanthaveerappa TR and Bourne GH: Perineural epithelium: a new concept of its role in the integrity of the peripheral nervous system. *Science* 154:1464–1467, 1966.

Shepherd GM: *The Synaptic Organization of the Brain: An Introduction.* New York, Oxford Univ. Press, 1974.

Shepherd GM: Microcircuits in the nervous system. *Sci Am* (2):92–103, 1978.

Sidman RL: Cell-cell recognition in the developing central nervous system. In Schmitt FO, Worden FG (eds): *The Neurosciences Third Study Program.* Cambridge, MIT Press, 1974, pp 743–758.

Sperry RW: Chemoaffinity in the orderly growth of nerve fiber patterns and connections. *Proc Nat Acad Sci USA* 50:703–710, 1963.

Uzman BG and Nogueira-Graf G: Electron microscope studies of the formation of nodes of Ranvier in mouse sciatic nerves. *J Biophys Biochem Cytol* 3:589–598, 1957.

Waxman SG: Membranes, myelin, and the pathophysiology of multiple sclerosis. *New Engl J Med* 306:1529–1533, 1982.

Weiss P (ed): *Genetic Neurology; Problems of the Development, Growth and Regeneration of the Nervous System and Its Functions.* Chicago, University of Chicago Press, 1950.

Weiss P and Hiscoe HB: Experiments on the mechanism of nerve growth. *J Exp Zool* 107:314–395, 1948.

Young JZ: The functional repair of nervous tissue. *Physiol Rev* 23:318–374, 1942.

Chapter 11

THE SPINAL CORD, CEREBELLAR CORTEX, AND CEREBRAL CORTEX

The central nervous system (brain and spinal cord) is a specialized epithelium containing various types of cell assemblies organized to perform neural functions. Groups of nerve cell bodies serving similar functions are termed *nuclei*. If linearly arranged (as in the spinal cord), such cell groups may be termed *columns*. Groups of nerve fibers interconnecting these neuronal groups are called *tracts*. Myelinated tracts form the *white matter* of the central nervous system (CNS). When neuronal cell bodies occupy layers at the surface of the brain, these areas are termed cortical regions or *cortex*. The CNS is surrounded by special connective tissue investments, the *meninges*, and is bathed, internally and externally, by a special fluid, the *cerebrospinal fluid* (CSF). The purpose of this chapter is to present the cytology of several typical CNS regions and to describe the connective tissue investments that act both as a subcompartment for the CSF and as a protective covering.

INVESTMENTS OF THE BRAIN AND CORD AND THE FLUID SPACES

The meninges of the brain and spinal cord are divisible into two more or less distinct connective tissue investments, the *dura mater* and the *pia-arachnoid*, the latter usually being subdivided into two layers, the *pia mater* and *arachnoid* (Figs. 11.1 and 11.2). The dura mater is sometimes referred to as the *pachymeninx* and the pia-arachnoid the *leptomeninx*, or *leptomeninges*.

The dura mater, which is the outer of the two investments, consists of dense fibrous tissue (Fig. 11.2). The *cerebral dura* serves both as an investing membrane for the

brain and as periosteum for the inner surfaces of the cranial bones. Its internal aspect is composed of dense connective tissue lined on its inner surface by a single layer of flat fibroblastic cells. The outer layer, which forms the periosteum, is similar in structure, but is much richer in blood vessels and nerves. The *spinal dura* corresponds to the inner cerebral dura; the vertebrae have their own separate periosteum. It contains more elastic tissue than the inner cerebral dura but otherwise resembles it in structure. The outer surface of the spinal dura is covered with a single layer of flat fibroblastic cells and is separated from the periosteum by the *epidural space*, which contains anastomosing, thin-walled veins lying in connective tissue rich in fat (Fig. 11.1). The inner surface of the spinal dura is also lined by a single layer of flat cells. Beneath the spinal dura, between it and the arachnoid, is the *subdural space*, a narrow cleft containing fluid. It has no apparent direct communication with the subarachnoid space.

The pia mater (Fig. 11.2) closely invests the brain and cord, extends into the convolutions of the brain, and protrudes into the ventricles at the thin-walled portions of the brain, where, in close proximity to modified ependymal cells, it contributes to the connective tissue and vasculature of the *choroid plexuses* (described below). The pia consists of fibrous tissue and contains the blood vessels that serve the neural tissues proper. The basal lamina of the CNS separates pial and perivascular connective tissue from the fibrous astrocyte end feet (*outer glia lamitans*) that comprise the basal surface of brain and spinal cord. Pial

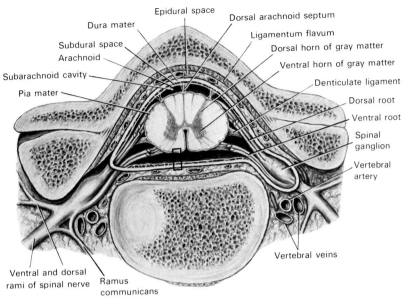

Figure 11.1. Diagram of a transverse section through the fourth cervical vertebra showing the coverings of the spinal cord and related structures. An area comparable to that within the *box* is shown at higher magnification in Figure 11.2. (From Rauber-Kopsch Lehrbuch und Atlas der Anatomie des Menschen, ed 13, vol 5, edited by F. Kopsch. Leipzig Georg Thieme Verlag, 1930.)

Figure 11.2. Photomicrograph illustrating the histology of the region outlined by the *box* in Figure 11.1. The white matter of the spinal cord (*sc*) shows a variety of neuroglia cells in the process of forming myelin. Many small myelin sheaths are seen in cross section. Immediately overlying the cord tissue is the pia mater (*p*), containing two blood vessels, one of which contains several red blood cells. The subarachnoid space between the pia mater and the arachnoid (*a*) contains the cerebrospinal fluid (*csf*). The heavy connective tissue layers of the dura mater (*d*) form the outermost investment. The arachnoid is shown in its normal close apposition to the dura; only in abnormal conditions does fluid accumulate in the potential space between these two investments. Kitten spinal cord.

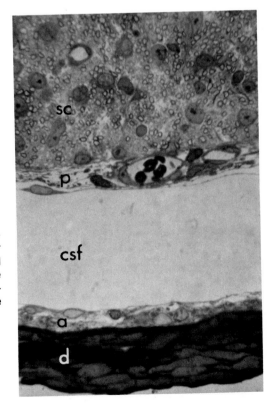

connective tissue is continuous with the perivascular connective tissue that accompanies vessels which loop into the walls of the CNS. That connective tissue comprises a narrow space (*perivascular space*) between CNS basal lamina on the one side and vascular endothelial basal lamina on the other. As a vessel extends more deeply into the CNS wall, the perivascular space narrows until it disappears, and the two basal laminae are fused around the deepest, smallest vessels.

The arachnoid (Fig. 11.2) passes over the convolutions of the brain without dipping into them. It is partly separated from the pia by a substantial space, across which *subarachnoid tabeculae* pass, connecting pia and arachnoid. This is the *subarachnoid space*, and it is filled with a clear fluid, the CSF. The trabeculae and arachnoid contain delicate strands of connective tissue covered with a layer of flat or low cuboidal cells which also extends discontinuously over the outer pial surface. This layer of cells is *epithelioid* and lines the subarachnoid spaces. The cells ordinarily have large, pale, oval nuclei. Recent evidence discloses that, like the cells of the perineurium, the outer arachnoid cells are attached by occluding junctions. Hence, they seem to serve as the outermost seal for the CSF-filled subarachnoid space. This cellular layer may be continuous with a perineurium at nerve roots. If so, a narrow continuity may exist between endoneurium and subarachnoid space or pial connective tissue.

The spinal dura and the inner layer of the cerebral dura are poor in blood vessels. The outer layer of the cerebral dura, forming as it does the periosteum of the cranial bones, is rich in blood vessels, which pass in to supply the bones. The pia is quite vascular, especially its inner aspect, from which vessels pass into the brain and cord. The arachnoid is nonvascular (Fig. 11.2).

The Cerebrospinal Fluid

The CSF in the subarachnoid space is in continuity with the CSF of the brain cavities (the *ventricles*) and the *central canal* of the spinal cord. This continuity is effected through an aperture in the caudal part of the thin roof of the fourth ventricle (the *foramen of Magendie*) and an aperture in each of the thin-walled lateral recesses of the fourth ventricle (the *foramina of Luschka*).

The CSF is a clear, colorless fluid which is slightly viscous and of low specific gravity (1.004 to 1.006). It contains small quantities of inorganic salts, chiefly sodium chloride and potassium chloride, as well as small amounts of dextrose and traces of proteins. It normally contains very few cells. Its quantity in an adult man is about 150 ml. The bulk of the CSF is probably formed by the activity of the epithelial cells lining the choroid plexus, from which it passes into the ventricles and thence by the foramina of Magendie and Luschka into the subarachnoid spaces. Because adjacent ependymal cells lining the walls of the ventricles and spinal cord are joined by junctions that do not appear to be everywhere tight, CSF probably also percolates between those cells and through the intercellular spaces of the brain and cord. Some workers believe that substantial amounts of the CSF or certain of its components are produced by cells of the neural tissue, to pass into the ventricles, spinal canal, or perivascular spaces. If so, CNS tissue may be considered to have not only its interior and exterior surfaces, but also its interstices and individual cell surfaces, bathed in CSF. The drainage of the fluid back into the bloodstream appears to be chiefly by passage through the walls of *arachnoid villi* (see below) and into the cerebral venous sinuses.

Choroid Plexuses

Certain parts of the wall of the brain are composed solely of modified ependymal cells forming a thin epithelial membrane, a *lamina epithelialis*, which is covered externally by a highly vascularized pia mater. These two layers together constitute the *telae choroideae*, which form the roof of the fourth ventricle, the roof of the third ventricle, and parts of the walls of the lateral ventricles. Projecting into the ventricles are complex folds and invaginations from the telae choroideae containing tortuous networks of small vessels and capillaries, the *choroid plexuses* (Fig. 11.3). The term "choroid plexus" is often used in referring to the entire mass of infolded membranes, rather than to the network of blood vessels alone.

The modified ependymal epithelium covering the choroid plexuses is a simple curboidal to low columnar type with a rather granular cytoplasm. In electron micrographs, the free surface of the cells appears to be thrown into fine irregular cytoplasmic projections, resembling a brush border. These cells play an important role in the production of the CSF. The cells of this modified ependyma, unlike ependyma elsewhere, are joined together along their lateral borders by occluding junctions. Thus, although the capillaries of this region are known to be quite "leaky" (as compared with capillaries elsewhere in the brain),

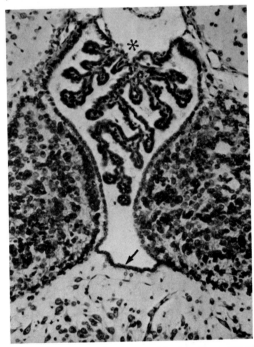

Figure 11.3. Photomicrograph showing tufts of choroid plexus protruding downward from the roof (*) of the third ventricle into the ventricular cavity. The *arrow* points to the ependymal cells that form the lining of the third ventricle. Rat brain (×130).

extravascular material is prevented from entering the CSF directly because of the seal along the lateral edges of the cells of the choroid plexus epithelium.

The Arachnoid Villi

In certain places, the arachnoid sends prolongations into the dura which protrude into a venous sinus or venous lacuna. The prolongations contain spaces, traversed by trabeculae, which may be regarded as continuations of the subarachnoid space. These arachnoidal outgrowths, which are covered with the usual layer of low cells, are known as *arachnoid villi* (Fig. 11.4). They are most numerous along the longitudinal fissure of the cerebral hemispheres, where they protrude into the superior sagittal venous sinus. They are also sometimes found along the transverse, cavernous, and superior petrosal sinuses. It is thought that these villi have small one-way valves which permit the intermittent flow of CSF from the subarachnoid space into the venous sinuses (which have a very low fluid pressure).

The Fluid Compartments and the Blood-Brain Barrier

As is pointed out in the above discussion, the CSF occupies both the cavities of the CNS and the spaces around the brain and spinal cord. Because neither the lining of the brain ventricles (the unspecialized ependyma) nor the covering of the brain surface (the pia) provides a tight barrier against the entry into or egress of fluids from the substance of the brain, the narrow extracellular clefts between neurons and glia of the CNS are also in continuity with CSF (Fig. 11.5). Clinical sampling of the CSF with analysis of its composition provides a useful index of cellular changes in CNS diseases.

Perivascular spaces are also thought to be in continuity with this fluid system (Fig. 11.5). Near the surface of the brain, where pial tissue is carried into brain substance with the penetrating blood vessels, this perivascular space is substantial and provides a common site of cell invasion in brain

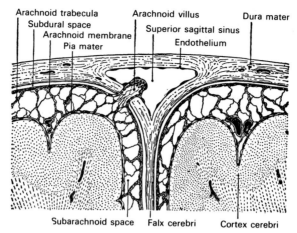

Figure 11.4. Schematic diagram of coronal section of meninges and cerebral cortex, to show relation of arachnoid villus to dural venous sinus. The potential subdural space is necessarily shown of greater size than is normal; the subarachnoid space is also increased in width to illustrate the character of the subarachnoid mesh. The nuclei of the cells lining the subarachnoid space are faintly shown. (Modified from L. H. Weed: The cytology of the cerebrospinal pathway. In Cowdry EV (ed): *Special Cytology*, vol 3, New York, Paul B. Hoeber, Inc. 1932, pp 1485–1521.)

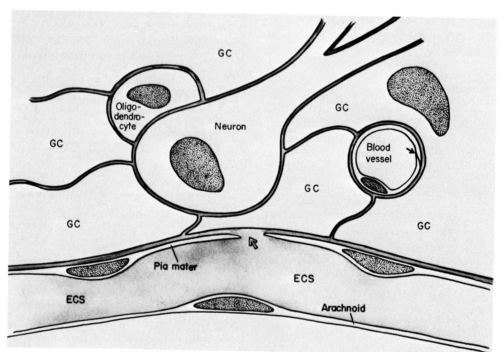

Figure 11.5. Diagram illustrating the continuity between the cerebrospinal fluid within the subarachnoid space and the fluid filling the extracellular space within the nervous tissue. Protein markers placed in the cerebrospinal fluid pass between the cells of the pia mater (*hollow arrow*) and into the narrow extracellular space of the nervous tissue. On the other hand, markers placed within the blood vessels of nervous tissue are confined to the vessel lumina by the presence of occluding junctions between the overlapping processes of endothelial cells (*solid arrow*). Thus the cerebrospinal fluid represents a type of extracellular fluid (*ECS*) for nervous tissue cells. *GC*, neuroglial cell. (Reprinted with permission from R. Bunge: *The Neurosciences: Second Study Program*, edited by F. O. Schmitt, p. 782, Rockefeller University Press, New York, 1970.)

disease. Deeper within the brain wall, the pericapillary spaces are scarcely larger than the other cleftlike intercellular spaces of nervous tissue. In these deeper areas, the basal lamina of the capillaries is often fused with basal lamina of the neural tissue border and surrounded by flattened cellular extensions of astrocytes, the outer *glia limitans*. This application of astrocytic processes to the capillary wall led to the suggestions that (*a*) these cells are avenues of nutrient passage or ion transport from blood vessel to neuron, and/or (*b*) the mosiac of applied cellular processes constitutes the barrier for the passage of materials from blood vessels to brain parenchyma (*the blood-brain barrier*).

The use of the electron microscope has demonstrated the precise site of the blood-brain barrier for certain types of molecules. When certain marker proteins (which can be rendered visible in the electron microscope) are injected into the vascular system, their entry into brain tissue is prevented by the minute occluding junctions between the lateral edges of the endothelial cells. When these protein markers are placed within brain substance, they pass between all cells (including the perivascular astrocyte processes and even through synaptic clefts) but do not enter blood vessels. Thus, the blood-brain barrier for these proteins is in the wall of the CNS capillaries and is not provided by the perivascular tissues (the astrocytic processes, connective tissue, or basal lamina). Whether the perivascular astrocytic feet function in nutrient transport is not known (see Chapter 10).

THE SPINAL CORD

In transverse section (Fig. 11.6), the spinal cord appears oval in shape and slightly more flattened on its ventral than on its dorsal surface. It is surrounded by the *pia mater spinalis*, which extends into the deep longitudinal *ventral median fissure*. Dorsally, the cord is partitioned longitudinally by the *dorsal median sulcus*, which is lined by astrocytic end feet and over which the pia matter passes with minimal amounts of its connective tissue actually entering. At the entrance of the dorsal root fibers on either side, there is a *dorsolateral groove* or *sulcus*.

The gray matter occupies the central part of the section, where it is arranged somewhat in the form of the letter H. Dorsally,

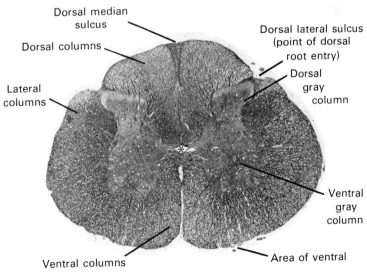

Figure 11.6. Photomicrograph of a cross section of the spinal cord in the lumbar region of a cat. The H-shaped central region is the gray matter, surrounded by the tracts of nerve fibers which form the white matter. *, central canal.

the gray matter extends almost to the surface of the cord as the *dorsal gray columns* (*posterior* or *dorsal horns*). The *ventral gray columns* (*anterior* or *ventral horns*) are shorter and broader and do not so nearly approach the surface of the cord. Surrounding the gray matter is the white matter, which, in each lateral half of the cord, is divided by the dorsal column into two parts. The part lying between the horn and the dorsal median septum is the *dorsal funiculus* (*dorsal* or *posterior white column*); the other part, comprising the remainder of the white matter, is the *ventrolateral funiculus* (*ventrolateral* or *anterolateral white column*).

The ventrolateral white column is again divided, rather indefinitely, by the ventral horn and nerve roots into a *lateral funiculus* (*lateral white column*) and a *ventral funiculus* (*ventral* or *anterior white column*). In the thoracic segments of the cord there is usually a lateral protrusion of the gray matter slightly dorsal to the dorsal boundary of the ventral horn. This region is called the *lateral horn*; it contains the nerve cell bodies of the CNS neurons of the thoracodorsal portion of the autonomic nervous system.

Gray Matter

In the cross portion of the H structure is seen the *central canal*, usually partially obliterated in the adult and represented only by a group of ependymal cells. The central canal divides the gray matter connecting the two sides of the cord into a *ventral gray commissure* and a *dorsal gray commissure*.

The components of the lateral portions of the H are, as noted above, the dorsal columns, which are primarily concerned with sensory input, and the ventral columns, which are concerned with motor activity. Between these two, and lateral to the gray commissures, is the *intermediate* (or *middle*) *gray*, which is associated largely with visceral innervation. The neuron cell bodies in all these regions of gray matter are arranged in longitudinal columns, each a linear aggregate of neurons specialized for a particular function.

The dorsal column contains three major

nuclear groups specialized for the reception of the sensory impulses carried into the spinal cord by the axons of dorsal root ganglia. The various modalities of somatic sensation are handled differently in this region, some of the incoming axons synapsing locally and others being carried upward toward the brain before synapsing. Thus the sensory information available to the organism via the *first order* sensory neurons of the dorsal root ganglia is carried to *second order* sensory neurons and is distributed widely throughout the CNS.

Visceral sensibilities, on the other hand, appear to be channeled primarily to the poorly defined nuclear columns of the intermediate gray. As has been noted, in certain regions of the cord this same intermediate zone contains motor neurons of the visceral system (in the lateral cell column). Thus, the visceral areas of the gray matter are generally more medially located than are the somatic regions.

The ventral column contains many motor cells (ventral or anterior horn cells) arranged in columns in relation to the portion of the body musculature that they innervate. Motor neurons providing fibers to trunk musculature are more medially disposed in ventral gray matter, and motor neurons to the muscles of the limbs are located laterally. Certain of these motor neurons are the largest neurons in the spinal cord. Their dendritic portions, which are generally multipolar, extend several millimeters up or down the cord to receive a variety of signals from local (spinal) interneurons as well as axons from distant (e.g., cortical) parts of the CNS. In higher animals, very few first order sensory neurons make direct contact with motor neurons. The large axons of the motor neurons can be seen passing out through the ventrolateral white matter to form, along with the fibers of the visceral motor neurons in the intermediate gray, the ventral spinal root at the surface of the cord.

White Matter

In order to carry nerve signals to and from gray matter at different levels of the spinal cord and to the higher centers in the brain, fibers must course up and down the long axis of the cord. These fibers (axons) leave the gray matter and form the more superficial white matter. The white matter is thus composed of myelinated and a few unmyelinated nerve fibers and neuroglia, along with blood vessels occupying inward continuations of the pia mater. White matter contains no neuron cell bodies or dendrites. If the section has been cut through a *dorsal (posterior) nerve root*, a small bundle of *dorsal root fibers* can be seen entering the white matter of the cord along the dorsal and medial side of the posterior column. Ventral to the anterior gray commissure is a bundle of transversely disposed myelinated fibers, the *ventral white commissure*. In the dorsal part of the dorsal gray commissure there are also fine, similarly disposed myelinated nerve fibers, the *dorsal white commissure*. Both of these commissures are composed of fibers crossing from one side of the spinal cord to the other.

THE CEREBELLAR CORTEX

General Structure

The cerebellum, connected with the rest of the brain by its three pair of peduncles, consists of two lateral lobes or hemispheres connected by a median lobe, the *vermis*. These are divided by transverse fissures into lobules, each lobule consisting of a median portion belonging to the vermis and two winglike extensions belonging to the hemispheres. The surfaces of the lobules are marked by folds (*laminae* or *folia*) running approximately parallel to the fissures and thus transversely to the longitudinal axis of the brain. The surface of the cerebellum is composed of gray matter, the cortex, which envelops the white matter.

In the *cerebellar cortex* there can be distinguished, with ordinary stains (hematoxylin-eosin, Nissl), an outer or *molecular layer* containing few cells and no myelinated fibers, an inner *granular layer*, and, between the two, a single row of large flask-shaped cells, the *cells of Purkinje* (Fig.

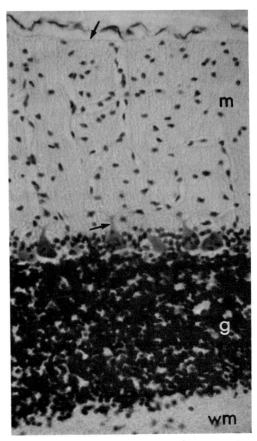

Figure 11.7. Photomicrograph showing the layers of neurons within the cerebellar cortex of a rat. The *upper arrow* indicates the surface of the cerebellum, which is covered by remnants of the pia. The *lower arrow* indicates the dendrite of a Purkinje cell. The soma of this cell and adjacent Purkinje cells are also visible. The molecular layer (*m*) contains a considerable number of capillaries. *g*, granule cell layer; *wm*, white matter. Compare with Figure 11.8.

11.7). Below the granular layer is an area of white matter containing the fibers that carry signals to or from the neuronal machinery of the cortex.

The major input of nerve fibers to the cerebellum arrives in the granule cell layer. With routine stains, this layer appears to be composed of closely packed cell nuclei, but there are clear spaces here and there which are called *islands* or *glomeruli*. The cell nuclei belong to small neurons, the *granule cells*, and the glomeruli are regions where the granule cell dendrites receive synapses from axons arriving from outside the cerebellum. The incoming fibers, which are highly branched, are called *mossy fibers* (Fig. 11.8). Each granule cell possesses three to six short dendrites for the reception of the mossy fiber input.

The granule cell sends its fine, unmyelinated axon to ascend into the molecular layer, where it divides into two branches running longitudinally along the folium and terminating in varicosities (Fig. 11.8). These are the *parallel fibers* of the molecular layer. They thus run at right angles to and through the dendritic expansions of the Purkinje cells, and their cross sections, together with the terminal dendritic arborizations of the Purkinje cells, give the molecular layer its punctate appearance. During their course in the molecular layer, the parallel fibers make synaptic contact (known to be excitatory) with dendrites from a number of different Purkinje cells.

The Purkinje dendrite also receives excitatory input from *climbing fibers*, many of which are recurrent collaterals from neurons of the deep cerebellar nuclei (see below). These climbing fibers, which entwine the dendritic trunk (Fig. 11.8), have a powerful excitatory influence on the Purkinje cell.

Other granule cell axons are known to make contact with smaller neurons, the *basket cells*, which are located in the region of the Purkinje layer. These cells are so named because their axons form basket-like skeins around the bodies and initial axonal segments of the Purkinje cells (Fig. 11.8). They are well disposed to exert an inhibitory influence on Purkinje cell activity. Thus there appear to be two excitatory inputs and one inhibitory input to the Purkinje cell.

The Purkinje cell possesses several main dendrites, which enter the molecular layer and form a remarkably rich arborization extending to the surface. The dendritic arborization is fan-shaped, extending at right angles to the laminae. The axon is given off from the end of the cell opposite to the dendrites and passes into the granular layer. Here axon collaterals may turn back to enter another part of the cerebellar cortex, but the main axon continues on to neurons deep within the cerebellum that

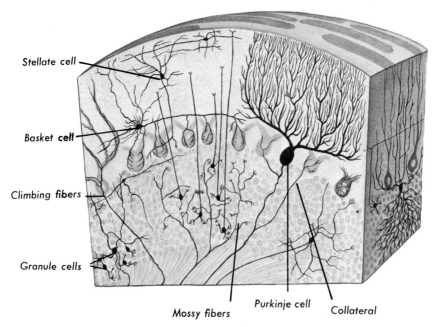

Figure 11.8. Schematic diagram of structure of cerebellar cortex. (After Bargmann W: *Histologie und mikroskopischen Anatomie des Menschen*, vol 15. Stuttgart, Georg Thieme Verlag, 1964.)

form the deep cerebellar nuclei. The influence of the Purkinje axons on the neurons of the deep cerebellar nuclei is thought to be inhibitory. It is the neurons of the deep cerebellar nuclei that have axons leaving the cerebellum to provide the cerebellar output to other regions of the nervous system.

As complex as the above interneuronal connections may appear at first reading, the cerebellar circuitry is actually more complex than this short review indicates. This complexity is achieved not by unique cytology but by repetition of basic neurocytological components (elaboration of the cell surface to provide a dendritic zone, development of basic synaptic types, extension of the cell as an axon with specializations at the axon terminal). The same statement can be made regarding the more complicated cerebral cortex discussed below.

Function

The cerebellum contributes to nervous system function by serving to modulate and coordinate skeletal muscle activity. Among other activities, it assists in preventing muscle "overshoot" so that a muscle contraction once started will not be carried too far; thus, fine movements are facilitated. The cerebellum is not involved in sensation or in intellectual processes.

Even a beginning understanding of how the cellular assemblies of the cerebellar cortex participate in this type of control must await the student's study of the origins of the fibers that enter the cerebellum and destinations of fibers that comprise the cerebellar output.

It is interesting that after aldehyde fixation, the cells known to provide inhibitory influences (e.g., the basket cell contacts with Purkinje cell bodies) have often been found to contain primarily flattened synaptic vesicles in their nerve endings, whereas cells known to provide excitatory influences (e.g., the climbing fiber contacts with Purkinje dendrites or granule cell contacts with Purkinje dendritic spines) contain primarily spheroid synaptic vesicles (see discussion of this point in Chapter 10).

THE CEREBRAL CORTEX

General Structure

The cerebral cortex (or *pallium*) is the external layer of gray matter covering the convolutions and fissures of the cerebral hemispheres. It has an area of about 200,000 mm^2 and varies in thickness from about 1.5 to 4.0 mm. It contains nerve fibers, neuroglia, and the bodies of nearly 14 billion neurons. The older, less elaborate olfactory cortex and hippocampus is termed the *allocortex*; the rest is the *neocortex* or *isocortex*.

The chief types of neurons found in the cortex are (*a*) *pyramidal cells*, (*b*) *stellate* or *granule cells*, (*c*)*horizontal cells*, and (*d*) *inverted* or *Martinotti cells* (Figs. 11.9 and 11.10). The pyramidal cells (Fig. 11.10) are characterized by a pyramid-shaped perikaryon with an apical dendrite directed toward the surface of the brain and an axon leaving the base of the perikaryon to course into the white matter as a projection or association fiber. These axons provide the principal output of the cortex. The stellate cells are characterized by their small size, numerous dendrites coursing in various directions, and a relatively short axon. Many of the axons providing an input to the cortex are thought to end on their dendrites. The horizontal cells, found mostly in the outer layer, are characterized by horizontally disposed dendrites and axons, which presumably serve to interconnect neighboring cortical regions. The inverted or Martinotti cells, located in the deeper cortical layers, have axons directed toward the surface, to be distributed entirely intracortically.

When viewed in a section cut perpendicular to the cortical surface, the most striking aspect of the cerebral cortex is the lamination of its cellular components in layers horizontal to the surface. The neocortex is characterized by six such layers (Fig. 11.9): (*a*) The outermost *molecular layer*, made up primarily of cell processes and of horizontal cells; (*b*) the *external granular layer*, composed mainly of small, triangular neurons; (*c*) the *pyramidal layer*, composed largely of relatively large py-

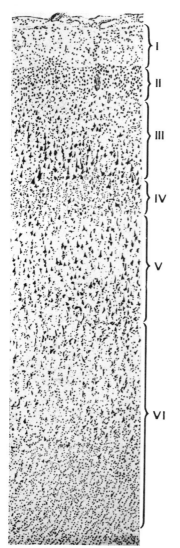

Figure 11.9. Photograph of cell layers of Nissl-stained preparations of cerebral cortex. (After Bargmann W: *Histologie und mikroskopischen Anatomie des Menschen,* vol 15. Stuttgart, Georg Thieme Verlag, 1964.)

ramidal cells plus many granule cells; (*d*) the *internal granular layer,* made up chiefly of the stellate or granule cells; (*e*) the *ganglionic layer* of large and medium-sized pyramidal cells; and (*f*) the *multiform layer,* containing neurons of widely varying shape, including Martinotti cells.

The laminar arrangement of cortical neurons so clearly visible in histological sections is deceptive in view of the known functional properties of certain cortical regions. The functional organization of some cortical areas receiving sensory stimuli (e.g., the visual cortex which receives signals from the visual system) involves *columns* of neurons oriented vertical to the cortical surface. Stimuli arriving in this cortical region activate a specific column of cells, each column 0.3 to 0.5 mm in diameter. The intrinsic morphological basis for these functional columns has not been clearly defined.

The thickness of the various cell layers differs considerably in different areas of the cerebral cortex. Some areas exhibit such marked modification in the layers of cells that they are known as *heterotypic,* in contrast with *homotypic* areas, which show all of the six layers outlined in Figure 11.9. On the basis of differences in structure and function, the cortex has been mapped into a number of areas. In some regions, the cytoarchitecture corresponds precisely to the functional modality known to be processed in that cortical region. This is true, for example, in cortical regions concerned with vision and with hearing. In other cases, cortical regions of different function have virtually identical cytological arrangements.

The input to the cortex comes from a great variety of sources. Many of the sensory modalities have representation in discrete cortical regions which provide surface representations for the different body parts. Other cortical regions are concerned with the initiation and/or control of motor activities; these regions are also *somatotopically* organized, each part of the body being represented in a discrete area of cortex. There are also discrete cortical regions associated with special faculties, e.g., speech. In the human, there are also substantial cortical areas, called *association areas,* which have connections with the motor and sensory regions of the cortex. These association areas provide additional orders of circuitry to assist in the analysis of sensory input and the programming of motor output.

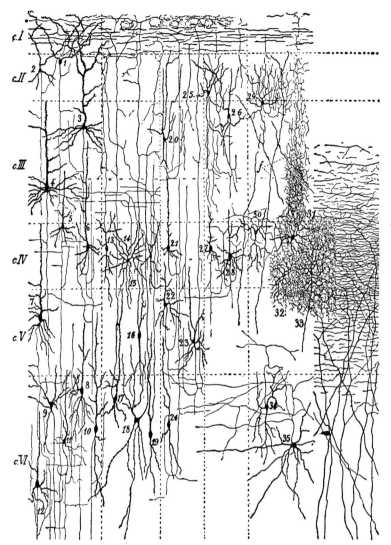

Figure 11.10. Various forms of nerve cells of the cerebral cortex. From various figures of Cajal, especially of the temporal cortex. *cI*, zonal layer of cortex; *cII*, external granular layer, *cIII*, pyramidal layer, *cIV*, internal granular layer; *cV*, ganglionic layer; *cVI*, multiform layer. *1* to *12*, cells, mostly pyramidal, whose axons enter the white matter (corticofugal cells); *13* to *35*, cells whose axons do not leave the gray matter (or cortex); *13* to *19*, cells with directly ascending axons; *20* to *24*, cells with arciform ascending axons; *25* to *28*, cells with short descending axons, with or without ascending collaterals; *29, 30*, short axon cells, properly speaking (Golgi's type II); *31* to *33*, cells with bushy axons (bipenicillate and neuroglia form), some forming terminal nests around the small granule cells; *34, 35*, large stellate cells of layer *VI* with extensively branching axons, especially extending horizontally; *f*, fibers of unknown origin. On the *right* are shown corticopetal fibers and their terminal plexus, especially dense in layer *IV*. (After Bonne C: L'écorce cérébrale. *Rev Gen Histol* 2: 1907; 4:1910.)

Function

The discussion of nervous tissue begins in Chapter 9 with the suggestion that higher animals use multiple sets of inter-

neurons to effect their more discriminating and exact behavior. Between the primary sensory neurons in various sensory ganglia and the motor neurons of the "final common path," there are interposed circuit upon circuit of neuronal "wiring." By these circuits, sensations reach cortical levels. This system provides for the convergence and association of many kinds of stimuli from all parts of the body. This cortical mechanism not only associates many stimuli before the performance of a motor activity, but it also dissociates, i.e., discriminates, and thus, by inhibition, it enables motor activity to be limited only to the necessary movements. There is also plasticity in cortical mechanisms, for the neurons are somehow changed by their activities. Whatever their nature, the acquired changes of the cortex, because of its plasticity and consequent capacity for "learning," affect the action of subsequent stimuli reaching the cortex and furnish the basis of memory, of personal experience, and of individually acquired neural mechanisms, as opposed to germinal or inherited neural mechanisms. Cortical mechanisms are also involved in the transmission, by educational processes using complex symbols, of acquired experience to the plastic cortex of other individuals. Animals other than man "learn," i.e., acquire and utilize individual experience, but it is doubtful that any animal other than man significantly *summates* experience, i.e., transmits it to other individuals and generations. The cortex is thus, in a sense, the organ of human culture and conduct. This supermaze of neuronal inter-connections provides for the origin and expression of the highest faculties of the mind. If it is possible for the human cerebral cortex to understand the mechanisms of its own function, the concentrated study of many generations will certainly be required to accomplish this task.

References

Brightman M W, Reese T S: Junctions between intimately opposed cell membranes in the vertebrate brain. *J Cell Biol* 40:648–677, 1969.

Carpenter M B, Sutin J: Neuroanatomy, ed 8. Baltimore, Williams & Wilkins, 1983.

Cervós-Navarro J, Artigas J, Mršulja BJ: Morphofunctional aspects of the normal and pathological blood-brain barrier. *Acta Neuropathol (Berl)* Suppl. VIII: 1–19, 1983.

Chow K L, Leiman A L: The structural and functional organization of the neocortex. *Neurosci Res Prog Bull* 8:157–220, 1970.

Crosby E C, Humphrey T, Lauer E W: *Correlative Anatomy of the Nervous System.* New York, Macmillan, 1962.

Eccles J C, Ito M, and Szentagothai J: *The Cerebellum as a Neuronal Machine.* New York Springer-Verlag, 1967.

Economo C: *The Cytoarchitectonics of the Human Cerebral Cortex.* London, Oxford University Press, 1929.

Hubel D H: The brain. *Sci Am* 241:44–53, 1979.

Lajtha A, and Ford D H (eds): Brain barrier systems. *Prog Brain Res* 29, 1968.

Peters A, Palay S L, and Webster H: *The Fine Structure of the Nervous System. The Neurons and Supporting Cells.* Philadelphia, W. B. Saunders, 1976.

Sholl D A: *The Organization of the Cerebral Cortex.* London, Methuen and Company, 1970.

Weed L H: Certain anatomical and physiological aspects of the meninges and cerebrospinal fluid. *Brain* 58:383–397, 1934.

Chapter 12

THE CIRCULATORY SYSTEMS

Complex organisms require the transport of nutrients, hormones, gases, and other vital materials over long distances, for example from points of synthesis, absorption, or release to points of utilization or conversion. Such transport requires directed, highly controlled flow, and the body actually as *two* circulatory systems which perform this function. These are the blood vascular system and a lymph vascular system. The *blood vascular system* consists of (*a*) the *heart*, which is a pump for propelling the blood, (*b*) the *arteries*, which are tubes for conveying the blood toward the organs and tissues, (*c*) the *capillaries*, which are anastomosing channels of small caliber with thin walls providing for much of the interchange of substances between the blood and tissue fluids, and (*d*) the *veins*, which in their initial segments also provide for blood-tissue fluid interchange but in addition serve for the return of blood to the heart. It is remarkable that a complete, but simple, blood vascular system is established in the embryo prior to definitive appearance of most organs.

The *lymph vascular system* consists of lymphatic capillaries and various-sized lymphatic vessels which ultimately drain into main trunks, the thoracic duct and the right lymphatic duct, which empty into the large veins in the neck.

THE BLOOD VASCULAR SYSTEM

The entire system—heart, arteries, veins, capillaries—has a common and continuous lining which consists of a single layer of *endothelial cells*. This single layer of cells forms the main component of the wall in the capillaries, but some additional cells and tissues are usually present. Accessory coats of muscle and connective tissue become prominent in the larger vessels and the heart. The portion of the system that is most intimately involved with tissue exchange, that is, capillary beds, the smallest branches of arteries (*arterioles*) and initial venous channels (*venules*), are now commonly referred to as the *microvasculature*. Because the structure of the capillary is simpler than that of the other parts of the system, it has become customary to describe the capillaries first.

Capillaries

The capillaries are thin walled tubes with an average diameter of about 7 to 9 μm. They branch extensively without much change in caliber, and the branches anastomose to form networks which vary in density and pattern in different tissues and organs. The tissues with the highest metabolic activity have networks of elaborately branched and closely packed capillaries. This is so in the lungs, liver, kidney, and most glands and mucous membranes. The capillaries of the network nearest to the arterioles supplying them are called arterial capillaries, and those nearest to the venules draining them are called venous capillaries.

The capillary network between arterioles and venules often contains a *central* or *preferential channel*, where the blood flow is continuous, in contrast with the branches of the network, where the flow tends to be intermittent (Fig. 12.1). The proximal portion of the central channel, i.e., the part just beyond the arteriole proper, is known as a *metarteriole* (from the Greek *meta*, beyond). The metarteriole has isolated smooth muscle cells dispersed at intervals along the outer surface of its endothelial cells. These smooth muscle cells are surrounded by a glycoprotein coat which is continuous with the basal lamina of the

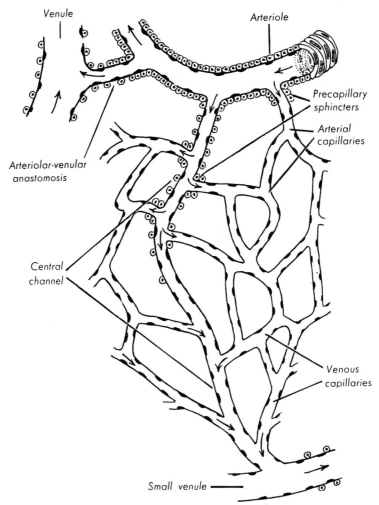

Figure 12.1. Diagram showing relationship of capillaries to arteriole and venule. The proximal portion of the central channel through a capillary bed is surrounded by scattered smooth muscle fibers and has been named the "metarteriole"; the distal portion of the central channel is structurally a true capillary.

endothelium. They have branching processes and tend to be oriented longitudinally on the vessel (Fig. 12.2), in contrast with the transversely oriented muscle cells of the arterioles proper (see Fig. 12.11). The venous end of the central channel resembles other capillaries except for its wider lumen.

The central channels differ from the branched portions of the capillary networks in their functional behavior, and they can be differentiated more readily in living than in fixed preparations. The preferential channels convey an active flow of blood at all times, although the amount of flow varies with vasoconstriction and vasodilation of the metarteriolar segment. Flow in the branches of the network is intermittent during relatively inactive metabolic periods; in other words, the branches do not all function at once, except when there is an increased demand. The amount of blood entering the branches is controlled by the state of contraction of smooth muscle cells of the *precapillary sphincters*, which are located where arterial capillaries arise from arterioles, whether from metarterioles or from arterioles proper. The number of preferential channels in proportion to the number of branched capillaries differs for different regions of the body; in skin, for example, the direct channels are numerous, whereas in skeletal muscle they are relatively infrequent in comparison with the branches of the meshwork.

The wall of the capillary is composed of a single layer of endothelial cells which

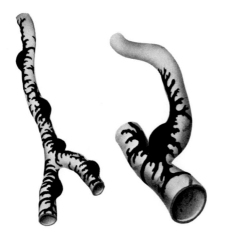

Figure 12.2. Modified smooth muscle cells on precapillary arterioles (metarterioles) of human heart. The cells and their processes are demonstrated by a chrome-silver impregnation method. *Left*, several muscle cells with their processes surrounding a metarteriole; *right*, higher magnification of one muscle cell at junction of metarteriole and capillary. (Redrawn and modified from Zimmermann KW: Der feinere Bau der Blutkapillaren. *Z Anat Entwicklungsmech* 68: 1923.)

rests on a basement membrane (basal lamina and lamina reticularis), plus a thin adventitia which consists of some connective tissue fibers along with a discontinuous layer of connective tissue cells. Two endothelial cells, and occasionally only one, generally suffice for the complete circumference of small capillaries, but three to five cells are often required for larger ones. In surface view, the endothelial cells are seen as a delicate mosaic when their cell boundaries are demonstrated by the precipitation of silver at the cell margins (Fig. 12.3). The cells usually have irregular borders and tend to be arranged with their long axes parallel with the long axes of the tubes. In routinely prepared sections for light microscopy, the cytoplasm appears clear or finely granular and the cells bulge into the lumen in the regions where the nuclei are located. This condition is generally accentuated by shrinkage of the vessels and their cells during fixation for light microscopy.

Electron micrographs of specially prepared tissue show that the endothelial cells have a thin glycoprotein layer over their luminal surface (*endocapillary layer*), some short microvilli, and the usual organelles, including a relatively small Golgi and some scattered mitochondria. They also have a variable number of specific granules of about 0.1 to 0.2 μm in diameter. These granules, like most organelles, are membrane-bounded and contain an electron-

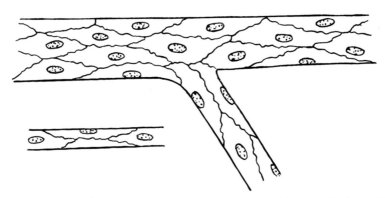

Figure 12.3. Surface view of large and small capillaries stained with silver nitrate and hematoxylin to show outlines of endothelial cells and their nuclei.

dense matrix which frequently contains some small tubular structures. The function of these granules has not been clearly defined. Electron micrographs also show that the capillary endothelial cells often have pinocytotic vesicles ranging in diameter from about 60 to 100 nm (see Fig. 12.5). Some of the vesicles are found entirely within the cell cytoplasm, whereas others are open either at the inner (luminal) surface or at the outer (tissue) side; the open vesicles are also known as *caveolae*. The view that pinocytotic vesicles function in transporting material, such as maromolecules, is supported by electron micrographs of tissues from animals which had received intravascular injections of colloidal particles which serve as markers. However, other mechanisms have a major role in the transport of substances across endothelium, as discussed below under "Structure and Function." It has also been proposed that caveolae may be involved in the elaboration of an endocapillary glycoportein substance and may serve as the site for enzymatic activation of angiotensin in the capillaries of the lung (see Chapters 17 and 18).

Adjacent endothelial cells may meet in a simple end-to-end pattern, but more often the edge of one cell overlaps that of another along an oblique course or in complicated S-shaped patterns. The walls of adjacent cells are separated from each other by about 20 nm along parts of their course, but at intervals they come into closer association by junctions which differ somewhat from the junctional complexes of simple columnar epitelium (Chapter 4). Fairly extensive areas of occluding junctions are present in cerebral capillaries and in the thymic cortex, but these junctions are less well developed in capillaries of other regions. Recent studies using freeze-fracture techniques show branching or staggered strands representing the occluding junctions, but no communicating (gap) junctions have been detected. The occluding junctions apparently do not form rings of complete occlusion at the adluminal ends of the cells.

Pericapillary cells are closely associated with the capillaries. This category includes *fibroblasts, macrophages* and *pericytes*. Fibroblasts and macrophages are present in the connective tissue associated with the capillaries in most parts of the body, but there are some locations where the capillaries are so closely related to the tissues with which they function that there is little or no intervening space for connective tissue. For instance, in the glomeruli of the kidney, the basal lamina of the endothelium is fused wtih the basal lamina of the epithelium of the visceral layer of Bowman's capsule. *Pericytes* are irregularly shaped, isolated cells distributed at intervals along the capillaries in a pattern resembling that of the modified muscle cells on metarterioles (Fig. 12.4). In transmission electron micrographs, the pericytes appear enclosed by the basal lamina of the endothelium because each pericyte is surrounded by an electron-dense coat which is continuous with the basal lamina portion of the endothelial cells (Fig. 12.5).

In the literature on capillaries, the term pericyte is sometimes used synonymously with Rouget cell. This is misleading because the cells described by Rouget (1875) as contractile units along vessels in the nictitating membrane of the frog eye in vivo were apparently smooth muscle cells on vessels that are now classified as metarterioles (Figs. 12.1 and 12.2). The cells currently identified as pericytes in electron micrographs are relatively undifferentiated in the sense that they apparently can develop into several different cell types, including smooth muscle. The endothelial cells themselves are contractile and can change their shape and reduce the diameter of the capillary lumen, but their contractility is not equivalent to that of smooth muscle.

Types of Capillaries

The vessels joining arterioles and venules can be divided into different categories on the basis of their ultrastructure and function as follows: (*a*) *continuous capillaries,*

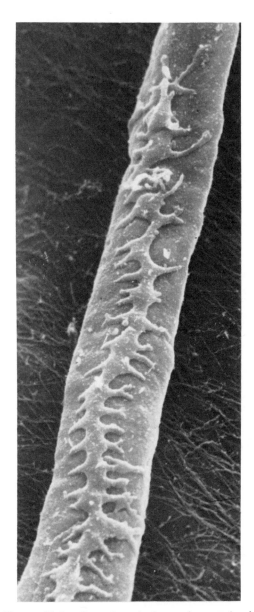

Figure 12.4. Scanning electron micrograph of pericytes on isolated capillary from rat skeletal muscle (×3700). (Courtesy of Dr. Rosemary Mazanet.)

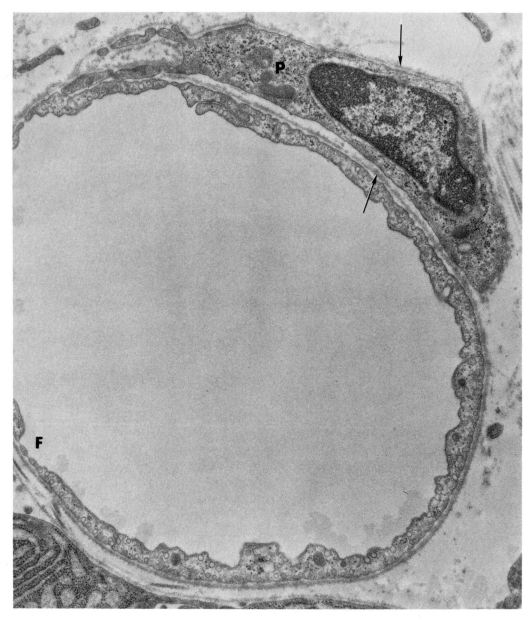

Figure 12.5. Electron micrograph of a capillary from monkey pancreas showing fenestrations (*F*) and a pericyte (*P*). Note the basal lamina on both sides of the pericyte (*arrows*) (×14,500).

(*b*) *fenestrated capillaries*, (*c*) *sinusoidal capillaries*, (*d*) *sinusoids*, and (*e*) *venous sinuses*.

In the *continous capillary*, there is a complete layer of cytoplasm throughout each endothelial cell (Fig. 12.6). This type is found in muscle and in many other locations. The *fenestrated capillary* differs from the continuous type in that its endothelial cells have numerous fenestrae of about 70 to 100 nm in diameter where the cytoplasm is absent and the cell wall consists solely of a porous diaphragm thinner than the cell membrane (Figs. 12.7 and 12.8). The fenestrae are not random in distribution but occur in patterns. This feature is best appreciated in freeze-fracture preparations where the fracture plane courses within the

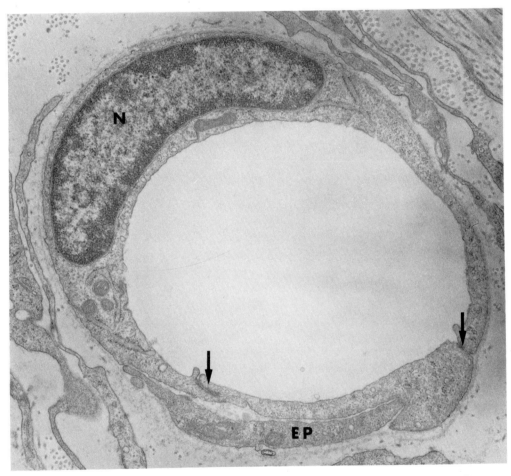

Figure 12.6. Electron micrograph of continuous type of capillary from the choroid tissue of hamster eye. The nucleus of an endothelial cell is at left (*N*). A process of overlapping endothelial cell appears at the bottom (*EP*) and junctions between endothelial cells are indicated at the *arrow* (×9,000). (Courtesy of Dr. Jen Yee Shen.)

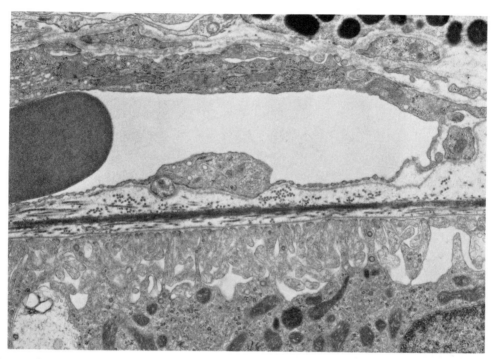

Figure 12.7. Section of a fenestrated capillary in the choriocapillaris of hamster eye. The pigment epithelium of the retina is at *bottom*. In this view the fenestrae are confined to the side of the capillary facing the pigment epithelium. A red blood cell is present in the capillary lumen. Pigment granules within a pigment cell of the choroid are seen at *upper right* (× 13,150). (Courtesy of Dr. Gregory Hageman.)

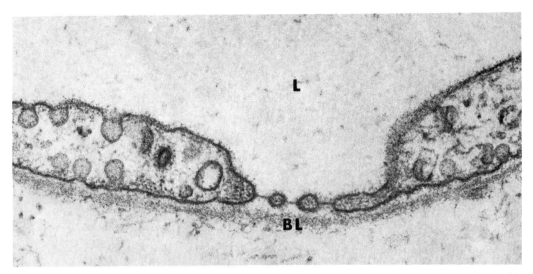

Figure 12.8. Electron micrograph of a fenestrated capillary wall showing fenestrae with a thin diaphragm and the continuous underlying basal lamina. L, lumen of capillary; BL, basal lamina (×67,500).

endothelial cell membrane to expose en face views of the fenestrae (Fig. 12.9). The cytoplasm of the endothelial cells of fenestrated capillaries also differs histochemically from that of the continuous capillaries of muscle in that it generally fails to show any alkaline phosphatase enzyme activity. The fenestrated type is found in locations known for their fluid transport, although fenestrae do not provide the only route for fluid transport. Good examples of this type of vessel are found in the intestinal villi, ciliary processes of the eye, and choroid plexuses. A special variety of the fenestrated type of endothelium is present in the glomerular capillaries of the kidney (Chapter 18).

Sinusoidal capillaries (in endocrine glands, carotid and aortic bodies) differ from both the continuous and fenestrated type in that they are wider and their basal and reticular laminae are less prominent (Fig. 21.6). Their fenestrae also may be somewhat larger than those of the fenestrated capillaries. They differ from sinusoids in that they have no intercellular gaps and no macrophages closely associated with their endothelial cells (Table 12.1).

The *sinusoids* of the liver and bone marrow differ from sinusoidal capillaries in a number of respects: they are wider, and their basal lamina is scanty and often absent (Fig. 12.10). The sinusoids of the liver also differ in that they have macrophages known as Kupffer cells closely associated with their endothelial cells (Chapter 16).

The *venous sinuses* of the spleen are wider than the sinusoids of the liver and differ in other respects, as listed in Table 12.1. They are described in detail in Chapter 14.

Correlation of Capillary Structure and Function

Exchange of substances between the blood vessels and surrounding tissues occurs chiefly in the capillaries and small venules. The passage of fluid across the capillary wall is partially dependent on the blood pressure within the capillaries and on the colloid osmotic pressure of the blood. The former factor promotes passage from the vessels to the tissues, and the latter factor favors reabsorption. The blood pressure in the arterial capillaries is normally higher than in the venous capillaries, and the blood pressure on the arterial side also exceeds the colloid osmotic pressure of the

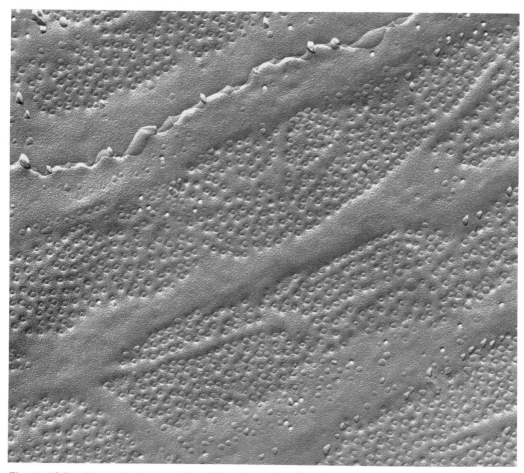

Figure 12.9. Freeze-fracture replica of fenestrated endothelium in the choriocapillaris of hamster eye. Irregular regions of thicker, nonfenestrated cytoplasm run between groups of fenestrae along the cell periphery where two adjacent endothelial cells abut. A boundary between two cells is seen running diagonally at the *upper left*. (×17,750). (Courtesy of Dr. Gregory Hageman.)

Table 12.1.
Diagnostic Properties of Blood Capillaries, Sinusoids, and Venous Sinuses

Parameter	Continuous Capillary	Fenestrated Capillary	Sinusoidal Capillary	Sinusoid	Venous Sinus
Cross sectional diameter	Small	Small	Intermediate	Large	Larger
Regularity of cross section	Regular	Regular	Variable	Irregular	Variable
Intercellular gaps	Absent	Absent	Absent	Present and variable	Variable
Fenestrations	Absent	Numerous	Numerous and larger	Variable	Absent
Basal lamina	Prominent and continuous	Prominent and continuous	Continuous	Scanty or absent	Dicontinuous
Lamina reticularis	Prominent	Prominent	Variable	Absent	Variable
Avid macrophages associated with endothelium	Absent	Absent	Absent	Common	Questionable

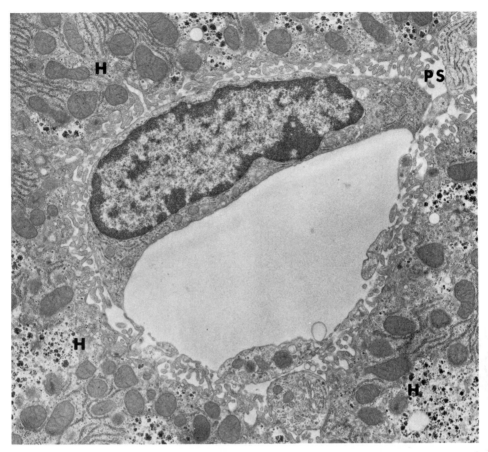

Figure 12.10. Electron micrograph of a portion of a hepatic sinusoid showing the discontinuous or fenestrated endothelial lining. There is no basal lamina beneath the endothelium in this region. *H*, hepatic cells; *PS*, perisinusoidal space (×7750).

blood plasma. Based on the pressure relationships, fluids normally pass by diffusion from the vessels to the tissues in the arterial part of the capillary bed and return to the vessels via the venous capillaries, small venules, and lymphatic channels. Pressure within the capillaries can be modified at the local level by vasoconstriction and vasodilation through contraction and relaxation of smooth muscle cells in the walls of arterioles, metarterioles, and precapillary sphincters (Fig. 12.1).

Electron microscope studies of tissues fixed after transfusion of substances of different molecular weight (e.g., horseradish peroxidase, molecular weight 40,000, and ferritin, molecular weight 500,000) have provided a better understanding of the permeability of vessels of different regions. It is known, for example, that the cerebral capillaries which have occluding junctions and relatively few pinocytotic vesicles are impermeable to macromolecules and also to horseradish peroxidase, which has a low molecular weight and a diameter of only about 5 nm. At the other extreme of permeability, there are the sinusoids of the liver and bone marrow and the venous sinuses of the spleen, which have relatively wide spaces between the cells, large and irregularly distributed fenestrations, and no or only an incomplete basal lamina; these permit the passage of larger molecules and even whole cells such as erythrocytes.

As already mentioned, the majority of the capillaries of the body lack well developed occluding junctions; in these, the exchange between the blood vessels and the surrounding tissue can occur via intercellular clefts plus pinocytotic vesicles, fenestrae, or both, according to the type of endothelium. Some authors assign a major role to the pinocytotic vesicles, but some studies have shown that the amount of fluid transported across the endothelium in a given period of time greatly exceeds the amount that can be accounted for by the number of pinocytotic vesicles present. Fluid exchange apparently occurs chiefly by the intercellular clefts. When vascular permeability is increased by injections of substances such as histamine and endotoxin, relatively large intercellular gaps appear in the endothelium of the venous capillaries and small venules. This is correlated with an even more sporadic occurrence of occluding junctions than is found in the nonstimulated capillaries. Under conditions of inflammation, substances pass from the blood to the surrounding tissues chiefly on the venous side of the capillary bed.

Lipid-soluble substances such as oxygen and carbon dioxide can readily diffuse through the endothelial cell membrane. Lipid-insoluble substances are transported across the endothelial cells by routes described by physiologists as a *small pore system* for low molecular weight substances such as water and a *large pore system* for macromolecules. The pinocytotic vesicles may represent the small pore system in part, but, as noted above, the amount of water transported over a given period of time in some tissues greatly exceeds the amount that could be accounted for by the number of pinocytotic vesicles present.

Considerable evidence has accumulated in support of the view that fluid transport across the capillaries of muscle, for example (continuous endothelium), is via the intercellular clefts of about 15 to 20 nm in width and that these correspond to the large pore system described by physiologists. The

equivalent of the small pore system is not known for capillaries with continuous endothelium. It has been reported, however, that in some vessels the pinocytotic vesicles may fuse to form patent transendothelial channels that could correspond to the small pore system. The cytological equivalents of the pore systems in fenestrated capillaries are more straightforward. The fenestrae are all permeable to smaller molecules (less than 10 nm) and a subpopulation of fenestrae seems to be permeable to larger molecules.

Despite the fact that the movement of many substances across capillary endothelium can be explained by invoking pore systems with specific limiting dimensions, the actual mechanisms for controlling permeability are undoubtedly far more complex. For example, recent studies show that chemically differentiated microdomains occur on the luminal and abluminal surfaces of certain endothelial cells and these apparently impart a degree of selectivity to the movement of components from vascular to interstitial space or vice versa. Subtle chemical alterations in these microdomains may be capable of producing marked differences in permeability without obvious morphological change. Thus, as more information on the molecular organization of endothelia becomes available, the controversy over pore system equivalency seems likely to subside in favor of consideration of regulating mechanisms at the molecular level.

Arteries

As mentioned previously, the walls of capillaries are composed mainly of endothelium, but scattered perivascular cells and a delicate connective tissue framework are also present. In larger vessels, the accessory cells and connective tissue become organized so that three tunics or coats become recognizable. These coats are most distinct in arteries of medium caliber. The innermost coat, the *intima*, consists of an endothelial lining continuous with that found in the walls of the capillaries, an intermediate layer of delicate connective tissue, which is absent in the smaller vessels, and an external layer of elastic fibers, the *internal elastic lamina*, which marks the boundary between the intima and media. The middle coat, or *media*, consists mainly of smooth muscle cells with varying numbers of elastic and collagenous fibers. The outer coat, *adventitia* or *externa*, is composed chiefly of connective tissue.

The structure and relative thickness of each of the tunics varies according to the size of the artery. Although the changes along the arterial tree are gradual and never abrupt, one may readily distinguish different types of arteries according to size, structure, and function. Following the blood vessels from the heart to the capillaries, it is customary to recognize (*a*) large, elastic arteries, (*b*) medium-sized, muscular arteries, and (*c*) small arteries and arterioles. Working backward from the capillaries which have been described, the structure of the arterioles will be considered first.

Arterioles and Small Arteries

The transition from a capillary to an arteriole is marked by the appearance of isolated smooth muscle fibers which are arranged spirally. These small arterioles of transitional type are called precapillary arterioles or metarterioles (Fig. 12.1). As the vessels become larger, the muscle cells increase in number and form a complete coat of one or two layers (Figs. 12.11 and 12.12). Outside of the muscle, the connective tissue is condensed to form a fibrous layer which is composed of flattened fibroblasts and

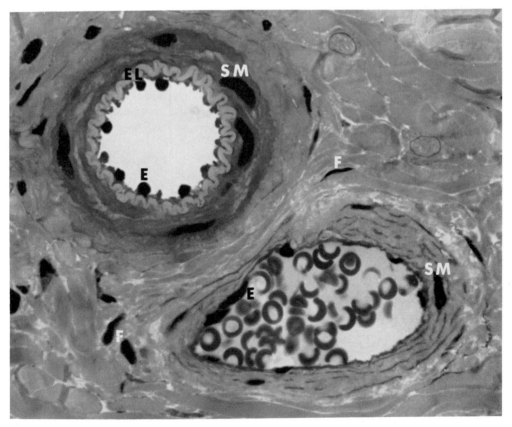

Figure 12.11. Light micrograph showing a cross section of an arteriole and venule from monkey connective tissue. The venule contains red blood cells in its lumen. *E*, endothelial nuclei; *SM*, smooth muscle nuclei; *EL*, internal elastic lamina; *F*, fibroblast nuclei (×1020).

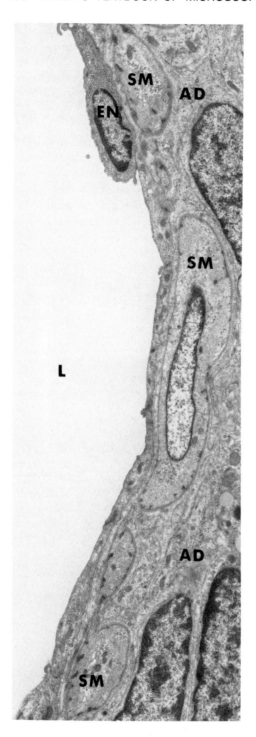

Figure 12.12. Portion of wall of an arteriole from hamster ovary. The lumen (*L*) is lined by endothelium; one edothelial cell nucleus (*EN*) is visible in this plane of section. Smooth muscle cell processes (*SM*) are sectioned obliquely. Adventitial cells underlie the smooth muscle (*AD*) (×6750). (Courtesy of Dr. Gregory Hageman.)

longitudinally arranged collagenous fibrils. Thus, in the walls of the arterioles, the three coats are already distinguishable: an endothelial intima, a muscular media, and an adventitia of connective tissue. Although a few scattered elastic fibers can be demonstrated in the walls of very small arterioles, an internal elastic membrane sufficiently thick to be visible under the light microscope does not begin until the vessels have reached a diameter of about 40 μm.

The endothelial cells often have footlike processes that extend through the basal lamina and the internal elastic lamina to make contact with the innermost layer of smooth muscle cells of the media; these are known as *myoendothelial junctions*. They are also present, but less numerous, in the medium-sized and large arteries. It has been suggested that they facilitate metabolic or informational exchange between the lumina of the vessels and the muscle cells of the media.

The coats of the vessels increase in thickness and become more organized as the vessels increase in caliber. In vessels of about 130 μm in diameter, the media has three or four layers of muscle cells and a more prominent elastic lamina. When the vessels reach a diameter of about 300 μm, their walls show all of the structural features of medium-sized vessels.

Some authors use the term arteriole for small arteries ranging in caliber from about 300 μm to the very small precapillary vessels. Under this definition, the term arteriole encompasses most of the small, unnamed arteries and consists of vessels in which the tunica media ranges in thickness from one to several layers of muscle cells. Other authors use the term arteriole for vessels which have only one or two layers of muscle cells (Fig. 12.1) and the term small artery, for vessels which connect the arterioles proper with the medium-sized or muscular arteries. The latter usage seems preferable.

The arterioles regulate distribution of blood to different capillary beds by vasoconstriction or vasodilation in localized regions. Widespread vasoconstriction or vasodilation of the arterioles alters the peripheral resistance to flow from the larger arteries and hence plays an important part in regulating blood pressure. The arterioles and small arteries are structurally adapted for vasoconstriction and vasodilation, because their walls are composed primarily of circularly arranged muscle fibers which are controlled by the autonomic nervous system. Elasticity is not as important in these vessels as in the larger arteries, in which the blood pressure is much higher. Arterioles are not directly involved in interchange between blood and tissue fluids, and the walls are relatively impermeable. This is accompanied by well developed occluding junctions between the endothelial cells. Hence, the sparseness of elastic tissue and the presence of well developed occluding junctions in arterioles are examples of correlation between structure and function.

Medium-Sized Arteries

These include all of the named arteries of gross dissections except the very large ones. There is a gradual transition between the branches of the medium-sized arteries and the small arteries described above. Examples of medium-sized arteries are the radial, tibial, popliteal, axillary, splenic, mesenteric, and intercostal arteries. The walls of these blood vessels are relatively thick, mainly as a result of the large amount of muscle in the media (Fig. 12.13). They are therefore called *muscular* arteries, in contrast with the *elastic* arteries like the aorta, in the wall of which elastic tissue predominates. The muscular arteries have also been called *distributing* arteries because they distribute the blood to different organs and, by contraction or relaxation, aid in regulating the supply to different regions in response to different functional demands.

The *intima* of the medium-sized arteries is composed of three layers: *endothelium*, *intermediate layer*, and *internal elastic lamina*. The endothelial layer is simlar to that described above for small arteries. The intermediate layer consists of delicate collag-

enous fibers and a few elastic fibers embedded in a connective tissue matrix. Isolated and longitudinally oriented smooth muscle fibers are present in the intermediate layer, especially in places where the vessels branch. Some of these were mistakenly identified by light microscopists as fibroblasts, but electron micrographs show practically no fibroblasts within the intima of normal vessels. Prominent bundles of longitudinally oriented smooth muscle fibers are present in the intima of some of the larger muscular arteries (femoral, popliteal, axillary, hepatic, splenic, renal, and coronary).

The *internal elastic lamina* of the medium-sized artery is a fenestrated band of closely interwoven elastic fibers. In the smaller vessels of this type, the internal elastic layer is prominent and often split into a double membrane. It is closely connected with the media and marks the boundary between the latter and the intima. This membrane often shows longitudinal folds in sections of fixed tissue; this is due chiefly to the postmortem contraction of the smooth muscle of the vessels.

The *media* is the thickest coat, consisting of 25 to 40 layers of circularly disposed muscle fibers. The thickness of the muscle coat is to some extent proportional to the size of the vessel, but there are considerable variations in arteries of the same size. Between the layers of muscle, there are small amounts of connective tissue composed of elastic, collagenous, and reticular fibers. Because there are apparently no fibroblasts within the media, it is assumed that the connective tissue fibers of this layer are formed by the smooth muscle cells. Furthermore, the intercellular proteoglycans are apparently also formed by the smooth muscle cells.

The smooth muscle cells of the medium-sized arteries, like those of other types of arteries, are in communication with each other by means of gap junctions, described in Chapters 4 and 8. Because most of the neuromotor nerve fibers terminate in the outermost part of the media and in the adjacent adventitia, the effect of the neu-

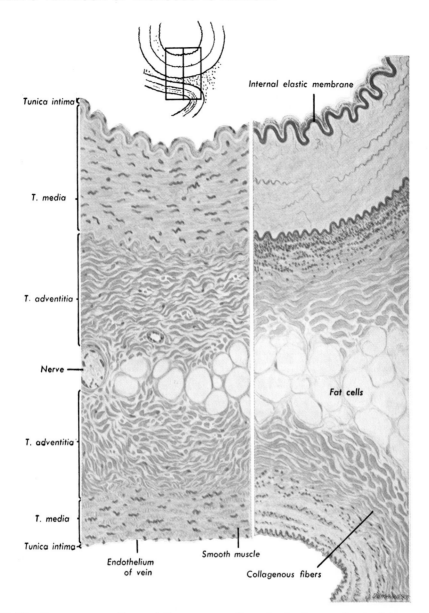

Figure 12.13. Two cross sections of the same medium-sized artery and vein (intercostal artery *above*, vein *below*). The *line drawing* at *upper left* gives orientation of regions drawn. Section on the *left* is stained with hematoxylin-eosin, that on the *right* with resorcin-fuchsin to show elastic tissue. *T*, tunica (×215).

rotransmitter substances on the innermost layers of the media may be via the gap junctions of the muscle fibers as well as by diffusion via intercellular substance.

The amount and distribution of elastic tissue in the media are closely correlated with the caliber of the vessel. In the smaller vessels, the elastic fibers are scattered be-

tween the muscle cells, but in the larger vessels they form circularly oriented elastic nets together with a few radially oriented fibers. In the larger vessels of the group there is a fenstrated membrane or network of elastic tissue, the *external elastic lamina*, at the junction of the media with the ad-ventitia (Fig. 12.13). The largest vessels of

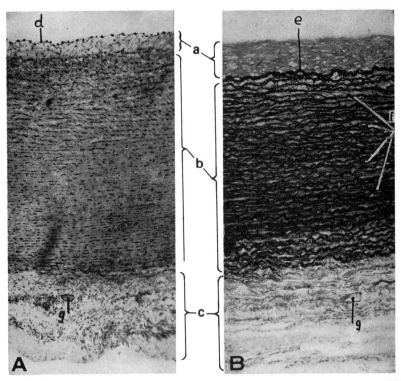

Figure 12.14. Cross section through internal carotid artery. Retouched photograph (×85). A stained with hematoxylin-eosin; B with resorcin-fuchsin; a, intima; b, media; c, adventitia; d, endothelium; e, internal elastic lamina; f, elastic lamina in media; g, vasa vasorum.

the group contain circularly disposed fenestrated membranes of elastic tissue (Fig. 12.14); hence, these vessels are transitional between the muscular and elastic types in structure.

The *adventitia* is a coat of considerable thickness, occasionally as thick as the media. It is composed of connective tissue containing collagenous and elastic fibers, most of which course longitudinally. The elastic fibers are concentrated in the inner layer of the coat, where they form a coarse network. The outer layer of the adventitia blends gradually with the surrounding connective tissue which attaches the artery to other structures.

A few longitudinal smooth muscle fibers are occasionally found in the inner layer of the adventitia, between the elastic fibers. In some arteries (splenic, dorsalis penis), bundles of longitudinally disposed muscle fibers occur in close proximity to the media.

Large Arteries

The large arteries belong to the *elastic* type. They have also been called *conducting arteries*, because they conduct the blood from the heart to the medium-sized distributing arteries. The walls of these vessels are relatively thin in proportion to their diameter; this is accompanied by an increase in elastic tissue and a decrease in smooth muscle. Whereas the various elements are generally arranged either circularly or longitudinally in the medium-sized arteries, they tend to follow a spiral course in the large arteries. The aorta is the chief representative of this group (Fig. 12.15). Other vessels of the type include the innominate, common carotid, subclavian, vertebral, and common iliac arteries. The transition in histological structure from large arteries to those of the medium-sized (muscular) type is gradual rather than abrupt.

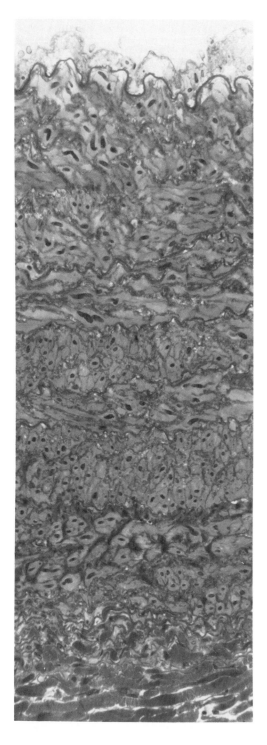

Figure 12.15. Cross section of wall of abdominal aorta showing entire thickness. The lumen and tunica intima are at the *top* and the adventitia is at the *bottom*. Smooth muscle fibers and elastic tissue are irregularly disposed in the thick tunica media occupying most of the field (×400).

The *intima* is thicker in large arteries than in the other types, and is lined by endothelial cells which tend to be short and polygonal in shape. The connective tissue immediately beneath the endothelium is composed of fine collagenous fibers together with some elastic fibers. The deeper portion of the intima contains connective tissue fibers and a few longitudinally oriented smooth muscle fibers (Fig. 12.15). The amount of elastic tissue and the character of the internal elastic lamina change with age. Because the inner elastic lamina is usually split into two or more lamellae which merge with other similar layers in both the intima and the media, it is difficult precisely to identify this lamina in the aorta.

The *media* is distinguished by numerous fenestrated elastic sheets which course spirally and anastomose to form complex nets. The elastic layer at the junction of the media with the adventitia does not differ from the elastic tissue found throughout the media; hence it is not as clearly demarcated as the external elastic lamina of medium-sized arteries. The narrow spaces between the lamellae are permeated by a finer elastic network, in the meshes of which the muscle fibers are contained. The muscle tissue is greatly reduced in amount, and its fibers are short, flat cells of irregular outline. They unite to form branching bands which, like the elastic lamellae, pursue a spiral course. The muscle fibers are surrounded and supported by a small amount of collagenous and reticular fibers.

The *adventitia* is a thin coat consisting of connective tissue composed mostly of collagenous fibers arranged in longitudinal spirals. It contains relatively few elastic fibers. A few longitudinally arranged smooth muscle fibers are occasionally found in the adventitia of some of the large arteries. A few ganglion cells are also occasionally present.

Because the blood is propelled through the blood vessels by the rhythmic contractions of the heart, the rate of flow is not uniform. When the heart contracts and forces blood into the aorta, the walls of the elastic arteries stretch and a part of the force of the beat is converted into potential energy in the form of increased elastic tension. During diastole of the ventricles, the potential energy of the expanded arterial walls is transformed into kinetic energy, which keeps the blood moving forward. Thus, the elasticity of the large arteries makes the blood flow less irreguarly than it would if the vessels were rigid tubes. The most marked irregularity is found at the beginning of the arterial system; the flow becomes more uniform in the terminal parts of the arterial system.

Special Forms of Arteries

There are certain arteries which exhibit pronounced structural peculiarities. The *cerebral* and *dural* arteries, which are protected from external mechanical forces, are thin-walled for their caliber. They have a well developed internal elastic lamina but almost no elastic fibers in the media. The adventitia is poorly developed and consists mainly of collagenous fiber bundles.

The arteries of the *lung* have thin walls, owing to a reduction of both muscle and elastic tissue. This is probably associated with the lower blood pressure in the pulmonary circulation.

In the *penile* and *pudic* arteries, a hyperplasia of the intima and media manifests itself after puberty, whereas the adventitia remains relatively thin. The intima especially becomes greatly thickened and contains many longitudinal muscle fibers in its outer layer.

The *umbilical* arteries have a media composed of two muscle layers, an inner longitudinal and an outer circular. The internal elastic lamina is indistinct and missing in some places. A true adventitia is lacking in the segment within the umbilical cord and is poorly developed in the intraabdominal segment.

Aging of the Arteries

The arteries undergo age changes which differ in type and degree in different vessels of the same individual. The elastic arteries, especially the aorta, show more changes than do the muscular arteries of the extremities such as the femoral or brachial. Particularly pronounced and early changes occur in the arteries of the brain and heart.

In a 4-month-old human fetus, the aorta has a tunica intima composed only of endothelium and one elastic lamina. By the end of fetal life, the internal elastic lamina has become thicker, and after birth it splits into two or more layers. Additional elastic and collagenous fibers develop between the endothelium and internal elastic lamina, and the elastic layers of the media also increase in number. The layers of the aorta are not completely differentiated until about 25 years of age. It is difficult to separate some of the final stages of differentiation from regressive changes resulting from use. In fact, some authors think that arteriosclerosis may be a physiological rather than a pathological process. In the aging process, the tunica intima becomes thicker, the elastic layers of the media change chemically and become less elastic, and fat gradually accumulates between the elastic and collagenous fibers.

The anterior descending branch of the left coronary artery furnishes another example of age changes. In this vessel, the internal elastic lamina is already split at the time of birth, definite hyperplasia of the elastic tissue occurs during the first decade, and calcification of the media begins in the third decade. Similar changes in another branch of the coronary arteries— the posterior descending branch of the right coronary—do not occur until considerably later. The calcification of the media is one of the main changes in the arteries of muscular type.

The Carotid and Aortic Bodies

These structures were once included with the endocrine system because their cells were erroneously thought to resemble those of the paraganglia and adrenal medulla. They have been described subsequently as chemoreceptors because their secretory activity changes in response to changes in O_2 and CO_2 in the blood.

The *carotid bodies* are small, paired organs located near or in the bifurcation of each common carotid artery. They have an abundant vascular supply and contain numerous sinusoidal capillaries. The *glomus cells* (principal cells of the globular shaped organs) show no particularly distinguishing characteristics in the usual hematoxylin and eosin-stained sections, but they have cytoplasmic granules which stain well with neutral red and with other basic dyes. Two main types of cells can be identified in electron micrographs. The *type I glomus cell* is the most numerous. It is relatively large and has a rounded nucleus and numerous membrane-bounded dense-cored granules that are relatively small. The *type II glomus cell* is less numerous and has an oval-shaped nucleus with rather densely staining heterochromatin and few or no cytoplasmic granules.

The type I cells are generally described as secretory units, with type II cells serving in a supporting role. However, there have been numerous questions about the manner in which the type I cells work. For example, because the type I cells lose their ability to respond to changes in O_2 tension and degenerate after the carotid body branch of the 9th cranial nerve is cut, it is evident that they are supplied with efferent nerve endings rather than solely with afferents as once believed. Furthermore, electron micrographs show that the nerve endings on the type I cells have the cytological characteristics of efferents. Recent electron microscope studies explain some of these supposed contradictions by showing that the nerve fibers of the type I cells have synapses of both afferent and efferent types. The nerve endings are cup-shaped and fit closely around the basal end of the cell. Whether the afferent or efferent synaptic endings predominate in function depends on the proportion of O_2 and CO_2 in the blood. When the blood vessels of the medullary region of the brain which function in respiratory control are carrying blood with a normal level of O_2 (normoxia), the glomus cells secrete dopamine at a high level. Under these conditions, the afferent synapses discharge spontaneously, i.e., they are en-

dogenously active, and their rate of discharge is controlled by an inhibitory feedback mechanism. When the O_2 tension of the blood is low (hypoxia), there is a decrease in the inhibitory feedback mechanism and also a stimulus of the efferent synapses which release a different neurotransmitter, perhaps acetycholine.

The *aortic bodies* have not been studied as extensively as the carotid bodies, but apparently they function in the same manner, i.e., as sensors for responding to changes in oxygen tension in the blood. In the rabbit, where the structure and innervation of these bodies has been studied in some detail, the right aortic body is in the angle formed by the subclavian and common carotid, whereas the left aortic body is closely applied to the roof of the arch of the aorta. The aortic bodies are innervated by a branch of the 10th cranial nerve.

The Carotid Sinus

This sinus is an enlargement at the bifurcation of each common carotid. In this region, the media of the wall of the artery is relatively thin and the adventitial layer has a rich supply of specialized sensory nerve endings derived from the carotid sinus branch of the glossopharyngeal nerve. The nerves have reticulated swollen endings in contact with the cells of the adventitial layer. They are stimulated by distention of the vessel wall (by an increase in blood pressure), and they bring about reflex dilation of splanchnic vessels, slowing of the heart, and a fall in systemic blood pressure.

Veins

The caliber of veins is as a rule larger than that of arteries, but their walls are much thinner because of a great reduction of the muscular and elastic elements. The collagenous connective tissue, on the other hand, is present in much larger amounts and constitutes the bulk of the wall. The relatively sparse circular muscle of the media is more loosely arranged and separated into layers by abundant collagenous fibers. The internal elastic lamina is not a compact fenestrated layer, but rather consists of a network of elastic fibers which becomes distinct only in the larger veins. The three coats—intima, media, and adventitia—are present, but their boundaries are often indistinct. The entire wall is flabbier and more loosely organized than in arteries, and it tends to collapse when not filled with blood.

A histological classification of veins is difficult, as their structure varies extensively. The variations are not always related to the size of the vessels, but rather depend on local mechanical conditions. A description of the venous wall can therefore enumerate only the most general features.

Small Veins

The transition from capillary to vein is gradual, the connective tissue elements appearing first and the smooth muscle cells somewhat later. The smallest veins (*venules*) are endothelial tubes surrounded by an outer sheath of collagenous fibrils with a few fibroblasts. A few intervening pericytes may occur. These vessels are highly permeable and are important sites of exchange between blood and tissue fluids. Occluding junctions are poorly developed between their endothelial cells. Postcapillary (high endothelium) venules have a special morphology and functional significance in many of the lymphatic tissues (see Chapter 14).

Isolated, circularly disposed muscle fibers make their appearance in vessels of 40 to 50 μm, although the presence of muscle fibers is variable and is not always dependent on caliber. In venules of 0.2 to 0.3 mm, the circular muscle fibers form a continuous layer and the adventitia is a relatively thick coat of longitudinally disposed collagenous fibers and a few scattered elastic fibrils.

Medium-Sized Veins

This category includes most of the veins of gross anatomy, with the exception of the main venous trunks (large veins) of the thoracic and abdominal cavities.

The *intima* is a thin layer (Fig. 12.13)

consisting of (*a*) an endothelial lining and (*b*) a delicate subendothelial zone of thin bundles of collagenous fibers interspersed with a few elastic fibers which form an internal elastic lamina in the larger vessels of this category.

The *media* is considerably thinner than that of a corresponding medium-sized artery and consists chiefly of circularly arranged smooth muscle fibers interspersed with collagenous fibers and a few elastic fibers. The latter are often arranged longitudinally and are particularly distinct in the outer portion of the media when the tissue is appropriately stained for elastic tissue (Fig. 12.13). The media is thickest in the veins of the lower extremity and thin in the veins of the head and abdomen.

The *adventitia* is well developed and forms the bulk of the wall. It consists of collagenous and elastic tissue and often contains a few bundles of longitudinally oriented muscle fibers.

Large Veins

In the large venous trunks of the thoracic and abdominal cavities the tunica media is relatively thin and poorly defined, whereas the adventitia is relatively thick. The media contains numerous collagenous fibers, a few elastic fibers, and scattered smooth muscle fibers that tend to be circularly arranged. The adventitia contains numerous bundles of longitudinally oriented smooth muscle fibers intermingled with irregularly distributed collagenous and elastic fibers (Figs. 12.16 and 12.17). Unusually stout bundles of longitudinally oriented muscle fibers are found in the portal vein and hepatic portion of the inferior vena cava. The category of large veins includes the superior and inferior venae cavae, the innominates, the internal jugulars, and the portal, splenic, azygos, superior mesenteric, renal, adrenal, and external iliac veins.

Special Features of Certain Veins

Very little or no muscle whatever is found in the following veins: the subpapillary veins ("giant capillaries") of the skin and nail bed, the trabecular veins of the spleen,

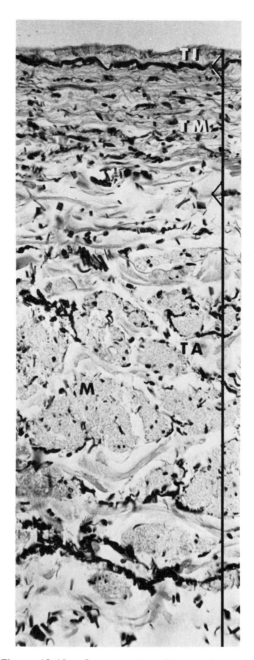

Figure 12.16. Cross section of human femoral vein stained for elastic tissue. The tunica intima (*TI*) (*top*) is separated from the tunica media (*TM*) by a fairly prominent internal elastic membrane. The tunica adventitia (*TA*) contains longitudinally oriented smooth muscle bundles (*M*) interspersed with elastic and collagenous fibers. The tunica media is poorly developed. The *open pyramids* (*top right*) indicate approximate boundaries of the tunica media (×395).

Smooth muscle   Leaflet of valve

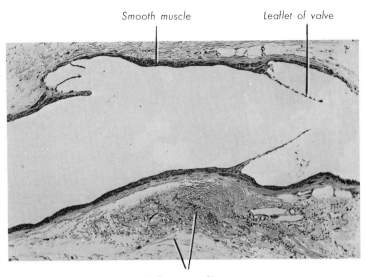

Collagenous fibers

Figure 12.17. Longitudinal section of a vein from human subcutaneous tissue showing valves. The valve at *upper left* is in a small tributary which curves out of the plane of the section. A part of the lower leaflet of the valve at *right* is enlarged in Figure 12.19. Photomicrograph (×84).

the dural sinuses, most pial and cerebral veins, the veins of the retina and of the bones, and the deeper veins of the maternal placenta.

Especially rich in muscle are the veins of the gravid uterus, which contain muscle fibers in all three coats. The umbilical vein has an inner longitudinal and outer circular muscle layer. The latter is occasionally interspersed with longitudinally oriented muscle fibers.

Longitudinal smooth muscle fibers are found in the intima of the saphenous, popliteal, femoral, basilic, cephalic, median, internal jugular, umbilical, and some mesenteric veins, and in the veins of the gravid uterus.

Near their entrance into the heart, the adventitia of the venae cavae and pulmonary veins is invested with a layer of cardiac muscle, the fibers coursing spirally or circularly around the tube.

Valves

Veins over 2 mm in diameter are provided at intervals with valves (Figs. 12.17 and 12.18). These are semilunar flaps or pockets which project into the lumen, their free margin being directed toward the heart. As the blood flows toward the heart, it flattens the flaps against the wall and thus passes without obstruction, but if it starts to flow in the reverse direction, the valves float up, approach each other, and occlude the cavity.

The valves are derived from the intima and consist of connective tissue covered by a layer of endothelium. Beneath the endothelium of the surface of the valve directed against the blood current is a rich network of elastic fibers continuous with the elastic tissue of the intima. The connective tissue of the side facing the wall of the vein is entirely free from or contains but few elastic fibers. Adjacent to the valve, on the side toward the heart, the wall of the vein is usually distended and thin; this region is called the *sinus of the valve*. The smooth muscle of the vein at the base of the valve and along the sinus region runs mostly in a longitudinal or spiral direction. Valves are especially numerous and strong in the larger veins of the lower extremities. They are absent from the veins of the brain and

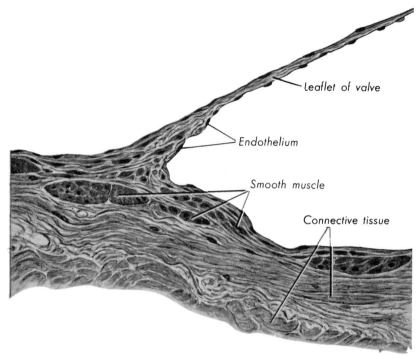

Figure 12.18. Higher magnification drawing of a part of the valve of the vein shown in Figure 12.14 (×447).

spinal cord and their meninges as well as from the umbilical vein, most of the visceral veins, with the exception of some branches of the portal, and the superior and inferior venae cavae and their branches.

Portal Vessels

In most parts of the body, arteries are connected with veins via capillary plexuses. Modifications of this pattern occur in some locations in adaptation to special functions. When capillaries lead to vessels which in turn supply a second set of capillaries (or sinusoids) before returning the blood to the systemic veins, the arrangement of vessels is known as a *portal system*. The liver is an example of an organ having a *venous portal system*. In this instance, the portal vein receives blood by its tributaries from the capillaries of most of the abdominal viscera and empties into the hepatic sinusoids that lead to the hepatic veins. The anterior pituitary gland is also served by a venous portal system. Capillaries from the infundibulum drain into veins which supply the sinusoidal capillaries of the anterior lobe.

The kidney glomerulus is an example of an *arterial portal system*, with a capillary plexus between arteries. In this case, afferent glomerular arterioles supply glomerular capillaries which drain into efferent glomerular arterioles and thence to a capillary plexus around the uriniferous tubules.

Arteriovenous Anastomoses

In addition to the capillary and sinusoidal connections of vessels already described, arteries sometimes empty directly into veins—*arteriovenous anastomoses*. Such connections may be found in pathological conditions resulting from injury, in vascular neoplasms, and in developmental anomalies. They also occur normally in certain parts of the body. They are especially numerous in the sole of the foot, in the palm of the hand, in the skin of the terminal phalanges, and in the nail bed. The arteriovenous anastomoses are usually surrounded by a connective tissue sheath, and the arterioles generally follow a convoluted course, forming a structure known as a *glomus* (Chapter 15). The smooth muscle fibers are modified in shape and structure and are epithelioid in appearance.

When the arteriovenous anastomoses are open, they shunt a considerable amount of blood directly into the veins and decrease the flow through adjacent arterioles leading to the capillary bed, but in the normal behavior of the peripheral vessels they are contracted a large part of the time.

Blood Vessels, Lymphatics, and Nerves of the Blood Vessels

Vasa Vasorum

Arteries and veins with a diameter over 1 mm are supplied with small nutrient blood vessels, the *vasa vasorum*. These vessels branch and form capillary networks within the adventitia. Branches also continue into the deepest layers of the media of the veins, whereas they penetrate only to the periphery of the media in arteries. The exchange of metabolites between the cells of the tunica media of arteries and the plasma of blood vessels is by diffusion through the interstitial material of the media. This exchange can be made with the blood within the capillaries of the tunica adventitia and also with the blood within the lumen of the artery itself.

Lymphatics

Lymphatics have been found in the adventitia of many of the larger arteries and veins. Extensive *perivascular lymph spaces* surround the thin-walled blood vessels of the pia-arachnoid of the brain and spinal cord.

Nerves

The walls of blood vessels have a rich nerve supply. The nerve fibers are mainly unmyelinated axons from sympathetic ganglia and are known as vasomotor nerves because they control the caliber of the blood vessel. The fibers form a plexus in the adventitia and terminate chiefly within the peripheral portion of the media, where they have delicate knoblike endings associated with the muscle fibers. Neurotransmitter substances released at the nerve endings may reach the more deeply situated muscle cells by diffusion through the intercellular material. The gap junctions between the muscle fibers may also transmit responses from the outer layers of muscle cells to those situated closer to the lumen.

Besides the vasomotor nerves, the blood vessels receive myelinated sensory nerve fibers which are the peripheral axons of spinal or cranial ganglion cells. The larger fibers run in the connective tissue surrounding the blood vessel. They enter the adventitia, divide repeatedly, lose their myelin sheaths, and terminate in free sensory endings.

The Heart

The heart is a pump for propelling the blood through the blood vessels. It is composed of four chambers in the following sequence in relation to blood flow: (*a*) the *right atrium* receives venous blood from the superior and inferior venae cavae and from the coronary sinus; (*b*) the *right ventricle* receives blood from the right atrium through the right atrioventricular (AV) orifice, which is guarded by the tricuspid valve, and it pumps blood into the pulmonary artery; (*c*) the *left atrium* receives blood from the pulmonary veins and opens into the left ventricle via the left AV orifice guarded by the bicuspid (mitral) valve (Fig. 12.19); and (*d*) the *left ventricle* pumps blood into the aorta.

Although the different chambers of the heart vary to some extent in their microscopic structure, the arrangement of tissues in each conforms to a general plan. The wall of each chamber consists of three layers: an inner layer or *endocardium*, a middle layer or *myocardium*, and an outer layer or *epicardium*. The myocardium forms the main mass of the heart.

Endocardium

The endocardium is a glistening layer covering the inner surface of the atria and ventricles. It is thick in the atria, especially in the left atrium, and thin in the ventricles; this explains the whiter color of the inside of the atria as contrasted with the red appearance of the inside of the ventricles, where the color of the cardiac muscle shows more obviously through the thin endocardium. At the arterial and venous orifices,

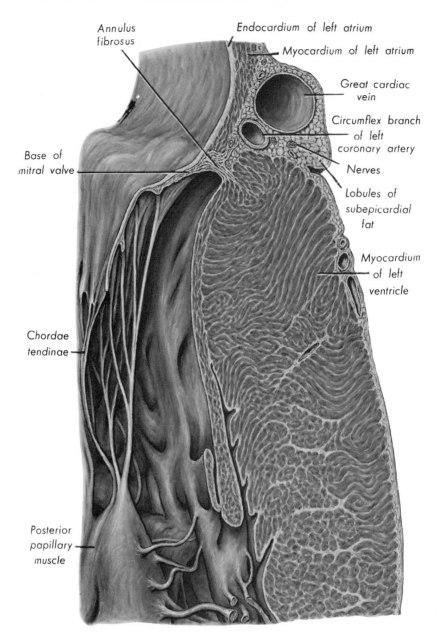

Figure 12.19. Low power three-dimensional view of the zone of junction of the left atrium with the left ventricle in the human heart. The region illustrated is from the posterior part of the heart and shows the posterior papillary muscle and the posterior cusp of the bicuspid (mitral) valve (×3.5).

the endocardium becomes continuous with the intima of the vessels, with which it is comparable in structure. It is lined by an endothelium of irregularly shaped, polygonal cells with oval or round nuclei. Beneath the endothelium is a thin layer of fine collagenous fibrils and, outside of this, a stouter layer containing abundant elastic tissue and varying numbers of smooth muscle cells. Smooth muscle is particularly prominent in some portions of the atria (Fig. 12.20). In most parts of the heart, the deepest layer of the endocardium is composed of loose connective tissue which binds the endocardium proper to the myocardium. This layer, often referred to as subendocar-

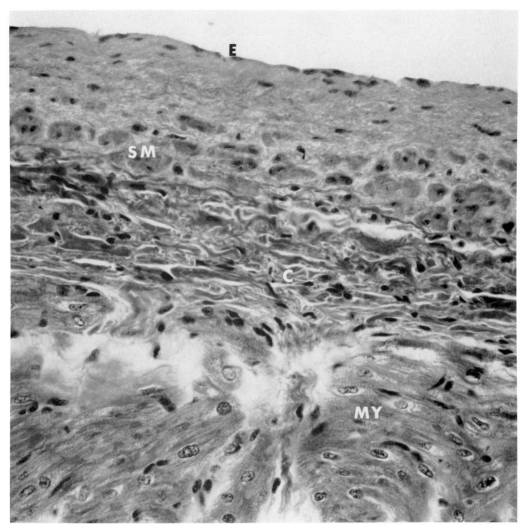

Figure 12.20. Section through the endocardium of the left atrium (human). Smooth muscle fibers (*SM*) and bundles of collagen (*C*) are prominent. *E*, endothelium; *MY*, cardiac muscle in myocardium (×475).

dium, contains collagenous fibers, elastic fibers, and blood vessels. In the ventricles, it also contains some of the specialized muscle fibers of the impulse-conducting system. This layer is absent from the papillary muscles and chordae tendinae.

Myocardium

As noted above, the myocardium forms the main mass of the heart. It consists of cardiac muscle cells (Chapter 8) arranged end-to-end into tracts that tend to run in bundles. Strands of connective tissue containing a rich vascular network lie between the tracts and bundles of cardiac muscle cells. The thickness of the myocardium varies in different parts of the heart; it is thinnest in the atria and thickest in the left ventricle. The atrial muscle tends to be arranged in fairly prominent bundles with intervening spaces where the connective tissue of the endocardium joins with that of the epicardium. The muscle bundles of the outer part of the atrial wall are oriented chiefly in a transverse or oblique direction and continue over both atria. The bundles in the deeper portions of the atrial wall are more independent for each atrium and are oriented approximately at right angles to the bundles of the outer layer. The innermost bundles stand out as ridges (pectinate muscles) in the auricular portions of the atria.

The disposition of the muscle tissue of the ventricles is much more complicated. It is described by gross anatomical dissection as composed of several layers of fiber bundles running in different directions and anchoring at the atrioventricular junction. This arrangement is important in providing for efficient pumping of the blood in a synchronized heart beat. It is important to keep in mind, however, that the term "fiber" in this context does not have the same meaning as it does for skeletal or smooth muscle. The gross anatomical cardiac muscle "fiber" consists of a linear chain of relatively short muscle cells, whereas cytologically a smooth or skeletal muscle "fiber" refers to an individual muscle cell.

The cardiac muscle of the atria is separated from that of the ventricles by strong fibrous rings, the *annuli fibrosi*, which surround the AV orifices. The fibrous rings are composed mainly of dense bundles of collagenous fibers. They also contain some elastic fibers, fibroblasts, and fat cells which become continuous with the accumulation of adipose tissue in the region of the coronary sulcus (Fig. 12.19).

The fibrous rings show structural variations in different persons and at different ages. They exhibit more marked variations in different species, e.g., they contain hyaline cartilage in sheep and bone in the ox.

The *annuli fibrosi of the atrioventricular orifices* form a part of a dense connective tissue supporting structure known as the *cardiac skeleton*. Other parts of this skeleton are: the *annuli fibrosi at the arterial foramina*, the *trigona fibrosa*, and the *septum membranaceum*.

Epicardium

The epicardium is the visceral layer of the pericardium. It is lined by a single layer of mesothelial cells, which may be flat or cuboidal, depending on the contractile state of the heart. Below the mesothelium is a layer of connective tissue containing a considerable number of elastic fibers in its deeper portion. At the venous and arterial openings, the connective tissue fibers pass over into the adventitia of the blood vessels. The deep layer of the epicardium contains blood vessels, nerves, and varying amounts of fat; it is often described as a subepicardium although it is a part of the epicardium. Fat is especially abundant in the subepicardial tissue of the atria and is particularly prominent near the AV junction (Fig. 12.19).

Valves of the Heart

The atrioventricular valves (tricuspid and mitral) are attached at their bases to the annuli fibrosi (Figs. 12.19 and 12.21). They consist of folds of endocardium covering a central plate of dense bundles of collagenous fibers which are continuous with the fibrous tissue of the annuli fibrosi and chordae tendinae. The endocardium is thicker on the atrial than on the ventricular side and contains more elastic tissue. Scattered bundles of smooth muscle extend into the endocardial layer on the atrial sides of the valve (Fig. 12.21). There are normally no blood capillaries beyond the region penetrated by the smooth muscles.

The semilunar valves of the pulmonary artery and aorta resemble the AV valves in their microscopic structure, but they are much thinner and contain no smooth muscle fibers. They also lack blood and lymphatic capillaries.

Impulse-Conducting System

Besides its ordinary musculature which furnishes the energy for the movement of the blood, the heart possesses a system of special muscle fibers whose function is to regulate the proper succession of contractions of atria and ventricles. It is known as the impulse-conducting system. A part of the system extending from the right atrium into the ventricles may be easily demonstrated by gross dissection and is known as the *atrioventricular bundle* or *bundle of His*. This bundle has its origin in the *atrioventricular node* which is found in the subendocardium of the median wall of the right

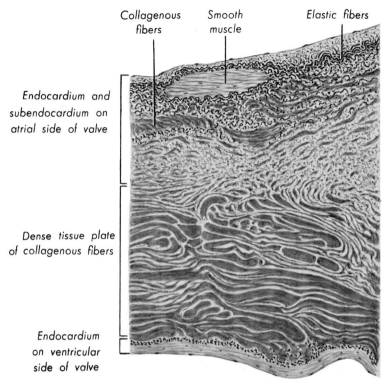

Collagenous fibers   Smooth muscle   Elastic fibers

Endocardium and subendocardium on atrial side of valve

Dense tissue plate of collagenous fibers

Endocardium on ventricular side of valve

Figure 12.21. Drawing of a cross section through a human mitral valve. The region shown is from the base of the valve, with the *right* side of the illustration facing the AV junction and annulus fibrosus. (Compare with Fig. 12.19 for orientation.) Weigert's elastic tissue and Van Gieson's stains to differentiate elastic fibers, collagenous fibers, and smooth muscle (×110).

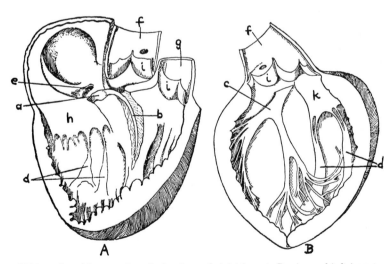

A   B

Figure 12.22. AV bundle of human heart. *A*, view of right heart; *B*, view of left heart. *a*, AV node; *b*, right trunk of bundle; *c*, left trunk of bundle; *d*, papillary muscles; *e*, coronary sinus; *f*, aorta; *g*, pulmonary artery; *h*, flap of tricupsid valve; *i*, semilunar valve; *k*, flap of mitral valve. (After Tandler.)

atrium close to the termination of the coronary sinus (Fig. 12.22). From the node, a common bundle or stem, the *crus commune*, is continued into the membranous septum of the ventricles, where it divides into two trunks which go, respectively, to the left and right ventricles. Small accessory bundles have also been described. Each trunk of the main bundle sends branches to the papillary muscles of its respective ventricle and divides to form an extensive network in the subendocardial tissue of each ventricle. Branches from the subendocardial plexus continue into the myocardium, where they continue to subdivide and eventually merge into regular cardiac muscle cells.

The modified cardiac muscle cells that make up the AV bundle and its branches are generally referred to as *Purkinje fibers.* In many organisms the Purkinje fibers differ markedly from ordinary cardiac muscle fibers, but these differences are less pronounced in humans. Nevertheless, they are usually readily distinguishable from ordinary cardiac muscle fibers (Fig. 12.23) by the following characteristics: their myofibrils are reduced in number and usually

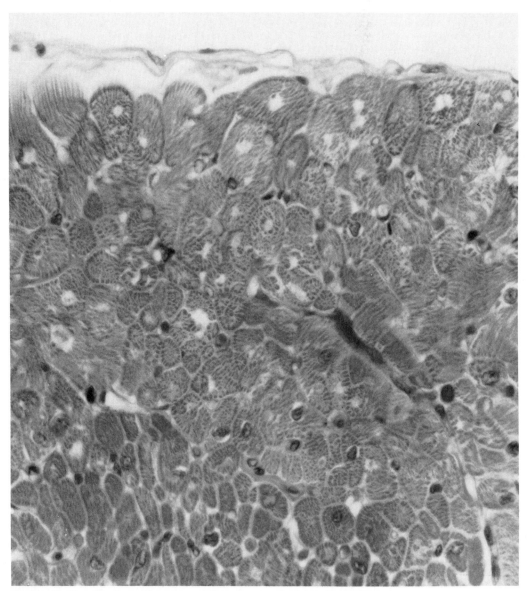

Figure 12.23. Section of human ventricle showing Purkinje fibers in cross section in the subendocardial region (*top*). Smaller diameter regular myocardial fibers appear in the *lower portion* of the micrograph (×625).

limited to the periphery of the fiber; they contain relatively more sarcoplasm; their nuclei are more rounded and more often in groups of two or more; they usually have a larger diameter, particularly in the peripheral branches of the system; they apparently lack the transverse tubules of cardiac muscle; they give a positive reaction for acetylcholinesterase; and they generally have more glycogen. The myofibrils resemble those of ordinary cardiac muscle in that they are cross-striated. Electron micrographs show that the Purkinje fibers are separate cells and that the intercalated discs seen under the light microscope are electron-dense areas along the membranes of cell junctions. The Purkinje fibers ultimately lose their specific characteristics and merge with ordinary cardiac muscle fibers (Fig. 12.24).

The AV node is composed of a group of irregularly arranged, branching fibers (*no-dal fibers*) which have a smaller diameter and fewer myofibrils than ordinary cardiac muscle fibers (Fig. 12.25). On the side of the AV node adjacent to the AV fibrous ring, the nodal fibers become continuous with Purkinje fibers of the AV bundle; on the opposite side of the node, they are continuous with other cardiac muscle fibers of the atrium. The junctions of the AV nodal fibers and Purkinje fibers occur at different levels ranging from those within the node itself (Fig. 12.25), to others within the AV bundle. In the latter instance, the nodal fibers are aligned longitudinally like the Purkinje fibers, but the two types are usually distinguishable by their morphology.

Another division of the specialized system, the *sinoatrial* (SA) *node* is found in the deep epicardium at the junction of the superior vena cava and right atrium in the region of the terminal sulcus (Fig. 12.26). This node is composed of slender, fusiform

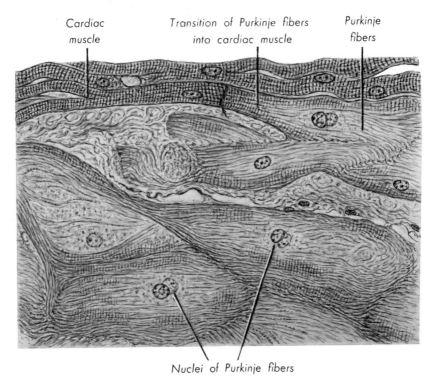

Cardiac muscle   Transition of Purkinje fibers into cardiac muscle   Purkinje fibers

Nuclei of Purkinje fibers

Figure 12.24. Drawing of a longitudinal section of beef moderator band showing transition of Purkinje fibers into cardiac muscle fibers in the myocardial portion of the band. The transition occurs near cell junctions and does not indicate a syncytium of cells. An intercalated disc can be identified in the region indicated by the *arrow*, although the discs are not stained in most parts of this preparation (×500). (Redrawn from preparation of R.C. Truex and W.M. Copenhaver.)

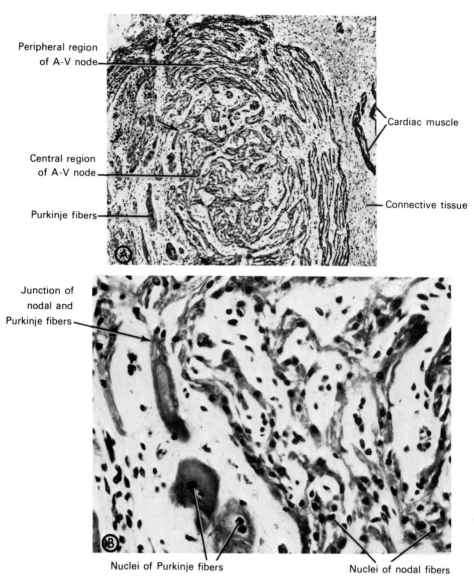

Peripheral region of A-V node

Central region of A-V node

Purkinje fibers

Cardiac muscle

Connective tissue

Junction of nodal and Purkinje fibers

Nuclei of Purkinje fibers

Nuclei of nodal fibers

Figure 12.25. Photomicrographs of a section through the AV node of a sheep heart. *A*, low magnification micrograph of an area from the wall of the right atrium medial to the opening of the coronary sinus and just above the origin of the AV bundle. Only a few atrial muscle fibers are seen in this section. The junctions of nodal fibers with atrial fibers occur chiefly in the preceding sections, at a greater distance above the origin of the AV bundle. *B*, higher magnification micrograph of a portion of the field seen in *A*. For orientation, note that the *arrows* to the junctions of nodal fibers with Purkinje fibers are directed to the same cells in *A* and *B*. The fibers of the AV node are very similar in size and structure to those of the SA node but are arranged in a different pattern. The presence of Purkinje fibers of large diameter in the AV nodal area is characteristic of hearts of ungulates; the special conduction fibers of the human heart do not attain the large diameter typical of ventricular Purkinje fibers until the branches of the AV system are reached. Hematoxylin and eosin. *A*, ×63; *B*, ×116. (From preparations of W. M.Copenhaver and R. C. Truex: *Anat Rec* 114: 1952.)

Connective tissue of epicardium   Artery

Fibers of sinoatrial node

Bundles of cardiac muscle fibers

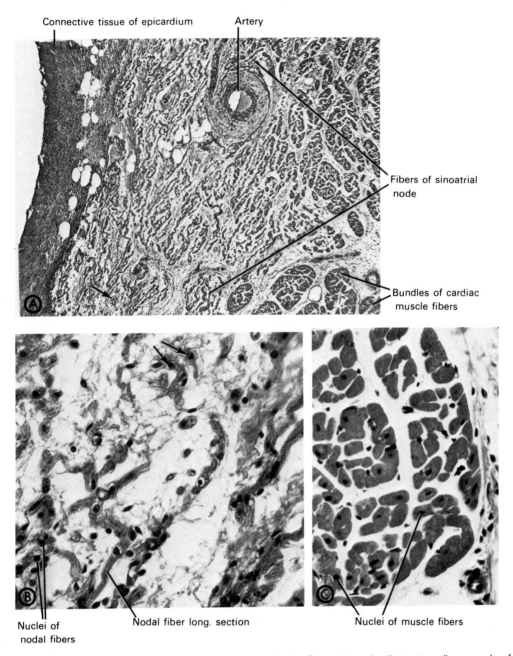

Nuclei of nodal fibers

Nodal fiber long. section

Nuclei of muscle fibers

Figure 12.26. Photomicrographs of a section through the SA node and adjacent cardiac muscle of a sheep heart. *A*, low magnification micrograph of an area from the wall of the right atrium near the junction of the atrium and the superior vena cava. *B*, a portion of *A* at higher magnification. For orientation, note that the *arrows* in *B* point to the same nodal cells that are indicated by the *arrow* in *A*. *C*, section of typical atrial myocardial fibers at the same magnification as that of the nodal fibers in *B*. Note that the diameter of the nodal fibers is less than that of the atrial muscle fibers. The nodal fibers are also interspersed with more loose connective tissue and course in a very irregular pattern. With higher magnification, one would also see that the myofibrils are less numerous and more irregularly arranged within the nodal fibers than they are in the atrial muscle fibers. Hematoxylin and eosin stain. *A*, ×63; *B* and *C*, ×146. (From preparations of W. M. Copenhaver and R. C. Truex: *Anat Rec* 114: 1952.)

fibers which have the general structure of the fibers of the AV node.

It is well established that the stimuli for cardiac contraction are normally initiated in the SA node. Because some of the fibers of this node come into close association with the typical cardiac muscle fibers and because the latter, as already described, are arranged as a meshwork of contiguous cells, the impulse initiated in the SA node may spread as a contraction wave over the typical cardiac fibers of both atria and then into the special fibers of the AV node. On the other hand, electrophysiological studies of canine and rabbit hearts indicate that the impulse initiated in the SA node is transmitted by special pathways to the AV node. The preferential atrial conduction pathways described from physiological and pharmacologial studies are located chiefly in regions which were at the junctions of the sinus venosus and atrium in the embryonic heart. They are also closely related with pathways of nerve fibers.

After the conduction impulse reaches the AV node, it is conducted at a relatively slow rate through the node to reach the AV bundle of His, where it travels rapidly to the ventricles. If this bundle is injured or destroyed, the normal rhythm in the succession of atrial and ventricular beats is lost. Branches of the bundle transmit the impulse at a relatively high velocity over both ventricles assuring their synchronous contraction.

Blood Vessels

Blood for the nutrition of the heart is supplied through the two coronary arteries. The distribution of the branches of the coronary arteries is quite variable; for example, the SA node of the human heart is supplied entirely by branches from the right coronary artery in about 70% of the cases studied, by the left coronary in a much lower percentage, and by both right and left branches in a few cases. However, regardless of variations in the blood supply for particular regions, the total amount of blood supplied by the left coronary greatly exceeds that supplied by the right coronary, in correlation with the greater work load and larger muscular mass on the left side.

The venous return is partly by venules that drain into the coronary sinus and partly by *venae cordae minimae* that empty directly into the heart chambers. Numerous vessels of this type, also known as Thebesian veins, open directly into the right atrium. Vessels of similar type also open into the left atrium and into both ventricular cavities. Retrograde flow, that is, flow from the ventricular cavities into the venae cordae, occurs under conditions of altered pressure relationships.

The AV valves apparently have only a few or no vessels in the dense, fibrous central plates. The supply in the subendothelial layers differs for the different leaflets of the valve: it is richer in the aortic cusp of the mitral valve than in others. The supply is also richer in infants than in normal adults.

The bundle of His is, according to some investigators, supplied by special fine branches of the coronary arteries. The capillary net is less dense than in the ordinary musculature of the heart.

Lymphatics

The heart is supplied with lymph channels which form networks in the endocardial, myocardial, and subepicardial layers.

Nerves

The heart receives nerve fibers from the vagus and the sympathetic division of the autonomic system. These fibers form an extensive cardiac plexus at the base of the heart. The vagus and sympathetic fibers have antagonistic functions; the former inhibits and the latter accelerates the action of the heart.

The efferent vagus fibers do not go directly to the cardiac muscle but arborize around parasympathetic ganglion cells scattered in the wall of the heart, chiefly in plexuses in the deep epicardium. These cells are especially numerous in the dorsal wall of the atria, in the coronary sulcus near the larger coronary vessels, and at the base of the aorta and pulmonary artery. The ganglion cells send out delicate, nonmyelinated nerve fibers which branch and end in terminal varicosities on the muscle fibers.

Some of the sensory nerve fibers are derived from the vagus; others have their cell bodies in the spinal ganglia of the first to the fourth thoracic nerves. The fibers of the latter group pass through the white rami, up the sympathetic trunk to the cervical sympathetic ganglia, and thence to the heart by way of the cardiac nerves.

THE LYMPH VASCULAR SYSTEM

Besides the blood vessels, the body contains a collateral system of endothelium-lined channels which collect tissue fluid and return it by a circuitous route to the bloodstream. The fluid in these vessels is called lymph. Unlike the blood, the lymph circulates in one direction only, from the periphery toward the heart. The *lymphatic capillaries* begin blindly in the tissues from which the lymph is collected (Fig. 12.27).

They, as well as the larger vessels which conduct the lymph to the bloodstream, freely anastomose along their course, gradually fuse to form fewer lymph channels, and are ultimately gathered into two main trunks, the large *thoracic duct* and the smaller *right lymphatic duct*. The thoracic duct empties into the left subclavian vein, and the right lymphatic duct drains into the right subclavian, in each case near the point where the subclavian joins with its respective internal jugular vein. In the pathways of the lymph vessels there are groups of lymph nodes containing lymph sinuses in which the lymph is filtered before reaching the thoracic and right lymphatic ducts.

Lymphatic capillaries and vessels occur in most tissues and organs. They have not been demonstrated in the central nervous system, the bone marrow, the intralobular portion of the liver, the coats of the eyeball, the internal ear, and the fetal placenta.

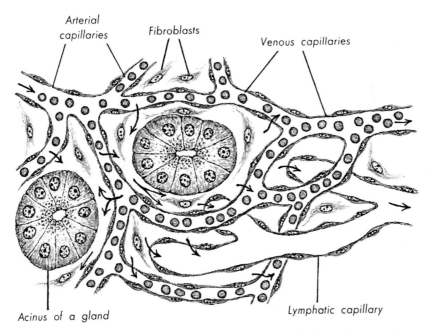

Figure 12.27. Diagram showing the relationship of lymphatic capillaries to blood capillaries and to the tissue fluids around the acini of a gland. Similar relationships exist in most of the organs of the body. *Arrows* indicate the direction of flow of fluid leaving the arterial capillaries, permeating the connective tissue spaces as tissue fluid, and reentering the blood capillaries on the venous side. The lymphatic capillaries supplement the venous capillaries in the drainage of fluid from the tissues to the circulatory system.

Lymph Capillaries

The lymph capillaries, like those of the blood, are delicate tubes with walls which consist of a single layer of endothelial cells. The tubes are larger, however, and instead of having a uniform diameter, they vary greatly in caliber within short distances. The exceedingly thin cells have a flattened, oval nucleus and an irregular outline which can be demonstrated with silver impregnations. Electron micrographs of lymphatic capillaries show no endothelial pores (fenestrae) but instead display fairly numerous micropinocytotic vesicles. Junctional complexes are rare and gaps readily appear between the cells under altered conditions. The basal lamina is usually absent or, at most, present only in spots. The outer surface of the endothelium is attached to the surrounding connective tissue at intervals by fine filaments that are perpendicular to the course of the capillary; these are known as *anchoring filaments*. They presumably aid in keeping the lumen from collapsing.

The lymph capillaries anastomose to form extensive networks in the spaces between the blood capillaries. In the skin and in the mucous and serous membranes, the lymph capillaries are usually more deeply placed than are the blood capillaries.

Lymph Vessels

The lymph vessels resemble the veins in structure, but their walls are as a rule thinner than those of veins of a corresponding caliber. In the smaller lymph vessels, the endothelium is surrounded by collagenous and elastic fibers and a few smooth muscle cells. In the larger ones, three coats may be distinguished: intima, media, and adventitia. The intima is composed of the endothelial lining, underneath which is a delicate network of elastic fibers disposed longitudinally. The media consists mainly of circularly disposed smooth muscle fibers and a few longitudinal ones. Between the muscle fibers are relatively few delicate, elastic fibrils. The adventitia, which is the thickest coat, is composed of longitudinally coursing collagenous fibers, among which are bundles of longitudinal muscle and elastic fibers.

The lymph vessels contain numerous valves which are usually arranged in pairs and whose free margins are always directed centrally, i.e., in the direction of the lymph flow. The valves are infoldings of the intima.

Thoracic Duct

The thoracic duct has a considerable amount of muscle tissue. The *intima* consists of an endothelial lining, a thin intermediate layer of fibroelastic tissue in which are bundles of longitudinal muscle fibers, and an internal elastic lamina composed of a longitudinal network of elastic fibers. The elastic lamina is best developed in the caudal portion of the duct and is much thinner or missing altogether in the cervical portion.

The *media* is the thickest coat and consists of longitudinal and circular muscle bundles, the former predominating. The muscle bundles are separated by abundant connective tissue composed mainly of collagenous fibers. Elastic fibrils are scarce in the inner layer of the media but become more numerous in the outer portion.

The *adventitia* is poorly defined. Near the media is a layer of coarse collagenous fibers, mainly longitudinally disposed and containing considerable elastic tissue and occasional longitudinal muscle fibers. The outer layer is more finely fibrillar and merges with the surrounding connective tissue.

DEVELOPMENT OF THE CIRCULATORY SYSTEM

Blood Vessels and Heart

The myocardium of the heart develops from bilaterally localized regions of splanchnic mesoderm. The endothelium of the heart and vessels differentiates from mesenchymal cells derived from mesoderm. The heart and the main trunks of its accompanying large vessels (e.g., aorta) develop independently of the peripheral vessels, with which they unite later. While the heart develops within the embryo, the earliest vessels and earliest blood cells develop from extraembryonic mesenchyme. The earliest vessels have the structure of capillaries. They appear first in the mesenchyme of the chorion and yolk sac. Here groups of cells known as "*blood islands*" differentiate from the rest of the mesenchymal cells. The superficial cells of these islands flatten to form the endothelium; the central cells develop into the primitive blood cells. The channels, which are at first unconnected, anastomose and give rise to a network of channels which are the earliest capillaries. These develop rapidly, and some of them increase in size to become arteries and veins, the smooth muscle and connective tissue of their walls being differentiated from the surrounding mesenchyme.This differentiation progresses toward the embryo where the vascular lumina unite with intraembryonic vessels which also have developed from mesenchyme in situ. After a primary system of closed vessels has been established and after the embryonic circulation has been initiated, new vessels develop as outgrowths from preexisting vessels. New vessels arise by a similar method in the adult, e.g., the outgrowth of new vessels into granulation tissue.

The *heart* in early human embryos (2 to 3 mm) consists of an *endothelial tube* surrounded by a layer of splanchnic mesoderm which forms the *myoepicardial mantle*. The two layers are at first separated by a considerable space filled with a gelatinous fluid (cardiac jelly). As development proceeds, the two layers become firmly united, the endothelium now forming the lining of the myoepicardial mantle. The endothelium and its underlying connective tissue form the endocardium. From the myoepicardial mantle are formed both myocardium and epicardium.

Lymphatics

The earliest lymphatic vessels arise by differentiation of mesenchymal cells into endothelium-lined spaces in situ. These spaces secondarily establish connections with venous plexuses, but the only connections which persist are via the thoracic duct on the left and the smaller right thoracic duct. In their development, the lymphatic plexuses arise first in the thoracic and abdominal regions and subsequently grow into the head and extremities.

References

Bennett HS, Luft JH, Hampton JC: Morphological classification of vertebrate blood capillaries. *Am J Physiol* 196:381–390, 1959.

Bundgaard M: Transport pathways in capillaries—in search of pores. *Annu Rev Physiol* 42:325–336, 1980.

Casely-Smith JR: Comparative fine structure of the microvasculature and endothelium. *Adv Microcirc* 9:1–44, 1980.

Clark ER, Clark EL: Observations on changes in blood vascular endothelium in the living animal. *Am J Anat* 57:385–438, 1935.

Copenhaver WM, Truex RC: Histology of the atrial portion of the cardiac conduction system in man and other mammals. *Anat Rec* 114:601–626, 1952.

Davies F, Francis ETB: The conduction of the impulse for cardiac contractions. *J Anat* 86:302–309, 1952.

French JE, Florey HW, Morris B: The absorption of particles by the lymphatics of the diaphragm. *Q J Exp Physiol* 45:88–103, 1960.

Hoffman BF: Physiology of atrioventricular transmission. *Circulation* 24:506–517, 1961.

Hogan PM, Davis LD: Evidence for specialized fibers in the canine right atrium. *Circ Res* 23:387–396, 1968.

Hollinshead WH: A cytological study of the carotid body of the cat. *Am J Anat* 73:185–215, 1943.

James TN, Sherf L, Urthaler F: Fine structure of the bundle-branches. *Br Heart J* 36:1–18, 1974.

Karnovsky MJ: The ultrastructural basis of capillary permeability studied with peroxidase as a tracer. *J Cell Biol* 35:213–236, 1967.

Landis EM, Pappenheimer JR: Exchange of substances through the capillary walls. In Hamilton WF, Dow P (eds): *Handbook of Physiology*, section 2, vol 2. Bethesda, American Physiological Society, 1963, pp 961–1034.

Leake LV, Burke JF: Ultrastructural studies on the lymphatic anchoring filaments. *J Cell Biol* 36:129–149, 1968.

Luft JH: Capillary permeability. 1. Structural considerations. In Zweifach BV, Grant L, McCluskey RT (eds): *The Inflammatory Process*, ed 2, vol 2. New York, Academic Press, 1973, pp 47–94.

Majno G, Shea SM, Leventhal M: Endothelial contraction induced by histamine-type mediators. An electron microscopic study. *J Cell Biol* 42:647–672, 1969.

Nonidez JF: The aortic (depressor) nerve and its associated epithelioid body, the glomus aorticum. *Am J Anat* 57:259–301, 1935.

Osborne MP, Butler PJ: New theory for receptor mechanism of carotid body chemoreceptors. *Nature* 254:701–703, 1975.

Palade GE, Bruns RR: Structural modulations of plasmalemmal vesicles. *J Cell Biol* 37:633–649, 1968.

Pappenheimer JR: Passage of molecules through capillary walls. *Physiol Rev* 33:387–423, 1953.

Phelps PC, Luft JH: Electron microscopical study of relaxation and constriction in frog arterioles. *Am J Anat* 125:399–428, 1969.

Raviola E, Karnovsky MJ: Evidence for a blood-thymus barrier using electron-opaque tracers. *J Exp Med* 136:466–498, 1972.

Reese TS, Karnovsky MJ: Fine structural localization of a blood-brain barrier to exogenous peroxidase. *J Cell Biol* 34:207–217, 1967.

Rhodin JAG: The ultrastructure of mammalian arterioles and precapillary sphincters. *J Ultrastruct Res* 18:181–223, 1967.

Rhodin JAG: Ultrastructure of mammalian venous capillaries, venules, and small collecting veins. *J Ultrastruct Res* 25:452–500, 1968.

Ross R: The arterial wall and atherosclerosis. *Annu Rev Med* 30:1–15, 1979.

Simionescu M, Simionescu N, Palade GE: Segmental differentiation of cell junctions in the vascular endothelium. The microvasculature. *J Cell Biol* 67:863–885, 1975.

Simionescu N, Simionescu M, Palade GE: Permeability of muscle capillaries to small heme peptides. Evidence for the existence of patent transendothelial channels. *J Cell Biol* 65:586–607, 1975.

Simionescu N, Simionescu M, Palade GE: Differentiated microdomains on the luminal surface of capillary endothelium. I. Preferential distribution of annionic sites. *J Cell Biol* 90:605–613, 1981.

Simionescu M, Simionescu N, Palade GE: Differentiated microdomains on the luminal surface of capillary endothelium: distribution of lectin receptors. *J Cell Biol* 94:406–413, 1982.

Sommer, JR, and Johnson, EA Cardiac muscle. A comparative study of Purkinje fibers and ventricular fibers. *J Cell Biol* 36:497–526, 1968.

Truex RC, Copenhaver WM: Histology of the moderator band in man and other mammals, with special reference to the conduction system. *Am J Anat* 80:173–201, 1947.

Walls EN: Dissection of the atrioventricular node and bundle in the human heart. *J Anat* 79:45–48, 1945.

Wearn JT: Morphological and functional alterations of the coronary circulation. *Harvey Lect* 35:243–269, 1940.

Williams MC, Wissig SL: The permeability of muscle capillaries to horseradish peroxidase. *J Cell Biol* 66:531–555, 1975.

Zimmerman J, Bailey CP: The surgical significance of the fibrous skeleton of the heart. *J Thorac Cardiovasc Surg* 44:701–712, 1962.

Chapter 13

DEVELOPMENT OF BLOOD CELLS (HEMOPOIESIS)

Although the earliest erythrocytes of the embryo develop from extraembryonic mesoderm of the yolk sac and subsequently in the liver and spleen (Chapter 12), erythrocyte and granulocyte development in the adult is normally limited to bone marrow. Hence, the erythrocytes and granular leukocytes are described as the *myeloid elements* of the blood. Considerable numbers of lymphocytes and perhaps some monocytes differentiate in the lymphatic organs; therefore, they are classified as *lymphoid elements.* These terms continue to have wide usage even though it is well established that large numbers of lymphocytes and monocytes also develop in marrow.

There is general agreement on most of the cytological characteristics and intercellular relationships of the cells illustrated in Figure 13.1, but numerous controversies have existed in regard to the precursors. According to the *monophyletic* (unitarian) theory, all blood cells are derived from a common stem cell (hemocytoblast). According to the *dualistic* theory, there is one stem cell for the granular leukocytes and erythrocytes and another stem cell for the lymphoid elements. These different theories were based on light microscope studies which indicated that in either case the primitive cell has a basophilic cytoplasm and a rounded nucleus with a prominent nucleolus.

Marked advances in our knowledge of the early stages of blood development have been achieved by the use of experimental methods. A major advance began with the discovery that rodents in which all blood cells were destroyed by total body X-irradiation would survive provided that they immediately received intravenous injections of bone marrow cells from a closely related animal. Similar results were obtained when one member of a surgically joined (parabiosed) pair received total body irradiation. These findings showed that a cell with the potency to form all types of blood cells circulates in the blood and is not confined to blood-forming organs as previously presumed.

The animals which were X-irradiated and transfused with marrow cells as outlined above frequently developed nodules on the surface of the spleen. The use of suspensions of marrow cells with "marker" chromosomes produced by irradiation showed that each spleen colony represents a clone; i.e., each colony of all types of marrow cells is derived from a single cell, known as a *stem cell.* Suspensions of marrow cells grown in vitro in an appropriate medium on agar plates produce colonies similar to those on the spleen; these are known as *colony-forming units* (CFU). A number of investigators noted a relationship between the number of colonies formed and the volume and concentration of marrow cells. This was verified by counting the number of cells plated as determined by hemocytometer counts of the marrow cells. The proportion of stem cells to the total number of nucleated marrow cells was found to be very low, normally about 1:1000.

The research outlined above provided information on the behavior of stem cells but gave no information on their morphology. A clue to the latter was obtained by differential sedimentation studies which showed that cells from the part of the sedimenting column that contains stem cells have a

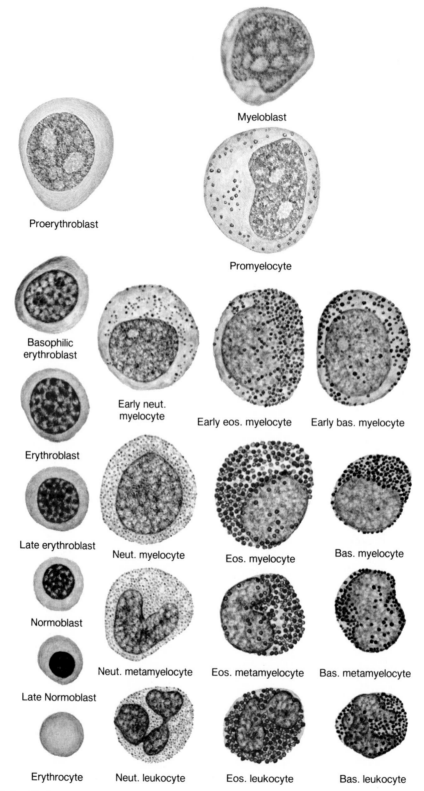

Figure 13.1. Various stages in blood development as seen in dried smears of human marrow. Wright's stain (×1560).

weight and size comparable with that of lymphocytes. In further studies, samples of cells from the part of the sedimentation column that has stem cell potency were examined by light and by electron microscopy. It was found that the sedimentation column cells have a nucleus which is more irregularly shaped than that of most lymphocytes. The mitochondria are smaller and more numerous than in lymphocytes, and free ribosomes but no rough-surfaced endoplasmic reticulum are present. The characteristics fit those which would be expected of a stem cell which maintains its own population for a lifetime and provides differentiating cells as they are required to replace the mature cells of blood and marrow.

The origin of the stem cell remains controversial. The view that the pluripotential cell arises from reticular cells of bone marrow is questionable. The earliest erythroblasts in the embryo develop from mesenchymal cells of the yolk sac in areas described as "*blood islands.*" There is evidence that undifferentiated cells from the yolk sac reach the liver and other blood-forming organs, where they survive as stem cells which proliferate and differentiate into all types of blood cells including monocytes.

BLOOD DEVELOPMENT IN BONE MARROW

Red bone marrow is composed of a framework or stroma of reticular cells and fibers plus free cells located within the meshwork. The stroma also contains a variable number of fat cells. The majority of the free cells are the immature developmental stages of the granular leukocytes and erythrocytes that normally develop only in marrow in the adult. Red marrow also contains megakaryocytes, mature erythrocytes, granular leukocytes, lymphocytes, monocytes and plasma cells. The structure and blood supply of marrow with its characteristic network of sinusoids have been described in Chapter 6.

The Granulocyte Series

The stages of granulocyte development, in order of differentiation, are: *stem cells,*

myeloblasts, promyelocytes, myelocytes, metamyelocytes, and *granular leukocytes.*

Myeloblasts

The myeloblasts develop from the pluripotential CFU stem cell, by way of at least two derivatives for the granulocyte line. The myeloblasts normally constitute about 2% of the nucleated cells of marrow. Because the stem cell is not specifically characterized by microscopy, it may be included in this number. However, the stem cells demonstrated by sedimentation studies are present in marrow in the proportion of less than 0.1%.

The myeloblasts are variable in size, ranging from 8 to 13 μm in diameter. They are characterized by a deeply basophilic cytoplasm and a relatively undifferentiated nucleus. The nucleus is round or ovoid and contains two or more coarse nucleoli. In dried smears treated with Wright's stain, the nucleoli are pale, and the arrangement of the granular chromatin frequently gives a characteristic sievelike appearance (Fig. 13.1). The nucleus of this same cell type has a very different appearance in sections stained with hematoxylin-eosin-azure (see myeloblasts, Fig. 13.2). Here the nucleoli are stained intensely, and the chromatin shows as a delicate reticulum enclosing pale-staining areas.

The cytoplasm is very basophilic both in sections and in dried smears, displaying a hue of blue similar to that typical of lymphocyte cytoplasm after Wright's stain. Electron micrographs show that the myeloblast cytoplasm contains an abundance of free ribosomes but relatively little rough endoplasmic reticulum. They also show numerous mitochondria which are spherical and relatively small.

The myeloblasts of the normal adult marrow arise chiefly by mitotic divisions of their own type and to a lesser extent by differentiation from stem cells. In some pathological conditions they become more numerous in the marrow and also appear in the circulating blood, as in myelogenous leukemia. Here the increase is by both accelerated mitotic activity of the myeloblasts

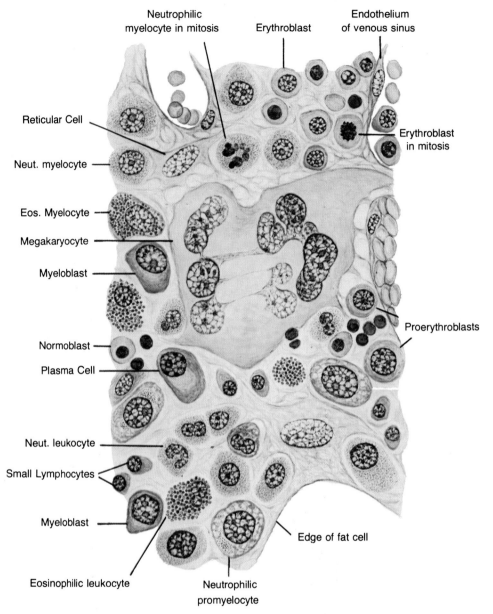

Figure 13.2. Various stages in blood development as seen in a section of marrow from a human rib. Hematoxylin-eosin-azure (×1365).

and increased rate of proliferation of stem cells.

Promyelocytes

The promyelocytes are more differentiated than the myeloblasts and are somewhat more numerous, about 5% of the nucleated marrow cells. They are usually larger, ranging up to 20 μm or more in

marrow smears. The nucleus is rounded or ovoid and occasionally indented. The chromatin is granular and frequently gives a sievelike appearance somewhat like that of the myeloblast. The nucleoli are still prominent. The cytoplasm is even more basophilic than that of the myeloblast and it contains *azurophilic granules*, a distinct difference from the nongranular cytoplasm of the myeloblast. Electron micrographs show an abundance of rough endoplasmic reticulum, plus free ribosomes, numerous mitochondria, and a well developed Golgi complex.

Myelocytes

The myelocytes constitute about 12% (range 5 to 20%) of the nucleated marrow cells. There are a number of mitotic divisions and several stages of differentiation within the myelocyte category. The earliest differential feature of the myelocytes is the initial appearance of *specific granules* which differ from the azurophilic granules that form only during the promyelocyte stage. With the appearance of specific granules at the myelocyte stage, the developing granulocytes are distinguishable as neutrophils, eosinophils, and basophils. Although the types of granules differ structurally and cytochemically, as outlined in Chapter 7, the course of differentiation is similar in the three types; the neutrophil will be described in more detail as an example.

Electron micrographs show an interesting difference in the manner in which the Golgi complex handles the packaging of the granules. The azurophilic granules form in the promyelocyte stage, arising by a coalescence of dense-cored vacuoles derived from the inner (adcentriolar) cisternae of the Golgi complex. The specific granules form only in the myelocyte stage and arise by fusion of dense-cored vacuoles derived from the outer cisternae of the Golgi complex (Figs. 1.36 and 1.37). Because the azurophilic granules form only in the promyelocyte stage, their number is reduced by each myelocyte division, and they are greatly outnumbered by the specific granules in the mature cell.

In addition to an increase in numbers of specific cytoplasmic granules during myelocyte maturation, the cytoplasm shows a decrease in basophilia in correlation with a decrease in free ribosomes and rough endoplasmic reticulum.

Maturation of myelocytes also involves changes in the nuclei. In the early myelocyte, the nucleus differs only slightly from that of the promyelocyte, but with successive divisions and maturation the nuclei become ovoid and irregular in shape, nucleoli disappear, and the chromatin becomes more dense and compact. The cells eventually reach a stage where they no longer divide, and then they are known as metamyelocytes.

Metamyelocytes

These cells constitute about 22% of the nucleated cells of marrow; the metamyelocyte is the most abundant cell of normal marrow. The nucleus continues its maturation, and in the *neutrophilic metamyelocyte* it becomes increasingly irregular and often assumes a shape known as a *band form*. With further maturation, the cytoplasm shows an increase in glycogen and a decrease in free ribosomes, rough endoplasmic reticulum, and mitochondria. The nucleus eventually becomes constricted into two to five lobes, frequently three. The *eosinophilic metamyelocytes* frequently form a nucleus of two lobes, although three or more are not particularly unusual. The chromatin of the nucleus is less dense and less compact than in the neutrophil (Fig. 13.1).

The *basophilic metamyelocyte* differs from the other types of metamyelocytes in the shape of its nucleus and the form of its specific granules. The nucleus does not differentiate into distinct lobes, as it generally does in neutrophils and eosinophils. Therefore, it is difficult to distinguish basophilic metamyelocytes from mature basophilic leukocytes in Wright's stained smears. Furthermore, the basophilic granules, like those of mast cells, are water-soluble and are generally not distinguishable in sections of material fixed in aqueous solutions.

General Considerations of Granulocytopoiesis

When the percentages of the different myelocyte stages are added to the number of mature granulocytes present in marrow (20% or more), it is found that the granular leukocyte line comprises approximately 60% of the cells in normal marrow. Lymphocytes, monocytes, reticular cells, plasma cells, and megakaryocytes may constitute another 10 to 20%, leaving only about 20 to 30% of the marrow cells in the erythrocyte line. Although the literature on differential counts for normal marrow gives an even greater range than that listed above, there is general agreement that the progenitors of the leukocytes outnumber those of the erythrocytes. The numerical preponderance of leukocytogenic over erythrocytogenic cells in marrow, in contrast with the opposite relationship in blood, can be explained partly by the fact that the leukocytes survive for a shorter time in the circulation than do the erythrocytes and also require a longer period for development and maturation in marrow.

Studies of bone marrow cells by the ultraviolet absorption method have shown that ribonucleic acid (RNA) is more abundant in the myeloblast than in any of the other developmental stages of the granulocyte line. The high concentration of RNA is responsible for the marked basophilia of the cytoplasm at the myeloblast stage. The high concentration of cytoplasmic RNA and the prominence of nucleoli are correlated with the rapid formation of cytoplasmic proteins during the early stages. It has been estimated that the total volume of all of the promyelocytes is about eight times the total volume of the myeloblast. This follows from the fact that the promyelocytes are more numerous and often larger than the myeloblasts. In the lineage from promyelocyte to myelocyte to metamyelocyte, the cells increase in number with a decrease in size, so that the total volume of all the metamyelocytes is only slightly greater than the total volume of the promyelocytes. Development during these later stages is dominated by differentiation rather than by cell growth. The rapid decrease in cytoplasmic basophilia during these later stages appears to be correlated with the decrease in RNA.

The life span of the granular leukocytes is approximately as follows: about 14 days for differentiation and maturation in bone marrow, about 6 to 10 hr in circulation, and about 1 to 2 days in the connective tissue. A loss of leukocytes from the circulation stimulates an increase in the rate of release of cells from the marrow and a severe loss of cells stimulates an increased rate of differentiation from the stem cell. Current evidence indicates that there are a number of specific factors which stimulate and regulate leukocyte production, most of which have obscure origins and modes of action. Differentiation of the CFU stem cell apparently proceeds through phases of gradually restricted potentiality before morphologically distinct cell types are established. For example, it is reported that one derivative of the CFU stem cell is a precursor for both the neutrophil and the monocyte-macrophage series, whereas another derivative gives rise to the eosinophil line. These cells, and perhaps a third type giving rise to basophils, would all fall into the category of myeloblasts as distinguished morphologically. With the intricacies of regulatory control that are operating, the wonder is not that abnormalities in hemopoiesis occur but that they occur in such a relatively low frequency.

The Erythrocyte Series

The stages of erythrocyte development are: *stem cells, proerythroblasts, basophilic erythroblasts, polychromatophilic erythroblasts, normoblasts* (orthochromatophilic erythroblasts), and *erythrocytes.*

Proerythroblasts

These are derived by differentiation from the pluripotential (CFU) stem cell by way of a derivative for the erythrocyte line (CFU-E). They are the earliest cells identifiable by light microscopy as a part of the erythrocyte series and they are relatively large, about 12 to 17 μm in diameter. Their nuclei are rounded and have a coarser chromatin structure than that of myeloblasts. Nucleoli are present but less prominent than in the myeloblast. In fresh preparations, or by special techniques, a small amount of hemoglobin can be detected in the cytoplasm of some of the cells, but it is obscured in stained preparations by the intense basophilia of the cytoplasm.

Basophilic Erythroblasts

After a few divisions, the proerythroblasts differentiate into the basophilic erythroblasts, in which the chromatin is somewhat more coarse and nucleoli are no longer discernible. The cytoplasm continues to be very basophilic because of free ribosomes and polyribosomes. Electron micrographs show little or no rough endoplasmic reticulum.

Polychromatophilic Erythroblasts

The basophilic erythroblasts undergo mitotic divisions and give rise to cells in which the hemoglobin is of sufficient quantity to be observed distinctly in stained preparations. There are many generations of erythroblasts and, with each mitotic division, there is a decrease in basophilia of cytoplasm and an increase in quantity of hemoglobin, which is acidophilic.

The cytoplasm of the different generations of cells takes varying amounts of the acid and basic components of Wright's stain; therefore, these cells show a "mixed color varying from purplish blue to lilac or gray" and are called polychromatophilic. A few of these stages are illustrated in Figure 13.1.

The nucleus of the polychromatophilic erythroblast has a denser chromatin network than that of the basophilic erythroblast, and the coarse chromatin bodies give a checkerboard appearance which is characteristic of developing erythrocytes, as contrasted with the more irregular arrangement of chromatin in the developing granulocytes. The polychromatophilic erythroblasts vary greatly in size but are on the average somewhat smaller than the basophilic erythroblasts. The size variation is related to the number of mitotic divisions any specific cell has undergone by the time of observation; there are several generations within the polychromatophilic stage.

Normoblasts (Orthochromatophilic Erythroblasts)

These cells have approximately the same amount of hemoglobin as the erythrocytes. The cells of this stage have usually stopped dividing and are in various stages of maturation. They are only slightly larger than the mature erythrocytes (Fig. 13.1). The chromatin is denser and more compact than in the polychromatophilic cells. Eventually the nuclei become pyknotic, assume bizarre shapes, and are extruded from the cells, usually along with a thin coat of cytoplasm and plasma membrane. Small fragments of the nucleus occasionally remain and give rise to deeply staining bodies (Howell-Jolly bodies).

Erythrocytes

The youngest erythrocytes (*reticulocytes*) contain a delicate reticulum which can be demonstrated by supravital staining with dyes such as cresyl blue (Fig. 7.1 *B*). Erythrocytes normally lose their reticular structure soon after leaving the marrow; the normal reticulocyte count of peripheral blood is less than 1% of the erythrocytes. Increased numbers may be called into circulation by repeated hemorrhages. Reticulocyte counts are used as an index of the effectiveness of therapy in pernicious anemia, an increase of reticulocytes after treatment being evidence of an increased production of young erythrocytes.

Normal marrow, in which erythrocytes develop through the stages as described above, is known as *normoblastic marrow*. This contrasts with *megaloblastic marrow*, which occurs in pernicious anemia and other macrocytic anemias.

As noted earlier, there is a lack of agreement on terminology for the developmental stages of blood cells. Use of the term normoblast is an example. If one uses normoblast only for cells which have acquired a sufficient amount of hemoglobin to give a cytoplasmic stain almost equal to that of a normal erythrocyte (i.e., for the immediate precursor of a normal erythrocyte), the terms apply as outlined in the preceding description. On the other hand, if one prefers to use the term normoblast for all stages of normal erythrocyte development in contrast with megaloblastic development in anemia, the names for the stages of development become: pronormoblasts, basophilic normoblasts, polychromatophilic normoblasts, orthochromatophilic normoblasts, reticulated erythrocytes, and mature erythrocytes.

General Considerations of Erythropoiesis

Ribonucleic acid is more abundant in the basophilic erythroblast than in the later stages of the erythrocyte line. The concentration of RNA is responsible for the marked basophilia of the cytoplasm in the early stages and is correlated with the active synthesis of cytoplasmic proteins during the stages which show the greatest increase in total cell volume.

The normal development of erythrocytes is dependent upon many different factors. Obviously, all of the parent substances which enter into the formation of hemoglobin must be present. The absence of one of these, iron, is responsible for a microcytic type of anemia. Certain additional substances are necessary for the normal maturation of the erythrocytogenic cells. The absence of one of these, vitamin B_{12}, produces pernicious anemia. Actually, the real defect in pernicious anemia is the lack of *intrinsic factor*, normally present in gastric secretion, which facilitates the intestinal absorption of vitamin B_{12}. After absorption, B_{12} is stored chiefly in the liver until it is utilized later in bone marrow.

The most potent stimulus for erythropoiesis is hypoxia, or cellular oxygen deficiency. Extracts from plasma of animals made anemic by experimental methods contain a factor which stimulates erythropoiesis when injected into normal animals. The plasma or humoral factor is known as *erythropoietin.*

Erythropoietin is a glycoprotein that is formed by the interaction of *erythrogenin* (a renal factor) and *globin* (hemoglobin protein). Erythrogenin usually forms in the kidney and is therefore known as a renal erythropoietic factor (REF), but it can also form in other locations as demonstrated by studies on animals after bilateral nephrectomy. Hypoxia stimulates the formation of REF and, therefore, increases circulating erythropoietin. Studies of fetal mouse liver cells in vitro indicate that erythropoietin increases the number of hemoglobin-forming cells (erythroblasts) by stimulating the stem cells (CFU-E) to multiply and differentiate into hemoglobin-synthesizing cells (proerythroblasts and erythroblasts).

Iron is present in hemoglobin as part of the heme moiety. Only a fraction of the iron used in erythrocyte development is obtained from absorption by the intestine; most of it is recycled in the body. Iron from degenerating senile erythrocytes is converted to ferritin or hemosiderin and is taken up by the macrophage system of the spleen and bone marrow where it is stored. It is released into the circulation as needed and is taken up by the erythroblasts of marrow by a process resembling pinocytosis. The utilization of the iron from ferritin in the synthesis of hemoglobin by erythroblasts is dependent on the presence of vitamin B_{12}, but the details of the process are not defined as clearly as are those related to erythropoietin.

Megakaryocytes and Platelet Formation

The megakaryocytes are giant cells (30 to 100 μm) derived from the CFU stem cell, and they give rise to blood platelets. In the normal adult, they are largely confined to the marrow. During embryonic development, however, they are present in other hemopoietic organs (liver, spleen) and may also appear in the placenta. During the differentiation of a megakaryocyte, the nucleus divides mitotically without accompanying division of cytoplasm. The nuclei usually separate to a late anaphase or early telophase stage and then reunite. In this way a polyploid nucleus is formed with $32N$-$64N$ chromosomes instead of the $2N$ number characteristic of most other cells. The polyploid nucleus is lobulated in a variable and complicated manner, often having only thin strands connecting different lobular units (Fig. 13.2). The megakaryocytes should not be confused with osteoclasts of marrow and foreign body giant cells, which are multinucleated and form by fusion of monocytes.

The cytoplasm of the megakaryocyte contains the usual organelles and numerous fine granules which apparently form in the Golgi complex. The cell has an irregular shape,with many pseudopodia. The peripheral regions of the cytoplasm become gradually subdivided by demarcation membranes into compartments, each subdivision having granules (Fig. 13.3). When the partitioning membranes become complete, the comparments separate from the parent cell to become free platelets, without rupture of the plasmalemma. The megakaryocytes are situated adjacent to sinusoids in the marrow. They release long strings of platelets which pass between endothelial cells of the sinusoids to enter the blood.

Megakaryocytes are limited in their life span, and stages of degeneration are not uncommon. The nucleus becomes smaller and stains more intensely, and the cytoplasm degenerates. Some of the fragmented nuclei may find their way into the blood vessels, to be carried through the right side of the heart into the lung capillaries where they degenerate. In pathological conditions, entire megakaryocytes may be carried into the lungs and form embolisms in the pulmonary vessels.

DEVELOPMENT OF LYMPHOID ELEMENTS

Lymphocytes

Studies with labeled cells have shown that an older view, that lymphocytes develop only in lymphatic organs, is incorrect. The lymphocytes develop in bone marrow *and* in lymphatic organs. They differentiate from stem cells and retain the ability to multiply after circulating and migrating to other locations. A relatively undifferentiated lymphocyte, known as a *lymphoblast*, is a relatively large cell with a large nucleus, prominent nucleoli, and very basophilic cytoplasm (Fig. 13.4).

The stages of differentiation resemble those of other leukocytes to the extent that the chromatin becomes more dense and compact, the nucleoli become less obvious, and a few azurophilic granules appear in the cytoplasm of some of the cells. Stages of differentiation are less obvious than in the other leukocyte types, because the nuclei do not become lobed or irregular in shape and there are no specific types of granules.

The lymphocytes which multiply and differentiate in the lymphatic organs previously were throught to arise from undifferentiated reticular cells, but this seems unlikely from present evidence. In accordance with recent findings on the origin of stem cells, the lymphocytes of lymphatic organs differentiate from stem cells which enter the circulation from bone marrow. The marrow stem cells for lymphocytes appear to be the same CFU stem cells already described, some of which secondarily take up residence in lymphatic tissue.

Monocytes

Studies by radioautography and by the chromosome marker technique indicate that the monocytes also develop from CFU stem cell precursors in the bone marrow. The fact that monocytes constitute only 1 to 2% of all of the nucleated cells in marrow adds to the difficulty in studying the differentiation of this cell type. The promonocyte is described as being 7 to 15 μm in diameter. It has a rounded or oval nucleus with dispersed chromatin and two or more nucleoli. Electron micrographs show that the cytoplasm contains an abundance of free ribosomes and polyribosomes. Some small granules, identifiable as the azurophilic granules of light microscopy, are present near the Golgi complex. The mature monocyte of marrow is about 9 to 11 μm in diameter, and its nucleus is smaller than that of the promonocyte. Electron micrographs show fewer ribosomes and more azurophilic granules.

The monocytes usually leave the marrow

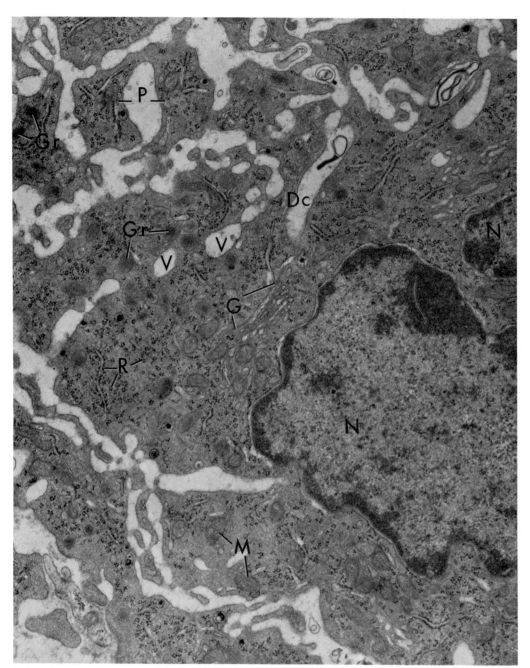

Figure 13.3. Electron micrograph of a portion of a megakaryocyte. The cell characteristically contains a large multilobed nucleus, but only portions of two nuclear lobes (*N*) are present within the field of the micrograph. A portion of one of the Golgi regions (*G*) is seen adjacent to one of the nuclear lobes. Most of the ribosomes (*R*) are distributed in clusters through the cytoplasm, and only a few are present along the cisternae of the endoplasmic reticulum. Electron-dense granules (*Gr*) are seen in the cytoplasm of the cell and within the platelets. They are somewhat smaller than the mitochondria (*M*), and they resemble lysosomes in that they contain acid phosphatase. In the process of platelet formation, portions of the megakaryocyte cytoplasm become partitioned off by membranes. First, membrane-lined vesicles (*V*) develop; later, platelet demarcation channels (*Dc*) arise by extension and fusion of the vesicles. Finally, the channels become continuous with one another, and membrane-bounded regions of the cytoplasm become detached as platelets. Precursor stage platelets (*P*), with only a few remaining attachments, are seen in the upper left portion of the micrograph. From the bone marrow of a mouse (×20,850). (Courtesy of Drs. K. R. Porter and M. A. Bonneville.)

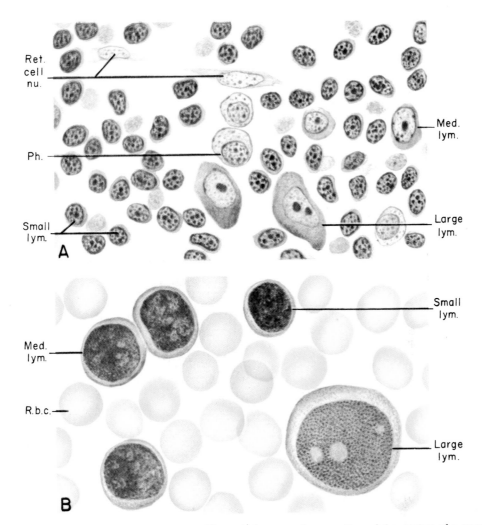

Ret. cell nu.

Ph.

Small lym.

A

Med. lym.

Large lym.

Med. lym.

R.b.c.

Small lym.

Large lym.

B

Figure 13.4. *A,* stages of lymphocyte differentiation seen in a section of the cortex of a monkey lymph node stained with hematoxylin-eosin-azure. Reticular cell nuclei (*Ret. cell nu.*) take a pale stain. Large lymphocytes (*Large lym.*) have prominent nucleoli in an otherwise pale nucleus, with very basophilic cytoplasm. Medium-sized lymphocytes (*Med. lym.*) are intermediate in staining characteristics between the large and the small lymphocytes (*small lym.*). A few phagocytes (*Ph*) are present. *B,* immature lymphocytes in a Wright's stained blood smear from a patient with lymphatic leukemia. The lymphoblast or large lymphocyte (*Large lym.*) has prominent nucleoli which are pale in this stain. Medium-sized lymphocytes, with nucleoli, are more numerous than the small lymphocytes. The size difference between the cells in *A* and *B* is due, in part, to differences in technique: *A* is from a section, *B* from a smear, which flattens the cells. Both figures ×1640.

about three days after beginning their differentiation and continue their maturation by forming additional azurophilic granules while they are in the blood. The azurophilic granules of promonocytes and monocytes give a positive peroxidase reaction, a characteristic difference from the azurophilic granules of lymphocytes, which give a negative peroxidase reaction. Once monocytes leave the blood and enter the connective tissue compartment they become macrophages. The time necessary for this transformation seems highly variable and some authorities simply adopt the arbitrary definition that for practical purposes a cell of this lineage situated in the connective tissue is a macrophage.

EMBRYONIC DEVELOPMENT OF BLOOD CELLS

Blood cell development in the human embryo begins with the formation of *blood islands* in the extraembryonic mesoderm of the yolk sac during the third week of development. The islands are composed of closely packed mesenchymal cells that differentiate along different lines. The peripheral cells become flattened and adherent, to form endothelium, while the central cells proliferate and differentiate into primitive cells which belong almost entirely to the erythroid line. In the earliest recognizable stage of differentiation observable by light microscopy, the cells have vesicular, pale-staining nuclei with prominent nucleoli and basophilic cytoplasm. They were described in the older literature as hemocytoblasts but are best termed simply stem cells. The cells identified as "primitive blood cells" and hemocytoblasts by light microscopy probably include the CFU stem cells and proerythroblasts.

The erythroid cells of yolk sac origin differ from bone marrow-derived erythroid cells in that they retain their nuclei throughout their life span. The yolk sac erythroid cells also have a type of hemoglobin that differs from that of the erythroid cells of all other blood-forming organs (liver, spleen, and marrow).

The *liver* becomes the second hemopoietic organ at about six weeks and is the most active site of hemopoiesis until the middle of fetal life. Then its activity begins to decrease and normally disappears at about the time of birth. The hemopoietic stem cells of the liver are seeded from those developing originally in the yolk sac. In the liver they differentiate into both nucleated and nonnucleated erythrocytes plus granular leukocytes and megakaryocytes. At seven weeks almost all of the circulating red cells are nucleated, but by 11 weeks most are nonnucleated. The mononuclear

precursors of macrophages probably arise initially from yolk sac stem cells but later arise from bone marrow precursors.

The *spleen* is an active blood-forming organ from the latter part of the second month until the eighth month. Erythropoiesis in the spleen ceases soon after birth, but lymphocytes continue to develop in the spleen throughout life.

Red bone marrow is the most important and permanent hemopoietic organ. It becomes functional in the 3rd fetal month. The sequence of differentiating cells in fetal marrow is similar to that described under "Blood Development". With the advent of marrow as a hemopoietic organ, the number of circulating normoblasts decreases and nonnucleated erythrocytes become predominant.

White (yellow) marrow is composed chiefly of fat cells, but it can readily change to red marrow when there is an increased demand for blood cells (Chapter 6).

References

Bainton DF, Ullyot JL, Farquhar MG: The development of neutrophilic polymorphonuclear leukocytes in human bone marrow. *J Exp Med* 139:907–934, 1971.

Barr RD, Whang-Peng J, Perry S: Hemopoietic stem cells in human peripheral blood. *Science* 190:284–285, 1975.

Becker AJ, McCulloch EA, Till JE: Cytological demonstration of the clonal nature of spleen colonies derived from transplanted mouse marrow cells. *Nature* 197:452–454, 1963.

Bennet M, Cudkowiz G: Functional and morphological characterization of stem cells; the unipotential role of "lymphocytes" of mouse marrow. In Yoffey JM (ed): *The Lymphocyte in Immunology and Haemopoiesis* (Bristol Symposium). London, Edward Arnold, 1967, pp 183–194.

Bloom W, Bartelmez GW: Hematopoiesis in young human embryos. *Am J Anat* 67:21–54, 1940.

Brahim F, Osmond DG: Migration of bone marrow lymphocytes demonstrated by selective bone marrow labelling with thymidine-H³. *Anat Rec* 168:139–159, 1970.

Downey H: The myeloblast. In Downey H (ed): *Handbook of Hematology*, vol 3. New York, Paul B. Hoeber, Inc, 1938, pp 1963–2041.

Everett NB, Tyler (Caffrey) RW: Lymphopoiesis in the thymus and other tissues: functional implications. *Int Rev Cytol* 21:205–237, 1967.

Fisher JW, Gordon AS: Conference: erythropoietin. *Ann NY Acad Sci* 149, 1968.

Gowans JL: Differentiation of the cells which synthesize the immunoglobulins. *Ann Immunol (Paris)* 125C:201–211, 1974.

Hudson G, Osmond DG, Roylance PJ: Cell-populations in the bone marrow of the normal guinea-pig. *Acta Anat* 53:234–239, 1963.

Linman JW, Bethell FH: *Factors Controlling Erythropoiesis.* Springfield, Ill., Charles C Thomas, 1960.

Marks P, Rifkind RA: Protein synthesis: its control in erythropoiesis. *Science* 175:955–961, 1972.

Metcalf D: Hemopoietic colonies—in vitro cloning of normal and leukemic cells. *Recent Results Cancer Res* 61:1977.

Micklem HS, Anderson M, Ross E: Limited potential of circulating hemopoietic stem cells. *Nature* 256:41–43, 1975.

Moore MAS, Metcalf D: Ontogeny of the hemopoietic system; yolk sac origin of in vivo and in vitro colony-forming cells in the developing mouse embryo. *Br J Hematol* 18:279, 1970

Nichols BA, Bainton DF: Differentiation of human monocytes in bone marrow and blood: sequential formation of two granule populations. *Lab Invest* 29:27–40, 1973.

Rifkind RA, Bank A, Marks PA, Nossel HL, Ellison RR, and Lindenbaum J: *Fundamentals of Hematology,* ed. 2. Chicago, Year Book Medical Publishers, 1980.

Roitt I: *Essential immunology* ed 4. London, Blackwell Scientific Publications, 1980.

Ropke C, Hougen HP, Everett NB: Long-lived T and B lymphocytes in the bone marrow and thoracic duct lymph of the mouse. *Cell Immunol* 15:82–93, 1975.

Vietta ES, Uhr JW: Immunoglobulin-receptors revisited. A model for the differentiation of bone marrow-derived lymphocytes. *Science* 189:964–969, 1975.

Weiss L: The hematopoietic microenvironment of the bone marrow: an ultrastructural study of the stroma in rats. *Anat Rec* 186:161–184, 1976.

Wintrobe M, Lee G, Boggs D, Bithell T, Foerster J, Athens J, Lukens J: *Clinical Hematology,* ed 8. Philadelphia, Lea & Febiger, 1981.

Chapter 14

LYMPHATIC ORGANS

Protection of the body against deleterious effects of invading foreign substances, cells, or microorganisms is a critical function which necessarily involves the activity of many organs and tissues. Components of the so-called "immune system" are spread over most parts of the body, in some regions being definable as discrete organs (*lymphatic organs*), in other areas spread throughout the connective tissue as *lymphatic tissue.* Lymphatic tissue is less highly organized and will be considered in each of the organs in which it appears.

Lymphatic (lymphoid) tissue is not one of the fundamental tissue types of the body. Rather, it is a special variety of reticular connective tissue that is regularly infiltrated with lymphocytes. With the exception of the thymic reticulum, lymphatic tissue seems solely derived from mesenchyme, and its cells and fibers are not separated from other connective tissue by a basal lamina. Regions where the lymphocytes are not closely packed are identified as *loose lymphatic tissue,* in contrast with *dense lymphatic tissue,* in which the lymphocytes are closely aggregated. There are numerous gradations between these two varieties of lymphatic tissue, and there is also a gradation between the loose lymphatic tissue and regions where widely scattered lymphocytes infiltrate into the connective tissue.

Regions where closely packed lymphocytes are in spherical aggregations are known as *lymphatic nodules* (lymphatic follicles). After birth, such nodules often have lighter-staining areas known as *germinal centers* (secondary nodules).

Solitary lymphatic nodules are widely scattered in the digestive, respiratory, and urinary tracts. Particularly prominent aggregations of nodules form the Peyer's patches found in the wall of the small intestine on the side opposite to the mesenteric attachment. The aggregations of lymphatic tissue that are identified as separate lymphatic organs include the lymph nodes, tonsils, thymus, and spleen. They are defined by the presence of a dense connective tissue capsule which isolates the enclosed lymphatic tissue from the surrounding tissues. The tonsils are examples of only partially encapsulated aggregations of nodules.

The chief characteristic common to all lymphatic organs is the presence of large numbers of lymphocytes pervading a framework of reticular cells and fibers. The lymph nodes are the only lymphatic organs located in the course of lymphatic vessels; that is, they are the only ones that have both afferent and efferent lymphatic vessels. They are also the only ones that contain lymphatic sinuses, and they are the only structures which filter the lymph. The spleen, thymus, and tonsils resemble most other organs in their relationship to lymphatic vessels. They have efferent lymph vessels draining from them, but they have neither afferent lymphatic vessels nor lymphatic sinuses.

THE LYMPH NODES

The lymph nodes are variable in number but are more or less constantly found in certain definite regions of the body such as the mesentery, axilla and groin. They are frequently in groups or in a series, as in the inguinal and axillary regions. They vary in size, ranging from minute bodies to as much as 2.5 cm in length. They are usually oval or bean-shaped, with an indentation, the *hilus,* on one side, where the blood vessels enter and leave the node. The lymphatic vessels leaving the node, the *vasa efferentia,* are also found at the hilus, but the entering vessels, the *vasa afferentia,* are found at various points along the convex surface of the node.

Lymph nodes are covered by a *capsule* of connective tissue which blends with the surrounding connective tissue. The capsule consists of bundles of collagenous fibers, scattered elastic fibers and a few smooth muscle fibers. At the hilus, there is a depression where the capsule is thickened and extends deep into the node. At various points over the surface of the node, the capsule gives off septa or *trabeculae* that extend into the substance of the organ. The trabeculae of connective tissue and the elements of the lymph tissue are arranged differently in the outer or cortical and the inner or medullary regions. However, there are also numerous similarities between the regions, and the structure of the organ can be understood best by considering the cortex and medulla together.

Cortex and Medulla

In the cortex, the trabeculae are more or less perpendicular to the surface, and they partly subdivide this region into compartments which are continuous centrally with the more irregularly arranged anastomosing subdivisions of the medulla (Figs. 14.1) and 14.2). The cortical compartments also communicate laterally with each other through spaces between the trabeculae. The degree of development of the trabeculae and of separation into compartments varies in nodes taken from different parts of the body and in nodes of different animals. In some of the other mammals (e.g., ox), the trabeculae are more highly developed than in man and mark off more distinct compartments.

The lymphocytes are closely packed in

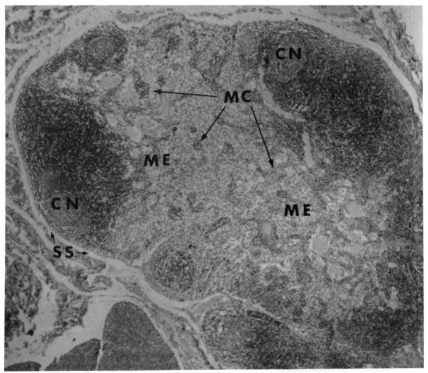

Figure 14.1. Section of a lymph node from monkey. *CN*, cortical nodules with germinal centers; *ME*, medulla with medullary sinuses; *MC*, medullary cords; *SC*, subcapsular sinus (artifactually expanded) (×42).

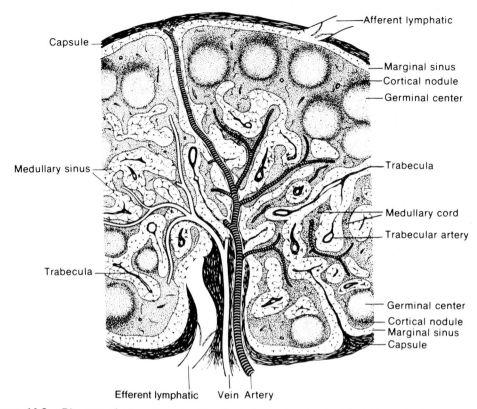

Capsule

Afferent lymphatic

Marginal sinus
Cortical nodule
Germinal center

Medullary sinus

Trabecula

Medullary cord

Trabecular artery

Trabecula

Germinal center
Cortical nodule
Marginal sinus
Capsule

Efferent lymphatic   Vein Artery

Figure 14.2. Diagram of a lymph node. (Modified after a drawing by M. Heidenhain, from Heudorfer K: Über den Bau der Lymphdrüsen. *Z Anat* 61: 365–401, 1921.)

the cortical regions of the nodes and often form spherical aggregations, the *cortical nodules* (*primary nodules* or *follicles*), which are continuous centrally with anastomosing cords of lymphatic tissue in the medulla known as *medullary cords*. The dense lymphatic tissue of the cortex is separated from the capsule by a lymphatic channel known as the *marginal sinus* (*subcapsular sinus*). This sinus is continuous around most of the circumference of the node except where it is interrupted by connective tissue trabeculae. The marginal sinus is continuous with other lymphatic channels, *trabecular sinuses*, which extend centrally between the connective tissue trabeculae and the aggregations of cortical nodules. In the deep cortical region, these latter channels continue as *paracortical (parafollicular) sinuses*. Paracortical sinuses become continuous with the anastomosing *medullary si-*

nuses, located between the medullary cords of lymphatic tissue and the connective tissue trabeculae (Fig. 14.2). There are generally several afferent lymphatic vessels leading into the marginal sinus along the convex surface of the node opposite the hilus, and usually only one or two efferent vessels that exit at the hilus.

Although the dense lymphatic tissue of the cortex commonly surrounds the medulla except at the hilus, it varies in thickness in nodes from different locations and also within the same nodes at different times. The nodules are often arranged in a single layer around the periphery, but they may also be found in layers where the cortex is thickened.

The cortical nodules often contain lighter-staining central areas known as *germinal centers* (secondary nodules, *reaction centers*). They were named germinal centers in recognition of the fact that they are more active in lymphocyte proliferation than are other parts of the node. It was also noted many years ago that the germinal centers appear during certain types of inflammation; hence the name reaction center. The framework of the center, like that of other parts of the node, is composed of reticular cells and reticular fibers. The reticular cells of the germinal centers are relatively large and have particularly long cytoplasmic processes; hence they are often described as *dendritic cells*. These cells have large, pale-staining nuclei and cytoplasm which is only lightly basophilic. The lymphocytes of the germinal center consist chiefly of the medium-sized and large varieties; these range up to 15 μm or more in diameter. The nuclei of these cells contain considerable euchromatin, which takes a relatively pale stain, thus counteracting the overall effect of the basophilic cytoplasm. The centers also contain a number of macrophages with cytoplasm that is only lightly basophilic. This combination of staining characteristics of the cells accounts for the light appearance of the germinal centers in

comparison with the more darkly staining borders of small lymphocytes that surround the centers (Figs. 14.1 and 14.3). The center itself often appears relatively dark on the side facing the medulla and lighter on the side facing the marginal sinus (Fig. 14.4). The darker-staining zone (cap) contains a higher proportion of dividing cells and more closely packed cells.

Germinal centers contain a number of plasma cells in addition to the other cell types described above. It is well established that plasma cells form antibodies and that they differentiate from lymphocytes of the B type (bursa-derived type, Chapter 7). It is also known that the lymphocytes of the germinal centers belong to the B type. Although plasma cells are not as numerous in the germinal centers as in the medullary cords (Fig. 14.5), it seems evident that the centers have a major role in the secondary response in antigen-antibody reactions. The centers do not appear until after birth, in response to antigen. They disappear in the absence of antigen and reappear in the same region after subsequent antigenic stimulation. When animals are kept in a

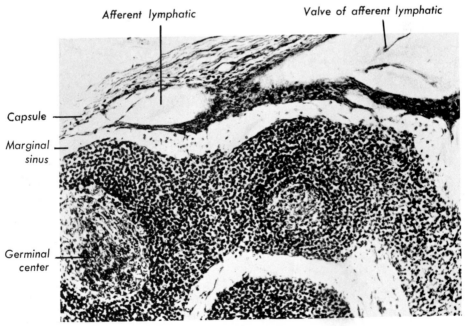

Figure 14.3. Portion of cortex of human lymph node. Photomicrograph (×260). (After Petersen.)

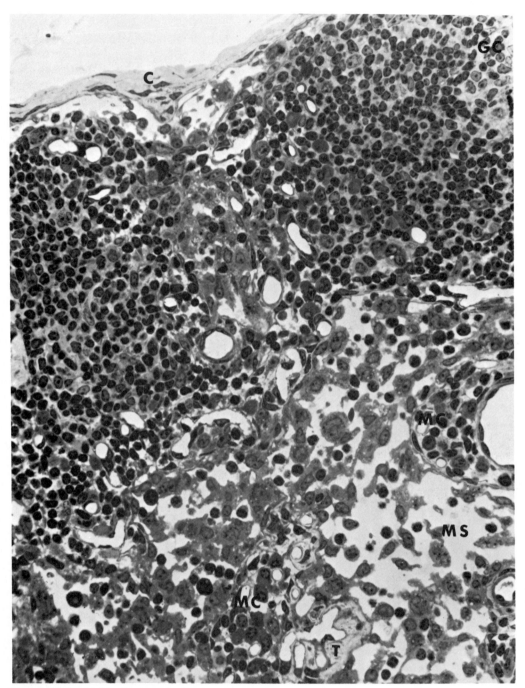

Figure 14.4. Light micrograph of a lymph node from monkey showing cortex and medulla. The capsule (C) in the *upper left* is underlain by marginal sinus. A germinal center (GC) of a cortical nodule is at the *upper right*. Medullary cords (MC), medullary sinuses (MS), and a trabecula (T) appear at the *lower right* (×400).

germ-free environment from the time of birth, the centers fail to develop. They also remain inactive in animals thymectomized at birth.

The interrelationships of reticular cells and endothelial cells lining the lymphatic sinuses have been studied extensively. It was once thought that the linings of the

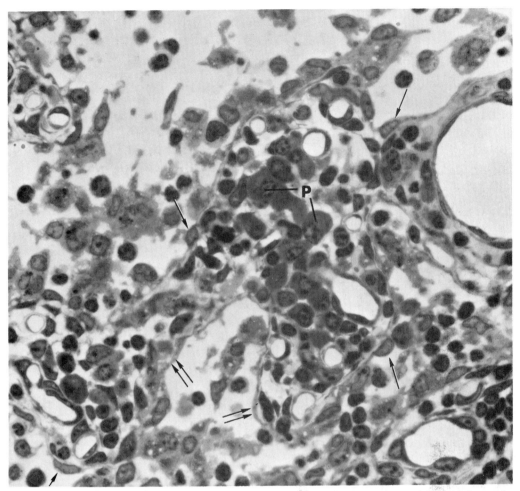

Figure 14.5. Light micrograph of a section through a medullary cord and medullary sinuses of a lymph node from monkey. Endothelial cells lining the medullary sinuses surrounding the cord, are indicated by the *arrows* (*single arrows* show nuclei and *double arrows* show thin cytoplasmic extensions). *P*, plasma cells (×640).

sinuses consist chiefly of reticular cells that are more flattened than those which form the framework of the cortical nodules and medullary cords of lymphatic tissue. However, more recent electron microscope studies indicate that the portions of the cortical and medullary sinuses that abut against the capsule and trabeculae, respectively, are lined by endothelial cells with gaps between them (Fig. 14.6). The walls of the cortical and medullary sinuses which abut, respectively, against cortical nodules and medullary cords (Figs. 14.5 and 14.6) are also lined by endothelial cells with intercellular gaps, but these endothelial cells are more frequently associated with reticular cells

and macrophages than are the cells on the capsular and trabecular sides of the sinuses.

The reticular cells which are associated with the endothelial cells of the sinus, as well as those which form a framework across the lymphatic cords and sinuses, are intimately associated with reticular (argyrophilic) fibers, and the protoplasmic processes of these cells form a thin, but complete, covering of the fibers. Electron microscope studies using transfused labeled cells indicate that the reticular cells are generally not very phagocytic, contrary to earlier views. Most of the macrophages seen in lymph nodes are apparently derived from monocytes which are closely associated

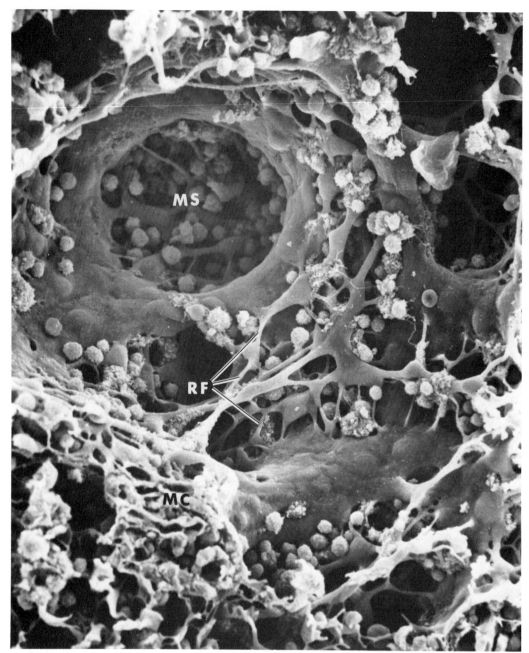

Figure 14.6. Scanning electron micrograph of a lymph node of dog, medullary region. Reticular fibers are covered with cell processes (either reticular cell or sinus lining cell). The lining of the medullary sinus (*MS*) and the medullary cord (*MC*) are covered with flattened lining cells. Most of the free cells have been washed out of this preparation, but a few lymphocytes and macrophages are still present (×830). (Courtesy of Dr. Masayuki Miyoshi.)

with the reticular cells of the framework and with the endothelial cells lining the sinuses. Although animals given repeated injections of colloidal dyes (e.g., trypan blue) for a relatively long period often show a few small vacuoles of ingested material in the reticular cells of their lymph nodes, the dye is not segregated and concentrated into large vacuoles, as it is in macrophages. The reticular cells and macrophages of lymph nodes differ from each other in their reaction to colloidal dyes in a manner rather similar to the difference exhibited by fibroblasts and macrophages in loose connective tissue (Fig. 5.3A and B).

Small lymphocytes are numerous in the node. Although they seldom divide, they may be readily stimulated to enlarge and become active mitotically. In studies using transfused labeled lymphocytes, it is found that the lymphocytes of the germinal centers and their caps consist entirely of the B type (bursa-derived type, Chapter 7). On the other hand, the lymphocytes of the deep (paracortical) region of the cortex belong to the T type (thymus-dependent type, Chapter 7). Other portions of the node contain mostly the B type.

Lymphatic Vessels and Sinuses

Several lymphatic vessels pierce the capsule on the convex side of the node and open into the marginal sinus which continues into the parafollicular and medullary sinuses. The lymph circulates slowly through the cortical and medullary sinuses, which afford a greatly enlarged area for circulating lymph in comparison with that provided by the afferent lymph vessels. From the medullary sinuses, lymph vessels course through the connective tissue of the hilus and form the efferent lymphatics, which are wider but less numerous than the afferent lymphatics.

The flattened lining cells of the sinuses become continuous at the periphery of the node with the endothelial cells lining the afferent and efferent lymph vessels. The lining cells lack a basal lamina and often have gaps between the cells. As mentioned earlier, the lining cells are closely associated with reticular cells, but they are apparently endothelial in nature and not flattened reticular cells as described in the earlier literature on this subject.

Blood Vessels

Arteries enter the nodes through the connective tissue at the hilus, and some of the arterial branches course in the trabeculae to the capsule. Other arterial branches leave the trabeculae soon after entering the node and course into the medullary cords. These supply capillaries to the medulla and continue into the cortex, where arterioles penetrate the cortical nodules, giving off capillaries to the lymphatic tissue. The vessels of the germinal centers apparently consist of capillaries only. The number of blood vessels in the germinal center is somewhat less than in surrounding areas. This is well shown in preparations washed free of lymphocytes and examined by scanning electron microscopy (Fig. 14.7). The venules that drain the cortex have a typical squamous endothelial lining in their course through the outer cortex but the venules from the deep (paracortical) cortex are lined by cuboidal endothelial cells (Fig. 14.8). These particular venules sometimes referred to as *high endothelial venules*, facilitate the passage of lymphocytes from the blood vessels into the lymphatic tissue for recirculation via the lymphatic and thoracic duct back to the blood vessels. The lymphocytes of the recirculating type selectively adhere to the endothelial cells of these venules at the site of migration. The migration has been described as occurring either by an intercellular route or by an intracellular (transcellular) course. Current evidence favors the intercellular route (Fig. 14.9).

The blood vessels draining the blood from all portions of the node other than the paracortical region consist of veins and venules lined by the usual squamous type of endothelium. They follow the same general course as the arteries and exit at the hilus.

Nerves

The nerves, which are not abundant, enter the node at the hilus and accompany the blood vessels. Some of them terminate in the trabeculae and capsule, whereas others form perivascular networks that follow the vessels into the lymphatic tissue.

Functions

The lymph nodes participate in the production of lymphocytes as evidenced by

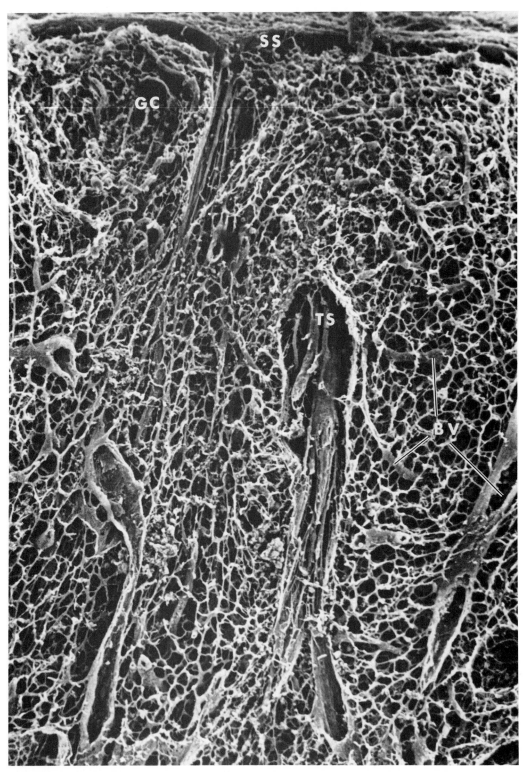

Figure 14.7.   Scanning electron micrograph of dog lymph node, cortical region. In this washed node the reticular fiber framework is well illustrated. *GC*, germinal center area; *SS*, subcapsular sinus; *TS*, trabecular sinus; *BV*, blood vessels (×250). (Courtesy of Dr. Masayuki Miyoshi.)

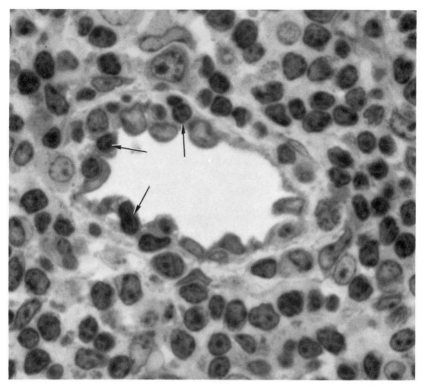

Figure 14.8.   Light micrograph of a high endothelial venule from the deep cortical region of monkey lymph node. Note the nuclei of endothelial cells bulging into the lumen particularly at the left side of the vessel. Dense nuclei of migrating lymphocytes appear at the *arrows*. (×975).

numerous mitoses of lymphoblasts within the node, particularly within the germinal centers. However, the presence of more lymphocytes in the efferent than in the afferent vessels is more closely related to the recirculation of lymphocytes. Studies with transfused labeled cells show that approximately 95% of the lymphocytes leaving the node belong to the recirculating type. These cells leave the high endothelial variety of postcapillary venules of the paracortical (juxtamedullary) region of the cortex and enter the lymph circulation, to be carried by the thoracic duct to the systemic circulation.

The lymph nodes also have an important role in phagocytosis of foreign material, which readily passes from the interstitial fluid of connective tissues into lymphatic capillaries via the gaps between their endothelial cells. The bronchial nodes are good examples of this. Inhaled carbon particles which pass through the epithelial lining of the alveoli of the lungs enter the connective tissue, then pass into lymphatic capillaries of the lung, and thence move on into bronchial lymph nodes by the afferent lymph vessels. The foreign material accumulates especially in the medullary regions of the node but may blacken the entire node after extensive and prolonged exposure. Because the lymphatic capillaries are permeable to large molecules and even to entire cells, the lymph node sinuses may contain erythrocytes that escape from blood vessels by internal hemorrhage. Unfortunately the great permeability of the endothelium of lymphatic capillaries also allows cancer cells to enter the lymph nodes; eventually these cells reach the blood circulation via the thoracic duct.

One of the major functions of lymph nodes is the production of antibodies. There are various ways in which antigens

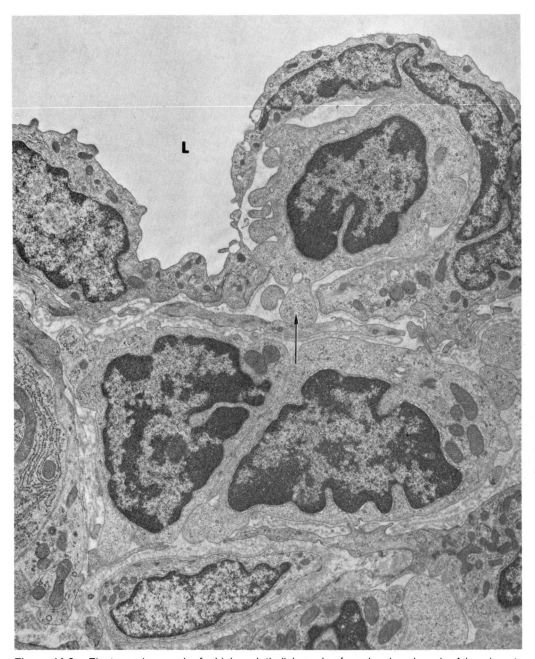

Figure 14.9. Electron micrograph of a high endothelial venule of monkey lymph node. A lymphocyte is seen nearly surrounded by cytoplasm of an attenuated endothelial cell. A process of the lymphocyte penetrates the basal lamina (*arrow*). From this micrograph it cannot be ascertained whether the lymphocyte has migrated between endothelial cells or through a single cell. Two other lymphocytes lie beneath the endothelium partially surrounded by basal lamina material. *L*, lumen of venule (×9200).

may be handled by the body. Some may be excreted, some may be taken up by macrophages and be subjected to degradative enzymes, and some may be processed by ad- herence to macrophages for reactions with lymphocytes. The lymph node is a major site for the interaction of "helper" T lymphocytes with reactive B lymphocytes for the initiation of humoral immune responses (see Chapter 7). In the lymph node, special processing of this type also occurs by the dendrite reticular cells in the germinal centers.

Development

Recent studies of well-fixed lymph nodes from human fetuses ranging from 26 to 245 mm in length have clarified the manner by which lymph nodes arise by partitioning of lymphatic sacs. Primordia of the nodes are first recognizable when some connective tissue, along with some blood vessels and lymphocytes, invaginates the endothelial walls of the sacs in certain locations (Fig. 14.10). Several nodes usually form from a single lymphatic sac; hence, the nodes are usually in groups. The invaginating connective tissue forms the capsule of the node

and surrounds it everywhere except where lymphatic vessels and blood vessels enter and exit. Connective tissue trabeculae are present at an early stage and become more pronounced as development progresses. The medullary region differentiates into its characteristic morphology earlier than the cortical region does. The latter does not attain its characteristic pattern until relatively late in fetal life. Germinal centers do not usually appear until after birth, and usually only after stimulation by antigen.

HEMOLYMPH NODES

In certain animals, structures have been described that are similar to lymph nodes, except that afferent and efferent lymphatic vessels are absent and the sinuses contain blood instead of lymph. True hemal nodes

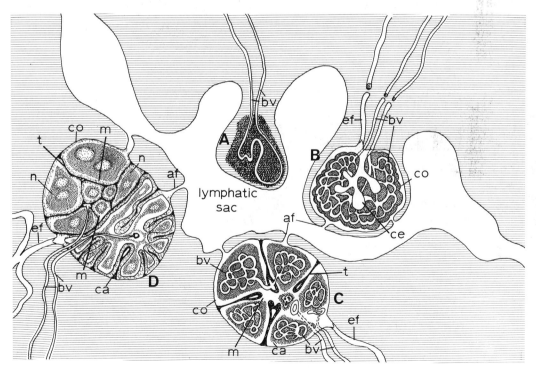

Figure 14.10. Diagram of several stages of lymph node differentiation. *A*, early stage, showing aggregation of lymphatic tissue around a capillary loop and invagination of the complex into the lymphatic sac lumen. *B*, later stage, showing formation of central and cortical lymphatic sinuses and the efferent drainage channel. *C*, later stage showing formation of trabeculae. *D*, final stage showing formation of definitive morphology. This mode of formation permits several nodes to form simultaneously in association with a single lymphatic sac and accounts for the usual grouping of nodes. *BV*, blood vessels; *CO*, cortical sinus; *CE*, central sinus; *CA*, capsule; *AF*, afferent lymphatics; *EF*, efferent lymphatics; *N*, nodules; *M*, medullary sinuses; *T*, trabeculae.

of this type occur in the sheep. In the pig, hemolymph nodes have been described which have sinuses connected with both lymphatic and blood vessels, so that they appear to be intermediate between lymph nodes and the hemal nodes of sheep. In man, the occurrence of organs of this type has been questioned and seems very doubtful. Normal lymph nodes usually contain a few red blood cells, some of which may have been brought in by the afferent lymphatics, whereas others probably enter from the blood vessels within the node by diapedesis. It is true that nodes may be found in man with considerable numbers of red blood cells, but there have been no descriptions of connections between the sinuses and the blood vessels. The presence of an unusual number of erythrocytes is most likely the result of hemorrhage from vessels either within the node or in the neighborhood of the afferent lymphatics.

THE TONSILS

The Palatine Tonsils

The palatine tonsils are paired, oval-shaped bodies located in the oropharynx between the glossopalatine and pharyngo-palatine arches. They consist of dense accumulations of lymphatic tissue in the connective tissue of the mucosa. They are covered on their free surface by a stratified squamous epithelium which is continuous with the epithelium of the rest of the pharynx. This epithelium has the same structure as elsewhere in the pharynx: flat surface cells, beneath which are irregular cells, whereas the deepest cells are cuboidal or more or less columnar and rest upon a basal lamina. A thin layer of fibrous connective tissue with papillae is usually found between the basal lamina and the underlying lymphatic tissue. At various places on the surface of the tonsil, deep indentations or pockets occur. These depressions, 10 to 20 in number, are known as the *crypts* of the tonsil (Fig. 14.11) and are lined by a continuation of the surface epithelium that becomes thinner as the deeper part of the

crypt is reached. Passing off from the bottoms and sides of the main or primary crypts are frequently several secondary crypts, also lined with the same type of epithelium.

Surrounding each crypt is a zone of varying thickness, consisting of a rather diffuse lymphatic tissue in which are embedded *nodules* of compact lymphatic tissue similar to those of the lymph nodes. The nodules, like those of lymph nodes, may contain *germinal centers* that consist of a lighter-staining central area and a surrounding zone of more closely packed cells.

There is a *capsule* of connective tissue over the attached or basal surface of the lymphatic tissue which is firmly adherent on the one side to the tonsillar tissue and on the other to the surrounding structures. From the capsule there are *septa* of loose connective tissue that separate the various crypts with their surrounding zones of lymphatic tissue from one another. Infiltrated into this connective tissue are various-sized lymphocytes, plasma cells, mast cells, and frequently, neutrophilic leukocytes.

At various points on the surface of the tonsil, and especially in the crypts, there occurs what is known as *lymphocytic infiltration of the epithelium* (Fig. 14.12). This consists of an invasion of the epithelium by the underlying lymphocytes. It varies from only a few lymphocytes scattered in the epithelium to an almost complete replacement of epithelium by lymphocytes. In this way, the lymphocytes may reach the surface and be discharged into the crypts. Such cells probably form the bulk of the so-called salivary corpuscles. In inflammation, the tonsillar tissue also contains numerous polymorphonuclear neutrophilic leukocytes which emigrate from the blood.

Small mucous glands, similar to those found in other parts of the pharynx, are numerous in the connective tissue adjacent to the tonsil. The bodies of these glands are separated from the tonsils by the capsule. Their excretory ducts usually open on the free surface, but occasionally they may open into the tonsillar crypts.

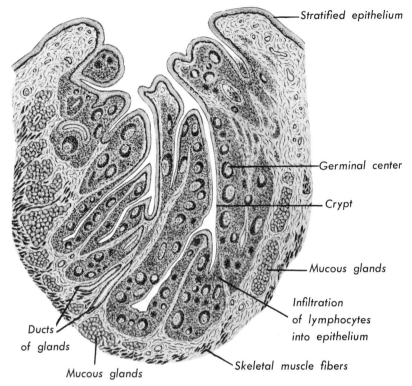

Figure 14.11. Drawing depicting a section through the palatine tonsil of man (×9).

The Lingual Tonsils

These are spherical aggregations of lymphatic tissue situated on the dorsum and sides of the back part of the tongue between the circumvallate papillae and the epiglottis (Fig. 16.4). They contain rather wide-mouthed, deep crypts, which may be branched and which are lined with a continuation of the surface stratified squamous epithelium. As in the palatine tonsil, each crypt is surrounded by an aggregation of lymph nodules containing germinal centers. In most crypts, there is marked lymphoid infiltration of the epithelium. Ducts of some of the mucous glands of the tongue frequently open into the crypts (Fig. 16.5).

The Pharyngeal Tonsil

There is a median aggregation of lymphatic tissue in the posterior wall of the nasopharynx which forms the pharyngeal tonsil. The lymphatic tissue is similar to that of the palatine tonsils. The epithelium over the free surface, as is characteristic for the nasopharynx and other respiratory passages, is largely pseudostratified columnar ciliated epithelium. There are patches of stratified squamous epithelium, which become more numerous in the adult. Hypertrophy of the pharyngeal tonsil, with consequent obstruction of the nasal openings is common, especially in children, constituting what are known as *adenoids.*

Blood Vessels of Tonsils

These have a distribution similar to that of the blood vessels of the lymph nodes, but they enter the organ along its entire attached side and not at a definite hilus.

Lymphatic Vessels

The tonsils have no afferent lymphatic vessels and no lymph sinuses. At the peripheral surface of the lymphatic tissue, there are plexuses of lymph capillaries which form the beginnings of efferent lymphatic vessels. The tonsils, therefore, unlike the lymph nodes, which are situated in

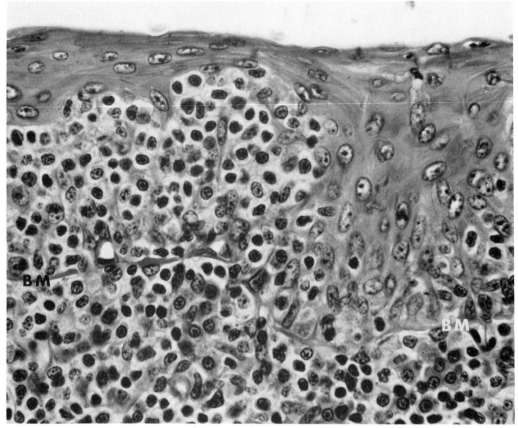

Figure 14.12. Section from a crypt in the palatine tonsil of a dog showing lymphocytic infiltration of the stratified squamous epithelium. The crypt lumen is at the top. *BM*, basement membrane (×640).

the course of lymphatic vessels, are situated at the beginnings of lymphatic vessels.

Nerves

The nerves of the palatine tonsils are derived from the glossopharyngeal nerve and from the sphenopalatine ganglion, and they enter the organ along its attached side.

Functions

Fairly numerous mitoses in the germinal centers show that the tonsils participate in lymphocyte development. The presence of plasma cells indicates that the tonsils also participate in antibody production. The tonsils are situated strategically for protecting the body against invasion by bacteria and foreign proteins. On the other hand, the lack of a complete epithelial lining in the deep tonsillar crypts may be a factor leading to general infections that

sometimes develop after invasion and proliferation of foreign microorganisms.

Development

The palatine tonsils make their appearance during the third month of development. Evaginations of endoderm grow into the underlying mesenchyme at the site of the second pharyngeal pouch and, at the same time, there is a subepithelial condensation of mesenchyme. The cells of the inner part of the mesenchymal condensation become arranged around the epithelium of the evaginations and gradually develop the reticulum and lymphocytes of the lymphatic tissue, whereas the endodermal evaginations become the crypts. At the outer part of the mesenchymal condensation, fibrous connective tissue develops into the capsule.

The lingual and pharyngeal tonsils begin their development during the later months of fetal life. In the pharyngeal tonsil, definite nodules appear at about the time of birth or during the 1st or second year. In the lingual tonsil, the nodules are not fully formed until the fifth or sixth year.

THE THYMUS

The thymus has a very important role in the immune mechanism of the body, and it becomes occupied with lymphocytes early in fetal development. It is a relatively large organ at the time of birth, weighing approximately 12 to 15 g, and its growth continues at a rapid rate until the end of the second year. After that time it grows at a somewhat slower rate until puberty, when it reaches a weight of 30 to 40 g. It subsequently becomes smaller in proportion to most other organs and eventually shows an actual decrease in size; i.e., it undergoes "age involution" and is partially replaced by fat and connective tissue (compare Figs. 14.13 and 14.14.)

The human thymus consists of two lobes which are closely applied to each other and joined in the midline by connective tissue. The lobes are surrounded by a connective tissue *capsule* which gives off relatively coarse *septa* or *trabeculae;* these partially subdivide each lobe into groups of lobules that are partially subdivided further into individual lobules by slender trabeculae (Fig. 14.13). Each lobule consists of a *cortex* and a *medulla*. In random sections, groups of lobules often appear to be completely separated from each other and individual lobules may also appear to be completely separated. However, serial sections show

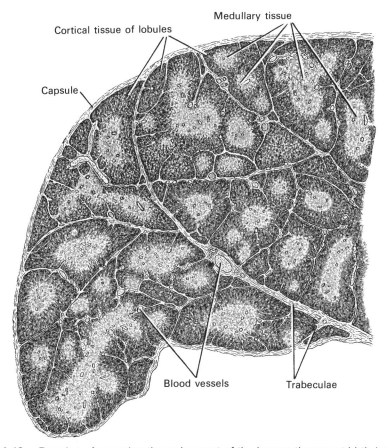

Figure 14.13. Drawing of a section through a part of the human thymus at birth (×12).

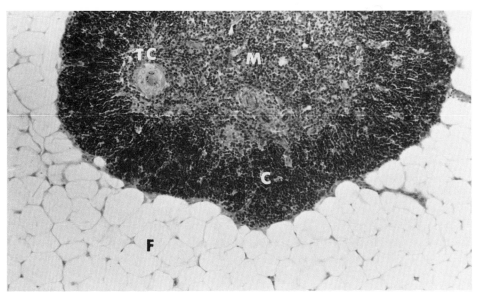

Figure 14.14. Photomicrograph of a portion of an adult human thymus. Cortical and medullary areas are still visible but much of the thymic tissue has been replaced by fat cells. *C*, cortex; *F*, fat cells; *M*, medulla; *TC*, thymic corpuscle (×35).

that at least until involution is well advanced, the medullary tissue is continuous from one lobule to another throughout each of the two lobes.

The thymus, like other lymphatic organs, is composed of lymphocytes and reticular cells. However, the latter differ in origin and structure from those of other lymphatic organs. They are derived from the endoderm of the third pair of pharyngeal pouches; hence they are designated as endodermal reticular cells or thymic *epithelial reticular* cells (see discussion in Chapter 4). The earliest lymphocytes associated with the thymus appear in the mesenchyme just outside the endodermal rudiment by the end of the second fetal month and are present within the organ shortly thereafter. These earliest lymphocytes are derivatives of stem cells of yolk sac origin which circulate to the thymus through the blood vessels via the liver and bone marrow. The epithelial reticular cells are close together and have relatively short processes before the initial entrance of lymphocytes into the organ. During the establishment of the lymphocyte population, the cell bodies of the reticular cells are pushed apart and are

left in contact with each other by long cytoplasmic processes.

The cortex consists of an abundance of lymphocytes which partially obscure the epithelial reticular cells. The lymphocytes, unlike those of lymph nodes, are not arranged in nodules, and, although mitoses occur, there are no germinal centers. The lymphocytes, known as T lymphocytes, vary in size and cytological characteristics, with the largest cells often located in the subcapsular region of the lobule. They proliferate at a rapid rate, and some of them enter the blood circulation and function in cell-mediated immunity. However, the vast majority of the newly formed lymphocytes degenerate within the thymus; the functional significance of this extensive degeneration is not fully understood.

The thymic cortex is unusual in that its blood vessels consist of capillaries only. The arteries to the thymus follow the connective tissue septa to the junction of cortex and medulla, where they send branches into the cortical and medullary tissues. The medulla receives small arteries and arterioles, which divide into capillaries, whereas the cortex receives capillaries only. The cortical capillaries consistute an important part of a *blood-thymic barrier,* which inhibits circulating macromolecules and particulate matter from entering the cortex. This allows the cortical lymphocytes to proliferate and differentiate in an environment free of circulating antigens. Studies of thymic tissues from rodents transfused with labeled macromolecules (cytochrome, peroxidase, catalase, and ferritin) show that none of these substances leave the vessels in the cortex, whereas ferritin, with a molecular weight of 462,000, and catalase, with a weight of 240,000, approximately that of IgG, readily leave the vessels in the medulla. The structures separating the blood from the cortical tissues are as fol-lows: endothelial cells joined by occluding junctions, basal lamina of the capillary endothelium, a thin compartment of connective tissue, basal lamina beneath a continuous border of the epithelial reticular cells, and the epithelial reticular cells. The latter are joined by desmosomes, particularly in the immature thymus.

The medulla resembles the cortex in that it is composed of lymphocytes and epithelial reticular cells, but the lymphocytes are less numerous and therefore the epithelial reticular cells are more obvious. The epithelial reticular cells of the medulla, like those of the cortex, have oblong pale-staining nuclei that are much larger than the lymphocyte nuclei (Fig. 14.15). Electron

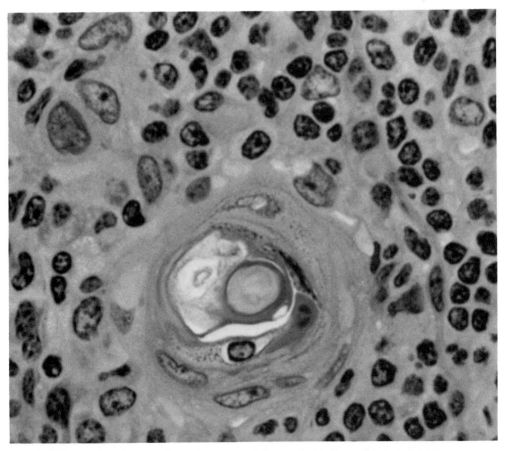

Figure 14.15. Light micrograph of thymic medulla from monkey showing Hassall's corpuscle, lymphocytes, and large, pale nuclei of thymic epithelial reticular cells. Note the flattened peripheral cells, some containing cytoplasmic granules resembling keratohyaline granules in the Hassall's corpuscle (×1000).

micrographs show that the epithelial reticular cells contain 10 nm filaments much like those of stratified squamous epithelium and that the filaments extend into the cell processes which are in contact by desmosomes. The cytoplasm contains a relatively small Golgi apparatus, some free ribosomes, and some rough endoplasmic reticulum.

The medulla also contains a number of spherical or oval bodies composed of concentrically arranged cells known as *thymic corpuscles* or *Hassall's corpuscles* (Figs. 14.14 and 14.15). They are characteristic of the thymus and begin to appear during the first half of fetal life. Their average diameter in the fully developed organ is 20 to 50 μm, but they vary considerably, and much larger corpuscles are often found. The cells are concentrically arranged in the corpuscle and range in shape from polygonal at the surface to flattened at the center. They take a bright red stain with hematoxylin and eosin. Some of the central cells may be completely degenerated. The cellular changes from periphery to center have been likened to the stages in cornification of stratified squamous epithelium.

Because the thymic epithelial reticular cells are endodermal in origin, it is not surprising to find that they are not generally associated with reticular fibers. The latter are sparse except in the connective tissue around blood vessels. In keeping with their origin, the endodermally derived reticular cells exhibit epithelial characteristics when grown in tissue culture. They also behave like epithelial cells in that they do not show much phagocytic activity for colloidal dyes (e.g., trypan blue), but this may be due at least in part to a failure of the colloidal dyes to penetrate the cortical blood-thymic barrier.

In addition to lymphocytes and epithelial-derived reticular cells, the thymus contains macrophages, particularly in the region of the corticomedullary junction. Plasma cells are not present within the cortex, but a few may be present in the medulla. The connective tissue of the septa and capsule contains fibroblasts plus some plasma cells and mast cells.

Blood Vessels

The thymus is supplied by branches of the internal thoracic and inferior thyroidal arteries. The arterial branches give off some vessels to the connective tissue of the septa and continue in the septa around the lobules to the corticomedullary junctions, where they send small arteries into the medulla and capillaries into the cortex. As noted above, the cortical capillaries are relatively impermeable to macromolecules. On the other hand, the postcapillary venules of the medulla are readily traversed by macromolecules and by lymphocytes. This is the route by which the lymphocytes proliferating in the thymic cortex enter the blood vessels. However, the endothelial cells of the postcapillary venules are not thickened like those of high endothelial venules of lymph nodes. The venules of the thymus converge in the medullary tissue to form larger veins that course in the connective tissue septa to accompany the arteries. They drain into the left innominate and thyroidal veins.

Lymphatics

There are no lymph sinuses in the thymus and no afferent lymphatic vessels; this condition is in contrast with that of lymph nodes but is similar to that of all other organs of the body. Lymphatic capillaries arise around the lymphatic tissue of the lobules and join to form larger lymphatic vessels that accompany the arteries in the connective tissue septa.

Nerves

Branches of the vagus and cervical sympathetics are distributed to the walls of blood vessels. A few fibers have been described as terminating freely in the cortex and medulla.

Functions

It has been known for many years that the thymus is active in lymphocyte proliferation, but the functional significance of this was not recognized before recent experimental studies. A better understanding of thymic function has been achieved by studies on the effects of thymectomy and by transfusions of labeled cells. It has been found that mice thymectomized on the first day after birth develop a wasting disease within a few months and die at an early age. There is also a marked deficiency in the development of other lymphatic organs, with few or no germinal centers appearing. The thymectomized mice also accept skin grafts from other strains of mice and rats, whereas normal mice reject foreign grafts. When thymectomized animals are given injections of lymphatic tissue from other strains and species, the injected cells react against the host, whereas normal animals reject the foreign cells. It is known that the rejection of foreign grafts (a part of cell-mediated immunity) is by thymus-derived lymphocytes (T lymphocytes) and that the formation of antibodies by plasma cells derived from B lymphocytes occurs with the help (or collaboration) of T cells (Chapter 7). As noted earlier, the thymus itself does not normally form antibodies.

Some studies have indicated that the implantation of thymic tissue (lymphocytes and epithelial reticular cells) into thymectomized mice restores the animal's ability to form antibodies. Furthermore, this is described as occurring when the implants are enclosed in Millipore filters, which should prevent the escape of cells. On this evidence, it has been proposed that the thymus may exert an influence on other lymphocytic tissues through a humoral factor, presumably produced by the epithelial reticular cells. At least two different thymic humoral factors have been isolated but their physiological roles are still controversial. However, some investigators claim that injection of a "purified" thymic product into individuals lacking normal immunological responses can result in establishment of nearly normal immunological function. In addition, there is evidence that a thymic factor is essential for the differentiation of T cells from precursor stem cells.

Development

The thymus arises as a paired endodermal outgrowth from the median and ventral portions of the third pair of pharyngeal pouches. Each outgrowth contains a narrow, cleft-like lumen at first, but this is soon obliterated by proliferation of the epithelial cells. In the thymus, the reticular cells are derived from epithelial cells and not from mesenchyme as in the other lymphatic organs. Transformation of epithelial cells into a reticulum begins at about the end of the second month in the central portion of the outgrowth. Studies of thymic glands fixed at successive stages of development show that lymphocytes are present in the mesenchyme around the gland earlier than in the epithelial reticulum. In embryos 50 to 60 mm in length, the medulla begins to become differentiated from the cortex as the lymphocytes become more densely aggregated in the peripheral regions of the gland and less numerous at the center. At about this same time, the lobules begin to form and become separated by the septa of connective tissue. As already stated, the connective tissue septa subdivide the cortical tissue but do not completely subdivide the medullary tissue.

Thymic corpuscles make their first appearance during the first half of fetal life. At first they are few in number and small in size, but they increase rapidly in diameter, and new ones continue to form until the time when thymic involution begins.

THE SPLEEN

The spleen is the largest lymphatic organ in the body. Unlike the lymph nodes, however, it has no afferent lymphatic vessels and no lymph sinuses.

At one point on the surface of the spleen a deep indentation occurs, which is known as the *hilus*. Except at the hilus, the spleen is covered by a serous membrane, the peritoneum. Beneath this is a *capsule* of fibrous tissue containing numerous elastic fibers and some smooth muscle. From the capsule (Figs. 14.16 and 14.17), dense connective tissue trabeculae extend into the interior of the organ. These branch and unite with one another to form very incomplete anastomosing chambers. The hilus marks the entrance and exit of the splenic vessels. Accompanying the vessels, broad strands of capsular tissue extend deep into the organ where they radiate and subdivide to form, with the smaller trabeculae extending in from other parts of the capsule, the connective tissue framework of the organ. Because of the abundance of elastic tissue, along with some smooth muscle, and because of the arrangement of fibrous connective tissue in wavy bundles, the spleen is distensible and capable of considerable change in volume.

The spaces within the connective tissue framework are filled with a soft, spongelike tissue known as the *splenic pulp*. On the basis of color differences seen in fresh preparations, different regions of the splenic pulp have been named *red pulp* and *white pulp*. Both types consist of lymphatic tissue (that is, reticular connective tissue and lymphocytes), together with other cell types described below under "The Splenic Pulp."

The red pulp is traversed by a plexus of *venous sinuses* (Figs. 14.17 through 14.21), by which it is subdivided into anastomosing cords known as *pulp cords* (*Billroth's cords*). The lymphatic tissue of the pulp cords is infiltrated with erythrocytes, the number of which varies under different conditions. The venous sinuses contain erythrocytes which are packed particularly close together when the sinuses are in a storage phase (see below). Thus, the red pulp (venous sinuses plus pulp cords) contains large numbers of erythrocytes which are responsible for its color in fresh preparations.

The white pulp is composed of compact lymphatic tissue arranged around certain divisions of the arteries in the form of a *periarterial sheath,* with ovoid enlarge-

ments at intervals which are known as *lymphatic nodules, splenic nodules,* or *Malpighian corpuscles.* The junction of a lymphatic nodule with the surrounding red pulp has characteristic features in the pattern of its vessels and reticulum and is known as the *marginal zone* (Fig. 14.16). Except for their larger blood vessels, the lymphatic nodules of the spleen are very similar to those found in lymph nodes and, like the latter, they may contain germinal centers. In children, a germinal center is usually found in each nodule, but in the adult spleen the germinal centers are less numerous.

The structure of the spleen depends largely upon the characteristic arrangement of the blood vessels, which are described before considering further the minute structure of the organ.

Blood Vessels

The arteries enter the spleen at the hilus and divide into branches which enter the trabeculae to become the *trabecular* or *interlobular arteries* (Fig. 14.17). These are accompanied by the trabecular branches of the splenic veins. After following the trabeculae for a short distance, the arteries leave the veins and the septa and pursue an entirely separate course through the splenic pulp. The adventitial coat of these smaller arteries takes on the character of reticular tissue and becomes infiltrated with lymphocytes, forming a thin periarterial sheath. At various points along the course of the vessels, the lymphatic tissue is increased in amount and forms the splenic nodules already mentioned. These arteries are called the *central arteries,* although they are eccentrically located with reference to the splenic nodules. When a nodule is located at a point where the artery divides, as frequently happens, two or more arteries are seen in a cross section of the nodule. In their passage through the white pulp, the central arteries give off capillaries which nourish the white pulp and continue as capillaries into the red pulp. In other words, there is no venous return directly from the white pulp. The central arteries

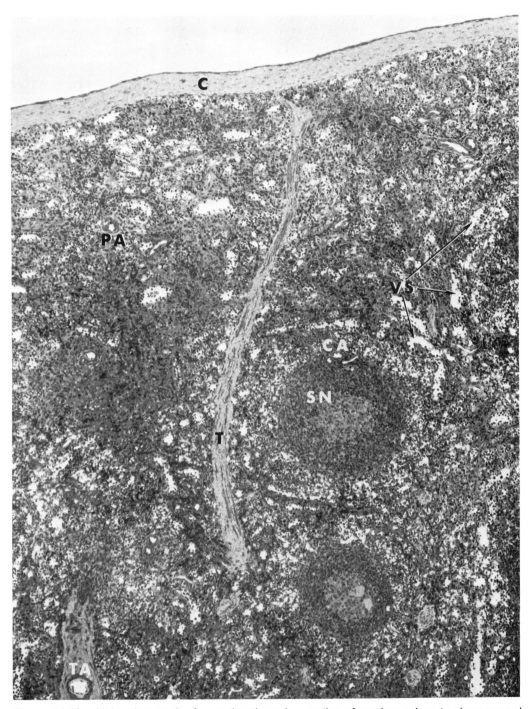

Figure 14.16. Light micrograph of a section through a portion of monkey spleen to show general topography. *C*, capsule; *CA*, central artery; *PA*, pulp artery; *SN*, splenic nodule; *T*, trabecula; *TA*, trabecular artery; *VS*, venous sinuses (×165).

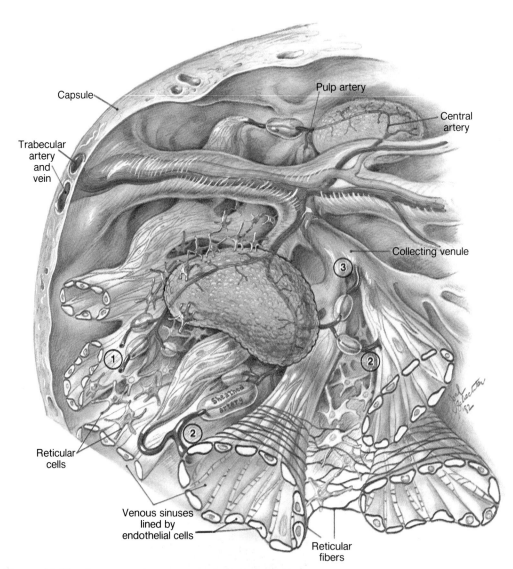

Capsule

Pulp artery

Central artery

Trabecular artery and vein

Collecting venule

Reticular cells

Venous sinuses lined by endothelial cells

Reticular fibers

Figure 14.17. Structure of the spleen. This diagram shows a trabecula extending inward from the capsule and carrying major vessels, the trabecular artery and vein. The artery exits the trabecula in close association with a periarterial sheath of lymphocytic tissue and continues into a splenic nodule as the central artery. The periarterial sheath and splenic nodule make up the white pulp. After giving off capillaries within the white pulp, the artery courses into the red pulp as an artery of the pulp. Here it usually branches and may terminate in the substance of the splenic cords (depicted at *1*), or run through a more or less developed "sheathed artery" to terminate in a venus sinus (sinusoid in some terminologies) (depicted at *2*), or directly in a collecting vein, bypassing the venus sinuses altogether (depicted at *3*). The splenic cords are comprised of reticular cells, reticular fibers, macrophages, and all elements of the circulating blood.

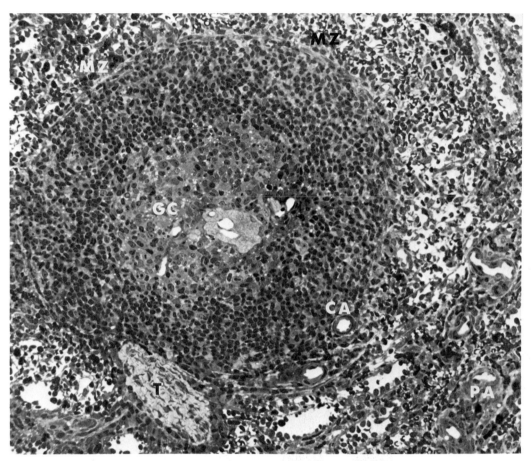

Figure 14.18. Light micrograph of a section of monkey spleen showing a splenic nodule and its marginal zone. *CA*, central artery; *GC*, germinal center, *PA*, pulp artery; *T*, trabecula; *MZ*, marginal zone (×420).

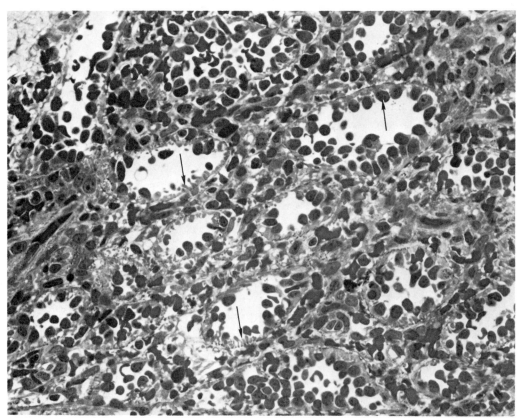

Figure 14.19. Light micrograph of a section of monkey spleen showing transverse sections of venous sinuses. Note the arrangement of endothelial cells (*arrows*). Compare with Figures 14.20 and 14.22 (×825).

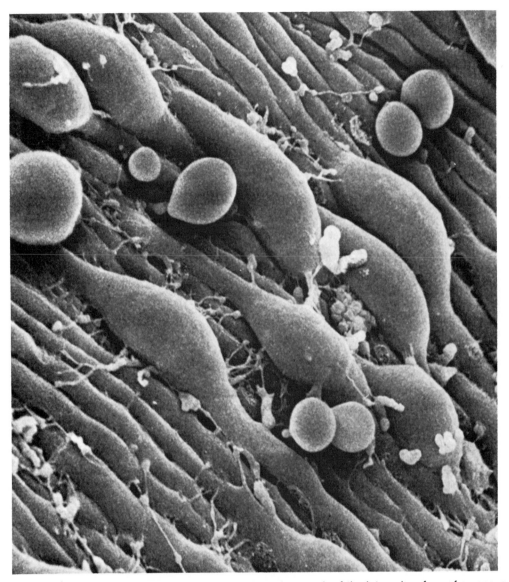

Figure 14.20. High magnification scanning electron micrograph of the internal surface of a venous sinus in human spleen. The elongate endothelial cells with bulging nuclei run diagonally in the field (×4800). (Courtesy of Dr. Masayuki Miyoshi.)

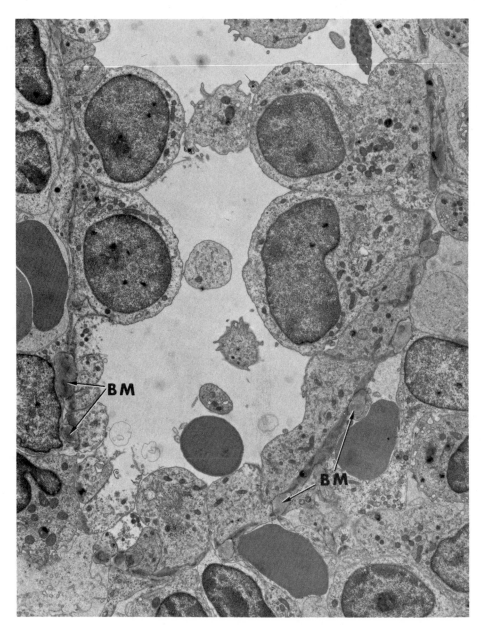

Figure 14.21. Electron micrograph of a venous sinus of monkey spleen showing the cuboidal appearance of endothelial cells, incomplete basement membrane (*BM*), and filamentous condensations in the bases of endothelial cells (×4300).

are lined by a *cuboidal* endothelium, and the capillaries given off to the white pulp also have cuboidal endothelium for a part of their course.

After a number of divisions within the white pulp, the central arteries reach the marginal zone (boundary between white and red pulp), where their sheaths of white pulp become reduced to only a thin layer of scattered lymphocytes. Within the marginal zone, each artery divides into a number of branches which are close together like the bristles of a brush or *penicillus.* These branches consist of three successive portions: *pulp arteries, sheathed arteries* (or *sheathed capillaries*), and *terminal arterial capillaries.* The pulp arteries are the longest of these segments; they qualify as arterioles, because their wall contains one or two layers of smooth muscle cells. The pulp arteries divide into several "sheathed arteries" that are actually capillaries because they no longer contain any smooth muscle. Their lumen is only about 8 μm in diameter, but their wall is thickened by the presence of concentric layers of reticular fibers and a number of interspersed cells which consist largely of macrophages. The sheath is not prominent in humans, as it is in some of the lower animals such as the dog and pig. On the other hand, some animals, such as rodents, lack this sheath.

Each of the sheathed arteries divides into two or more arterial capillaries, which may have conical enlargements (ampullae) at their terminations. The exact manner in which these vessels terminate has been a controversial subject. Some authors believe that the capillaries empty into intercellular spaces of the red pulp reticulum and that the blood finds its way from the pulp spaces into the venous sinuses through perforations in the walls of the sinuses (Fig. 14.17, *1*). Other authors believe that the capillaries empty directly into the venous sinuses (Fig. 14.17, *2*). However, openings of terminal arterioles into the intercellular spaces of the red pulp can be seen in electron micrographs, and it is evident that at least some of the arterioles terminate in

this manner. There is also evidence that some of the capillaries bypass the splenic sinuses altogether and empty directly into collecting venules (Fig. 14.17, *3*).

The *venous sinuses* form an anastomosing plexus throughout the red pulp, dividing it into pulp cords. The endothelial cells of the venous sinuses differ from ordinary endothelial cells in that they protrude prominently into the vascular lumen (Fig. 14.19), are more elongated than ordinary endothelial cells, and are arranged paralleling each other in a rather uniform pattern (Fig. 14.20). An incomplete basement membrane of variable thickness lies beneath the cells (Figs. 14.21 and 14.22).

The outer part of the sinus wall contains relatively coarse, circularly arranged reticular fibers, which are obvious in silver-stained preparations under the light microscope. Electron micrographs show that these fibers are embedded in a perforated layer of ground substance. Although the perforations of the basement membrane and the intercellular clefts between the endothelial cells seen with the light microscope (Fig. 14.19) are exaggerated by shrinkage of cells during standard light microscope preparation of tissues, their presence has been confirmed by electron microscope studies (Figs. 14.20 and 14.22). Erythrocytes and other blood cells pass readily through the walls of the sinuses, producing interchange between the cords and sinuses.

The terminal veins or venous sinuses unite to form larger *pulp veins,* or *collecting venules.* They enter the trabeculae to become the *trabecular* or *interlobular veins,* which follow the trabeculae toward the hilus, where they unite to form the splenic veins (Fig. 14.17).

Union of Arteries and Veins

The question of whether the splenic circulation is "open" or "closed" has been long debated. The view that the splenic circulation is closed received its strongest support from studies of blood flow in living animals. Using a quartz rod method of transillumi-

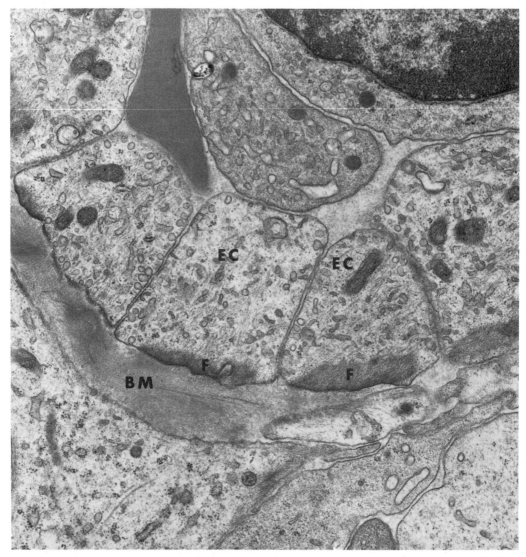

Figure 14.22. Electron micrograph of a portion of the wall of a venous sinus of monkey spleen showing processes of endothelial cells (*EC*) containing dense basal filaments (*F*) and part of the discontinuous basement membrane (*BM*) (×19,000).

nation, Knisely observed arterial capillaries emptying directly into the venous sinuses and also into the collecting venules of the red pulp. He observed cyclic activity in the venous sinuses with conducting and storage phases. Although the method made significant contributions to an understanding of splenic function, it could not provide adequate resolution to resolve the question. More recent studies using electron micros-copy show clearly that most of the terminal capillaries open into intercellular spaces in the red pulp (Fig. 14.17, *1*) and that relatively few vessels open directly into venous sinuses. It seems likely that the degree to which the splenic circulation may be open or closed is dependent on physiological conditions, but one way or another, all of the components of the blood have ready access to the extravascular splenic cords.

The Splenic Pulp

As already stated, the splenic pulp fills all of the spaces between the connective tissue trabeculae; it has been subdivided into white pulp, consisting of compact lymphatic tissue surrounding the central arteries, and red pulp, containing an abundance of erythrocytes (Fig. 14.23).

A meshwork of reticular connective tissue extends throughout both the red and white pulp, although its density and arrangement vary in different parts. The reticular cells and fibers are more numerous and more closely arranged around the arteries and at the marginal zone of the lymphatic nodule than they are elsewhere (Fig. 14.24).

The *reticular cells* resemble those described for lymph nodes. For example, their nuclei are relatively pale-staining in comparison with the densely chromatic nuclei of small lymphocytes, and their cytoplasm stains lightly with most techniques. The processes of reticular cells form a covering for the reticular fibers, as they do in lymph nodes. Although the reticular cells of the spleen were once thought to be very phagocytic, more recent studies using transfused labeled cells and electron microscopy indicate that most of the splenic macrophages are derivatives of monocytes.

Lymphocytes of large, medium, and small sizes are closely packed in the white pulp, with the first two types particularly numerous in the germinal centers. The lymphocytes are much less numerous and more randomly dispersed in the red pulp. A high percentage of the lymphocytes of the spleen belong to the recirculating type. They tend to localize in specific regions of the white pulp, with T lymphocytes aggregated around the central arteries and B lympho-

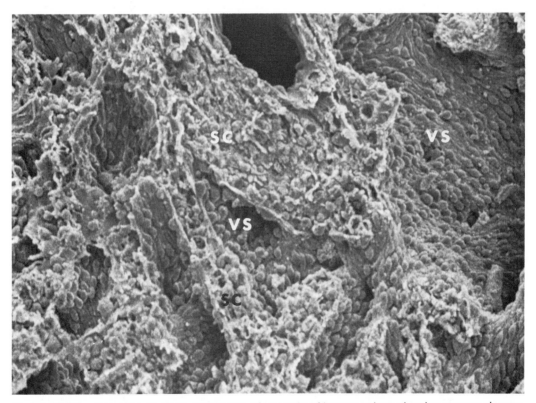

Figure 14.23. Scanning electron micrograph of red pulp of human spleen showing venous sinuses (*VS*) and splenic cords (*SC*) (×480). (Courtesy of Dr. Masayuki Miyoshi.)

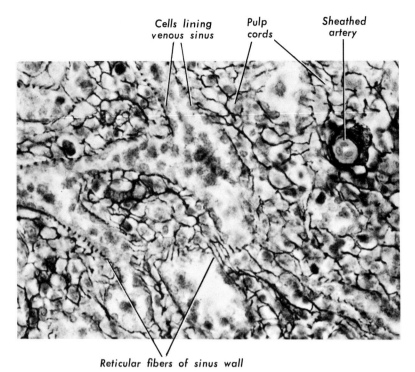

Cells lining   Pulp   Sheathed
venous sinus   cords   artery

Reticular fibers of sinus wall

Figure 14.24. Light micrograph of spleen of rhesus monkey. Stained with Bielschowsky-Foot silver for reticular fibers and with hematoxylin-eosin-azure for cell types (×540).

cytes aggregated around the germinal centers of the lymphatic nodules (periarterial sheath).

Monocytes, macrophages, and *plasma cells* are also fairly numerous. Monocytes are brought into the spleen by the blood vessels and also form by proliferation and differentiation within the organ. The macrophages of the spleen are generally similar to those found in other parts of the body. However, they more frequently contain reddish or brownish pigment granules of hemosiderin that are derived from the hemoglobin of phagocytized erythrocytes.

The red pulp also contains the various types of *granular leukocytes* and a variable number of *erythrocytes.* Because of the thinness of the walls of the sinuses and the presence of some erythrocytes outside the sinuses, it is frequently difficult in ordinary sections to distinguish between the sinuses and pulp cords.

Giant cells or *megakaryocytes,* similar to those of bone marrow, are found in the splenic pulp of a number of animals (e.g.,

cat, rat). They are present in man during fetal life but are usually absent in the adult.

Lymphatics

Efferent lymphatic vessels are present in the connective tissue of the capsule and trabeculae. Deep efferent lymphatic vessels are also present in the white pulp, coursing parallel with the arteries.

Nerves

These are mainly nonmyelinated, although a few myelinated fibers are present. The latter are probably sensory in function. The nonmyelinated fibers—axons of sympathetic neurons—accompany the arteries, around which they form plexuses. From these plexuses, terminals pass to the muscle cells of the arteries, to the septa, to the capsule, and to the splenic pulp.

Functions

The spleen is not essential for life and can be removed because various other organs, particularly the bone marrow, readily take over its functions.

The spleen acts as a filtering organ for the blood in much the same way as the lymph nodes function as organs of lymph filtration. The phagocytic cells of the spleen remove foreign particles, including bacteria, degenerating leukocytes, etc., from the circulating blood.

The macrophages also remove fragmented and whole erythrocytes, and in this way the spleen functions as an organ for blood destruction. Many of the engulfed cells have already begun to fragment in the peripheral circulation, but the spleen is thought to play a role in making the cells more fragile. Regardless of what initiates the fragmentation or determines which erythrocytes are to be destroyed, the spleen is of importance as an organ for the removal and phagocytosis of the cells.

Engulfed erythrocytes are digested by the phagocytic cells, and iron is recovered from the hemoglobin and temporarily stored in the cells. In this way the spleen plays a part in the iron metabolism of the body. The stored iron is given up as needed and is utilized by the body in the formation of new hemoglobin.

The spleen functions as an organ for blood development during a part of fetal life, but after birth the only blood cells normally formed in the spleen are lymphocytes and monocytes. In certain pathological conditions, the splenic pulp reassumes its earlier function as a blood-forming organ for all types of cells and becomes similar to bone marrow in appearance, containing all types of myelocytes, erythroblasts, and megakaryocytes.

As already described, the framework of the spleen includes elastic fibers and smooth muscle, and it is able to make rapid changes in volume. Contraction of the spleen expels erythrocytes and increases the number of these corpuscles in the general circulation. Contraction and decrease in volume occurs under many different conditions (e.g., during exercise, after hemorrhage), and, although this reservoir function of the spleen is not necessary for life, there are a great variety of conditions, both normal and pathological, in which it may be of considerable value.

The white pulp of the spleen has an important role in the formation of antibodies and in the immune reaction. In response to an antigen entering the body for the first time, i.e., a primary response, lymphoblasts proliferate in numerous portions of the spleen. After four or five days, there is also an obvious increase in the numbers of plasma cells associated with the lymphatic sheaths along the periarterial vessels of the nodules and along those of the penicilli. Slightly later, changes are seen in the germinal centers, with an increased proliferation of lymphoblasts and with macrophages containing ingested lymphocytes. In the case of the primary response, the centers continue to show some evidence of an increased activity for about one month. In a subsequent or secondary response to the same antigen, the germinal centers respond more rapidly.

Development

The spleen arises as a thickening in the mesenchyme in the left side of the dorsal mesogastrium during the fifth or sixth week of fetal development (10-mm embryo). With continued growth, the primordium becomes elevated from the mesentery and the attachment is reduced to a narrow band of tissue surrounding the splenic vessels. The primordium is composed of reticular cells of mesenchymal origin and is invaded by lymphocytes which apparently differentiate from stem cells of yolk sac origin before their transportation via the blood vessels to the liver, bone marrow, and spleen.

The fetal spleen participates in the development of lymphocytes, monocytes, granular leukocytes, erythrocytes, and megakaryocytes. However, erythropoiesis decreases at about the eighth month and generally ceases at about the time of birth. Granular leukocyte development usually ceases soon after birth. The spleen remains active in lymphocyte and monocyte development throughout life and has the ability to revert to erythrocyte development in young individuals when there is an unusual demand.

The enlargements of white pulp to form definite nodules does not occur until late in fetal life, and germinal centers usually do not appear until after birth and after stimulation by foreign antigens.

SUMMARY OF THE "IMMUNE SYSTEM"

As noted at the beginning of this chapter, the immune system involves the activity of cells, tissues, and organs spread over the entire body. Two main types of immune reaction occur: (*a*) the *humoral response* (the production of free, circulating antibody); and (*b*) *cell-mediated response* (the production of sensitized cells which themselves act in the response). Lymphocytes are involved with both types of response. B lymphocytes, originating in the bone marrow in adult mammals (Bursa of Fabricius in birds) are responsible for the humoral response, and T lymphocytes, which have a thymus-dependent phase in their development, are responsible for the cell-mediated response.

Although the triggering of an immune response may be the result of a highly localized invasion of a foreign substance, the response itself involves much more than an activation of local cells. A broader reaction is promoted by the release of enzymes and chemotactic agents by some of the local cells. These factors attract other cells to the site, affect local vascular permeability and activate phagocytic activity, all of which serve to amplify the reaction.

The relative numbers and types of cells in the circulating blood at any point in time reflect the status of the immune system, but the primary site of the immunological response is the connective tissue. Noncirculating neutrophils are highly phagocytic, particularly for certain classes of bacteria. Macrophages (derived from monocytes) are even more phagocytic. Moreover, macrophages have the capacity to process some of their ingested material so as to make key components available at the cell surface for recognition by both T and B lymphocytes. Other specialized cells of less certain origin located in lymph nodes and mucosa-associated lymphatic tissues also appear to be capable of processing antigens and presenting them to lymphocytes. Thus, the sensitivity and efficiency of the immune response may be further amplified.

The cell-mediated immune response is distinct from the humoral response; only T lymphocytes can participate directly in cell-mediated responses. It is abundantly clear, however, that B lymphocytes are not independent effectors. An interaction with a helper class of T lymphocytes is essential before the B lymphocyte is activated to produce plasma cells and humoral antibodies.

The cellular interactions involved in immune responses can occur anywhere in connective tissue, but the most effective response occurs in the lymph nodes and spleen. This is because the structure of these organs provides an opportunity for lymph and blood filtration at sites especially enriched in appropriate cell populations.

A crucial factor for understanding the operation of the immune system is the realization that the seemingly separate lymphatic tissues and organs are in fact in constant communication with each other. The communication is accomplished by a traffic of cells circulated by lymphatic and blood vascular channels. The bone marrow produces a continuous supply of granulocytes, monocytes and B lymphocytes and houses an undifferentiated stem cell (*CFU stem cell*). This pluripotent stem cell, or various of its partially committed differentiation products, has access to the lymphatic tissues and organs through their vascular supplies. For example, pre-T lymphocyte stem cells produced in the bone marrow apparently continue to seed the thymus throughout life. T lymphocytes, in turn, home to thymic-dependent areas of lymph nodes, spleen, and mucosa-associated lymphatic accumulations and are thus appropriately positioned to interact with macrophages and B lymphocytes. The B lymphocytes, elaborated by the germinal centers in these same tissues, are continually seeded by programmed B lymphocytes emanating from the bone marrow. A significant proportion of both T and B lymphocytes continually recirculate, entering lymphatic or blood vascular drainage in local areas eventually to be combined by the merging of the two drainage systems, and then reentering lymphatic tissue by migration across capillary or venular walls. A primary route for the latter migration in lymph nodes (and some of the other lymphatic tissues as well) is high endothelial (postcapillary) venules, where special recognition sites for the recirculating lymphocytes may exist.

In addition to direct cellular interaction (cell-mediated response) and the production of circulating antibodies (humoral response), certain B lymphocyte-derived plasma cells produce a type of antibody that is released into the intestinal lumen and onto other mucosal surfaces after the addition of a specific portion to the molecule by the local epithelium. This *secretory IgA* is of major importance in reducing adherence of foreign antigens to mucosal cell surfaces, thereby reducing their uptake and serving as one of the first lines of defense in the immune mechanism.

The regulation of all of the activities of the immune system is as delicate and finely tuned as that of neural and endocrine integrations, and, as with those systems, the details of regulatory mechanisms are only now beginning to be elucidated.

References

Ackerman GA, Hostetler JR: Morphological studies of the embryonic rabbit thymus. *Anat Rec* 166:27–46, 1970.

Barcroft J, Stephens JG: Observations on the size of the spleen. *J Physiol* 64:1–22, 1927.

Barr RO: Hemopoietic stem cells in human peripheral blood. *Science* 190:284–285, 1975.

Bradfield JWB, Born GVR: The migration of rat thoracic duct lymphocytes through spleen. *Br J Exp Pathol* 54:509–517, 1973.

Chen LT, Weiss L: The role of the sinus wall in the passage of erythrocytes through the spleen. *Blood* 41:529–538, 1973.

Clark SL, Jr: The penetration of proteins and colloidal materials into the thymus from the blood stream. In Defendi V, Metcalf D (eds): *The Thymus*, Wistar Institute Symposium Monograph 2. Philadelphia, Wistar Institute Press, 1964, pp 9–32.

Coons AH, Leduc EH, Connolly JM: Studies on antibody formation. *J Exp Med* 102:49–60, 1955.

Everett NB, Tyler (Caffrey) RW: Lymphopoiesis in the thymus and other tissues: functional implications. *Int Rev Cytol* 22:205–237, 1967.

Farr A, Debruyne PH: The mode of lymphocyte migration through post-capillary venule endothelium in lymph node. *Am J Anat* 143:59–00, 1975

Feldman M, Rosenthal A, Erb P: Macrophage-lymphocyte interactions in immune induction. *Int Rev Cytol* 60:149–179, 1979.

Ford CE, Micklem HS, Evans EP, Gray JG, Ogden DA: The inflow of bone marrow cells to the thymus. Studies with part-body irradiated mice injected with chromosome marked bone marrow and subjected to antigen stimulation. *Ann NY Acad Sci* 129:283–296, 1966.

Hartmann A: Die Milz. In von Möllendorff (ed): *Handbuch der mikroskopischen Anatomie des Menschen*, vol 6, part 1. Berlin, Springer-Verlag, 1930, pp 397–563.

Hayes TG: The marginal zone and marginal sinus in the spleen of the gerbil. A light and electron microscopy study. *J Morphol* 141:205–216, 1973.

Helmann T: Die Lymphknötchen und die Lymphknoten. In von Möllendorff (ed): *Handbuch der mikroskopischen Anatomie des Menschen*, vol 6, part 1. Berlin, Springer-Verlag, 1930, pp 233–396.

Kalpaktsoglou PK, Yunis EJ, Good RA: The role of the thymus in development of lympho-hemopoietic tissues. The effect of thymectomy on development of blood cells, bone marrow, spleen and lymph nodes. *Anat Rec* 164:267–282, 1969.

Knisely MH: Spleen studies. *Anat Rec* 65:23–50, 131–148, 1936.

MacKenzie DW, Whipple AO, Wintersteiner MP: Studies on the microscopic anatomy and physiology of living transilluminated mammalian spleens. *Am J Anat* 68:397–456, 1941.

Peck HM, Hoerr NL: The intermediary circulation in the red pulp of the mouse spleen. *Anat Rec* 109:447–478, 1951.

Pettersen JC, Rose RJ: Marginal zone and germinal center development in the spleens of neonatally thymectomized and non-thymectomized young rats. *Am J Anat* 123:489–500, 1968.

Raviola E, Karnowsky MJ: Evidence for a blood-thymus barrier using electron opaque tracers. *J Exp Med* 136:466, 1972.

Song SH, Groom AC: Scanning electron microscopic study of the splenic red pulp in relation to the sequestration of immature red cells. *J Morphol* 149:437–450, 1974.

Waksman BH, Arnason BG, Jankovic BD: Role of the thymus in immune reactions in rats. III. Changes in the lymphoid organs of thymectomized rats. *J Exp Med* 116:187–206, 1962.

Weiss L: The structure of the intermediate vascular pathways in the spleen of rabbits. *Am J Anat* 113:51–92, 1963.

Yoffey JM (ed): *Bristol Symposium: The Lymphocyte in Immunology and Haemopoiesis*. Baltimore, Williams & Wilkins, 1967.

Chapter 15

THE INTEGUMENT

The integument is the body's most massive organ. It is composed of the skin that covers the entire body, together with certain accessory organs which are derivatives of the skin, such as nails, hair, sweat and sebaceous glands. These derivatives originate as invaginations of the embryonic surface ectoderm, developments which result from regional inductive interaction between the ectoderm and underlying mesoderm.

The skin performs more important functions than are usually appreciated. It protects the body from injurious substances and desiccation, helps in the regulation of the body temperature, excretes water, fat, and some other substances, and constitutes the most extensive sense organ of the body for the reception of tactile, thermal, and painful stimuli.

THE SKIN

The skin or cutis consists of two main parts: (*a*) the *epidermis*, a stratified epithelial layer derived from the ectoderm, and (*b*) the *dermis, corium*, or cutis vera, a connective tissue derivative of the mesoderm. Below the dermis is a layer of loose connective tissue, the *subcutaneous tissue* (superficial fascia), which attaches the skin to the underlying organs (Fig. 15.1). In certain places this layer is richly infiltrated with fat and is called the subcutaneous adipose tissue. The subcutaneous tissue provides mobility for the skin, and where this layer is slight or absent, as in the soles, palms, and fingertips, the skin is more dense.

The thickness of the skin varies considerably in different parts of the body. The relative proportions of epidermis and dermis vary also, and a thick skin is found in regions where there is a thickening of either or both layers. On the interscapular region of the back, where the dermis is particularly thick, the skin may be more than 5 mm in thickness, whereas on the eyelids it may be less than 0.5 mm; the usual thickness is 1 to 2 mm. The skin is generally thicker on the dorsal or extensor surfaces of the body than on the ventral or flexor surfaces, but this is not true for the hands and feet; the skin of the palms and soles is thicker than on any dorsal surface except the interscapular region. The palms and soles have a characteristically thickened epidermis, in addition to a thick dermis (Fig. 15.1). The epidermis of these regions also differs structurally from the thin epidermis present elsewhere.

The whole surface of the skin is traversed by numerous fine furrows which run in definite directions and cross each other to bound small rhomboid or rectangular fields. These furrows correspond to similar ones on the surface of the dermis so that, in section, the boundary line between epidermis and dermis appears wavy. On the thick skin of the palms and soles, the fields form long, narrow ridges separated by parallel coursing furrows, and in the fingertips these ridges are arranged in the complicated loops, whorls, and spirals that give the fingerprints characteristic for each individual. In those regions where the epidermis is thickest, these ridges are more prominent.

Where there is an epidermal ridge externally there is a narrower projection, the *rete peg*, on the dermal surface. On either side of each rete peg, *dermal papillae* project irregularly into the epidermis (Figs. 15.1 and 15.2). In the palms and soles, the dermal papillae are numerous, tall, and often

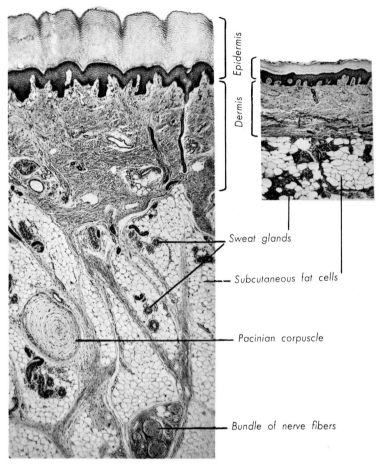

Figure 15.1. Low power photomicrographs of vertical sections of skin. Thick skin from fingertip at *left*; skin of medium thickness from dorsal surface of finger at *right*. The fields shown do not include the total thickness of the subcutaneous tissue (×30).

branched, varying in height from 0.05 to 0.2 mm. They are likewise numerous and tall in the lips, clitoris, penis, labia minora, and nipples. Where mechanical demands are slight and the epidermis is thinner, as on the abdomen, chin, and face, the papillae are low and few in number.

The Epidermis

The stratified squamous epithelium of the epidermis contains four distinct cell types. The predominant cell is the *keratinocyte*, so named because of its high content of the protein keratin. The other cells are *melanocytes*, *Langerhans cells*, and *Merkel cells*. Keratinocytes and Merkel cells develop from embryonic ectoderm but mela-

nocytes and Langerhans cells originate elsewhere and secondarily take up residence in the epidermis.

Keratinocytes are continually replaced by mitotic proliferation in the basal layers of the epithelium. When mitosis occurs, one daughter cell moves upward and begins to differentiate, while the other remains undifferentiated. Differentiation involves the accumulation of keratin, secretion of a membrane-coating material, the loss of nucleus and cytoplasmic organelles, and a change in shape from cuboidal to squamous. This process of transformation gives rise to a series of morphologically identifiable strata representing phases in the turnover of keratinocytes. The turnover time

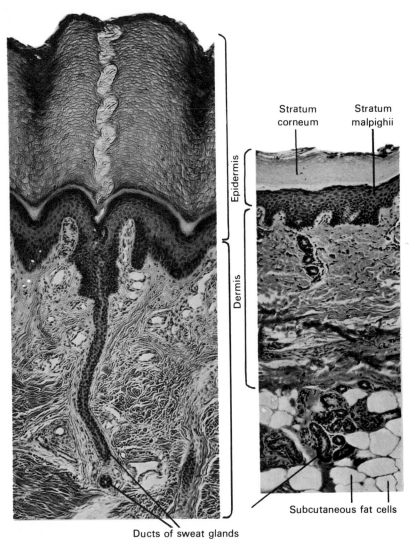

Figure 15.2. Photomicrographs of vertical sections of skin, showing thick epidermis from fingertip, at *left*, and thinner epidermis from dorsal surface of finger, at *right* (×94).

varies from a few weeks to several months, depending on the region of the body. The process is greatly accelerated after injury.

The thickness of the epidermis varies in different body regions. The various strata are most easily identified in the thick epidermis of the surfaces of the palms, soles, and volar surfaces of the digits. In these regions five different strata are visible: (*a*) the *stratum basale* (*stratum cylindricum*), (*b*) *stratum spinosum*, (*c*) *stratum granulosum*, (d) *stratum lucidum*, and (*e*) *stratum corneum* (Figs. 15.2 and 15.3). The stratum

basale and stratum spinosum together compose the *stratum Malpighii.*

The *stratum basale* consists primarily of columnar or high cuboidal keratinocytes arranged in a single layer which rests on a well-defined basement membrane. The lamina reticularis portion of this basement membrane is relatively thin in mammals but thicker and more complex in some of the lower animals. Electron micrographs show that the border of the cell and of its underlying basal lamina follow an irregular course (Fig. 15.4). Slender strands of con-

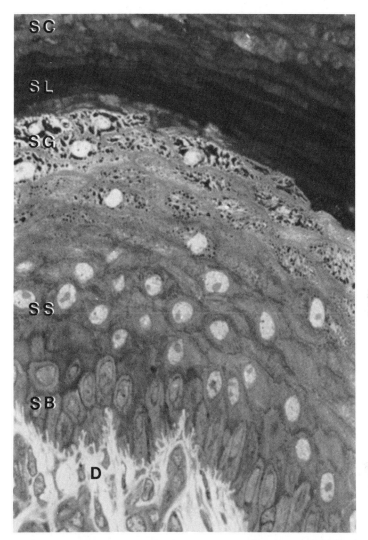

Figure 15.3. Section of thick epidermis from human fingertip. The field includes only a small portion of the stratum corneum (*SC*) but shows the entire thickness of the viable strata. *D*, dermal connective tissue; *SB*, stratum basale; *SG*, stratum granulosum; *SL*, stratum lucidum; *SS*, stratum spinosum (×640) (Courtesy of Dr. Mary Bell.)

nective tissue penetrate spaces between in-foldings of the cell membrane, and hemi-desmosomes are frequent along the base of the cells. Adherence between the epithelium and its underlying connective tissue is aided by the irregularity of the boundary between the two tissues and by the hemi-desmosomes.

The nuclei of the keratinocytes of the stratum Malpighii are deeply chromatic. Their shape varies with that of the cells,

being ovoid in the stratum basale and round in the stratum spinosum. The cytoplasm of these keratinocytes is basophilic in its staining reaction, particularly in the deepest cell layer. This is correlated with the ribosomal content of the cytoplasm and hence with active protein synthesis (Fig. 15.4). The cytoplasm of the cells contains numerous intermediate filaments. Bundles of the filaments are distributed throughout the cytoplasm, and they are found consis-

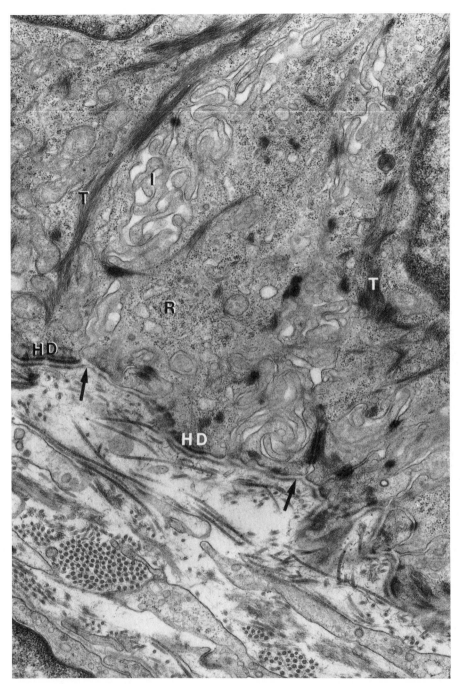

Figure 15.4. Basal epidermal cells from a fetal rhesus monkey at the dermoepidermal junction. The basal lamina (*arrows*), hemidesmosomes (*HD*) and interdigitated lateral plasma membranes (*I*) are obvious. The basal cell cytoplasm contains bundles of tonofilaments (*T*) and numerous free ribosomes (R) (×18,600). (Courtesy of Dr. Mary Bell.)

tently in the cytoplasm adjacent to the desmosomes, often coursing toward these points of cell adhesion (Figs 15.4 and 4.3). Aggregates of the filaments are visible with the light microscope and, as such, they were originally described by light microscopists as *tonofibrils*. In keeping with this terminology, the individual filaments seen with the electron microscope are often called *tonofilaments.* The epidermal filaments of the deeper cells subsequently mature to become the fibrous elements of the filament-matrix complex of the stratum corneum.

The keratinocytes of the stratum spinosum contain a variable number of rounded or ovoid granules that are membrane-bounded; these are relatively small and are known as *membrane-coating granules* (Figs. 15.5 and 15.9). It is thought that their contents are secreted into the intercellular space where they contribute to a thickening of the cell membrane that occurs by the time the cells reach the stratum lucidum.

Keratinocytes of the stratum Malpighii contain variable numbers of *melanin pigment granules.* These granules are more numerous in black than in white individuals and they are also distributed differently. In black individuals melanin granules remain separate and do not localize to any particular cellular region, whereas in Caucasians the granules occur in clumps closely associated with the nucleus. Melanin granules are not produced by keratinocytes but are formed in *melanocytes* and transferred secondarily to keratinocytes.

Melanocytes differentiate from *melanoblasts,* which are of neural crest origin and migrate to their definitive position at the dermoepidermal junction during embryonic development. Subsequent differentiation involves a change in cell shape from round to stellate, and the formation of melanin granules through a series of intermediate steps. First, membrane-bounded, lamellar bodies called *premelanosomes* are formed. These accumulate protyrosinase, but this proenzyme does not initiate melanin synthesis until it is activated to *tyrosinase.* Once tyrosinase is formed and melanin synthesis begins, the membrane-bounded bodies are referred to as *melanosomes.* As melanin pigment accumulates in melanosomes, the latter are transformed into mature melanin granules. The differentiation of melanosomes is accompanied by a change in position in the cell: the premelanosomes

appear in the region of the Golgi complex, the melansomes appear in the basal portions of the long dendritic processes, and the mature melanin granules are chiefly in the peripheral portions of the dendritic processes. Thus, the body or perikaryon of the melanocyte appears relatively clear in routine preparations. The melanocyte processes insinuate between keratinocytes of the stratum Malpighii where transfer of the melanin granules occurs. Transfer occurs by a process of endocytosis involving entire tips of the dendritic processes of melanocytes.

African and Mongoloid races have a somewhat higher number of melanocytes than Caucasians, but the difference in skin color is due chiefly to the manner in which the pigment is dispersed. In Caucasians the total amount of melanin is concentrated primarily within the cells of the stratum basale and is situated in membrane-bounded melanosome complexes, whereas in black individuals larger melanin granules are spread throughout the Malpighian layer.

Melanocytes can be identified by their reaction to the "*dopa*" reagent, dihydroxyphenylalanine: they oxidize the solution and stain black. The intracellular substance responsible for the reaction is tyrosinase, the oxidative enzyme responsible for synthesis of melanin from tyrosine. The dopa reaction does not occur for the fully formed melanin granules within keratinocytes or in dermal chromatophores because the mature melanin granules lack tyrosinase.

The cell bodies of the melanocytes are normally confined to the basal layer of the epidermis, near their place of origin from the primitive melanoblasts (Fig. 15.6). However, melanocyte processes extend for some distance between epidermal cells. When melanin formation is stimulated, e.g., by ultraviolet radiation, or by X-irradiation, the cell bodies of melanocytes also appear in the suprabasal layers of the epidermis.

The melanocytes supposedly wear out and slough off with the epidermal scales,

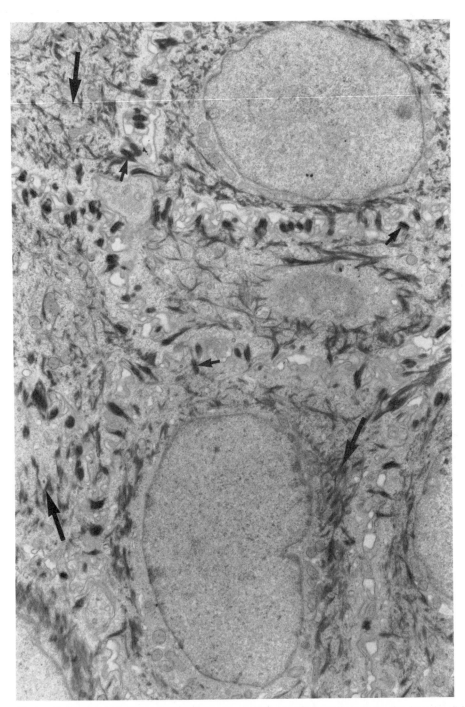

Figure 15.5. Cells of the spinous layer of human epidermis. Cells adjacent to the basal cell layer (*bottom*) are oriented perpendicularly to the plane of the epidermis, whereas cells higher up are becoming oriented parallel to that plane. Desmosomes (*small arrows*) and tonofibrils (*large arrows*) are numerous (×7800). (Courtesy of Dr. Mary Bell.)

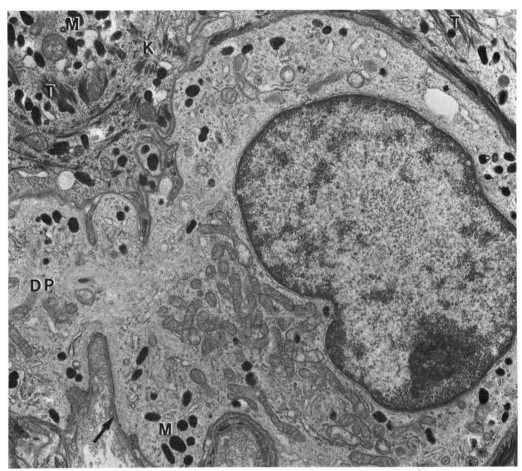

Figure 15.6. Melanocyte and adjacent keratinocyte from the skin of a black individual. There are no desmosomes attaching these cells. *Arrow*, basal lamina; *DP*, dendritic process of melanocyte; *K*, keratinocyte; *M*, melanosomes; *T*, tonofibrils (×13,600). (Courtesy of Dr. Mary Bell.)

but their number is maintained by proliferation of cells which are presumably melanocytes in an active phase of melanogenesis.

Another cell type, the *Langerhans cell*, is also present in the stratum Malpighii (Fig. 15.7). These cells were once thought to represent effete melanocytes, but recent evidence demonstrates that they are a form of phagocyte of bone marrow origin. They function in the processing of antigens in much the same way as connective tissue macrophages or dendritic cells of lymphatic nodule germinal centers. The unusual feature of the Langerhans cell is that it is a macrophage normally residing in an epithelium. Cytologically, the Langerhans cell is characterized by a lack of tonofibrils, the presence of an unusual raquet-shaped cytoplasmic organelle, and the absence of desmosomal attachments to adjacent keratinocytes (Fig. 15.7).

The fourth cell type of the epidermis is the *Merkel cell*. It lies basally and stains differently from the keratinocyte, melanocyte or Langerhans cell, but it is not readily distinguished in routine preparations. It also has a somewhat restricted regional distribution and is always associated with axons. Merkel cells appear to be specialized epithelial cells involved with slowly adapting mechanoreception. The cells contain a

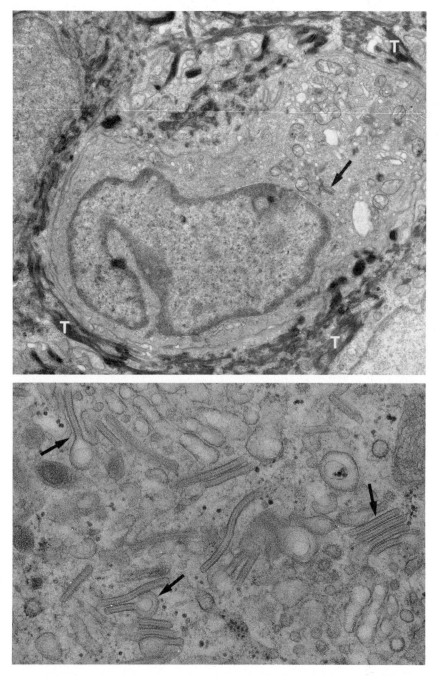

Figure 15.7. Langerhans cell of human epidermis. Adjacent keratinocytes have prominent tonofibrils (*T*) but the two cell types are not attached with desmosomes. The lower figure is higher magnification of a portion of cytoplasm of a Langerhans cell showing the characteristic racquet-shaped inclusions (*arrows*) (×52,500). (Courtesy of Dr. Mary Bell.)

lobulated nucleus and characteristic electron-dense cytoplasmic granules and are adjoined to adjacent keratinocytes by desmosomes (Fig. 15.8). In addition, speciali-

zations of the membranes of both the Merkel cell and apposed axon terminals have been reported.

The *stratum spinosum* is composed of

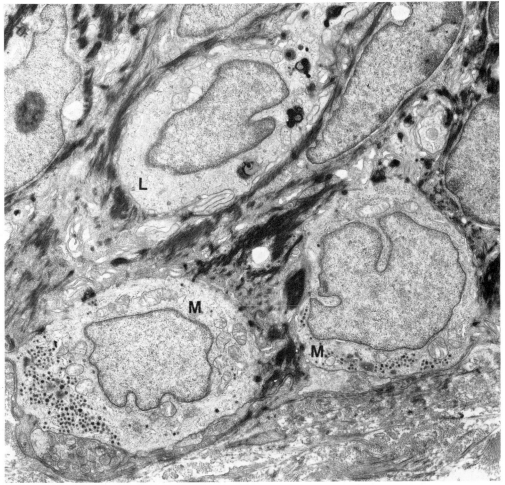

Figure 15.8. Merkel cells (*M*) and a Langerhans cell (*L*) in the epidermis of rhesus monkey (×7300). (Courtesy of Dr. Mary Bell.)

keratinocytes of polygonal shape. The plasma membranes of adjacent cells are normally in close apposition throughout most of their extent, but they tend to pull apart, except in the region of the desmosomes (Figs. 15.5 and 4.5), when the cells shrink during preparation of routine sections. Thus, the cells in sections have an irregular outline, with delicate processes or spines projecting from their surfaces. They are often called "prickle cells." Before electron microscope studies, it was thought by some histologists that the spinous processes formed cytoplasmic connections between cells. Electron micrographs now show that the points of apposition are not bridges of cytoplasmic continuity but are processes of separate cells joined by typical *desmosomes* (Fig. 4.4).

The *stratum granulosum* consists of two to five rows of flattened, rhombic cells with their long axes parallel with the surface of the skin (Figs. 15.3, 15.9 and 15.10). The cytoplasm contains numerous *keratohyalin* granules that stain intensely with hematoxylin. Electron micrographs show that these granules are actually irregularly shaped masses of electron-dense material in close association with bundles of filaments. They are relatively rich in proline and in sulfur-containing amino acids and serve as the precursors of the amorphous portion of the

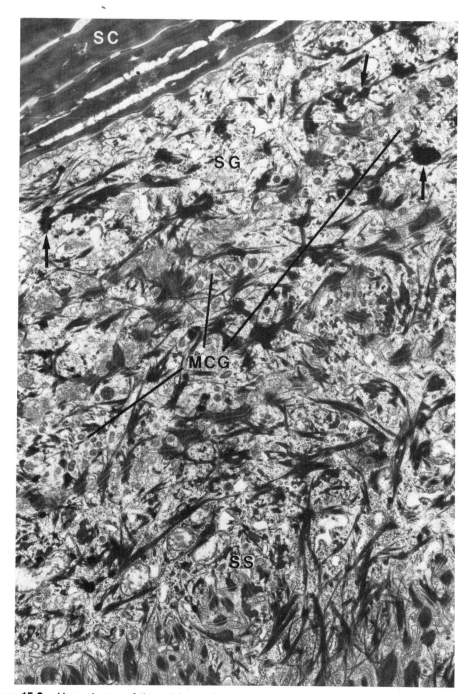

Figure 15.9. Upper layers of the epidermis from skin of rhesus monkey. The stratum granulosum (SG) contains small keratohyalin granules (*arrows*) and numerous membrane-coating granules (*MCG*). *SC*, stratum corneum; *SS*, stratum spinosum (×14,900). (Courtesy of Dr. Mary Bell.)

extensive filament-matrix complex of stratum corneum (discussed below).

The *stratum lucidum* is a thin usually lightly staining zone, located between the stratum granulosum and the cornified surface layer. The lucidum is readily seen in the epidermis of the palms and soles but is usually not identifiable in other parts of the

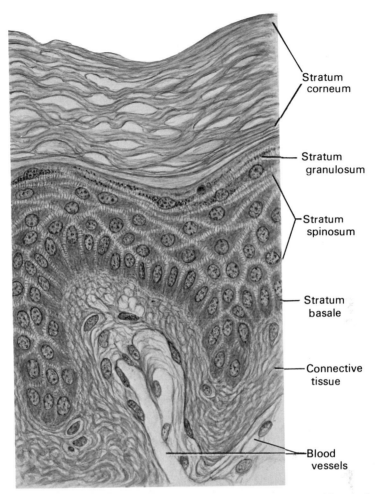

Stratum
corneum

Stratum
granulosum

Stratum
spinosum

Stratum
basale

Connective
tissue

Blood
vessels

Figure 15.10. Drawing of a vertical section through the relatively thin epidermis from the median side of the lower extremity. The field includes the total thickness of the stratum corneum which is much thinner than that of the fingertip. The stratum lucidum is barely discernible (×700). (Compare with Figure 15.3.)

body. The nuclei begin to degenerate in the outer cells of the granulosa layer and disappear in the lucidum. Tonofilaments seen in electron micrographs are aggregated and arranged in a more orderly fashion than in the granulosum cells and the cell membranes are increased in thickness. There is also an increased amount of intercellular material.

The *stratum corneum* is very thick in the palms and soles and is composed of clear, dead, scalelike cells which become more and more flattened as the surface is approached, the most peripheral layer containing flat, horny plates which are con-

stantly desquamated. The cells have a thickened membrane, as noted above, and they are closely interdigitated. The nuclei have disappeared, but some of the spaces that they occupied can be seen.

The former cytosol of these dead cells is greatly shrunken and almost totally occupied by filaments tightly packed in orthogonal arrays that lie parallel to the skin surface and embedded in an opaque, electron-dense, interfilamentous material. Desmosomes, although modified, persist and are thought to play a role in spatial stabilization. As the cells move outward from the stratum basale to the cornified layer, the keratinization process is characterized by a number of changes including aggregation of filaments, formation of keratohyalin granule precursors of the interfilamentous matrix material of keratin, and the loss of cell organelles after the keratohyalin granules have reached their maximal size. The emergence of the keratin complex (tonofilaments plus keratohyalin-derived interfilamentous matrix) is characterized by formation of disulfide groups in keratin from sulfhydryl groups in the filaments of the deeper layers.

The thickened membranes or husks which envelop the keratinized cells are resistant to keratinolytic agents and provide integrity for the filament-matrix complex: The filamentous portion of the complex provides for flexibility and elastic recovery of the cell content. The amorphous portion of the filament-matrix complex is primarily responsible for the chemical resistance of the keratinized cells.

The cornified layer of the epidermis is composed of "*soft keratin,*" as contrasted with "*hard keratin,*" found in the nails and in the cortex of the hairs. Hard keratin contains relatively more sulfur, is less elastic, and is more permanent, in the sense that it does not desquamate, as does the epidermis.

The peripheral region of the stratum corneum which is constantly being desquamated is often referred to as the *stratum disjunctum.*

Epidermis of the General Body Surface

The epidermis of most of the body is considerably thinner than that of the palms, soles, and volar surfaces of the digits. All layers of the epidermis are reduced, and the stratum corneum and stratum Malpighii are the only layers that are constantly present. A thin stratum granulosum, composed of only one or two cell rows, is frequently present, but a definite stratum lucidum is generally absent. The structure varies with the region studied. On the leg, for example, where the epidermis is thicker than that of abdominal or pubic skin yet much thinner than that of the fingertip, a faint stratum lucidum may be found. The reduction in the thickness of layers in thin epidermis is probably due to the fact that keratinization is far less marked and occurs not as a continuous process, but only at certain times.

The Dermis or Corium

The dermis varies from 0.2 to 4 mm in thickness and is composed of dense, irregularly arranged connective tissue. It contains the three types of connective tissue fibers plus fibroblasts and macrophages. Two layers can be distinguished, although they blend without distinct demarcation. The deeper one is relatively thick and is known as the reticular layer. The superficial layer is thinner and is named the subepithelial or papillary layer.

The *reticular layer* is characterized by coarse collagenous fibers and fiber bundles which often unite to form secondary bundles of considerable thickness (nearly 100 μm in diameter). The fibers cross each other to form an extensive feltwork with rhomboid meshes, the direction of the fibers generally being parallel to the surface of the skin. The elastic fibers form complex elastic nets permeating the entire dermis. Here too the course of the main fibers is parallel with the surface, although vertical and oblique fibers are present in considerable number. The elastic fibers form basket-like, capsular condensations around the hair bulbs, and sweat and sebaceous glands.

The *papillary* or *subepithelial layer* is similar in structure to the reticular layer, but the fibers are finer and more closely arranged.

Although the connective tissue fibers of the dermis form complex nets and meshes, those bundles which course parallel with the lines of tension of the skin are more numerous and better developed than the others. The lines of skin tension, which are caused by the direction of the predominant fibers, are known as *Langer's lines*. These lines have different directions in the various parts of the body. Their direction is of surgical importance because incisions made parallel with the lines gape less and heal with less scar tissue than do incisions made across the lines.

As has been mentioned, the surface of the dermis is studded by numerous papillae that indent the underside of the epidermis. Seen in sections, some are simple; others are branched. Some contain loops of capillary blood vessels (vascular papillae); others contain special nerve terminations (nervous papillae) (Fig. 10.53).

In addition to the usual types of connective tissue cells, the dermis of certain regions may contain a few branched, pigmented connective tissue cells, the *dermal chromatophores*, which resemble the pigmented cells of the choroid coat of the eye. The dermal chromatophores are normally scarce in white individuals. They occur chiefly in regions where the epidermis itself is richly pigmented, and their pigment is apparently obtained from melanogenic cells of neural crest origin.

Smooth muscle is found in the skin in connection with the hair (*arrector pili* muscles). Smooth muscles fibers also occur in considerable number in the skin of the nipple, prepuce, glans penis, scrotum (tunica dartos), and parts of the perineum. The fibers are arranged in a network parallel to the surface, and contraction of the fibers gives the skin of these regions its wrinkled appearance. In the face and neck, skeletal muscle fibers from the mimic musculature likewise penetrate the dermis. Both smooth and skeletal fibers end in delicate, elastic bands that are continuous with the general elastic network of the dermis.

Glands of the Skin

Two kinds of glands occur in the skin: sweat glands and sebaceous glands.

Sweat Glands (Glandulae Sudoriferae)

Most of the sweat glands are of the eccrine (merocrine) type; i.e., the product of the cell is secreted by exocytosis. Eccrine sweat glands are found over the entire body surface, excepting the margin of the lips, the ear drum, the inner surface of the prepuce, and the glans penis. They are most numerous in the palms and soles and are the only glands found in these places. They are simple, coiled, tubular glands. The deepest portion of the sweat gland is secretory and hence is known as the *secretory tubule*. It is quite coiled and it frequently, but not invariably, begins in the subcutaneous tissue. The secretory tubule drains into the *coiled duct* which continues into a *straight* or *oblique duct* that passes through the dermis to contact the epidermis between two dermal papillae (Fig. 15.2). The *intraepidermal channel* takes a spiral course to the surface, where it opens via a minute pit just visible to the naked eye.

Although the nuclei of the cells of the secretory portion of the sweat gland are located at different levels (Fig. 15.11), the epithelium is classified as simple columnar because all cells extend from the basal lamina to the lumen or to intercellular canaliculi continuous with the lumen. Two types of cells have been described: *clear* and *dark*. The *clear cells* are somewhat pyramidal in shape, with a broad base on the basal lamina, whereas the *dark cells* are broader at the luminal surface and slender toward the basal lamina. Electron micrographs show that both types of cells have irregularly arranged and short cytoplasmic processes at the luminal surface and around the cell, including the basal portion (Fig 15.12). The cytoplasm of the clear cells contains a considerable amount of smooth endoplasmic reticulum, numerous mitochondria, and an abundance of glycogen, but very few ribosomes. On the other hand, dark cells have very few mitochondria but numerous ribosomes and a number of secretory vacuoles which contain proteoglycans (Fig. 15.12).

The secretory portion also contains *myoepithelial cells* (Figs 15.11 and 15.12). These cells are stellate in shape, are contractile, and have processes which bear some ultrastructural resemblance to smooth muscle cells (Fig. 15.12). They differ from smooth muscle in being ectodermal

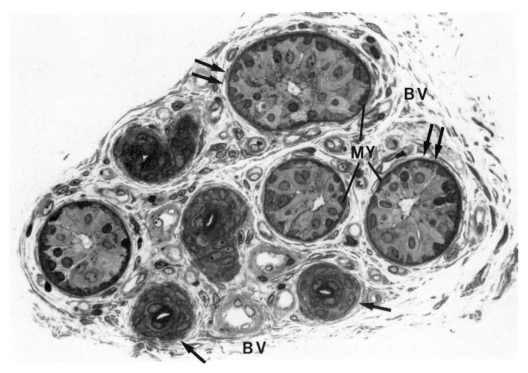

Figure 15.11. Section through a human eccrine sweat gland showing portions of the secretory coil (*double arrows*) and the sweat duct (*single arrows*) surrounded by condensed connective tissue and numerous small blood vessels (*BV*). *MY*, myoepithelial cells (×400). (Courtesy of Dr. Mary Bell.)

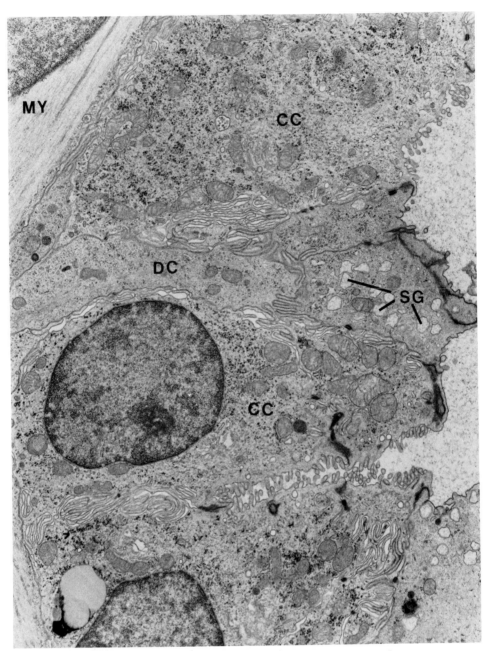

Figure 15.12. Portion of a human eccrine sweat gland showing clear cells (*CC*) containing glycogen granules, dark cells (*DC*) containing ribosomes and glycoprotein secretion granules (*SG*), and the edge of a myoepithelial cell (*MY*). The lumen is to the *right* (×6600). (Courtesy of Dr. Mary Bell.)

in origin and in not being surrounded completely by an external lamina. It is assumed that their contractions aid in movement of secretions toward the duct.

The chief components of the sweat released by the secretory tubule are water and sodium chloride plus urea, ammonia, uric acid, and proteoglygans. The clear cells apparently function in releasing water, sodium chloride, urea, etc., whereas the dark cells apparently secrete proteoglycans.

The *duct* of the sweat gland has a wall composed of a two-layered stratified cuboidal epithelium resting on a basal lamina surrounded by connective tissue cells and fibers (Figs. 15.11 and 15.13). It does not have myoepithelial cells. The cells of the inner layer of the duct have an apical border which is acidophilic and is composed of irregularly shaped microvilli. They are particularly numerous in the coiled portion of the duct. The microvilli contain closely packed microfilaments that project downward in the cytoplasm in a manner similar to that of the terminal web of many other epithelial cells (Chapter 4). After the duct reaches the epidermis, it loses its own wall and becomes a channel through the epidermis (Fig. 15.2). The ducts have an important function in addition to that of conduction: they resorb sodium without water following. Thus, sweat becomes hypotonic as it passes through the duct.

Particularly large sweat glands of a special type are located in the axilla, mammary areola, labia majora, and circumanal regions. These are known as *apocrine or odoriferous* glands (Figs. 15.14 and 15.15). The *ceruminous glands* of the external auditory meatus and the *glands of Moll* in the margins of the eyelid also belong to this general type. The apocrine glands received their name because some light microscope studies gave the erroneous impression that some of the secretion is produced by the apical ends of the cells breaking off. These results were probably artifacts of poor fixation.

The *apocrine gland secretory tubules* differ from those of merocrine glands in a number of respects. They are wider, they branch, and their myoepithelial cells are more prominent. Electron micrographs indicate that there is probably only one parenchymal cell type in the apocrine glands and that it resembles the dark cells of merocrine glands more than the light ones (Fig. 15.15). Its microvilli are more numerous and prominent than those of merocrine glands; it has numerous mitochondria, lysosomes that contain lipofuscin, and vacuoles which contain considerable proteoglycan. The *ducts* of the apocrine glands resemble those of the merocrine glands in that they lack myoepithelial cells, but they differ in that they open into the cavity of the hair follicle rather than by an intraepidermal channel. Their secretion is also more viscous than that of the ordinary sweat glands.

The apocrine glands become functional at about the time of puberty, apparently as a result of the influence of sex hormones. Their secretion is odorless when it is released but quickly develops a characteristic odor after contamination by bacteria. The apocrine glands respond to adrenergic stimuli, whereas the merocrine glands respond chiefly to cholinergic stimuli.

Sebaceous Glands

These are usually associated with the hair follicles and are described in that connection.

THE HAIR

The hairs are elastic, cornified threads developed from the epidermis. They are placed in deep narrow pits or pockets that traverse the dermis to varying depths and usually extend into the subcutaneous tissue (15.16). Each hair consists of a *shaft* that projects above the surface and a *root* that is imbedded within the skin. At its lower end, the root of the hair is expanded into a knoblike structure known as the *hair bulb* which is composed of a *matrix* of epithelial cells that are beginning to differentiate along different lines. The hair bulb is indented on its undersurface by a *papilla* of

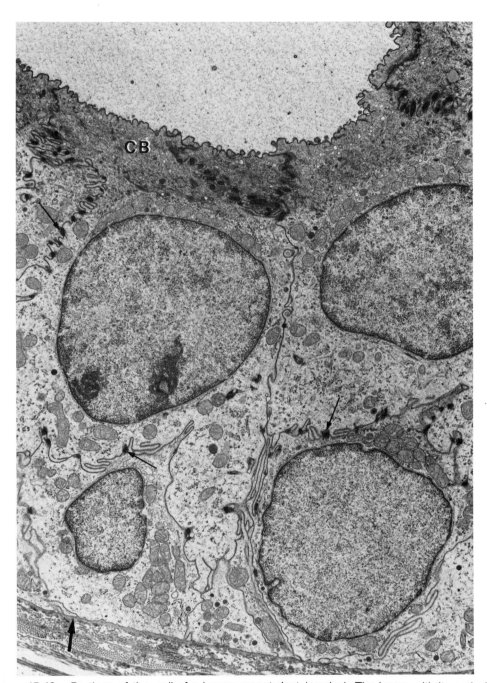

Figure 15.13. Portions of the wall of a human sweat duct (eccrine). The lumen with its cuticular border (*CB*) is at the top of the field. *Large arrow*, basal lamina; *small arrows*, desmosomes (×6600).(Courtesy of Dr. Mary Bell.)

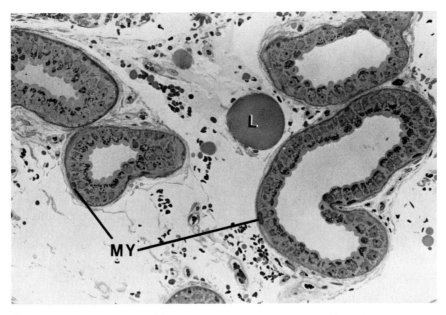

Figure 15.14. Light micrograph of human apocrine sweat gland. Nuclei of myoepithelial cells can be distinguished (*MY*). *L*, lipid within a fat cell (×224). (Courtesy of Dr. Mary Bell.)

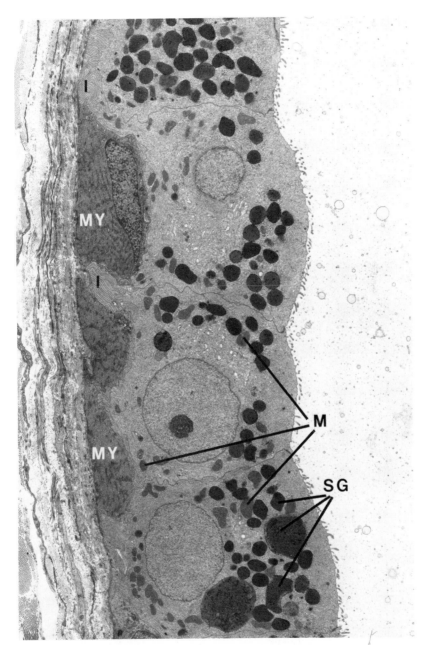

Figure 15.15.   Electron micrograph of human apocrine gland showing myoepithelial cells (*MY*), basal membrane interdigitations (*I*), secretory granules (*SG*), and mitochondria (*M*). The lumen is at *right* (×3800). (Courtesy of Dr. Mary Bell.)

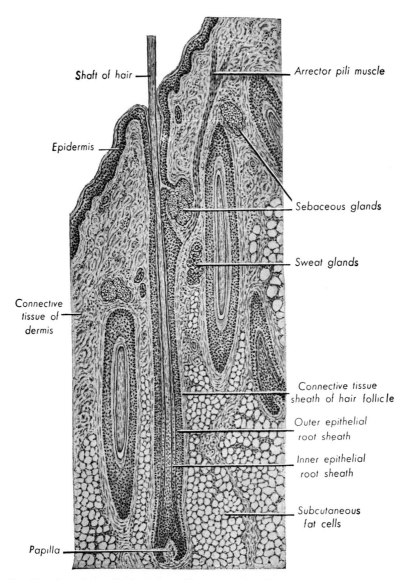

Shaft of hair

Epidermis

Connective
tissue of
dermis

Papilla

Arrector pili muscle

Sebaceous glands

Sweat glands

Connective tissue
sheath of hair follicle

Outer epithelial
root sheath

Inner epithelial
root sheath

Subcutaneous
fat cells

Figure 15.16. Drawing of a vertical section of human scalp, showing a longitudinal section of a hair and its follicle. Reconstructed from serial sections to show a complete follicle cut through its longitudinal axis (×36).

connective tissue. The hair root is enclosed by the *hair follicle,* which consists of an epidermal (epithelial) portion and an outer, dermal (connective tissue) portion.

Structure of the Hair

The hair is composed entirely of epithelial cells, which are arranged in three definite layers: the medulla, cortex, and cuticle.

The *medulla* forms the central axis of the hair, varying in thickness from 16 to 20 μm.

It consists of two or three layers of cells which vary in appearance in different parts of the hair. In the lower portion of the root of the hair, the cells are cuboidal and have rounded nuclei (Fig. 15.17). In the shaft, the cells of the medulla are cornified and shrunken and the nuclei are rudimentary or absent (Fig. 15.18*A* and *B*). The intercellular spaces are usually filled with air. The medulla is absent from the finer, shorter (lanugo) hairs and also from some

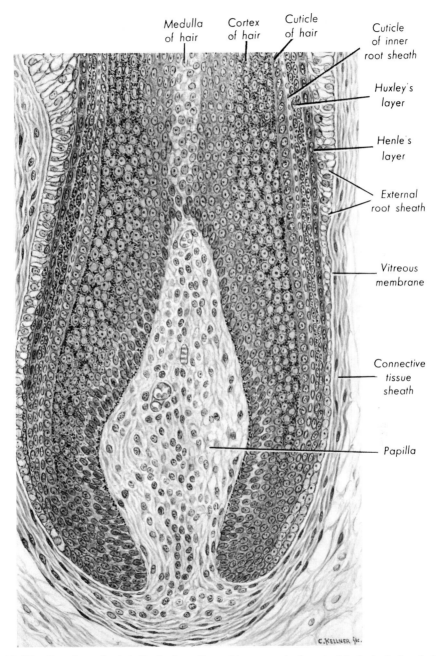

Figure 15.17. Drawing of a longitudinal section of lower end of root of hair, including hair follicle and connective tissue papilla (×310).

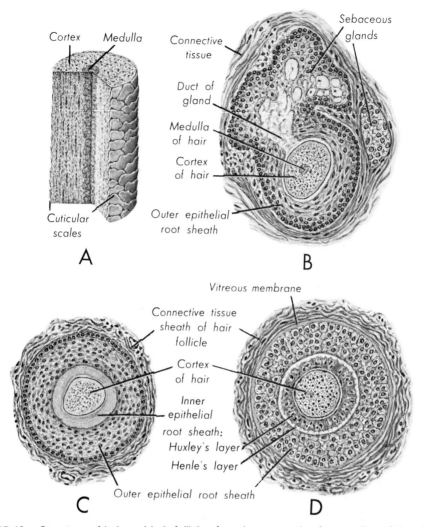

Figure 15.18. Structure of hair and hair follicles from human scalp. *A,* a portion of the shaft of a hair reconstructed from a surface view and from longitudinal sections. *B, C,* and *D,* drawings of cross sections of hairs and their follicles at various levels: *B,* at the level of the sebaceous glands; *C,* midway between epidermis of scalp and papilla of hair root; *D,* through the lower one-third of follicle. No medulla was present in the hairs illustrated in *C* and *D (A,* ×280; *B, C,* and *D,* ×175).

of the hairs of the scalp. It frequently fails to extend the whole length of the hair.

The *cortex* makes up the main bulk of the hair and consists of several layers of cells. In the lower part of the root of the hair, the cortex is composed of cuboidal cells with nuclei of normal appearance (Fig. 15.17). The cells become progressively flattened and modified at higher levels. In the upper part of the root and in the shaft, the cortex is composed of cornified, elongated cells with longitudinally striated cytoplasm and shrunken, degenerated nuclei (Fig.

15.18). In colored hair, pigment granules are found in and between the cells. Air also accumulates in the intercellular spaces.

The *cuticle* of the hair is exceedingly thin and is composed of a single layer of clear cells. In the deeper part of the hair root, the cuticular cells are nucleated (Fig. 15.17). In the upper part of the root and on the shaft, the cuticular cells are clear, scale-like, and nonnucleated (Fig. 15.18). The cells overlap like shingles on a roof, giving the surface of the hair a serrated appearance.

The color of the hair is determined primarily by the amount and distribution of pigment but to some extent also by the presence of air, because the latter appears white in reflected light. Hair in which the pigment has faded and the medulla has become filled with air appears silvery white.

Hair Follicle

The hair follicle consists of the inner and outer epithelial root sheaths, derived from the epidermis, and the connective tissue sheaths, derived from the dermis.

The *inner epithelial root sheath* is composed of three distinct layers: the cuticle of the root sheath, Huxley's layer, and Henle's layer.

The *cuticle of the root sheath* lies against the cuticle of the hair and is similar to the latter in structure (Fig. 15.17). It consists of thin, scalelike, overlapping cells, nucleated in the deeper parts of the sheath and nonnucleated nearer the surface. The free edges of the scales project downward and interdigitate with the upward projecting edges of the hair cuticle.

Huxley's layer lies immediately outside the cuticle of the root sheath and consists of several rows of elongated cells whose protoplasm contains eleidin-like granules (trichohyalin). In the deeper portion of the hair follicle, these cells contain nuclei (Fig. 15.19). Nearer the surface the nuclei are rudimentary or absent (Fig. 15.18C).

Henle's layer is a row of rectangular, somewhat flattened, clear cells. The cytoplasm contains longitudinal horny fibrils, and nuclei are present only in the deepest portions of the follicle (Figs. 15.17 and 15.19). Between the cells are sometimes

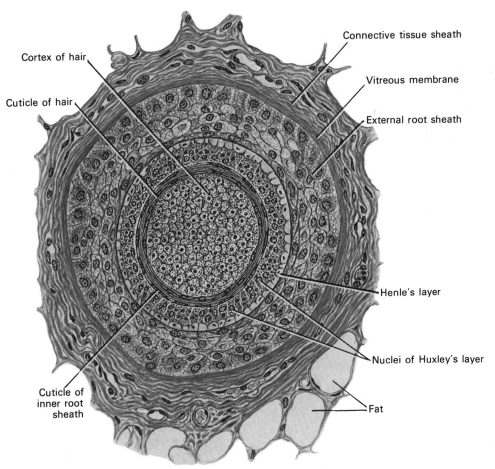

Figure 15.19. Drawing of a transverse section through root of hair and hair follicle (×334).

seen short, wedgelike processes which extend from the cells of Huxley's layer.

The *outer epithelial root sheath* is a direct continuation of the Malpighian layer of the epidermis, to which it corresponds in structure. The outermost cells, adjacent to the connective tissue, are tall and arranged in a single row. The rest of the cells are more polygonal in shape. They have spinous processes and resemble the prickle cells already described for the stratum spinosum of the skin.

The *connective tissue sheath* is derived from the dermis and consists of an inner, a middle, and an outer layer.

The inner layer is a distinctive basement membrane. It has classically been termed the *hyaline* or *vitreous membrane,* and is closely applied to the cells of the outer root sheath. The middle layer is thickest and is composed of fine connective tissue fibers which are arranged circularly. The outer layer is poorly defined and consists of rather coarse, loosely woven bundles of white fibers which run in a longitudinal direction.

In the deeper portion of the root, some little distance above the bulb, all of the layers of the hair and its follicles can be seen distinctly. The differentiation of the layers becomes less marked as one passes in either direction. At the level of entrance of the ducts of the sebaceous glands (Fig. 15.16), the inner epithelial root sheath disappears and the outer root sheath passes over into the Malpighian layer of the epidermis. The connective tissue follicle ceases as a distinct structure at about the level of insertion of the *arrector pili* muscles.

Marked changes are also noted as the bulb is approached. The outer root sheath thins down to two and finally to one layer of rather flat cells and then disappears. The layers of the inner root sheath retain their identity until the neck of the papilla is reached, at which point the different layers merge.

The bulbous thickening of the hair root which surrounds the papilla is not organized into layers but constitutes a matrix of growing, multiplying cells that superficially become transformed into the hardened cells of the hair and the inner root sheath. Laterally, the cells of the bulb become continuous with the outer root sheath, which, like the Malpighian layer of the epidermis, grows by mitosis of cells in the deeper layers, i.e., the external layers of the root sheath. Thus, the growth of the outer root sheath is radial, whereas the hair and inner root sheath grow upward from the thickened base of the follicle. The hair papilla, although much larger, is similar in structure to other dermal papillae and contains delicate elastic and collagenous fibrils, cellular elements, blood vessels, and nerves.

Muscles and Glands of the Hair Follicle

The erectors of the hairs (*arrectores pilorum*) are oblique bands of smooth muscle fibers, from 50 to 220 μm in diameter, which arise in the subepithelial tissue and are usually inserted in the connective tissue follicle of the hair, about the middle of the follicle or a little above. Each muscle, at its origin, is attached to several delicate connective tissue strands, runs for a distance as a compact bundle, and then divides into several bundles that go to the individual hairs of a hair group. The muscles usually arch around the sebaceous glands which fill the angle between the muscle and hair, although large sebaceous glands occasionally penetrate the muscle. The thickness of the muscle bands corresponds roughly to the thickness and length of the hair. They are poorly developed in the hairs of the axilla and in certain parts of the face, where the muscles of facial expression apparently take over the function of erectors. The eyebrows, eyelids, and lashes have no erectors.

The hairs and hair follicles are not perpendicular to the skin but slope distinctly. The *arrector pili* muscle is situated in the obtuse angle between the hair follicle and surface. When the muscle contracts, the hair becomes more vertical to the surface and, at the same time, a small groove appears in the skin at the place where the muscle is attached. This gives rise to the so-called "goose flesh."

The *sebaceous* glands are with few exceptions connected with the hair follicles (Fig. 15.20). They are simple or branched alveolar (saccular) glands. Their size varies considerably and bears no relation to the size of the hair, the largest glands being frequently connected with the smallest hairs. The glands are spherical or ovoid in shape, and each is encapsulated in connective tissue. The excretory duct is wide and empties into the neck of the follicle. It is lined with stratified squamous epithelium continuous with the outer root sheath and the Malpighian layer of the epidermis. The lower end of the duct opens into several simple or branched alveoli, at the mouths of which the epithelium becomes thinner. The alveoli themselves are completely filled with a stratified epithelium.

The most peripheral cells are rather small and cubical in shape (Figs. 15.20 and 15.21) and occasionally show mitotic figures. Toward the interior the polyhedral or spheroidal cells become progressively larger as a result of the accumulation of numerous fat droplets in their cytoplasm (Figs. 15.20 and 15.22). Their secretion, an oily substance called *sebum,* appears to be the direct product of disintegration of the alveolar cells (holocrine mode of secretion), and all of the stages of the process are seen in the various layers of cells. The smaller peripheral cells contain only a few small fat droplets or none at all (Fig. 15.21). The most central ones and those in the lumen of the duct show the most marked changes. Their cytoplasm is almost wholly converted into fat, and their nuclei are shrunken or disintegrated (Fig. 15.22). In the middle zone are cells showing intermediate stages.

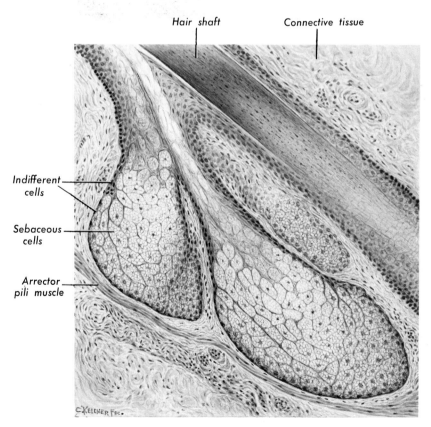

Figure 15.20. Drawing of a sebaceous gland from scalp (×130).

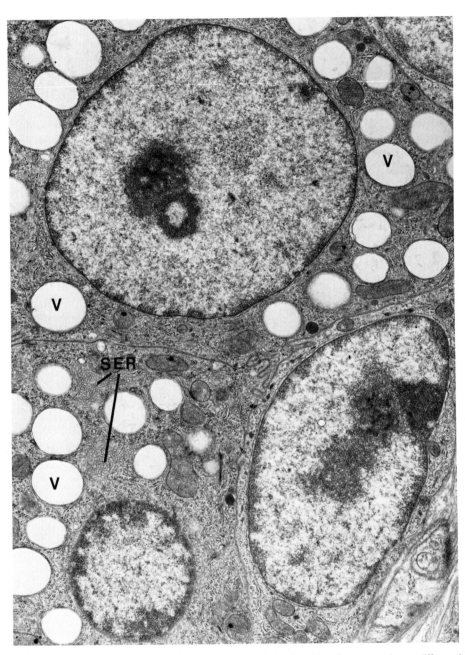

Figure 15.21.   Peripheral differentiating cells of sebaceous gland from mouse. An undifferentiated cell is at *lower right*. Other cells show accumulations of smooth endoplasmic reticulum (*SER*) and forming lipid vesicles (*V*). These are clear because the lipid has been extracted during specimen preparation (×13,600). (Courtesy of Dr. Mary Bell.)

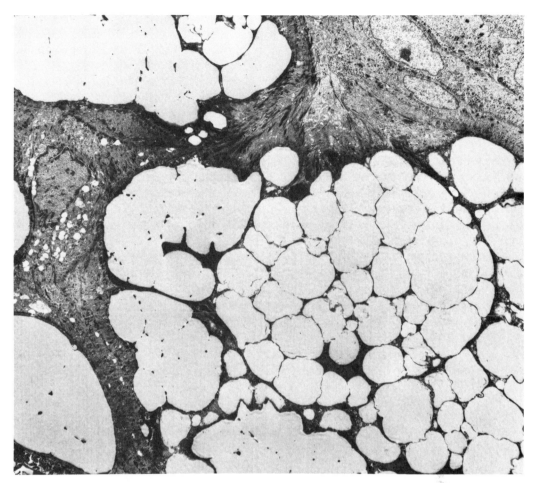

Figure 15.22. Portion of a human sebaceous gland near the pilosebaceous duct. Most of the field shows remnants of degenerating cells. Part of the duct wall appears at upper right (×2400). (Courtesy of Dr. Mary Bell.)

The replacement of cells lost in secretion is accomplished chiefly by mitotic divisions of the indifferent cells at the periphery of the gland (Fig. 15.20). The stages in this process, as well as the proliferation of new alveoli from the cells of the excretory ducts, can be demonstrated in animals in which the growth of the sebaceous glands is stimulated experimentally. In fetal development, the glands and their ducts arise by proliferation and differentiation from the outer epithelial root sheath of the hair follicle (see Fig. 15.26).

Sebaceous glands unconnected with hair follicles occur along the margin of the lips, in the nipple, in the glans and prepuce of the penis, and in the labia minora.

Replacement of Hairs

Shedding of hair takes place in most mammals at regularly recurring periods. In man there is constant although gradual loss and replacement of hairs. The scalp hairs have the longest duration of life, from two to five years, whereas those of the eyebrows and ears last only from three to five months. Even shorter is the age of the eyelashes.

When a hair is about to shed, proliferation of cells above the papilla slows down and finally ceases. The bulb develops into a solid, club-shaped mass and becomes completely keratinized; its lower end splits brushlike into numerous fibers. The club-shaped bulb, firmly fused with the lower ends of the inner root sheath, which likewise cornifies, becomes detached from the papilla and is slowly shifted toward the surface of the skin to about the level of the entrance of the sebaceous ducts. There it may remain for some time, until pulled out or shed or pushed out by a replacing hair. Such hairs are called *club hairs* to distinguish them from hairs that possess papillae.

The papilla atrophies and may completely disappear. The outer root sheath collapses and forms a cord of cells extending between the atrophied papilla and the lower end of the shedding hair.

The formation of a new hair starts with the proliferation of cells of the outer root sheath in the region of the old papilla. The papilla becomes larger and invaginates the cell mass or, according to some authors, a new papilla is formed. From this new matrix or "hair germ," the new hair develops in a manner similar to embryonal hair formation. The new hair grows toward the

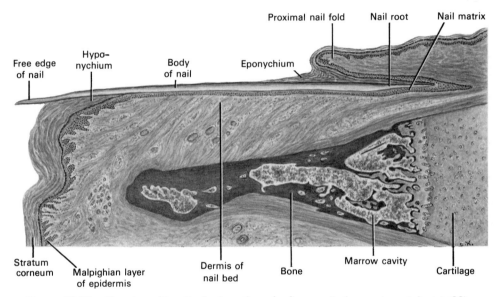

Figure 15.23. Drawing of longitudinal section of a fingernail of a newborn infant (×22).

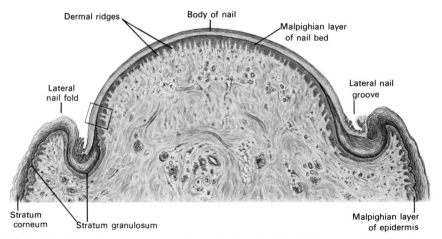

Figure 15.24. Drawing of a transverse section of nail and nail bed. Human adult. The area marked by the *square* is enlarged in Figure 15.25. (×20).

surface, under or to one side of the dead hair, which it finally replaces.

THE NAILS

The nails are composed of flat, cornified scales which form protective coverings for the distal phalanges of the fingers and toes. Each nail consists of (a) a *body,* the attached uncovered portion of the nail, (b) a *free edge,* the anterior unattached extension of the body, and (c) the *nail root,* the posterior or proximal part of the nail which lies beneath a fold of the skin (Fig. 15.23). Most of the body of the nail is pink because it is sufficiently translucent to transmit the color from the underlying vascular tissue. The proximal part of the nail is whitish and is called the *lunula* because of its shape.

The fold of skin which extends around the proximal and lateral borders of the nail constitutes the *nail fold,* and the skin which lies beneath the nail forms the *nail bed.* The furrow between the nail bed and nail fold is the *nail groove* (Figs. 15.23 and 15.24).

The nail itself is hard and consists of several layers of clear, flat cells that contain shrunken and degenerated nuclei. The striated appearance observed in sections cut perpendicular to the surface is produced by the arrangement of the cells in layers.

The nail bed consists of epithelium and dermis continuous with the epidermis and dermis of the skin of the nail folds. The epidermis of the nail folds usually has the zones characteristic of palmar skin, although the stratum lucidum may be thin or absent in some cases. The stratum corneum of the proximal nail fold turns into the nail groove, spreads over the upper surface of the nail root, and continues for a short distance onto the surface of the body of the nail as the *eponychium* (Fig. 15.23). The stratum corneum of the lateral folds ends in the lateral grooves in contact with the borders of the nail (Figs. 15.24 and 15.25). The stratum granulosum and lucidum terminate in the lower part of the grooves.

The epithelium of the nail bed corresponds to the Malpighian layer of the skin

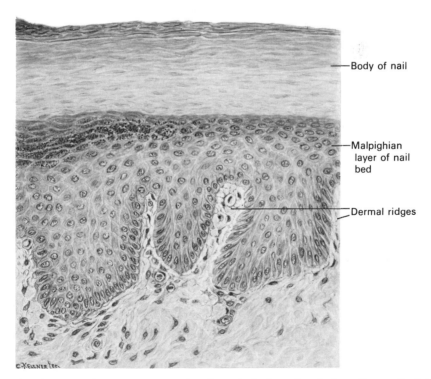

Body of nail

Malpighian layer of nail bed

Dermal ridges

Figure 15.25. Drawing of a transverse section through the lateral part of a nail, near the lateral nail groove, as outlined in Figure 15.24 (×365).

and, like the latter, consists of polygonal prickle cells and a stratum basale resting upon a basement membrane. The epithelium of the posterior part of the nail bed, the part that lies beneath the root and the proximal portion of the body corresponding to the lunula, is thicker than elsewhere and is called the matrix because if functions for nail growth. Growth of the nail takes place by a transformation of the more superficial cells of the matrix into true nail cells. In this process, the outer, harder layer is pushed forward over the Malpighian layer, the latter remaining always in the same position. The nails generally increase in length by about 0.5 mm/week.

Under the distal free edge of the nail, the epithelium of the nail bed becomes continuous with the Malpighian layer of the skin, and the other layers characteristic of the epidermis begin. The stratum corneum of the skin beneath the free edge of the nail is thickened and is known as the *hyponychium* (Fig. 15.23).

The dermis of the nail bed differs somewhat from that of ordinary skin. Its connective tissue fibers are arranged partly longitudinal to the long axis of the nail and partly in a vertical plane extending from the periosteum to the nail. Dermal papillae are found beneath the proximal part of the nail root but disappear beneath the distal part of the root, to be replaced by longitudinal dermal ridges which, increasing in height as they pass forward, continue to the distal end of the nail bed. Because the dermal ridges run longitudinally, the boundary between the epithelium and connective tissue appears smooth in longitudinal sections and irregular and papilla-like in cross sections (Fig. 15.24).

BLOOD VESSELS, LYMPHATICS, AND NERVES OF THE SKIN

Blood Vessels

From the larger arteries in the subcutaneous tissue, branches penetrate the reticular layer of the dermis, where they anastomose to form cutaneous networks. The latter give off branches that pass to the papillary layer of the dermis and there form a second series of networks, the subpapillary, just beneath the papillae. From the cutaneous networks arise two sets of capillaries, one supplying the fat lobules, the other supplying the region of the sweat glands. From the subpapillary networks are given off small arteries that break up into capillary networks for the supply of the papillae, sebaceous glands, and hair follicles. The return blood from these capillaries first enters a horizontal plexus of veins just under the papillae. This communicates with a second plexus just beneath the first. Small veins from this second plexus pass alongside the arteries of the deeper part of the dermis, where they form a third plexus with larger, more irregular meshes. Into this plexus pass most of the veins from the fat lobules and sweat glands, although one or two small veins from the sweat glands usually follow the duct and empty into the subpapillary plexus. The blood next passes into a fourth plexus in the subcutaneous tissue, from which arise veins of considerable size. These accompany the arteries.

As noted in Chapter 12, arteriovenous anastomoses are especially numerous in the dermis of the fingers and toes. In these areas, the arterial part of the anastomosis often forms a part of a specific organ known as a glomus. The artery is coiled or ball-like and its media contains epitheloid cells. The internal diameter of the narrowest part of the anastomosis is usually 20 to 40 μm; thus, the anastomoses convey much more blood than capillaries do. By contraction or relaxation, they influence the amount of blood flowing through localized regions. They play an important role in conserving heat and in regulating the temperature of peripheral areas. In this respect, their high degree of development in the feet of penguins is noteworthy.

Small arteries from the plexuses of the skin and subcutis pass to the hair follicle. The larger arterioles run longitudinally in the outer layer of the follicle. From these are given off branches which form a rich plexus of small arterioles and capillaries in the middle vascular layer of the follicle. Capillaries from this plexus also pass to the sebaceous glands, the arrectores pilorum muscles, and the papillae.

Lymphatics

The lymphatics of the skin begin as capillaries within the dermal papillae and continue into a horizontal network of capillaries and small lymphatic vessels within the papillary layer of connective tissue. The lymphatics from the dermis join larger lymphatic vessels that accompany the blood vessels within the subcutaneous tissue. These become afferent lymphatic channels to lymph nodes, as described in Chapter 14. For details on the course of the lymphatic vessels in different regions, reference should be made to textbooks of gross anatomy.

Nerves

The nerves of the skin are mainly sensory. Efferent sympathetic axons supply the smooth muscle of the walls of the blood vessels, the arrectores pilorum, and the secretory cells of the sweat glands. The sensory nerves are peripheral processes of somatic ganglion cells. The larger trunks lie in the subcutis, giving off branches which pass to the dermis, where they form a rich subpapillary plexus of both myelinated and nonmyelinated fibers. From the subcutaneous nerve trunks and from the subpapillary plexus are given off fibers which terminate in more or less elaborate special nerve endings (Chapter 11). Their location is as follows. (*a*) *In the subcutaneous tissue: lamellar (Pacinian) corpuscles.* They are most numerous in the palms and soles. (*b*) *In the dermis: tactile corpuscles of Meissner* are found in the papillae, especially of the fingertip, palm, and sole. *Krause's end bulbs* are usually in the dermis just beneath the papillae, more rarely in the papillae themselves. (*c*) *In the epithelium:* free nerve endings are found within intercellular spaces.

Branches of the cutaneous nerves supply the hair follicles, which are important in sensory reception. As a rule, only one nerve passes to each follicle, entering it just below the entrance of the duct of the sebaceous gland. As it approaches the follicle, the nerve fiber loses its myelin sheath and divides into two branches, which further subdivide to form a ringlike plexus of fine fibers encircling the follicle. From this ring, small varicose fibrils run for a short distance up the follicle, terminating mainly in slight expansions on the vitreous membrane.

DEVELOPMENT OF THE SKIN AND ITS APPENDAGES

The *epidermis* develops from the ectoderm and consists at first of a single layer of cuboidal cells. By the second month it has differentiated into two layers. The outer layer, the *periderm* or *epitrichium,* consisting of flattened cells, is a transient structure and is lost shortly before or after birth. The inner layer, composed of irregular cells with large nuclei and abundant cytoplasm, gives rise to the entire epidermis. The cells multiply by mitosis and soon form a stratified epithelium. True keratinization, however, begins only in the fifth month.

The *dermis* develops from the parietal mesoderm and consists at first of typical mesenchyme. In the second month, cell differentiation begins, some of the cells becoming fibroblasts. Toward the end of the second month, fibrils make their appearance, at first reticular and collagenous, and, soon after, elastic as well. Some time later the whole mass shows a differentiation into two layers, an upper, denser one, giving rise to the dermis proper, and a deeper, looser one that forms the subcutaneous tissue.

Hair appears in human embryos at the end of the second month, the first places being the brows, upper lips, and chin. By the seventh month, lanugo hairs are distributed all over the body.

Each hair develops as a thickening of the germinative layer that grows down obliquely into the dermis, forming a slender solid cord of cells, the *hair germ* or *hair plug* (Fig. 15.26). The connective tissue cells of the dermis surrounding the cord condense to form the dermal follicle, and an invagination of connective tissue into the lower end of the hair germ forms the papilla.

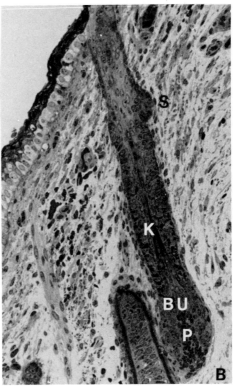

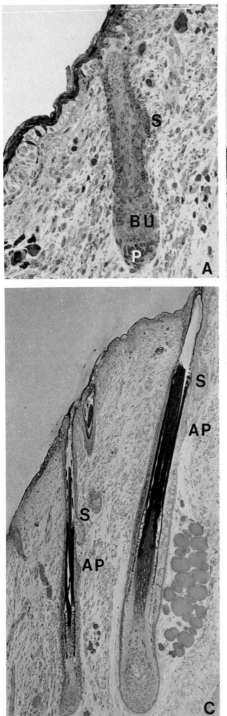

Figure 15.26. Stages in the differentiation of hair follicles in rhesus monkey. *A*, early stage showing hair bulb (*BU*), condensing tissue of dermal papilla (*P*), and anlage for sebaceous gland (*S*). *B*, later stage showing hair bulb (*BU*) encircling the dermal papilla (*P*), the anlage for a sebaceous gland (*S*), and beginning keratinization of the hair shaft (*K*). *C*, later stage showing nearly mature hair follicles. In addition to sebaceous glands (*S*) there are bulges in the root sheath corresponding to attachment of arrector pili muscles (*AP*) (*A* and *B*, ×224; *C*, ×90). (Courtesy of Dr. Mary Bell.)

The cells surrounding the papilla become differentiated into two zones, a central conical mass whose apex is directed toward the surface (the hair bulb) and an outer layer of epithelial cells which becomes the outer root sheath. The cells of the hair bulb grow toward the skin, the axial cells forming the hair and the peripheral cells giving rise to the inner root sheath. The various sublayers are formed from these by subsequent differentiation. Above the apex of the cone, the axial cells of the hair plug cornify and disintegrate, and a channel is formed that penetrates the epidermis. The hair grows into this channel and, when first formed, lies wholly beneath the surface. As the hair reaches the surface, its pointed extremity pierces the surface epithelium and emerges as the hair shaft.

The *sebaceous* gland develops from the outer root sheath and appears first as a thickening in the upper portion of the hair germ (see above). It soon develops into a flask-shaped, solid mass of cells which later differentiate to form the ducts and alveoli of the gland.

The *sweat* glands first appear as solid ingrowths of the epithelium into the underlying dermis. The lower end of the ingrowth becomes thickened and convoluted to form the coiled portion of the gland, and somewhat later the central portion becomes channeled out to form the lumen. The myoepithelial cells, which lie within the epithelium and rest on the basal lamina, are derived from the ectodermal cells of the ingrowth and not from mesoderm.

References

Braverman IN, Yen A: Ultrastructure of the human dermal microcirculation. II. The capillary loops of the dermal papillae. *Invest Dermatol* 68:53–60, 1977.

Breathnach AS: Identification of keratohyalin in freeze-fracture replicas of rat buccal epithelium. *J Pathol* 123:203–212, 1977.

Breathnach AS: The cell of Langerhans. *Int Rev Cytol* 18:1–28, 1965.

Cairns J: Mutation selection and the natural history of cancer. *Nature* 255:197–199, 1975.

Cummins H: Dermatoglyphics; a brief review. In Montagna W, Lobitz WC Jr (eds): *The Epidermis.* New York, Academic Press, 1964, pp 375–386.

Dahl MV: *Clinical Immunodermatology.* Chicago, Year Book Medical Publishers, 1981.

Ellis RA: Fine structure of the myoepithelium of the eccrine sweat glands of man. *J Cell Biol* 27:551–563, 1965.

Frelinger JG, Litabod S, Hill S, Frelinger JA: Mouse epidermal Ia molecules have a bone marrow origin. *Nature* 282:321–323, 1979.

Giroud A, Leblond CP: The keratinization of epidermis and its derivatives, especially the hair, as shown by x-ray diffraction and histochemical studies. *Ann NY Acad Sci* 53:613–626, 1951.

Katz SI, Tamaki K, Sachs DH: Epidermal Langerhans cells are derived from cells originating in bone marrow. *Nature* 282:324–326, 1979.

Laidlaw GF: The dopa reaction in normal histology. *Anat Rec* 53:399–413, 1932.

Lerner AB, Fitzpatrick TB: Biochemistry of melanin formation. *Physiol Rev* 30:91–126, 1950.

Lewis T: *The Blood Vessels of the Human Skin and Their Responses.* London, Shaw and Sons, 1937.

MacKenzie IC: Spatial distribution of mitosis in mouse epithelium. *Anat Rec* 181:705–710, 1975.

Masson P: Pigment cells in man. The biology of melanomas. *N Y Acad Sci* (special publ.) 4:15–51, 1948.

Matoltsy AG, Matoltsy MN: The chemical nature of keratohyalin granules of the epidermis. *J Cell Biol* 47:593–603, 1970.

Menton DN: The effects of essential fatty acid deficiency on the fine structure of mouse skin. *J Morphol* 132:181–206, 1970.

Menton DN, Eisen AZ: Structure and organization of mammalian stratum corneum. *J Ultrastruct Res* 35:247–264, 1971.

Montagna W: *The Structure and Function of Skin.* New York, Academic Press, 1962.

Montagna W, Lobitz WC (eds): *The Epidermis.* New York, Academic Press, 1964.

Moyer FH: Genetic effects on melanosome fine structure and ontogeny in normal and malignant cells. *Ann N Y Acad Sci* 100:584–606, 1963.

Munger BL: The ultrastructure and histophysiology of human eccrine sweat glands. *J Biophys Biochem Cytol* 11:385–402, 1961.

Odland GF: Tonofilaments and keratohyalin. In Montagna W, Lobitz WC Jr (eds): *The Epidermis.* New York, Academic Press, 1964, pp 237–249.

Seiji M, Shimao K, Birbeck MSC, Fitzpatrick TB: Subcellular localization of melanin biosynthesis. *Ann N Y Acad Sci* 100:497–533, 1963.

Starico RG: Amelanotic melanocytes in the outer sheath of the human hair follicle and their role in the repigmentation of regenerated epidermis. *Ann N Y Acad Sci* 100:239–255, 1963.

Trotter M: Classification of hair color. *Am J Physiol Anthropol* 25:237–260, 1939.

Turner DF: The morphology and distribution of merkel cells in primate gingival mucosa. *Anat Rec* 205:197–205, 1983.

Willier BH, Rawles ME: The control of feather color pattern by melanophores grafted from one embryo to another of a different breed of fowl. *Physiol Zool* 13:177–199, 1940.

Zelickson AH (ed): *Ultrastructure of Normal and Abnormal Skin.* Philadelphia, Lea and Febiger, 1967.

Chapter 16

THE DIGESTIVE SYSTEM

Whereas the simpler microscopic organisms can effectively absorb nutritive materials directly into their cells from the surrounding medium, this has become impossible as size and complexity have evolved. Higher invertebrates and all vertebrates are therefore equipped with a tubular system specialized to process and absorb, in sequential fashion, the foodstuffs captured from the external environment. This digestive tube is established very early in embryogenesis through interaction of endodermal epithelium and splanchnic mesoderm (see Chapter 3). Through the establishment of a mouth and an anus, the lumen of the tube becomes an internalized extension of the external environment, and it is regionally differentiated for the sequence of events constituting the process of digestion. The main tube is termed the *alimentary tract* or canal, but a variety of appendages of the tube are also important parts of the digestive system.

The alimentary tract is conveniently divided by structural variations and topographical locations into a series of regions: mouth, pharynx, esophagus, stomach, small intestine, and large intestine, including the rectum and anal canal. The structural modifications of the various regions are associated with the function of the tract, namely, the forwarding of the food through the tube, where in transit it can be mechanically altered and acted on by enzymes, a portion of it absorbed, and the residue eliminated as feces.

GENERAL FEATURES OF THE ALIMENTARY CANAL

The innermost layer of the alimentary canal is a *mucous membrane* or *mucosa*. This has two constantly occurring components, an *epithelial lining* and a surrounding stratum of connective tissue, the *lamina propria*. The lamina propria is formed of interlacing connective tissue fibers, which are usually fine. It contains fibroblasts and macrophages, is frequently infiltrated with lymphocytes, and may also contain plasma cells and eosinophils. Beginning with the esophagus, a thin stratum of smooth muscle (*muscularis mucosae*) appears subjacent to the lamina propria and forms a third component of the mucosa.

A *submucosa*, formed of loose connective tissue, is invariably present beneath the mucosa from the beginning of the esophagus to the lower end of the anal canal. This layer is absent from parts of the mouth and pharynx. It contains rather coarse collagenous fibers which are usually loosely interwoven and among which are elastic and reticular fibers and connective tissue cells. The submucosa attaches the mucosa to the underlying firm structures but allows considerable movement in much the same way that superficial fascia allows movement of the skin. In regions where no definite submucosa is present, the mucosa attaches directly to the firm underlying structures, as, for example, in the gums.

Throughout most of the alimentary canal, there is a rather thick layer of muscle (*muscularis externa*) which has a regular arrangement. In the mouth the muscle layer has no uniform arrangement and it is absent in certain regions.

Beginning with the pharynx, there is an external layer composed of connective tissue (*fibrosa*) or of connective tissue and mesothelium (*serosa, serous membrane*).

During embryonic development, the epithelial lining of the digestive system and its numerous attached glands have originated from the endoderm or, in the oral region, from stomodeal ectoderm. All of the surrounding connective tissue and muscular and vascular investments have arisen from splanchnic mesoderm or mesenchyme of the head.

The Mouth

The *mouth* or oral cavity is an irregularly shaped structure which is bounded by and contains a number of different parts, such as the lips, cheeks, teeth, gums, tongue, and palate. Except over the surface of the teeth, the mouth is lined throughout by stratified squamous epithelium; the lamina propria is rather dense, and a submucosa is present only in certain regions.

Lips and Cheeks

The lips may be divided into three rather distinct regions: the *cutaneous area*, the *red area*, and the *oral mucosa*. The cutaneous area of the lips is covered by typical thin skin with cornified epithelium, hair follicles, and sebaceous and sweat glands. The red area is covered by noncornified, relatively translucent stratified squamous epithelium which is indented by tall vascular connective tissue papillae (Fig. 16.1). The red color of the lip is due to the blood in the vessels of the tall papillae and the translucency of the epithelium. Glands are absent in the red area, except for an occasional sebaceous gland. The red area is continuous with the skin externally and with the mucous membrane of the lips internally.

The inner surfaces of the lips and cheeks are similar in structure. However, the epithelium is not cornified, and connective tissue papillae of moderate length indent it. The lamina propria is rather compact and is connected by a submucosa to the underlying skeletal muscle (orbicularis oris in the lips, buccinator in the cheeks). The submucosal fibers are thick and are so arranged that they closely bind the mucosa to the underlying structures, preventing the formation of folds and thus reducing the chance of biting the mucous membrane during mastication. In the area where the mucosa of the lips and cheeks becomes continuous with that of the gums, the submucosa is very loose, allowing movement.

Numerous glands of a mixed (mucous and serous) type and a purely mucous type are present in the submucosa of the lips and cheeks, and they also penetrate into the buccinator muscle.

Gums

The epithelium of the *gums* or *gingivae* is cornified to a variable degree. Cornification is most pronounced in those areas which are subject to the greatest amount of abrasion from mastication or brushing, i.e., on the free margin of the gums. Numerous long vascular papillae deeply indent the epithelium and are responsible for its pink color. At the gingival sulcus, the epithelium of the gums is continuous with the epithelial attachment of the tooth (see "The Teeth" and Fig. 16.7). The lamina propria of the gums is formed of coarse, interweaving collagenous fibers which bind it closely to the periosteum of the alveolar processes of the maxillae and mandible. The lamina propria is also attached to the gingival fibers of the periodontal membrane. No submucosa and no glands are present in the gingiva.

Hard Palate

The epithelium of the *hard palate* is much like that of the gums. It has a cornified layer in which the cells are hard and scalelike (Fig. 16.2), and it usually has a stratum granulosum. Long vascular papillae indent it deeply, giving a pinkish color. Except in the area adjacent to the gums and in the midline, a submucosa is present. Its fibers are coarse and run largely in a vertical direction, thus binding the lamina propria firmly to the periosteum of the hard palate. In the anterior region of the hard palate, a considerable amount of fat is present in the submucosa (the fatty zone); in the posterior two-thirds are many mucous glands (the glandular zone). In the narrow longitudinal zone of the raphe,

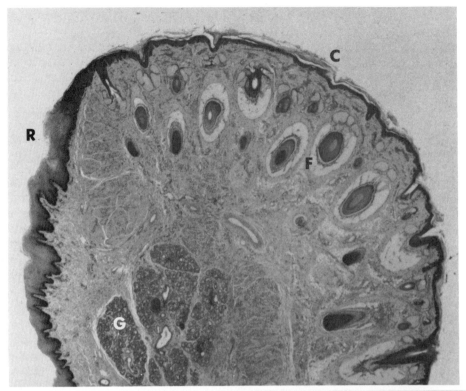

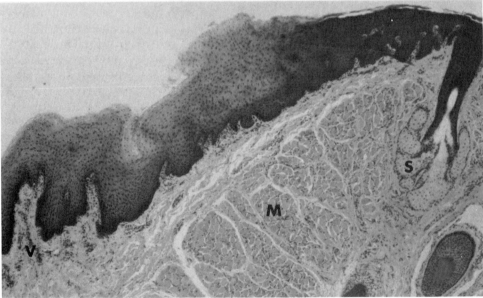

Figure 16.1. Transverse section of the lip of an infant. The upper view shows the cutaneous area (C) with hair follicles (F) at the *right* and the red part of the lip (R) at the *left*. Labial glands appear at the *lower left (G)*. The transition between cutaneous and red parts of the lip is shown at higher magnification in the *lower figure.* Note the skeletal muscle fibers of the orbicularis oris (M), the sebaceous gland associated with the hair follicle (S), and the rich vascularity (V) of the connective tissue papillae in the red part of the lip (*upper figure*, ×20; *lower figure*, ×73).

Cornified layer of stratified squamous epithelium

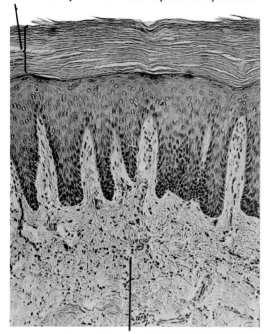

Lamina propria

Figure 16.2. Mucous membrane from anterior region of hard palate. Human (×110).

glands are absent. Spherical or ovoid aggregations of flattened, concentrically arranged epithelial cells occasionally occur near the midline. They are remnants of the embryonic fusion of the palatine processes. Structures of this type are called epithelial pearls.

Soft Palate

The oral surface of the *soft palate* and *uvula* is lined by noncornified stratified squamous epithelium. This type of epithelium extends over the free margin and for a variable distance onto the pharyngeal surface, where it becomes continuous with pseudostratified ciliated columnar epithelium. The submucosa is loose and contains many glands: mucous on the oral side and mixed (mucous and serous) on the upper (respiratory) side. A number of small skeletal muscles enter into the formation of the soft palate and uvula.

Floor of the Mouth

The *floor* of the *mouth* is lined by a noncornified epithelium. The submucosa is loose and contains the sublingual glands.

The Tongue

The main bulk of the tongue, particularly of the anterior two-thirds, is skeletal muscle. The interlacing muscle fibers course chiefly in three directions, longitudinally, transversely, and vertically, an arrangement which gives maximal mobility and physical control. In the posterior one-third of the tongue, there are aggregations of lymphatic tissue, the lingual tonsils (Fig. 16.3).

The *lower surface* of the tongue is covered by a stratified squamous epithelium which is not cornified. The lamina propria is thin and closely bound to the underlying muscle.

The *dorsal surface* of the tongue is divided into an anterior two-thirds and a posterior one-third by a V-shaped row of circumvallate papillae (Fig. 16.3). Some structural features are very different in the two regions. On the *anterior two-thirds*, there are numerous projections, the *lingual papillae*. These papillae are virtually small organs and should not be confused with the connective tissue papillae which indent stratified squamous epithelium. The lingual papillae are formed of a central core of connective tissue and a covering layer of stratified squamous epithelium (Figs. 16.4 to 16.6). The connective tissue core may give rise to small (connective tissue) papillae which indent the epithelium. According to their shape, the lingual papillae are divided into three types: *filiform, fungiform,* and *circumvallate (vallate)*.

The *filiform papillae* are by far the most numerous and are quite evenly distributed over the dorsal surface of the anterior two-thirds of the tongue. Each consists of a slender vascular core of connective tissue covered by stratified squamous epithelium which is cornified. The epithelium forms one or more secondary projections which taper into thread-like points (Fig. 16.6).

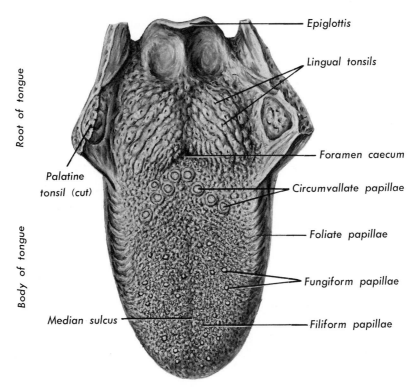

Figure 16.3. Dorsum of human tongue. (Redrawn after Spalteholz W: *Atlas of Human Anatomy*, ed 13. Leipzig, S. Herzel Verlag, 1933.)

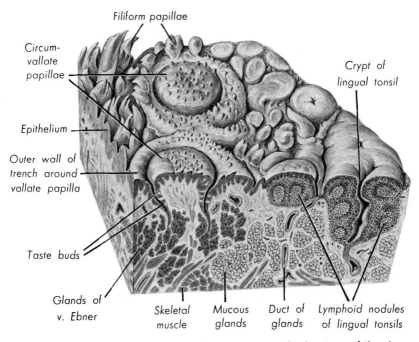

Figure 16.4. Reconstruction of the surface of the tongue at the juncture of the dorsum and root (×13). (Redrawn from Braus H: *Anatomie des Menschen*. Berlin, Julius Springer, 1924.)

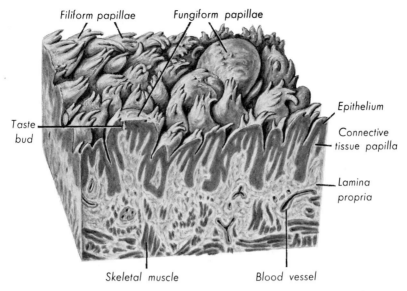

Filiform papillae *Fungiform papillae*

Epithelium

Connective tissue papilla

Taste bud

Lamina propria

Skeletal muscle *Blood vessel*

Figure 16.5. Reconstruction of the surface of the dorsum of the tongue. The *front* surface represents a sagittal section, with the root of the tongue at *right* (×16). (Redrawn from Braus H: *Anatomie des Menschen*. Berlin, Julius Springer, 1924.)

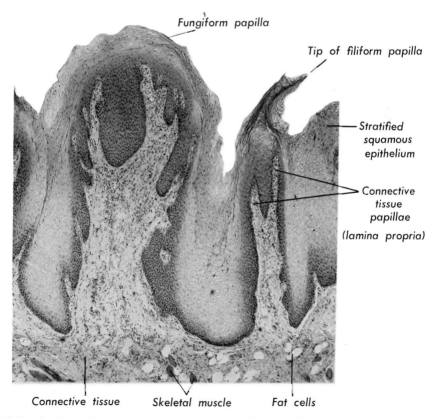

Fungiform papilla

Tip of filiform papilla

Stratified squamous epithelium

Connective tissue papillae

(lamina propria)

Connective tissue *Skeletal muscle* *Fat cells*

Figure 16.6. Section of human tongue showing a fungiform papilla (*left*) and a filiform papilla (*right*) (×56).

The *fungiform papillae* are relatively few in number and are interspersed among the filiform papillae. Their summits are rounded and are broader than the bases. They are covered by noncornified epithelium which is indented with connective tissue papillae. The connective tissue core is highly vascular. This and the thinness of the epithelium are responsible for their red color.

The *circumvallate papillae*, usually 9 to 12 in number, are arranged along a V-shaped line, the apex of the V pointing posteriorly. They resemble the fungiform papillae but are much larger and are surrounded by a trench and a wall; hence their name, vallate or circumvallate. The wall is somewhat lower than the papilla, thus allowing the latter to project slightly above the surface. Connective tissue papillae indenting the epithelium are limited to the upper surface; the sides are devoid of them. The circumvallate papillae, the trench, and the wall are covered by noncornified stratified squamous epithelium. In the epithelium of the lateral wall and sometimes in that of the trench also, are small oval bodies, *taste buds* (Figs. 16.4 and 22.46), which serve as receptor organs of taste (see Chapter 22).

Along the posterolateal border of the tongue there are folds of the mucous membrane, sometimes called the foliate papillae (Fig. 16.3). They are not well developed in man.

The *dorsal surface* of the *posterior third* of the tongue is free of papillae but has mucosal ridges and *lingual tonsils*. The latter appear as low eminences caused by the underlying aggregations of lymphatic nodules (Figs. 16.3 and 16.4). Each tonsil usually has a centrally placed pit or crypt lined by stratified squamous epithelium. The epithelium is infiltrated with lymphocytes.

No submucosa is distinguishable on the dorsum of the tongue.

Glands of the Tongue

The glands of the tongue can be divided into three main groups according to their structure and location.

A paired group of mixed mucous and serous glands are located in the anterior part of the tongue near the apex. They are embedded in the muscle but are closer to the ventral than to the dorsal surface. They have several ducts which open on the ventral surface.

A group of serous glands located in the region of the vallate papillae are known as the *glands of von Ebner*. They extend into the muscle and their ducts open into the trenches of the vallate papillae (Fig. 16.4).

Mucous glands of the root of the tongue are the most numerous. They lie in the posterior third of the tongue and extend far enough forward to mingle with the serous (von Ebner's) glands. Their ducts open into the crypts of the lingual tonsils and into depressions between the tonsils.

Nerve Supply

The *nerve supply* of the oral cavity is complex. The skeletal muscle (having arisen embryonically from mesenchyme of the second branchial arches—the hyoid arches) of the lips and cheeks is supplied by the seventh cranial nerve. Skeletal muscle of the tongue originates from somitic myotomes of the embryonic cervical region, hence receives its innervation from the 12th cranial nerve. The fibers carrying ordinary sensation are from the lingual branch of the fifth nerve and from the ninth nerve, which serve derivatives of the first and third branchial arches, respectively. The fibers carrying the special sense of taste are from the seventh nerve (through the chorda tympani) and from the ninth nerve.

The Teeth

A *tooth* has three anatomical divisions, *crown*, *root*, and *neck* or *cervix* (Fig. 16.7).

The *clinical crown* refers to that part which is visible with the tooth in situ. In early life the gums cover a part of the enamel so that the clinical crown consists of only a part of the anatomical crown. More of the enamel normally becomes exposed with the aging process, so that later in life the clinical crown includes all of the

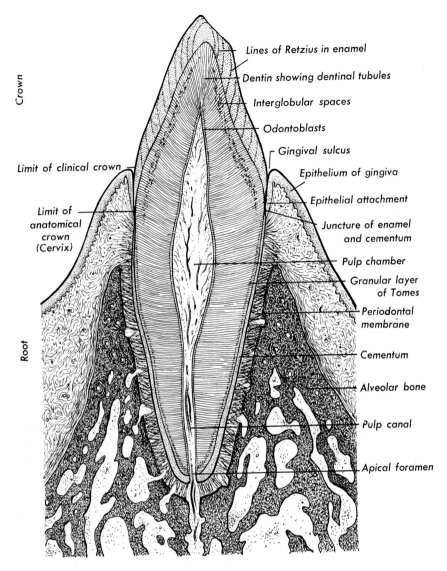

Figure 16.7. Diagram of a section through an incisor tooth and surrounding structures. The enamel at the tip of the crown shows some abrasion.

anatomical crown and even a part of the anatomical root.

The root is embedded in a cavity (the *alveolus* or *socket*) in the alveolar process of either the mandible or the maxilla, and is firmly attached to the bony wall of its socket by connective tissue, the *periodontal membrane* or *ligament*.

Structurally, a tooth has four components: *enamel, dentin, cementum,* and *pulp*.

Enamel

Enamel is the hardest substance in the body and, by weight, is composed largely (96%) of inorganic salts, of which the greater part (about 90%) is calcium phosphate. By volume, however, the organic component of enamel is considerable, nearly equaling the inorganic element. Enamel is somewhat brittle but, because of the support of the underlying dentin and also because of its internal structural arrangement, it does not fracture from the amount of stress produced by the contact relation (occlusion) of opposing maxillary and mandibular teeth during normal mastication. Enamel is present in greatest amounts on the cusps of the permanent bicuspids and molars, where it is 2 to 2.5 mm in thickness.

Structurally, enamel is composed of *enamel rods* or *prisms* and *interprismatic substance.*

The *enamel rods* are elongated columns, each of which extends throughout the thickness of the enamel layer from the dentinoenamel juncture to the surface of the anatomical crown. They have been deposited, and gradually built up in length, during tooth development before eruption, by the activity of an ectodermally derived epithelium, the *ameloblast layer* (see discus-

sion below). When seen in cross section, some rods are hexagonal, oval, or polygonal, but most are arcade- or scale-shaped with a depression on one side (Fig. 16.8). The average diameter of the enamel rods is about 5 μm, i.e., about one-half that of a red blood cell. The diameter of the rods increases as they course toward the periphery, because the area of the outer surface of the enamel is greater than that at the dentinoenamel juncture.

Each enamel rod is composed of submicroscopic crystals of inorganic substance embedded in a sparse framework of organic material. A thin peripheral region, the *rod sheath*, contains a higher proportion of organic material than does the bulk of the rod (Fig. 16.9). Between the rods is a small amount of a calcified organic substance, the *interprismatic* or *interrod substance*, which appears to act as a cementing substance.

Enamel rods are transversely striated,

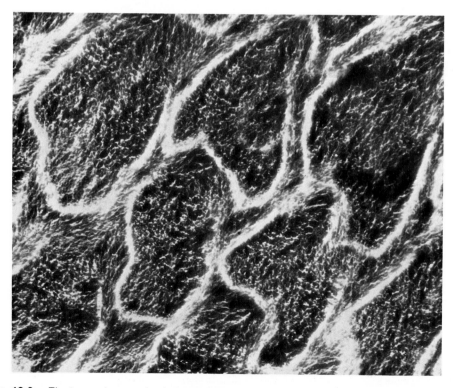

Figure 16.8. Electron micrograph of demineralized enamel. The field includes cross sections of several enamel rods. Note the submicroscopic fibrillar network of the organic matrix and the more dense peripheral rod sheaths. Human (×5000). (Courtesy of Dr. D. B. Scott.)

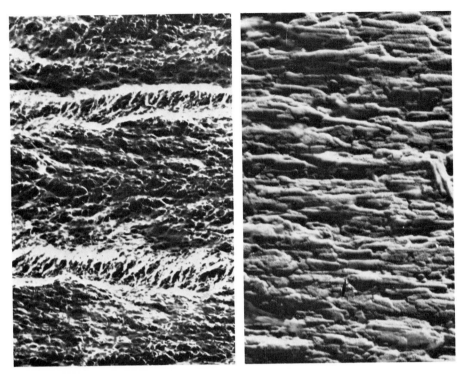

Figure 16.9. Electron micrographs of longitudinal sections of mature enamel. *Left*, demineralized enamel. The field shows the entire width of one enamel rod and parts of two adjacent rods. Note the submicroscopic fibrillar network of enamel rods and rod sheaths. Extending crosswise between the rods (prisms) are interprismatic fibrils (×10,000). *Right*, pseudoreplica of acid-etched, ground longitudinal section of mature enamel. The field shows the surface layers of crystallites and the crystalline pattern within a single enamel rod (×21,000). (Courtesy of Dr. D. B. Scott.)

the striations being evenly spaced at intervals of about 4 μm (Fig. 16.10). This is due to the rhythmic longitudinal growth of the rods during development. In addition to the closely spaced striations on the individual rods, there are more widely and somewhat more variably spaced continuous lines in the enamel, the *incremental lines of Retzius* (Fig. 16.7). In coronal sections through the crown, these appear as concentric circles. In longitudinal sections, they form arches over the apex of the dentin. In the deciduous teeth and in the first permanent molar, an especially prominent line, the *neonatal line*, marks the boundary between the enamel formed before and after birth. The incremental lines are due to variations in the rate of enamel deposition and are roughly analogous to the growth rings of a tree. The neonatal line is an accentuated

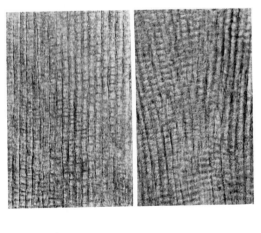

A   B

Figure 16.10. Photomicrographs of ground section through enamel of human bicuspid tooth. *A*, lateral area in which the prisms are regularly arranged. *B*, cuspal area in which the prisms entwine (×380).

incremental line resulting from a disturbance in the deposition of enamel at the time of birth.

The course of the enamel rods is usually wavy, or, especially on the occlusal surfaces, the rods may entwine, forming *gnarled enamel*. This is a functional adaptation which adds strength to the enamel by reducing the danger of cleavage between the rods.

An awareness of the direction and course of the enamel rods in different regions of a tooth is important in preparation of fillings from the standpoint of maintaining the strength of the surrounding wall.

A membrane, *Nasmyth's membrane* or *enamel cuticle*, covers the exposed surface of the crown for a short time after eruption.

Dentin

Dentin is hard, yellowish, and elastic. It forms the bulk of a tooth and also gives the main strength to it. Chemically, it contains more mineral than bone but less than enamel (69% of weight, as compared with 46 and 96%, respectively). Morphologically, it resembles bone in that it is composed of collagenous fibers in a calcified ground substance. It differs from bone in that it contains no cells but has only processes of cells (odontoblasts) whose bodies lie adjacent to the dentin in the pulp cavity.

Mesenchymally derived cells responsible for the deposition of dentin, the *odontoblasts*, are arranged in an epithelium-like layer on the inner surface of the forming dentin. Unlike osteoblasts, the odontoblasts do not become imprisoned but retreat progressively as the layers of dentin are deposited, each one leaving a single branching process embedded in the dentin matrix. These *odontoblastic processes* or *dentinal fibers* (of Tomes) become increasingly elongated as the odontoblasts recede with the formation of successive layers of dentin. The dentinal fibers thus occupy narrow, tubular channels within the dentin, the *dentinal tubules*. The dentinal fibers branch and anastomose somewhat, but in general they run parallel to one another in

a slightly wavy course through the dentin. This is well shown in ground sections of dentin in which the dentinal tubules are filled with air and thus appear dark in transmitted light (Fig. 16.11). The odontoblastic processes probably completely fill the dentinal tubules in the living tooth; the spaces which appear between the processes and the walls of the tubules in fixed sections are probably artifacts (Fig. 16.12). The rim of dentin matrix bordering on the tubule stains darker than the remainder of the dentin and is known as *Neumann's sheath*.

In each layer of dentin, the meshwork of collagenous fibers in the matrix runs perpendicular to the long axis of the tubules, i.e., parallel or tangential to the outer surface of the tooth. The mineral salts are in the form of crystals and have two types of arrangement: (*a*) the long axes of the crystals are parallel to the collagenous fibers, and (*b*) the crystals radiate out from a center in spherulitic arrangement. The ground substance of dentin is composed of glycosaminoglycans.

In certain regions of the tooth, there are areas which have less inorganic material than elsewhere, as a result of a failure of the individual areas of calcification to meet and fuse. The matrix in such regions shrinks in ground (dried) sections, and a space is formed which becomes filled with air and so appears dark in transmitted light. One such constantly occurring region is in the root of the tooth close to the dentinocementum juncture. It has a granular appearance and is known as the *granular layer of Tomes* (Figs. 16.7 and 16.11*A*). A second location, the *interglobular spaces* (Fig. 16.11*B*), occurs chiefly in the crown (Fig. 16.7) but may be present in the root also. It lies a short distance from the dentinoenamel (or dentinocementum) juncture. Each area is irregular in shape and much larger than the areas forming the granular layer of Tomes.

Parallel incremental growth lines (*contour lines of Owen, imbrication lines of von Ebner*) which are due to the deposition of

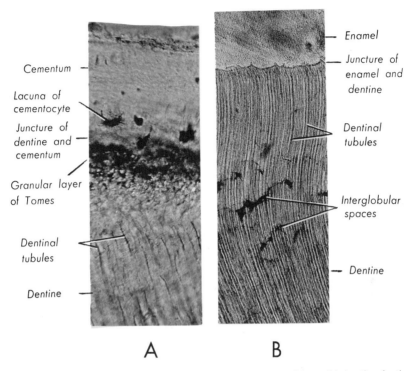

Cementum

Lacuna of cementocyte

Juncture of dentine and cementum

Granular layer of Tomes

Dentinal tubules

Dentine

Enamel

Juncture of enamel and dentine

Dentinal tubules

Interglobular spaces

Dentine

A   B

Figure 16.11. Photomicrographs of ground section of human bicuspid tooth; *A*, through root, showing dentin and adjoining cementum; *B*, through crown, showing dentin and adjoining enamel. The dark areas in the enamel are not due to pigment or discoloration but to refraction of the rods (×265).

dentin in successive lamella-like layers are present. In cross sections of a tooth, they appear like annual rings of a tree.

Dentin, unlike enamel, forms throughout life. The dentin that forms before the completion of root development is known as *primary dentin* in contrast with that which arises subsequently, the so-called *secondary dentin*. The former consists of relatively straight dentinal tubules, whereas the latter has tubules which follow a more wavy course. The distinction between the two types is somewhat arbitrary. The dentin that arises after severe stimuli, such as caries or erosion, is composed of elements that are very irregularly arranged; it is known as *reparative dentin*. The deposition of dentin induced by stress may be so extensive that it obliterates the pulp chamber and even part of the root canal. It is an important protective response.

Dentin is sensitive to a number of painful stimuli. Despite this well known fact, nerve fibers have not been demonstrated penetrating its matrix to any appreciable extent. The odontoblastic processes presumably convey impulses to the pulp, where many nerve endings are located.

Cementum

Cementum is similar to bone both in morphology and in composition. It is darker than enamel but lighter in color than dentin. It forms a thin sheath on the surface of the dentin of the anatomical root of the tooth (Fig. 16.7). It is usually somewhat thicker at the apex of the root, and sometimes it covers the inner surface of the dentin for a short distance at the apical foramen.

Cementum may either be free from cells, *acellular cementum*, or it may be *cellular,*

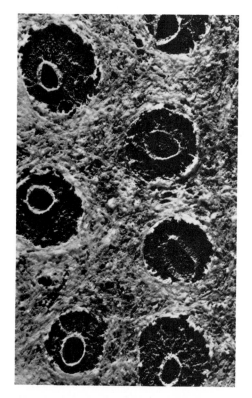

Figure 16.12. Electron micrograph of thin section of demineralized dentin, showing organic matrix and cross sections of dentinal tubules with their enclosed odontoblastic processes (dentinal fibers). The space between each process and the rim of organic matrix (Neumann's sheath) is probably largely artifact. Human (×5500). (Courtesy of D. B. Scott.)

containing cells similar to osteocytes (*cementocytes*) which lie in irregularly shaped lacunae in the matrix (Fig. 16.11*A*). Except at the apex of the root, the acellular type is usually adjacent to the dentin. The ground substance of cementum resembles that of bone. Collagenous fibers of the matrix extend into the surrounding connective tissue (periodontal membrane) and, as in bone, are known as *Sharpey's fibers*. Cementoblasts on the surface continue to form cementum throughout life. The added layers are irregular in thickness and may be either cellular or acellular. Hypertrophy of cementum frequently occurs in response to unusual stress or movement of a tooth.

Although the bond between dentin and cementum is a firm one, the mode of attachment is not clear. Cementum forms a protective covering over the dentin and serves to attach the tooth to the surrounding structures. Movement of teeth without injury to the tooth structures is possible in orthodontic procedures because cementum is more resistant to resorption than is the alveolar bone.

Periodontal Membrane

The *periodontal membrane* or *ligament* is composed of connective tissue which surrounds the root of the tooth. It attaches the root to: (*a*) the wall of its alveolus, (*b*) the gingival connective tissue, and (*c*) the more superficial parts of the roots of adjacent teeth. Fibers extending into the cementum of the tooth interweave with those extending into the alveolar bone, thus binding the tooth to the bone. The fibers do not course in the same direction at different levels (Fig. 16.7) but are arranged in a way that makes them most effective in maintaining the tooth in position and in serving as a suspensory ligament. The fibers are collagenous, but, because of their waviness, some temporary movement of a tooth is possible without morphological alterations in its root and socket.

In the periodontal membrane are fibroblasts, osteoblasts, and cementoblasts. There are also groups of cells which are remnants of Hertwig's epithelial root sheath, a derivative of the enamel organ. Blood vessels and nerve fibers, particularly proprioceptive endings, are present.

The density and strength of a periodontal ligament varies with the stress to which a tooth has been subjected. Thus, if there is no opposing tooth, the fibers of the membrane become more delicate, a change which is accompanied by a rarefaction of the bone of the alveolus. When this is allowed to occur, restorative measures become more difficult.

Pulp Cavity and Dental Pulp

The shape of the *pulp cavity* is quite similar (in minature) to that of the tooth in which it occurs. It consists of an expanded *pulp chamber*, which lies in the crown portion and adjacent part of the root, and a narrow *pulp canal* or *root canal* in each root (Fig. 16.7). The pulp cavity is much larger in teeth of young than of old individuals, for there is a continuous deposition of dentin throughout life. A root canal communicates with the periodontal tissues through one or more foramina at or near the apex, the *apical foramina.*

The *dental pulp* is essential to the nourishment and vitality of the tooth. It consists of fine connective tissue, which fills the pulp cavity. In addition to fibroblasts and macrophages, it contains the specialized connective tissue cells, odontoblasts, which are responsible for dentin formation.

The pulp is richly vascular. An arteriole entering at the apical foramen forms a profuse capillary network close to the odontoblast layer, the blood being returned by one or more venules.

The dental pulp contains both myelinated and unmyelinated nerve fibers. The sensory fibers terminate as free nerve endings among the odontoblasts. They are pain receptors (eliciting a sensation of pain regardless of the type of stimulus).

Attachment of Gingiva to Teeth

The gums are attached to the teeth in two ways. One, the attachment of the subepithelial connective tissue to the cementum, has been described under "Periodontal Membrane." The other is a direct attachment of the gingival epithelium to the tooth, the *epithelial attachment* (Figs. 16.7 and 16.19). At the gum line the epithelium turns inward and follows along the surface of the tooth, to which it is attached. Although the structural features of this attachment are not clear, it is certain that there is a definite adhesion of the epithelium to the tooth. In contrast with the epithelium of the exposed part of the gums, the epithelium of this zone of attachment is not indented by connective tissue papillae.

With advancing age, an increasing proportion of a tooth becomes exposed; i.e., the clinical crown increases in size. This is due to a continued but slow rate of eruption and also to a normal recession of the gums. As more of the crown becomes exposed, the epithelial attachment gradually grows apically for a short distance over the surface of the anatomical root. Thus, in young individuals, the epithelial attachment is on the enamel only; with increased exposure of the crown. it is partly on the cementum; late in life, it may attach to the cementum only. Mild mechanical stimulation, such as massage and brushing, strengthens the epithelium at its attachment by increasing keratinization of its surface layers.

Development of the Teeth

In man there are normally two sets of natural teeth, the *primary dentition* or *deciduous teeth* and the *secondary dentition* or *permanent teeth.* Each tooth develops from a *tooth germ* which is derived from ectoderm and mesoderm. One part of this complex, the *enamel organ*, derived from the ectodermal oral epithelium, forms the enamel. The *dental papilla*, a condensation of mesenchyme which becomes partially enclosed by the enamel organ, gives rise to the dentin and pulp. The sac of connective tissue that surrounds the enamel organ and papilla, the *dental follicle*, produces the cementum and periodontal membrane.

The first indication of tooth development in man occurs during the sixth or seventh week of intrauterine life, at which time the embryo measures slightly over 1 cm in length. Tooth development appears to be initiated by an inductive influence of the mesenchyme on the overlying epithelium. This mesenchyme is of neural crest origin. The epithelium folds into the underlying mesenchyme as the *dental lamina* along the future dental arch of each jaw. Slightly external to this lamina, but in close association with it, a second epithelial ingrowth occurs, the *labiogingival lamina*, in which a groove (Fig. 16.13) and then a deep separation will form (Fig. 16.14). This will divide the dental arch from the lips and cheeks. The dental lamina is of nearly uni-

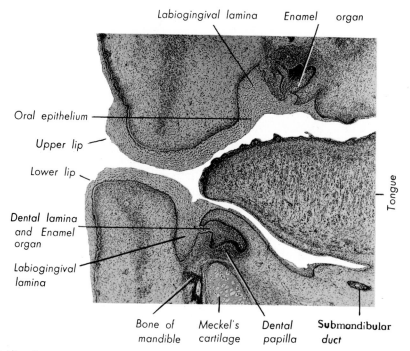

Figure 16.13. Sagittal section through developing upper and lower medial deciduous incisor teeth of a 50-mm human embryo. Age about 10 weeks (×34).

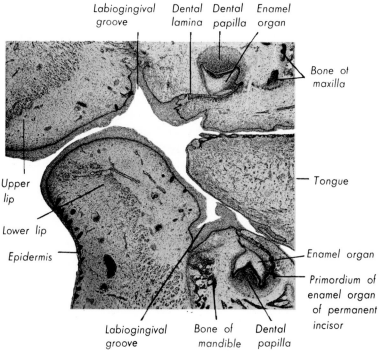

Figure 16.14. Sagittal section through developing upper and lower medial deciduous incisor teeth of an 86-mm human embryo. Age about 3 months (×34).

form thickness at first, but proliferations soon form at intervals on its outer side close to the oral epithelium. These proliferations are the primordia of the *enamel organs* of the deciduous teeth. They develop into cap-shaped and then into bell-shaped structures (Figs. 16.13 and 16.14). Within and beneath the concavity of an enamel organ, a proliferation and condensation of the mesenchyme take place, forming the *dental papilla*, the primordium of the pulp. Its peripheral cells, i.e., those adjacent to the enamel organ, will become odontoblasts. The mesenchymal differentiation is dependent on the presence of the epithelial component. Experiments with lower organisms have shown that epithelium transplanted from other areas of the embryo are induced to form enamel organs by the jaw mesenchyme. In reciprocal experiments, however, it was found that only the jaw mesenchyme differentiates into dental papillae, and it is this mesenchyme that specifies the type of tooth (molar, incisor, etc.) that will develop.

Somewhat later in development, there appear the primordia of the enamel organs of those permanent teeth that will correspond in position to the milk teeth. Each primordium arises as an inner or lingual growth from the dental lamina at a point coexistent with the enamel organ of a milk tooth. Later, as the dental arch lengthens, the dental lamina also grows dorsally, and from this dorsal extension arise the primordia of the enamel organs of the molars. The primordium of the last molar (wisdom tooth) does not form until the fourth or fifth year. The developmental pattern of the permanent teeth is the same as that of the deciduous teeth.

During the development of an enamel organ, the dental lamina, which connected the enamel organ with the oral epithelium, disintegrates. The developing tooth thus becomes entirely separated from the oral epithelium and does not again come into relationship with it until eruption.

The mesenchyme surrounding the enamel organ and dental papilla plays a role in tooth development. It thickens and forms a capsule-like structure named the *dental sac* or *dental follicle*. From the relationship in the developing tooth, it is evident that the segment of the dental sac adjacent to the papilla has the position of the future periodontal membrane. From it arise the cells associated with the deposition of cementum. Its peripheral part serves as the periosteum of the wall of the future alveolus.

All of the teeth do not show the same degree of development at any one time. The most anterior ones are usually the most advanced in development. In any one tooth, the future occlusal area develops more rapidly than do the more apically situated regions. Thus, at the time of eruption, the crown is fully formed but the root is still in the process of development.

Formation of Dentin

Dentin is the first hard substance formed in a developing tooth. Preceding its actual deposition, several changes occur in the dental papilla. Reticular fibers form in the papilla, particularly in the peripheral zone adjacent to the enamel organ. The outer portions of these fibers fuse with the delicate basal lamina which separates the papilla from the enamel organ, and the thickened membrane thus formed is known as the *membrane preformativa*. The mesenchymal cells closest to the membrane enlarge and form a continuous layer of columnar cells, *odontoblasts*. The reticular fibers which lie between the odontoblasts enlarge and change their direction so that they become largely parallel to the membrana preformativa. Around them is deposited a gel-like ground substance. The organic matrix of collagen and ground substance is referred to as *predentin*. The final stage in the formation of dentin is the deposition of lime salts in the organic matrix. The organization of the organic matrix controls the deposition of inorganic salts so that fully formed dentin appears to be deposited in

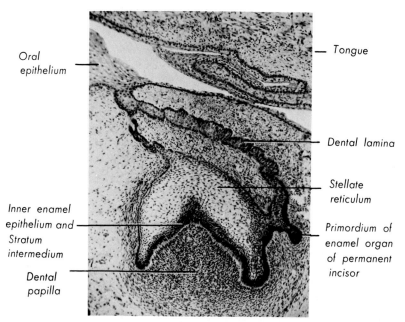

Oral epithelium

Tongue

Dental lamina

Stellate reticulum

Inner enamel epithelium and Stratum intermedium

Primordium of enamel organ of permanent incisor

Dental papilla

Figure 16.15. Higher magnification of the developing lower incisor tooth shown in Fig. 16.14 (86-mm human embryo) (×73).

lamellae. The incremental or growth lines are known as *contour lines of Owen* or *imbrication lines of von Ebner.*

The odontoblast is an extremely active cell metabolically. It synthesizes and secretes both the collagen and ground substance components of the organic matrix of dentin. The synthesis of these products is carried out in an orderly sequence involving well developed rough endoplasmic reticulum and Golgi material. The odontoblasts secrete collagen in the form of procollagen by means of small Golgi-derived granules which fuse with the cell surface in much the same manner by which zymogen granules are produced and released by pancreatic acinar cells (see Chapter 1). The apical ends of the odontoblasts prior to the deposition of dentin were in contact with the membrana preformativa. As dentin is deposited, the odontoblasts are not imprisoned but remain on the advancing surface of the dentin. Each, however, leaves a process, the *odontoblastic process* (fiber of Tomes), in the path of its retreat. As more and more dentin is deposited, these processes increase in length, for they extend

through the entire thickness of the dentin. The processes branch and contact each other. Communicating (gap) junctions have been seen at some of these contact points. The odontoblasts remain functionally active throughout the life of a tooth.

Enamel Organ and Deposition of Enamel

Developing as a continuous epithelial sac which has invaginated basally upon itself, the enamel organ* becomes structurally rather complex (Figs. 16.15 to 16.19). Four layers are usually described which, from its concavity outward, are as follows: (*a*) the *inner enamel epithelium,* a single layer of columnar cells, the future *ameloblasts.* A basal lamina separates these from the dental papilla; (*b*) the *stratum intermedium,*

---

* Some authors prefer to substitute the term *epithelial dental organ* for enamel organ, since this structure, although primarily concerned with enamel formation, does contribute to the form and development of the entire tooth, particularly in the formation of root dentin by means of Hertwig's epithelial root sheath. Similarly, there is some justification for the use of the terms *inner* and *outer dental epithelium* in place of inner and outer enamel epithelium.

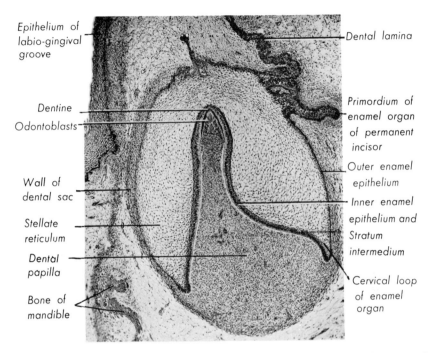

Epithelium of labio-gingival groove

Dentine

Odontoblasts

Wall of dental sac

Stellate reticulum

Dental papilla

Bone of mandible

Dental lamina

Primordium of enamel organ of permanent incisor

Outer enamel epithelium

Inner enamel epithelium and Stratum intermedium

Cervical loop of enamel organ

Figure 16.16.   Sagittal section of medial deciduous incisor tooth of an 111-mm human embryo. Age about 14½ weeks (×57).

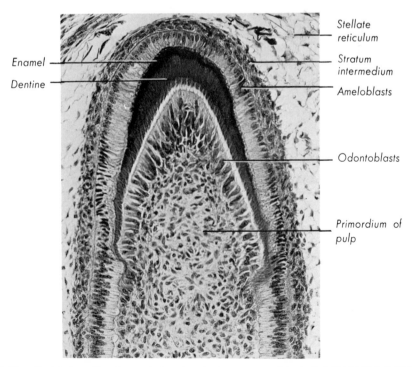

Enamel

Dentine

Stellate reticulum

Stratum intermedium

Ameloblasts

Odontoblasts

Primordium of pulp

Figure 16.17.   Sagittal section through the developing crown of a medial deciduous incisor tooth of a 170-mm human fetus. Age about 5 months (×180).

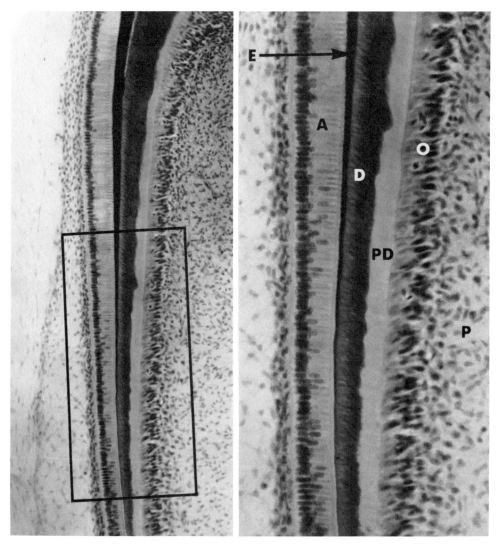

Figure 16.18. Parasagittal section through a developing molar tooth of a cat. The apex of the tooth is oriented upward. The boxed area in the figure at *left* is shown at higher magnification at *right*. A, ameloblasts; D, dentin; E, enamel; O, odontoblasts; PD, predentin; P, pulp primordium (left, ×137; right, ×275). (From a preparation by Dr. Sol Bernick.)

composed of two or more layers of squamous or cuboidal cells; (c) the *stellate reticulum* (*enamel pulp*) composed of loosely arranged branching cells; and (d) the outer enamel epithelium, a single layer of cuboidal cells, adjacent to which is a rich vascular plexus in the connective tissue. The basal lamina outside this layer is actually continuous with that of the inner enamel epithelium. Each of these layers retains many of its epithelial characteristics.

The margin of the bell-shaped enamel organ is called the *cervical loop* (Fig. 16.16). After completion of the crown, the inner and outer enamel epithelial layers of the cervical loop grow apically (i.e., toward the future root apex) to form *Hertwig's epithelial root sheath*. This structure determines the shape of the future root or roots and stimulates the differentiation of odontoblasts from the underlying mesoderm. The root sheath later disintegrates, leaving nests of cells in the periodontal membrane.

Deposition of enamel begins only after a

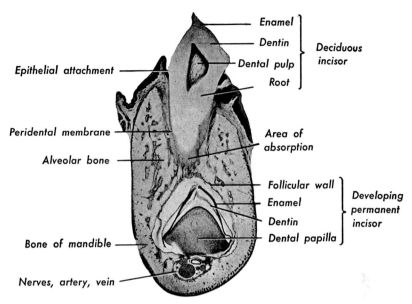

Figure 16.19. Section through the mandible of a kitten, showing deciduous tooth and developing permanent tooth germ (×18).

layer of dentin is formed. At this time, the cells of the inner enamel epithelium elongate and differentiate into *ameloblasts*. Enamel is elaborated in the form of rods or prisms cemented together by an interprismatic substance. A short segment at the dentinal end of each ameloblast becomes more granular. This part of the cell is then known as *Tomes' process*. This part of the cell is where the organic material produced by the ameloblast is released from the cell surface to form enamel rod matrix. The deposition of the organic matrix by ameloblasts appears to be more precisely controlled than is the deposition of predentin by odontoblasts. The process also differs significantly in that the ameloblast recedes synchronously with matrix deposition so nothing comparable to odontoblastic processes occurs in enamel. The organic matrix froms the framework of enamel prisms. As the enamel prisms increase in length, there is a progressive mineralization, an uncalcified segment always remaining next to the ameloblast. The interprismatic substance between the processes also becomes calcified. The amount of mineral deposited at this time, however, is only about one-fourth

that of mature enamel. Complete calcification takes place after the rods have reached full length. At that time, *maturation* of the enamel matrix takes place, water is withdrawn and there is a crystallization and further deposition of salts. Maturation always begins at the occlusal region and progresses toward the gingival attachment.

After completion of enamel formation, the ameloblasts deposit on its surface a thin (0.2 μm), homogeneous, protective covering, the *primary enamel cuticle*. The enamel organ then regresses but remains as a few layers of cuboidal cells, the *reduced enamel epithelium*. As the tooth erupts, it is covered by a thicker (up to 10 μm) keratinous layer, the *secondary enamel cuticle*, produced by the reduced enamel epithelium. These two cuticles together form a thin membrane, which covers the surface of the enamel until it is worn off by mastication or brushing. When the tooth erupts, the reduced enamel epithelium fuses with the oral epithelium at the gingival margin and forms the *epithelial attachment* or *attached epithelial cuff*. As the tooth continues to erupt and more of the crown becomes exposed, the epithelial attachment gradually separates from the exposed enamel. Concomitantly, the epithelial attachment grows apically on the tooth so that the extent of the attachment does not materially decrease.

Deposition of Cementum

The developing tooth is surrounded by a condensation of embryonal connective tissue which forms the *dental follicle* or *dental sac.* That portion of the follicle adjacent to the dental papilla occupies the position of the future periodontal membrane. It is separated, however, from the papilla by the apically directed extension of the enamel organ, Hertwig's epithelial root sheath. Following the first deposition of dentin in the root, the epithelial root sheath disintegrates. At this time, cells of the dental sac differentiate into *cementoblasts,* following which cementum is deposited on the surface of the root. Mesenchymal cells in the outermost zone of the dental sac differentiate into osteoblasts of the periosteum of the alveolus. Collagenous fibers also develop in the follicular tissue. Some are attached to the cementum, others to the alveolar bone or gingival connective tissue. Together they form the fibrous component of the *periodontal membrane* or *ligament.*

Salivary Glands

All of the major extrinsic glands of the digestive system are presented below under the heading "Extrinsic Digestive Glands."

The Pharynx

The *pharynx* extends from the level of the base of the skull to the level of the cricoid cartilage, where it becomes continuous with the esophagus. It is 5 to 6 inches in length. Its cavity is continuous with the cavities of the nose, mouth, and larynx. Superiorly and laterally, the auditory tubes open into it. The cavity of the pharynx is incompletely divided by the soft palate and uvula into upper (pars nasalis) and lower (pars oralis and pars laryngea) regions.

The *wall of the pharynx* consists of three coats: mucosa, muscularis and fibrosa or adventitia. There is no submucosa except in the superior lateral region and near the juncture with the esophagus.

The *epithelium* lining the pharynx is not the same throughout. That lining the nasopharynx is the ciliated pseudostratified columnar type, except near the juncture with the oropharynx where the soft palate and uvula come in contact with the posterior wall. There the epithelium changes to a stratified squamous type which continues through the lower region. The *lamina propria* of the pharynx is a tough, collagenous connective tissue layer, subjacent to which is a strongly developed layer of elastic fibers which course mainly in a longitudinal direction. Fibers from it penetrate between the underlying skeletal muscle bundles and thus bind the lamina propria to the muscularis.

The *muscle* of the pharynx, having originated from mesenchyme of the embryonic branchial arches, is skeletal and is quite irregularly arranged. The *fibrosa* is a tough, fibroelastic layer which, with varying degrees of firmness, attaches the pharynx to the surrounding structures.

In the *nasopharynx,* lymphatic tissue is abundant, being arranged both diffusely and as aggregations. These aggregations, the *pharyngeal tonsils,* frequently become enlarged and are then known as adenoids. Mixed glands which often penetrate deeply into the muscular layer are present. (See also Chapter 17, under "Nasopharynx.")

In the *oral* and in the *laryngeal pharynx,* scattered nodules of lymphatic tissue occur. The glands are a mucous type and are few in number.

Plan of the Esophagus, Stomach, and Intestines

Except for the mucosa, no layer is constantly present throughout the mouth and pharynx. Beginning with the esophagus, however, four layers are constantly present through the remainder of the alimentary tract (Fig. 16.20): *mucosa, submucosa, muscularis externa* and *fibrosa* or *serosa* (peritoneum). The chief structural modifications in the different segments of the tract occur in the mucosa, and these modifications are closely correlated with differences in function. An additional component, the

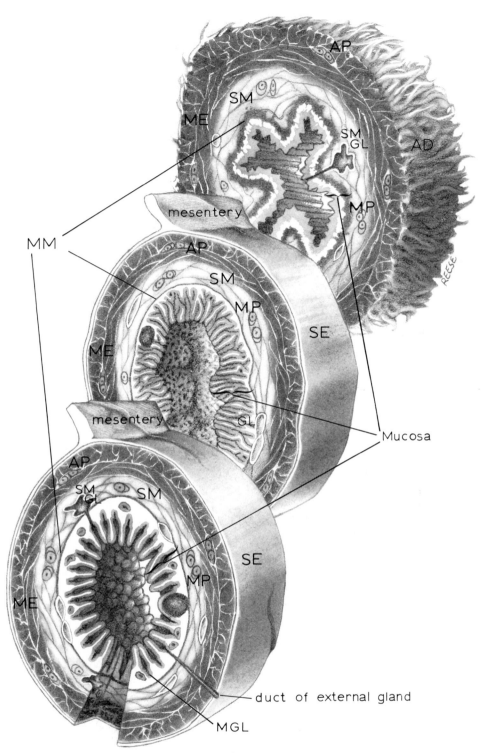

Figure 16.20. Diagram to illustrate the basic structural plan of three portions of the alimentary tract: esophagus (*top*), stomach (*middle*), and intestine (*bottom*). The wall consists of a mucosa separated from a submucosa (*SM*) by a muscularis mucosae (*MM*), a muscularis externa (*ME*), and either an adventitia (*AD*) or a serosa (*SE*). Glands (*GL*) occur in the mucosa, submucosa, or completely externally. Nerve plexuses occur in both the submucosa (*MP*) or between muscle layers of the muscularis external (*AP*). The muscle of the muscularis externa typically is arranged in inner circular and outer longitudinal layers; additional less distinctly oriented layers may also occur. The muscularis mucosae is usually disposed longitudinally in the esophagus and circularly along the remainder of the canal. Most of the canal is suspended from the dorsal body wall by a mesentery.

527

muscularis mucosae, appears for the first time at the beginning of the esophagus. This is composed of smooth muscle, most of the fibers running in a longitudinal direction. The submucosa differs somewhat in successive segments of the alimentary tract, chiefly as regards the presence or absence of glands. The muscularis externa (so named in contradistinction to the muscularis mucosae) is formed of two very regularly arranged layers, an *inner circular* and an *outer longitudinal*, except in the stomach. As in other saccular organs, the muscle of the stomach is irregularly arranged, especially in the upper, more expanded part. Three rather indistinct layers have been described, largely by exposing the muscle through dissection.

Two nerve plexuses from the autonomic nervous system are present, beginning with the esophagus. One of these, the *myenteric (Auerbach's) plexus*, is readily seen in most sections of the tract. It is located between the two layers of the muscularis externa. The other, the *submucous (Meissner's)* plexus, is in the submucosa. It is more difficult to find.

A knowledge of these general features will be helpful in the more detailed descriptions which follow.

The Esophagus

The *esophagus* begins at the level of the cricoid cartilage and extends to slightly below the diaphragm where it becomes continuous with the stomach, a distance of 10 to 12 inches.

There is no sharp structural demarcation between the esophagus and pharynx, although a greater regularity in the muscularis externa and also the beginning of the muscularis mucosae soon become evident. The esophagus is the most muscular segment of the alimentary tract. Except during the passage of food or water, the lumen is small and irregular in shape as a result of the contraction of the inner layer of the muscularis externa, with a consequent formation of longitudinal folds (Fig. 16.20).

Mucosa

The *mucous membrane* (Figs. 16.20 to 16.22) is lined with a stratified squamous epithelium and, as in the pharynx, it is not cornified in man. The lamina propria is formed of fine interlacing connective tissue fibers interspersed with fibroblasts, macrophages and, frequently, areas of infiltration with lymphocytes. The *muscularis mucosae* is formed of smooth muscle running in a longitudinal direction but with some inner circular fibers. It occupies a position corresponding to that of the elastic stratum of the pharynx, with which it is continuous. The muscularis mucosae is thicker in the esophagus than in any other segment of the digestive tube.

Submucosa

The *submucosa* is composed mainly of coarse, loosely interweaving collagenous fibers which permit the formation of extensive folds of the mucous membrane. It contains a plexus of the larger blood vessels, lymphatics and occasional autonomic (parasympathetic) ganglion cells and nerve fibers.

Muscularis

The *muscularis externa* of the first quarter or even less of the esophagus is composed of skeletal muscle and, from the juncture with the pharynx, it becomes progressively more regularly arranged into inner circular and outer longitudinal layers. This muscle is of branchiomeric origin† and its contraction is involuntary. Innervation is through cranial nerves IX and X via special visceral efferent fibers. The presence of typical motor end plates coupled with an involuntary control make these muscle fibers highly unusual. Some smooth muscle soon appears in each of the layers and gradually increases in amount. Skeletal

---

† This term refers to derivatives of mesenchymal cells of the embryonic branchial arches. Many of the cells which give rise to branchiomeric derivatives are now known to be of neural crest origin. Some recent evidence raises a question about the validity of the concept of branchiomeric musculature.

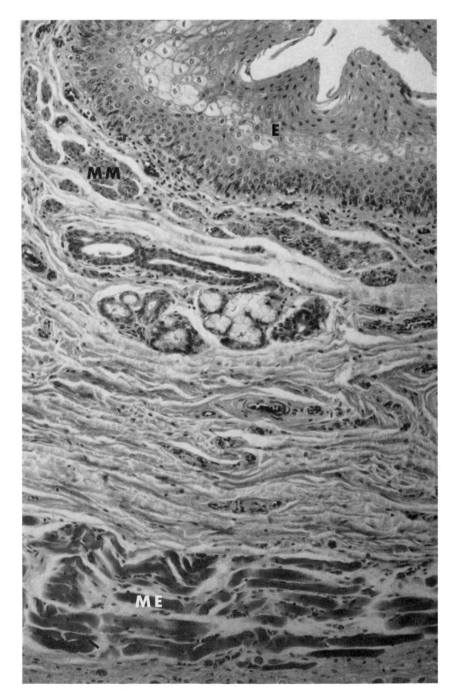

Figure 16.21. Transverse section through a part of the wall and lumen of the upper third of the esophagus. *E*, stratified squamous epithelium; *MM*, muscularis mucosae; *GL*, submucosal gland with duct; *ME*, skeletal muscle fibers of muscularis externa (×273).

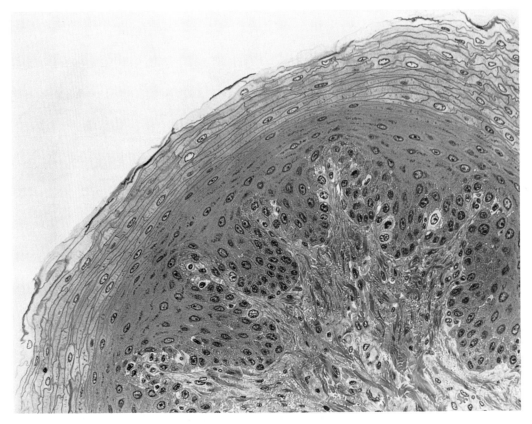

Figure 16.22. Section of the lining epithelium of the esophagus (×308).

fibers extend for a variable distance, but in the human they are rarely present below the juncture of the upper and lower halves of the organ and may be replaced entirely by smooth muscle at a higher level. Small groups of autonomic ganglion cells, part of Auerbach's plexus, are frequently found in the connective tissue between the inner and outer layers of muscle, especially in the lower half of the organ.

Fibrosa

The *fibrosa* is composed of loosely arranged connective tissue which binds the esophagus to surrounding structures. The short segment of esophagus that extends below the diaphragm lies in the peritoneal cavity and is covered by a *serosa*.

Glands of the Esophagus

Glands occur in the submucosa (*submucosal glands*) and in the mucosa (*mucosal* or *cardiac glands*). The number of *submucosal glands* is extremely variable in man. In some animals, e.g., the dog, they are numerous. The submucosal glands are composed of typical mucous alveoli such as those in the tongue (Fig. 16.21). Several alveoli may open by short ducts into a main duct which, in its course through the submucosa and muscularis mucosae, may be dilated, forming an ampulla. In the lamina propria, the walls of the duct change from a simple cuboidal to a stratified epithelium, the surface cells being either squamous or columnar.

The *mucosal glands* (*cardiac*) of the esophagus occur in its uppermost and lowermost regions and lie in the lamina propria. The upper group is frequently absent. The cardiac glands are structurally similar to the glands in the upper or cardiac region of the stomach (Fig. 16.23). They are

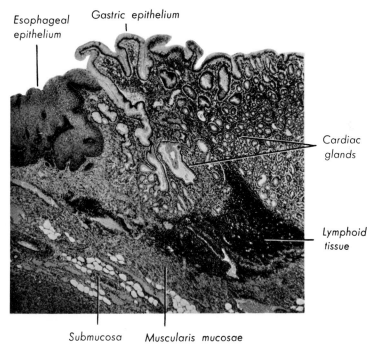

Figure 16.23. Longitudinal section through juncture of human esophagus and stomach (×26).

branched tubular glands which secrete a mucous substance.

The Stomach

The stomach extends from the esophagus to the duodenum. In the empty state, it is almost tubular in shape except for the upper part, which has a pear-shaped bulge superiorly and to the left. A frequently assumed shape when the organ is moderately distended is shown in Figure 16.24. As regards motor activity, the stomach is divisible into upper and lower halves. The upper half acts as a reservoir and has no—or only slight—peristaltic contractions. The lower half has peristaltic contractions which increase in intensity toward the pylorus. It is in this part that the various constituents of the food are thoroughly mixed with each other and with the secretions of the glands of the stomach. Associated with this motor activity is an increase in musculature, especially in the pyloric canal.

At the junction of the esophagus and stomach, the epithelium changes abruptly from stratified squamous to simple columnar. The transition is seen strikingly in fresh specimens where the smooth, whitish mucosa of the esophagus gives way to the

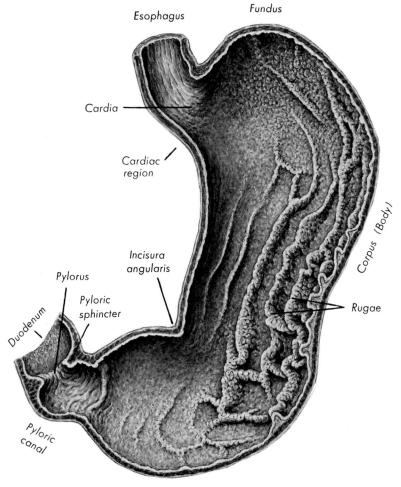

Figure 16.24. Drawing of a cast of human stomach. The organ has been moderately distended in situ with formalin (×⁴/₉). (Preparation and drawing made by Mr. Kellner.)

more irregular, pinkish mucosa of the stomach. The pink color of the stomach mucosa is due to the thinness of the epithelium and the proximity of the richly vascular lamina propria to the surface.

In the deeper structures, the line of demarcation is not as clear; the muscularis mucosae of the esophagus is continuous with that of the stomach, and glands of the stomach type extend up under the stratified epithelium of the esophagus.

Mucosa

The *mucous membrane* of the stomach has numerous ridges or *folds*, also known as *rugae* (Figs. 16.20 and 16.24), which vary in height and number with the degree of distention of the organ. When the stomach is fully distended, they almost disappear. The epithelial surface is also divided by grooves into small irregular areas, 1 to 5 mm in diameter, the *mamillated* or *gastric areas* (Fig. 16.20).

The entire surface of the mamillated or gastric areas is studded with minute depressions, the *gastric pits* or foveolae (Fig. 16.20). In the fundus, they are comparatively shallow, extending through about one-fifth the thickness of the mucosa; in the pyloric region, the pits are much deeper, extending through one-half or more of the thickness of the mucous membrane. The glands open into the bottoms of the gastric pits.

The Surface Epithelium

The epithelium that lines the inner surface of the stomach and gastric pits is made up of columnar cells which differ structurally and functionally from the cells of the gastric glands. The characteristics of the stomach lining cells also differentiate them from the lining cells of all other parts of the digestive tract. The apical end of every surface cell has a deep, cup-shaped zone filled with mucigen. Since the mucigen is not preserved and stained in ordinary histological preparations, the cells show a clear distal zone (Fig. 16.25). The nucleus is oval or spheroidal, depending on the shape of the cell and the amount of mucigen in the cytoplasm. These mucous lining cells differ from goblet cells in shape and in the chemical constitution of their mucigen. Electron micrographs show that the mucigen droplets of the stomach lining cells are smaller, more discrete and more electron-dense than are those of the goblet cells.

The epithelium lining the stomach, in contrast with that of the intestine, has no striated free border as seen with the light microscope. However, electron micrographs do show microvilli on the free surface of these cells. The absence of an obvious striated border aids in delimiting the epithelium of the stomach from that of the intestine at the stomach-duodenal junction.

As the epithelium extends deeper into the gastric pits, the cells become progressively shorter and have a narrower apical zone of mucigen. This gradual transition correlates with evidence that desquamated cells of the surface of the stomach are replaced by a migration of cells up the walls of the foveolae. Radioautographic studies using tritium-labeled thymidine, show that the surface cells arise by differentiation from cells which multiply in the isthmus or neck region of the glands. From the latter regions most cells move upward to replace the worn-out surface cells, whereas a few move downward to differentiate into the various cell types of the gastric glands (see below).

Lamina Propria

The lamina propria (Figs. 16.25 and 16.26), in which the glands are located, consists of delicate, interweaving connective tissue fibers plus connective tissue cells and occasional smooth muscle cells. In most regions the glands are so numerous that connective tissue fibers are reduced to thin strands. There is a diffuse infiltration of lymphocytes throughout the lamina propria; in addition, there are scattered lymphatic nodules, or "solitary follicles," which occur most frequently in the pyloric region (Fig. 16.31).

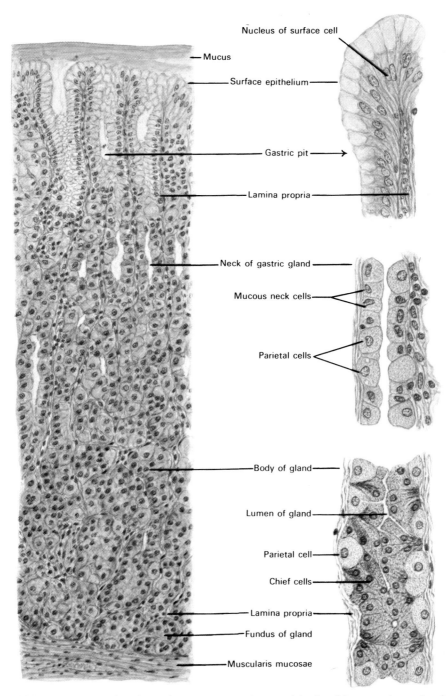

Nucleus of surface cell

Mucus

Surface epithelium

Gastric pit

Lamina propria

Neck of gastric gland

Mucous neck cells

Parietal cells

Body of gland

Lumen of gland

Parietal cell

Chief cells

Lamina propria

Fundus of gland

Muscularis mucosae

Figure 16.25. Vertical section through mucous membrane of body of human stomach, showing surface epithelium, gastric pits and gastric glands. Hematoxylin-eosin stain (*left*, ×250; figures at *right*, ×500).

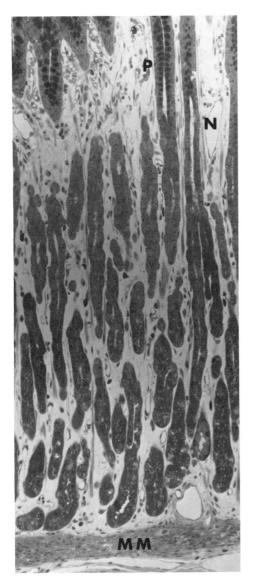

Figure 16.26. One-micrometer section of gastric glands from the monkey stomach. The lumen of the stomach is just out of view at the top and the muscularis mucosae is seen at the bottom (*MM*). A gastric pit lined with mucous surface cells is seen at *P*, and the neck of a branched tubular gland is seen at *N* (×110).

Muscularis Mucosae

The muscularis mucosae consists of a thin layer of smooth muscle in which the fibers usually course in both the circular and longitudinal directions. Strands of smooth muscle extend into the lamina propria between the glands.

Glands of the Stomach

The glands extend from the bottoms of the gastric pits, and their epithelium is continuous with that of the pits (Fig. 16.25). There are three types of glands: (*a*) *gastric, fundic* or *oxyntic, glands*,‡ distributed through the greater part of the gastric mucosa; (*b*) *pyloric glands*, confined to the region immediately above the pylorus; and (*c*) *cardiac glands*, found in the cardiac region of the stomach near its junction with the esophagus.

The gastric glands produce the essential digestive elements of the gastric juice, and the pyloric and cardiac glands function largely as mucous glands.

The Gastric Glands

The gastric glands (Fig. 16.25) are simple, sometimes branched, tubular glands; three to seven open into each gastric pit. They extend downward through the entire thickness of the lamina propria to the muscularis mucosae.

Each gland consists of (*a*) a *mouth* opening into the pit, (*b*) a constricted portion, (*c*) the *body* or main portion of the tubule, and (*d*) a slightly dilated and bent blind extremity, the *base* (Fig. 16.26).

In the glands proper, one can distinguish three types of cells in most preparations. These are (*a*) *chief cells*, (*b*) *parietal cells*, and (*c*) *mucous neck cells* (Fig. 16.25). A fourth type, the *enteroendocrine cell*§ is

‡ The terminology is not entirely satisfactory. For example, the term *gastric glands* might be thought to indicate that these glands occur throughout the stomach, whereas they are absent from a narrow zone around the cardia and from the lower part of the pyloric region. A synonym, *fundic glands*, is even more misleading for it indicates that these glands are limited to the fundic region of the stomach, whereas they are much more widely distributed. Oxyntic refers to the presence of parietal cells and is reasonably satisfactory, but in some species parietal cells may occur in significant numbers in pyloric or cardiac regions.

§ Several names have been applied to these cells reflecting their stainability with silver or dichromate-containing solutions. It is clear from recent studies that there is a diverse population of cells involved rather than one or two types as implied by the names argentaffin and enterochromaffin. Present information indicates that there are at least 10 cell types and 12 hormones produced by these cells in the gut mucosa.

present but may be difficult to identify except in special preparations.

The *chief cells* (zymogenic cells), as the name indicates, are the most numerous cells of the gastric glands. They are large pyramidal-shaped cells (Figs. 16.25 through 16.27) whose bases lie against the basal lamina and whose apical borders face the lumen of the gland. The nucleus lies in the basal half of the cell. In the usual histological preparations, the apical region appears as a delicate cytoplasmic meshwork enclosing clear, vacuolated spaces, which represent the position of the unpreserved zymogen granules. With proper fixatives and stains, these zymogen granules can be preserved and stained in situ.

In the base of the cell, below and lateral

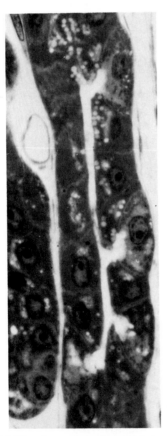

Figure 16.27. A portion of one of the gastric glands shown in Figure 16.26 showing the continuity of intracellular canaliculi of parietal cells with the gland lumen (×750).

to the nucleus, there is an accumulation of basophilic substance that consists of rough endoplasmic reticulum and unattached ribosomes. The high concentration of rough endoplasmic reticulum in the gastric chief cell is correlated with the function of the cell in synthesizing the proteins of the zymogen granules, in this case, predominantly *pepsinogen.*

Mitochondria tend to be concentrated in the basal region of the cell also, and they are largest and most numerous when the cell is active in replenishing its secretory granules. The Golgi complex occupies a position between the nucleus and the apical border of the cell as is typical for secretory cells.

The stages in the formation of secretions by exocrine glands have been described in detail in chapter 1. The same processes occur in the chief cells. The pepsinogen becomes activated after release and is converted into *pepsin.*

In addition to forming pepsinogen, in some animals the chief cells appear to be responsible for forming *intrinsic factor* which enhances the absorption of vitamin B_{12} by the lower portion of the small intestine. Recent studies show conclusively that in the human it is not the chief cell, but the parietal cell that elaborates intrinsic factor.

The *parietal cells* were the earliest described cells of the gastric glands and have retained their nondistinctive name. They are also referred to as the HCl cells because they secrete the hydrochloric acid of the gastric juice. The cells are oval or polygonal in shape and are often larger than the chief cells (Figs. 16.25 and 16.27). The nuclei are spherical and centrally located. Binucleate or multinucleate cells are occasionally seen. Unlike the chief cells, the parietal cells have frequently been reported to divide. The cytoplasm of the parietal cells is finely granular throughout. It stains intensely with acid aniline dyes, with the result that, in stained specimens, these cells contrast sharply with the chief cells. In fresh, unstained preparations, the cytoplasm appears clearer than that of the chief cells. In electron micrographs, it is seen that the cytoplasm contains an abundance of large mitochondria with numerous cristae (Fig. 16.28). These are apparently responsible for the acidophilia and granular appearance of the cytoplasm seen with the light microscope.

The parietal cells are numerous in the neck region of the gland, where they are interspersed among the neck mucous cells. Here their inner margins reach the glandular lumen. In the body and especially in the base of the gland, the parietal cells are pushed away from the lumen by the crowding chief cells, so that they come to lie peripherally against the basal lamina. However, they actually maintain a connection with the lumen of the gland (Figs. 16.27 and 16.28). Good cytological preparations and electron micrographs reveal bay-like surface involutions, termed *intracellular canaliculi*. The extensiveness of these canaliculi and the numbers of accompanying microvilli appear to vary directly with the functional state of the cell. Under conditions of active HCl secretion, both the can-

aliculi and microvilli of the parietal cell are maximally developed. When acid secretion is reduced, the number of microvilli is diminished and the canaliculi may lose their direct communication with the lumen of the gastric gland (thus becoming truly intracellular). The cytoplasm surrounding the canaliculi is replete with tubulovesicular profiles in the latter condition. During active secretion of HCl the tubulovesicular structures fuse with the plasmalemma, releasing their content and adding membrane to the cell surface. In the usual preparations of stomach mucosa, parietal cells having either of the above morphologies and others with various intermediate configurations are commonly seen. This indicates that not all parietal cells assume the same functional state simultaneously. The tubulovesicular profiles may also be involved with the sequestration and release of intrinsic factor.

The mechanism of acid secretion by parietal cells remains somewhat obscure. Since free acid is not found within the parietal cells, investigators have presumed

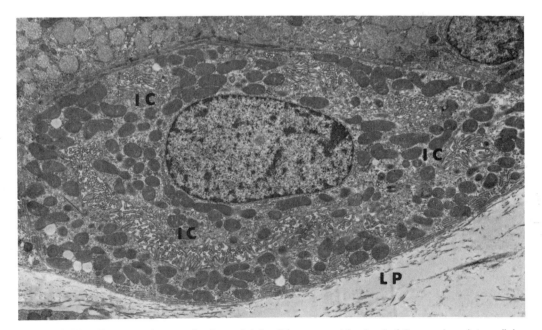

Figure 16.28. Electron micrograph of a parietal cell from a gastric gland of the monkey. Intracellular canaliculi (*IC*) and numerous mitochondria are obvious. Portions of chief cells are seen at the top of the micrograph and a part of the lamina propria is seen at the bottom (*LP*) (×5000).

that it must either be present in the form of bound acid or be formed in the vicinity of the cell membrane. In microdissection studies of living gastric mucosa, using a variety of indicator dyes, it has been found that, although the cytoplasm of the parietal cell gives a somewhat alkaline reaction, the intracellular canaliculi and the lumen of the gastric gland contain free acid. It appears, therefore, that the membrane of these cells is a highly selective structure which plays an important part in segregating and secreting both H^+ and Cl^- ions. Present evidence indicates that although the two ions are secreted simultaneously, they are transported independently.

The secretion of HCl into the lumen of the stomach is accompanied by an equivalent release of bicarbonate into the blood draining from the stomach. *Carbonic anhydrase*, an enzyme present in the parietal cell canalicular microvilli, apparently plays an important role by bringing about the formation of carbonic acid from water and carbon dioxide. Although the energy requirements for HCl secretion by parietal cells have been well delineated, not all of the membrane transport activities involved have been clarified.

Certain cells which differ from the pepsinogen cells are found mainly in the neck region of the gland, where they occur in groups interspersed among the parietal cells. The *mucous neck cells* are cuboidal or low columnar in shape, with a finely granular cytoplasm which, in routine preparations, is paler than that of the chief cells but not as pale as the mucous surface cells. With special fixation and staining, it may be seen that the cells contain many small mucigen granules. The nucleus is situated basally and is frequently oval, with its long axis perpendicular to the long axis of the cell. The upper surface of the nucleus is sometimes indented (Fig. 16.25).

The mucus of the neck cells differs in several respects from that of the surface cells. Histochemical staining reactions indicate that the mucigen in the neck cells is more acidic in nature than that in the sur-face mucous cells. The droplets of mucigen are distributed differently, being dispersed throughout the cytoplasm in the neck cells and confined to the apical region of the surface cell. The mucus produced by the two types differs in consistency, that of the neck cells being less viscous. The mucus secreted by the neck cells, however, is apparently similar to that formed by the cardiac and pyloric glands. It has been suggested that the secretion of the mucous neck cell has a role in protecting the gastric gland itself from attack by HCl and proteolytic enzymes released from the other cell types.

A small population of *undifferentiated cells* is described for the neck region of the gastric glands, interposed between mucous neck cells. The undifferentiated cells are believed by some investigators to give rise to both the surface mucous cells and the cells of the gastric glands. Other workers have shown intermediate stages in the formation of surface mucous cells from neck mucous cells so the undifferentiated cells may in fact give rise only to the cells of the gastric glands. The various cell types have different turnover times. Surface mucous cells appear to be replaced most rapidly and chief cells most slowly.

The *enteroendocrine cells* are not easily recognizable in routine histological preparations but frequently they can be identified by their basal location in the epithelium and by their clear cytoplasm. The classical methods of silver and chromate staining that first delineated these cells and gave rise to the names argentaffin, argyrophil and enterochromaffin have provided an additional source of confusion for the modern histologist. Cell types recognizable by electron microscopy and immunocytology must now be equated with those described by the nonspecific earlier techniques (Figs. 16.29 and 16.30). Evidence is mounting that as many as 10 to 12 different endocrine cell types may exist in the epithelium of the human gastrointestinal tract, and as many as 6 have been described in the stomach alone by some investigators.

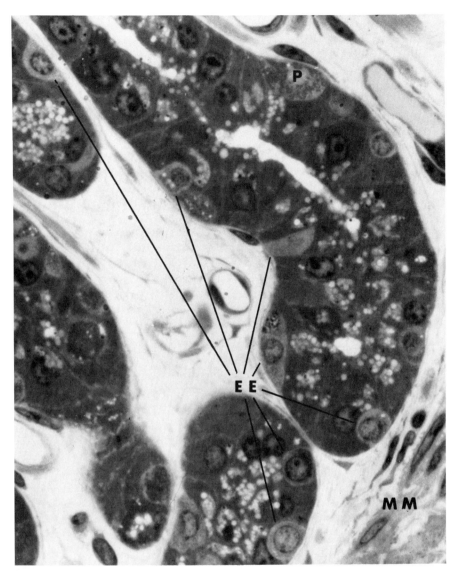

Figure 16.29. Deep portion of the gastric glands from monkey showing a number of enteroendocrine cells (*EE*). A portion of a parietal cell is at *P* and the cells with prominent secretory granules are chief cells. Smooth muscle of a muscularis mucosae is at the lower right (*MM*) (×900).

Endocrine products known to be elaborated in the stomach include: *serotonin, histamine, gastrin, enteroglucagon, somatostatin, endorphin, VIP, bombesin,* and *substance P.* It appears that some of these products may be produced by separate enteroendocrine cell types, but there is evidence that some individual cells elaborate several of these secretions simultaneously.

Electron microscopy shows that some of the enteroendocrine cells reach the glandular lumen but all except the gastrin cell contain granules concentrated basally and their secretions are released toward the blood vessels of the lamina propria rather than into the gut lumen. Some investigators believe that the gastrin cell releases its secretion into the lumen of the stomach and should be classified as a type of exocrine cell.

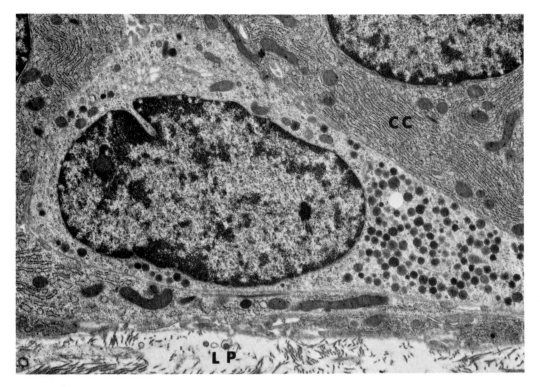

Figure 16.30. Electron micrograph of an enteroendocrine cell in the wall of the gastric gland of the monkey. This cell lies near the base of the epithelium wedged between chief cells (*CC*). The lamina propria (*LP*) with collagenous fibers is at the bottom (×8500).

There is considerable evidence that some of the enteroendocrine cells have intimate direct associations with each other and with other epithelial cells in the gastric epithelium. It is believed that some of the secretion products act primarily on cells in their immediate environment. This type of secretion is referred to as *paracrine* and it represents a specialized form of endocrine activity.

The Pyloric Glands

These are simple, branched, tubular glands, several of which open into each of the deep *pyloric pits*. These pits occupy a much greater proportion of the thickness of the mucous membrane than do the pits of the gastric glands (compare Figs. 16.25 and 16.31), and the proportionate depth occupied by the glands themselves is correspondingly less. The pyloric glands, although short, are quite tortuous, so that in section the tubules are seen cut mainly transversely or obliquely. Most of the pyloric gland cells resemble the mucous neck cells of the gastric glands in that their secretion protects against autodigestion. They differ morphologically from the neck cells in that they are taller and their ovoid nuclei are generally oriented parallel with the long axes of the cells. Parietal cells are found only occasionally in the pyloric glands.

The transition from the gastric to the pyloric type of stomach gland is not abrupt but is marked by a "transitional border zone" in which gastric and pyloric glands are intermingled and in which are also found single glands which combine the characteristics of both types.

Cardiac Glands

The transition zone between esophagus and stomach contains glands that resemble those in the lamina propria of the lower end of the esophagus (Fig. 16.23). Because of their location they have been designated *cardiac glands*. Those nearest the esophagus are lined with clear cells which resemble closely the cells of the pyloric glands and the mucous neck cells of the gastric

glands. As one passes farther from the gastroesophageal junction, parietal cells and then chief cells make their appearance and become more and more numerous. There is, thus, a gradual transition between cardiac glands and typical gastric glands. It should be noted that on occasion there may

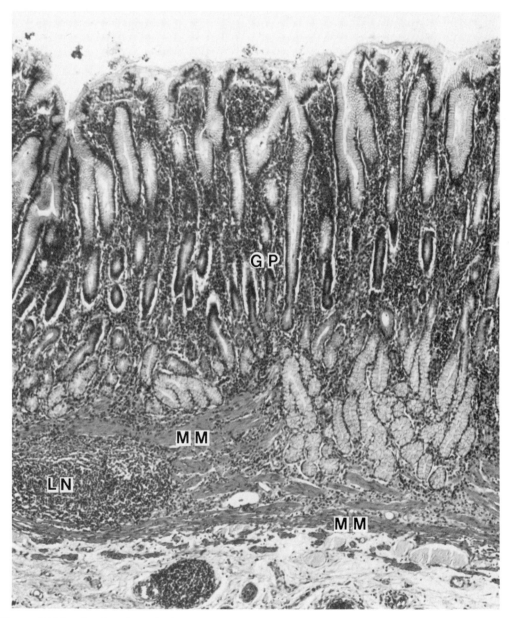

Figure 16.31. Section through the mucosa of the pyloric canal of human stomach. Note the long gastric pits (*GP*) and the irregular nature of the muscularis mucosae (*MM*). A lymphatic nodule (*LN*) appears at lower left. The lamina propria contains many free lymphocytes (×94).

be patches of gastric mucosa in the esophagus or patches of intestinal mucosa in the stomach of normal individuals.

Submucosa

The *submucosa* consists of coarse, loosely arranged connective tissue. It contains the larger blood vessels and nerves, including the plexus of Meissner.

Muscularis

The *muscular coat* of the stomach is usually described as consisting of three layers, an inner oblique, a middle circular and an outer longitudinal. In the fundus, however, the muscle bundles run in various directions, so that a separation of the muscular coat into layers having definite directions is difficult. The inner and middle layers of the pylorus are thickened to form the sphincter pylori. In the connective tissue which separates the longitudinal and circular muscles, there are groups of parasympathetic nerve cells and fibers which, while much less distinct, are homologous to Auerbach's plexus of the intestine.

Serosa

The *serous coat* consists of a layer of loosely arranged connective tissue which is covered by mesothelium.

Blood vessels, lymphatics and nerves are so similar throughout the stomach and intestines that they are described together at the close of the sections on the intestines.

The Small Intestine

The small intestine, which extends from the pylorus of the stomach to the colon, is commonly divided into three regions, an upper, the *duodenum*; a middle, the *jejunum*; and a lower, the *ileum*. The subdivisions of the small intestine are not demarcated by abrupt structural changes as is the case where the duodenum joins the stomach and where the ileum joins the colon. Changes occur gradually along the small intestine and the differences between different divisions are not as obvious as are the similarities. Therefore the divisions will be described together, pointing out the general characteristics first, and directing attention to certain distinctive features as they occur. However, it may be helpful to understand at the outset that some areas are readily differentiated in routine histological preparations. For example, the first part of the duodenum is easily identified by the presence of Brunner's glands in the submucosa, and the lower part of the ileum is characterized by aggregates of lymphatic tissue known as Peyer's patches. Structural changes along the remainder of the tract (lower duodenum, jejunum, and upper ileum) occur gradually and are more obscure.

If the small intestine is opened by a longitudinal incision through its wall, a series of definite folds will be seen on its inner surface. They are in general parallel to one another and pass in a circular or oblique manner partly around the lumen of the tube. These folds are known as *plicae circulares* (*circular folds*) or *valves of Kerckring*. They are absent in the upper region of the duodenum, tallest in the jejunum and much less prominent in the ileum as it nears the colon. These folds involve the entire mucosa, and a portion of the submucosa (Fig. 16.32). Unlike the folds of the stomach, the plicae cannot be completely flattened out by distention of the intestine.

The mucosa is further carried up into finger-like projections, the *villi*, which cover not only the surface of the plicae but the entire surface of the small intestine (Fig. 16.20 and 16.32). The villi differ in shape in the different parts of the small intestine, being leaf-shaped in the duodenum, rounded in the jejunum and club-shaped in the ileum. The plicae and the villi are characteristic of the small intestine. It is important to note that, while the pits of the stomach are *depressions in* the mucous membrane, the intestinal villi are *projections above* the general intestinal surface. By means of its folds and projections, the absorbing and secreting surface of the intestinal mucosa is enormously increased. Opening between the villi and extending

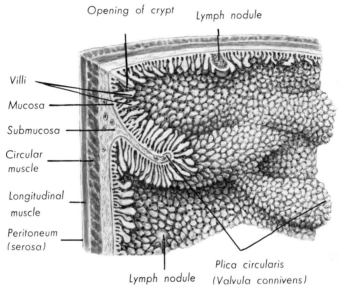

Figure 16.32. Reconstruction of a portion of the wall of small intestine (×17). (After Braus H: *Anatomie des Menschen*. Berlin, Julius Springer, 1924.)

into the mucosa as far as the muscularis mucosae are simple glandular pits, the *crypts (of Lieberkühn)* or *intestinal glands.* All of the above modifications are treated in detail in a discussion of the mucosa.

The wall of the intestine consists of the same four coats that constituted the wall of the stomach: *mucosa, submucosa, muscularis externa* and *serosa.*

Mucosa

The mucosa is composed of its lining *epithelium*, a *lamina propria* with its connective tissue and glands, and a limiting *muscularis mucosae* below. The most characteristic feature of the small intestinal mucosa is the *villus* (Figs. 16.32 to 16.35).

The villi are mucosal projections barely visible to the naked eye. Situated close together and covering the entire mucosal surface, they give the interior of the intestine a soft, velvety appearance grossly.

Each villus consists of a core of delicate, loose connective tissue and an epithelial covering. The connective tissue, the lamina propria, is infiltrated with lymphocytes to a variable extent and contains occasional isolated smooth muscle cells.

A single small lymphatic vessel (lacteal) with definite endothelial lining traverses the center of each villus, beginning at the tip in a slightly dilated, blind extremity. Since this *central lacteal* is usually collapsed in ordinary preparations, it is often difficult to see. It appears most frequently as two closely approximated rows of flat cells with bulging nuclei. During absorption of fat from the intestinal lumen, the lacteals become distended with fat droplets and are then clearly visible. The blood capillaries of the villus form a network which lies, for the most part, away from the lacteal, just beneath the basal lamina of the intestinal epithelium (Fig. 16.36).

Observations of the villi in the living condition have revealed that they continually change in length and undergo waving motions. This is possible because of the presence of smooth muscle in them. These movements bring the villi into contact with new material to be absorbed and aid in the circulation of the villus, particularly in the movement of fluid in the lymph vessels (lacteals).

Epithelium

The *epithelium* covering the villi is a single layer of columnar cells attached to a delicate basement membrane (i.e., basal lamina plus lamina reticularis). The epithelium consists mainly of two quite different kinds of cells, *columnar absorbing cells* and *goblet cells.* Enteroendocrine cells are also present in small numbers. The columnar absorbing cells are quite plastic and, although generally long and narrow, they vary in length and breadth as they adapt themselves to movements of the intestine. Their various shapes can best be studied in dissociated (macerated) epithelium. The cytoplasm is finely granular by light microscopy; its appearance changes somewhat in different phases of absorption. It frequently contains fat droplets. The nucleus is ovoid and is usually situated in the lower half of the cell (Figs. 16.36 and 16.37).

One of the most striking and distinguishing features of the columnar absorbing cells is their *striated free border* (brush border). With low magnification, this is seen as a nearly homogeneous, refractile layer (Figs. 1.11*C*, and 16.37) covering the apical surface of the cell but, with greater magnification, it appears finely striated. By means of phase contrast and electron microscopy, it is seen that the striated free border is actually composed of a great many very fine, closely packed *microvilli* (Figs. 16.38 and 16.39). The length of the microvilli varies in cells of different regions, being greatest (1 to 1.5 μm) on cells at the tips of the villi (Fig. 16.40). High resolution electron micrographs show that the outer leaflet of the plasmalemma over the microvilli has very slender branching filaments which form a coat of fuzzy appearance. This surface coat gives staining reactions of acid glycoproteins and ranges in thickness from

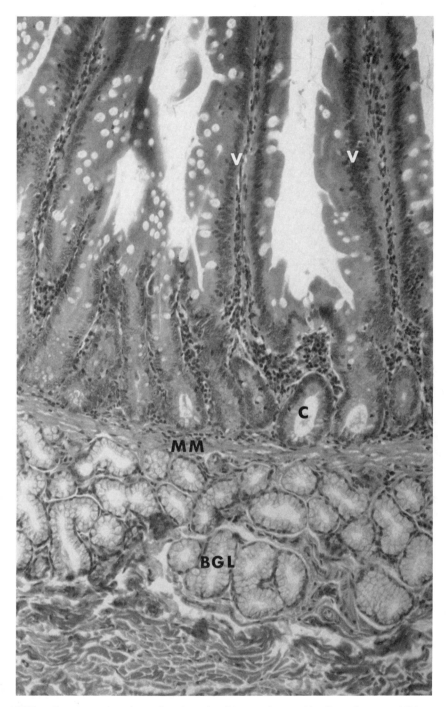

Figure 16.33. Cross section through upper duodenum of man. *V*, villus; *C*, crypt; *MM*, muscularis mucosae; *BGL*, submucosal glands (Brunner's) (×273).

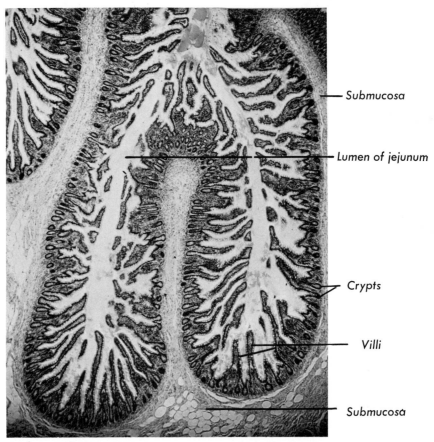

— Submucosa

— Lumen of jejunum

— Crypts

— Villi

— Submucosa

Figure 16.34. Longitudinal section of mucosa of jejunum. The section shows plica circularis in the *center* of the field, and on either side of it part of a taller plica. The entire luminal surface is covered with villi; submucosal connective tissue forms the core of each plica. Hematoxylin-eosin stain (×32).

Goblet cells   Striated border

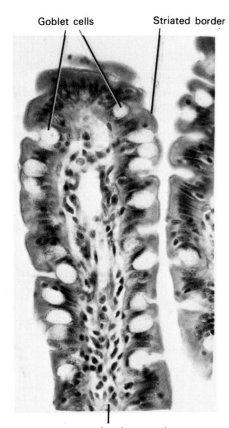

Lamina propria

Figure 16.35. Light micrograph of a longitudinal section of the upper portion of a villus of the jejunum of a cat. The double border appearance at the tip of the villus is caused by the relationship between the plane of the section and irregularities in the contour of the surface of the villus. The central lacteal is dilated somewhat because the animal was actively absorbing fat prior to the time of autopsy (×390).

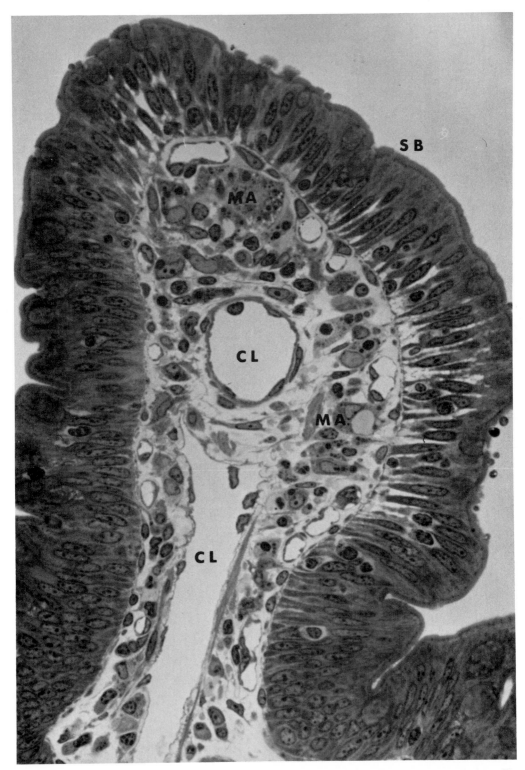

Figure 16.36. Light micrograph of a 1-μm section of an intestinal villus from the monkey. The epithelium shows numerous goblet cells and a prominent striated border (*SB*). The villar core shows profiles of the central lacteal (*CL*) and numerous cells, including macrophages (*MA*). Blood capillaries are distributed peripherally immediately beneath the basal lamina of the epithelium (×550).

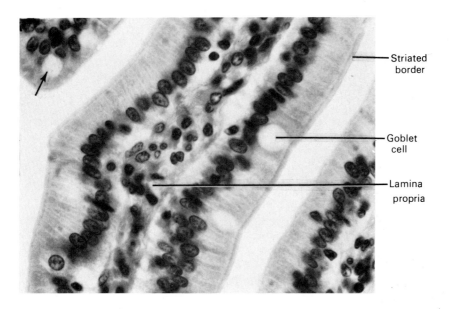

Striated
border

Goblet
cell

Lamina
propria

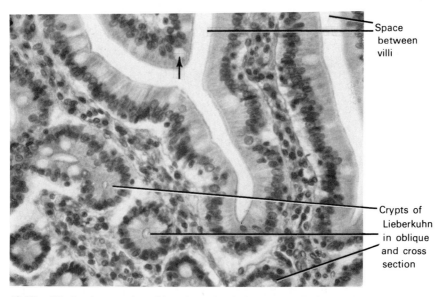

Space
between
villi

Crypts of
Lieberkuhn
in oblique
and cross
section

Figure 16.37. Photomicrographs of basal portions of villi and subjacent portions of crypts from a section of human jejunum. Some of the crypts are seen in transverse section. The *upper* figure is a higher magnification micrograph that includes the upper portion of the field shown in the *lower* figure. As an aid in orientation, an *arrow* is directed to the same goblet cell in each photograph (*upper*, ×650; *lower*, ×390).

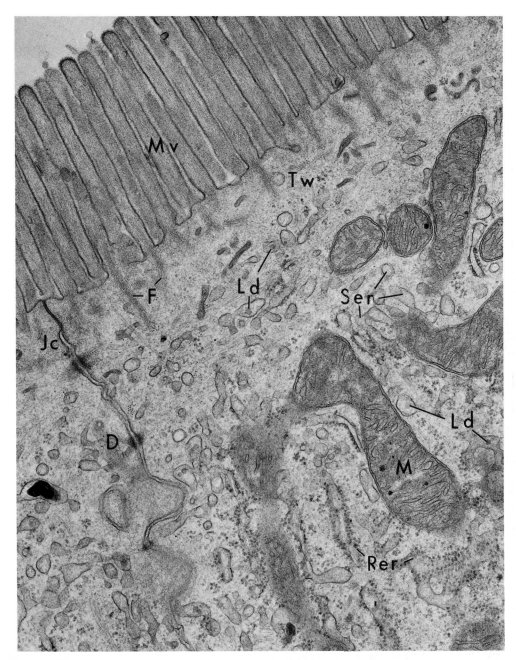

Figure 16.38. Electron micrograph of a portion of the apical region of a columnar absorptive cell from the jejunum of a rat. The area of the adluminal surface of the cell is increased by microvilli (*Mv*). Fine filaments in the core of each microvillus are continuous with filaments (*F*) in the subjacent cytoplasm, in a region known as the terminal web (*Tw*). Filaments of the terminal web also loop into portions of the junctional complex (*Jc*). The complex consists, from above downward, of a zonula occludens, a zonula adherens, and a macula adherens (desmosome) as described in chapter 4. Other desmosomes (*D*) are seen at irregular intervals along the course of apposing membranes of adjacent cells. Tubules of smooth endoplasmic reticulum (*Ser*) become continuous with rough endoplasmic reticulum (*Rer*). Some small lipid droplets (*Ld*) are seen within tubules of the *Ser*. This is explained by the fact that the animal was given fat by stomach tube 45 min before autopsy. *M*, mitochondrion. ×35,000. (Reprinted with permission from R. R. Cardell, Jr., S. Badenhausen, and K. R. Porter: *J Cell Biol* 34: 1967.)

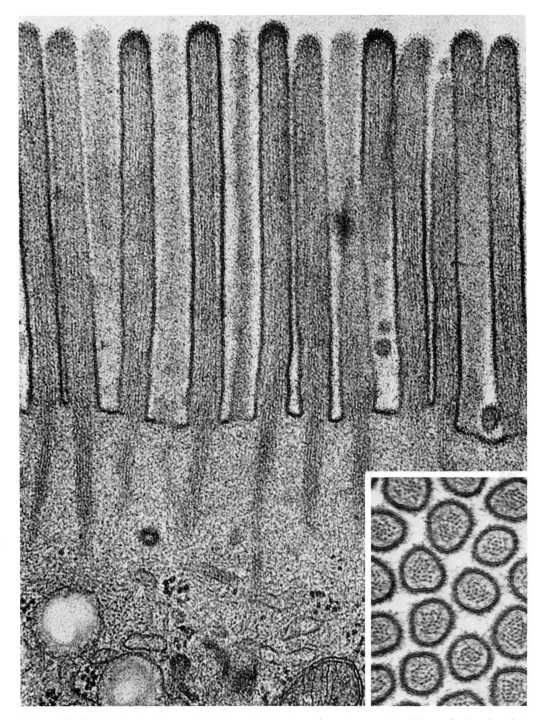

Figure 16.39. Electron micrograph of the apical region of a columnar absorbing cell, showing the microvilli and the terminal web region of the cytoplasm at higher magnification than in the preceding figure. Note the prominent core of filaments in each microvillus. The adluminal surface of the plasmalemma of each microvillus is covered with a fuzzy coat. The *inset* at lower right shows the microvilli in transverse section. Small intestine of a rat (×75,000). (Courtesy of Drs. Mary Bonneville and Keith Porter.)

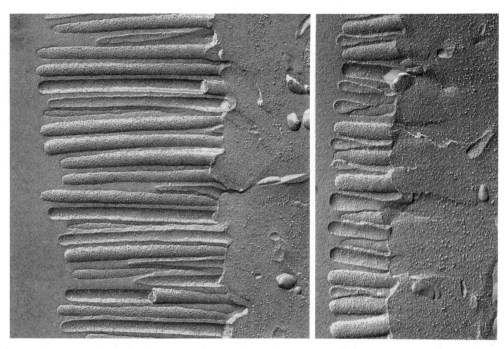

Figure 16.40. Freeze-fracture replicas of microvillous borders in rat ileum. At the *left* is a field of microvilli from the tip of the villus, and at the *right*, a similar field from the lumen of a crypt (×32,705).

0.1 to 0.5 μm. The central portion of each microvillus contains fine filaments oriented longitudinally and extending into a feltwork of filaments, the *terminal web*, in the cytoplasm just beneath the level of the microvilli. It has been presumed for some time that the filaments in the microvilli serve a structural function, but their size and reactivity with heavy meromyosin indicate that they contain actin and may also be contractile in nature (see discussion in Chapter 4). The terminal web zone is free of cell organelles and is rich in filaments which course chiefly in a direction perpendicular to the long axis of the cell. The filaments of the web connect laterally with electron-dense material in the subplasmalemmal region of the intermediate junctions and appear to be both structural and contractile.

The striated border region contains a number of enzymes, including alkaline phosphatase, maltase, adenosine triphosphatase and aminopeptidase. At least some of these enzymes appear to be integral components of the plasma membrane itself. Thus, the border not only provides an increase in the luminal surface of the cell for absorption but also contains enzymes of importance for the final stages of the digestive process.

The *mitochondria* (Fig. 1.11C) are distributed above and below the nucleus. In both regions they are rod-shaped or filamentous. Those in the basal portion of the cell are particularly numerous.

The *Golgi apparatus* lies between the nucleus and the free surface of the cell. Its possible significance in the absorption of foodstuffs is discussed below under "Cytological Changes During Absorption."

The *endoplasmic reticulum* is chiefly of the smooth variety in the apical part of the cell and mostly of the rough variety in the deeper portion. Free ribosomes are also fairly numerous in the basal part of the cell.

The *intercellular junctions* at the adluminal ends of the cells are typical junctional complexes as described in Chapter 4. Desmosomes are also found at deeper levels, but in contrast with most epithelia, gap junctions are rare between cells of the intestinal epithelium. It will be recalled that potential intercellular space is sealed around the adluminal ends of the cells by zonular occluding junctions and that the width of the intercellular space in most other regions is about 10 to 20 nm. In the deeper regions of the intestinal epithelium the intercellular space may reach a width of 200 nm or more. This is correlated with the important role these spaces play in the normal movement of absorbed substances across this epithelium (see below).

The occluding junctions normally vary in their degree of complexity from the crypt to the villar tip. This is presumed to be related to variations in degree of paracellular permeability in different regions of the epithelium. Support for this view comes from studies on junctional morphology in celiac sprue, a pathological condition in which the epithelium has an increased permeability to macromolecules. In this disease the villar occluding junctions are structurally abnormal and reduced in complexity. It should not be concluded, however, that the relative permeability is necessarily uniform through all paracellular pathways in the intestinal epithelium. In fact, recent evidence indicates that the occluding junctions associated with a subpopulation of villar goblet cells may serve as focal sites of high ionic permeability in comparison to the majority of such junctions between absorptive cells.

Goblet cells, unicellular mucous glands, are dispersed among the columnar absorptive cells. In the early stages of the secretory process, only a few mucigen droplets are present in the cytoplasm adjacent to the Golgi region. As more droplets form, the apical portion of the cell becomes distended to the typical goblet shape, and the nucleus, together with most of the remaining cytoplasm, is displaced into the narrow basal region or stem. These cells differ from the absortive cells in a number of respects, including shape and staining. The mucigen droplets are dissolved by routine methods of preparing sections for light microscopy;

thus, the upper portion of the goblet cell appears relatively empty. When the mucigen droplets are preserved by special methods, they are found to be basophilic, metachromatic, and periodic acid-Schiff-positive. Electron micrographs show that microvilli are short and sparse on goblet cells (Fig. 16.41). Because of the regular cellular turnover in the epithelium, it is likely that the goblet cells normally secrete continuously during their brief life span. More details on the goblet cells are given in Chapter 4.

The number of goblet cells is small in the duodenum and becomes progressively greater in the jejunum, ileum, and colon.

Crypts or *intestinal glands* occur throughout the small intestine. They are simple tubular glands located in the mucous membrane that open between the villi and extend through the lamina propria to the muscularis mucosae. The epithelium of the crypt is continuous at its opening with the surface epithelium of the villi. In general, the columnar cells which lie near the base of the gland are less differentiated and somewhat shorter than the columnar absorbing cells of the villi. The striated border of the cells deep in the glands is poorly developed with microvilli less than 0.5 μm in length (Fig 16.40). There is a gradual increase in the height of the microvilli of the striated border on the columnar cells from the base toward the mouth of the crypt (Fig 16.40). This fact, together with the presence of numerous mitoses in the crypts (Fig. 16.42), correlates well with the results obtained by thymidine labeling studies which show conclusively that the intestinal surface cells arise from cells in the crypts.

Recent studies have elucidated the interrelationships of the various cell types in the crypts and on the villi. *Primitive cells* (undifferentiated) located in the bases of the crypts are maintained as a propulation of stem cells. These have the capacity to differentiate and form all of the other cell types. Thymidine labeling indicates that intermediate stages in formation of all the

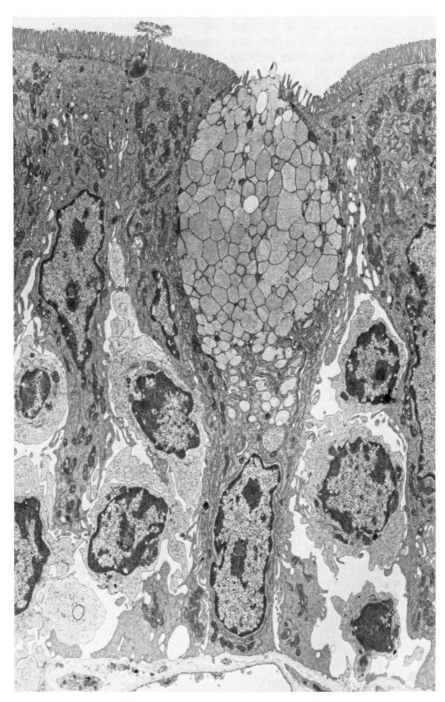

Figure 16.41. Mucous goblet cell in the mucosal epithelium of rat ileum. Migratory lymphocytes are present in the basolateral extracellular spaces (×4400). (Courtesy of Dr. David Chase.)

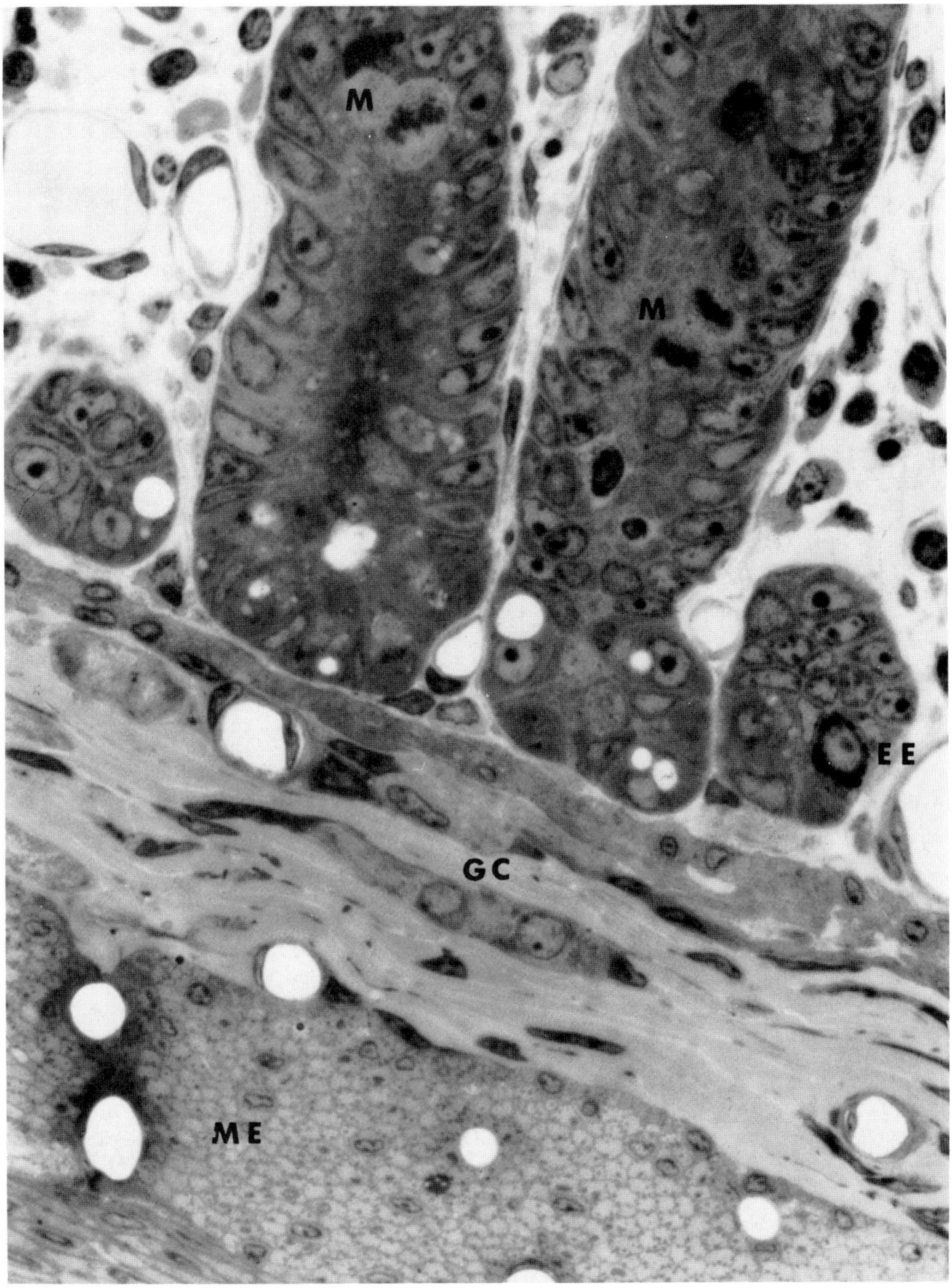

Figure 16.42. Light micrograph of a 1-μm section of intestinal crypts from the monkey. This is a longitudinal section and the smooth muscle of the internal layer of the muscularis externa appears in cross section (*ME*). Mitotic figures (*M*) and an enteroendocrine cell (*EE*) are apparent in this view. The collagen bundles of the submucosa appear nearly homogeneous in this preparation and two nuclei of ganglion cells from the submucosal plexus are seen at *GC*. Capillaries are expanded because the animal was fixed by vascular perfusion (×800).

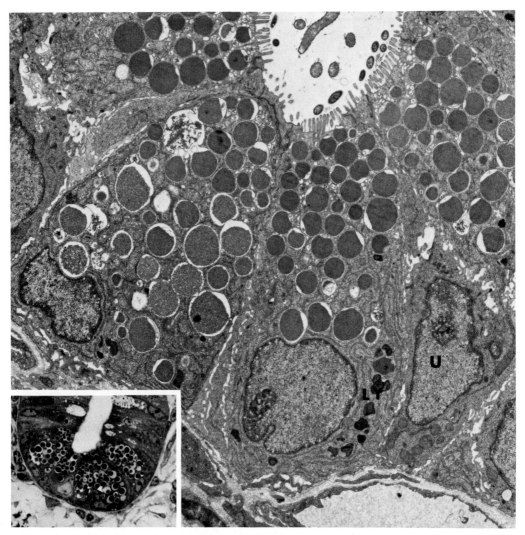

Figure 16.43. Electron micrograph of Paneth cells in the base of a crypt in mouse ileum. The *inset* shows a comparable area by light microscopy. The lumen of the crypt contains bacteria. *Ly*, lysosomes; *U*, undifferentiated crypt cell (×5100; *inset*, ×400). (Courtesy of Dr. David Chase.)

epithelial cell types lie in the midcrypt region. *Oligomucous cells* that give rise to *goblet cells*, and the early *absorptive cells* are still capable of mitosis, but their progeny are committed to their respective cell lines. On the other hand, there are also coarsely granular cells in the bases of the crypts, the *cells of Paneth*, that differentiate from the primitive cells but remain in bases of the crypts. It appears that Paneth cells do not divide, but they degenerate and are replaced at about the same rate as the other cell types. Paneth cells have prominent acido-philic granules and appear secretory in organization but their precise function is not understood. There is evidence that they contain bacteriocidal enzymes and are phagocytic at least in rats (Fig. 16.43). The earlier speculation that they elaborate important digestive enzymes has not been confirmed. Their failure to migrate out of the crypts with other differentiating cells has not been explained. Paneth cells occur mainly in the crypts of the small intestine but occasionally they may be present in the large intestine as well.

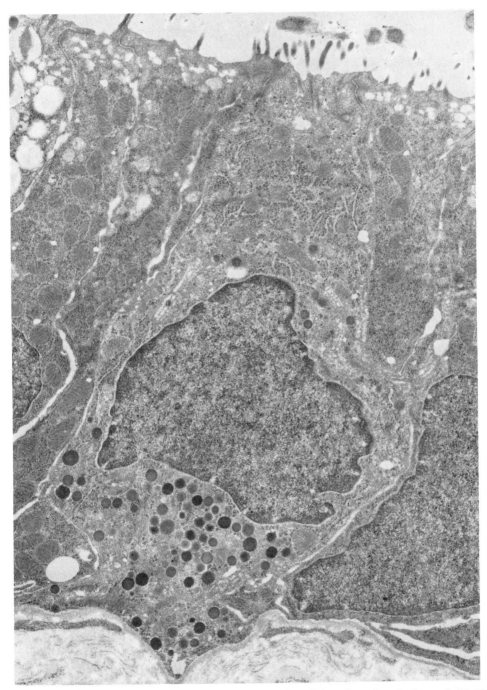

Figure 16.44. Enteroendocrine cell in an intestinal crypt of rat. This cell reaches the lumen (×12,600). (Courtesy of Dr. David Chase.)

Enteroendocrine cells also rise in the intestinal crypts (Figs 16.42 and 16.44). The suggestion by some investigators that these cells may be of neural crest origin has not been verified. In fact, thymidine labeling studies provide strong evidence that these cells also differentiate from the basal primitive cells. Nevertheless, because of the wide diversity of cell types and products, there is still a possibility that some of these cells have a neural crest origin. The enteroendocrine cells do not appear to be capable of division once they attain clearly recognizable morphology. They are most numerous in the proximal duodenum and the appendix, although they are present throughout the small intestine and colon. Again, the reader is reminded that several cell types are actually represented. These cells are thought to produce the intestinal hormones important in controlling gastric and intestinal motility, release of stomach contents, release of bile from the gall bladder, and release of pancreatic secretions. In addition, as in the gastric mucosa, one of these cell types produces serotonin and another is thought to secrete enteroglucagon. Again, there is evidence for paracrine secretory activity for some enteroendocrine cells and further evidence that some of the hormones have a broader physiological action than simply digestive regulation. A trophic action on the gastrointestinal epithelium has been demonstrated, and some of these cells have been implicated in causing the release of other hormones. Thus, their metabolic effects may turn out to be of major importance.

All of the intestinal epithelial cells turn over at about the same rate, the total life span in humans being four to six days. Thus, millions of cells are lost daily and minor disruptions in the normal proliferative events can have profound consequences on intestinal function. *It is clear that the major importance of the crypts in the small intestine is not that they represent conventional glands, but that they are responsible for continual renewal of the epithelial cell population.*

Cytological Changes During Absorption

The epithelium of the gastrointestinal tract has two main functions: (*a*) The *secretion* of substances necessary in digestion (dealt with in connection with the description of the various secretory cells), and (*b*) the *absorption* of the products of digestion.

With regard to the latter function, the epithelium of the intestines is involved in uptake of all three classes of food—carbohydrates, proteins and fats.

The absorption of fats has been studied extensively by biochemical methods and by electron microscopy. Breakdown of dietary fats in the intestine is effected by pancreatic lipase with the aid of bile salts. About one-fourth of the ingested fat is hydrolyzed completely to fatty acids and glycerol, and the remainder is hydrolyzed to monoglycerides and diglycerides. Most of the fat is absorbed in the form of fatty acids and monoglycerides and these are recombined to form triglycerides within the intestinal mucosa.

The cellular pathway and organelles involved in fat absorption can be followed by electron microscopy because unsaturated lipids are blackened by the osmium tetroxide commonly used in fixation. Within a relatively short time after fat is introduced directly into the digestive tube, small lipid droplets appear within apical smooth endoplasmic reticulum (SER) of absorptive cells, which is the site of reesterfication of fatty acids (Figs. 16.38 and 16.45). As the droplets accumulate, they form aggregates that include some protein and some carbohydrate (added by the RER and Golgi, respectively). These become visible by light microscopy and migrate to the lateral cell surface where the contents are released into extracellular space (Fig. 16.46). At this stage the free droplets are referred to as *chylomicrons.*

The chylomicrons pass through the basal lamina and into the intercellular connective tissue spaces and thence to lymphatic capillaries. Diagrammatic summaries of the sequence of events in fat absorption, as revealed by electron microscopic and histochemical studies, are shown in Figure 16.47.

The pathway from the epithelial cells to the vascular system proceeds primarily by the lymphatics. Neutral fats (triglycerides) pass from the connective tissue underlying the epithelial cells into lymphatic capillaries and eventually reach the blood vessels

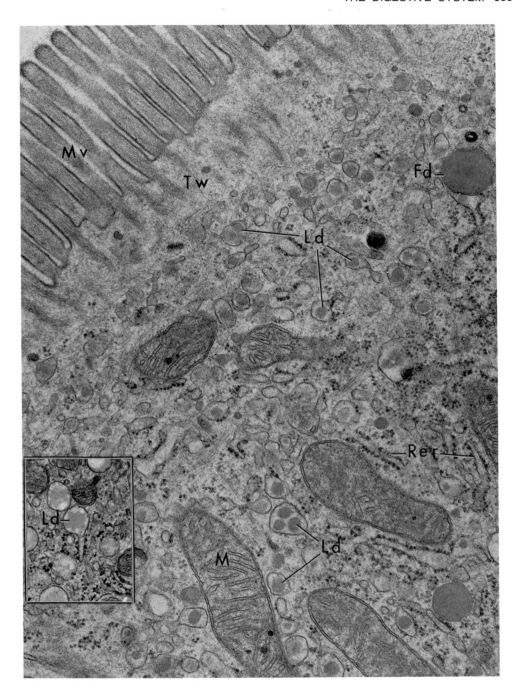

Figure 16.45. Electron micrograph of the apical portion of an intestinal absorptive cell fixed during active fat absorption. Numerous lipid droplets (*Ld*) are present within tubules of the smooth endoplasmic reticulum. The latter is hypertrophied and is often seen in continuity with the rough endoplasmic reticulum (*Rer*). Lipid droplets are often seen in bulbous expansions of the reticulum (*Ld* of *inset*). Free lipid droplets (*Fd*) within the cell can be distinguished from the droplets in stages of absorption by their diameter and by the absence of an enveloping membrane. *M*, mitochondrion; *Mv*, microvilli; *Tw*, terminal web area. From rat jejunum fixed 40 min after intubation of corn oil; *inset*, from rat jejunum fixed at 60 min after intubation of corn oil. ×31,500. (Reprinted with permission from R. R. Cardell, Jr., S. Badenhausen, and K. R. Porter; *J Cell Biol* 34: 1967.)

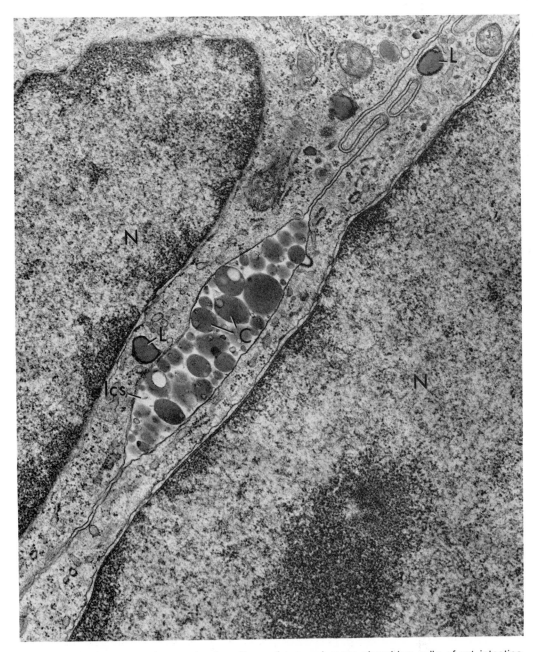

Figure 16.46. Electron micrograph of portions of two columnar absorbing cells of rat intestine subsequent to the intubation of corn oil. Intercellular spaces (*Ics*) are generally enlarged during fat absorption and they contain chylomicra (*C*) which are similar to the largest lipid droplets (*L*) in the cytoplasm. The chylomicra pass downward through the intercellular spaces and through the basal lamina of the epithelium to reach the subepithelial connective tissue where they enter lymphatic capillaries. *N*, nuclei (×23,225). (Reprinted with permission from R. R. Cardell, Jr., S. Badenhausen, and K. R. Porter: *J Cell Biol* 34: 1967.)

via the thoracic duct. Most of the absorbed fatty acids which are more than 10 carbon chains in length are resynthesized with glycerol to form triglycerides and enter the lymphatics. Fatty acids with short carbon chains (less than 10 or 12 carbons) pass directly into the blood capillaries of the intestine and thence to the portal vein. The bile salts which were combined with the fatty acids during the absorptive process become free and they are absorbed directly into the blood to return by the portal vein to the liver where they are excreted into the bile for a role in another cycle of fat absorption.

The uptake and transport of sugars and amino acids is less well documented morphologically. It is clear, however, that some of the final degradation to monosaccharides and amino acids takes place at the surface of the absorptive cell and that these lower molecular weight substances are transported and released so that they are taken up predominantly by blood capillaries rather than lymphatics. During their cotransport with Na^+, sodium is actively pumped at the basolateral side of the absorptive cells where it accumulates, drawing water osmotically from the lumen to expand the basolateral extracellular compartment.

Lamina Propria

The loose connective tissue, besides forming the centers of the villi, fills in the spaces between the crypts and between the latter and the muscularis mucosae. It is composed of interweaving reticular and delicate collagenous fibers, with a considerable number of elastic fibrils. It also contains fibroblasts, eosinophils, plasma cells, mast cells and some smooth muscle cells. Lymphocytes are abundant and in many places they are so numerous as to give the appearance of diffuse lymphatic tissue. Here and there the lymphatic cells are more closely packed together to form distinct lymph nodules. These are known as solitary nodules to distinguish them from groups of lymph nodules which occur in the lower sections of the small intestine and are

known as Peyer's patches (see below). Solitary nodules are more numerous in the small intestine than in the stomach but they are identical in structure.

The lamina propria of the intestine appears to be the prime site for production of secretory immunoglobulin (sIgA), a dimeric form of IgA. Plasma cells synthesize sIgA and release it into the connective tissue spaces. The adjacent epithelial cells recognize sIgA, take it up, and couple it to a glycoprotein (secretory component, or SC) produced by the epithelial cells. The entire complex is then secreted into the intestinal lumen. The SC is believed to serve as both the specific receptor molecule and the transporting molecule for sIgA and also confers resistance to proteolysis after secretion into the intestinal lumen. Secreted sIgA coats the luminal surface of the epithelial cells and apparently helps to control the penetration of antigens by preventing their attachment to the epithelial cells.

Secretory IgA produced by plasma cells in the intestinal lamina propria also circulates and is transported across other mucosal epithelia in the body by a mechanism similar to that in intestinal epithelium. The secretory component is produced by other epithelia as well, such as hepatocytes and salivary gland epithelium. Thus, sIgA elaborated in the intestinal lamina propria has importance for local immunological responses throughout the body.

Aggregated Lymph Nodules (Peyer's Patches)

These are aggregations of lymph nodules found mainly in the ileum, especially near its junction with the colon. They always occur on the side of the gut opposite the attachment of the mesentery. Each patch consists of from 10 to 70 nodules, which lie side by side and are so arranged that the entire patch has an oval shape, its long diameter lying lengthwise of the intestine. The dome-shaped apices of the nodules are directed toward the lumen and project almost through the mucosa. They are not covered by villi; a single layer of columnar epithelium alone separates them from the

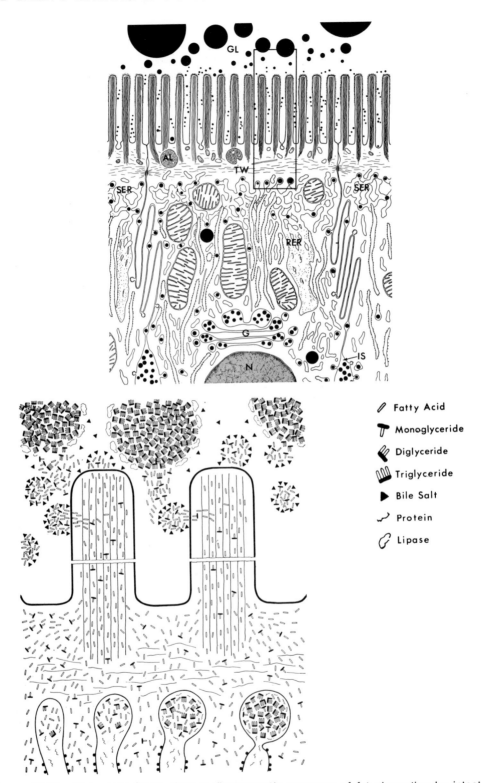

Figure 16.47. The *upper figure* gives a diagrammatic summary of fat absorption by intestinal epithelial cells as interpreted from results of electron microscopic and biochemical studies. Fat in the gut lumen (*GL*) is broken down to small lipid droplets seen above and between the microvilli. Fat diffuses through the cell membrane in the form of monoglycerides and fatty acids. These enter the

lumen of the gut, where their smooth surfaces can readily be seen in gross dissection (Figs. 16.48 and 16.49).

The epithelium covering the nodules contains typical absorptive cells but lacks goblet cells. Instead, there are specialized cells, termed *M cells* (*membranous cells*), that maintain an intimate relationship with intraepithelial lymphocytes. There is evidence that M cells incorporate luminal antigens and present them to the associated lymphocytes. The latter can be transported to mesenteric lymph nodes where they proliferate and differentiate before being distributed to other lymphoid tissues. Thus, the presence of these antigens within the body at a later time can elicit an immediate protective secondary immune response.

The bases of the nodules are not confined to the lamina propria but extend into the submucosa. The relation of the patch to the mucosa and submucosa can be best appreciated by following the course of the muscularis mucosae. This is seen to stop abruptly at the circumference of the patch, appearing throughout the patch as isolated groups of smooth muscle cells. Sometimes the individual nodules that make up a Peyer's patch are quite discrete and well defined. More frequently, however, the nodules tend to coalesce except at their apices, so that the individual nodules can be definitely outlined only at their apices and identified to some extent by their germinal centers. As in other nodules, there is a mantle of small B lymphocytes around each germinal center and a more peripheral T cell-dependent region. In addition, high endothelium venules may be present. Peyer's patches are most prominent in children. In

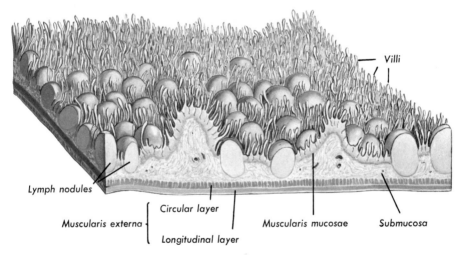

Figure 16.48. Low power, three-dimensional view of a segment of human ileum, showing part of an aggregate of lymph nodules (×15).

tubules of the smooth endoplasmic reticulum (*SER*) where they are resynthesized to form droplets of triglycerides. The membrane-bounded droplets are transported either directly or via the Golgi complex (*G*) to intercellular spaces (*IS*) at the level of the nucleus (*N*). *AI*, apical lysosomes; *RER*, rough endoplasmic reticulum; *TW*, terminal web. The enclosed area is enlarged in the *lower figure* to show the biochemical events in the initial phases of fat absorption. Triglycerides and diglycerides, in the presence of bile salts in the gut lumen, are hydrolyzed by pancreatic lipase to form micelles of monoglycerides and fatty acids. The monoglycerides and fatty acids diffuse from the micelles into and through the cell membrane to enter the cell cytoplasm where they encounter a network of smooth endoplasmic reticulum. Within the tubules of SER, they are resynthesized to triglycerides that form droplets, along with phospholipids and cholesterol, in a protein solution. By the synthesis and sequestration of triglycerides within the cell, an inward diffusion gradient of monoglycerides and fatty acids is maintained. (Reprinted with permission from R. R. Cardell, Jr., S. Badenhausen, and K. R. Porter: *J Cell Biol* 34: 1967.)

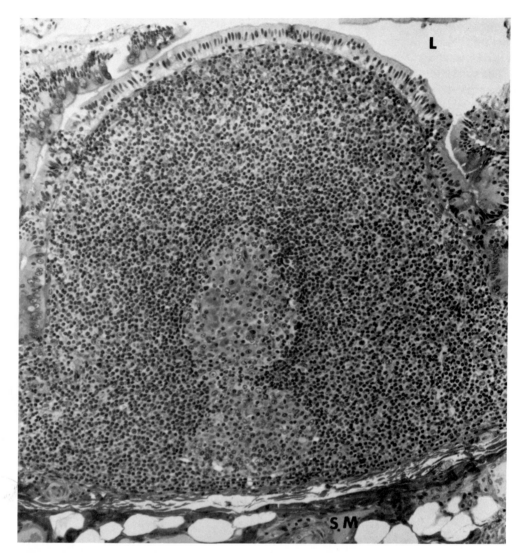

Figure 16.49. Lymph nodule of Peyer's patch in the lamina propria of the ileum. Note the simple columnar epithelium covering the luminal surface (*L*) and the prominent germinal center in the nodule. *SM*, submucosa (×160).

the adult and in old age, the lymphatic tissue gradually undergoes regression and involution. This correlates with a gradual decrease in efficiency of the immune response with aging.

Muscularis Mucosae

The muscularis mucosae is thin, consisting of an inner circular and an outer longitudinal layer of smooth muscle. Small groups of muscle fibers extend from the muscularis mucosae into the cores of the villi.

Submucosa

The *submucosa* (Fig. 16.48) consists, as in the stomach, of loosely arranged connective tissue, and it contains the larger blood vessels and lymphatics. Autonomic nerve fibers and parasympathetic ganglion cells are present in scattered groups. They form a plexus (*Meissner's*) that interconnects with the *myenteric* (*Auerbach's*) plexus of the muscularis externa. The submucosa is free from glands except in the duodenum, where it contains *duodenal glands* (*of Brunner*) (Fig. 16.33).

Duodenal glands are the most distinguishing characteristic of the *upper* duodenum and are absent in its inferior part. Duodenal glands are generally classified as branched and compound tubular glands, although the lumen of the terminal portion of the tubule is frequently enlarged to approach a tubuloalveolar form (Fig. 16.33). They are lined with a columnar epithelium similar to that of the pyloric glands. The ducts are also lined with simple columnar epithelium and pass up through the muscularis mucosae and lamina propria and empty usually into a crypt. Occasionally they empty on the surface between the villi. In the region of the juncture between the pylorus and duodenum, there is a zone in which the glands of the two segments merge imperceptibly. Glands of similar structure lie partly in the lamina propria and partly in the submucosa, with strands of the muscularis mucosae present among the alveoli. The juncture of the stomach and duodenum thus is not sharply demarcated by the position of the glands. Duodenal glands, like the pyloric glands, secrete an alkaline mucoid substance.

Muscularis

The *muscular coat* (Figs. 16.20 and 16.48) consists of two well defined layers of smooth muscle, an inner circular and an outer longitudinal. Connective tissue septa divide the muscle cells into groups or bundles, while between the two layers of muscle is a connective tissue septum which varies greatly in thickness at different places and contains the myenteric plexus of nerve fibers and parasympathetic ganglion cells.

Serosa

The *serous coat*, as in the stomach, consists of loose connective tissue covered by a layer of mesothelium.

The Large Intestine

The large intestine is divided topographically and to some extent structurally into three main segments: colon, rectum, and anal canal. Throughout the length of the large intestine, the wall consists of the same four coats that have been described for the stomach and small intestine, viz., mucosa, submucosa, muscularis, and serosa (or fibrosa).

The Colon

There is an abrupt change at the ileocecal juncture from the small intestine to the *colon*. The greater diameter of the colon is perhaps the most striking difference grossly. Other differences of structure are noted in the description of the various coats.

Mucosa

The *mucous membrane* of the colon has a comparatively smooth surface, for *there are no plicae or villi* as in the small intestine. Long, straight, tubular glands extend from the surface down through the entire thickness of the mucosa. These glands are *crypts* as in the small intestine (Figs. 16.50 and 16.51).

The surface *epithelium* is tall columnar. The absorbing cells have a striated border but it is much less prominent than that on the cells of the small intestine. Goblet cells are interspersed among the columnar absorbing cells. As the epithelium continues down into the tubular glands, the columnar cells become lower and goblet cells become exceedingly numerous. In fact, the walls of the glands frequently appear to be composed almost entirely of goblet cells. Primitive cells at the base of the crypts differentiate into goblet, absorptive, enteroendocrine and occasionally Paneth cells in a manner similar to that in the small intestine. Enteroendocrine cells (Figs. 16.51 and 16.52) are normally present although rare, but one type may become numerous and form a carcinoid tumor. This tumor is characterized by production of excessive amounts of serotonin.

The mucous membrane of the colon has two chief functions which are attributed to the columnar absorbing and goblet cells, respectively: namely, the absorption of water and the copious production of mucus. This mucous secretion lubricates the sur-

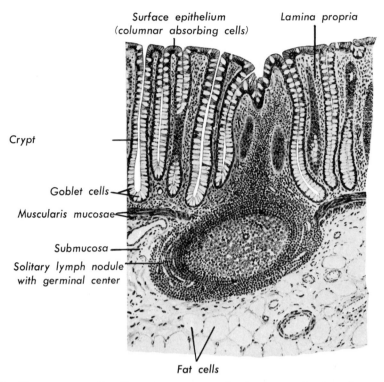

Figure 16.50. Transverse section through mucosa and submucosa of colon of man (×70). (After Braus H: *Anatomie des Menschen.* Berlin, Julius Springer, 1924.)

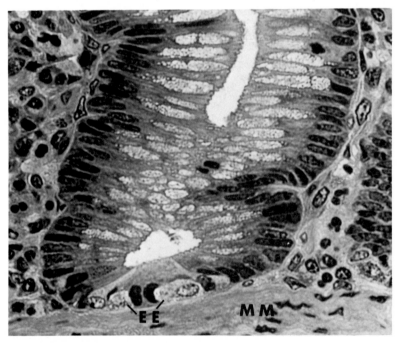

Figure 16.51. Light micrograph of the base of a crypt in the colon showing enteroendocrine cells (*EE*), *MM*, muscularis mucosae (×600).

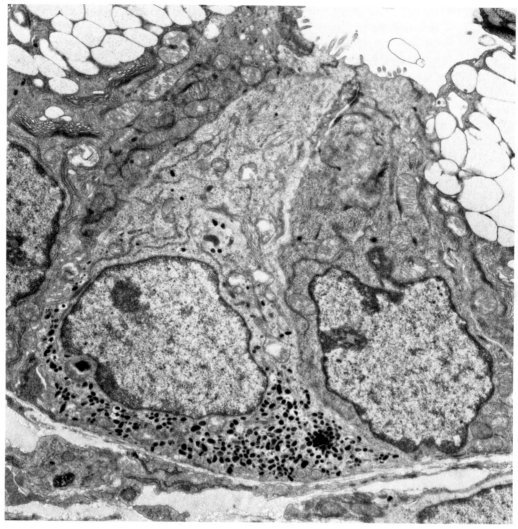

Figure 16.52. Enteroendocrine cell in a crypt from colon of rat. This cell extends to the crypt lumen (*top*) but the secretory granules are basal in position (×8800). (Courtesy of Dr. David Chase.)

face of the colon and facilitates the forwarding of the gradually dehydrated feces.

The connective tissue of the *lamina propria* extends up between the glands but is reduced to a minimum because of the close proximity of the tubular glands. Solitary lymph nodules are present in the mucosa and push through the muscularis mucosae into the submucosa. The lamina propria of the colon contains numerous lymphocytes, plasma cells and eosinophils.

The *muscularis mucosae* consists of an inner circular and an outer longitudinal layer of smooth muscle.

Submucosa. The *submucosa* is composed of loosely arranged connective tissue. It contains large blood vessels and the submucosal nerve plexus (of Meissner.) Solitary lymph nodules, although properly considered as structures of the lamina propria from which they originate, lie mainly in the submucosa.

Muscularis

The *muscularis externa* in the colon shows some variation from its arrangement in the small intestine. The inner circular layer is complete and prominent, but the longitudinal muscles become arranged into three strong, flat, equidistant, longitudinal bands, the *lineae coli* (taenia coli). Between these thick strands the longitudinal muscle coat becomes thinned but is rarely entirely absent. Nerve cell and fiber components of the myenteric plexus lie as usual in the connective tissue just external to the circular muscle layer.

Serosa

The *serous coat* is composed of a thin connective tissue layer covered by mesothelium. In certain regions, the mesothelial covering is absent. Here the connective tissue *fibrosa* binds the colon firmly to adjacent structures.

The Vermiform Appendix

The *vermiform appendix* is a diverticulum from the cecum. Its walls are continuous with those of the latter and closely resemble them in general structure. There are the same four coats: mucosa, submucosa, muscularis, and serosa.

The *mucosa* has its usual characteristic structures: the epithelium, crypts, lamina propria and the muscularis mucosae. The surface epithelium is simple columnar with a striated apical border. It continues into the glands or crypts where the border gradually becomes thinner. The glands frequently have many goblet cells, some Paneth cells and a number of enteroendocrine cells. In the embryo, the mucosal surface is lined with villi, but these disappear early in childhood. The lumen is often thrown into deep, pocketed folds, and in many adults it is nearly or completely obliterated.

The most characteristic histological feature of the appendix is the lymphatic tissue. Not only is the lamina propria infiltrated with lymphocytes, but it is often conspicuously occupied by a complete ring of solitary lymphatic nodules. These closely resemble the nodules that surround the crypts of the palatine tonsils. The nodules do not remain confined to the mucosa but push through the muscularis mucosae and invade the submucosa. In fact, the lymphatic development frequently makes it difficult to follow the muscularis mucosae and to separate the mucosa from the submucosa (Fig. 16.53). The *submucosa* contains numerous fat cells. It should be mentioned that, in some instances, more commonly after middle age, the mucosa and portions of the submucosa are largely replaced by fibrous connective tissue.

The *muscularis externa* varies greatly, both in thickness and in the amount of admixture of fibrous tissue. The inner circular layer is usually thick and well developed. The outer longitudinal layer differs from that of the large intestine in having no arrangement into lineae, the muscle tissue forming a continuous layer. The muscular layers are covered as usual by the *serosa*.

The Rectum

The *rectum* is usually divided into two parts. The *upper part* (the rectum proper), measuring 5 to 7 inches in length, is structurally similar to the colon. The crypts are longer than in the colon, however, and are lined almost entirely by goblet cells. The longitudinal layer of the muscularis externa is thicker on the front and back than it is on the sides. This retroperitoneal segment of the gut has no mesentery, and the serous coat is incomplete.

The *lower part* (*anal canal*) is 1 to 1½ inches in length. It pierces the pelvic floor and is closed except during defecation. Its mucous membrane has a number of permanent longitudinal folds, the *rectal columns* (*anal columns, columns of Morgagni*) which terminate distally about ½ inch from the anal orifice. These contain strands of smooth muscle and usually an artery and a vein. The bases (distal ends) of these columns are connected by transverse folds of the mucosa, the *anal valves* (Fig. 16.54).

Above the anal valves, the mucosa is lined by simple columnar epithelium like that of the rectum proper, composed of columnar absorbing cells, interspersed with many goblet cells. Crypts are present.

At the level of the anal valves, the epithelium becomes a stratified squamous

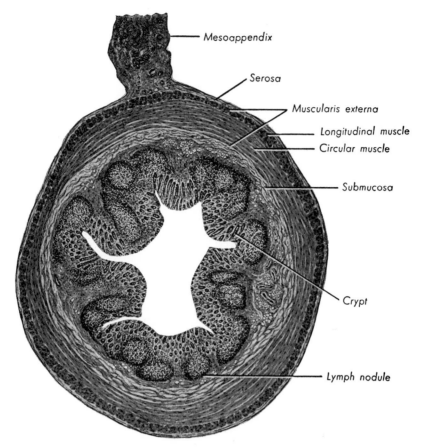

Figure 16.53. Transverse section of human vermiform appendix (×14).

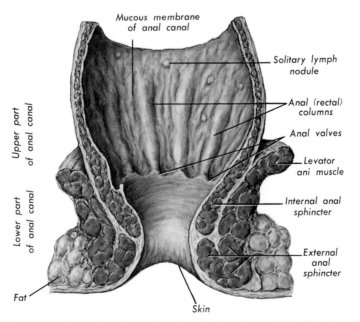

Figure 16.54. Mucous surface of anal canal (redrawn). (Courtesy of Wyeth Laboratories, Philadelphia, Pa.)

type, the surface cells of which are not cornified. No crypts are present below the juncture. The noncornified stratified squamous epithelium extends nearly to the anal orifice, where it changes to epidermis. Hairs, sebaceous glands and sweat glands appear at the anal orifice.

The sweat glands are of two types. One type has the characteristic structure of the general body sweat glands (Chapter 15). The other type (*circumanal glands*) are very large and are structurally similar to the axillary sweat glands. Their secretory cells contain granules, and inside the basal lamina are prominent myoepithelial cells.

At about the level of the anal valves, the muscularis mucosae subdivides into diverging strands which soon disappear.

The submucous coat of the anal canal has a rich plexus of blood vessels. The veins are often tortuous. Their size and arrangement and the absence of valves are conducive to the formation of hemorrhoids.

The circular layer of the smooth muscle of the anal canal is thick and forms the *internal anal sphincter*. The longitudinal layer of smooth muscle continues over the sphincter and attaches to connective tissue. The *external anal sphincter* is formed of skeletal muscle. It lies just inside the levator ani muscles which also act as a sphincter (Fig. 16.54).

The Peritoneum

The *peritoneum* is a serous membrane which lines the walls of the abdomen (parietal peritoneum) and is reflected over the contained viscera (visceral peritoneum). It consists of two layers, a loose connective tissue and a mesothelium. The connective tissue is arranged into loose bundles which interlace in a plane parallel to the surface. There are numerous elastic fibers, especially in the deeper layer of the parietal peritoneum, and comparatively few connective tissue cells. The mesothelium consists of a single layer of flat, polygonal cells with bulging nuclei. The cells have irregular, wavy outlines which are easily demonstrated with silver preparations. The shapes of the cells vary considerably according to the direction in which the tissues are stretched.

Over some parts, e.g., the liver and intestine, the peritoneum or serosa is thin and very closely attached. In places where the peritoneum is freely movable, a considerable amount of loose connective tissue, rich in elastic fibers and containing varying numbers of fat cells, connects the peritoneum with the underlying tissue. This is known as the "subserous tissue." The peritoneum is well supplied with blood vessels and lymphatics. The former give rise to a rich capillary network.

The *mesentery* is a sheet-like attachment between the visceral organs and the posterior abdominal wall. Its surfaces are covered by a mesothelium which is continuous with that of the parietal peritoneum lining the abdominal cavity, and the visceral peritoneum enclosing or covering each visceral organ. Between its two mesothelial layers, the mesentery also contains a layer of loosely arranged connective tissue. Here may be found numerous lymph nodes and adipose cells. The connective tissue core of the mesentery also houses the blood vessels, lymphatic channels and nerves which serve each visceral organ. Portions of the mesentery are quite long, allowing freedom of visceral organ movement. Other parts are short, firmly fixing certain organs into position. In some cases (e.g., rectum) a mesentery is nonexistent, the organ being so intimately applied to the posterior abdominal wall, that peritoneum covers only a small portion of its surfaces. Such organs or segments of them are said to be "retroperitoneal."

Mesenteric attachments to the anterior body wall have disappeared during embryonic development, except in a few isolated regions such as the falciform ligament of the liver. Other tough mesenteric continuities (*visceral ligaments*) are also found interconnecting many of the visceral organs and the intestine. In embryonic and fetal life, certain parts of the mesentery and visceral ligaments fuse or expand disproportionately, adding greatly to the complexity of the mesenteric "system." The *greater omentum* is an enormously expanded sacculation of the dorsal mesentery of the stomach (*dorsal mesogaster*). During development its surfaces fuse with each other and enshroud the anterior aspect of most of the coiled intestine. Its connective tissue may become the repository of considerable amounts of stored fat.

Blood Vessels of the Stomach and Intestines

The arteries reach the gastrointestinal tract through the mesentery, give off small branches to the serosa and pass through the musclar coats to the submucosa, where they form an extensive plexus of large vessels (Heller's plexus). Within the muscular coats, the main arteries give off small branches to the muscle tissue. From the plexus of the submucosa, two main sets of vessels arise, one passing outward to form the main supply of the muscular coats, the other inward to supply the mucous membrane (Fig. 16.55). Of the former, the larger vessels pass directly to the intermuscular septum, where they form a plexus from which branches are given off to the two muscular tunics. Of the branches of the submucous plexus which pass to the mucous membrane, the shorter supply the musclaris mucosae, while the longer branches pierce the latter to form a capillary plexus among the glands of the lamina propria. These capillaries are most numerous around the bodies and necks of the glands. They pass over into a dense network of capillaries just beneath the surface epithelium. From the capillaries, small veins take origin which pierce the muscularis mucosae and form a close-meshed venous plexus in the submucosa. These in turn give rise to larger veins, which accompany the arteries into the mesentery. A significant portion of the venous return from the intestine is into the vessels of the hepatic portal system for distribution to the sinusoids of the liver (see below).

In the small intestine, the distribution of the blood vessels is modified by the presence of villi (Fig. 16.56). Each villus receives one small artery or, in the case of the large villi, two or three small arteries.

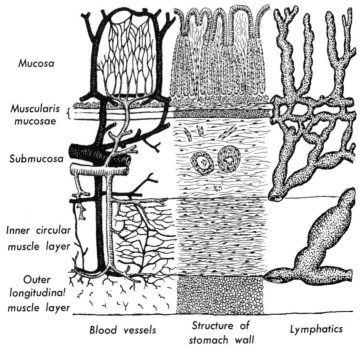

Mucosa

Muscularis mucosae {

Submucosa

Inner circular muscle layer

Outer longitudinal muscle layer

Blood vessels   Structure of stomach wall   Lymphatics

Figure 16.55. Three sections of stomach wall placed side by side to show relationship of blood vessels and lymphatics to the different layers. (Redrawn after Mall.)

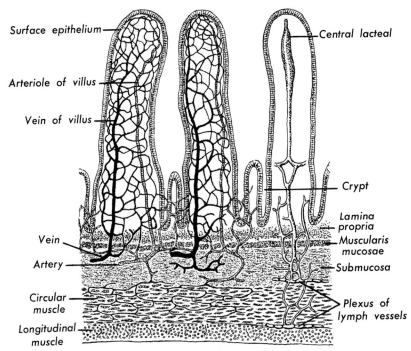

Figure 16.56. Scheme of blood vessels and lymphatics of human small intestine. (Redrawn from Böhm AA, von Davidoff M: *Lehrbuch der Histologie des Menschen.* Wiesbaden, 1903. After Mall.)

The artery passes through the long axis of the villus close under the epithelium to its summit, giving off a network of fine capillaries which for the most part lie just beneath the epithelium. From these, one or two small veins arise which usually lie on the opposite side of the villus from the artery.

Lymphatics of the Stomach and Intestines

Small lymph or chyle capillaries begin as blind canals in the lamina propria of the mucous membrane among the tubular glands (Fig. 16.55). In the small intestine, a lymph capillary (lacteal) occupies the center of the long axis of each villus, ending in a blind extremity beneath the epithelium of its summit (Fig. 16.56). The walls of the lymph capillaries are made up of a single layer of large endothelial cells. Although the lymph capillaries are considerably larger than the blood capillaries, they are usually collapsed and inconspicuous. These vessels unite to form a narrow-meshed

plexus of lymph capillaries in the deeper part of the lamina propria, lying parallel to the muscularis mucosae. Vessels from this plexus pass through the muscularis mucosae and form a wider meshed plexus of larger lymph vessels in the submucosa. In this region they often expand into sinuses surrounding the lymphatic nodules. A third lymphatic plexus lies in the connective tissue which separates the two layers of muscle. From the plexus in the submucosa, branches pass through the inner muscular layer, receive vessels from the intermuscular plexus and then pierce the outer muscular layer to pass into the mesentery in company with the arteries and veins. The larger lymph vessels are provided with definite valves, and their walls are also supported by a thin tunic of smooth muscle cells. In their course through the mesenteries, they are associated with numerous mesenteric lymph nodes. These relations are well demonstrated in the cat by the injection of 1% Berlin blue into the intestinal wall.

Although the primary function of the lymphatic system is the return of tissue fluids to the blood stream, the vessels of the small intestine form channels through which absorbed fats are drained. During digestion, the lymph fluid, carrying a rich emulsion of fat (chyle), gives to the vessels a white appearance and renders them clearly visible.

Nerves of the Stomach and Intestines

The nerves to the stomach consist of preganglionic parasympathetic fibers (branches of the vagus nerve) and postganglionic sympathetic fibers. They reach the intestinal walls through the mesentery. In the connective tissue between the two layers of muscle, these fibers are associated with groups of parasympathetic ganglion cells to form the *myenteric plexus* (*of Auerbach*). Within this plexus, the preganglionic parasympathetic fibers synapse with the ganglion cells. The axons are grouped together in small nonmyelinated bundles which pass, together with the sympathetic fibers, into the muscular coats. There they form intricate plexuses, from which are given off club-shaped terminals to the smooth muscle cells. From the myenteric plexus, fibers pass to the submucosa, where they form a similar but finer meshed and more delicate plexus which is also associated with other groups of parasympathetic ganglion cells, the *submucosal plexus* (*of Meissner*; see Fig. 16.42). Both fibers and cells are smaller than those of the myenteric plexus. From the submucosal plexus, delicate nerve fibers pass to their terminations in submucosa, muscularis mucosae and mucous membrane. Some fibers appear to end within the epithelium itself, but their functional role in that location is not fully understood.

EXTRINSIC DIGESTIVE GLANDS

The smaller tubular and tubuloalveolar glands which form a part of the mucous membrane and submucosa of the alimentary tract have been described. There remain to be considered certain larger compound tubuloalveolar glands, the development of which is similar to that of the smaller glands but which come to lie wholly outside the alimentary tract, connected with it by their main excretory ducts. Functionally, they are an important part of the digestive system. These structures are the *salivary glands*, the *pancreas*, and the *liver*.

The Salivary Glands

Associated with the oral cavity there are a number of glands which secrete a seromucous fluid, the *saliva*. The smaller of these glands are situated within the oral mucous membrane, whereas the larger glands are paired structures located outside the oral cavity proper but connected to it by excretory ducts. These *major salivary glands* include the *parotid, submandibular* and *sublingual* glands. Embryonically, the parenchyma of these glands arises as evaginations of the epithelium lining the oral cavity. Since both ectoderm and endoderm contribute to this lining, salivary gland epithelium arises from both germ layers, ectoderm for parotid and endoderm for submandibular and sublingual. The duct system in all cases develops first and gives rise secondarily to the secretory alveoli. In the adult the ducts may still proliferate mitotically and give rise to new alveoli, but the alveolar cells can also divide independently.

In the human the major function of the salivary glands is to produce a copious hypotonic saliva that keeps the oral mucosa moist and provides a medium for softening and lubricating food that is to be swallowed. Minor quantities of lipase, amylase, kallekrein, and other enzymes are present, but their roles in the digestive process are minimal because of their low concentrations and the short time a bolus of food is retained in the mouth. Saliva also contains secretory IgA and bacteriocidal compounds that aid in the natural control of oral flora. The specific composition of saliva is determined by the activity of both the secretory alveoli and the intralobular duct cells (see below).

The major salivary glands are tubuloalveolar in organization. In the human, the parotid has only serous alveoli, but the submandibular and sublingual are mixed glands, containing both serous and mucous alveoli.

Structure of the Salivary Glands

Each gland consists of a glandular epithelium (*parenchyma*) and a supporting connective tissue framework (*stroma*). The parotid and submandibular glands possess a definite connective tissue capsule which encloses the gland and blends with the connective tissue of surrounding structures. The sublingual gland has no distinct capsule. Connective tissue septa divide each gland into *lobes* and *lobules*. In these septa are found the larger ducts, the blood vessels, and occasional ganglion cells.

The Serous Alveoli

The serous alveoli are lined with pyramidal epithelial cells which rest upon a basal lamina and surround a narrow lumen. The cell boundaries are indistinct by light microscopy. The appearance of these cells varies according to their particular phase of activity as well as the mode of preservation. In a "resting" condition, the cytoplasm is filled with a number of small, highly refractile secretory droplets, the zymogen granules.

There is an abundance of *basophilic material* (rough endoplasmic reticulum) in the basal portion of the cells and a prominent Golgi region between the nucleus and the apex of the cell. Protein synthesized by ribosomes is combined with polysaccharides in the Golgi region to form membrane-bounded glycoprotein secretory droplets. The latter move into the apical region of the cell for storage as zymogen granules until the time of secretion (Fig. 16.57).

By employing the Golgi silver technique, using thin plastic embedded sections, or by electron microscopy, one can demonstrate fine *intercellular secretory canaliculi* between adjacent cells of the serous alveoli.

Although not obvious in routine histological preparations, peculiar stellate-shaped cells may be demonstrated by special techniques in the region between the secreting cells and the basal lamina. They lie in close contact with the secreting cells, and their processes form a sort of basketwork around the alveolus. These are the *basket cells* (Fig. 16.58), and they are a type of *myoepithelial cell*. They also occur in intralobular ducts. By their contraction, they assist in the discharge of the secretion products into the main excretory ducts.

Mucous Alveoli

In ordinary hematoxylin-eosin preparations, the purely mucous alveoli stain a light bluish purple, in contrast with the deep reddish purple of serous alveoli (Fig. 16.59). Usually the lumen is fairly large and may contain masses of mucin. The mucous cells rest on a basal lamina, and their boundaries are usually quite distinct. When the cell becomes filled with secretory droplets, the nucleus becomes flattened in the basal part of the cell. Most of the cell is occupied by a network of cytoplasm with spaces that, in the living state, were occupied by secretory droplets. The mucigen droplets are dissolved out by most of the routine methods used for light microscopy, leaving only a network of cytoplasm and remnants of some of the secretory droplets. After the cell discharges its secretion, the nucleus resumes a spherical or oval shape. Mitochondria are present, but rough endoplasmic reticulum is sparse. There is a well developed Golgi apparatus. Intercellular canaliculi are not seen in the mucous alveoli.

In the mixed glands, several types of terminal alveoli may be seen. Some alveoli may be composed entirely of serous cells, others entirely of mucous cells. An alveolus may contain both kinds of cells, in which case the serous cells are more likely to occupy the blind end of the alveolus, with the mucous cells nearer the exit (Fig. 16.59). In this instance, crescent-shaped groups of serous cells, are termed *demilunes* (Fig. 16.59). These may have direct access to the lumen of the alveolus, but more often they communicate with it by means of intercellular secretory canaliculi which pass

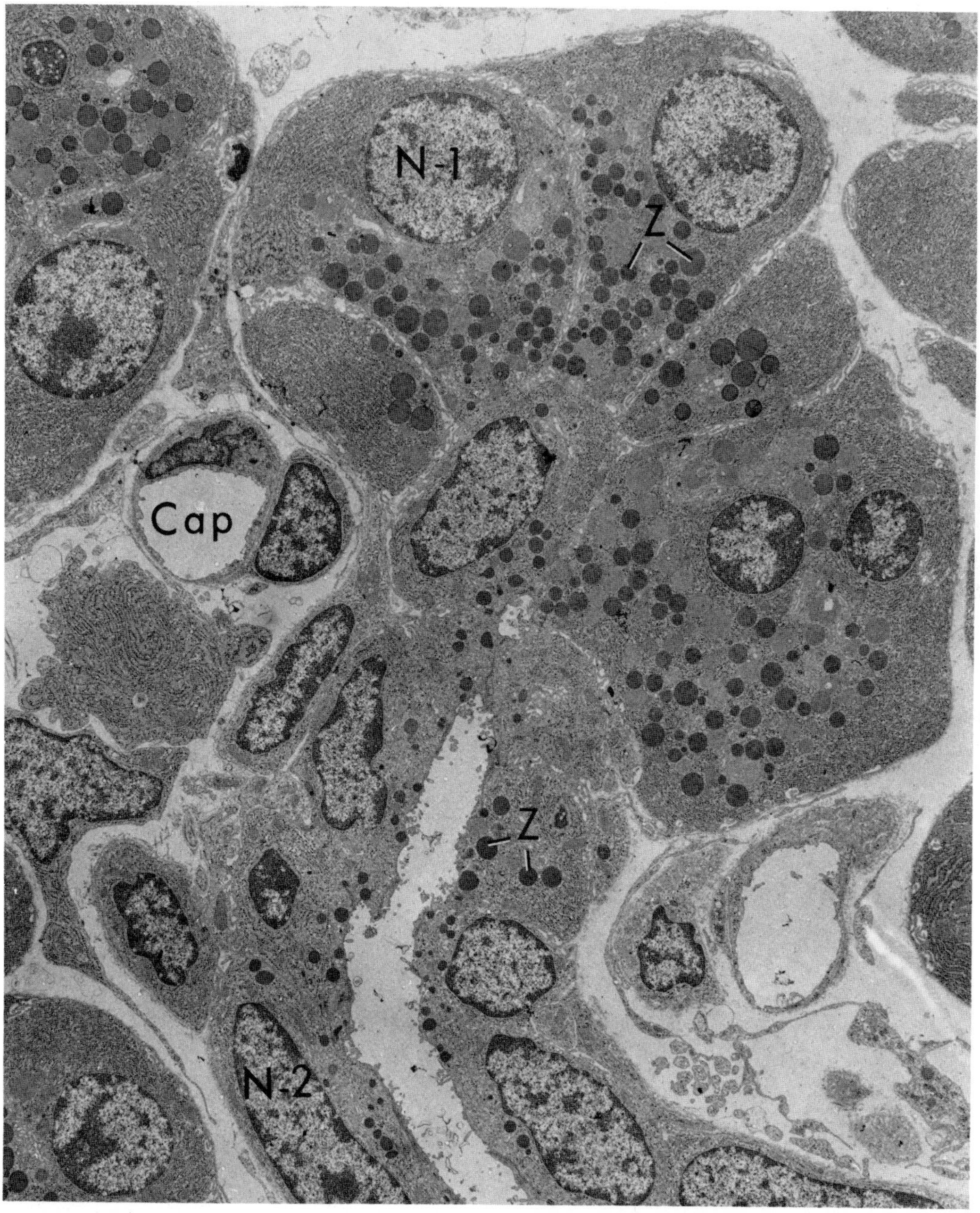

Figure 16.57. Electron micrograph of a rat parotid gland showing the junction of an intralobular intercalated duct with an acinus composed of parenchymal cells. The cells lining the junctional region of the duct have ultrastructural characteristics that are intermediate between those of acinar and duct cells. They have some zymogen granules and they also have more rough endoplasmic reticulum than do typical duct cells. *Cap*, capillary; *N-1*, nucleus of acinar parenchymal cell; *N-2*, nucleus of duct cell; *Z*, zymogen granules (×2250). (Courtesy of Dr. I. Joel Leeb.)

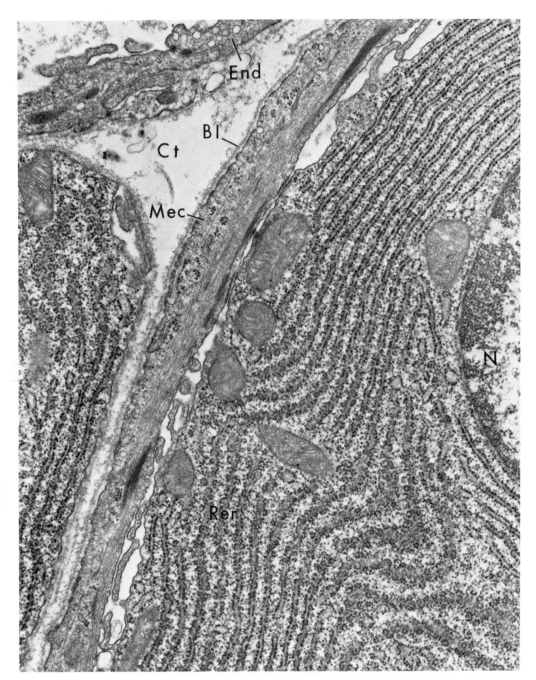

Figure 16.58.   Electron micrograph of portions of two cells of adjacent acini of the rat parotid gland. A portion of a myoepithelial (basket) cell (*Mec*) is seen between the basal end of an acinar cell and the basal lamina (*Bl*) of the acinar cells. The basket cells resemble the smooth muscle cells of other parts of the body in that they have a number of fine filaments and are contractile. *Ct*, connective tissue space; *End*, endothelium lining a small blood vessel; *N*, nucleus of acinar cell; *Rer*, rough endoplasmic reticulum (×22,500).

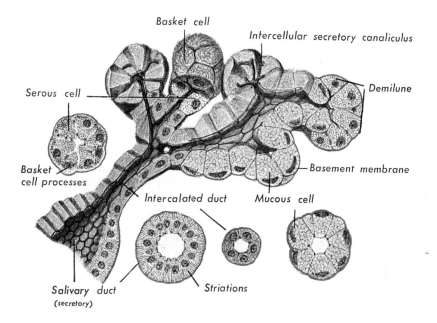

Figure 16.59. Reconstruction of terminal ramification of human submandibular gland, showing salivary and intercalated ducts and several alveoli. (From Braus H: *Anatomie des Menschen*. Berlin, Julius Springer, 1924. After a reconstruction by A. Vierling.)

between the mucous cells and branch among the serous cells of the demilune.

Duct System

From the alveoli the primary secretion products pass to the main excretory ducts by way of a hierarchy of ducts of increasing diameters (Fig. 16.60). Those immediately connected with the alveoli have a squamous or cuboidal epithelium and are of variable length, depending on the particular gland. They are referred to as *intercalated ducts* because they lie between the alveoli and the more prominent *secretory* or *striated ducts* (Figs. 16.57 and 16.59). Intercalated ducts are more readily seen by light microscopy in the parotid and submandibular glands. Striated ducts are lined with columnar epithelial cells that have numerous basal plasmalemma infoldings and rows of interposed mitochondria that result in a striated appearance when viewed by light microscropy. These ducts modify the composition of the alveolar secretion by transporting ions, secreting additional products and resorbing some materials. The salivary glands are excellent examples of the complexity of glandular secretion.

Consideration is now given to the more important characteristics of the particular glands.

The Parotid Gland

The *parotid gland* is the largest of the salivary glands and, in man, dog, cat and rabbit, it is entirely *serous* (Fig. 16.61). Its duct system is complex. The main excretory duct (Stenson's) opens into the oral cavity opposite the second upper molar tooth. It is lined with pseudostratified or stratified columnar epithelium, with occasional goblet cells. The main duct divides into the interlobar ducts which, in turn, divide to form interlobular ducts, the various branches following the connective tissue septa. Except in the larger of these ducts, the epithelium becomes reduced to a simple columnar type. All of these ducts are often referred to simply as excretory ducts. From the interlobular ducts, branches are given off which penetrate the lobules.

Most of the large intralobular ducts are of the striated variety. They are lined by a single layer of columnar cells in which the nucleus is spheroidal and centrally located. The cytoplasm is acidophilic. The basal portion of the cell presents a characteristic striated appearance (Figs. 16.59 and 16.61).

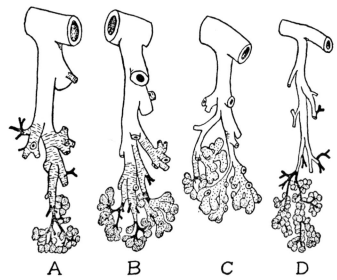

A B C D

Figure 16.60. Schematic drawing to illustrate the structure of the salivary glands and pancreas. *A*, parotid; *B*, submandibular; *C*, sublingual; *D*, pancreas. Excretory ducts, white; salivary ducts, cross striped; intercalated ducts, black; mucous alveoli, coarse stipple; serous alveoli, fine stipple. (Redrawn, slightly modified, after Braus H: *Anatomie des Menschen*. Berlin, Julius Springer, 1924.)

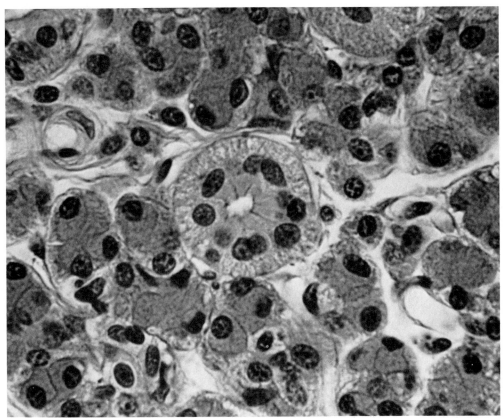

Figure 16.61. Section of dog parotid gland. Basal striations are apparent in the secretory duct (*center of field*) (×1,025).

The rodlike mitochondria are oriented perpendicular to the base of the cell, and electron micrographs show deep infoldings of the basal and basolateral plasma membrane into the cytoplasm, a configuration somewhat like that in the distal tubules of the kidney. This arrangement is characteristic of regions active in transport of sodium from the lumen to the interstitium and it has been shown that this segment is responsible for the lowered sodium and overall hypotonicity of saliva. The *intercalated ducts*, connecting the salivary ducts and the terminal alveoli are of small diameter (Figs. 16.57, 16.59, and 16.60) and are lined by low cuboidal epithelium. In the parotid, they are fairly long.

The gland is covered by a thick connective tissue capsule, from which branches extend inward around the lobes and their lobular subdivisions. Fine connective tissue

fibers also envelop each alveolous. Fat cells are frequent in the connective tissue of the parotid, and they tend to increase in number with age.

The Submandibular Gland

The *submandibular* (submaxillary) in man and most mammals is a *mixed gland*, but the proportion of serous and mucous alveoli varies. In man, it is preponderantly serous (Fig. 16.62). The main duct (Wharton's) opens into the mouth beneath the tongue. It is lined by pseudostratified columnar epithelium and has, in addition, a richly cellular stroma and longitudinally disposed smooth muscle cells. The main duct branches in the manner described for the parotid, the pseudostratified epithelium continuing into the larger interlobular ducts. The intralobular ducts are of the same types as in the parotid gland. The

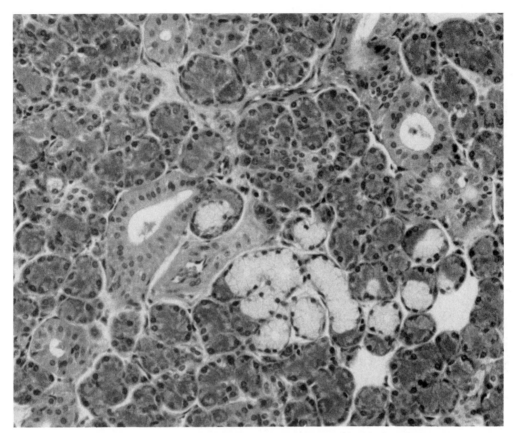

Figure 16.62. Section of human submandibular gland. Striated ducts are prominent. Mucous alveoli, some with serous demilunes, are apparent at *lower center* (see Fig. 16.63) (×280).

striated ducts are longer and more numerous than in the parotid; the intercalated ducts are short and narrow.

The mucous alveoli frequently are capped by serous demilunes. (Figs. 16.62 and 16.63) Some mucous alveoli also have serous cells lining their terminal portions. The connective tissue within the lobules and in the capsule is well developed.

The Sublingual Gland

The *sublingual gland* is also a *mixed gland* in man, dog, cat, rabbit and sheep. It is the smallest of the large salivary glands and in man is preponderantly mucous. A series of ducts opens into the mouth at the side of the frenulum of the tongue, near the opening of Wharton's duct. The pseudostratified epithelium that lines the larger ducts is replaced by simple columnar epithelium in the smaller ones. There are relatively few intralobular ducts. Typical striated ducts are rare. However, patches of striated cells may occur in the walls of intralobular ducts with an otherwise unmodified simple columnar epithelial lining. Intercalated ducts are likewise reduced in number so that most of the terminal alveoli, which are often quite elongated, either open directly into the larger intralobular ducts or into the interlobular ducts at the periphery of the lobule. Some investigators believe that typical intercalated ducts are entirely lacking.

The terminal alveoli are mostly of the mucous type. Serous cells occur mostly in the form of demilunes around mucous alveoli. Such demilunes are numerous and large.

The connective tissue septa are well developed in the sublingual, but the gland does not have a distinct capsule, as do the parotid and submandibular glands.

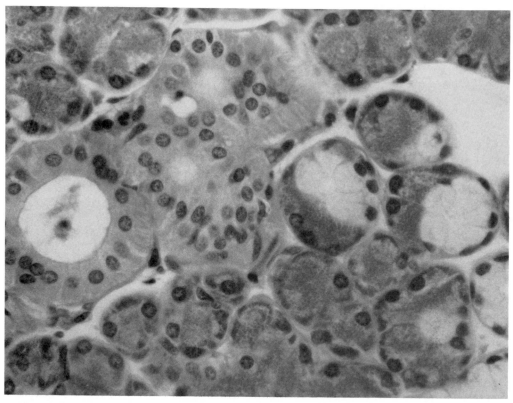

Figure 16.63. A portion of the field shown in Figure 16.62 at higher magnification. The basal striations of a striated duct are visible at *left* and serous demilunes on mucous alveoli are seen at *right* (×682).

Blood Supply

The salivary glands have a relatively rich blood supply. The larger arteries run in the connective tissue septa with the ducts, giving off branches which accompany the divisions of the ducts to the lobules. There is a particularly rich capillary bed around the striated ducts and alveoli. These give rise to veins which follow the course of the arteries.

Lymphatics

Relatively few in number, the lymphatics begin as minute vessels in the smaller connective tissue septa and empty into lymph vessels which accompany the arteries.

Nerve Supply

The sensory innervation of the salivary glands is by the trigeminal nerve. The motor innervation is derived from both sympathetic and parasympathetic systems. Preganglionic sympathetic fibers run in the thoracocervical trunk to terminate in the superior cervical ganglion. Here they form synapses with postganglionic fibers which course in the walls of the branches of the carotid artery to the respective glands.

The parasympathetic supply to the parotid is by way of preganglionic fibers of the ninth cranial nerve to the otic ganglion, from which postganglionic fibers pass to the gland. The parasympathetic innervation of the submandibular and sublingual glands is by way of preganglionic fibers in the chorda tympani nerve to the mandibular ganglion, which usually lies within the glands. Short postganglionic fibers pass to the elements of the gland. Nerve endings are seen to penetrate the basal lamina and lie within the epithelium itself.

Other Functions

The salivary glands of many lower organisms have important secondary functions, and may be sexually dimorphic. They have been shown to be a source of *nerve growth factor* in rodents, although this factor probably is not important in nerve growth but in the healing of licked wounds. There is no evidence that human salivary glands elaborate any of these products.

The Pancreas

The pancreas is both a gland of *external secretion*, furnishing the pancreatic juice which is conveyed to the duodenum and a gland of *internal secretion*, elaborating substances which, circulating in the blood, play an essential role in the regulation of the carbohydrate metabolism of the body. Serving the former function, it has a system of excretory ducts and terminal secreting *acini*, the arrangement of which somewhat resembles that of the parotid gland. For the performance of its endocrine function, there are highly vascularized aggregations of secreting cells, the *islets of Langerhans.*

Embryonically, the pancreas arises between the third and fourth week of gestation as a pair of evaginations of endodermal epithelium from the primitive gut into the surrounding mesenchymal bed. The two epithelial buds commence dichotomous branching under the influence of the mesenchyme and eventually fuse into a single organ. Groups of endocrine cells are distinguishable early in this differentiation sequence and they become isolated from the main epithelial bud to form primitive islets by seven or eight weeks of development. However, individual endocrine cells may appear in the exocrine ducts and acini, even in the adult organ. The proliferating epithelial evaginations assume a tubular form and give rise to the entire exocrine pancreas, ducts and acini. The surrounding mesenchyme differentiates into the supporting connective issue framework and the rich vascular bed which characterizes the entire adult pancreas.

The adult pancreas is a compound tubuloacinar gland, lying behind the stomach and extending transversely from the spleen to the loop of the duodenum. The broader portion of it, the *head*, lies in the concavity

of the latter organ. The head is joined to the *body* of the gland by a slightly constricted portion, the *neck*. The body tapers gradually into an extremity, the *tail*.

The pancreas has no distinct connective tissue capsule but is covered with a thin layer of loose tissue from which septa pass into the gland, subdividing it into many small lobules. In some of the lower animals (as, for instance, the cat), these lobules are well defined, being completely separated from one another by connective tissue. A number of these *primary lobules* are grouped together and surrounded by connective tissue which is considerably broader and looser in structure than that separating the primary lobules. These constitute a *lobule group* or secondary lobule. It is difficult to distinguish lobes and lobules in sections of human pancreas because the connective tissue septa are incomplete.

The main excretory duct of the pancreas, the *pancreatic duct* or *duct of Wirsung*, extends almost the entire length of the gland, giving off short lateral branches, one of which courses to each lobule. As the ducts enter the lobules, their epithelium becomes low cuboidal. They have characteristics similar to intercalated ducts of other glands, and it should be noted that these ducts of narrow caliber are the only intralobular ducts present in the pancreas; there are no striated ducts as in the salivary glands. The intralobular intercalated ducts are long, and they branch many times before terminating in the serous acini. The terminal cells of the duct system are usually surrounded by acinar cells and are referred to as centroacinar cells (Figs. 16.64 and 16.65). It is to be noted that intercalated duct cells of the pancreas do not contain secretory granules as they do in some of the duct cells of the salivary glands.

In addition to the main excretory duct, there is also a secondary excretory duct, the *accessory pancreatic duct* or *duct of Santorini*. It may have an independent opening into the duodenum; otherwise, it communicates with the main duct.

The interlobular and main ducts are

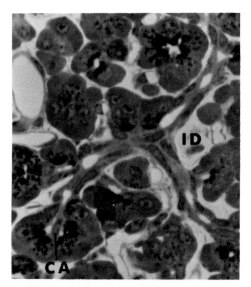

Figure 16.64. One-micrometer section of monkey pancreas showing branching of intercalated ducts (*ID*) to several acini. The acinus at the lower left shows a prominent centroacinar cell (*CA*) (×300).

lined with a simple high cuboidal to columnar epithelium which rests upon a basal lamina (Fig. 16.66). Occasional goblet cells and enteroendocrine cells are present in this epithelium. Outside of the epithelium is a connective tissue coat, the thickness of which is directly proportional to the size of the duct. In the accompanying connective tissue of the main duct and its larger branches, there are small mucous glands. As the ducts decrease in size, the epithelium becomes lower until, in the intercalated ducts, it is low cuboidal.

The *acini* are all of the serous (serozymogenic) type. They are lined by irregularly pyramidal epithelial cells resting on a basal lamina. In each cell, there may be distinguished a juxtalumenal zone and an intensely staining zone toward the basal lamina. The first contains numerous *zymogen granules* (Figs. 16.64 and 16.65). These granules vary in number with the functional activity of the cell, and they are the intracellular antecedents of the enzymes.

The nucleus lies in the basal zone of the cell. It is spherical and characteristically contains one or more distinct nucleoli. Bi-

nucleate cells may occur, but this is infrequent in man.

The basal zone is *basophilic*; electron micrographs show this region to contain a highly developed rough endoplasmic reticulum (Fig. 16.65). The surfaces of its membranes are studded with ribosomes, which accounts for the basophilic staining. The striated appearance in the basal region of the cell is accentuated by the presence of numerous elongated mitochondria between the lamellae of endoplasmic reticulum.

Pancreatic Islets

As mentioned earlier in this discussion, the pancreas also has an *endocrine* function, which is carried on by cellular aggregations interspersed irregularly among the acini or along the ducts. These cell groups are the *pancreatic islets* ("islands" of Langerhans); their secretion is released into the interstitial spaces where it has immediate access to the bloodstream, the islets have no functional communication with the duct system of the gland.

In ordinary preparations, the islets appear as more or less spheroidal masses of pale staining cells, arranged in the form of irregular anastomosing cords (Fig. 16.67). Between the cords, closely applied to the epithelial cells, are numerous blood capillaries. Only a few fine connective tissue fibers are present within the islets. The islets may be more or less closely surrounded by pancreatic acini (Fig. 16.67), or they may lie in the interlobular connective tissue septa.

The size of the islets varies from those having only a few cells to islets which are macroscopically visible. Isolated islet cells are also found occasionally among the cells lining the ducts of the exocrine pancreas. The number of islets varies in different portions of the gland as well as in different individuals. They are more abundant in the tail of the pancreas than in the head.

In routine histological preparations, all of the islet cells appear to be similar (Figs. 16.67 and 16.68); by special methods, however, a total of six types of cells have been distinguished in the human pancreas. The

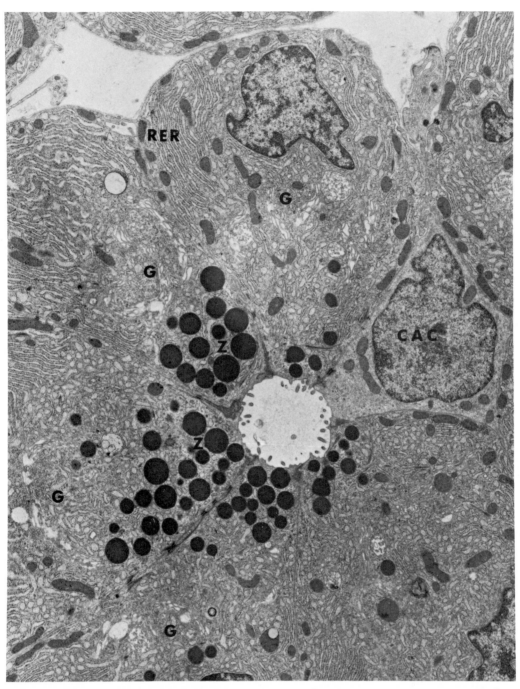

Figure 16.65. Part of pancreatic acinus from monkey. The prominent rough endoplasmic reticulum (*RER*), Golgi complexes (*G*) and zymogen granules (*Z*) are seen. A centroacinar cell (*CAC*) also borders the secretory lumen of the acinus (×6,250).

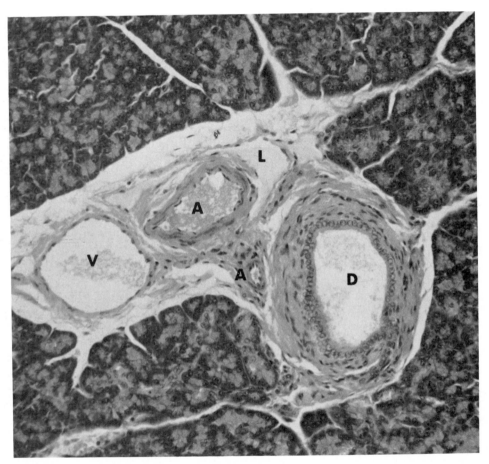

Figure 16.66. Interlobular duct and accompanying vessels in human pancreas. *D*, duct; *A*, arterioles; *V*, venule; *L*, lymphatic vessel (×280).

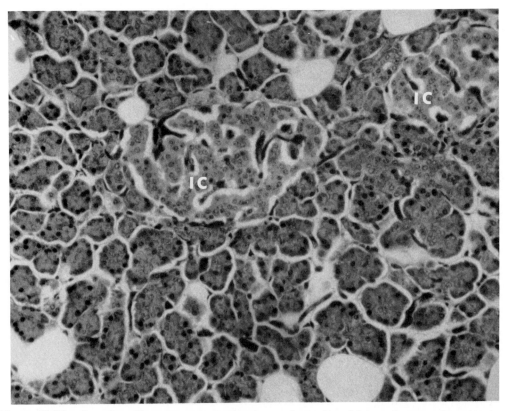

Figure 16.67. A section of human pancreas showing portions of two islets and surrounding exocrine tissue. Note the cord-like groups of islet cells (*IC*) separated by vascular channels. Masson's trichrome stain (×250).

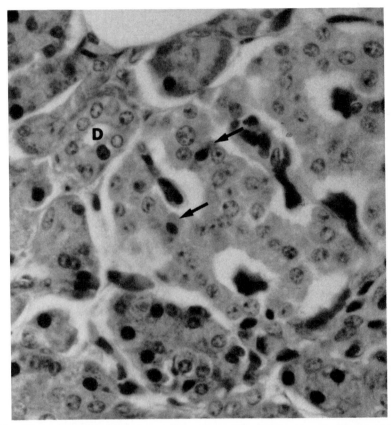

Figure 16.68. Higher magnification of a portion of one of the islets shown in Figure 16.67. Note the denser, more homogenous staining of both nucleus and cytoplasm in two A cells (*arrows*). An intralobular duct lies close to this islet (*D*). Masson's trichrome stain (×890).

most common ones are A or *alpha cells*, B or *beta* cells and D or *delta* cells. The A and B cells are by far the most numerous.

The granules of the A and B cells differ from each other in solubility and in staining reactions. The A cell granules are preserved by alcohol, whereas those of the B cells are soluble in alcohol. Of the various staining methods used for differentiating the cells (e.g., Masson's trichrome, chrome hematoxylin-phloxine, aldehyde fuchsin), the chrome hematoxylin and phloxine method is the one most common. With this technique (Fig. 16.69) the A cells are seen to contain numerous fine, red-staining granules in contrast with blue-staining granules of B cells. Electron micrographs show that the granules are enclosed by membranes. The A cell granules are highly opaque (electron-dense), relatively uniform in size and distributed evenly in the cytoplasm. The granules of the B cells are less opaque than those of the A cell, they are more variable in cytoplasmic distribution, and each granule is characteristically separated from its enclosing membrane by a prominent clear space. The B cell granules vary in shape in different species; in man, dog, and cat, they appear as crystalloids.

Although the relative numbers of A and B cells vary in different islets, the B cells are generally more numerous. B cells may

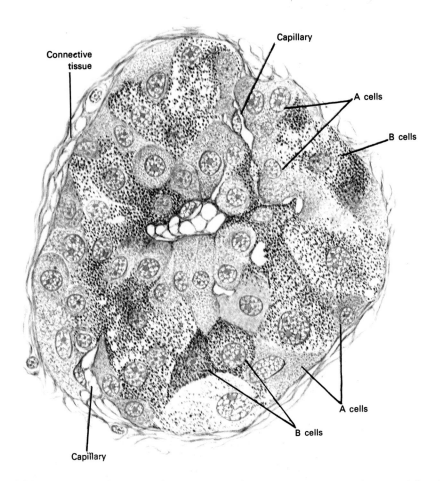

Figure 16.69. A section of an islet of Langerhans of human pancreas showing A and B cells. A 3-μm section of a surgical specimen. The relative proportions and distributions of the A and B cells are unusual in the particular section illustrated. The B cells are generally about three times as numerous as the A cells and the latter are usually found toward the periphery of the islet. Chrome hematoxylin and phloxine stain (Gomori) (×113).

also occur outside the islets, either singly or as small groups, in association with fully developed ducts or with acini. Estimates of the percentages of the various cell types indicate that B cells comprise 60 to 90% of all of the islet cells in the human pancreas.

The D cells are differentiated by Mason's triple stain (Fig. 1.11*B*), which also selectively colors the A cells. There are few D cells in the human. Immunochemical studies have demonstrated recently that there are three other cell types present in small numbers. In experimental animals, both zymogen granules and beta-type granules have been observed to occur in the same cell under some conditions. It is not known whether this can also occur in human pancreas.

Secretions of the Pancreas

The *external secretion* of the pancreas is an alkaline liquid, the pancreatic juice, the important constituents of which are certain enzymes. Among these are *trypsin*, a powerful proteolytic enzyme which breaks down proteins into amino acids, *amylase*, which converts starches into maltose, and *lipase*, which splits fats into glycerol, and fatty acids. It is interesting to note that, although these several chemically dissimilar enzymes are elaborated by the pancreatic acini, the acinar cells are apparently cytologically similar.

Secretory pathways have been studied extensively in pancreatic acinar cells. These are described in some detail in Chapter 1.

The pancreas may be stimulated to activity either by nervous impulses from the vagus or by the action of the hormones, *secretin* and *pancreozymin*, formed in the duodenal mucosa (probably by separate types of enteroendocrine cells) and carried to the pancreas in the bloodstream. Secretin appears to be formed whenever acid substances, such as the acid contents of the stomach or acid bile, come in contact with the duodenal mucosa. It stimulates intercalated duct cells to secrete bicarbonate. Pancreozymin stimulates release of zymogen granules from the acinar cells.

The *internal secretion* of the pancreas includes two major hormones. One of these, *insulin*, is known to play an important role in carbohydrate metabolism. Without this hormone, the cells of the body are unable to utilize the available glucose and allow formation of glycogen stores. The clinical condition resulting from a deficiency of insulin, *diabetes mellitus*, is thus marked by hyperglycemia and glycosuria of variable severity.

Insulin is produced in the islets, specifically by the B cells. Evidence for this is available from various sources, both clinical and experimental. Impaired sugar assimilation results from removal of the entire pancreas but not from ligation of the pancreatic duct, which destroys the acinar tissue but leaves the islets intact. Furthermore, it has been amply demonstrated, as in the first successful extractions of insulin by Banting and Best, that insulin is present in such a duct-ligated pancreas. In man, functional tumors of the B cells produce hypoglycemia, the effect being comparable to that caused by the administration of insulin. Removal of the tumor restores the patient to a normal condition. Experimentally, diabetes can be produced in many animals by the selective destruction of the B cells by injection of the drugs alloxan or streptozotocin. Also, in certain species the repeated injection of crude extracts of the anterior pituitary gland results in B cell injury and diabetes.

The islets also secrete another hormone known as *glucagon*, a hyperglycemic-glycogenolytic factor. This hormone is formed by the A cells and it has an effect which is, in some respects, antagonistic to that of insulin. It causes an elevation of blood sugar. Like insulin, it is present in pancreatic tissue following duct ligation. Unlike insulin, it is present in the pancreas of a duct-ligated, alloxan-treated animal.

At least one other peptide hormone, *somatostatin*, is found in islet tissue and can be localized to the D cell by immunocytochemistry. The function of this hormone and other peptides that have been described in islet tissue is not fully understood, but a paracrine suppressor effect on the secretion of insulin and glucagon is reported.

Blood Supply

The pancreas receives its blood supply from the superior and inferior pancreaticoduodenal arteries and from pancreatic rami of the splenic artery. The vessels course in the interlobular connective tissue and give off branches which enter the lobules. These form capillary networks among the acini and in the islets. The islets have an extremely rich vascular network, a characteristic which they share with other endocrine tissues. Also in common with other endocrine tissues, the capillaries have a fenestrated endothelium with diaphragms spanning the pores. The extensiveness of the capillary network within the islets is not usually appreciated in sections but can be demonstrated in injected specimens. The blood leaves the pancreas by the pancreaticoduodenal veins to the superior mesenteric and portal veins and by several small pancreatic veins to the splenic vein.

Lymphatics

The lymph vessels lie mainly in the interlobular connective tissue. They drain chiefly into the celiac lymph nodes.

Nerve Supply

The nerves to the pancreas are from the splanchnic (sympathetic) and the vagus (parasympathetic). The former are nonmyelinated. The latter are myelinated preganglionic fibers; the cell bodies of their postganglionic fibers lie within the substance of the gland. The terminal fibers of the nerves are distributed about the secreting acini, some penetrating the basal lamina to lie within the epithelium, on the walls of blood vesels and within the islets in close association with both vessels and endocrine cells. Pacinian corpuscles are occasionally found in the interlobular connective tissue of the gland.

The Liver

The liver is the largest gland of the body. Its organization differs from that of the other major digestive glands because most of its functions relate to producing chemical changes in the blood rather than exocrine secretion. The liver does secrete bile, which is conveyed to the intestine by a system of ducts, but even this function is as much excretory as digestive in nature. The liver is involved in processing or storage of all of the major categories of food materials, fats, carbohydrates, proteins and vitamins, performs an essential function in the removal of waste products from the blood and synthesizes serum proteins, lipoproteins and clotting factors. Because of its role in releasing products directly into the blood stream it has been considered an endocrine organ, by broad definition of the term endocrine. Current concepts of endocrine function center around the elaboration of hormones, however, and the liver does not produce true hormones. Despite the multiplicity and diversity of its functions, the liver has no groups of cells cytologically specialized for the performance of one function or the other, as is the case, for example, in the pancreas.

The unique organization of the liver has its origins in its mode of development. Rather than forming from a branching primary duct system as do typical exocrine glands, the liver arises from an initial diverticulation of the foregut and a secondary mass of proliferating endodermal epithelial cells that invade the mesenchyme of the embryonic septum transversum. These latter cells interdigitate with mesenchymally derived primary vascular spaces (vitelline venous channels). They form cords or sheets that help to subdivide the vascular channels into endothelium-lined sinusoids and the epithelial cells remain intimately associated with these sinusoids throughout life. Intrahepatic bile ducts arise secondarily by dedifferentiation of partially differentiated hepatic parenchymal cells and these ducts then join the extrahepatic duct system. The latter, along with the gall bladder, develops from the original gut diverticulum.

The adult liver is situated in the upper and right part of the abdominal cavity, immediately below the diaphragm to which it is attached. Several fissures partially divide it into four *lobes*. It is incompletely invested by an outer *tunica serosa*, derived from the peritoneum, within which is a delicate connective tissue capsule, the *capsule of Glisson*. This capsule, which contains a fair abundance of elastic fibers, covers the entire surface of the organ. At the *porta hepatis* (transverse fissure, hilus), it surrounds the entering blood vessels and follows into the gland, forming a framework and dividing it into innumerable small *lobules*. In some animals, e.g., the pig and camel, each lobule is completely invested by connective tissue. In man, the connective tissue is sparse and the lobular investment is incomplete. It is apparent mainly at points where three or more lobules meet (Fig. 16.70). The lobules are cylindrical or

irregularly prismatic in shape and approximately 1 mm in breadth and 2 mm in length. Except just beneath the capsule, where they are frequently arranged with their apices directed toward the surface, the lobules are irregularly arranged.

The *hepatic lobule*, which may be considered the anatomical unit of structure of the liver, has two main constituents: an epithelial parenchyma and a system of anastomosing blood sinusoids. The parenchyma is made up of hepatic cells arranged in irregular, branching, interconnected plates. Since in sections the sheets of cells often give the appearance of cell cords (Fig. 16.70), they have frequently been called the *hepatic cords*. However, reconstructions which portray the interrelationships of the cells in three dimensions clearly show that the cells are aligned in broad plates or

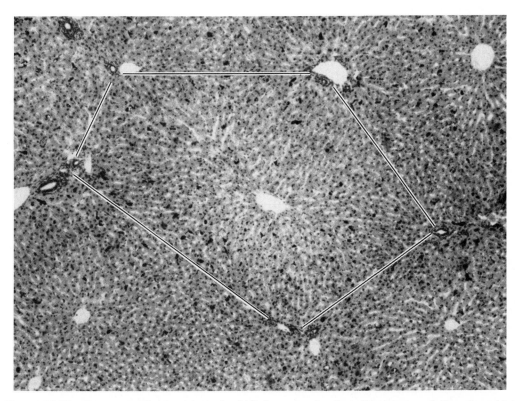

Figure 16.70. Low magnification view of rabbit liver showing hepatic plates, radiating sinusoidal spaces, and the lack of distinct boundaries to hepatic lobules. The *line* indicates a rough outline of a lobule whose central vein lies in the *center* of the micrograph. The black deposits on this micrograph are due to carbon particles phagocytized by Kupffer cells in the sinusoids (×75).

sheets (Fig. 16.71). The plates tend to be arranged in a radiating manner around the central blood vessel of the lobule.

The hepatic plates or laminae form the secretory portions of the gland and are thus analogous to the secretory tubules of other glands. The hepatic plates are arranged in a definite manner relative to the blood

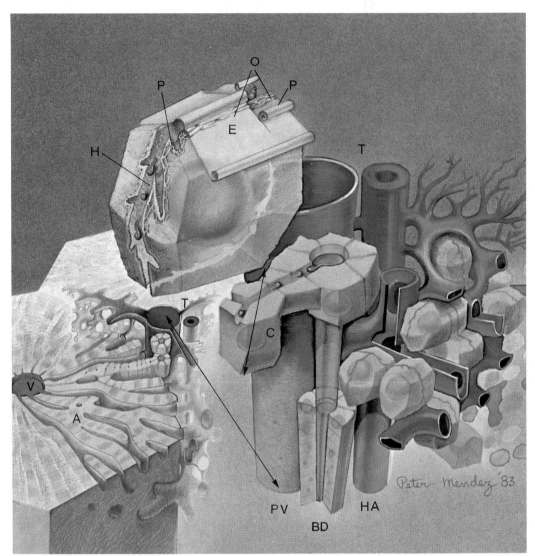

Figure 16.71. Diagram illustrating relationships of the major components of liver. A lobule containing a central vein (*V*) and anastomosing plates of hepatocytes (*A*) is shown at *lower left.* A portal triad area (*T*) has been enlarged and dissected at *right*, offset as indicated by the *long arrow.* A peripheral hepatocyte is isolated along with plasma membrane of a neighboring hepatocyte at *top left center,* having been elevated as indicated by the *short arrow.* The portal triad consists of branches of the portal vein (*PV*), hepatic artery (*HA*), and bile ducts (*BD*). As depicted at *right*, the venous blood (*blue*) mixes with arterial blood (*red*) to supply the sinusoids. Bile (*green*) is secreted by individual hepatocytes into an intercellular canaliculus (*H*) bounded by apposed hepatocyte surfaces. The canalicular space is segregated from other intercellular space by occluding junctions (*O*), shown here as they would appear in freeze-fracture replicas. The E face of the plasma membrane of an overlying cell (*E*) displays anastomosing grooves, and the P face of the membrane of the isolated hepatocyte (*P*) shows complementary anastomosing ridges. Bile flows within canalicular spaces to the periphery of the lobule and empties into bile ducts by way of a short connecting ductule (*C*).

channels, forming partitions between them. The blood vessels may therefore conveniently be considered first.

Blood Supply

The blood supply of the liver is peculiar in that, in addition to the ordinary arterial supply and venous return which all organs possess, the liver receives venous blood in large quantities through the portal vein. There are thus *two afferent vessels*, the *hepatic artery* and the *portal vein*, the former carrying arterial blood, the latter venous blood from the intestines and spleen. Both vessels enter the liver at the porta and divide into large *interlobar branches* which follow the connective tissue septa between the lobes. From these are given off *interlobular branches* which run in the smaller connective tissue septa between the lobules.

From the interlobular branches of the portal vein arise veins which are still interlobular at the portal terminals. These terminals send branches into the lobular periphery where they subdivide and anastomose to form a specialized capillary bed, the hepatic *sinusoids* (Figs. 16.71 to 16.73). The sinusoids all converge toward the center of the lobule, where they empty into the *central vein*. The central veins are the smallest radicles of the *hepatic veins*, the efferent vessels of the liver. As it passes through the center of the long axis of the lobule, the central vein constantly receives blood from sinusoids from all sides and, increasing in size, leaves the lobule at its base. Here it unites with the central veins of other lobules to form a *sublobular vein*, which is a branch of a hepatic vein.

The hepatic artery accompanies the portal vein, following the branchings of the latter through the interlobar and interlobular connective tissue (Fig. 16.73). Some of the interlobular arterioles break up into capillary networks which supply the interlobular structures and then empty into the smaller branches of the portal veins. Other arterioles empty peripherally into the hepatic sinusoids.

Intrahepatic Ducts

The duct system of the liver serves to convey the external secretion, the *bile*, to the duodenum. The smallest branches of the duct system are the narrow, intralobular *bile canaliculi* which form a ramifying network of channels between the parenchymal cells of the hepatic plates (Fig. 16.71). Like the plates in which they lie, the canaliculi radiate outward from the central axis of the lobule. Most of the canaliculi drain into small *interlobular bile ducts* found at the periphery of a lobule. The short connections between the hepatic cells and the interlobular bile ducts are called *terminal ductules, cholangioles* or ducts of Hering. They are lined by cuboidal cells which are smaller and paler staining than the hepatic cells. The lumen is little if at all larger than that of a bile canaliculus (Fig. 16.74). A few of the terminal ductules extend to variable depths within the lobule.

Each interlobular duct joins with others, forming progressively larger ducts lined by cuboidal or columnar epithelium. As the ducts increase in size toward the porta of the liver, the epithelium becomes high columnar and the connective tissue layer becomes thicker, with many elastic fibers and a few scattered smooth muscle cells.

In their ramifications through the connective tissue septa, the interlobular bile ducts always accompany the branches of the portal vein and the hepatic artery. These three structures are often referred to as the *portal triad*. Together with the interlobular connective tissue which marks the point of separation of three or more lobules, they occupy the *portal canal* or *portal area* (Fig. 16.73). A network of lymphatic vessels accompanies the branches of the portal vein in the portal area and in the interlobular connective tissue. However, the lymphatic vessels tend to collapse and are not obvious in sections prepared by routine methods.

Extrahepatic Ducts

The right and left hepatic ducts join to form the *hepatic duct* which, after its juncture with the *cystic duct*, becomes the com-

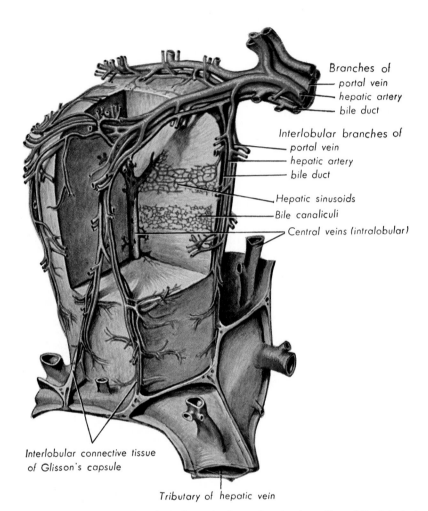

Branches of
- portal vein
- hepatic artery
- bile duct

Interlobular branches of
- portal vein
- hepatic artery
- bile duct

Hepatic sinusoids

Bile canaliculi

Central veins (intralobular)

Interlobular connective tissue
of Glisson's capsule

Tributary of hepatic vein

Figure 16.72. Reconstruction of a lobule from the liver of a pig. A portion of the lobule is cut away to show the hepatic sinusoids and bile canaliculi. (Redrawn and slightly modified from Braus H: *Anatomie des Menschen*. Berlin, Julius Springer, 1924. After a reconstruction by A. Vierling.)

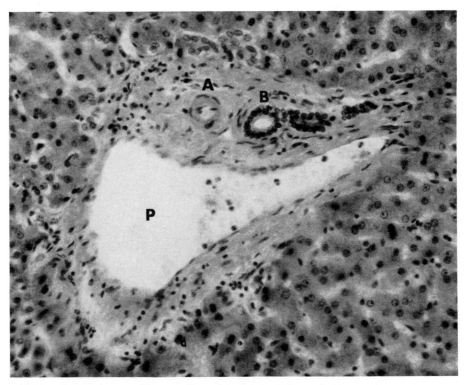

Figure 16.73. A portal area of human liver showing branches of the portal vein (*P*), the hepatic artery (*A*), and an interlobular bile duct (*B*) lying in interlobular connective tissue (×280).

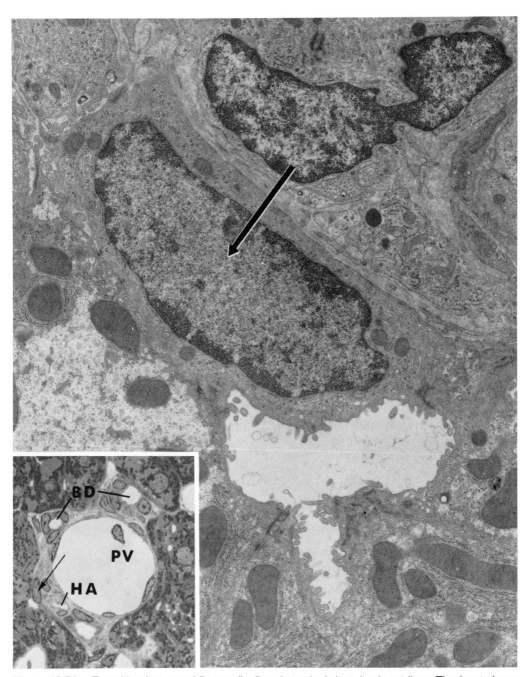

Figure 16.74. Transition between bile canaliculi and terminal ductules in rat liver. The *inset* shows a 1-μm section of a portal area with branches of the portal vein (*PV*), bile ducts (*BD*) and the hepatic artery (*HA*). The *arrow* indicates a region of transition between a bile ductule and a bile canaliculus. The electron micrograph is from an adjacent thin section. The *large arrow* is on the nucleus of the transition ductule cell. Electron micrograph ×10,500; *inset* ×980.

mon bile duct (ductus choledochus) and conveys the bile to the duodenum. The hepatic ducts, the cystic duct and the common bile duct are referred to as the *extrahepatic ducts* of the liver, in contrast with the intrahepatic system of ducts. The extrahepatic ducts are lined by high columnar epithelium which rests on a connective tissue lamina propria containing smooth muscle and elastic fibers. The epithelium and underlying lamina propria are thrown into numerous folds. Goblet cells occur in the epithelium, more abundantly in the lower portion of the common bile duct. Small multicellular glands may be seen extending into the lamina propria. In the cystic duct, the smooth muscle fibers are disposed in transverse, longitudinal and diagonal directions. They are less abundant in the hepatic ducts and the common duct, except in the duodenal end of the latter, where they form a sphincter.

The Hepatic Lobule

It is apparent that the hepatic lobule, the *anatomical unit* of structure of the liver, differs markedly from the lobules of glands such as the pancreas or salivary glands. In the latter, the lobule is surrounded by interlobular connective tissue and comprises a group of secreting tubules drained by the terminal branch of an interlobular duct. Thus, the unit of structure and the unit of function are identical.

In the liver, the parenchyma comprising one hepatic lobule is drained of its secretion by several interlobular bile ducts lying in the adjacent portal canals. As a result, a single interlobular bile duct carries off the secretions of portions of several adjacent hepatic lobules. This area of hepatic tissue, drained by a single interlobular bile duct lying in the axis of the area, has been designated a *portal lobule*. According to another interpretation, (usually ascribed to Rappaport and his colleagues), a *functional unit* of liver tissue is defined as a small parenchymal mass (*acinar unit*) that surrounds a terminal branch of a portal vein, accompanied by a hepatic arteriole and a

bile ductule. A diagrammatic representation of this unit is shown in Figure 16.75. This interpretation differs from the portal lobule in that it includes only the parenchymal tissue around a terminal branch of a portal vein rather than all of the parenchyma around all branches of a portal vein located at an axis. The diagram of acinar units also calls attention to the fact that triads (composed of portal veins, hepatic arteries and bile ducts), are present in only two or three of the portal canal areas of hexagonal shaped lobules. The hexagonal lobule is readily identified in the liver of the pig and a few other mammals, but this is not the case in man and in most other mammals. Acinar units are of particular interest in relation to certain pathological lesions. In many cases the pathological changes occur in a pattern corresponding to the units of parenchyma around terminal branches of the portal venules. In some cases, however, the changes appear in patterns corresponding more to the classically described hepatic lobule. Therefore, the concepts of lobulation should be considered as complementary, not mutually exclusive. It is also important to realize that lobulation is only found in mammals and does not appear until after birth. This relates to the fact that mammals have evolved a high degree of specialization in liver function, mostly involving direct exchange of substances between hepatocytes and sinusoidal blood.

The Hepatic Plates or Laminae

The parenchymal cells of the liver were described in the older literature as being arranged in elongated, anastomosing cords made up of two rows of cells, with the main channel of the bile canaliculus extending throughout the length of the cord and its branches. This interpretation was based largely on studies of the liver of lower vertebrates. In sections of liver of man and other mammals, the cord appears to be either one cell thick or two or more cells thick, depending on the plane of the section. Since the cords radiate from the pe-

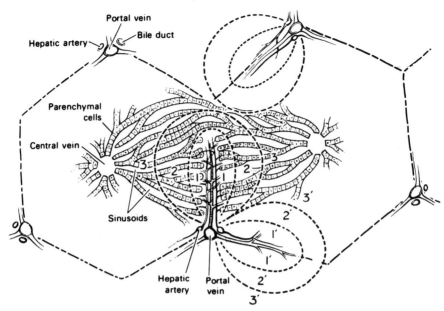

Figure 16.75. Diagram of the arrangement of liver parenchymal cells contained in two lobules (*dot-dash lines*) and showing functional units (acinar units, *dashed lines*) around terminal afferent blood vessels and terminal bile ductules. The oxygen tension and nutrient level of the blood is highest in zone 1 and lowest in zone 3. Zones labeled as *1′*, *2′*, and *3′* represent corresponding regions of an adjacent acinar unit. (Adapted from A. M. Rappaport, Z. J. Borowy, W. M. Lougheed, and W. N. Lotto: *Anat Rec* 119:1954.)

riphery of the lobule to the center with the cells of a row frequently arranged in a vertical relationship to each other (i.e., in a plane parallel to the course of the central vein), cross sections of a lobule often show the cord as a single row of cells. Cords of two rows of cells, as outlined above, are found in some embryonic livers and in livers of some of the lower vertebrates. However, a modified arrangement is present in man and other mammals where the cells are arranged in sheets known as *hepatic plates* or *hepatic laminae*. This understanding of the cell arrangement resulted from a study of reconstructions showing the structure of the liver lobule in three dimensions.

Bile Canaliculi

Between the hepatic cells are minute intercellular channels, the *bile canaliculi*. These branch and have a very irregular course (Fig. 16.71). Short side branches of the canaliculi frequently extend between the liver cells toward the surface of a plate.

They ramify throughout the hepatic parenchyma, anastomosing with the canaliculi of adjacent anastomosing plates (Fig. 16.76), but they seldom approach the surface of a plate.

Each canaliculus lies midway along the interface between adjacent hepatic cells and is formed by the somewhat modified cell membranes of the two opposing cells. They can be demonstrated in light microscope preparations particularly well by the Golgi silver impregnation method or histochemical staining for certain phosphatase enzymes. They are difficult to distinguish in ordinary preparations. Electron micrographs show that the membranes of the hepatic cells which form the canaliculi have short microvilli projecting into the lumen (Figs. 16.71 to 16.78). The canalicular space is separated from the remaining intercellular space by a junctional complex. However, the occluding junction close to the lumen is not highly developed and resembles those of other areas in the body

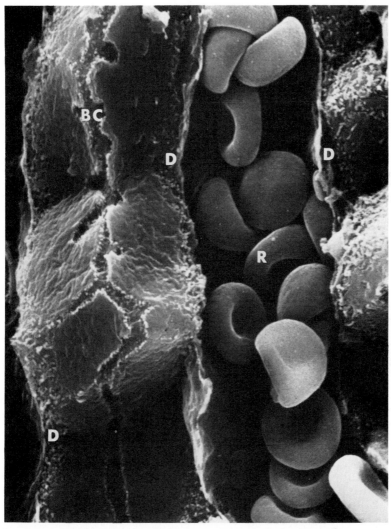

Figure 16.76. Scanning electron micrograph of hepatic plates and sinusoids in hamster liver. The tissue has been fractured so as to reveal a bile canalicular channel (*BC*), a sinusoid filled with red blood cells (*R*), and perisinusoidal spaces of Disse (*D*). The thin endothelial lining of sinusoids is also apparent. Compare this specimen with Figure 16.71 (×3070).

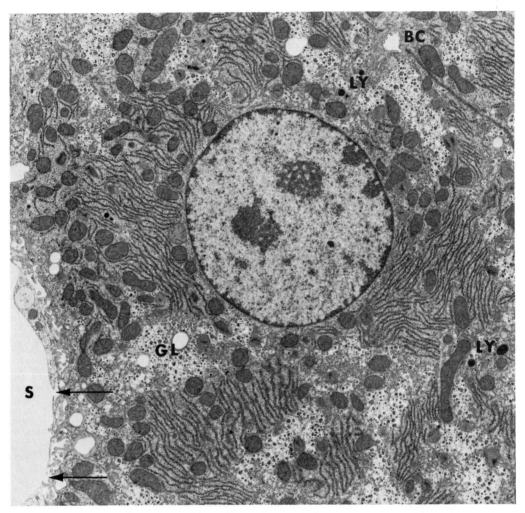

Figure 16.77. Low magnification electron micrograph of a liver cell of mouse showing relationships to bile canaliculus (*BC*) and the blood sinusoid (*S*). Gaps in the sinusoidal endothelium are shown at the arrows. *LY*, lysosomes; *GL*, glycogen. Clumps of rough endoplasmic reticulum characteristic of liver cells are seen (×5500).

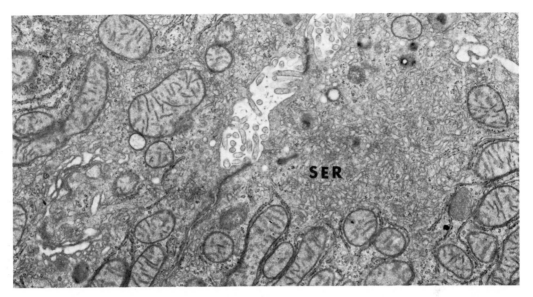

Figure 16.78. Electron micrograph of portions of two hepatic cells bounding a bile canaliculus with a prominent Golgi zone in the cell at the left. This animal had been treated experimentally and smooth endoplasmic reticulum (SER) is increased in amount (×10,850).

that are only moderately tight. Their organization is especially well seen in freeze-fracture preparations (Fig. 16.79).

Hepatic Cells

The hepatic cells which make up the hepatic plates are polyhedral in form and, under normal conditions, their boundaries are sharply defined. Each cell has a central nucleus with a distinct nuclear envelope and one or more prominent nucleoli. Multinucleate hepatic cells are occasionally seen, the usual variation being the binucleate condition.

Binucleate cells result from mitotic division of the nucleus of a mononucleate cell without accompanying division of the cytoplasm. Each of the two nuclei is of approximately normal size and possesses the normal (diploid) number of chromosomes; the cytoplasmic portion of the cell may be large. Large hepatic cells with either one or two unusually large nuclei also occur. These result from mitotic division of the above mentioned binucleate cells in which all of the chromosomes merge on one spindle, with the formation of either (*a*) two large mononucleate cells, each with an unusually large nucleus containing a tetraploid number of chromosomes, or (*b*) one large cell with two large tetraploid nuclei. Further divisions of this type may produce mononucleate cells with still larger nuclei having a further increase in chromosome number.

The mitochondria of the hepatic cells are spherical, rod-shaped, or filamentous, depending on the location of the cell within the lobule and on the functional state. The Golgi apparatus lies either near the edge of the cell beneath the bile canaliculus, or close to the nucleus. The cytoplasm contains clusters of free ribosomes plus ribosomes attached to the cisternae of rough endoplasmic reticulum. There are also numerous areas of smooth endoplasmic reticulum which becomes continuous in places with the rough reticulum (Fig. 16.80). Lysosomes are present, and another organelle known as a *microbody* or *peroxisome* is present. The peroxisomes vary in morphology in different species. In most species, but not in man, they have a dense core or nucleoid (Figs. 16.80 and 16.81). They contain oxidative enzymes, including urate oxidase and catalase. The urate oxidase is localized to the nucleoid and the absence of

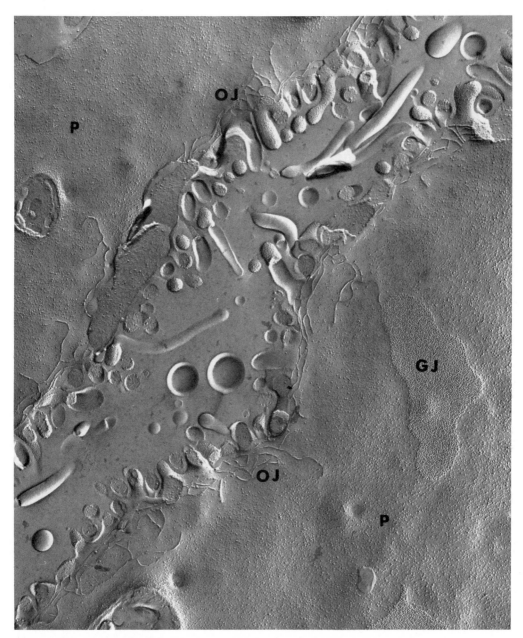

Figure 16.79. Freeze-fracture replica of mouse liver showing a bile canaliculus and adacent structures. Strands of occluding junctions (*OJ*) are apparent beneath the microvillar border and a gap junction (*GJ*) profile is seen at *right center*. The hepatocyte membranes fractured so as to reveal P fracture faces (*P*). Compare with Figure 16.78 (×35,000).

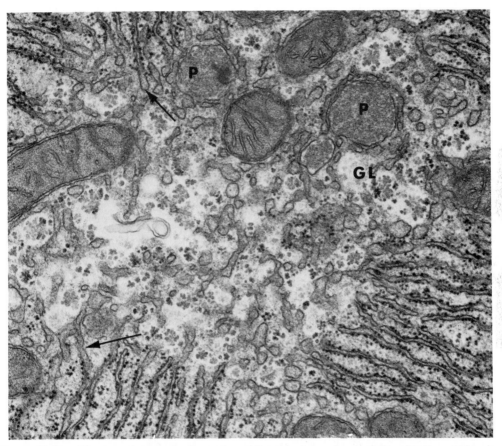

Figure 16.80. Electron micrograph of a portion of the cytoplasm of an hepatic cell in the rat showing continuity between rough endoplasmic reticulum and smooth endoplasmic reticulum (*arrows*). *P*, peroxisomes; *GL*, glycogen (×34,000).

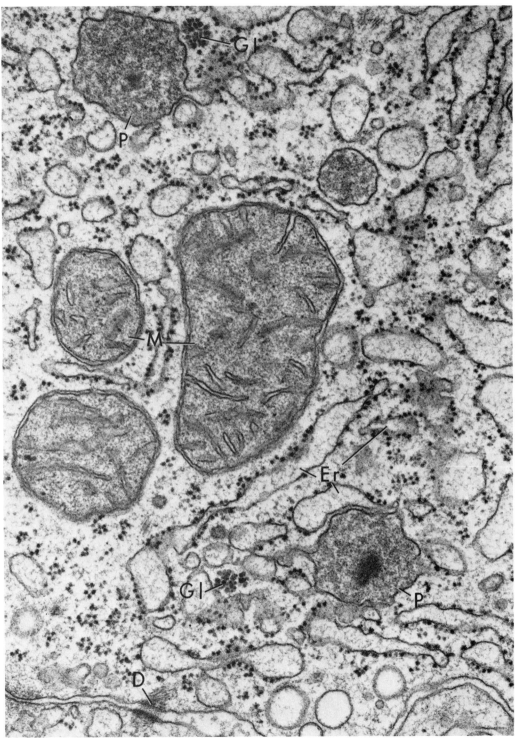

Figure 16.81. Electron micrograph showing peroxisomes (microbodies) in a liver parenchymal cell of a fetal rat. The peroxisomes (*P*) of the rat liver (and of most mammals other than man) contain electron dense cores (nucleoids) in which liver urate oxidase is localized. Outpouchings are seen at the surface of two of the peroxisomes present in the field illustrated. This suggests that new peroxisomes form either as buds from other peroxisomes or as vesicles derived from the smooth endoplasmic reticulum. *GL*, glycogen; *M*, mitochondria; *D*, desmosome; *Er*, rough endoplasmic reticulum (×50,000).

this component of the peroxisome in man is correlated with the lack of liver urate oxidase. The origin of these organelles is not entirely clear but they are thought to be involved in some manner with lipid metabolism. They were once believed to be continuous with the endoplasmic reticulum, from which they derived their constituent enzymes. Current evidence indicates, however, that at least the catalase is formed independently of the ER. The mechanism by which the enzymes enter the peroxisome is still not known.

Scattered throughout the cytoplasm in ordinary preparations are small clear areas. These represent areas of *glycogen* which can be seen with the light microscope only after appropriate methods of fixation and staining. Electron micrographs show glycogen in liver cells in the form of rosettes of dense granules (Figs. 16.77, 16.80 and 16.81). *Fat droplets* may also appear as inclusions in the cytoplasm, particularly after fasting or after ingestion of an excess of fats. The amount of fat which may be demonstrated in the hepatic cells varies inversely with the amount of glycogen. Pigment granules (bile pigments) are occasionally seen in the cytoplasm.

As in other gland cells, the appearance of the cytoplasm varies with the functional state of the cell. Both glycogen and the basophilic material are markedly reduced after a prolonged period of fasting, and they reaccumulate in the cytoplasm with refeeding. Glycogen is more abundant in the hepatic cells after digestion of a carbohydrate meal. It represents stored carbohydrate, which is returned to the blood as glucose when the needs of the body demand it.

In addition to the cell junctions associated with bile canaliculi already described, apposed liver cell membranes frequently have desmosomes and gap junctions. The latter are correlated with physiological evidence that hepatic cells are electrically coupled.

The classical liver lobule may be divided into three zones on the basis of structural and functional differences: an inner, hepatic zone around the central vein, an outer, portal zone at the periphery of the lobule and an intermediate zone between the central and peripheral regions. The mitochondria differ in appearance in the different zones, probably in relation to functional activity. The basophilic substance also differs in the different zones. The zones differ metabolically as exemplified by their storage and release of glycogen. When the livers of rats and mice are depleted of glycogen by prolonged fasting, feeding results in the deposition of glycogen in the peripheral region first, progressing centrally until the lobule is filled. After completion of the period of digestion, glycogen is usually given up from the peripheral region of the lobule first, leaving a central region with stored glycogen. Metabolic zonation is also describe for Rappaport's liver acinus. In either case, the areas most closely associated with the blood supply are the most active metabolically.

The membranes of the hepatic cells which border on the sinusoids show short, irregular microvilli (Figs. 16.76 and 16.77); in most areas the processes are covered by the lining cells of the sinusoids, but they occasionally protrude into the sinusoidal lumen.

Hepatic Sinusoids

The hepatic sinusoids make up the intralobular system of blood capillaries which course centripetally through the lobule and convey the blood from the interlobular branches of the portal vein and the hepatic artery to the central vein. They have relatively wide lumina, they anastomose irregularly and everywhere they separate the hepatic plates one from another. It thus follows that the hepatic cells have one or more surfaces always adjacent to blood sinusoids (Figs. 16.76 and 16.82).

The sinusoids appear to be lined by two morphologically recognizable types of cells. It has long been debated whether these constitute two separate cell types or are merely functional states of a single cell. The evidence now indicates that the sinusoids are lined primarily by *endothelial cells* similar to those of other blood vessels (Fig.

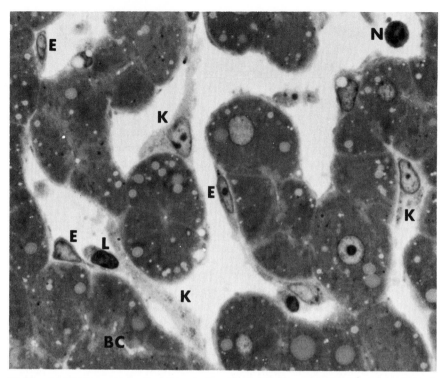

Figure 16.82. Light micrograph of a 1-μm section of monkey liver showing liver plates and sinusoids. The difference in morphology between endothelial cells (*E*) and Kupffer cells (*K*) can be seen. A lymphocyte (*L*) and a neutrophil (*N*) are also present in the sinusoidal lumen. A bile canaliculus is at lower left (*BC*) (×800).

16.82). The nucleus is dark and the cytoplasm is attenuated. In most mammals, including man, the lining cells form a discontinuous layer which is remarkable in that it is not underlain by a complete basal lamina (Fig. 16.77). The other principal sinusoidal cell has branching pseudopodial processes and is highly phagocytic. It is commonly called a *Kupffer cell* and its origin is from monocytes (Figs. 16.82 to 16.84). Kupffer cells normally lie on the luminal side of the endothelial cells and may extend processes through some of the endothelial discontinuities. However, they occasionally appear to be interposed between endothelial cells and thus may form a minor portion of the sinusoidal wall. Even more frequently they are seen to span the sinusoidal lumen, appearing stellate in shape (Fig. 16.82). Neither endothelial cells nor Kupffer cells develop obvious junctional complexes at their points of intercellular contact. The porosity of the sinusoidal lining is also enhanced by numerous fenestrations in the endothelial cells (Figs. 16.84 and 16.85). Intercellular gaps, cellular fenestrations and the lack of a complete basal lamina permit blood plasma to have direct access to the hepatic parenchymal cell surfaces. This has obvious advantages for efficiency in nutrient uptake and the release of synthesized products directly into the blood stream.

Perisinusoidal Space

Between the sinusoidal lining cells and the hepatic cells is a connective tissue space of variable dimensions. In early light microscopy this space was frequently exaggerated by the preparation techniques and it was termed the *space of Disse*. It is now recognized that the space is normally rather small, but nonetheless real. Besides the microvilli of hepatic cells it contains reticular

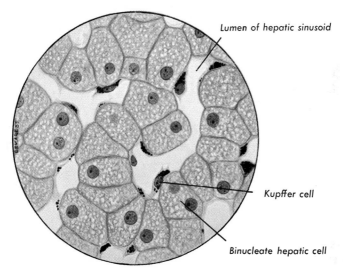

Lumen of hepatic sinusoid

Kupffer cell

Binucleate hepatic cell

Figure 16.83. Section of liver from a monkey which had received several intraperitoneal injections of trypan blue. Most of the Kupffer cells have taken in some of the dye by phagocytosis. Azocarmine and metanil yellow stain (×720).

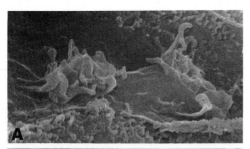

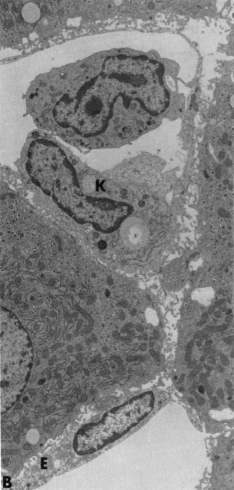

Figure 16.84. *A*, scanning electron micrograph of a Kupffer cell in mouse liver (×5400). *B*, transmission electron micrograph of a Kupffer cell (*K*) and endothelial cells (*E*) in rat liver. The Kupffer cell forms part of the true sinusoidal lining along part of its surface. The free cell in the upper sinusoid is believed to be a monocyte (×3700).

fibers and occasional perisinusoidal cells differing from either the endothelial or the Kupffer cells. The perisinusoidal cells often contain lipid droplets and have been referred to as *fat storage cells*. Their function is not well understood. Typical fibroblasts are not common in the perisinusoidal space, but still may be in sufficient numbers to account for the synthesis of the reticular fibers found in this space. Direct evidence that the endothelial cells give rise to the reticular fibers has not been obtained. However, there is evidence that hepatocytes may be capable of collagen synthesis, particularly type IV collagen. This suggests that the scanty basal lamina is synthesized at least in part by hepatocytes.

Connective Tissue

Ordinary sections of the human liver reveal scant amounts of connective tissue. The interlobular connective tissue concentrated in the portal areas has already been described. Silver stains and electron micrographs show that there is a framework of reticular (argyrophilic) fibers within each lobule (Fig. 16.86). They form a network which envelops each sinusoid and radiates outward from the region of the central vein. As mentioned previously these reticular fibers lie in the perisinusoidal space.

Lymphatics

The lymph vessels of the liver form a rich plexus in the capsule of Glisson and in its connective tissue septa within the gland. Lymph vessels enmesh the larger blood vessels and ducts, and there are anastomoses between lymphatics which surround the portal veins and those which surround hepatic veins. Anastomoses between lymphatics of neighboring portal canals enclose the hepatic lobules in a network of small lymph vessels but, so far as can be determined, no lymphatic vessels penetrate the lobules themselves. Since the lobules comprise the bulk of the liver tissue, it is puzzling that more lymph flows from the liver than from any other organ of the body. It has been postulated that the lymph is formed in the perisinusoidal space; this

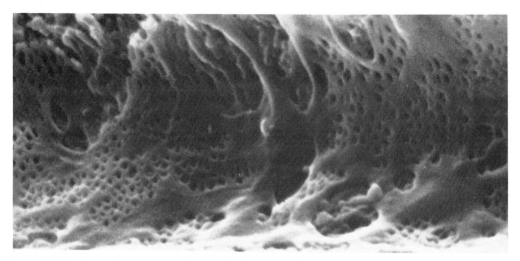

Figure 16.85. Scanning electron micrograph of part of a sinusoidal wall of mouse liver. Fenestrations of various sizes are obvious (×16,380).

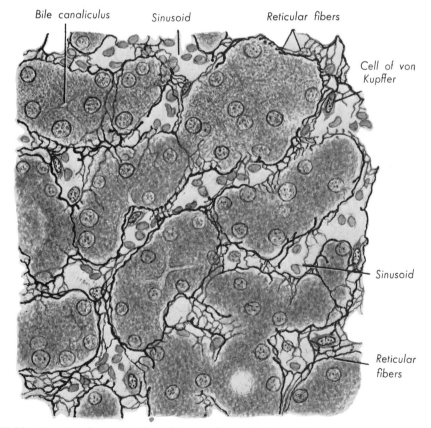

Bile canaliculus   Sinusoid   Reticular fibers

Cell of von Kupffer

Sinusoid

Reticular fibers

Figure 16.86. Drawing from a section of human liver, showing reticular tissue in a lobule. Reticular fibers do not extend through the lumen of the sinusoid, although tangential sections through the wall of the sinusoid may give this impression. Foot's silver technique (×700).

space should not, however, be confused with a lymphatic vessel as it is not an endothelium-lined space.

Nerve Supply

The nerves of the liver are mainly non-myelinated fibers of the sympathetic system. They accompany the blood vessels and bile ducts, around which they form plexuses. These plexuses give off fibers which terminate on the blood vessels and bile ducts but do not appear to penetrate the lobule.

Functions of the Liver

The exocrine function of the liver is concerned with the production of bile, which is carried by the system of bile ducts into the duodenum.

Bile is a product of the hepatic cells and is partly a secretion important in the absorption of fats and partly an excretion carrying off waste products which are eliminated with the feces. Among the constituents of bile are: bile acids, bile pigments, cholesterol, lecithin, neutral fats and soaps, traces of urea, and water and *bile salts*. The bile salts, as emulsifying agents, facilitate the absorption of fats in the intestine. They are themselves reabsorbed in part from the intestine and are again secreted by the hepatic cells. The *bile pigments* are derived from the breakdown of hemoglobin; this apparently does not take place in the liver, although the Kupffer cells may play a part. The bile pigments are removed from the blood by the liver and excreted in the bile as a waste product. Cholesterol is also excreted in the bile.

Claude Bernard was the first to show that the liver stores glycogen and gives it up as glucose. The liver not only stores reserve sugars, but it is essential for the transformations which are necessary before some of the sugars can be utilized by the body. Conversion of fats and perhaps also of proteins to carbohydrates is accomplished in the liver (*gluconeogenesis*). Through its diversified chemical processes, the liver is able to maintain a constant blood sugar level under widely different dietary conditions.

The liver has other important functions. It is involved in protein metabolism and is the chief site of deaminization of amino acids, with the production of urea as a byproduct. Fats are likewise metabolized and stored in the liver. Some of the plasma proteins (fibrinogen, prothrombin, albumin) are synthesized in the liver. The liver is also an important place of storage for many vitamins, chiefly A, D, B_2, B_3, B_4, B_{12} and K, which are essential to the body. The liver also plays an important role in the detoxification of a number of lipid soluble drugs, e.g., barbiturates. The enzymes which perform the detoxification are in smooth endoplasmic reticulum (Fig. 16.78). This organelle increases markedly on challenge of the liver with such drugs. The increased amount of smooth reticulum makes drug metabolism more efficient and is responsible for the development of drug tolerance. The same basic set of enzymes is involved with alcohol degradation and this overlap in function accounts for the potential danger of combining alcohol imbibition with certain kinds of drug therapy.

Regeneration of Liver

Whan a part of the liver is removed by operation or when there is partial destruction by toxic agents (chloroform, etc.), the organ regains its normal weight within a relatively short time. In the rat, surgical removal of as much as 75% of the gland is followed by complete weight restitution within one month. The repair is accomplished by mitotic multiplication of parenchymal cells throughout the remaining portion of the organ and by cell enlargement. Differentiation of new liver cells from budding interlobular bile ducts may also play a part. In restored liver tissue, there is an increased number of the mononucleated cells which have large nuclei containing a multiple number of chromosomes. These are produced by division of binucleated cells. There is also a general increase in nuclear size of all of the parenchymal cells.

Recent studies have shown that in rat, partial hepatectomy elicits a marked temporary reduction in communicating (gap) junctions between the remaining hepatocytes. Nevertheless, the degree of ionic coupling between those cells is not significantly altered. Furthermore, gap junctions are reassembled extremely rapidly after a lapse of 38 to 40 hours. This experimental system is proving to be useful for studies on the lability and mode of formation of vertebrate gap junctions.

The liver also variably regenerates after toxic injury. If the injury is singular and not immediately fatal, complete regeneration may be possible. If the toxic condition is chronic, the regeneration is only partial and gradual impairment of function usually ensues. Under these conditions normal lobulation is lost, there is an increase in fibrous tissue (fibrosis) and *cirrhosis of the liver* may eventually develop.

The Gall Bladder

The gall bladder is a hollow, pear-shaped organ lying obliquely on the inferior surface of the liver. It may be regarded as a diverticulum of the bile duct. It consists of a *fundus*, which is the blind end, a *body* and a *neck* which passes into the cystic duct.

The wall of the gall bladder is composed of three layers: *mucosa*, *muscularis* and an *adventitia* or *serosa*. The mucosa is thrown into numerous folds which divide the surface roughly into irregular polygonal areas (Fig. 16.87). The epithelium is composed of tall columnar cells with oval nuclei situated in the middle or the basal zones (Fig. 16.88). A thin, striated border can be seen on the apical surface of the cells. It is less prominent than that of the intestinal cells, so that it is seen well only with special preparation (Fig. 16.89) or by electron microscopy (Figs 16.90 and 16.91). Intercellular spaces occur between the epithelial cells (Figs. 16.90 and 16.91). These change in dimension in response to physiological activity in water absorption. The lamina propria consists of connective tissue containing extensive vascular plexuses and a few scattered muscle cells derived from the muscularis. Near the neck of the gall bladder, small tubuloalveolar glands occur in the mucosa.

Small diverticula of the mucosa which extend down into the muscular and peri-

muscular layers are known as the *Rokitansky-Aschoff sinuses*. Their epithelium is a continuation of the surface epithelium.

The muscular layer of the gall bladder is formed of interlacing bundles of smooth muscle fibers. Bundles of longitudinal fibers occur nearer the lamina propria, coursing the length of the bladder and curving over the fundus. The remainder of the muscle bundles, which form the greater part of the muscularis, are circularly disposed. Connective tissue, with an abundance of elastic fibers, occurs between the muscle bundles.

The external connective tissue layer is usually thick but shows wide individual differences. Just external to the muscularis, it consists of fibrous connective tissue sufficiently distinct to be designated the *perimuscular layer*. Outside this is a subserous layer of connective tissue containing blood and lymph vessels and nerves. On its free surface, the gall bladder is covered by the peritoneum; the connective tissue of its attached surface merges with that of the liver.

Lymph nodules occur in the wall of the gall bladder. One may also find duct-like structures, lined with epithelium, which have no connection with the lumen of the bladder, although they have occasionally been described as having connections with the bile ducts. These are known as *Luschka ducts* (Fig. 16.88). They are interpreted as aberrant embryonic bile ducts.

The gall bladder functions as a reservoir for the bile produced by the liver. By the reabsorption of large quantities of water and mineral salts through its mucosal layer, it also serves to concentrate the bile.

The Bile Ducts

There are three main ducts associated with the gall bladder. These are (*a*) the *cystic duct*, (*b*) the *hepatic duct*, and (*c*) the common bile duct (*ductus choledochus*). The hepatic duct conducts bile from the liver to a point where the cystic duct from the gall bladder meets with it and forms the common bile duct leading to the duodenum. The bile normally passes through the cystic duct into the gall bladder for concentration and storage. Contraction of the gall bladder

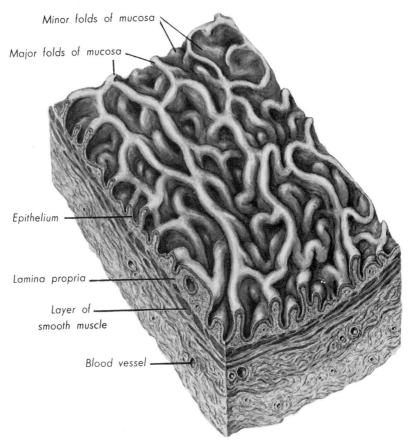

Minor folds of mucosa

Major folds of mucosa

Epithelium

Lamina propria

Layer of smooth muscle

Blood vessel

Figure 16.87. Low power, three-dimensional drawing of a portion of the wall of a human gall bladder (×24).

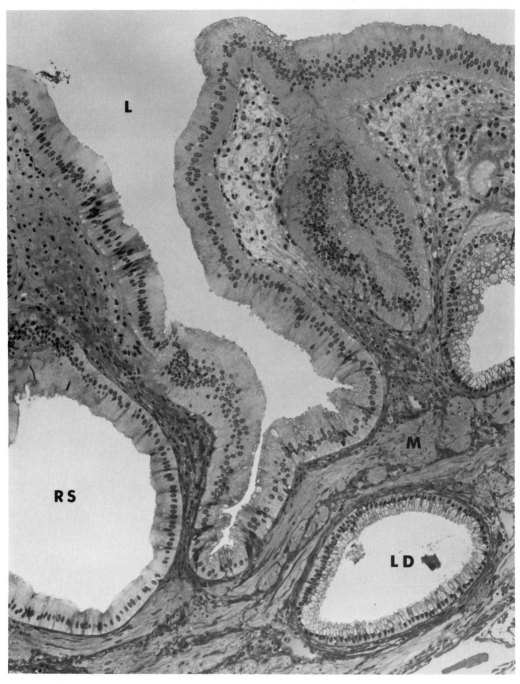

Figure 16.88. Light micrograph of a 1.5-μm section from gall bladder of the monkey. The luminal surface is lined with tall columnar epithelium. A mucosal diverticulum appears at the *lower left (RS)*. The space at the *lower right* lies in the muscular wall (*M*) and may represent a portion of a duct of Luschka. *L*, lumen; *M*, muscularis; *RS*, sinus of Rokitansky-Aschoff; *LD*, Luschka duct (×140).

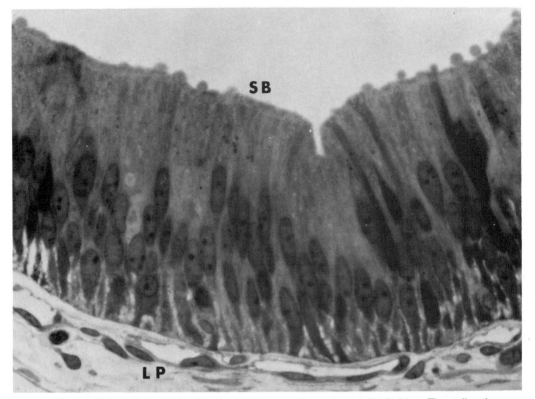

Figure 16.89. Light micrograph of a 1-μm section of monkey gall bladder. The tall columnar epithelium shows intercellular spaces basally and a striated border at the apex. *SB*, striated border, *LP*, lamina propria (×1,100).

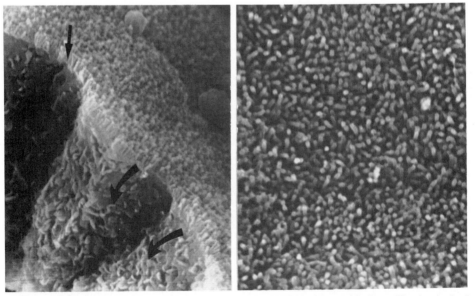

Figure 16.90. Scanning electron micrographs of mouse gall bladder epithelium. The luminal microvillous border is apparent at left (*straight arrow*) and the mucosa has been broken to reveal lateral cell surfaces with interdigitating folds (*curved arrows*). At *right* is a higher magnification view of the luminal microvilli (*Left*, ×5280; *right*, ×12,900).

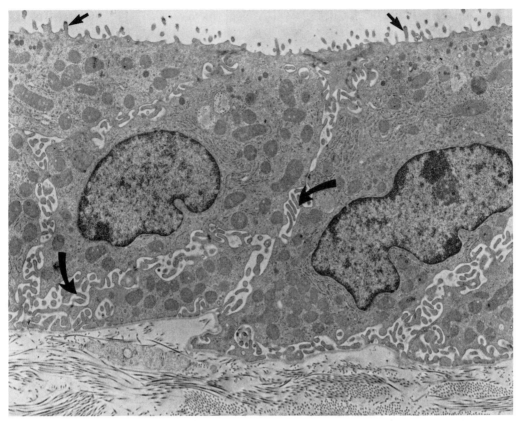

Figure 16.91. Transmission electron micrograph of a portion of the same mouse gall bladder seen in Figure 16.90. The basolateral interdigitating folds (*curved arrows*) and apical microvilli (*plain arrows*) are apparent. The epithelial cells have a cuboidal rather than columnar shape because the organ was full of bile at the time of fixation (×7750).

forces the bile back through the cystic duct and thence through the common bile duct to the intestine. As the ductus choledochus passes obliquely through the wall of the duodenum, it lies side by side with the ductus pancreaticus. In their course through the submucosa of the duodenum, the associated pancreatic and bile ducts are surrounded by layers of smooth muscle which form the *sphincter of Oddi*. A portion of this muscular sheath which encircles only the bile duct is known as the *sphincter choledochus*. While this sphincter remains contracted (as for example during fasting), pressure is maintained in the duct system, and bile from the liver is forced into the gall bladder for storage. Upon the ingestion of food, especially fats or proteins, the sphincter of Oddi relaxes, the gall bladder is stimulated to contract and the bile traverses the cystic duct and common bile duct to the duodenum.

The ducts are lined with a columnar epithelium similar to that of the gall bladder. Most of the bile ducts have epithelial-lined outpouchings which simulate irregularly distributed glands. Mitosis of epithelial cells occurs chiefly in these outpouchings, and the cells move upward to replace worn-out cells of the luminal surface much like the replacement cells in the intestine by mitosis of cells in the crypts. After removal of the gall bladder surgically, the common bile duct expands and assumes some of the storage functions of the gall bladder. The muscularis of the ducts is not as prominent as in the gall bladder. The arrangement of muscle fibers into layers is not definite, but they tend to be circularly arranged in the hepatic duct and longitudinally disposed in the cystic and in the common bile duct.

DEVELOPMENT OF THE DIGESTIVE SYSTEM

In the development of the digestive system, all of the germ layers are involved. Mesoderm and endoderm are the layers most involved, however, as the ectoderm forms the lining of only a part of the mouth, the epithelium of some of the salivary glands and a part of the anal canal.

The primary gut, composed of endoderm and its surrounding mesoderm, is at first a *blind tube*, except for its temporary opening to the yolk stalk. Connections to the exterior occur later by oral and anal invaginations of ectoderm which extend inward and open into the ends of the hitherto imperforate gut. The epithelial lining of the gut and the parenchyma of all glands (except some salivary) connected with it are derived from endoderm. The muscle, the connective tissue and the mesothelium of the serosa are developed from mesoderm.

The mesodermal elements show little variation throughout the gut, the peculiarities of the several anatomical divisions being dependent mainly on special differentiation of the endoderm (epithelium). Beneath the endodermal cells is a narrow layer of loosely arranged tissue which later separates into lamina propria, muscularis, mucosae and submucosa. Outside this, a broader mesodermal band of firmer structure represents the future muscularis.

The *stomach* first appears as a spindle-shaped dilation about the end of the first month. Its endodermal cells, which had consisted of a single layer, increase in number and arrange themselves in short, cylindrical groups. These are the first traces of tubular glands. They increase in length and extend downward into the mesodermal tissue. The cells lining the gastric glands are apparently alike before about the fourth month when differentiation into chief cells and parietal cells take place.

In the *intestines* a proliferation of the epithelium and of the underlying connective tissue results in the formation of *villi*. These appear about the 10th week, in both small and large intestines. In the former they increase in size, while in the latter they atrophy and ultimately disappear. The simple tubular glands of the intestines develop in a manner similar to those of the stomach.

The mesothelium of the serosa is derived from the mesodermal cells of the primitive body cavity.

The *development of the larger glands* connected with the digestive tract takes place in a manner similar to the formation of the simple tubular glands. All originate as extensions of endodermal cords into the surrounding splanchnic mesodermal tissue. From the lower ends of these cords, branches extend in all directions to form the complex systems of tubules found in the compound glands.

The *salivary glands*, being developed from the oral cavity, originate as similar invaginations of both ectodermal and endodermal tissue.

As noted earlier the *pancreas* arises as two separate outgrowths from the embryonic duodenum. The dorsal outgrowth forms a part of the head and all of the body and tail of the adult pancreas. The ventral outgrowth forms the remainder of the head of the pancreas. The duct of the ventral outgrowth enlarges to form the main pancreatic duct (duct of Wirsung) which drains the acini derived from both outgrowths. A small accessory duct often persists at the site of the dorsal outgrowth. The islets of Langerhans develop as buds from a system of fine tubules which are derived from the ducts and which form a network around the ducts. Many of the islets become secondarily detached, but some of them retain their attachment to the tubules in the adult.

The *liver* and *gallbladder* develop during the third week of gestation from an evagination of endodermal epithelium of the foregut into the mesenchyume of the *septum transversum*. The result of interaction of the epithelial bud with this special mesenchymal bed differs significantly from what occurs with pancreas and salivary glands. The primary liver diverticulum differentiates into the gall bladder, cystic duct, and common bile ducts. Solid cords of epithelial cells proliferate from the cranial pole of the diverticulum into a rapidly expanding capillary network (from the vitelline veins) in the septum transversum. The vascular channels are subdivided by the epithelial cords establishing anastomotic *sinusoids* intimately associated with the cords of *hepatic parenchymal cells*. The adult pattern of single-cell-thick anastomotic sheets of hepatic cells (hepatic plates) intermingled with sinusoidal spaces is not fully formed until after birth. The mesenchyme of the septum transversum forms the connective tissue stroma and capsule as well as the mesothelial covering of the adult liver. The connective tissue area lying between sinusoids and hepatocytes (*perisinusoidal space*) becomes the major site of hemopoiesis in the second trimester of development.

Intrahepatic biliary channels begin to appear by six weeks of development; bile canaliculi arise as specializations of extracellular space between hapatocytes. Intrahepatic bile ducts and ductules seem to be derived by dedifferentiation of hepatic plates lying adjacent to developing portal canals. Bile is secreted quite early and appears in both the gall bladder and the duodenum by 4 to 4½ months of gestation.

During the differentiation of extrahepatic bile ducts, the original epithelial diverticulum loses it lumen and then recanalizes. Failure of proper canalization is a primary cause of *congenital biliary atresia*. A secondary form of biliary atresia may result from improper differentiation of ductule connections between canaliculi and intrahepatic bile ducts.

References

Beams HW, King RL: The origin of binucleate and large mononucleate cells in the liver of the rat. *Anat Rec* 83:281–297, 1942.

Bjerknes M, Cheng H: The stem cell zone of the small intestinal epithelium, I-V. *Am J Anat* 160:51–112, 1981.

Boas A, Wilson TH: Cellular localization of gastric intrinsic factor in the rat. *Am J Physiol* 206:783–786, 1963.

Cardell RR, Jr, Badenhausen S, Porter KR: Intestinal triglyceride absorption in the rat. An electron microscopical study. *J Cell Biol* 34:123–155, 1967.

Cheng H, Leblond CP: Origin, differentiation and renewal of the four main epithelial cell types in the mouse small intestine. V. Unitarian theory of the origin of the four epithelial cell types. *Am J Anat* 141:537–562, 1974.

Cohen P J: The renewal areas of the common bile duct epithelium. *Anat Rec* 150:237–242, 1964.

De Duve C: Glucagon. The hyperglycemic-glycogenolytic factor of the pancreas. Lancet 2:99–104, 1953.

Dieglemann RF, Guzelian PS, Gay R, Gay S: Collagen formation by the hepatocyte in primary monolayer culture and in vivo. *Science* 219:1343–1345, 1983.

Dockray GJ: Evolutionary relationships of the gut hormones. *Fed Proc* 38:2295–2301, 1979.

Eckman CA, Holmgren H: The effect of alimentary factors on liver glycogen rhythm and the distribution of glycogen in the liver lobule. *Anat Rec* 104:189–216, 1949.

Elias H: A re-examination of the structure of the mammalian liver. I. Parenchymal architecture. *Am J Anat* 84:311–333; II. The hepatic lobule and its relation to the vascular biliary system. *Am J Anat* 85:379–456, 1949.

Erlandson, S. L. Types of pancreatic islet cells and their immunocytochemical identification. *Int Acad Pathol Monogr* 21:140–155, 1980.

Friend DS: The fine structure of Brunner's glands in the mouse. *J Cell Biol* 25:563–576, 1965.

Gale RP, Sparkes RS, Goloe DW: Bone marrow origin of hepatic macrophages (Kupffer cells) in humans. *Science* 201:937–938, 1978.

Higgins GM, Anderson RM: Experimental pathology of the liver. I. Restoration of the liver of the white rat following partial surgical removal. *Arch Pathol* 12:186–202, 1931.

Hirokawa N, Tilney LG, Fujiwara K, Heuser JE: Organization of actin, myosin, and intermediate filaments in the brush border of intestinal epithelial cells. *J Cell Biol* 94:425–443, 1982.

Hoedemaker PJ, Abels J, Wachters JJ, Arends A, Nieweg HO: Investigations about the site of production of Castle's gastric intrinsic factor. *Lab Invest* 13:1394–1399, 1964.

Hoedemaker PJ, Ito S: Ultrastructural localization of gastric parietal cell antigen with peroxidase-coupled antibody. *Lab Invest* 22:184–188, 1970.

Hunt TE, Hunt EA: Radioautographic study of proliferation in the stomach of the rat using thymidine-H[3] and compound 48/80[1,2]. *Anat Rec* 142:505–517, 1962.

Ito S: The enteric surface coat on intestinal microvilli. *J Cell Biol* 27:475–491, 1965.

Ito T, Nemoto M: Über die Kupfferschen Sternzellen und die "Fettspeicherungszellen" ("fat storing cells") in der Blutkapillarenwand der menschlichen Leber. *Folia Anat Jpn* 24:243–258, 1952.

Johnson LR: Gastrointestinal hormones and their functions. *Annu Rev Physiol* 39:135–158, 1977.

Jones AL, Fawcett DW: Hypertrophy of the agranular

endoplasmic reticulum in hamster liver induced by phenobarbital (with a review of the functions of this organelle in liver). *J Histochem Cytochem* 14:215–232, 1966.

Kagnoff MF: Immunology of the digestive system. In Johnson LR (ed): *Physiology of the Gastrointestinal Tract*, vol II. New York, Raven Press, 1981, pp 1337–1359.

Kaye GI, Wheeler HO, Whitlock RT, Lane N: Fluid transport in rabbit gall bladder. A combined physiological and electron microscope study. *J Cell Biol* 30:237–268, 1966.

Kraehenbuhl JP, Campiche MA: Early stages of intestinal absorption of specific antibodies in the newborn. *J Cell Biol* 42:345–365, 1969.

Ladman AJ, Padykula HA, Strauss EW: A morphological study of fat transport in the normal human jejunum. *Am J Anat* 112:389–419, 1963.

Lechago J, Bencosme S: The endocrine elements of the digestive system. *Int Rev Exp Pathol* 12:119–201, 1973.

Legg PG, Wood RL: New observations on microbodies. A cytochemical study on CPIB-treated rat liver. *J Cell Biol* 45:118–129, 1970.

Madara JL, Trier JS: Structural abnormalities of jejunal epithelial cell membranes in celiac sprue. *Lab Invest* 43:254–261, 1980.

Madara JL, Trier JS, Neutra MR: Structural changes in the plasma of epithelial cells in human and monkey small intestine. *Gastroenterology* 78:963–975, 1980.

Madara JL, Trier JS: Structure and permeability of goblet cell tight junctions in rat small intestine. *J Memb Biol* 66:145–157, 1982.

Meyer DJ, Yancey SB, Revel J-P: Intercellular communication in normal and regenerating rat liver: a quantitative analysis. *J Cell Biol* 91:505–523, 1981.

Moog F: The lining of the small intestine. *Sci Am* 245:154–176, 1981.

Owen RL, Jones AI: Epithelial cell specialization within human Peyer's patches: an ultrastructural study of intestinal lymphoid follicles. *Gastroenterology* 66:189–203, 1974.

Palay SL, Revel J-P: The morphology of fat absorption. In Meng H C (ed): *Lipid Transport*. Springfield, Ill. Charles C Thomas, 1964.

Rappaport AM, Borowy ZJ, Lougheed WM, Lotti WN: Subdivision of hexagonal liver lobules into a structural and functional unit. Role in hepatic physiology and pathology. *Anat Rec* 119:11–34, 1954.

Rappaport AM: Acinar units and the pathophysiology

of liver. In Rouiller C (ed): *The Liver; Morphology, Biochemistry, Physiology*, vol 1. New York, Academic Press, 1963, pp 265–328.

Reiser R, Bryson MJ, Carr MJ, Kuiker KA: The intestinal absorption of triglycerides. *J Biol Chem* 194:131–138, 1952.

Scott DB: Recent contributions in dental histology by use of the electron microscope. *Int Dent J* 4:64–95, 1953.

Selzman HM, Liebelt RA: Paneth cell granules of mouse intestine. *J Cell Biol* 15:136–139, 1962.

Senior JR: Intestinal absorption of fats. *J Lipid Res* 5:495–521, 1964.

Solcia E, Capella C, Vassallo G, Buffa R: Endocrine cells of the gastric mucosa. *Int Rev Cytol* 42:223–286, 1975.

Spicer SS, Staley MW, Wetzel MG, Wetzel BK: Acid mucosubstance and basic protein in mouse Paneth cells. *J Histochem Cytochem* 15:225–242, 1967.

Strauss EW: Electron microscopic study of intestinal fat absorption *in vitro* from mixed micelles containing monoolein, and bile salt. *J Lipid Res* 7:307–323, 1966.

Sulkin NM: A study of the nucleus in the normal and hyperplastic liver of the rat. *Am J Anat* 73:107–125, 1943.

Trotter N: Electron opaque, lipid-containing bodies in mouse liver at early intervals afer partial hepatectomy and sham operation. *J Cell Biol* 25:41–55, 1965.

Walker WA: Antigen binding by the gut. *Arch Dis Child* 53:527–531, 1978.

Weinstock M, Leblond CP: Synthesis, migration and release of precursor collagen by odontoblasts as visualized by radioautography after H^3-proline administration. *J Cell Biol* 60:92–127, 1974.

Wilson JW, Leduc EH: Role of cholangioles in restoration of the liver of the mouse after dietary injury. *J Pathol Bacteriol* 76:441–450, 1958.

Wisse E: Observations on the fine structure and peroxidase cytochemistry of normal rat liver Kupffer cells. *J Ultrastruct Res* 46:393–426, 1974.

Wisse, E: Kupffer cell reactions in rat liver under various conditions as observed in the electron microscope. *J Ultrastruct Res* 46:499–520, 1974.

Wisse E, Knock DL (eds): Kupfer cells and other liver sinusoidal cells. In *Proceedings of the International Kupffer Cell Symposium*. Amsterdam, Elsevier/North Holland, 1977.

Yamada E: The fine structure of the gall bladder epithelium of the mouse. *J Biophys Biochem Cytol* 1:445–458, 1955.

Chapter 17

THE RESPIRATORY SYSTEM

The evolution of larger and complex terrestrial vertebrates has necessitated elaboration of an efficient, internalized air-blood gaseous exchange mechanism—the lungs. These and their associated complex of airways have evolved through diverticular development from the digestive tube. Collectively these are termed the respiratory system. During embryogenesis the system develops, largely in tree-like branching fashion, from the foregut, giving rise to two main divisions. These are:(a) an *air conducting division* composed, in sequence, of the nasal cavity, nasopharynx, oropharynx (which serves for conduction of air as well as food), larynx, trachea, bronchi and bronchioles, and (b) a *respiratory division* specialized for the exchanges of gases between air and blood. The latter is composed of respiratory bronchioles, alveolar ducts, alveolar sacs and alveoli. These divisons of the respiratory system perform their functions with the aid of a ventilation mechanism that includes the rib cage, the intercostal muscles, the diaphragm and the elastic tissue of the lungs.

THE NASAL CAVITY AND NASOPHARYNX
Nasal Cavity

The nasal cavity extends from the nares (nostrils) to the choanae, through which it opens into the nasopharynx. The cavity of the nose is divided into lateral halves or *fossae* by a median cartilaginous and bony septum. The inferior region of each fossa is somewhat expanded and is named the *vestibule* (Fig. 17.1). This leads into the major cavity, which is named the respiratory region in contrast with the olfactory region in the upper part of each fossa, which has receptor cells for the sense of smell.

The medial wall of each fossa (the septum) is smooth, but the lateral wall has an irregular contour because of the presence of horizontal scroll-shaped structures, the *conchae* (Figs. 17.1 and 17.2). Each concha is attached along its upper margin to the lateral wall, and the space beneath each concha is known as a *meatus*. The lacrimal duct and some of the nasal sinuses open into the meatuses.

The main current of air passing through the nose comes in contact with the mucosa of the septum and the medial surfaces of the conchae. Therefore, these surfaces are subjected to more cooling and drying than are the less exposed surfaces of the meatuses and the even less exposed mucous membranes of the sinuses.

The nasal passages function for the conduction of air and also as efficient air conditioning and filtering units. By the numerous blood vessels beneath the epithelium of some areas, the inhaled air is warmed before being transmitted to the lungs. By the mucous and serous glands, the moisture content of the air is maintained at a proper value and the epithelium itself is protected from excessive drying. The mucous coat over the epithelium, combined with ciliary action, traps a portion of the particulate matter of the inspired air and moves it to the oropharynx to be expectorated or swallowed.

The lining of the anterior part of the vestibule is similar to the epidermis of the nose. However, it has long thick hairs and associated sebaceous glands. Sweat glands are also present. The junction of the anterior part of the vestibule with the major or respiratory region of the nasal cavity is known as a transitional zone. The latter has stratified squamous epithelium like that of the anterior part of the vestibule,

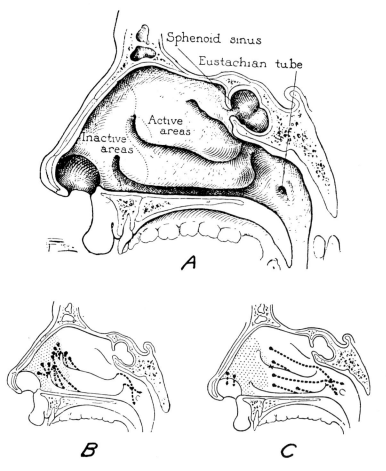

Figure 17.1.   Lateral wall of right nasal fossa and nasal pharynx. The superior, middle and inferior nasal conchae are seen, together with the opening of the sphenoid sinus into the sphenoethmoidal recess above the superior nasal concha. The right frontal sinus opening, which opens usually into the middle meatus in back of the middle concha, is not seen. *A*, the areas of the lateral wall where ciliary movements are active and relatively inactive. *B*, the course of mucous drainage of the inactive area. *C*, the course of mucous drainage of the active area. (After Hilding AC: The physiology of drainage of nasal mucus. *Arch Otolaryngol* 15:92–100; 16:9–17, 1932.)

Ciliated pseudostratified
columnar epithelium

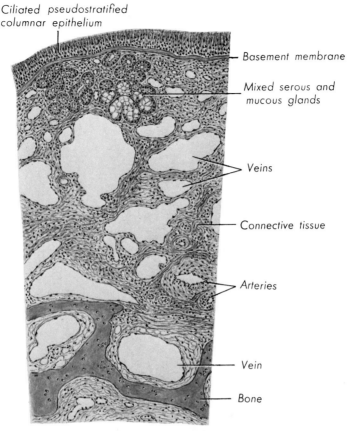

- Basement membrane

- Mixed serous and
  mucous glands

- Veins

- Connective tissue

- Arteries

- Vein

- Bone

Figure 17.2. Drawing of a section through the medial portion of an inferior nasal concha of a woman 47 years of age. Blood which filled the veins is not shown. (×67).

but it lacks sweat glands, sebaceous glands and hair follicles. It has mixed mucous and serous glands like those of the respiratory region.

The *respiratory region* is lined by a ciliated pseudostratified columnar epithelium which is the characteristic type for the conducting division of the respiratory system. In the more exposed areas, the epithelium is thick, goblet cells are numerous and the basement membrane is prominent (Fig. 17.3) by reason of a thick lamina reticularis. In the meatuses, the epithelium is thinner, goblet cells are fewer and the basement membrane is not prominent. Intraepithelial glands (mucous crypts) are present in a few individuals. These glands are depressions in the epithelium and are lined by a continuous layer of goblet cells.

The *olfactory mucosa* occupies a small area in the upper part of the respiratory region. For details of the structure of the olfactory region, see Chapter 22.

The nasal epithelium changes its character with increased ventilation. If all of the air is made to pass through one side of the nose by occluding the other nostril, the epithelium of the side subjected to the increased ventilation at first hypertrophies and then changes by metaplasia to a stratified squamous type.

The lamina propria contains numerous mucous and serous glands, particularly in the more exposed regions. Lymphocytes are usually present in both the epithelium and the lamina propria (Fig. 17.3).

The lamina propria of the nasal mucosa is quite vascular everywhere, but on the

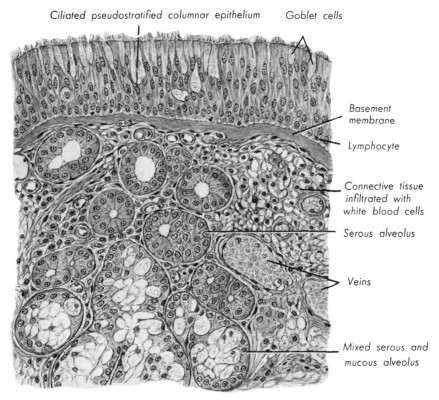

Ciliated pseudostratified columnar epithelium   Goblet cells

Basement membrane

Lymphocyte

Connective tissue infiltrated with white blood cells

Serous alveolus

Veins

Mixed serous and mucous alveolus

Figure 17.3. Drawing of a section through the epithelium and subjacent part of the lamina propria of inferior nasal concha. Human, 49 years old, with no history of nasal inflammation (×286).

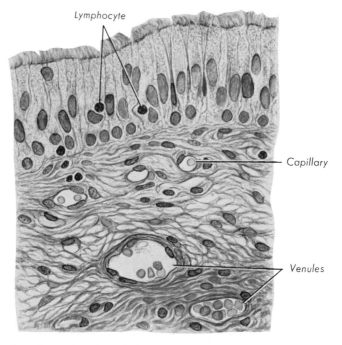

Lymphocyte

Capillary

Venules

Figure 17.4. Drawing of a section through the mucous membrane of maxillary sinus of man (×665).

medial surfaces of the middle and inferior conchae, and to a degree on the apposed surface of the septum, it is so vascular as to be distinctive. There are many large veins (Fig. 17.2) which may become engorged with surprising rapidity. With their engorgement, the mucosa becomes swollen and turgid, obstructing the flow of air through the nasal cavities, e.g., in allergic reactions.

The *paranasal sinuses*—maxillary, ethmoid, frontal, sphenoid—are lined by an epithelium which is continuous with that of the nasal passages. It is a pseudostratified columnar ciliated epithelium (Fig. 17.4), but is only about half as thick as that which lines the nose, having two or three rows of nuclei instead of four or five as in the nasal epithelium. Goblet cells and glands are also less numerous. In contrast with the nasal and tracheal epithelium, the basement membrane is very thin. The lamina propria is thin and is attached to the periosteum.

Nasopharynx

In the *nasopharynx*, both stratified squamous and pseudostratified ciliated columnar epithelia are found. The distribution of these two types here and in the other respiratory passages is correlated with the attrition to which the surface is subjected. When surfaces are frequently brought in contact with each other, they are lined by stratified squamous epithelium. Those passages which usually remain open are lined by pseudostratified epithelium. Since, in the occlusion of the upper part of the nasopharynx from the oropharynx, the soft palate and its appendage (the uvula) are brought in contact with the posterior wall of the nasopharynx, these surfaces are lined by stratified squamous epithelium.

In the deeper stratum of the subepithelial connective tissue of the posterior and lateral walls of the pharynx, there is a layer of elastic tissue; near the juncture with the esophagus, it disappears. In the superior lateral region, but not elsewhere in the pharynx, a submucosa can be distinguished beneath the elastic stratum.

Glands are present throughout the naso-

pharynx. In the regions covered by stratified squamous epithelium, they are mucous and lie beneath the elastic layer. In the other areas, they are mixed serous and mucous, as in the other parts of the respiratory passages, and they lie more superficially.

Lymphatic tissue is especially abundant in the superior part of the nasopharynx. In addition to the general lymphatic infiltration of the connective tissue, there are, in the posterior wall, aggregations of lymph nodules known as the *pharyngeal tonsils*. Lymphatic aggregations also occur behind the openings of the Eustachian tubes, forming the *tubal tonsils*.

The *muscle* of the pharynx, which is striated, is deficient near the base of the skull.

Ciliary Action

The epithelium lining the paranasal sinuses, nasal passages and nasopharynx is coated with a mucous film. The cilia lie mostly underneath the mucous film. The viscosity of the mucous coat would greatly hinder the movement of cilia if it were to fill the interstices between them. In fact, the watery proteinaceous secretions of serous glands provide the medium that enables the cilia to remain motile. Since the cilia of the paranasal sinuses beat toward the openings of these cavities into the nose, and since the cilia on the epithelium lining the nose and nasopharynx beat toward the oropharynx, there is a continuous movement of this mucous coat toward the oropharynx. The surfaces are thus freed of particulate matter that has impinged on and adhered to the mucous covering. In the posterior three-fourths of the nose, the movement is more rapid than it is in the anterior part, which has led to the characterization of these two portions as active and inactive parts. The path of movement of the mucus is shown in Figure 17.1.

THE LARYNX

The wall of the larynx consists of a mucosa, a poorly defined submucosa, a series of irregularly shaped cartilages connected by joints of relatively dense fibroelastic tissue and a group of intrinsic skeletal muscles which act upon the cartilages.

Each lateral wall of the larynx has two prominent folds, between which is a deep recess or *ventricle*. The superior pairs of folds, the *ventricular folds*, are also known as the false vocal cords; the inferior pair, the *vocal folds*, are the true vocal cords. The *epiglottis* is a broad, flat structure projecting upward from the anterior wall of the larynx. During swallowing, there is active constriction of the pharyngeal wall, with a depression of the epiglottis and an upward movement of the larynx, trachea, and pharynx. The latter movement plays an important role in closure of the *glottis*, preventing food from entering the larynx and trachea.

The lidlike action of the epiglottis appears relatively unimportant, inasmuch as surgical removal of the tip of the epiglottis does not interfere with swallowing.

Two types of epithelium line the walls of the larynx, pseudostratified ciliated columnar and stratified squamous. These are distributed in accordance with the principle discussed in connection with the nasopharynx. At the juncture of these two types of epithelium, a third type—ciliated stratified columnar—is frequently present (Fig. 17.5). The wall of the aperture of the larynx, including the epiglottis down nearly as far as its tubercle or cushion, is lined by stratified squamous epithelium. This is succeeded by the ciliated pseudostratified type

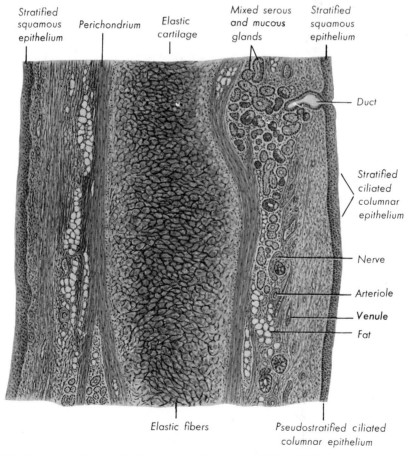

Figure 17.5. Drawing of the epiglottis of a boy 13 years old. The middle part of the free portion, cut in a sagittal plane, is illustrated. The lingual surface is at *left*. Stained with elastin H, Delafield's hematoxylin and eosin (×45).

that lines the remainder of the laryngeal wall, except for the vocal folds, which have the stratified squamous variety.

The lamina propria is rich in elastic fibers. It is infiltrated with lymphocytes, and lymphatic nodules occur in the stroma surrounding the ventricles. There is no sharp demarcation between the mucosa and the submucosa. The latter is structurally less dense and more cellular than the lamina propria. Over the vocal folds and epiglottis, the mucosa is more closely adherent to the underlying framework than it is in the other parts of the larynx. Mixed glands are present except in the vocal folds and are especially numerous in the ventricular folds (false vocal cords).

Most of the cartilages composing the framework of the larynx are hyaline. The *epiglottic*, the *corniculate* and the *cuneiform cartilages* are elastic, and this variety of cartilage is said also to occur inconstantly

in the apex and vocal process of each arytenoid cartilage. Calcification in the *thyroid* and *cricoid cartilages* begins in males during the second decade of life and at a somewhat later period in females.

THE TRACHEA AND CHIEF BRONCHI

The layers composing the larynx continue, with certain modifications, into the trachea and bronchi. The chief changes are in the cartilaginous framework and musculature (Fig. 17.6).

The trachea and chief bronchi are lined by pseudostratified columnar ciliated epithelium which rests on a distinct basement membrane (Figs. 4.21, 17.7, and 17.8). Several types of cells can be identified. The tall *ciliated columnar* cells are the most numerous. *Goblet cells* are fairly numerous and exhibit the characteristics already described in Chapter 4. Nonciliated columnar cells (brush cells) which have microvilli

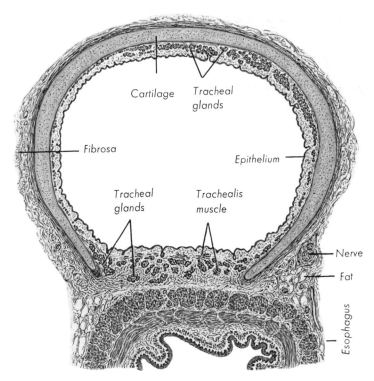

Figure 17.6.   Drawing of a transverse section through midregion of trachea and adjacent part of esophagus. The section is through a cartilage ring. Woman, 35 years old (×5).

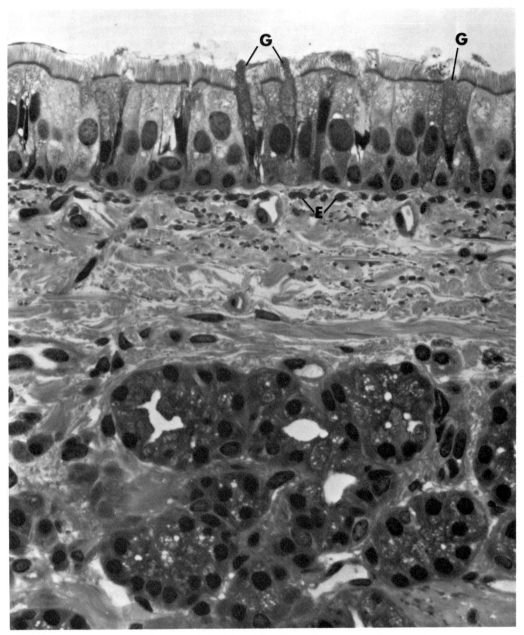

Figure 17.7. Light micrograph of transverse section through mucosa and submucosa of monkey trachea. The pseudostratified epithelium with cilia and goblet cells (G) is underlain by a basement membrane, elastic fibers (E), and bundles of collagen. A mixed gland lies in the submucosa at the bottom of the field (×610).

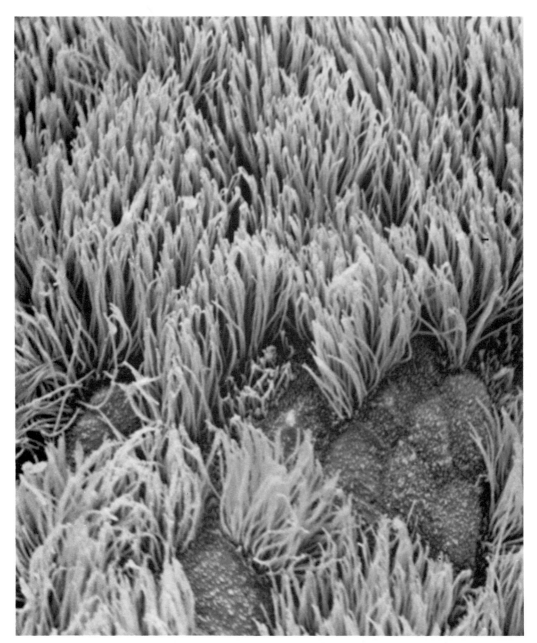

Figure 17.8. Scanning electron micrograph of lumenal surface of human tracheal epithelium. Most of the surface cells are ciliated. Nonciliated cells with short microvilli presumably represent goblet cells (×4500). (Courtesy of Drs. A. Zaitsu and M. Miyoshi.)

may represent an inactive stage of the goblet cell (Fig. 17.8). There are a number of *short cells*, more or less pyramidal in shape, which rest on the basal lamina but do not extend to the lumen as do the other cell types. The lamina propria contains many elastic fibers, which are especially numerous in the deeper zone. The submucosa consists of loose connective tissue and contains fat and mixed glands, the latter often penetrating into or even through the muscle layer (Fig. 17.6).

The framework of the trachea and chief bronchi consists of a series of regularly spaced, C-shaped hyaline cartilages. The open segment points posteriorly. The cartilages vary in width and thickness; their ends may bifurcate, and they may have bars that fuse with an adjoining cartilage. The lowest tracheal cartilage (carinal cartilage) especially varies in shape.

A fibroelastic layer, which blends with the perichondrium of the cartilages, extends across their open segments and connects adjacent cartilages to each other, thus forming a tube. Posteriorly, in the cartilage-free zone, smooth muscle is imbedded in the fibroelastic layer. Most of these muscle fibers run transversely. Some, however, run longitudinally and obliquely. The transverse fibers attach largely to the inner surface of the ends of the cartilage rings and to a lesser extent to the intervening fibroelastic layer. This is often called the "trachealis" muscle.

Localized areas of stratified squamous epithelium have been described in the trachea and bronchi of individuals suffering from chronic coughs. This change to a stratified squamous type of epithelium is possibly because of the capacity of the pseudostratified epithelium of the respiratory passages to undergo metaplasia and to change to the more resistant type when subjected to attrition, as has been pointed out in the description of the nasopharynx.

THE LUNGS

The lungs are paired structures which, together with the mediastinum, fill the thoracic cavity. On the right side, the lung is divided by two deep clefts into three lobes; on the left side, it is divided by a single deep cleft into two lobes. Entering the *hilus*, and forming the *root* of each lung, are a *bronchus*, a *pulmonary artery* and *vein*, *bronchial arteries* and *veins*, lymphatics and nerves. These structures are embedded in connective tissue.

The surface of the lungs is covered by a serous membrane, the *visceral pleura*, which dips into the interlobar fissures and covers the interlobar surfaces. At the hilus, the visceral pleura becomes continuous with the *parietal pleura*.

The surface of the lungs is pinkish in early life but later become grayish in color as a result of the inspired particulate matter which is in the pulmonary tissue. On the surface of the lungs, small, irregularly shaped areas (1 to 2 cm) are delineated by dark lines. The dark lines are due to deposits of inspired particulate matter in the delicate interlobular connective tissue. Each of these units is designated a *secondary lobule*, to distinguish it from smaller *primary lobules*. Each of the latter is made up of a *respiratory bronchiole* and its branches (Fig. 17.9).

Plan of the Lungs

A main bronchus, the primary division from the trachea, enters the root of each lung. There it divides, one secondary bronchus going to each lobe. Thus there are three branches to the right and two to the left lung. Each *lobar* (secondary) *bronchus* divides, the number of branches varying from two to five in the different lobes. Each of these bronchi supplies a portion of a lobe known as a *segment* or *bronchopulmonary segment*. There are 10 segments in the right lung and eight in the left lung. These segments are of considerable importance from a surgical standpoint. The segmental bronchi divide a number of times within the lung, with a progressive reduction in diameter and a gradual decrease in cartilage (Fig. 17.10). When the tubes reach a caliber of about 1 mm, the cartilage is lacking and the tubes are known as *bronchioles*. The bronchioles continue to divide and, when their branches have been reduced to a caliber of about 0.5 mm (or less), they become devoid of glands and goblet cells and are known as *terminal bronchioles* (Figs. 17.11 to 17.13). There are a number of terminal bronchioles within a secondary lung lobule. The terminal bronchioles, as their name implies, are the terminal segments of the purely conducting division of the respira-

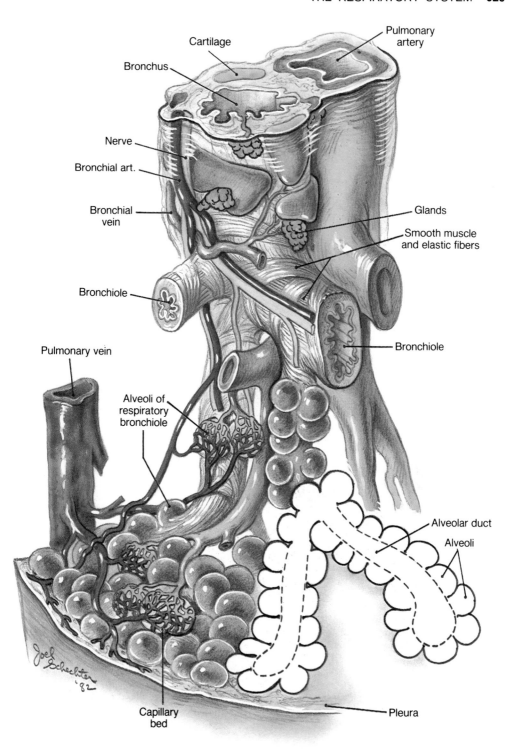

Figure 17.9. A portion of a lung lobule. (Modification from Braus H: *Anatomie des Menschen*. Berlin, Julius Springer, 1924.)

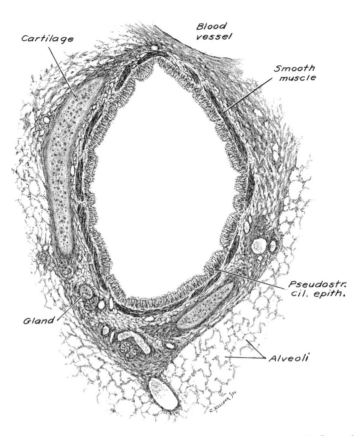

Figure 17.10. Drawing of a section through a bronchus approximately 2 mm in diameter.

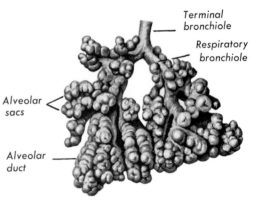

Figure 17.11. Cast of a terminal bronchiole and its branches. (From Braus H: *Anatomie des Menschen*. Berlin, Julius Springer, 1924.)

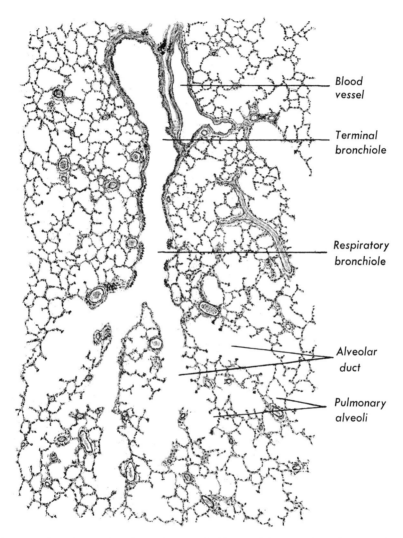

Figure 17.12. Drawing of a section through a terminal bronchiole, together with part of the system arising from it. Camera lucida drawing. Human lung (×19).

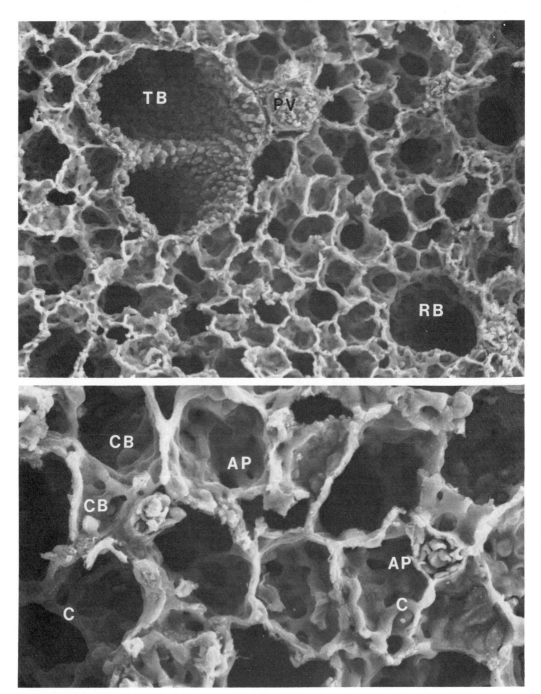

Figure 17.13. Scanning electron micrographs of terminal air passages in mouse lung. *Top*, a branched terminal bronchiole (*TB*) with associated pulmonary vessel (*PV*) is at *upper left* and a respiratory bronchiole (*RB*) is at *lower right*. Alveolar sacs are partially expanded because fixation was accomplished by injecting fixative into air passages. *Bottom*, higher magnification view of alveolar sacs showing alveolar pores (*AP*), anastomosing capillary profiles (*C*), and cell bodies of either type II alveolar cells or dust cells projecting into the alveolar spaces (*CB*) (*top*, ×275; *bottom*, ×740).

tory system. Each of them terminates by branching into two or more *respiratory bronchioles* (Figs. 17.11 to 17.13). As noted earlier, each respiratory bronchiole and its subsidiary divisions make up a functional unit known as the *primary lobule*. Each respiratory bronchiole undergoes further divisions into *alveolar ducts*. These in turn may branch further, terminating after a relatively long course in *alveolar sacs*. The smallest units or subdivisions are the *pulmonary alveoli*, small outpocketings that form the lining of the alveolar ducts and alveolar sacs and in whose walls the interchange of gases between air and blood takes place.

Pulmonary alveoli are confined to the respiratory division of the lung. They first appear, in the branching system outlined above, in the respiratory bronchioles, which have characteristics of both the conducting and respiratory divisions. The alveolar ducts and alveolar sacs have continuous pulmonary alveoli forming their walls. The pulmonary alveoli of one system interdigitate with those of neighboring systems, so that two adjacent alveoli have a common capillary bed, an arrangement which gives a maximal surface area for the exchange of gases.

Changes in the Lungs during Ventilation

An understanding of the changes that occur during ventilation gives a better appreciation of the distribution of elastic tissue, smooth muscle and cartilage within different parts of the respiratory system. The existence of a subatmospheric pressure within the pleural cavities is the first item to consider. The lungs fill the pleural cavities in early embryos and subatmospheric pressure is not present at first. However, as the pleural cavities enlarge and as elastic tissue and smooth muscle develop within each lung, tending to contract each toward its hilus, a subatmospheric intrathoracic pressure develops. This exerts an expanding or stretching action on the lungs. The presence of an elastic recoil mechanism is clearly demonstrated by the fact that the

lung collapses and retracts toward its hilus when air is allowed to enter the pleural cavity through a hole in the chest wall, producing *pneumothorax*, and when fluid increases in the cavity, producing *hydrothorax*. The retraction of the lung tissue is brought about by the recoil of the stretched elastic tissue and by contraction of the spirally arranged smooth muscle fibers in the walls of the conducting divisions and parts of the respiratory divisions of the lungs.

During ventilation, the volume of the lung changes in correlation with changes in intrathoracic pressure, and the latter in turn varies in association with changes in intrathoracic volume. In inspiration, the volume of the thoracic cavity is increased by muscular movements which elevate the ribs to increase the cross sectional area of the thoracic cavity and by contraction of the diaphragm to increase the cephalocaudal dimension. This reduces intrathoracic pressure, and the lungs expand. In expiration, the elastic forces of the lungs are usually sufficient to expel the air and allow the chest to return passively from its expanded state in a person at rest. Muscular movements play a greater part in expiration during strenuous exercise, when there is an increase in rate and amplitude of ventilatory movements.

The presence of hyaline cartilage in the form of separate plates in the walls of the bronchi (Fig. 17.10) gives strength without hindering changes in length and diameter. The presence of smooth muscle, coursing in a spiral direction around the bronchi and bronchioles and onto the alveolar ducts, provides for active reduction of both length and breadth of these passages. Elastic tissue is present in the form of a dense feltwork of longitudinally oriented fibers in the lamina propria of the conducting divisions and as a network around all of the respiratory divisions. This permits expansion of lung tissue when the intrathoracic pressure is decreased during inspiration, but rapid contraction of the lung tissue during expiration. The epithelium lining the conducting and respiratory divisions shows particularly important functional adaptations. These can best be considered in connection with a more detailed description of structure.

Structure of the Lungs
The Conducting Division

Modifications in the structure of the bronchi appear in the root of the lungs and continue with each subsequent branching. A comparison of a terminal segment (terminal bronchiole) with a main bronchus reveals the eventual great cumulative effect of the series of gradual changes.

The epithelium, although continuing as a pseudostratified columnar type through most of the conducting division, nevertheless decreases in height as the tubes become progressively smaller. In the terminal bronchiole, it becomes a single layer of columnar or cuboidal cells, many of which still bear cilia (Fig. 17.14). Goblet cells and glands (seromucous) become fewer, and both cease to be present before the terminal bronchioles are reached.

The lamina propria also decreases in thickness as the conducting divisions decrease in caliber, and elastic fibers form a feltwork, with the majority of them coursing in a longitudinal direction. Smooth muscle increases in relative amounts along the conducting divisions and is arranged in bundles that follow a spiral course around the bronchi, interior to the cartilage plates (Fig. 17.10). The smooth muscle is relatively most abundant in the terminal bronchioles, where it forms a prominent component of the wall (Fig. 17.14).

With the first branching of the primary bronchi, the cartilage ceases to occur as C-shaped rings and becomes distributed in irregularly shaped plates. As the bronchi continue to branch and decrease in diameter, the cartilaginous plates are replaced by islands of cartilage. As noted earlier, cartilage disappears completely when the bronchioles are reached, at a diameter of about 1 mm.

Terminal bronchioles (0.5 mm or less in caliber) are lined by simple columnar or cuboidal cells, both ciliated and nonciliated. There are no goblet cells or glands. Elastic tissue and smooth muscle are closely associated, and the amount of muscle in proportion to the diameter of the tubule is higher than in the other divisions of the system.

It is significant that the cilia extend farther down the tubes than do the mucous secreting elements. If the reverse were the case, accumulations of mucus might occlude the passageways.

The Respiratory Division

Each terminal bronchiole divides into two or more respiratory bronchioles (Fig.

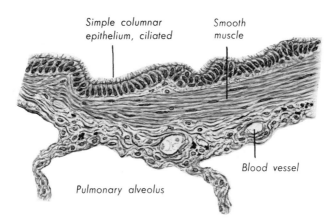

Figure 17.14.   Drawing of a transverse section through a portion of the wall of a terminal bronchiole and adjacent pulmonary alveoli. Human lung (×320).

17.11) which may further branch so that respiratory bronchioles of the first and second order are formed. The *respiratory bronchioles* bear pulmonary alveoli on those portions of their walls which are not in contact with the accompanying pulmonary artery (Figs. 17.12 and 17.13). The alveoli are few in number proximally but become more numerous distally. Between the alveoli, the wall of the respiratory bronchiole is lined by cuboidal epithelium; cilia are present in the proximal part but not distally. The nonciliated cells are secretory in appearance and have been referred to as *Clara cells* or *nonciliated bronchiolar epithelial cells.* Smooth muscle and elastic fibers are well developed in the respiratory bronchiole, although they do not form as thick a layer as in the terminal bronchiole. Collagenous fibers are also present. The smooth muscle bundles and the elastic fibers course obliquely, i.e., in a spiral direction, but they branch and anastomose, thus forming a loose elastic and contractile network. In sections through the opening of an alveolus into a respiratory bronchiole, the muscle fibers are seen to be cut obliquely or transversely.

The walls of the alveolar ducts are formed by pulmonary sacs and alveoli with only a few squamous to low cuboidal epithelial cells intervening. Small smooth muscle bundles which branch and anastomose are concentrated around the openings of the alveoli. Reticular, elastic and delicate collagenous fibers are also present (Figs. 17.15 to 17.17). The alveolar ducts terminate in a variable number of alveolar sacs.

The *alveolar sacs* are thin-walled structures which are studded with pulmonary alveoli. The walls of the alveolar sacs contain little smooth muscle but have elastic and reticular fibers. Some authorities do not distinguish alveolar sacs, as their walls cannot be distinguished from those of the pulmonary alveoli.

The Pulmonary Alveoli

Pulmonary alveoli (air cells) are cup-shaped structures through whose thin walls the interchange of gas between the blood

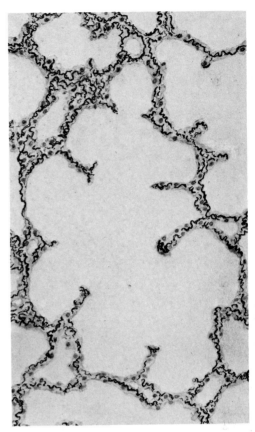

Figure 17.15. Drawing of a section through an alveolar duct, showing the reticular fibers (*black*). Lung of rhesus monkey. Foot-Hortega silver carbonate method and Orth's carmine (×240).

and air takes place. The mouth of each alveolus opens into the lumen of a respiratory bronchiole, an alveolar duct or an alveolar sac (Figs. 17.9 and 17.12). Because of the interdigitating arrangement of the alveoli, a single wall, or *interalveolar septum*, is usually formed between adjacent alveoli (Figs. 17.15 and 17.16).

An interalveolar septum is composed of the lining cells of adjacent alveoli and the structures interposed between the alveoli. Capillaries occupy a major portion of the septum, and they are shared by the lining cells of the adjacent alveoli (Figs. 17.17 and 17.19). The capillaries have wide lumina and they anastomose so freely that the volume of the vascular network exceeds that of the intervening spaces (Fig. 17.18). The meshes of the capillary network con-

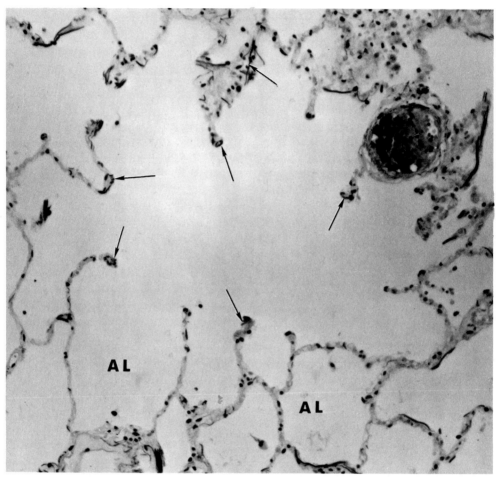

Figure 17.16. Light micrograph of an aveolar duct. Elastic fibers (*black*) are obvious in alveolar septa, especially in the expanded terminations (*arrows*). Red blood cells are also stained black. AL, pulmonary alveoli. Human lung, Verhoeff's stain (×195).

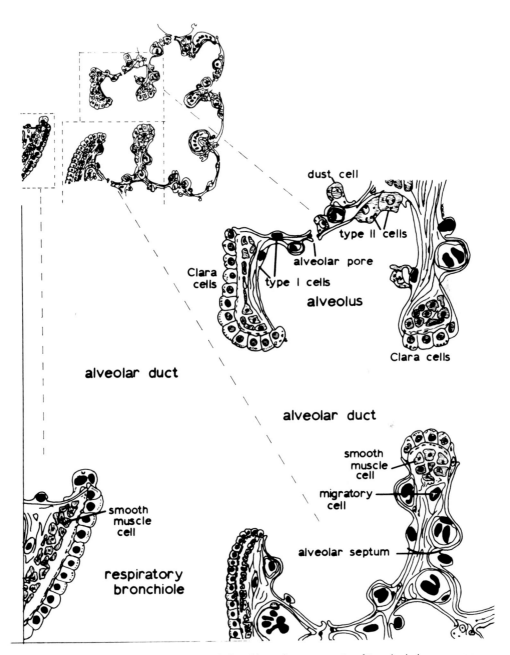

Figure 17.17. Diagram showing relationships of components of terminal air passages.

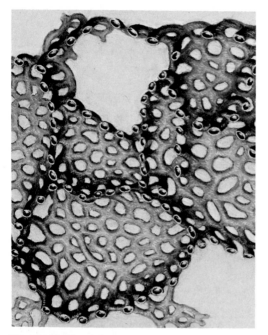

Figure 17.18. Injected lung, showing capillaries in walls of pulmonary alveoli. Dog. Preparation by Mr. Kellner (×400).

tain reticular and elastic fibers arranged in a manner to permit expansion and contraction of the alveolar wall. The intercapillary spaces also contain a few fibroblasts, some wandering leukocytes, macrophages and occasional smooth muscle cells (Fig. 17.17).

The interalveolar septa are interrupted in places where adjacent alveoli not only make contact but open to each other to form *alveolar pores* (Fig. 17.13 and 17.17). The pores are about 10 to 15 μm in diameter in the expanded lung. In certain pathological conditions, they become more prominent and contain strands of fibrin extending from one alveolus to another. It has been suggested that, by providing intercommunication, they prevent the overdistention of some alveoli and the collapse of others when small bronchioles of a functional unit are occluded.

The alveolar lining cells have been studied extensively. Prior to the advent of electron microscopy, there was considerable controversy as to whether the alveoli were completely lined by epithelium. It was

known from light microscope studies that the entire pulmonary system is lined by epithelium in early stages of fetal development, but this was questionable as applied to late fetal- and postnatal life when the walls of the alveoli thinned out. Electron microscope studies showed that the alveoli are completely lined by epithelium, but that the cells have regions which are so attenuated that they lie at the limits of resolution provided by the light microscope.

The alveolar lining consists of *type I alveolar cells* (*squamous* cells) and *type II alveolar cells* (*surfactant* cells).

The *type I alveolar cells* have low or flat nuclei, much like those of the cells of mesothelium. The cytoplasm becomes very thin or attenuated beyond the perinuclear region (Figs. 17.17 and 17.19). These cells have junctional attachments laterally with each other and with the type II alveolar cells. Because of the lateral extent of these cells, they are actually much larger than the type II cells and form the vast majority of the alveolar surface.

The *type II alveolar cells* have an irregular, cuboidal shape. They are fairly numerous, taller than the squamous cells and can be seen more readily with the electron microscope. They have characteristic cytoplasmic structures which look like vacuoles under the light microscope (Fig. 17.20), but which are seen in electron micrographs as osmiophilic bodies with internal concentric lamellae. These *lamellar bodies* are 0.2 to 1.0 μm in diameter. They are periodic acid-Schiff-positive, and also stain with Sudan black. The lamellar contents are secreted into the alveoli where the phospholipid constituents coat the air-water interface, lowering the surface tension and thus permitting expansion of the alveoli. Early investigations provided some confusion between bronchiolar Clara cells and type II alveolar cells, but more recent studies indicate that the two cell types are probably unrelated. There is no evidence that Clara cells form surfactant. Infants born prematurely may fail to produce adequate surfactant material and exhibit *respiratory distress syn-*

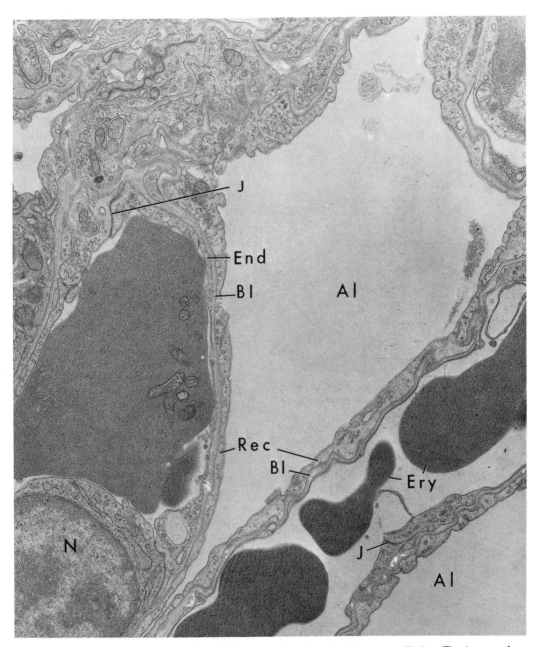

Figure 17.19. Electron micrograph of pulmonary alveoli and adjacent capillaries. The lumen of an alveolus (*Al*) is separated from the lumen of the capillaries by a thin layer of tissue composed of: small alveolar cells (*Rec*) that line the alveolus; a basal lamina (or laminae, *Bl*); and endothelial cells (*End*) that line the capillaries. The basal lamina of the endothelium appears to be fused with that of the squamous respiratory cells along a considerable portion of the interalveolar septum. The respiratory cells are very attenuated in regions where they are apposed to the endothelial cells, but they form a continuous layer. Likewise, the endothelial cell is attenuated except in the region around the nucleus (*N*). *Ery*, erythrocytes in the capillaries; *J*, intercellular junctions of endothelial cells. From the lung of a mouse. (×16,000). (Courtesy of Drs. K. R. Porter and M. A. Bonneville.)

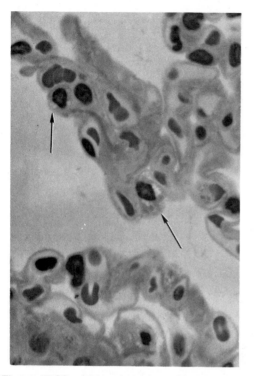

Figure 17.20. Light micrograph of monkey lung showing vacuolated type II alveolar cells (*arrows*). The thinness of the wall between alveolar space and capillary lumina is well shown. There are no obvious cell bodies of type I alveolar cells in this field (×765).

drome. These individuals do not have normally developed type II alveolar cells but have normal appearing Clara cells.

The *alveolar membrane* may be defined as the barrier through which gases must pass in exchange between air and blood (Fig. 17.19). This membrane consists of the *type I alveolar cell* together with its underlying *basal lamina* and the *capillary endothelial cell* with its *basal lamina*. The basal laminae of epithelium and endothelium are fused in some areas and are separated in many other areas only by a few elastic or reticular fibers. The endothelium of the capillaries is relatively thin, is not fenestrated, but has numerous caveolae. Besides the exchange of gases, the capillary bed of the lungs is involved in the metabolism of certain vasoactive substances, such as *angiotensin* and prostaglandins. There is evi-

dence suggesting that activation of angiotensin by peptidase activity may occur in association with the caveolae of the endothelial cells.

Alveolar macrophages or *dust cells* are found within the alveolar wall and also in the alveoli resting on the alveolar surface often in contact with type II cells. They are highly phagocytic cells and received the name dust cells because they remove inspired particles that reach the alveoli. In clinical disorders in which the pulmonary vessels become congested with blood, the macrophages ingest some of the erythrocytes and become filled with brownish granules of hemosiderin.

There is evidence that more than one type of dust cell may occur. One type makes its appearance embryonically and is capable of mitotic proliferation. However, the major population of dust cells in the adult arises from monocytes of bone marrow origin. The macrophages of the interstitial connective tissue are also of monocytic origin but do not appear to interchange with alveolar dust cells.

Inspired Particulate Matter

Many particles of dust are present in the air which is inspired, and the number of particles is greatly increased in smoky or dusty environments. Many of the inspired particles are removed by lodging on the mucous film of the nose, nasopharynx, larynx, and trachea. The mucous film and adherent particles are constantly being moved by ciliary action to the oropharynx.

The bronchi and bronchioles in the lung also play a role in the removal of particulate matter. As repeated branchings take place, with only a slight increase in cross section area, the total surface of the walls is greatly increased. Because of the increased area, particles are more likely to impinge on the mucous coat than in the upper, larger passages. As in the trachea and nasal passages, ciliary action carries the particles lodged on the mucous film to the oropharynx.

Many of the smaller particles, however, reach the alveoli of the lungs, and their removal by ciliary action is not possible. A different mechanism operates whereby these particles are removed by alveolar macrophages or dust cells.

Some particles are digested, others pass with the alveolar macrophages into the terminal bronchioles and up the bronchociliary ladder. However, when larger amounts of insoluble particulates are present, some of the particles are deposited, perhaps after passage through several cells, in the connective tissue of the lungs or in the lymphatic tissue. In this transport of the particles, the lymph vessels play an important role. The connective tissue may increase greatly in amount (fibrosis) and may encapsulate masses of the particles. The degree of connective tissue overgrowth is influenced by the type of the inhaled dust. Siliceous dust and asbestos, for instance, cause a marked fibrosis, whereas coal dust, even when present in large amounts, induces a very slight reaction, or none at all, of the connective tissue. The condition which results from the dust is termed *pneumoconiosis*, special names (*anthracosis, silicosis, asbestosis*, etc.) being used to designate the reactions to the various types of dust.

Endocrine (Neuroendocrine) Cells

Within the epithelial lining of the respiratory system there also exists a diverse population of specialized cells with a morphology similar to some of the enteroendocrine cells of the digestive tract. Immunocytochemical studies show that these cells in lung are capable of converting amine precursors to dopamine or serotonin, and also contain peptide hormones such as bombesin and calcitonin. The origin and functional significance of these cells have been subjects of considerable interest and speculation. Their presence is rationalized in part by the common endodermal origin of the lining epithelium of lung and digestive tracts. As with enteroendocrine cells, suggestions that the lung endocrine cells have a neural crest origin have not been confirmed experimentally. It appears that

many, if not all, arise from undifferentiated cells of the epithelium itself.

Lung endocrine cells may occur singly or in groups and in either configuration they may or may not be associated with nerves. Larger aggregates may form distinct entities referred to as *neuroepithelial bodies*. The number of endocrine cells varies widely in lungs of different species. Normally, they are not numerous in human lung. The reasons for such variability are as unclear as is their functional significance. It is known, however, that certain categories of these cells can proliferate abnormally and give rise to pulmonary neoplasms such as oat cell carcinoma.

The Pleura

The pleura is a mesothelial serous membrane which completely lines the pleural cavity. The visceral portion invests and is closely adherent to the lungs. It is continuous with the parietal pleura at the root of the lungs. Beneath the mesothelial lining of the pleura is a fibroelastic connective tissue which contains smooth muscle. In the connective tissue are blood capillaries and a rich plexus of lymph vessels.

Continuous with the connective tissue of the pleura are delicate septa that extend between the lobules, anastomosing with each other and with the peribronchial connective tissue. The septa are composed of fibrous and elastic connective tissue, and they contain smooth muscle, lymph and blood vessels and macrophages.

The Blood and Lymph Circulation of the Lungs

Blood Vessels

The lungs receive blood from two sources: venous blood, to be purified, through the *pulmonary arteries*, and arterial blood, for the nutrition of the walls of the conducting system and blood vessels, through the *bronchial arteries*. This blood is returned to the systemic circulation through the pulmonary and bronchial veins. The former, in contrast with the latter, are devoid of valves.

The pulmonary artery enters the lung with the corresponding chief bronchus. It branches with and follows the bronchial tree to the termination of the respiratory bronchioles. As the alveolar duct is reached, the artery gives rise to the capillary plexus in the walls of the alveoli (Figs. 17.18 and 17.21). Veins arise from these capillaries. They do not immediately join the bronchioles but course in the septa. Later they join the bronchioles and course along them to the root of the lung.

The bronchial arteries likewise accompany the bronchi. Along their course they give origin to capillaries which supply the walls of the bronchi, arteries, veins and the peribronchial and septal connective tissue. The bronchial arteries do not extend beyond the respiratory bronchioles. The cap-

illaries arising from them in that segment anastomose with the pulmonary capillary plexus. Part of the blood carried by the bronchial arteries passes into the pulmonary veins through this anastomosis. The remainder returns through the bronchial veins.

The pleura, in man, is supplied by the bronchial arteries. This blood returns through the pulmonary veins.

Lymphatics

There are two sets of lymphatic vessels in the lung: a superficial set in the pleura and a deep set in the substance of the lung. The superficial (pleural) lymph vessels are particularly numerous near the juncture of the interlobular septa with the pleura, and thus they outline the lobules (Fig. 17.21).

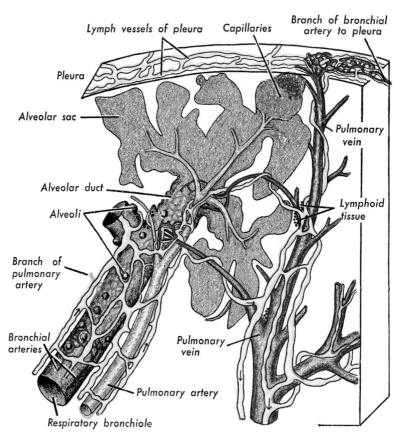

Figure 17.21. The blood supply and lymph drainage of a portion of a lung lobule and the pleura. (Reprinted with permission or from W.S. Miller: *The Lung.* Springfield, Ill., Charles C Thomas, 1947.)

There are numerous anastomoses between the vessels of the superficial and deep plexuses at the surface of the lung. These serve as afferents to the superficial vessels; numerous valves in the latter prevent the backflow of lymph. The efferents of the superficial plexus course first in the pleura and then in the connective tissue along the larger bronchi to the root of the lung.

The vessels of the deep plexus are found chiefly around the bronchi and bronchioles, around the branches of the pulmonary artery and in the interlobular connective tissue associated with the branches of the pulmonary veins. There are no lymphatics in the interalveolar septa; they begin in the connective tissue around the respiratory bronchioles and blood vessels. Although some of the lymph from the deep plexus enters the superficial vessels by channels of anastomosis over the lung surface, a considerable portion of the lymph of the deep plexus is carried by larger vessels which follow the bronchi and blood vessels to the hilus, where the main vessels of the two sets of lymphatics join. There are no valves in the deep lymphatics, except in a few of the larger trunks.

Lymphatic tissue in the form of lymph nodes or solitary nodules with germinal centers occurs along the larger bronchial branches. The amount of lymphatic tissue is said to increase with age. It becomes infiltrated with the inspired particulate matter. There is also a lymphocytic infiltration of the walls of the bronchi.

Nerves

The bronchi are accompanied by sympathetic and parasympathetic nerves. The latter come from the vagus. Ganglion cells are present in the walls of the bronchi. Sympathetic fibers mediate dilation of the air tubes, whereas parasympathetic fibers mediate constriction.

DEVELOPMENT OF THE RESPIRATORY SYSTEM

The epithelium of the respiratory system develops from endoderm. The rudiment of the larynx, trachea and lungs appears as a ventral, groove-like evagination in the floor of the primitive pharynx. This evagination grows caudally and becomes cut off by constriction from the digestive tube except in its superior part, and its apex bifurcates. The portion which does not bifurcate, together with the surrounding mesenchyme, forms the larynx and trachea. The bifurcated part is the anlage; its endodermal epithelium forms the simple columnar, coboidal or squamous linings of the rapidly branching, tree-like passages, while the surrounding mesenchyme provides muscular, connective tissue, and vascular components. The main right branch subdivides into three branches corresponding to the three lobes of the future right lung, and the left divides into two branches corresponding to two lobes of the left lung. By repeated branching of these tubules, the entire bronchial system of the lungs is formed. This process is similar to the development of a compound gland. The last to develop are the respiratory bronchioles and the alveolar ducts and sacs, structures that are characteristic of the lung. During fetal life, the alveoli are lined by a cuboidal epithelium. At the time of birth, these cells become extremely thin, so thin that over most of their extent, they are not individually resolved by light microscopy.

During gestation, as well as following birth, there is a continued growth of the lung. The bronchioles increase in length, and new respiratory units are formed. The increase in the length of the bronchioles, while to a small degree caused by an interstitial growth of the existing bronchioles, is mainly due to the transformation of the respiratory bronchioles, alveolar ducts and alveolar sacs into bronchioles. The lengthening of the respiratory division takes place by a terminal budding and growth of the air sacs.

References

Adams FH: Fetal and neonatal cardiovascular and pulmonary function. *Annu Rev Physiol* 27:257–284, 1965.

Bertalanffy FD, Leblond CP: The continuous renewal of the two types of alveolar cells in the lung of the rat. *Anat Rec* 115:515–542, 1953.

Boyden EA: *Segmental Anatomy of the Lungs. A Study of the Patterns of the Segmental Bronchi and Related Pulmonary Vessels.* New York, McGraw-Hill, 1955.

Boyden EA, Tompsett DH: The changing patterns in the developing lungs of infants. *Acta Anat* 61:164–192, 1965.

Cutz E: Neuroendocrine cells of the lung. An overview of morphologic characteristics and development. *Exp Lung Res* 3:185–208, 1982.

Fishman AP, Pietra GG: Handling of bioactive materials by the lung. *N Engl J Med* 291:884–890, 1974.

Gil J: Alveolar wall relations. *Ann N Y Acad Sci* 384:31–43, 1982.

Hayek H von: *The Human Lung* (Krahl VE, trans) New York, Hafner Publishing, 1960.

King RJ: The surfactant system of the lung. *Fed Proc* 33:2238–2247, 1974.

Kolata G: Cell biology yields clues to lung cancer. *Science* 218:38–39, 1982.

Krahl VE: Anatomy of the mammalian lung. In *Handbook of Physiology*, section 3, vol 1. Washington, D.C. American Physiological Society, 1964, p 213.

Lauweryns JM, De Bock V, Verhofstad AAJ, Steinbusch HWM: Immuno-histochemical localization of serotonin in intrapulmonary neuroepithelial bodies. *Cell Tissue Res* 226:215–223, 1982.

Lenfant C (ed): *Lung Biology in Health and Disease*, vols 1–18. New York, Marcel Dekker, 1976–1981.

Loosli CG: Interalveolar communications in normal and pathological mammalian lungs. *Arch Pathol* 24:743–776, 1937; *Am J Anat* 62:375–425, 1938.

Low FN: The pulmonary alveolar epithelium of laboratory mammals and man. *Anat Rec* 117:241–264, 1953.

Low FN: The extracellular portion of the blood-air barrier and its relation to tissue space. *Anat Rec* 139:105–123, 1961.

Plopper CG, Hill LH, Mariassy AT: Ultrastructure of the nonciliated bronchiolar epithelial (Clara) cell of mammalian lung. III. A. Study of man with comparison of 15 mammalian species. *Exp Lung* 1:171–180, 1980.

Pratt SA, Finley TN, Smith MH, Ladman AJ: A comparison of alveolar macrophages and pulmonary surfactant (?) obtained from the lungs of human smokers and nonsmokers by endobronchial lavage. *Anat Rec* 163:497–508, 1969.

Said S: The lung in relation to vasoactive hormones. *Fed Proc* 32:1972–1976, 1973.

Smith U, Ryan J: Electron microscopy of endothelial and epithelial components of the lungs: correlations of structure and function. *Fed Proc* 32:1957–1966, 1973.

Sorokin SP: A morphologic and cytochemical study of the great alveolar cell. *J Histochem Cytochem* 14:884–897, 1966.

Thurlbeck WM: Structure of the lungs. In Widdicombe JG (ed): *International Review of Physiology*, vol 14: *Respiratory Physiology II*. Baltimore, University Park Press, 1977, pp 1–36.

Tobin CE: Lymphatics of the pulmonary alveoli. *Anat Rec* 120:625–636, 1954.

Weibel ER: Morphogenetics of the lung. In *Handbook of Physiology*. Washington, D.C., American Physiological Society, 1964.

Will JA, DiAugustine RP (eds): Lung neuroendocrine cells and regulatory peptides: distribution, functional studies and implications. *Exp Lung Res* 3:185–418, 1982.

Chapter 18

THE URINARY SYSTEM

The urinary system consists of paired *kidneys*; their ducts leading to the bladder, the *ureters*; the *bladder* and its duct leading to the exterior, the *urethra*. The urinary system is closely associated both developmentally and phylogenetically with the reproductive system, especially in the male. With the need to conserve water in land animals (amniotes), there is a change from a kidney that is supplied by blood vessels with a relatively low pressure and that produces copious quantities of hypotonic urine, to a system supplied by vessels at higher pressures that is capable of producing urine hypertonic to the blood and interstitial fluid.

THE KIDNEY

The kidney is a compound tubular gland which separates urea and other nitrogenous waste products from the blood. It is also a major homeostatic organ that has an important role in regulating the composition of the extracellular fluid which bathes the cells and tissues of the body. It is enclosed by a firm connective tissue capsule composed of collagenous fibers and a few elastic fibers. In many of the lower animals and in the human fetus, septa extend from the capsule into the gland, dividing it into a number of lobes. In human adults, the lobated character is obscured by the great reduction of the interstitial connective tissue and the apparent blending of the peripheral parts of the different lobes. Rarely, the fetal divisions persist in adult life, such a kidney being known as a "lobated kidney." In some animals, such as the guinea pig and rabbit, the entire kidney consists of a single lobe.

On the mesially directed border of the kidney is a depression known as the *hilus*. This serves as the point of entrance for the *renal artery* and of exit for the *renal vein* and *ureter*.

In sections, the kidney is seen to consist of *cortex* and *medulla* partially surrounding a cavity—the *renal sinus*—which opens at the hilus (Fig. 18.1). The renal sinus contains: (*a*) the upper, expanded portion of the ureter which is known as the *renal pelvis*, (*b*) subdivisions of the pelvis that form two or three *major calyces* and about eight *minor calyces*, (*c*) branches of the renal arteries, veins and nerves, and (*d*) loose connective tissue and fat. In fresh, unfixed kidneys, the outer or cortical zone of the kidney is dark brown in color and granular in appearance. It contains many convoluted tubules and numerous round, reddish bodies, the *renal* or *Malpighian corpuscles*, which are barely visible to the unaided eye. The inner, medullary zone of the kidney is radially striated in appearance because its tubular and vascular elements run in parallel radial lines.

The cortex, in addition to forming the outer zone of the kidney parenchymal tissue, penetrates inward between portions of the medulla to the margin of the renal sinus as the *renal columns*. The main medullary mass consists of 8 to 18 *medullary* or *Malpighian pyramids*, the number corresponding to the number of lobes in the fetal kidney. The broad base of each pyramid is in contact with the cortex, and the rounded apex projects into a minor calyx (Fig. 18.1). As a rule, two or sometimes three pyramids unite to form a single *papilla*; hence, the number of papillae is less than that of the pyramids. The tip of the papillary surface presents a sieve-like appearance, *area cribrosa*, as a result of the presence of 10 to 25 pores, which are the openings of the

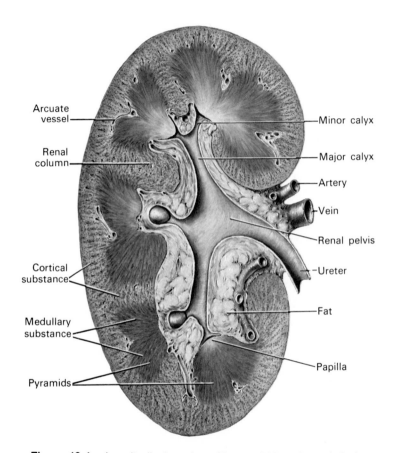

Arcuate vessel

Renal column

Cortical substance

Medullary substance

Pyramids

Minor calyx

Major calyx

Artery

Vein

Renal pelvis

Ureter

Fat

Papilla

Figure 18.1. Longitudinal section of human kidney (actual size).

major collecting ducts or *papillary ducts* into the minor calyx. Even in gross preparations, two zones may be distinguished in the medulla: an outer, more deeply colored zone in contact with the cortex, and an inner, somewhat paler papillary zone.

The cortical region is subdivided into many radiating, slender columns composed of straight tubules alternating with regions containing glomeruli and convoluted tubules (Figs. 18.2 and 18.3). The columns of straight tubules radiate outward from the medulla and hence are named *medullary*

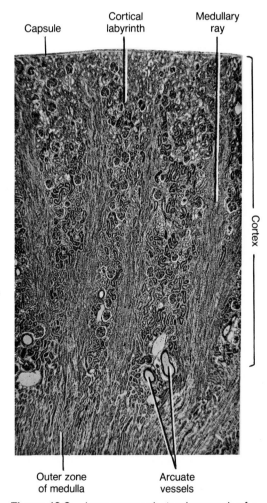

Capsule   Cortical labyrinth   Medullary ray

Cortex

Outer zone of medulla   Arcuate vessels

Figure 18.2. Low power photomicrograph of a section of a kidney from an infant of eight months, showing topography of the cortex and a part of the outer zone of the medulla (×28).

rays. The regions between the rays contain glomeruli and convoluted tubules and are called *cortical labyrinths.* A medullary ray and the adjacent cortical tissue whose tubules drain into the collecting tubules of the ray constitute a *lobule.*

The Uriniferous Tubules

The lobules are composed of closely packed uriniferous tubules. Each uriniferous tubule consists of an initial unbranched portion, the *nephron,* and a branched portion, the *collecting tubule,* that connects the nephron to the pelvis (Fig. 18.4). This subdivision of the uriniferous tubule also separates the portion of the tubule derived from the metanephric blastema (the nephron) from the part derived from the ureteric bud (the collecting tubule). The uriniferous tubules are entirely derived from epithelialized mesodermal tissue and constitute the parenchyma of the kidney. Between the tubules are numerous blood vessels and scanty interstitial connective tissue.

The Nephron

Each of the approximately 1,000,000 nephrons per kidney is a single unbranched tubular structure. The nephron begins as a double walled, epithelial cup, *Bowman's capsule,* which surrounds a tuft of capillaries, the *glomerulus.* Bowman's capsule and the glomerulus together form the *renal* or *Malpighian corpuscle* (Fig. 18.5).

The glomerulus will be discussed as a portion of the renal vascular system, but it should be noted here that the glomerulus is the source of the ultrafiltrate of the blood that enters Bowman's capsule and that is subsequently modified by the rest of the nephron to produce urine.

Bowman's capsule consists of two simple epithelial layers, an inner or *visceral layer* covering the glomerulus, and an outer or *parietal layer* (Figs. 18.5 and 18.6). The visceral layer of Bowman's capsule closely invests the glomerulus, largely taking its shape from the underlying capillaries. It is continuous with the parietal layer at the rim of the opening to the renal corpuscle. This region where the vessels enter and

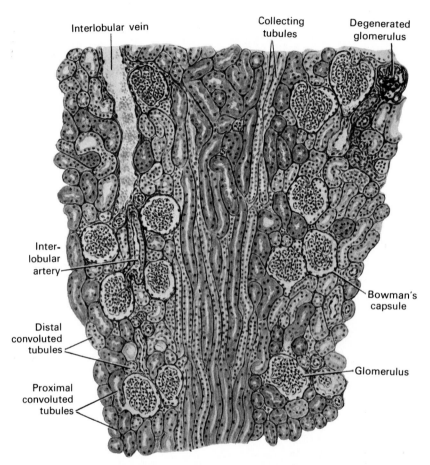

Figure 18.3. Section through a part of the cortex of a human kidney, showing the structure of a medullary ray *(central part of the figure)* and of adjacent cortical labyrinths *(lateral parts of figure)* (×55).

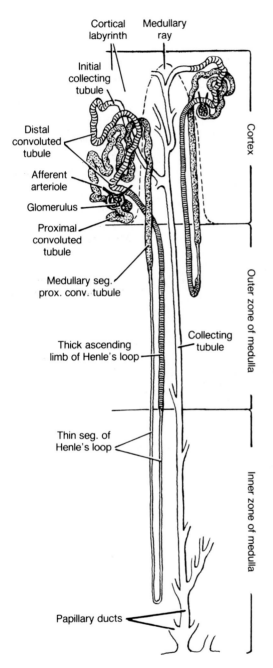

Figure 18.4. Diagram of the subdivisions of the uriniferous tubules to show their relations and locations in a section extending from the capsule to the tip of a renal pyramid. (Redrawn and modified from Peter K: *Untersuchungen über Bau und Entwicklung der Niere.* Jena, 1927.)

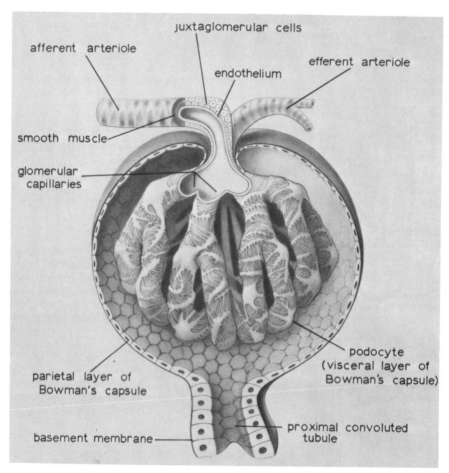

Figure 18.5. Diagram of structure of renal corpuscle, showing relationship of Bowman's capsule to glomerular capillaries. (Redrawn and modified from Bargmann W: *Histologie und Mikroskopische Anatomie des Menschen*, 0.5). Stuttgart, Georg Thieme Verlag, 1964.)

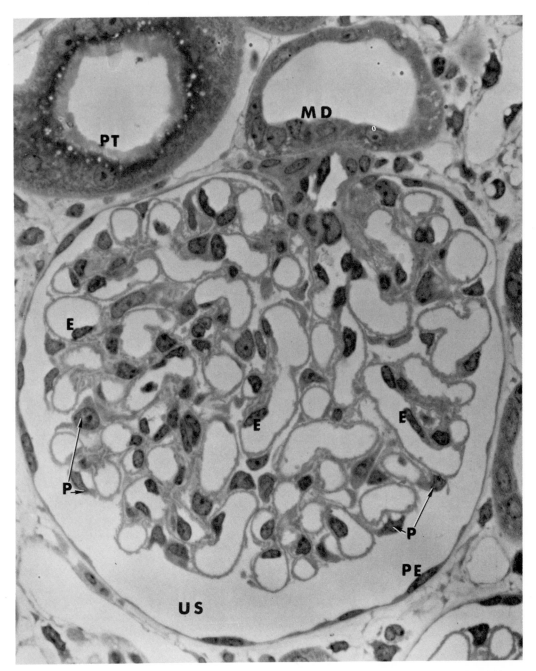

Figure 18.6. Light micrograph of a 1-μm section of a glomerulus from perfused monkey kidney. *MD,* macula densa; *PT,* proximal tubule; *PE,* parietal epithelium of Bowman's capsule; *P,* podocytes (visceral epithelium of Bowman's capsule); *E,* endothelial cell nuclei; *US,* urinary space ($\times$700).

leave the glomerulus is the *vascular pole of the corpuscle*. The parietal layer reflects smoothly over the entire structure and is in turn continuous with the first tubular part of the nephron, the proximal tubule, at the *urinary pole of the corpuscle*, which is roughly opposite the vascular pole. Where the parietal layer becomes continuous with the wall of the proximal segment of the tubule, there is often a short transitional zone called the neck. It is here at the urinary pole that the capsular space within

Bowman's capsule is confluent with the lumen of the proximal tubule.

The cells constituting the visceral epithelium of Bowman's capsule, the *podocytes*, are extraordinary. The nucleus and surrounding cytoplasm protrude into the capsular space and rest on processes that extend from the cell body, branching one or more times to form a series of slender processes on the basal lamina (Figs. 18.7 and 18.8). These terminal processes, which are known as *foot processes* or *pedicels*, inter-

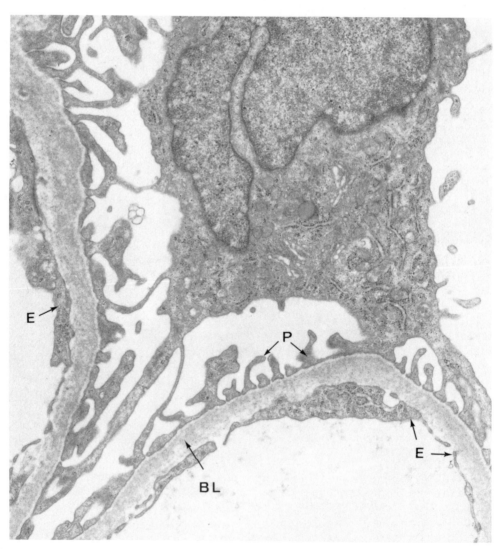

Figure 18.7. Electron micrograph of a rhesus monkey kidney glomerulus showing podocyte processes (*P*), fenestrated endothelium (*E*), and the interposed thick basal lamina (*BL*) (×12,500).

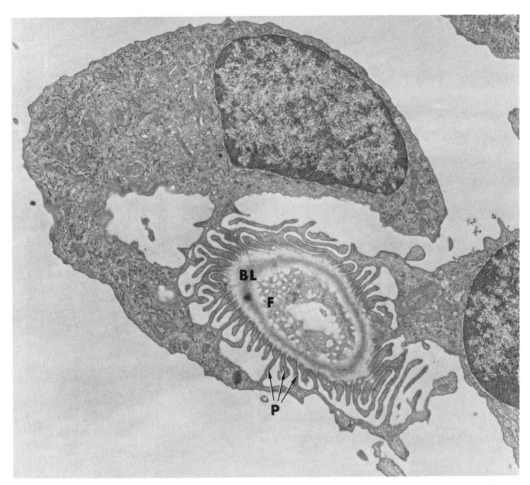

Figure 18.8. Electron micrograph of mouse kidney glomerulus showing interdigitated podocyte processes on the surface of a capillary in tangential section. *P*, podocyte processes; *F*, fenestrated endothelium; *BL*, basal lamina (×9200).

digitate with the pedicels of neighboring podocytes, leaving a series of slits between the pedicels (Figs. 18.9 and 18.10). The slits range in width from 0.02 to 0.04 μm and are spanned by an electron-dense membrane, the *slit membrane* or *slit diaphragm*, which is about 5 nm thick. Studies of the substructure of the slit membrane indicate that it is filamentous in nature with an arrangement of pores ranging from 4 to 14 nm. Substances in the glomerular capillaries pass through the single *glomerular basement membrane* (an unusually thick basal lamina) between the endothelium and podocytes, then through the slit membrane before entering the urinary space within Bowman's capsule.

The *parietal layer of Bowman's capsule* begins where the visceral layer is reflected at the vascular pole (Figs. 18.5 and 18.6). It is composed of simple squamous epithelium resting on a thin basal lamina, surrounded by a thin layer of connective tissue. In marked contrast to the elaborate structure of the podocytes, the epithelial cells of the parietal layer are more uniform in thickness and have the type of abbreviated occluding junction found in mesothelia. The cells increase in height and become cuboidal in the neck region.

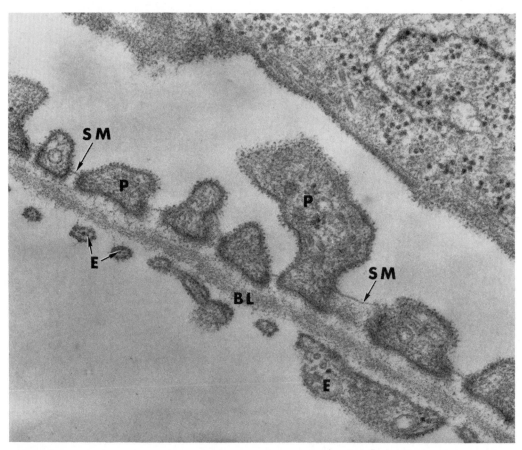

Figure 18.9. Mouse kidney glomerulus showing podocyte processes (*P*), basal lamina (*BL*), fenestrated endothelium (*E*) and filtration slit membranes (*SM*). Part of a podocyte cell body is at the *upper right* (×57,500).

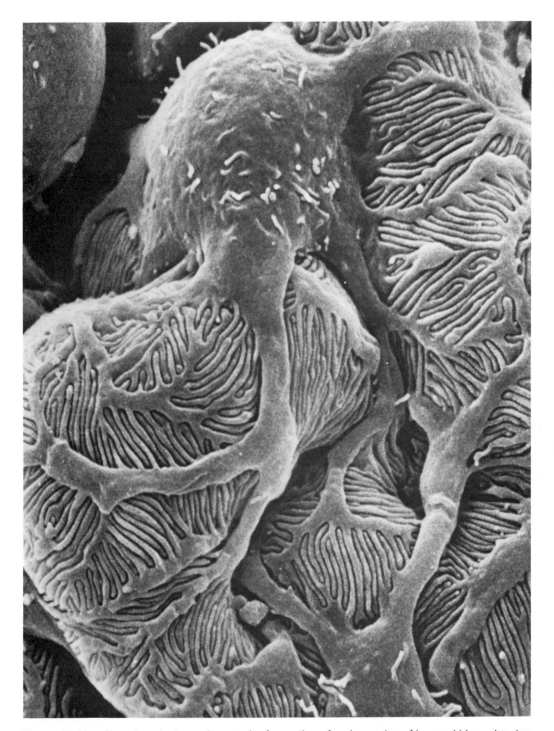

Figure 18.10. Scanning electron micrograph of a portion of a glomerulus of human kidney showing the interdigitation of podocyte cell processes over the surfaces of capillary loops (×9800). (Courtesy of Dr. Masayuki Miyoshi.)

The Tubular Portion of the Nephron

The tubular portion of the nephron is composed of a *proximal tubule*, which has a convoluted and a straight portion, a *thin segment*, and a *distal tubule*, again with a straight and a convoluted portion. The straight portions of the proximal and distal tubules, together with the thin segment, are arranged in a hairpin loop extending a variable distance into the medulla. The three segments together are called the *loop of Henle*. The convoluted portion of the distal tubule joins the arched (initial) collecting tubule which begins the system of ducts or collecting tubules.

The *proximal convoluted tubule* is the longest and most convoluted segment of the nephron, and it forms a major portion of the cortical substance. It has a length of about 14 mm, an overall diameter of about 50 to 60 μm, and a lumen whose diameter varies in proportion to the amount of provisional urine formed by its renal corpuscle. Typically it coils toward the renal capsule before coiling back toward the medulla, where the straight portion of the tubule forms the thick descending limb of the loop of Henle, entering a medullary ray and extending into the medulla.

The proximal convoluted tubule is lined by a single layer of low columnar or pyramidal cells with round nuclei and granular cytoplasm which stains deeply with eosin (Fig. 18.11). The cell boundaries are difficult to make out in ordinary preparations. In silver impregnations, they appear irregularly serrated, with processes which interdigitate with those of adjacent cells.

An important characteristic of the proximal convoluted tubule is the *brush border* at the apical surface of the cells (Fig. 18.11). Because this region undergoes rapid postmortem change, it often has a ragged appearance in routine histological preparations. Electron micrographs of well fixed material show that the brush border is composed of microvilli about 1.2 μm in length and about 0.03 μm in width (Fig. 18.12).

The cell surface available for resorption is thus greatly increased. Histochemical studies show that the border has a high concentration of alkaline phosphatase and ATPases. The border also contains proteoglycans, as indicated by its intense staining with the PAS reagent. In electron micrographs, invaginations are often seen between the bases of the microvilli, and vesicles and vacuoles are present in the apical cytoplasm. The supranuclear cytoplasm also contains mitochondria of variable shape and size (Fig. 18.12) and the usual organelles such as ribosomes. Peroxisomes and lysosomes are present and the latter apparently fuse with vacuoles during the breakdown of resorbed proteins into amino acids. The Golgi complex of the proximal convoluted tubule cells is usually on the adluminal side of the nucleus. Rough endoplasmic reticulum is present throughout the cell but is sparse.

The subnuclear portions of the cytoplasm of the proximal tubule cells appears striated in light microscope preparations. Electron micrographs show that this appearance is due to deep infoldings of the plasmalemma at the base of the cell (Fig. 18.13) and to the longitudinal arrangement of numerous rod-shaped mitochondria. There are also irregular infoldings and interdigitations of the lateral cell borders and this explains why the intercellular boundaries cannot be followed in ordinary preparations under the light microscope. The adluminal portions of the lateral borders of the cells are relatively straight, and there are junctional complexes that include a few strands of occluding junction.

The *straight portion of the proximal tubule*, or thick descending limb of the loop of Henle, is a direct continuation of the convoluted portion of the proximal tubule and is not sharply delimited from it. As the proximal tubule leaves the cortical labyrinth and enters the medullary ray, it assumes first a spiral and then a straight course. It is lined by cells that appear structurally similar to those of the convoluted portion of the proximal tubule as seen in

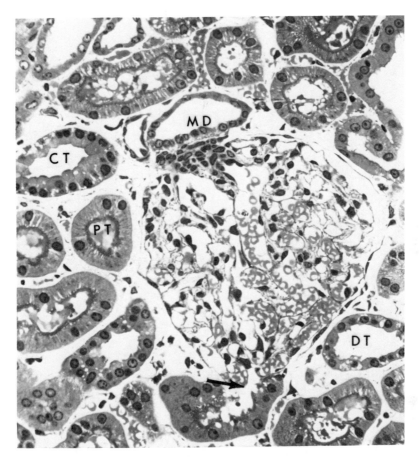

Figure 18.11. Portion of a glomerulus and adjacent tubules from the cortex of a rhesus monkey kidney. One of the segments of a distal convoluted tubule shows a modification, known as the macula densa (*MD*), where it borders the vascular pole of the glomerulus. At the opposite pole, the urinary pole, Bowman's capsule is continuous with the proximal convoluted tubule (*arrow*). In other regions proximal tubules (*PT*), distal tubules (*DT*), and collecting tubules (*CT*) are seen (×360).

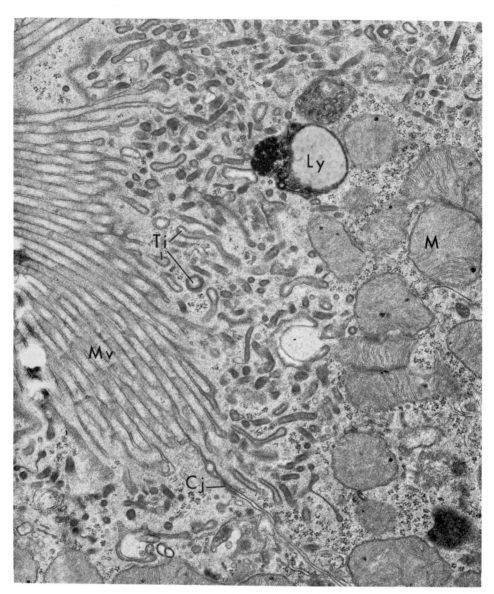

Figure 18.12. Electron micrograph of adluminal portions of two epithelial cells of a proximal convoluted tubule of a mouse kidney. The adluminal surface of each cell is increased in area by numerous microvilli (*Mv*). Invaginations, arising from clefts between the basal portions of the microvilli, penetrate downward into the cell to form tubular invaginations (*Ti*) that are also known as apical canaliculi. The invaginations become continuous with vesicles in the cytoplasm and they apparently function in the resorption of large molecules, such as proteins. *Cj*, junction of apposing cells; *Ly*, lysosomes; and *M*, mitochondrion (×23,250). (Courtesy of Drs. K. R. Porter and M. A. Bonneville.)

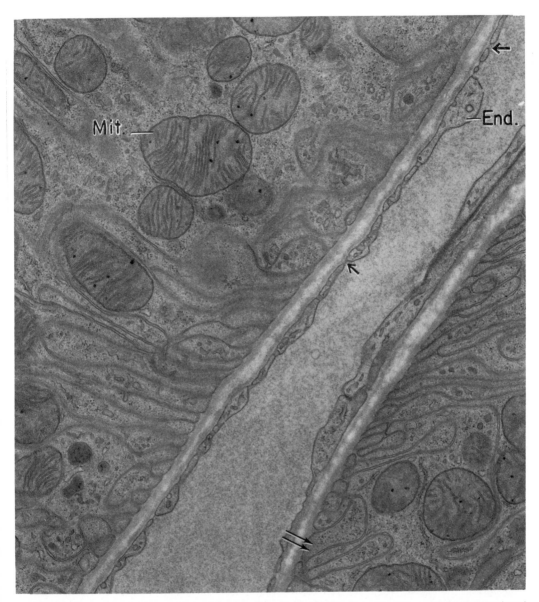

Figure 18.13. Electron micrograph of the basal portions of epithelial cells of two proximal convoluted tubules and a blood capillary within the connective tissue between the tubules. The plasmalemma of the basal surface of each proximal tubule cell has numerous infoldings which partially partition the cytoplasm of the basal region into cylindrical columns around the mitochondria (*Mit*). Isolated cell processes (*double arrows*) are seen along the basal lamina of each tubule. Processes of different epithelial cells apparently interdigitate along the basal lamina in a manner somewhat like that of podocytes of glomerular epithelium. The endothelial cells (*End*) of the capillaries around the tubules are attenuated and have "pores" or fenestrae (*arrows*). The basal lamina of the endothelium is separated from the basal lamina of the proximal tubule by only a narrow space. Section of a kidney of a bat (×27,000). (Courtesy of Dr. Keith Porter.)

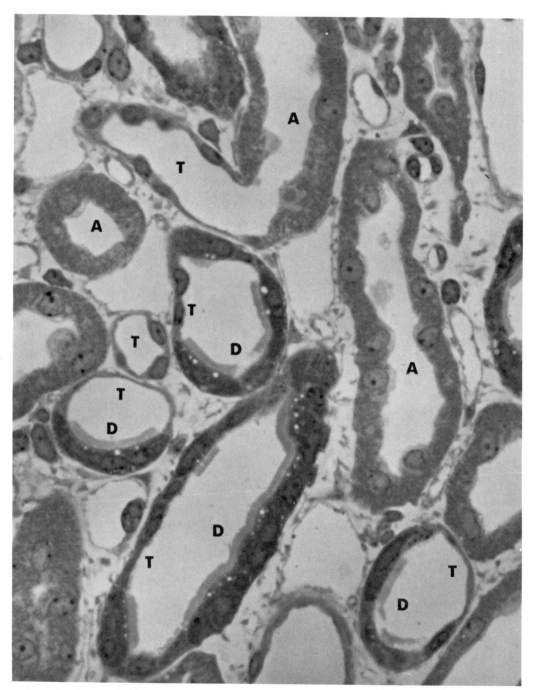

Figure 18.14. Light micrograph of monkey kidney medulla showing transition in morphology of the tubule epithelium in the loop of Henle. Descending thick limbs with brush border (*D*) grade into thin limbs (*T*) which in turn grade into ascending thick limbs with a morphology characteristic of the distal tubule (*A*) (×740).

Table 18.1.
Locations of Portions of Uriniferous Tubules

Location in Kidney		Portion of Tubule
Cortex		
	Cortical labyrinth	Renal corpuscles Proximal convoluted tubules Distal convoluted tubules Arched collecting tubules
	Medullary ray	Thick descending limb of loop of Henle Straight segments of proximal tubules Thick ascending limb of loop of Henle Straight collecting tubules
Medulla		
Outer zone	Outer stripe	Thick descending limb of loop of Henle Thick ascending limb of loop of Henle Thin segment and crests of short loops Straight collecting tubules
	Inner stripe	Thick ascending limb of loop of Henle Thin descending segments of loop of Henle Straight collecting tubules
Inner zone		Thin segments of Henle's loops Crests of long loops Straight collecting tubules Fusions of straight collecting tubules Papillary ducts

preparations stained with hematoxylin and eosin; that is, the cells have a brush border, an acidophilic granular cytoplasm and the other characteristics described for the convoluted segment. However, electron micrographs show that the cells of the straight segment, in comparison with the convoluted segment, have fewer intercellular interdigitations, mitochondria and lysosomes. These findings indicate that the straight portion of the proximal segment does not participate in transcellular transport to the same extent that the convoluted segment does.

The *thin segment of Henle's loop* is about 15 µm in diameter and is lined by a single layer of flattened epithelial cells with nuclei that bulge into the lumen (Fig. 18.16). In the primate kidney, the cells of the thin segment are somewhat less flattened than are the endothelial cells of the adjacent blood vessels (Fig. 18.14). However, they are much lower than either of the thick segments of the loop, and there is a sharp transition from thick descending limb to thin limb, and from thin to thick ascending

limbs. Electron micrographs show only sparse microvilli, simple junctional complexes with few strands in the occluding junctions, and simple infoldings of the basal cell membrane. The cells have fewer mitochondria and lysosomes than those of other segments of the nephron.

The thin ascending limb of the loop is composed of cells with more extensive junctional complexes than the descending limb. As the thin ascending limb approaches the transition to the thick portion, the cell borders become more irregular so that processes of more cells are seen in a given cross section.

The extent of the thin segment, the level at which it is located, and the length of the entire loop, all vary with the location of the renal corpuscle (Figs. 18.4 and 18.17). The distribution of the segments gives rise to a partitioning of the medulla into inner and outer medulla, and of the latter into inner and outer stripe (see Table 18.1). The tubules whose renal corpuscles are located near the corticomedullary junction have long loops of Henle that extend into the inner zone of the medulla. The nephrons of corpuscles that are located in the outer part of the cortex have short loops with the thin segment confined to a small part of the descending limb, and the loops extend only as far as the outer stripe of the outer medulla. The transition from the inner medulla to the inner stripe of the outer medulla occurs where the thick ascending portions of the longer loops begin. Thus short loops of Henle and both thick ascending and thick descending portions of long loops of Henle are found in the outer stripe of the outer medulla. Thick ascending portions and thin descending portions of the loop are encountered in the inner stripe of the outer medulla, and the only portions of the loop of Henle in the inner medulla are the thin segments of loops of nephrons with juxtamedullary corpuscles.

The *straight portion of the distal tubule*, or thick ascending limb of the loop of Henle, is about 9 mm long and 30 μm in diameter. In the short loops, it may begin in the lower part of the proximal limb (Fig. 18.4). It ascends to the cortex and closely approaches the vascular pole of the same corpuscle from which the nephron began, a region with which the tubule has maintained a close association throughout its development. At this level, it becomes continuous with the distal convoluted tubule. It is lined by cuboidal cells that are lower than are those of the thick segment of the proximal limb of the loop. In comparison with the proximal segment, the cells of the distal segment are narrower and therefore their nuclei appear closer to each other in sections. No brush border is observable under the light microscope, although a few short microvilli can be seen in electron micrographs (Fig. 18.15). The cells are characterized by abundant mitochondria in the basal part of the cell, where folds of the basal cell membrane and projecting flanges from adjacent cells produce a region extremely rich in oriented mitochondria and paired cell membranes (Fig. 18.15). The nuclei of the cells tend to be displaced apically and there are few microvilli, resulting in a cuboidal epithelium that tends to show pronounced striations in the basal portion of the cells in light microscopic preparations.

The *distal convoluted tubule* begins near the vascular pole of the glomerulus and terminates by becoming continuous with the arched collecting tubule (Fig. 18.4). It is much less convoluted than the proximal tubule and is only 4.5 to 5 mm in length. It has an irregular outline, and its diameter varies from 22 to 50 μm. It is lined by cuboidal cells containing a granular cytoplasm which stains less intensely with acid dyes than does the cytoplasm of the proximal convoluted tubules. The basal striations are less pronounced than those of the distal ascending limb, and no brush border is observable under the light microscope. Electron micrographs show fewer mitochondria and basal infoldings in the cells of the distal convoluted tubule than in the distal ascending limb. The distal convoluted segment resembles the thick ascending limb in that its cells are not as large as those which line the proximal convoluted tubules, and the nuclei are irregularly spaced (Fig. 18.11).

The cells of the distal tubules show special cytological characteristics where the tubule contacts the vascular pole of the glomerulus. This is also the approximate point at which the distal ascending segment becomes continuous with the distal convoluted portion. A specialized group of cells on the side of the tubule adjacent to the afferent arteriole forms a plaque called the *macula densa*. The cells are taller and more slender than elsewhere in the distal tubules. The nuclei are closer together and the cells have few basal infoldings (Figs. 18.6, 18.11 and 18.18). The Golgi complex of these cells is in a subnuclear position, in contrast with its supranuclear position in other portions of the tubules.

Collecting Tubules

The *arched* (initial) *collecting tubules* in the cortical labyrinth empty into the *straight collecting tubules* (Fig. 18.4). The

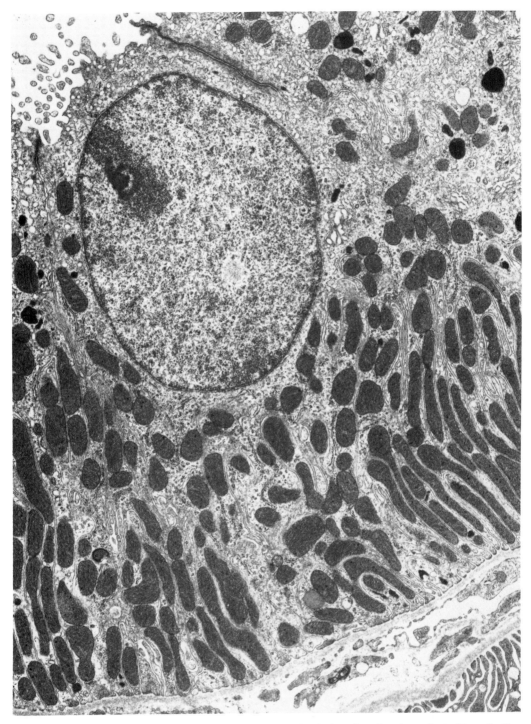

Figure 18.15. Electron micrograph of distal convoluted tubule cells, showing oriented basal mito-chondria and foldings of the basal and basolateral cell membranes. Note the relatively small apical portion of the cell and the apical location of the nucleus (×17,000). (Courtesy of Dr. Barry F. King.)

straight tubules receive a number of arched tubules (7 to 10) as they pass down through the medullary rays of the cortex, the outer zone of the medulla, then to the inner zone of the medulla, where they unite with other straight tubules, and, after a number of fusions, form the *papillary ducts.* The papillary ducts open on the area cribrosa of the papilla. It appears that about seven successive confluences occur before the papillary ducts are formed.

The caliber of the collecting tubules ranges from about 40 μm for those located in the medullary rays to over 200 μm for the papillary ducts of the medullary pyramids. The lining cells range in height from cuboidal in the initial collecting tubule to tall columnar in the papillary ducts. The intercellular borders are more distinct than in any other portions of the uriniferous tubule (Fig. 18.16). This correlates with electron microscope studies which show only a few or no intercellular projections and invaginations.

Two types of cells are seen: those with extensive microvilli or microplicae, and those with relatively few of these structures. Generally the former are more abun-

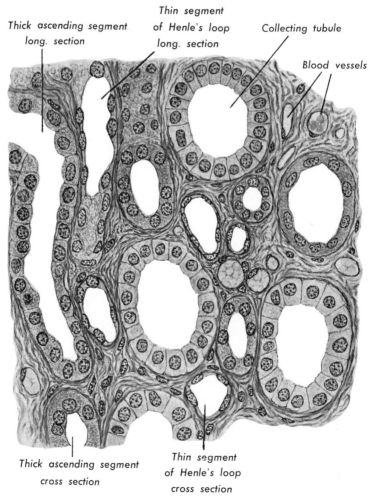

Figure 18.16. Drawing of a section from the medulla of a human kidney (×575).

dant in the cortical region of the collecting tubules, and they disappear entirely before the area cribrosa. Cortical collecting tubule cells have basal mitochondria, although fewer than the distal tubule cells, and some infoldings of the basal cell membrane, again considerably fewer than the distal convoluted tubule cells.

The largest collecting ducts, the papillary ducts, are composed of simple columnar cells with little basal folding and a paucity of organelles. The collecting ducts, like the distal convoluted tubules, have broad areas of occluding junctions that display multiple lattices in freeze-fracture replicas.

The length of the collecting tubule from its beginning in the medullary ray to its opening on the papilla is 20 to 22 mm; that of the nephron is 30 to 38 mm. The entire uriniferous tubule thus measures from 50 to 60 mm, the variations depending mainly on the length of Henle's loop.

A summary of the locations of the various portions of the uriniferous tubules is given in Table 18.1. The epithelium of all parts of the uriniferous tubule rests on a thick basal lamina, the urinary basement membrane. The interstitial connective tissue is scanty in the cortical region but more developed in the medulla (Figs. 18.11, 18.14 and 18.16). It consists of a fine network of fibers, together with the usual connective tissue cells, chiefly fibroblasts.

Blood Vessels (Fig. 18.17)

The *renal* artery divides into an anterior and a posterior branch; these divide further into a series of segmental vessels that pass through the hilus into the sinus, where branches lie between the calyces as the *interlobar arteries*. These pass to the boundary zone of medulla and cortex where they give rise to the *arcuate arteries*, which tend to run parallel to the surface. The arcuate arteries divide into a large number of finer branches, the *interlobular arteries*, which ascend perpendicularly through the cortical labyrinths toward the capsule. The interlobular arteries give off numerous short lateral branches, the *afferent glomer-*

ular arterioles, that pass to the individual renal corpuscles. Interlobular arteries terminate as a final afferent arteriole, except for a few that provide the blood supply to the renal capsule.

The *glomerulus* consists of a number of capillary loops connecting an afferent glomerular arteriole with an *efferent glomerular arteriole*; in other words, *the entire vascular system of the glomerulus is arterial.* The arterioles lie close together at the *vascular pole* where they enter and leave the glomerulus (Figs. 18.6 and 18.18).

As it enters the glomerulus, the afferent arteriole divides into four or five relatively large capillaries. Each of the latter vessels subdivides into a number of smaller capillaries that follow an irregularly looped course in their pathway from the afferent to the efferent arteriole. The looped capillaries arising from each main branch of the afferent arteriole tend to be grouped together, giving the glomerulus a lobulated appearance. Carefully injected preparations show that there are numerous anastomoses between the capillaries within each lobule, as well as occasional anastomoses between those of different lobules. All of the capillaries of the different lobules eventually reunite to form the efferent arteriole, which is always smaller in caliber than is the afferent arteriole.

The *endothelial cells of the glomerular capillaries* are extremely thin, with the exception of the regions where the nuclei are located. Most of the endothelial cell cytoplasm extends along the basal lamina in the form of a *fenestrated plate* with transendothelial pores that have an average diameter of about 80 nm (Figs. 18.8 and 18.9). These pores lack diaphragms and thus differ from the pores of fenestrated capillaries in other parts of the body. Between endothelium and podocytes is a single thick basal lamina composed of an electron-dense central layer, the *lamina densa*, sandwiched between two electron-lucent layers, the internal and external *lamina rara*. This is often referred to as a basement membrane, but it lacks the lamina reticularis component of basement membranes of most other types of epithelium (Chapter 4). The lamina varies in thickness from 0.08 to 0.12 μm, and is observable under the light microscope in sections stained with the periodic acid-Schiff (PAS) technique.

The arrangement is such that the endo-

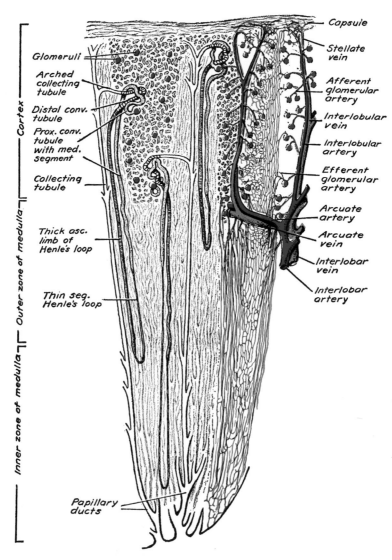

Figure 18.17. Diagram of the structure of the human kidney. The cortical labyrinth is indicated by the presence of convoluted tubules and glomeruli, and the medullary ray is marked by the parallel arrangement of tubules. The medullary ray with adjacent regions of cortical labyrinths represents the lobule. Note that the straight medullary (*med.*) segment of the proximal tubule forms the upper part of Henle's loop and that these loops extend varying distances into the medulla. The thick ascending (*asc.*) limb of the loop is sometimes subdivided into a proximal opaque portion (stippled) and a distal more clear portion (closely cross-lined). Electron microscope studies show that the portion described by light microscopists as opaque has more mitochondria and more basal infoldings. For clearer illustration, the convoluted tubules are simplified and all segments of the tubules are magnified more in width than in length. (Blood vessels are redrawn and modified from Braus H: *Lehrbuch der Anatomie.* Berlin, Julius Springer, 1924.) and tubules are modified from Peter K: *Untersuchungen über Bau und Entwicklung der Niere.* Jena, 1927.)

thelial pores only filter out cellular blood constituents, while the basal lamina forms the primary filter of macromolecules. Both size and charge limit passage of substances. Molecules that are not highly charged and have a molecular weight of less than 60,000 can pass readily into the intracapsular space. The smallest molecule regularly retained by the glomerulus is serum albumen.

At the vascular pole of the glomerulus, there is an association of three structures called the juxtaglomerular complex. The *juxtaglomerular complex* consists of (*a*) *juxtaglomerular* (JG) *cells* (granular and nongranular) in the wall of the afferent arteriole, (*b*) a group of *extraglomerular mesangial cells,* between the afferent and efferent arterioles at the vascular pole of the renal corpuscle and (*c*) the *macula densa* of the distal tubule (Fig. 18.18). The extraglomerular mesangial cells are separated from the macula densa by a basal lamina, but are directly contiguous to the smooth muscle cells of the arterioles and to cells situated within the glomerulus, the *intraglomerular mesangial cells* (Fig. 18.19). The cytological characteristics of both intra- and extraglomerular mesangial cells are largely those of pericytes (see Chapter 12). The *granular juxtaglomerular cells*, together with a few nongranular cells, form a collar on the afferent arteriole in the position of the tunica media in this part of the vessel, and they are derived from the smooth muscle cells of this layer (Fig. 18.20). The JG cells are larger and more epithelioid than other smooth muscle cells, but contain some myofilaments. Granules may accumulate in JG cells in any part of the arteriolar wall which is adjacent to extraglomerular mesangial cells or macula densa. The JG cells are separated from the blood in the afferent arterioles only by an endothelium and basal lamina, and from the macula densa only by a thin basal lamina. The position of the JG cells suggests that they might respond either directly to afferent arteriolar blood pressure or indirectly to changes in the composition of the fluid in the distal tubule at the level of the macula densa.

It has been known for many years that the kidney secretes a proteolytic enzyme known as *renin*. Evidence from the use of fluorescent antibody techniques shows that renin is secreted by the granular JG cells under conditions of reduced blood pressure. Renin acts on a plasma constituent called *angiotensinogen* (an α_2-globulin), releasing a decapeptide fraction called *angiotensin I*, which is inactive but is converted in the lungs to an octapeptide, *angiotensin II*. Angiotensin II is an effective vasoconstrictor and causes release of the steroid hormone *aldosterone* from the zona glomerulosa of the adrenal cortex. Aldosterone in turn promotes sodium reabsorption by the distal convoluted tubule.

In addition to the role of JG cells in regulating blood pressure, it is thought that the JG complex participates in the tubuloglomerular feedback mechanism. With increased salt content in the distal tubule at the level of the macula densa, the filtration rate in that renal corpuscle is reduced. The diminished flow of fluid in the nephron enables the transport mechanism to reduce the salt level. The cells of the macula densa apparently respond to luminal salt concentrations; whatever message they produce is transmitted to the afferent arteriole, probably by the extraglomerular mesangial cells, and results in contraction of the smooth muscle of the wall of the afferent arteriole.

The efferent glomerular arteriole is considerably smaller than the afferent arteriole, since it is carrying less than 85% of the volume of blood due to the loss of ultrafiltrate into the capsule.

The efferent glomerular arteriole divides into a *second* system of capillaries, the *peritubular plexus*, which forms a dense network around the tubules of the cortex. (Figs. 18.17 and 18.21).

The arterial supply of the medulla is furnished by the efferent glomerular vessels of those renal corpuscles which lie close to the medulla (Figs. 18.17 and 18.21). These vessels pursue a straight course into the outer medulla and give rise to clusters of capillaries composed of both descending and ascending vessels that extend to the

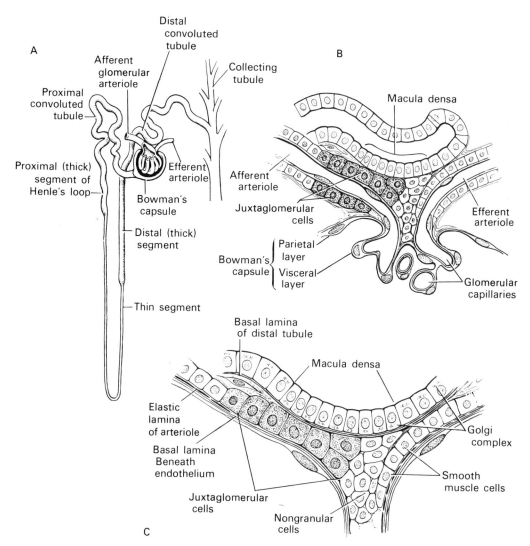

Figure 18.18. Diagrams of a uriniferous tubule and its glomerular arterioles to show the location and structure of the juxtaglomerular cells and macula densa. *A,* a diagram of the relationship between the glomerular arterioles and the uriniferous tubule at the point where the distal segment of Henle's loop continues into the distal convoluted tubule. *B,* a portion of the region at higher magnification. The *macula densa* in the wall of the distal tubule is apposed to portions of the afferent and efferent glomerular arterioles and is particularly close to the *granular juxtaglomerular cells. C,* an enlargement of a portion of *B* showing the apposition of the macula densa to juxtaglomerular cells as well as to the extraglomerular mesangial cells *(nongranular cells)* and the efferent arteriole. The internal elastic lamina of the arteriole and most other connective tissue elements are absent from the region where the macula densa cells and granular juxtaglomerular cells are apposed.

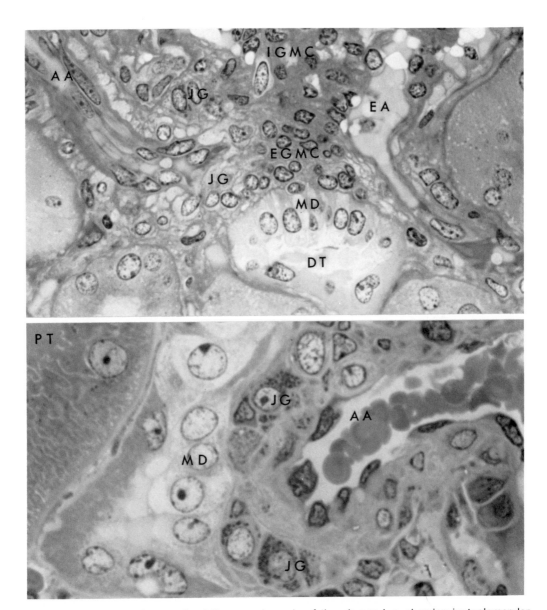

Figure 18.19. Light micrograph of the vascular pole of the glomerulus, showing juxtaglomerular cells (*JG*) in the wall of the afferent arteriole (*AA*), extraglomerular mesangial cells (*EGMC*) between the afferent arteriole and the efferent arteriole (*EA*) and adjacent to the macula densa (*MD*) of the distal tubule (*DT*). Some intraglomerular mesangial cells (*IGMC*) are present within the glomerulus (×580).

Figure 18.20. JG cells with numerous granules are seen in the muscular layer of the afferent arteriole (*AA*) adjacent to the macula densa (*MD*). *PT,* proximal tubule (×1250).

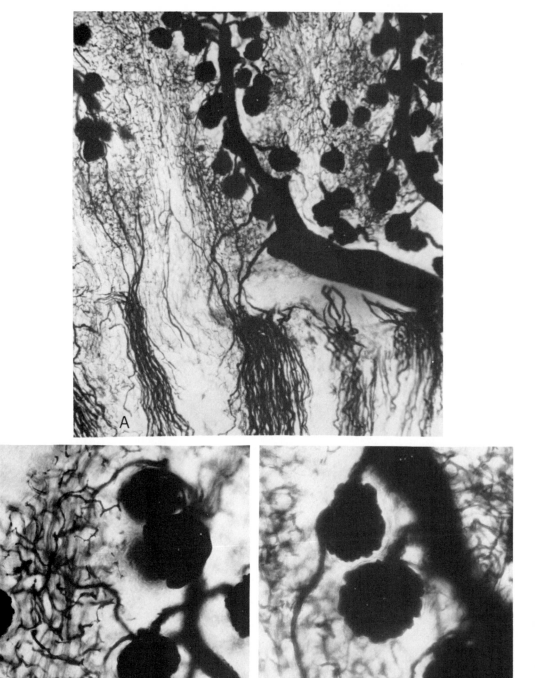

Figure 18.21. Vascular injection of a kidney. *A,* a large arcuate artery, an interlobular artery, and numerous glomeruli. Vessels from the efferent arterioles of the juxtamedullary glomeruli aggregate in bundles of straight vessels entering the medulla. *B,* interlobular artery gives off afferent branches to a number of glomeruli. Note that the efferent artery from the central glomerulus divides immediately into two branches that give rise to the peritubular capillaries (*left*). *C,* the glomerulus at the top has a short afferent arteriole; a long slender efferent arteriole is proceeding down toward the medulla. (*A,* ×36; *B,* ×100; *C,* ×100)

apex of the pyramids. These vessels are known as the *vasa recta*. The clustered arrangement not only shortens the diffusion distance by placing the vessels close together, but also places vessels with opposite directional flow adjacent to one another, forming a *countercurrent exchange* unit. This type of association of vessels is sometimes called a *rete mirabile*. The vasa recta are closely associated with the loops of Henle and are arranged in patterns seen best in specimens with intravascular injection (Fig. 18:21) or in sections cut perpendicular to the long axis of the pyramids (Figs. 18.22 and 18.23). The endothelium of the venule limb of the vasa recta is of the attenuated (fenestrated) type. The looping pathway and association of vessels is significant. There is a progressive increase in tonicity of the interstitial fluid in the medulla, reaching as high as 1200 milliosmoles at the tip of the papilla (Fig. 18.24). The association of vessels in the rete mirabile allows the blood in descending vessels to become increasingly hypertonic, and that in the ascending vessels to become decreasingly hypertonic, thus supplying blood to the medulla in a manner least likely to diminish the gradient of hypertonicity. The hypertonicity of the medulla plays an important role in urine concentration (see below).

The blood from the peripheral portion of the cortex is collected into small venules that unite beneath the capsule; from these arise the *interlobular veins*, which accompany the corresponding arteries and empty into the *arcuate veins*. The latter also receive short interlobular veins from the deeper portions of the cortex. Straight veins collect the blood from the capillary nets of the medulla and terminate in the arcuate veins. From the arcuate veins the large *interlobar veins* pass down between the medullary pyramids and unite to form the renal vein.

Lymphatics

The lymph capillaries are arranged in two systems: a superficial system which ramifies in the capsule, and a deeper system which lies in the glandular tissue. The capsular lymph is collected by superficial lymph vessels that communicate with the lymphatics of adjacent organs. The lymph from the parenchyma is collected by a number of lymphatic trunks which accompany the blood vessels. They leave the kidney at the hilus to enter lymph nodes that are situated on both sides of the aorta.

Nerves

The kidneys are richly supplied with nerves, the majority of which are unmyelinated. They are derived from the celiac plexus and from the 10th to the 12th thoracic nerves. It is probable that branches from the vagus also supply the kidney. The nonmyelinated fibers follow the blood vessels and terminate by numerous endings in the vascular wall, particularly in the glomerular arterioles. Delicate terminals have been described as ramifying in the basement membrane of the tubules or even between the epithelial cells. Sensory myelinated fibers are distributed within the capsule, the smooth muscle of the pelvis and the adventitia of the renal vessels.

Regional Function of the Renal Corpuscle, Nephron, and Collecting Ducts

The kidney participates in the maintenance of homeostatic conditions in the blood and interstitial fluid through a number of mechanisms. First, an ultrafiltrate is formed in the renal corpuscle, then small molecules such as glucose and amino acids are reclaimed by selective reabsorption through the wall of the uriniferous tubules. The content of these tubules is modified further by secretion of both endogenous and exogenous compounds into the nephron. In addition, ions from the luminal fluid can be transported actively to the interstitium, and, through the process of differential permeability, these ions subsequently contribute osmotic work. The kidney both responds to hormones and produces hormones and hormone-like substances (erythropoietin, renin).

Procedures for determining the rates at

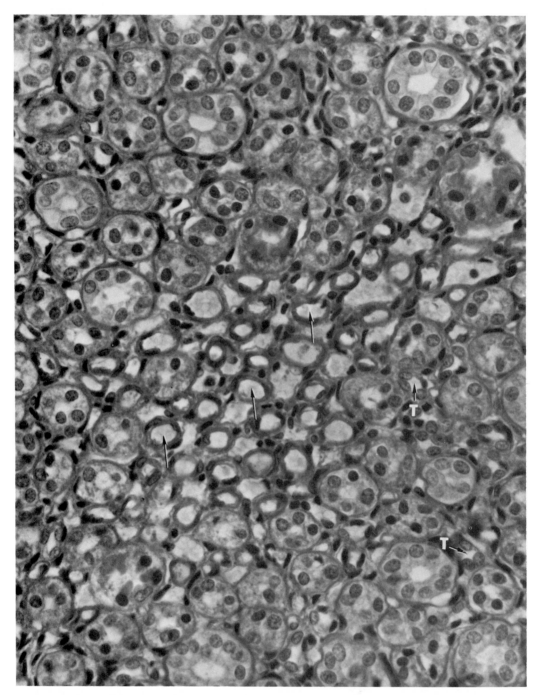

Figure 18.22. Light micrograph of human kidney medulla showing vasa recta. Thicker-walled vessels (*arrows*) are descending (arterial) segments and thinner-walled vessels are ascending (venous) segments. Thin limbs of Henle's loop are difficult to distinguish among the vasa recta in this preparation, but some are seen close by (*T*) (×475).

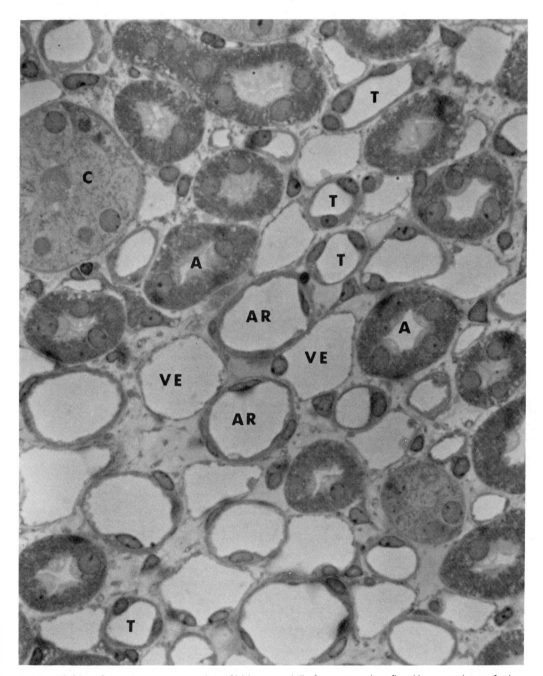

Figure 18.23. One-micrometer section of kidney medulla from a monkey fixed by vascular perfusion. The thicker-walled arterial segments (*AR*) of the vasa recta are clearly distinguished from the thinner-walled venous segments (*VE*) and the thin limbs of Henle's loop (*T*). *A,* ascending thick segment of Henle's loop; *C,* collecting duct (×800).

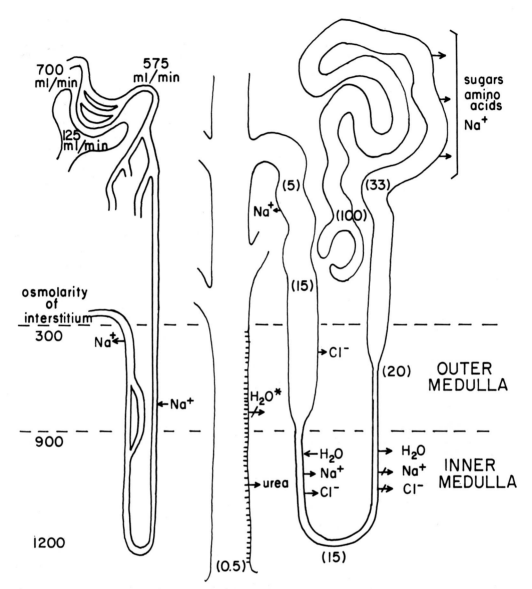

Figure 18.24. Diagram of vascular and nephron relationships in the medulla. The figures on the *left* represent total kidney filtration rates (*upper*) and osmolarities (*lower*). The figures in *brackets* on the *right* indicate percentage of the filtrate remaining in the tubule. *, this portion of the collecting duct is permeable to water in response to ADH, but otherwise is largely water-impermeable.

which different substances are "cleared" from the blood by excretion into the urine have contributed greatly to our knowledge of the function of the human kidney. *para*-Aminohippuric acid (PAH) and the polysaccharide inulin are particularly useful chemicals for clearance studies. PAH is filtered in the glomeruli and is eliminated in addition by tubular excretion. It is cleared completely from the plasma in one passage through the kidney when injected in low concentrations. Therefore, by measuring the amount of PAH in the urine in a unit of time and knowing the initial concentration in the plasma, one can readily calculate the renal blood flow. By this method, it has been found that the average normal flow through the two kidneys is about 1220 cc per min, or about 1750 liters of whole blood in a 24-hr period.

Inulin is eliminated solely by glomerular filtration, and none is reabsorbed in the tubules. Therefore, by simultaneous measurements of the plasma level of inulin and the amount of inulin excreted in the urine in a unit of time, one can calculate the glomerular filtration rate. Studies of this type show that about 175 liters of fluid are filtered daily through the two kidneys under normal conditions.

The 175 liters of *capsular* or *provisional urine* become concentrated to 1 liter or less of actual urine and become altered in composition by the resorption of water and other constituents during passage through the uriniferous tubule. In the process of resorption, substances pass through the tubular epithelium to the surrounding connective tissue and thence to the peritubular capillaries and venules. The proximal tubules and their capillaries come into close association at many points where only a minimal amount of connective tissue separates the basal lamina of the tubular epithelium from that of the capillary endothelium (Fig. 18.14). Although some resorption occurs by diffusion through the tubular epithelium, the resorption of most substances is dependent upon work done by the cells.

The formation of the ultrafiltrate is made possible not only by the structure of the renal corpuscle but also by the fact that the glomerulus is an arteriolar portal system. When the kidney or portion of kidney has reduced blood pressure the JG cells release renin, which tends to increase blood pressure both by the direct pressor effects of angiotensin II and by sodium reabsorption from the distal convoluted tubule under the influence of aldosterone.

The ultrafiltrate originally entering the proximal convoluted tubule contains nitrogenous wastes, conjugated metabolites and other "waste" products. It contains relatively little protein under normal conditions, but is rich in sugars, especially glucose, amino acids, and other small molecules. Resorption of some of these compo-

nents from the filtrate is facilitated by the extensive surface area provided by the great length of the proximal tubule and by the multitude of closely packed, slender microvilli that form the brush border. The increased surface is available for diffusion and for binding sites such as those for different classes of amino acids, and it is the site of a number of enzymes (dipeptidyl peptidase II, endopeptidase, glutamyl transferase, trehalase, alkaline phosphatase).

Proteins in small amounts that appear in the ultrafiltrate are rapidly reabsorbed into the intermicrovillous canaliculi and caveolae of the proximal convoluted tubule cells (Fig. 18.12). Small vesicles coalesce to form larger vacuoles which fuse with lysosomes that initiate degradation. Normal levels of glucose in the blood produce levels of glucose in the ultrafiltrate that can be removed in the first third of the proximal tubule. If the levels of glucose become unusually high, the glucose uptake system can be saturated and glucose will appear in the urine. Glucose passes through the proximal convoluted tubule epithelium in a co-transport system with sodium. The sodium is actively pumped at the basolateral surface of the cells and glucose and chloride follow. Since the epithelium is relatively water-permeable, the luminal content remains nearly isotonic despite the active pumping of sodium. In this fashion generally 75 to 80% of the volume of the filtrate is removed in the proximal tubule (Fig. 18.24). The flanges of the basal side of the proximal convoluted tubule cells and their leaky occluding junctions are particularly suited to the sodium type co-transport system.

The isotonic ultrafiltrate leaving the proximal tubule passes from the thick portion of the descending loop to the thin portion. There is experimental evidence to suggest that the descending portion of the loop is water-permeable but not sodium- or urea-permeable, whereas the ascending portion has largely reversed permeabilities. However, there is little evidence of any active ion pumping by these segments.

Where the thin loop of a juxtamedullary nephron reverses direction near the tip of the papilla, it is situated in an environment that may be as high as 1200 milliosmoles (nearly four times normal plasma), largely due to the presence of large amounts of sodium chloride and urea. When the luminal content enters the thick ascending loop it comes to a portion of the nephron that is relatively water- and urea-impermeable, but in which a combination of coupled transport and co-transport systems, at the apical and basal membranes, and an active pump, situated at the basolateral membrane of these cells, results in chloride transport from the tubular lumen into the peritubular interstitium. Micropuncture studies indicate that when the intraluminal fluid reaches the macula densa it is only 100 milliosmoles with highly reduced chloride and sodium but appreciable urea. The convoluted portion of the distal tubule is thought, both from tubular isolation experiments and from micropuncture studies, to transport sodium ions actively, but the amount of pumping depends on the level of aldosterone. The acidification of the urine and some of the exchanges that occur in the distal convoluted tubule have no particular morphological correlates, unlike the salt pumping which dominates those cells, and which relies upon folded and interdigitating basal regions and associated mitochondria.

The fluid leaving the nephron and entering the collecting duct is hypotonic and low in sodium chloride. Some minor pumping of sodium may be possible by the cortical collecting tubule cells. However, it is the differential permeability of the walls of the medullary portion of the collecting ducts that is most important for water loss or retention. When there is ample water in the interstitial fluid of the body and there is little circulating antidiuretic hormone (ADH), the walls of the collecting tubule, including the papillary ducts, are relatively water-impermeable and hypotonic urine is produced (Table 18.2). When ADH levels are elevated the walls of the collecting tubules become permeable and water is drawn from the lumen of these tubules into the interstitium of the medulla, resulting in a hypertonic urine.

The way in which the osmotic gradient is maintained is generally described as a *countercurrent multiplier*. That is, not only is there exchange between fluids flowing in different directions in separate tubules, but in addition energy is put into the system by active transport at some position. Since the tonicity of fluid in the medulla is known to be a gradient it was originally thought that there was a pump throughout the loop.

Table 18.2.
Permeability and Transport Properties of Nephron Segments

	Permeability			Active Salt Transport
	H₂O	Urea	NaCl	
Thin descending loop of Henle	++++	±	±	0
Thin ascending loop of Henle	0	+++	++++	0
Thick ascending loop of Henle	0	0±	0±	++++
Distal convoluted tubule	±	0±	0±	+++
Cortical collecting tubule	+++[a]/+[b]	0	0±	++
Outer medullary collecting duct	+++[a]/+[b]	0	0±	+
Inner medullary collecting duct	+++[a]/+[b]	+++	0±	+

[a] With ADH.
[b] Without ADH.
Modified from Kokko (1981).

However, only the thick ascending portion has demonstrable major ionic pumping activity. It is apparently this portion that is the major energy-producing segment, pumping salt from the tubule.

To achieve a gradient from the tip of the papilla to the outer medulla rather than a sharp transition at the border between the inner and outer medulla, another factor must come into play. The lower portion of the papillary duct is apparently permeable to urea. Thus urea contributes a major part of the osmotic sink in the following fashion. Chloride is transported out of the thick ascending tubule leaving behind urea. The hypotonic fluid that then enters the collecting duct is low in sodium and chloride but high in urea. When it reaches the permeable segment some of the urea diffuses out of the tubule into the interstitium. Thus the activity of the cells of the thick ascending portion of the loop of Henle situated in the outer medulla results both in the addition of Na^+ and Cl^- to the interstitium at this level. It is also responsible for the concentration of urea which does not diffuse out of the uriniferous tubules until it reaches the permeable papillary duct in the inner medulla. There may also be some back diffusion of urea from the minor calyces through the walls of the papilla itself, a process that is certainly more important in some desert rodents (with their long papillae and 4800 milliosmolar urine) than it is in man.

THE RENAL PELVIS AND URETER

The renal pelvis with its subdivisions (the calyces) and the ureter constitute the *main excretory duct* of the kidney. The walls of the renal pelvis and ureter consist of three coats: an inner mucous, a middle muscular, and an outer fibrous.

The *mucosa* of the calyces and ureter is lined by transitional epithelium which varies in thickness, depending on the state of distension of the ureter (Figs. 18.25 and 4.27). In the collapsed state, the cells of the basal layers are cuboidal, almost columnar. The superficial layer consists of large cu-

boidal cells with lighter cytoplasm, often containing two or more nuclei. A basement membrane is not discernible with the light microscope, but a basal lamina and a thin lamina reticularis can be seen in electron micrographs. Diffuse lymphatic tissue frequently occurs in the lamina propria, especially of the pelvis. Occasionally the lymphatic tissue takes the form of small nodules. There is no distinct submucosa, although the outer part of the stroma is sometimes referred to as such.

The *muscularis* consists of an inner longitudinal and an outer circular layer (Fig. 18.26). In the lower part of the ureter, a discontinuous outer longitudinal layer is also present.

The *fibrosa* consists of loosely arranged connective tissue and contains many large blood vessels. It is not sharply limited externally but blends with the connective tissue of surrounding structures and serves to attach the ureter to the latter.

The larger *blood vessels* run in the fibrous coat. From these, branches pierce the muscular layer, give rise to a capillary network among the muscle cells and then pass to the mucosa, in the stroma of which they break up into a rich network of capillaries. The veins follow the arteries.

The *lymphatics* follow the blood vessels, being especially numerous in the stroma of the mucosa.

Plexuses of both myelinated and nonmyelinated *nerve fibers* occur in the walls of the ureter and pelvis. The nonmyelinated fibers pass mainly to the cells of the muscularis. Myelinated fibers enter the mucosa, where they lose their myelin sheaths. Terminals of these fibers have been traced to the lining of epithelium.

THE URINARY BLADDER

Except for the increased thickness of the muscular coat, the walls of the bladder are similar in structure to those of the ureter. The mucosal membrane is thrown up into folds or is comparatively smooth, according to the degree of distention of the organ. The epithelium is of the same general type–

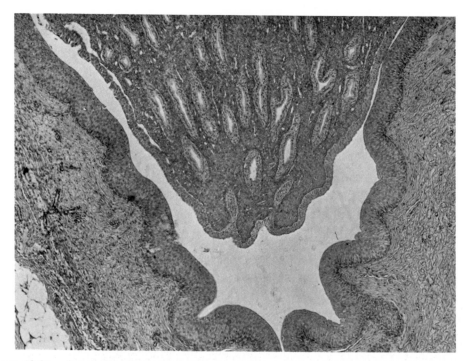

Figure 18.25. Survey light micrograph of a minor calyx and renal papilla of monkey kidney. Papillary ducts open at the tip of the papilla with their lining epithelium becoming continuous with that on the surface of the papilla. This columnar epithelium grades into transitional epithelium that lines the calyx and continues into the ureter and bladder (×60).

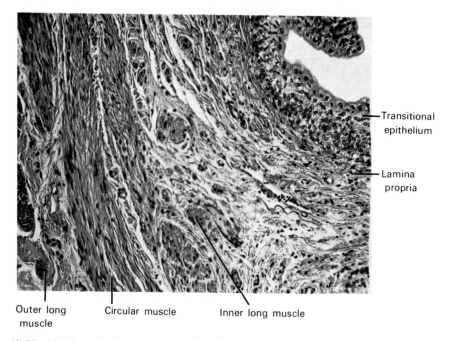

Figure 18.26. Portion of a transverse section of a human ureter. The inner and outer longitudinally (long) oriented smooth muscle fibers do not form continuous layers (×145).

transitional—as that of the ureter and, as already described for the ureter, the surface cells may have two or more nuclei. The ultrastructural characteristics of transitional epithelium have been introduced under "Transitional Epithelium" in Chapter 4. The apical portions of the epithelial cells are characterized by the presence of surface ridges and by fusiform vesicles. Apparently these vesicles participate both in addition and in removal of relatively water-impermeable cell membrane to the surface of the cells during expansion and contraction of the bladder (Figs. 18.27 and 18.28). The number of layers of cells and the shapes of the cells depend largely upon whether the bladder is full or empty. In the moderately distended bladder, the superficial cells be-

come flatter and the entire epithelium thinner than in the contracted organ. In the distended organ, there is further flattening of the superficial cells, and the entire epithelium may have a thickness of only two or three cells. The stroma consists of fine, loosely arranged connective tissue containing many lymphocytes and sometimes small lymph nodules. There is no distinct submucosa and, as in the ureter, there are no glands.

The three muscular layers of the lower part of the ureter continue onto the bladder, where the muscle bundles of the different layers anastomose but still retain some indication of three layers—inner longitudinal, middle circular and outer longitudinal.

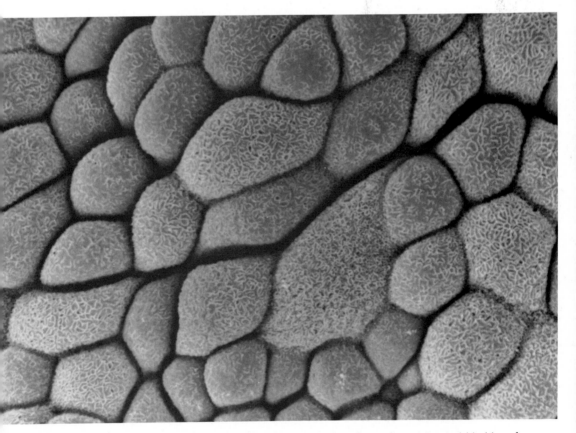

Figure 18.27. Scanning electron micrograph of the luminal surface of a contracted bladder of a rhesus monkey. Note the pronounced pattern of ridges (microplicae) on the surface of the bulging cells (×1,700). (Courtesy of Dr. Barry F. King.)

The fibrous layer, which is similar to that of the ureter, attaches the organ to the surrounding structures.

The blood and lymph vessels have a distribution similar to that in the ureter.

Sensory myelinated nerve fibers pierce the muscularis, branch repeatedly in the stroma, lose their myelin sheaths and terminate among the cells of the lining epithelium. Sympathetic fibers form plexuses in the fibrous coat, where they are interspersed with numerous small groups of gan-

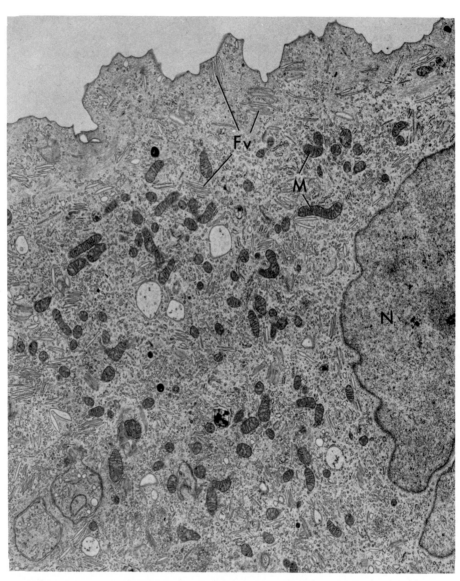

Figure 18.28. Electron micrograph of a portion of a surface cell of transitional epithelium of the urinary bladder. The free adluminal surface has an irregular contour, showing a number of crests and hollows. The cytoplasm just beneath the adluminal surface contains a meshwork of fine filaments but is generally free of mitochondria (*M*). Fusiform vesicles (*Fv*) are found throughout the cytoplasm of the surface cells. They are lined by trilaminar membranes similar to the plasmalemma. *N*, nucleus. From a section of the urinary bladder of a mouse (×8650). (Courtesy of Drs. K. R. Porter and M. A. Bonneville.)

glion cells. Axons of these sympathetic neurons penetrate the muscularis. Here they form plexuses, from which terminals are given off to the narrow interstitium surrounding individual muscle cells.

THE URETHRA

The male and female urethrae differ from each other in many respects. The short female urethra is the terminal urinary passage conducting urine from the bladder to the vestibule. The relatively long male urethra constitutes a urogenital duct conducting both urine and seminal fluid to the exterior.

The Male Urethra

The male urethra has a length of about 20 cm and is divisible into three portions, prostatic, membranous and cavernous. The *prostatic portion*, about 3 to 4 cm in length, is surrounded by the prostate gland. From the dorsal wall of this portion a conical elevation, the *verumontanum* or *colliculus seminalis*, extends into the lumen. On the apex of the colliculus is the small opening of a blind tubule, the *utriculus prostaticus*, a remnant of the embryonic Müllerian duct. On either side of the utricle are the slitlike openings of the ejaculatory ducts, the terminal portions of the ductus deferens (see Chapter 19 on the male reproductive system). Also in this part of the urethra are the numerous small openings of the ducts of the prostate gland.

The *membranous* portion is the narrowest and shortest, measuring about 1 cm in length.

The *cavernous* portion is about 15 cm long and extends through the penis to open on the end of the glans. At its beginning, the lumen is enlarged to form the *bulb* of the urethra. Then it continues with a uniform diameter to the glans penis, where the lumen is again enlarged in a dorsoventral direction and is known as the *fossa navicularis*. Throughout its course this portion is surrounded by a cylindrical mass of erectile tissue, the *corpus cavernosum urethrae* (Figs. 18.29 and 19.27).

The structure of the mucous membrane varies in the different portions. The prostatic urethra is lined by a transitional epithelium similar to that of the bladder. In the membranous and cavernous portions, the epithelium is stratified columnar or pseudostratified, up to the fossa navicularis. There it changes to stratified squamous which, at the external urethral opening, becomes continuous with the epidermis of the skin. More or less extensive areas of stratified squamous epithelium are often seen throughout the whole course of the urethra.

The epithelium rests on a thin basement membrane, beneath which is a stroma of loose connective tissue rich in elastic fibers and containing in its deeper portion a plexus of capillaries and thin walled veins. Smooth muscle fibers, both longitudinally and circularly disposed, are found in the prostatic and membranous portions. A definite submucosa cannot be distinguished.

The prostatic urethra is surrounded by the fibromuscular tissue of the prostate which, under ordinary conditions, keeps the urethral lumen closed. The membranous portion is encircled by a sphincter of skeletal muscle fibers from the deep transverse perineal muscle.

The mucosa of the cavernous portion contains very little muscle and is surrounded by a cylindrical mass of erectile tissue, the corpus cavernosum urethrae. The latter consists of a network of large, irregular, venous spaces, or lacunae, which are lined by endothelium and are separated from each other by trabeculae of fibroelastic tissue containing numerous smooth muscle fibers running both longitudinally and circularly. These lacunae connect with the plexus of veins in the mucosal stroma. The corpus spongiosum is enclosed in a connective tissue capsule containing numerous elastic fibers and, on its inner surface, smooth muscle cells.

The lumen of the urethra shows a number of deep, irregular outpocketings or *lacunae*. These continue into branched tubular glands, the *glands of Littré*, which

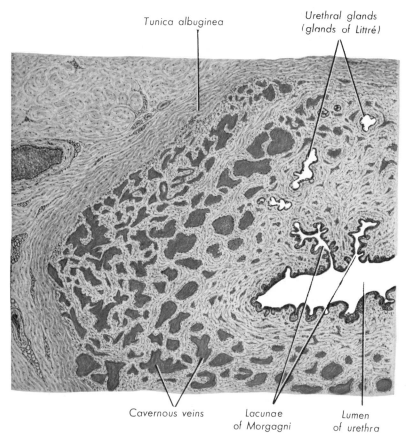

Tunica albuginea

Urethral glands
(glands of Littré)

Cavernous veins

Lacunae
of Morgagni

Lumen
of urethra

Figure 18.29. Drawing of a transverse section of a part of the cavernous portion of the urethra. See Figure 19.27 for lower magnification, showing complete section of penis (×19).

extend deep into the stroma and may even penetrate into the corpus spongiosum. They are most numerous in the dorsal part of the cavernous portion of the urethra (Figs. 18.29 and 18.30). Most of the cells lining the gland tubules are clear staining, mucous secreting cells. Isolated mucous cells or groups of them (intraepithelial glands) are likewise found interspersed in the epithelium lining the lacunae.

The Female Urethra

The female urethra is a short tube 3 to 5 cm long. The epithelium varies considerably in different individuals. Near the bladder it is usually transitional. The remainder of the urethra is lined mainly by stratified squamous epithelium, with areas of stratified columnar or pseudostratified epithelium. The mucosa is thrown into longitudinal folds. Glands of Littré, although fewer in number than in the male, open into the lacunae between the folds.

The abundant stroma is rich in elastic fibers and contains a plexus of numerous thin walled veins.

The rather indefinite muscularis contains both longitudinal and circular smooth muscle fibers, many of which penetrate into the stroma between the veins. An outer layer of skeletal muscle fibers forms a urethral sphincter.

A definite fibrosa is absent, the outer connective tissue fusing with that of the vagina.

DEVELOPMENT OF THE URINARY SYSTEM

During development, three generations of urinary structures make their appearance. These in order of their succession are known as the *pronephros*, *mesonephros* and *metanephros*. The first two are present only in the embryo in higher animals, but are important in furnishing the efferent duct system of the male reproductive organs. Most adult aquatic and marine vertebrates possess functional mesonephroi as the end point of their kidney development. Emergence of terrestrial forms has been paralleled by the evolution of the true kidney, or metanephros, a more compact, lightweight and efficient urinary organ common to all reptiles, birds and mammals.

All three kidney generations arise from the *intermediate mesoderm* or *nephrotome*, a mesodermal mass which is situated between the primitive somites and the lateral plates. In man, only the cranial portion of the intermediate cell mass shows any degree of segmentation corresponding to that of the primitive somites, and it is this region that is believed to correspond to a pronephros. Below the 10th somite, the segments of the nephrotome are so close together as to form a continuous cord of mesoderm, the *nephrogenic cord*, extending to the sacral region of the body. The upper, longer portion of the cord (mesonephric cord) furnishes the mesonephros. The uriniferous tubules of the permanent kidneys are formed from the lower portion (metanephric cord).

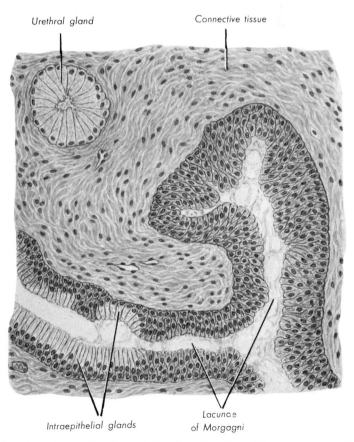

Figure 18.30. Drawing of a section through the dorsal portion of the corpus cavernosum urethrae, showing clear, mucous-secreting cells in a tubule of the urethral glands (glands of Littré) and groups of similar cells (intraepithelial glands) in the lacunae (×294).

The *pronephros* in man is a variable and rudimentary structure which has no urinary function whatever. In some embryos it may be entirely missing. It arises in the cranial segments of the nephrotome in the form of a variable number of ridge-like condensations which may or may not acquire a lumen. The most anterior ridge or tubules are the most rudimentary and soon undergo involution. The caudal ones become somewhat longer and fuse at their lateral ends to form a duct, the pronephric duct, which grows caudally beyond the territory of the pronephros and ultimately empties into the cloacal portion of the intestine. The pronephric duct is situated in the lateral aspect of the nephrotome. The greatest extent of the pronephros is seen in embryos of about 2.5 mm, while in embryos of 5 mm involution of the tubules has definitely begun. All of the tubules gradually disappear, leaving only the pronephric duct.

The *mesonephros* begins its development in embryos of 2.5 mm, just caudal to the pronephros. Cellular condensations appear in the mesonephric cord and soon become vesicular by developing lumina. The vesicles elongate and are transformed into S-shaped tubules, which then connect at one end with the pronephric duct. The latter is now called the *mesonephric* or *Wolffian duct*. The distal end of each tubule becomes invaginated to form a two-layered capsule which encloses a tuft of blood vessels, the glomerulus, derived from a branch of the aorta. The capsule, together with the enclosed glomerulus, constitutes a renal corpuscle.

The mesonephric tubules develop progressively from the front backward and finally form a series extending from the cervical to the pelvic region of the embryo. By increase in number and length of the tubules, each mesonephros comes to form a large structure projecting into the dorsal part of the body cavity. The greatest extent is reached during the fifth or sixth week when the more cranial nephrons are beginning to degenerate, while the more caudal nephrons are still proliferating.

From the sixth week on, the mesonephros gradually atrophies, leaving finally only certain parts which differ in the two sexes. In the male, 8 to 15 tubules in the cephalic portion persist as the *efferent ductules*, the functional connection of the rete testis to the epididymis. The mesonephric duct is transformed into the *ductus epididymidis*, *ductus deferens* and *ejaculatory duct*. In the female, the mesonephric tubules largely disappear leaving only a few nonfunctional remnants.

Each *metanephros* or kidney begins in embryos of about 5 mm as a hollow bud (the *ureteric bud*) evaginating from the dorsal side of the mesonephric duct near its opening into the cloaca. This bud, the anlage of the ureter, grows dorsally and cranially into the metanephric portion of the nephrogenic cord, the *metanephric blastema*, where it ends in a terminal dilation or ampulla, the primitive pelvis. The pelvis elongates in a cranioventral direction and forms four to six branches that likewise terminate in ampullae. These branches are the primordia of the primary calyces. Each ampulla then divides into two to four secondary ampullae, and this process is repeated progressively until the whole system of collecting tubules is formed.

The nephrons, or uriniferous tubules proper, originate from the mesenchymal metanephric tissue which forms caplike condensations around the growing ampulae and the collecting tubules (Fig. 18.31). This development is the result of reciprocal inductive interactions between the epithelium of the ampullae and the mesenchyme of the metanephric blastema. Portions of the condensations acquire a lumen and detach themselves from the nephrogenic cap. Each vesicle elongates into an S-shaped tubule which secondarily establishes a communication with the collecting tubule (Fig. 18.31). The blind end of the S-shaped tubule enlarges and becomes invaginated as Bowman's capsule. The curve of the S ad-

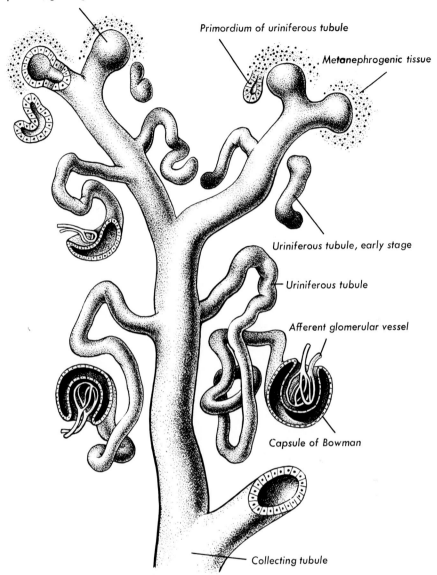

Expanded, growing end of collecting tubule

Primordium of uriniferous tubule

Metanephrogenic tissue

Uriniferous tubule, early stage

Uriniferous tubule

Afferent glomerular vessel

Capsule of Bowman

Collecting tubule

Figure 18.31. Diagram of the development of kidney tubules. Early differentiation of uriniferous tubules from metanephrogenic tissue is shown in the *upper part* of figure; later stages are shown in the *lower portion* of the diagram. (Redrawn and modified from Corning.)

jacent to the capsule enlarges greatly, growing toward the cortex and looping into the medulla to form both the proximal tubule and part of the loop of Henle. Where the loop curves back past the forming glomerulus, it remains in association with the vascular pole, and it is here that the macula

densa of the distal tubule develops. The remaining part of the S-shaped tubule forms the convoluted portion of the distal tubule which joins the arched or junctional collecting tubule. In this fashion, the nephrons are derived from the metanephric blastema (metanephric cord). The ureter, pelvis, calyces, and all of the collecting tubules are formed from the ureteric bud. Thus, it can be seen that all components of the kidney and its predecessors, the pro- and mesonephros, are developed entirely from mesoderm.

References

Andrews PM, Porter KR: A scanning electron microscope study of the nephron. *Am J Anat* 140:81–116, 1974.

Barajas L: The juxtaglomerular apparatus: anatomical considerations in feedback control of glomerular filtration rate. *Fed Proc* 40:78–86, 1981.

Bell PD, Navar LG: Cytoplasmic calcium in the mediation of macula densa tubulo-glomerular feedback responses. *Science* 215:670–673, 1982.

Brenner BM, Rector FC Jr (eds): *The Kidney*, vols 1 and 2. Philadelphia, W.B. Saunders, 1981.

Brenner BM, Bayliss C, Deen WM: Transport of molecules across renal glomerular capillaries. *Physiol Rev* 56:502, 1976.

Bulger RE, Siegel FL, Pendergrass R: Scanning and transmission electron microscopy of the rat kidney. *Am J Anat* 139:483–502, 1974.

Evan AP, Dail WG Jr: Efferent arterioles in the cortex of the rat kidney. *Am J Anat* 187:135–146, 1977.

Gottschalk CW, Mylie M: Micropuncture study on the mammalian urinary concentrating mechanism: evidence for the countercurrent hypothesis. *Am J Physiol* 196:927–936, 1959.

Graham RC, Karnovsky MJ: The early stage of absorption of injected horseradish peroxidase in the proximal convoluted tubules of mouse kidney: ultrastructural cytochemistry by a new technique. *J His-tochem Cytochem* 14:291–302, 1966.

Kanwar YS, Linker A, Farquhar MG: Increased permeability of the glomerular basement membrane to ferritin after removal of glycosaminoglycans (heparan sulfate) by enzyme digestion. *J Cell Biol* 86:688–693, 1980.

Karnovsky MJ, Ryan GB: Substructure of the glomerular slit diaphragm in freeze-fractured normal rat kidney. *J Cell Biol* 65:233–236, 1975.

Kenny AJ, Maroux S: Topology of microvillar membrane hydolases of kidney intestine. *Physiol Rev* 62:91–128, 1982.

Kokko JP: Renal concentrating and diluting mechanisms. *Hosp Pract*, Feb.: 110–116, 1979.

Latta H, Johnston WH, Stanley TM: Sialoglycoproteins and filtration barriers in the glomerular capillary wall. *J Ultrastruc Res* 51:354–376, 1975.

Orci L, Humbert F, Brown D, Perrelet A: Membrane ultrastructure in urinary tubules. *Int Rev Cytol* 73:183–242, 1981.

Rodewald R, Karnovsky MJ: Porous substructure of the glomerular slit diaphragm in the rat and mouse. *J Cell Biol* 60:423–433, 1974.

Smith HW: *Principles of Renal Physiology*. New York, Oxford University Press, 1956.

Strum JM, Danon D: Fine structure of the urinary bladder of the bullfrog. *Anat Rec* 178:15–40, 1974.

Sullivan LP, Grantham JJ: *Physiology of the Kidney*. Philadelphia, Lea & Febiger, 1982.

Taugner R, Schiller A, Kaissling B, Kriz W: Gap junctional coupling between the JGA and the glomerular tuft. *Cell Tissue Res* 186:279–285, 1978.

Ullrich KJ: Sugar, amino acid, and Na+ cotransport in the proximal tubule. *Ann Rev Physiol* 41:181, 1979.

Walker F: The origin, turnover and removal of glomerular basement membrane. *J Pathol* 110:233–244, 1973.

Chapter 19

THE MALE REPRODUCTIVE SYSTEM

The reproductive system of the male consists of the testes, the various excretory ducts, the accessory reproductive glands—seminal vesicles, prostate, and bulbourethral glands—and the penis (Fig. 19.1). The testis performs two main functions: (*a*) production of the male gamete, the spermatozoon, and (*b*) production of androgens (male sex hormones, principally testosterone), which are necessary for both the production of spermatozoa and the maintenance of the differentiated state of the various excretory ducts and accessory glands.

The *testes* are ovoid bodies that have the organization of compound tubular glands. Each testis is enclosed in a dense fibrous capsule, the *tunica albuginea*, underneath which there is a looser layer of connective tissue rich in blood vessels, the *tunica vasculosa*. A closed serous sac, the *tunica vaginalis*, surrounds the anterior and lateral surfaces of the testis. This cleft-like sac is a detached diverticulum from the peritoneal cavity. The testes have approximately the same relationship with this sac as they had with the peritoneal cavity before their descent into the scrotum. The visceral layer of the tunica vaginalis adheres as a smooth membrane to the tunica albuginea; the parietal layer lines the inner surface of the scrotum. Both layers are lined by mesothelial cells. Posteriorly where the serous sac is lacking, structures from within the testis (blood vessels, ducts, etc.) communicate with other scrotal constituents.

The tunica albuginea of the posterior portion of the testis is greatly thickened to form the *mediastinum testis*, from which connective tissue septa radiate into the organ and are continuous with the tunica

albuginea (Fig. 19.1). In this way, the interior of the testis is subdivided into approximately 250 pyramidal lobules, with bases directed toward the periphery and apices at

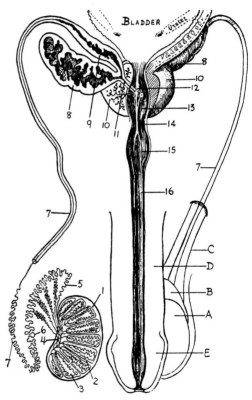

Figure 19.1. Sketch of male genital organs. *A,* testis; *B,* head of epididymis; *C,* spermatic cord; *D,* penis, *E,* glans penis; *1,* tunica albuginea; *2,* septum of testis; *3,* seminiferous tubule; *4,* mediastinum with rete testis; *5,* efferent ductules; *6,* epididymis; *7,* ductus deferens; *8,* seminal vesicle; *9,* ampulla of ductus deferens; *10,* prostate gland; *11,* ejaculatory duct; *12,* colliculus seminalis; *13, 14* and *16,* prostatic, membranous and penile portions of urethra; *15,* bulb of urethra. (After Dickinson.)

the mediastinum. The septa do not form complete partitions; the lobules anastomose with each other in numerous places.

Behind the testis and outside of its tunica albuginea is an elongated body, the *epididymis*. In addition to being the site of sperm concentration and storage, the epididymis provides a favorable environment for further sperm maturation. Three regions of the epididymis may be distinguished: (*a*) an upper expanded portion, the *head* or *caput*, which projects above the upper pole of the testis, (*b*) a narrower *body* or *corpus*, and (*c*) a somewhat thickened lower portion, the *tail* or *cauda*. At the lower pole of the testis, the tail of the epididymis turns sharply and becomes continuous with the main excretory duct, the *ductus deferens* or *vas deferens*.

Within the testis, each lobule contains several highly coiled tubules, the *seminiferous tubules*, surrounded and supported by intertubular connective tissue (Figs. 19.2 and 19.3). They have a length of as much as 70 cm. Although the diameter of the tubules varies from 150 to 300 μm, it is relatively constant in the same individual.

The tubules do not end blindly but form single or double loops. Both limbs of a loop are not always in the same lobule, but may pass through the incomplete interlobular septa. Toward the apex of a lobule, the coiling of the seminiferous tubules diminishes, and there is a short transition portion followed by the narrow *straight tubules*, which are only 30 μm in diameter. The straight tubules pass into the mediastinum and there empty into an irregular network of thin-walled channels, the *rete testis* (Fig. 19.16). The straight tubules and rete testis form the beginning of the genital duct system.

From the rete testis 10 to 15 tubules, the *efferent ductules*, pass into the head of the epididymis and there converge to join the *duct of the epididymis* (Fig. 19.1). The efferent ductules start as straight tubules but, soon after leaving the mediastinum, they pursue a tortuous spiral course, each tubule with its surrounding connective tissue

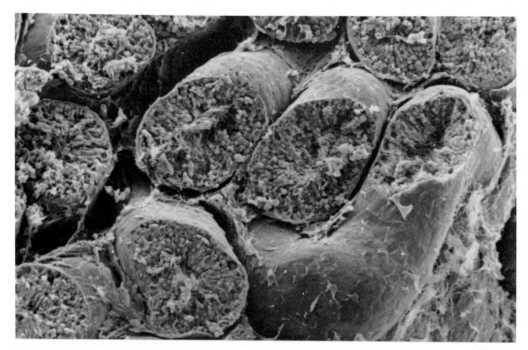

Figure 19.2. Scanning electron micrograph of seminiferous tubules dissected from a testis of an adult rhesus monkey (×210).

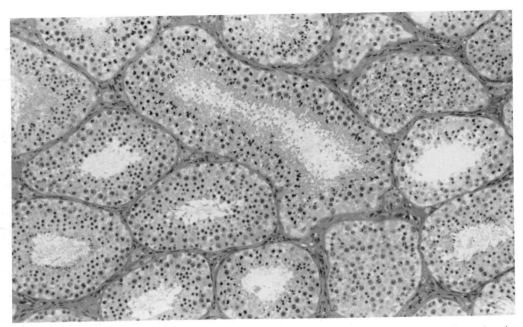

Figure 19.3. Cross section of seminiferous tubules of the testis of an adult rhesus monkey, showing the basic organization of the tubules surrounded by interstitial tissue (×220).

forming a conical lobule. The length of the efferent tubules is 8 to 10 cm. The most anterior ductule becomes directly continuous with the duct of the epididymis, which then receives the remaining efferent ductules at shorter or longer intervals.

The duct of the epididymis is an enormously convoluted tubule having a length of over 4 m. At the caudal pole, it turns sharply upon itself and passes without any definite demarcation into the *ductus deferens*. The ductus deferens, after passing through the prostate, joins the urethra, thus allowing sperm to be ejaculated from the penis.

THE TESTIS

The Seminiferous Tubule

The seminiferous tubules continually produce immature spermatozoa from a stem population of germ cells. The tubules are composed of a complex stratified epithelium surrounded by a thick basal lamina and by alternate layers of collagen and flattened cells called *myoid cells*. The myoid cells have actin filaments disposed in a manner similar to that in smooth muscle cells, but the cells are more sheet-like than fusiform. Peripheral to the myoid cells, in addition to collagen, one or more layers of typical fibroblasts are usually found.

The adult seminiferous epithelium consists of two types of cells, the supporting or *Sertoli cells* and the spermatogenic cell line, the *spermatogonia* and their derivatives, *primary spermatocytes, secondary spermatocytes*, and *spermatids*.

The *Sertoli cells* (Figs. 19.4 and 19.5) are some of the largest cells of the body, 70 to 90 μm tall and about 30 μm wide, and extend from the basal lamina to the lumen. Their lateral borders are difficult to see in the light microscope without special methods because of their close association with the various spermatogenic cells (Figs. 19.6 and 19.7).

The Sertoli cells form the major structural components of the seminiferous tubules, and they serve a number of functions, including: (*a*) mediating movement of spermatogenic cells from the basal lamina to the lumen, and release of the late spermatids into the tubule lumen; (*b*) compart-

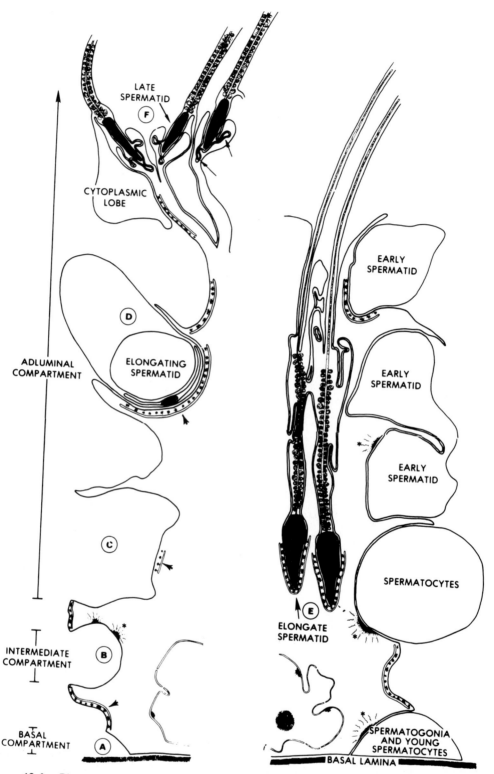

Figure 19.4. Diagram showing the relative positions of the developing spermatogenic cells in relation to the surface of a Sertoli cell. The cytoplasm of the Sertoli cell occupies the center of the figure and is split to portray its two lateral surfaces in close proximity. At level *A*, spermatogonia and young spermatocytes are covered by adjacent Sertoli cells that meet above them to form occluding junctions of the blood-testis barrier. At level *B*, cells leaving the basal compartment are removed from the basal

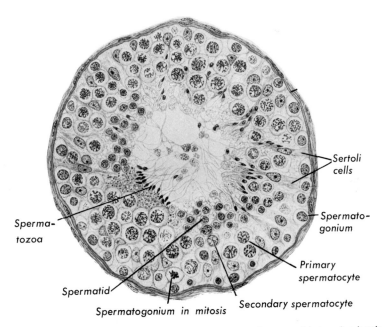

Figure 19.5. Section through a seminiferous tubule of a man 19 years old showing basic organization (×360). (After Stieve H: In von Möllendorf W (ed): *Handbuch der mikroskopischen Anatomie des Menschen*, vol 7, part 2. Berlin, Julius Springer, 1930.)

lamina, and Sertoli cells form junctional complexes below them. At level *C*, once the Sertoli junctions above the spermatocyte dissociate, the germ cell is in the adluminal compartment. At level *D*, elongating spermatids become situated within a narrow recess of the Sertoli cell. At level *E*, this recess deepens as the spermatid elongates. At level *F*, the germ cell moves toward the lumen, where only its head region is related to the Sertoli cell. Specialized contacts: *arrowheads*, ectoplasmic specialization; *∗*, desmosome-gap junctional complex. (Reprinted with permission from L. D. Russell: *Gamete Res.* 3:1980.)

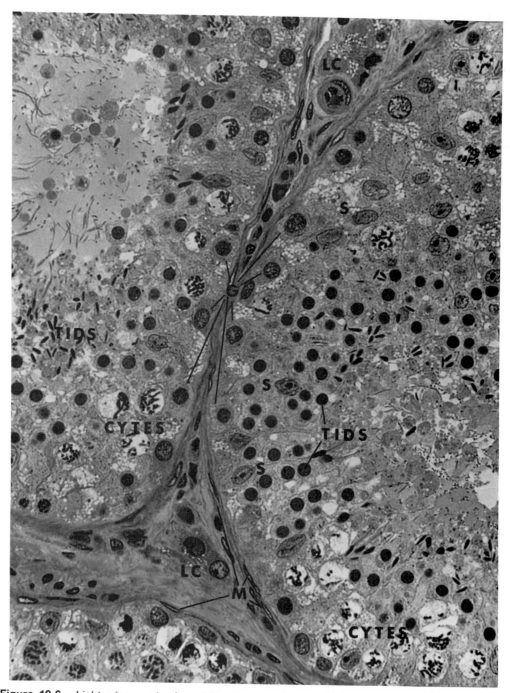

Figure 19.6. Light micrograph of seminiferous tubules of the monkey testis. The progression of maturation of the germ cells is from spermatogonial cells (*G*) to spermatocytes (*CYTES*) to spermatids (*TIDS*). Early spermatids are indicated in the tubule to the *right* and late spermatids in the tubule to the *left*. Myoid cells (*M*) are seen at the surfaces of the tubules and Leydig cells (*LC*) appear in the interstitial regions (×1300).

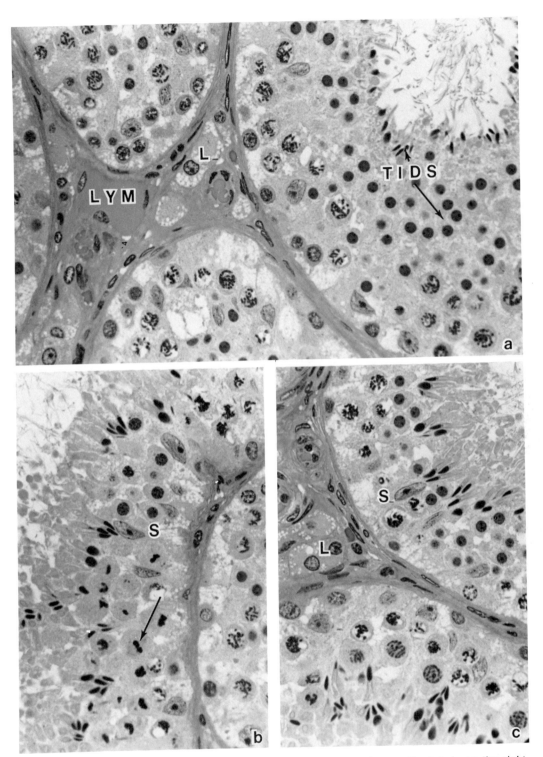

Figure 19.7. Sections of several seminiferous tubules from a monkey. *a*, the tubule on the *right* shows two populations of spermatids and one population of primary spermatocytes. The spermatogonia, with slightly darker cytoplasm, are adjacent to the myoid layer. In the interstitium, in addition to Leydig cells (*L*), there is a large lymphatic (*LYM*). *b*, the association of later spermatids with a Sertoli cell (*S*) is seen. The *arrow* indicates a dividing primary spermatocyte. *c*, the seminiferous tubule above shows two ages of spermatids and one of primary spermatocytes, whereas in the seminiferous tubule below there are two stages of primary spermatocytes and only one of spermatids (×590).

mentalizing the epithelium into *basal* and *adluminal* compartments, thus forming part of the blood-testis barrier; (*c*) phagocytizing of degenerating germ cells and residual bodies left after release of spermatozoa; (*d*) producing steroids from pregnenolone and progesterone; (*e*) secreting fluid, including androgen binding protein and inhibin in the adult and Müllerian inhibiting hormone in the fetus; (*f*) receptor-mediated binding of testosterone and its metabolism to dehydrotestosterone (and aromatization to estrogens); (*g*) serving as the conduit for passage of nutrients from the blood vascular system to the spermatocytes and spermatids.

The fine structure of the Sertoli cells reflects its varied functions, and thus has both generalized and specialized features. The nuclei are usualy ovoid with finely dispersed chromatin and an unusually prominent nucleolus; they often contain indentations. The mitochondria are typically thin but extremely long. The cytoplasm also contains numerous basal lipid droplets, glycogen and, in man, spindle-shaped crystalloids of unknown function. As might be expected of a cell with both protein and steroid synthetic functions, there are patches of rough endoplasmic reticulum and *annulate lamellae* (a rare form of endoplasmic reticulum), in addition to extensive areas of smooth endoplasmic reticulum. Tracts of microtubules and intermediate filaments associated with the lateral margins of the cells are thought to participate in the progression of spermatogenic cells from the basal to the adluminal compartments.

There are also a variety of specialized junctions between Sertoli cells, and between Sertoli cells and germ cells (Fig. 19.4). Extensive regions of occluding junctions between Sertoli cells constitute a portion of the *blood-testis barrier*. This junctional formation prevents the movement of blood-borne substances, such as IgG, from diffusing between cells into the adluminal compartment. Freeze-fracture studies reveal the extensive nature of the occluding

junctions (Fig. 19.8). Interspersed between these occluding junctions are small communicating junctions that are thought to allow some exchanges between adjacent Sertoli cells. Between Sertoli cells and germ cells are desmosome-like junctions; these junctions first become conspicuous between Sertoli cells and pachytene stage spermatocytes, and disappear by the late spermatid stage. In addition, there are junctions between Sertoli cells and some of the spermatogenic cells called Sertoli ectoplasmic specializations (Fig. 19.4). At these sites, filaments within the Serotoli cell are interposed between the cell membrane and saccules of endoplasmic reticulum, but there is no morphologically distinct junctional specialization within the germ cell. These specializations are believed to be concerned with the association of the germ cells with the Sertoli cells, and seem to maintain a fixed relation between the two cells as the germ cell migrates along the Sertoli cell lateral surface towards the tubule lumen. In the basal compartment exchange of nutrients between the interstitial vasculature and the primitive spermatogonia takes place as in any epithelium, but the adluminal compartment is isolated from direct exchanges. Thus the Sertoli cells control the availability of substances presented to the more differentiated stages of the developing germ cells. Not only are immunoglobulins and lymphocytes barred from the adluminal compartment but, in addition, the lumen of the seminiferous tubule has an unusually high potassium content and a different amino acid composition from plasma.

Sertoli cells have receptor sites for FSH and respond to this hormone by increased synthesis and secretion of androgen-binding protein into the luminal compartment. They also are believed to be the source of *inhibin*, a polypeptide hormone that enters the blood and acts as a feedback inhibitor of FSH in the hypophysis and of gonadotropin-releasing factor in the hypothalamus.

The *spermatogenic cells* are interspersed

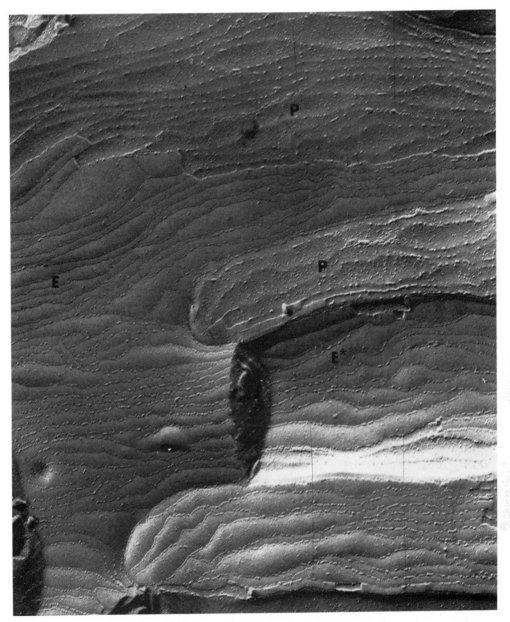

Figure 19.8. Freeze-fracture replica of occluding junctions between Sertoli cells in the mouse. Granular material occurs on the ridges and in the grooves of the fractured membrane surfaces. *E*, fracture face adjacent to cell exterior; *P*, fracture faces adjacent to cell cytoplasm; *E**, E fracture face of a second cell process (×47,000). (Courtesty of Dr. Toshio Nagano.)

between the Sertoli cells, with which they are intimately associated (Figs. 19.5 and 19.6). In the undeveloped testis, only the primitive germ cells or spermatogonia are present. With the onset of sexual maturity, the spermatogenic cells are represented in

all stages of differentiation and are arranged in several more or less distinct associations (Fig. 19.5).

The primitive germ cells, or *spermatogonia*, have a diploid number of chromosomes and have not yet entered meiosis.

From these cells the *primary spermatocytes* (first stage of meiosis) are derived. The primary spermatocytes divide and form the *secondary spermatocytes* (second stage of meiosis), which in turn divide to form the postmeiotic haploid cells, the *spermatids.* Spermatids undergo morphogenesis into spermatozoa. The spermatogonia are located adjacent to the basal lamina and are spherical or cuboidal in shape, with a diameter of about 12 μm. They have a spherical nucleus with granular chromatin. They divide to maintain their own number and to provide the cells that differentiate into spermatocytes.

There are two major types of spermatogonia: *type A*, which is subdivided by nuclear characteristics into type A dark and type A pale, and *type B*. Experimental studies using local injection of tritiated thymidine have demonstated that the dark type A spermatogonia constitute resting cells with little DNA synthesis and little fluctuation in cell number. Consequently they are considered a population of reserve stem cells. The pale type A spermatogonia readily incorporate tritiated thymidine and are therefore considered to be the renewing spermatogonia that undergo mitosis to yield both more proliferating pale type A cells and type B cells.

As is characteristic of stem cells, spermatogonia have few distinctive cytological features. However, the spherical mitochondria with septate cristae typical of mammalian germ cells are present both in spermatogonia and in oogonia.

Type B spermatogonia divide mitotically to form *primary spermatocytes.* The newly formed primary spermatocytes are initially similar to type B spermatogonia but with slightly smaller nuclei, and are briefly in interphase before entering meiosis. The primary spermatocytes then enter the prolonged prophase of meiosis during which they remain large rounded cells with few distinguishing cytological characteristics, while both their nuclei and cytoplasmic size greatly increase. At the end of the first meiotic division, primary spermatocytes divide to form appreciably smaller *secondary spermatocytes*; these rapidly divide with little or no further growth to form the small, round *spermatids* that differentiate into spermatozoa (Figs. 19.6, 19.9, and 19.10).

An interesting feature of division of spermatogonia is that there is incomplete division of the cytoplasm, and a cytoplasmic bridge remains in the region of the midbody at the close of mitosis. These intercellular bridges persist throughout meiosis and differentiation of the spermatids until just

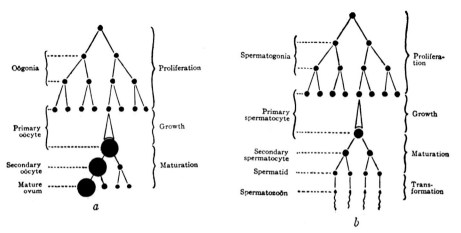

Figure 19.9. Diagrams comparing stages of (a) oogenesis and (b) spermatogenesis. (Modified from Boveri.)

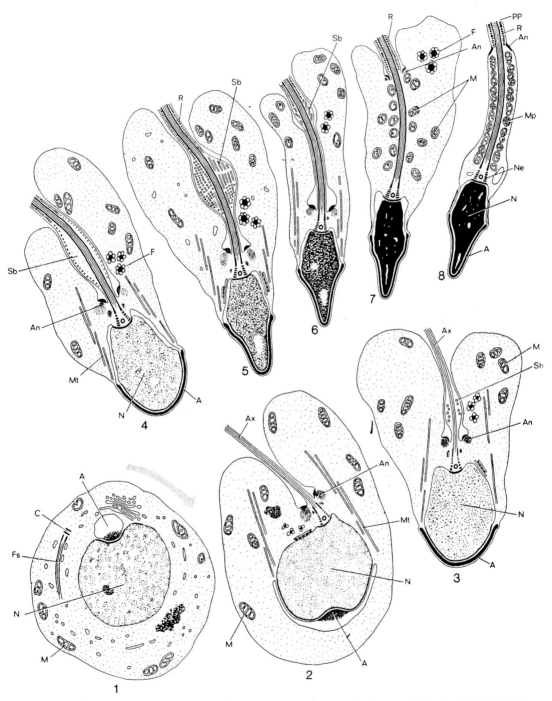

Figure 19.10. Progressive changes in the spermatid during spermiogenesis, illustrating condensation of the nucleus (*N*), formation of the acrosome (*A*), formation of the axoneme (*Ax*), the fibrous sheath (*R*), and the association of mitochondria (*M*) in the midpiece. (Courtesy of Dr. E. C. Roosen-Runge.)

before release of the mature spermatozoon. Thus large groups of differentiating spermatogenic cells are linked together.

Meiosis

In order to understand further development of spermatocytes, it is necessary to consider briefly the events of meiosis. This subject is covered in more detail in textbooks of genetics.

Meiosis results in: (a) the *reduction* of the number of chromosomes from the diploid number of 46 to the haploid number of 23; (b) the *redistribution* of chromosomes of maternal and paternal origin; and (c) the exchange of genetic material between some of these chromsomes (*crossing over*). Two nuclear divisions are involved. As in mitosis, replication of the DNA occurs during the interphase prior to the division, but unlike mitosis it occurs only prior to the first division, and no DNA duplication occurs prior to the second division. During the first meiotic division, which occurs in primary spermatocytes, there is a prolonged prophase in which the homologous chromosomes become associated along their entire length, and crossing over (exchange of segments of chromatids between homologous chromosomes) takes place. During the subsequent metaphase, the homologous pairs are organized on an equatorial plate with the homologous chromosomes associated with one or the other pole of the spindle, rather than the *kinetochores* of the individual chromatids being so associated. As a result, during the first anaphase the homologous chromosomes are separated rather than the chromatids, and only one set of chromosomes goes to each telophase nucleus. The results of this division are (a) the reduction in chromosome numbers to half the original number and (b) the exchange of regions of the chromatids, where crossing over has occurred, between homologous chromosomes.

The secondary spermatocytes formed as a result of division of the primary spermatocyte has the haploid number of chromosomes but they have already replicated their DNA. No further DNA synthesis occurs and there is no interphase step. The chromosomes associate on the equatorial plate at metaphase in the usual fashion. In anaphase the daughter chromatids separate, and after the subsequent telophase, spermatids with a haploid number of chromosomes and haploid amount of DNA are the final product.

The prophase of the first meiotic division is extensive and the events have been divided into a series of stages. As soon as there is some condensation of the chromosomes so they can be visualized as threads, it is considered that the primary spermatocyte has entered the *leptotene stage* of prophase. At the end of this stage there is a cluster of threads toward one side of the nucleus. With continuing condensation it can be seen that there is a pairing of homologous chromosomes (*synapsis*); this is the *zygotene stage* of meiosis. By the end of this stage the chromosomes are associated by the *synaptonemal complex* and are attached to the nuclear envelope.

As the primary spermatocyte continues through the *pachytene stage*, the chromosomes become shorter and each of the homologous chromosomes can be seen to consist of two chromatids. There is a considerable increase in both nuclear and cellular volume during the pachytene stage. During the subsequent short *diplotene stage*, a slight separation of the homologous chromosomes allows the morphological evidence of crossing over, the *chiasmata*, to be seen. During the last stage of prophase, *diakinesis*, the homologous chromosomes move further apart and the chiasmata move toward the ends of the chromosomes.

The metaphase and anaphase of meiosis I separate the homologous chromosomes rather than separating the two chromatids of each chromosome, thus halving the chromosomal number. This *reduction division* results in two secondary spermatocytes, each with 23 chromosomes.

Although originally a set of autosomes was derived from each parent to make up the 44 autosomes of the diploid mitotic cell, when the reduction division occurs the distribution of the maternally or paternally derived member of each autosomal pair to one or the other pole is random. Consequently any secondary spermatocyte may have a variable number of autosomes derived from either paternal or maternal origin.

Occasional failure of separation of the homologous pairs (*nondysjunction*) can result in abnormal numbers of chromosomes (trisomy, etc.).

As previously mentioned, the second division, meiosis II, is of short duration. There is no DNA replication and after a brief prophase the chromosomes are organized on the equatorial plate, and the centromeres divide as they do in mitosis. However, since there are already only half the number of chromosomes, the cells resulting from the subsequent anaphase and telophase (spermatids) are haploid.

A similar reduction in number of chromosomes and in DNA content occurs during the maturation of the oocytes. Fertilization restores the diploid number of chromosomes with the characteristic amount of DNA.

The members of one pair of chromosomes (the sex chromosomes) are dissimilar in the male. One is known as the *X chromosome* and is of maternal origin. The other is the *Y chromosome*, of paternal origin. When the members of homologous pairs of chromosomes separate during the meiotic division of the primary spermatocytes, one half of the secondary spermatocytes receive an X chromosome, whereas the other half recieve a Y chromosome. This differs from the condition in the female, in which each ovum contains an X chromosome. Consequently, when a sperm carrying an X chromosome fertilizes an ovum, an XX combination is established and a female develops. On the other hand, when a sperm bearing a Y chromosome fertilizes an ovum, an XY combination is produced and the embryo develops as a male.

Spermiogenesis

Whereas sperm*ato*genesis refers to the entire process of forming spermatozoa from spermatogonia, sperm*io*genesis refers only to the differentiation of spermatozoa from spermatids. This occurs without further division and without DNA replication. It is the process by which a small round nondescript cell is transformed into a highly specialized cell, with an inactive condensed haploid nucleus, that on further maturation will become capable of coordinated swimming motions and fertilization.

During spermiogenesis, the *acrosome* is formed and comes to cap the nucleus, the nucleus condenses, a flagellum is developed, and excess cytoplasm is removed. These processses are illustrated in Figure 19.10. First the Golgi complex associates with one side of the nucleus, and the centrioles migrate to the opposite side (*1*). A vesicle, the acrosome, derived from the Golgi, spreads over a portion of the nucleus forming the acrosomal cap (*2* to *4*). The cap end of the nucleus becomes oriented toward the base of the seminiferous tubule, and the nucleus becomes more condensed as it assumes its definitive shape (*4* to *7*). While the nucleus is condensing, mitochondria orient along the forming flagellum in the portion of the tail called the midpiece; the distal centriole organizes the axoneme of the flagellum (*7* to *8*). After these changes are accomplished, the residual cytoplasm of the spermatid is phagocytized by the Sertoli cell except for a small cytoplasmic droplet, and the spermatozoa are subsequently released into the lumen of the seminiferous tubule. The result of these events is the formation of a morphologically nearly mature spermatozoon (Fig. 19.11), although it is not capable of appropriate swimming motions until after its sojourn in the epididymis.

The Mature Spermatozoa

The spermatozoa are slender, motile, flagellate bodies having a total length of 55 to 65 μm. They are formed in enormous numbers. From 200 to 600 million sperm may be present in a single ejaculation. In the seminiferous tubules and ducts of the testis, sperm are quiescent. When expelled by the peristaltic action of the ductus def-

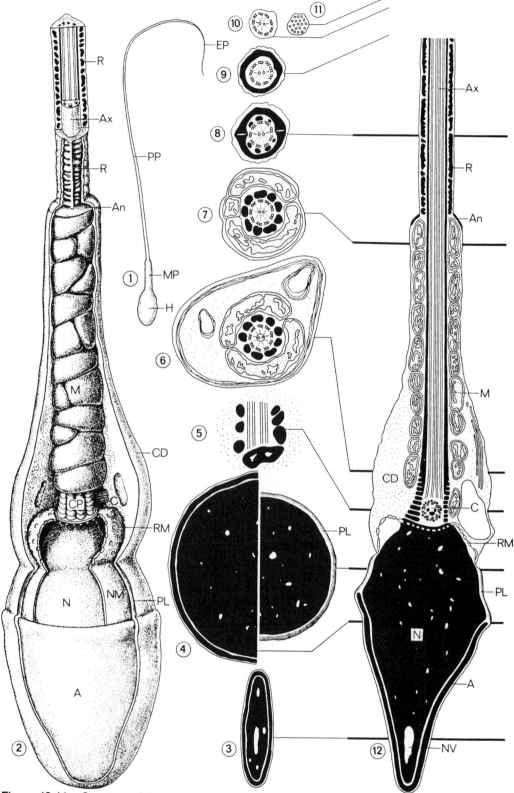

Figure 19.11. Structure of the mature spermatozoon. *1*, the relative size of the head (*H*), midpiece (*MP*), principal piece (*PP*) and end piece (*EP*) is shown. *2*, a three-dimensional cutaway drawing showing the acrosome (*A*), nuclear envelope and nucleus in the head, the connecting piece (*CP*) of the neck, the mitochondria (*M*) in the midpiece, fibrous sheath (*R*), and axoneme (*Ax*) of the principal piece. *3* to *11*, cross sections at the level indicated on diagram *12*. (Courtesy of Dr. E. C. Roosen-Runge.)

erens and duct of the epididymis, they are activated into movement by the secretion of the accessory genital glands, especially the prostate. By the undulatory motion of the tail, they can move independently, and when fully active they can cover a distance of 1 to 3 mm/min. In the favorable environment of the male genital tract, the spermatozoa remain alive for some time after leaving the testis. Living spermatozoa have been found in the epididymis several weeks after the experimental ligation of the ductuli efferentes. In the female reproductive tract, their life is short.

The mature spermatozoon consists of a *head* and a tail. The tail is composed of three parts in sequence: a *middle piece*, a *principal piece* and an *end piece*. The junction between the head and tail is known as the *neck*.

The *head* of the human spermatozoon is a flattened, oval body with a length of 4 to 5 μm and a maximal width of about 3 μm. The anterior portion is thinner than the posterior so that in profile it is pear-shaped (Fig. 19.11). The head consists chiefly of a nucleus with compact, deep staining chromatin enclosed within the nuclear envelope. The anterior two-thirds of the nuclear envelope is covered by the acrosomal cap, and the entire cell is covered by the cell membrane or plasmalemma.

The *neck* is a short region connecting the head of the sperm with the middle piece. The proximal centriole is modified and is located against the basal end of the nucleus at an angle to the axis of the tail. The peripheral portion of the neck region contains coarse fibers that are continuous with the longitudinally oriented dense fibers of the middle piece. Electron micrographs show that some of the coarse fibers are fused in the neck region, and they also appear cross banded due to electron-lucent segments.

The *middle piece* of the tail is about 5 to 9 μm in length and about 1 μm in width. It has a core with the typical structure of a flagellum or elongated cilium, i.e., a central pair of single microtubules surrounded by nine doublets, the axoneme (Figs. 19.11 and 19.12). Peripheral to the axoneme, there is a ring of nine longitudinally oriented, dense fibers. A sheath of mitochondria oriented end to end in a tight coil spirals around the dense fibers of the middle piece.

The *principal piece* is the longest portion of the tail, being 40 to 45 μm in length. It lacks the mitochondrial sheath of the middle piece, and the outer coarse fibers are surrounded by a fibrous sheath composed of rib-like circumferential fibers attached to two longitudinal columns or thickenings of the sheath. These longitudinal columns are in turn associated with two of the coarse fibers (Fig. 19.12).

The coarse fibers become reduced in size, as does the outer diameter of the tail proceeding along the principal piece. At the end of the principal piece the fibrous sheath ends abruptly.

The *end piece* is a short terminal segment lacking any components other than the microtubules of the axoneme inside the plasmalemma.

Cycle of the Seminiferous Epithelium

The entire process of spermatogenesis from a pale spermatogonial cell to a released spermatozoon takes more than two months in man. During the time that one population of spermatozoa is developing, several others are initiated in the same area of the seminiferous tubule. Since the duration of the stages of spermatogenesis remains relatively constant, it has been found that rather than a random distribution of different stages within the seminiferous tubule, there are specific cell associations. That is, a cell in one given stage is always found in association with certain other stages. An examination of the seminiferous tubules of man show that six different associations can be discerned. Since the frequency with which a given stage in cell development will appear depends both on the number of such cells and duration of this stage, some stages can be expected to be seen more frequently. For example, the pachytene stage of prophase lasts about 15

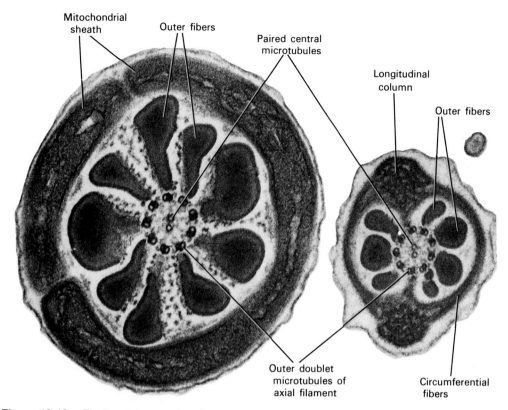

Figure 19.12. Electron micrographs of transverse sections of the tail of a mature spermatozoon of a Chinese hamster. At the *left*, micrograph of a section through the middle piece; at the *right*, through the principal piece. (Courtesy of Dr. Don W. Fawcett.)

to 16 days, whereas the secondary spermatocyte stage lasts only about 0.8 day. Consequently in a cross section of a seminiferous tubule pachytene stages of prophase of primary spermatocytes are more common than secondary spermatocytes, despite the fact that each primary spermatocyte forms two secondary spermatocytes.

In the human testes the cellular associations occur as a mosaic of patches in any given tubule and in a cross section of a single tubule three or more different associations may be encountered. The picture is further complicated in human seminiferous tubules by the fact that active areas of germ cell proliferation appear to be intermingled with inactive areas.

Tunica Albuginea

The *tunica albuginea testis* is a tough, fibrous membrane that encapsulates the testis (Fig. 19.13). It is about 0.5 mm in thickness. Externally it is covered by mesothelium.

Beneath the basal lamina of the simple squamous epithelium there is a layer of rather fine, closely woven collagenous fibers that blends with a deeper layer of interweaving, coarse collagenous fibers. This deeper layer forms the tunica albuginea. The inner part of the tunic is composed of looser connective tissue, which is highly vascular and is called the *tunica vasculosa*. The tunica vasculosa, as its name implies, contains numerous large blood vessels. The connective tissue on the interior of the tunica vasculosa extends into the testis surrounding the seminiferous tubules.

The surface epithelium of the testis and the subjacent connective tissue is often called the *visceral layer* of the *tunica vaginalis*. At the posterior part of the testis, this

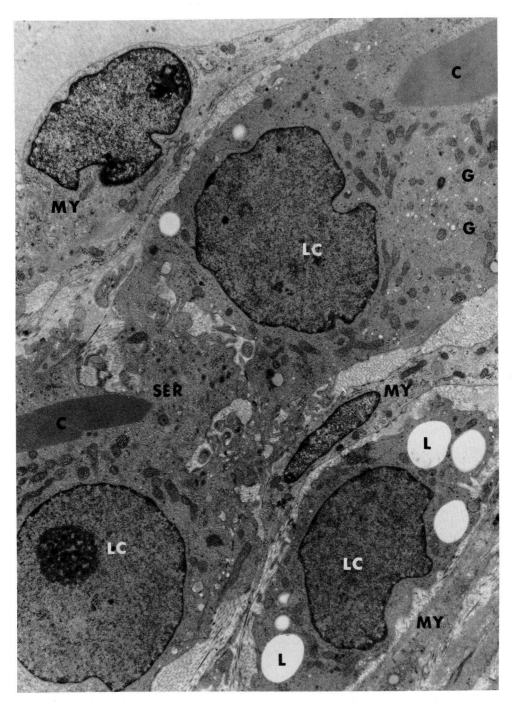

Figure 19.13. Low-power electron micrograph of three human Leydig cells (*LC*). Most of the cytoplasm is filled with smooth endoplasmic reticulum (*SER*); there are also mitochondria, extracted lipid droplets (*L*), and Reinke crystals (*C*). A basal lamina is present on the right side of the upper Leydig cell, but not on its left surface. Two myoid cells (*MY*) with characteristic microfilaments are separated from the general myoid layer (*MY*, *lower right*) that surrounds an adjacent seminiferous tubule. Bundles of collagen are present between various cells (×8,000). (Reprinted with permission from A. K. Christensen: Leydig cells. In Hamilton DW, Greep RO (eds): *Endocrinology*, section 7, vol 5: *Male Reproductive System: Handbook of Physiology*. Washington, D.C., American Physiological Society, 1975.)

layer is continuous with the parietal layer of the tunica vaginalis.

Interstitial Cells (Leydig Cells)

Besides the usual connective tissue elements, the stroma between the seminiferous tubules contains characteristic cells known as the *interstitial cells* or *Leydig cells*. These cells are the principal source of androgens, especially testosterone, the major male steroid hormone.

The interstitial cells occur in groups of various sizes and are quite distinct in the human testis (Figs. 19.6 and 19.13). Small blood vessels are usually present in the groups. The interstitial cells are large and are ovoid or polygonal in shape. They have a large nucleus which is frequently eccentrically located. The cytoplasm of the interstitial cells is granular and fairly dense near the nucleus but peripherally it is vacuolated, and in usual preparations it stains

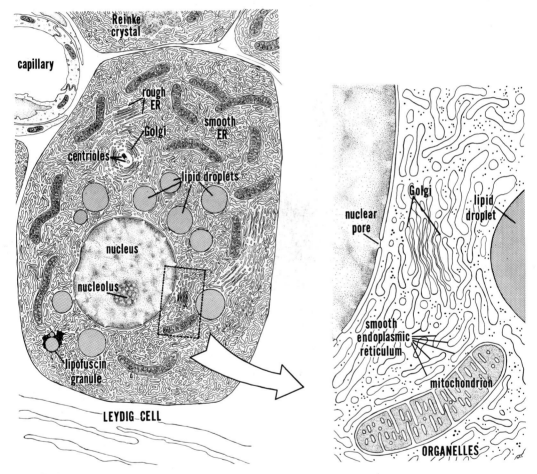

Figure 19.14. Within the cytoplasm of a Leydig cell, the most abundant organelle is the smooth endoplasmic reticulum, although patches of rough endoplasmic reticulum also occur. Mitochondria are common. The Golgi complex consists of Golgi elements that are clustered at one pole of the nucleus but also extend elsewhere in the cytoplasm. Lipofuscin pigment granules and other lysosomal stages are present, as are peroxisomes (not illustrated). (Reprinted with permission from A. K. Christensen: Leydig cells. In Hamilton DW, Greep RO (eds): *Endrinology*, section 7, vol 5: *Male Reproductive System: Handbook of Physiology*. Washington, D.C., American Physiological Society, 1975.)

quite lightly. This is largely due to the extraction of lipid droplets during tissue preparation. The interstitial cells also contain lipochrome pigment granules and crystalloids. The pigment granules increase in number in older men.

The ultrastructure of Leydig cells typifies that of steroid-secreting cells (Figs. 19.13 and 19.14). The cytoplasm of the Leydig cell is filled with an extensive branched tubular interconnecting smooth endoplasmic reticulum. In addition there are small patches of rough endoplasmic reticulum. Mitochondria with both lamellar and tubular cristae, lipid droplets composed largely of fatty acids, lysosomes, peroxisomes, and residual bodies (containing lipochrome pigments) are present. In the human a variable number of proteinaceous crystals, *Reinke's crystals*, are also found.

Interstitial cells are capable of synthesizing cholesterol from fatty acids as well as synthesizing androgens from cholesterol. Since many of the enzymes involved are associated with the smooth endoplasmic reticulum, the abundance of smooth endoplasmic reticulum is not surprising. Enzymes in the ground cytoplasm (cytosol) are also involved in cholesterol synthesis, and enzymes in mitochondria are involved with the formation of acetyl coA from fatty acids, and formation of pregnenolone from cholesterol. Since the smooth endoplasmic reticulum contains many of the enzymes necessary for the total synthetic pathway this organelle is particularly striking. It has been estimated that a Leydig cell may have as much as 4,000 μm^2 of membrane surface.

The production of testosterone by the Leydig cells is apparently under the influence of the pituitary gonadotropin luteinizing hormone (LH) which not only increases the production of testosterone by individual cells, but also increases the number of Leydig cells by differentiation, possibly from peritubular myoid cells or undifferentiated stem cells. Mature Leydig cells do not undergo division, and replacement does not keep up with loss. It has been estimated that the total number of such

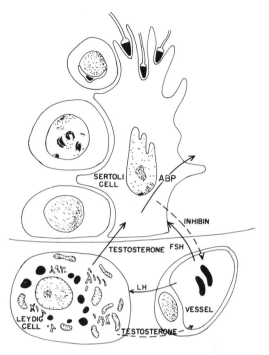

Figure 19.15. Diagram of some of the major hormonal relationships between the cells of the testis and blood-borne pituitary hormones.

cells is reduced from 700 million to approximately 200 million between the ages of 20 and 80.

The androgens produced by the Leydig cells are essential for maintenance of secondary sexual characteristics and are directly responsible for spermatogenesis. They also act in negative feedback regulation of LH production by the pituitary (Fig. 19.15).

Vasculature, Lymphatics, and Innervation of the Testis

Arteries and nerves proceed to the testis, and lymphatics and veins exit from the testis via the spermatic cord. The arrangement of the blood vessels is unusual in that there is a plexus of veins (*pampiniform plexus*) surrounding the coiled testicular artery. This arrangement permits heat exchange between arteries and veins so that blood entering the testis is cooled and that leaving it is warmed. Therefore the pampiniform plexus is thought to be partially responsible for controlling scrotal temperatures. Whatever the mechanism of cooling, the scrotal temperature is 1.5 to 2.5°C cooler than the abdominal cavity. Tempertures above normal scrotal temperatures inhibit spermatogenesis.

Branches of the spermatic artery ramify in the mediastinum and in the tunica vasculosa. Arteries from both locations penetrate into the testis to form the rich capillary beds in the interstitium among the seminiferous tubules. The interstitium also has a rich lymph drainage. In man the lymph capillaries are normal-sized vessels, not large sinusoidal structures. The difference in structure is significant, since it has been suggested that, in species with sinusoidal vessels, the lymphatics form a pathway for local distribution of testosterone synthesized by the interstitial cells.

THE GENITAL DUCTS

Straight Tubules and Rete Testis

At the juncture of a seminiferous tubule with a straight tubule, there is an abrupt change in structure. The junctures occur at varying distances from the rete. Close to the juncture, the developing germ cells of a seminiferous tubule decrease in number and finally disappear. The Sertoli cells change somewhat in structure, their cytoplasm becoming more vacuolated and their nuclei more dense. They increase in number and finally form a continuous epithelial layer which protrudes into the enlarged initial portion of the straight tubule (Fig. 19.16). The epithelial lining then changes abruptly into the columnar type characteristic of the straight tubules; subsequently there is a transition to the cuboidal cells lining the rete.

The rete testis is composed of wide, anastomosing channels, the general course of which is upward toward the ducts. The spaces of the rete are lined by a simple epithelium that varies somewhat in height but is characteristically cuboidal (Fig. 19.16). Occasional cells have a single cilium (flagellum) that is connected to a basal body. In contrast with Sertoli cells, the

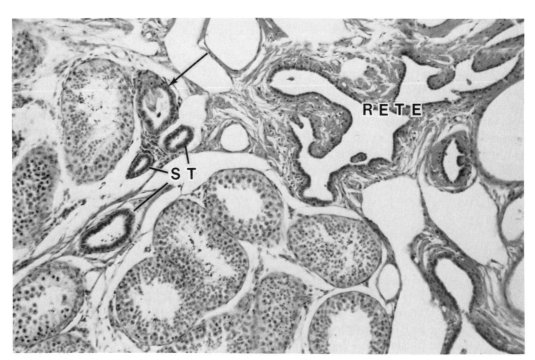

Figure 19.16. Section through a testis, showing a part of the mediastinum and rete testis and the adjacent seminiferous tubules. The juncture of a seminiferous with a straight tubule (ST) is shown in the *upper left* of the figure (*arrow*). (×150).

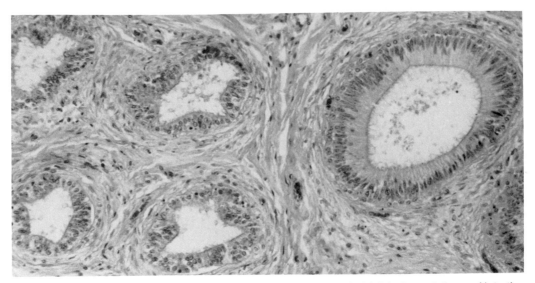

Figure 19.17.   Section of the efferent ductules (*left*) and epididymis (*right*) of an adult man. Note the smooth contour of the lumen of the epididymis and the extensive apical region of the cells (×180).

nuclei stain deeply and the cell membrane is well defined. The tubules of the rete have no definite lamina propria that is distinct from the connective tissue comprising the mediastinum. Myoid cells are associated with the straight tubules, but no smooth muscle per se is present around either these tubules or the rete testes. There are, however, some scattered bundles of smooth muscle in the connective tissue between the rete channels. Whether such muscle could assist sperm transport is questionable.

Ductuli Efferentes

The epithelium of the efferent ductules consists mainly of groups of high columnar cells alternating with groups of low columnar cells. Some of the columnar cells are ciliated, and both the ciliated and nonciliated cells often contain lipid droplets and pigment granules. The variation in height of the cells gives the inner surface of the tubule a characteristic irregular contour, with the low cells lining crypt-like depressions or pockets (Fig. 19.17). The basal border of the tubule is not affected by the alternating height of the cells and has a relatively smooth contour. In addition, to the various columnar cells, rounded cells that do not extend to the lumen occasionally occur at intervals along the basal lamina; hence, the epithelium, strictly speaking, belongs to the pseudostratified type.

The epithelium rests on a distinct basement membrane, surrounded by a lamina propria of connective tissue containing many capillaries and some circular smooth muscle fibers.

The efferent ductules not only are the conduit for sperm from the rete testis to the epididymis, but in addition are the site of resorption of much of the potassium- and bicarbonate-rich fluid from the seminiferous tubules. The resorption of fluid probably facilitates passage of spermatozoa out of the seminiferous tubules, and both cilia and the smooth muscle may contribute to the passage of sperm through the efferent ductules into the epididymis.

Epididymis

The epididymis is a single elongated duct composed of a head, body, and tail. The tortuosity of the duct can be appreciated when one considers that it is 4 to 5 m long, and yet occupies an area at the posterior of the testis only about 5 cm long. Spermatozoa are immotile within the epididymis, and take about two weeks for transit through this structure. The time varies somewhat since the epididymis and especially the tail of the epididymis, is the principal storage area of sperm. During transit through the epididymis, sperm undergo androgen-dependent maturation such that they become capable of appropriate swimming motions by the time they reach the tail.

In contrast to the efferent ductules, the epithelium of the epididymis presents a smooth internal as well as external contour (Fig. 19.17). The epithelium consists of two cell types: a tall columnar *principal cell* and intermittent *basal cells* (Fig. 19.18). The columnar cells are relatively uniform in

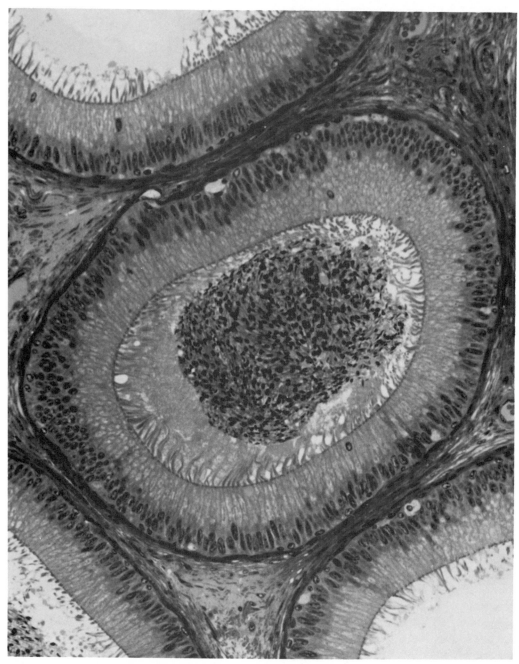

Figure 19.18. Light micrograph of the epididymis of monkey. Tall, columnar cells with apical stereocilia and intermittent basal cells characterize this epithelium. A clump of spermatozoa appears in the center of the tubule (×300).

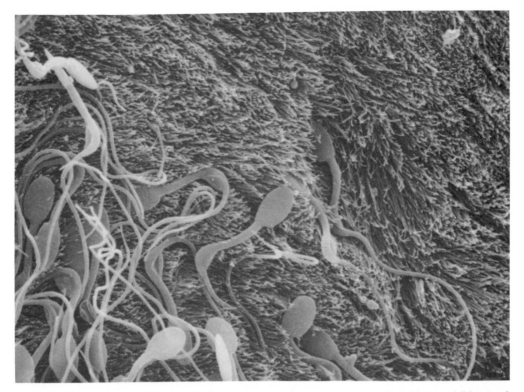

Figure 19.19. Scanning electron micrograph of sperm on the luminal surface of the epididymis of a monkey, illustrating the relative sizes of sperm as compared to the stereocilia of the epididymal epithelial cells (×2,600).

height and have numerous long branching microvilli sometimes called "stereocilia," although they entirely lack the microtubules and basal bodies of cilia (Fig. 19.19). The basal cells are low cuboidal cells, situated adjacent to the basal lamina.

The nurture and maturation of the spermatozoa involves both secretory and absorptive activity by the principal cells of the epididymis. The head region of the epididymis appears to be particularly active in fluid resorption, and the tail region forms a storage compartment that can contract vigorously during ejaculation. Morphological maturation of sperm during movement along the epididymis includes loss of the residual cytoplasmic droplet. A number of other features of functional maturation can be shown biochemically such as an increase in disulfide bonding and deposition of a surface glycoprotein. It is not surprising therefore that cytological differentiation in the principal cells of the epididymis can be

shown along the epididymis. In general, the principal cells are characterized by both rough and smooth endoplasmic reticulum, large apical Golgi complexes, and an extensive lysosomal system including multivesicular bodies and vesicles. Progressing along the duct within the head of the epididymis, the principal cells become taller and the microvilli longer; subsequently, cell height and length of microvilli diminish and the nuclear envelope becomes increasingly folded from the body through the tail.

The epithelial tubules are surrounded by layers of smooth muscle and by connective tissue that is especially rich in elastic fibers. The smooth muscle coat is roughly divided into inner and outer longitudinal and middle circular layers.

Ductus Deferens

The ductus deferens is a direct continuation of the duct of the epididymis. Its proximal portion, which runs along the ep-

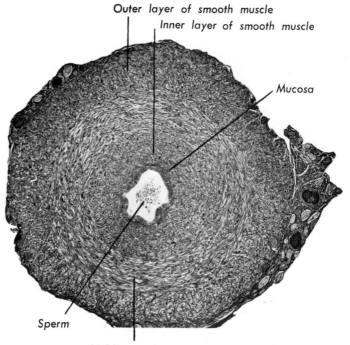

Outer layer of smooth muscle
Inner layer of smooth muscle
Mucosa
Sperm
Middle circular layer of smooth muscle

Figure 19.20. Transverse section through ductus deferens. Adult man (×38).

ididymis, is coiled. Then it straightens and, as part of the spermatic cord, passes into the abdominal cavity to terminate in the prostatic portion of the urethra. Shortly before reaching the prostate, the ductus deferens shows a spindle-shaped dilation, the *ampulla,* which gradually narrows to form the thin *ejaculatory duct.* The two ejaculatory ducts penetrate the prostate gland and empty into the urethra on either side of the prostatic utricle. When fully straightened, the duct is about 0.5 m in length.

The wall of the ductus deferens consists of three coats: mucosa, muscularis and adventitia (Fig. 19.20).

The *mucosa* is lined by a pseudostratified columnar epithelium somewhat similar to that of the duct of the epididymis. The surface cells are lower, however, and the stereocilia show a variable distribution, being absent on some cells and present on others. Cytoplasmic granules are not as numerous as they are in the epithelium of

the epididymis. The epithelium is surrounded by a connective tissue exeedingly rich in elastic fibers and in the deeper portion, numerous blood vessels. Due to the abundant elastic tissue and strong muscularis, the mucosa is thrown into several longitudinal folds, so that in transverse section the lumen may appear star-shaped.

The *muscularis* is by far the thickest coat (1 to 1.5 mm) and consists of three smooth muscular layers: an inner longitudinal, a middle circular and an outer longitudinal. The middle and outer coats are strongly developed layers. The inner longitudinal layer is relatively thin (Fig. 19.21).

The adventitia consists of fibrous connective tissue containing numerous blood vessels, nerves, and often scattered bundles of smooth muscle fibers. It merges without definite demarcation with the surrounding connective tissue.

In the *ampulla* of the ductus deferens, the mucosa shows numerous folds forming crypts, many of which extend as tubular

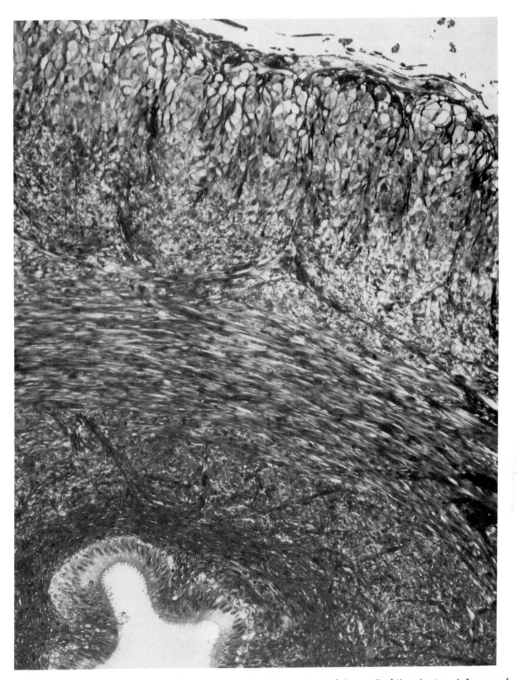

Figure 19.21. Light micrograph of a cross section of a portion of the wall of the ductus deferens of the monkey. The lumen at the lower left is lined with epithelium similar to that of the epididymis (Fig. 19.18). The layering of smooth muscle in the wall is prominent. Some of the most external muscle cells are consideralby swollen in this preparation (×190).

structures into the underlying connective tissue. These are glandular structures lined by a cuboidal or columnar epithelium of a secretory character; the cells frequently contain yellow pigment granules.

The *ejaculatory ducts* have a thin mucous membrane thrown into numerous fine folds, with glandular recesses like those of the ampulla. The epithelium is simple columnar or pseudostratified and becomes transitional near the urethral opening. Beneath the epithelium is a rich network of elastic fibers. A distinct muscularis is present only at the beginning. In the prostatic portion, the muscularis disappears and is replaced by the fibromuscular tissue of the prostate gland.

ACCESSORY GENITAL GLANDS
The Seminal Vesicles

The seminal vesicles are elongated, convoluted sacs that open into the ductus deferens at the junction of ampulla and ejaculatory duct. They contribute about 2 ml of a thick yellowish fluid that is concentrated within the last portion of the ejaculate. The mucosa is folded in a complicated manner, forming numerous irregular chambers or crypts (Fig. 19.22). The epithelium varies somewhat but is usually pseudostratified, being composed of cuboidal or columnar cells that reach the surface, and irregularly shaped basal cells similar to those described in the genital ducts. The borders

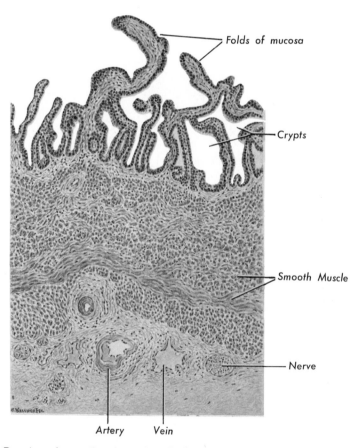

Figure 19.22. Drawing of a section through wall of seminal vesicle. Human, 34 years old, Mallory-azan stain. (×65).

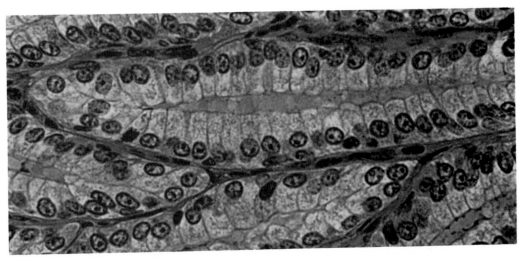

Figure 19.23. Light micrograph of the seminal vesicle of an immature monkey. The epithelial cells are columnar and contain granular secretory material. Basal cells are also obvious (×600).

of the surface cells are very distinct (Fig. 19.23). The cytoplasm of these cells contains secretion granules and a yellowish lipochrome pigment. The pigment appears at sexual maturity and increases with age.

The lamina propria is rich in elastic fibers and forms a continuous layer around the vesicle. The connective tissue of the folds is likewise rich in elastic fibers and contains some smooth muscle cells. Outside of the lamina propria is smooth muscle, which may display indistinct inner circular and outer longitudinal layers, both layers being thinner than in the ductus deferens.

Spermatozoa in varying numbers are often seen in the seminal vesicles. Their presence there is accidental, however. The seminal vesicles are not storehouses for sperm but are glandular structures contributing a slightly alkaline, viscid secretion to the seminal fluid. The secretion is rich in fructose which serves an an energy source for the sperm.

The Prostate Gland

The prostate gland (Figs. 19.24 and 19.25) is an indented sphere of about 20 g situated in contact with the bladder and surrounding the urethra. It contributes a watery secretion that tends to be concentrated in the early portion of the ejaculate. Embryologically it is derived from a series of small periurethral glands and a larger series of lobules that form the greater bulk of the prostate. It can be separated into a *central portion* of short glands proximal to the urethra, and a more *peripheral portion* composed of 30 to 50 tubuloalveolar glands converging to 15 to 30 ducts opening into the urethra. Benign prostatic hypertrophy generally involves the central portion of the gland, whereas prostatic carcinoma commonly involves the peripheral portion. The prostate is dependent on the hormonal secretion of the testis for maintenance of its secretory activity.

The gland is surrounded by a vascular capsule of fibroelastic tissue containing numerous smooth muscle fibers in its inner layer. From the capsule, broad septa penetrate into the interior and become continuous with the abundant connective tissue, separating the scattered tubules or alveoli. This fibromuscular tissue may constitute one-third or more of the mass of the prostate.

The epithelium varies from low columnar to pseudostratified. The peripheral lobules usually have a somewhat simpler epithelium with few basal cells, but are larger in

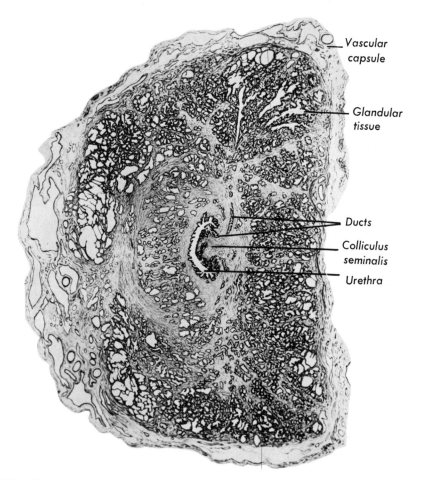

Vascular capsule

Glandular tissue

Ducts

Colliculus seminalis

Urethra

Figure 19.24. Transverse section through the prostate at the level of the colliculus seminalis. Man, 19 years old. (×4). (After Stieve, H. In von Möllendorf W (ed): *Handbuch der mikroskopischen Anatomie des Menschen*, vol 7, part 2. Berlin, Julius Springer, 1930.)

diameter. The cells in the central zone are more irregular in height and are crowded. The ducts are lined by a simple columnar epithelium that changes to transitional epithelium near their confluence with the urethra. The raised central portion where the ejaculatory ducts and ducts of the peripheral prostatic tubules enter the urethra is called the *verumontanum* or *colliculus seminalis*. Within the prostate is also found a small vesicle that is the remnant of the Müllerian duct, the *prostatic utricle*.

Prostatic secretion is acidic, and is rich in proteolytic enzymes which contribute to the liquifaction of the seminal clot. It is particularly rich in citric acid, acid phos-phatase, and zinc. A small amount of the secretion is discharged with the urine, but the major bulk of secretion is discharged by the contraction of the smooth muscle during ejaculation.

The fine structure of the epithelium of the glands is that to be expected of a tissue secreting large amounts of glycoprotein. There is a great abundance of slightly dilated rough endoplasmic reticulum and a well-developed Golgi complex. The numerous secretion granules tend to be somewhat flocculent.

Characteristic of the normal human prostate is the accumulation of concretions within the alveoli of the gland (Fig. 19.25).

Typically, they are spherical bodies about 250 μm in diameter, but there is considerable variation in size. In the fresh condition, they are fairly soft and light yellowish brown in color. In sections, concentric layers that stain with different intensities are evident. They are composed of protein and carbohydrates. The concretions increase in number with age. They may become calcified and then are known as *calculi*, some of which reach a very large size.

The *blood vessels* of the prostate ramify in the capsule and connective tissue trabeculae. The small arteries give rise to a capillary network that surrounds the tubules. From these arise small veins that accompany the arteries in the septa and form venous plexuses in the capsule.

The *lymphatics* begin as clefts in the trabeculae and follow the general course of the blood vessels.

The *nerves* of the prostate are both motor and sensory; the majority are unmyelinated. Many of them come from groups of autonomic ganglion cells which are found underneath the capsule and in the larger trabeculae. Axons of these cells pass to the smooth muscle of the trabeculae and blood vessels and probably also to the epithelium of the tubules.

The Bulbourethral Glands

The bulbourethral glands or *glands of Cowper* (Fig. 19.26) are two small glandular structures close to the bulb of the urethra. During erotic stimulation, the gland secretes a glairy substance resembling mucus into the urethra. This probably serves as a lubricant for the epithelium.

The bulbourethral glands are compound tubuloalveolar glands whose tubules and ducts have a very irregular diameter. The terminal portions may be tubular or alveo-

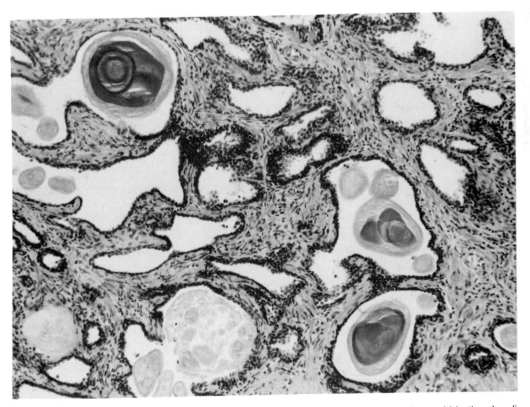

Figure 19.25.   Section of human prostate gland showing characteristic concretions within the alveoli (×150).

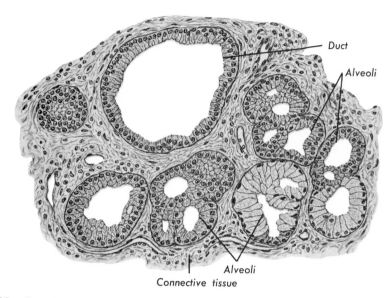

Figure 19.26. Drawing of a section through a lobule of the bulbourethral (Cowper's) gland. Human, 23 years old (×200).

lar or in the form of cyst-like dilations. They are lined by a simple epithelium whose height varies from columnar to low cuboidal and which may even be flat in distended alveoli. Most of the columnar cells are of the mucous type, with the nuclei basally placed, and the cytoplasm containing mucinogen droplets. Other cells stain darker with eosin and have a granular appearance, often containing fibrillar or spindle-shaped inclusions.

The smaller ducts are lined by a simple epithelium and seem to be secretory in character. They unite to form two main ducts that run parallel to the urethra for a variable distance and then open into the latter. The main ducts have a stratified columnar epithelium.

The connective tissue with a few muscle fibers forms the septa between epithelial lobules. Smooth and skeletal muscle fibers are, however, quite numerous in the septa. Externally, the glands are enclosed by a layer of skeletal muscle fibers from the deep perineal and bulbocavernosus muscles.

THE PENIS

The penis (Fig. 19.27) is composed of three cylindrical masses of erectile tissue,

the dorsally paired *corpora cavernosa* and the unpaired *corpus cavernosum urethrae*. The latter surrounds the urethra and terminates distally in a conical enlargement, the *glans penis*. The three cylindrical bodies are enclosed in a common fascia of loose, irregularly arranged connective tissue rich in elastic fibers, to which the covering skin is loosely attached. In the glans, the loose connective tissue is lacking and the skin adheres firmly to the underlying erectile tissue.

Each corpus cavernosum is surrounded by a dense capsule or *tunica albuginea* composed of collagenous fibers (an inner circular and outer longitudinal layer). Elastic fibers are quite numerous. Between the cavernosa, the capsules fuse to form a median septum which is thickest and most complete near the root of the penis. Distally it becomes thinner and contains numerous slit-like spaces that permit a communication between the two bodies (Fig. 19.27). Directly underneath the albuginea is an irregular plexus of small veins.

The interior of each body consists of a network of large spaces or lacunae lined by endothelium (cavernous veins). These are separated by fibrous trabeculae rich in smooth muscle fibers which are disposed both circularly and longitudinally. The lacunae are large and trabeculae are thin in the central portion. At the periphery is a layer of narrower spaces which communicate with the venous plexus on the inner surface of the albuginea. In the flaccid organ, the lacunae are kept closed by the tonus of the trabecular muscle and appear as mere slits.

The corpus cavernosum urethrae has a similar structure, but the albuginea is thin and contains many elastic fibers, so that the organ is not highly resistant to expansion. The trabeculae are thin, the lacunae are quite uniform in size and a peripheral layer of smaller lacunae is absent. Toward the urethra the lacunae become continuous with the mucosal plexus of veins; at the periphery they communicate with the venous network of the albuginea.

In the glans, the erectile tissue has the character of a dense, venous plexus. An albuginea is lacking, the skin being firmly attached to the erectile tissue.

The skin of the penis is characterized by tall dermal papillae and a thin epidermis containing considerable pigment in the basal layer. Coarse hairs are found only at the root, but fine lanugo hairs are distributed over all of the shaft. Only the glans and inner surface of the prepuce are entirely hairless.

The *prepuce* is a fold of skin that overlies the glans. It consists of connective tissue containing bundles of muscles fibers and is covered by a very thin epidermis. On its inner surface, and on the glans as well, are

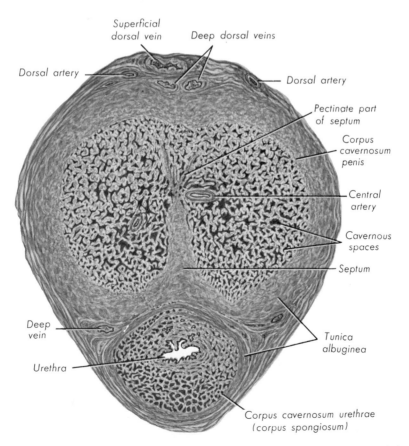

Figure 19.27.   Cross section of penis of adult man. The section is at the juncture of the proximal two-thirds and the distal one-third of the organ. The skin has been removed (×4.5).

found a number of modified sebaceous glands.

Blood Vessels

The penis has a complicated blood supply that can respond to varying functional states. The organ is supplied chiefly by the *dorsal artery* and the *deep artery* which are branches of the *penile artery.* The dorsal artery sends twigs to the albuginea and the larger cavernous trabeculae, where they break up into capillaries. Leaving the capillaries, the blood enters the lacunae and is drained by the plexus of albugineal veins. This is the course of most of the blood during the flaccid state.

The principal vessels for filling the lacunae during erection are the deep arteries (*central arteries*), one of which runs lengthwise in each corpus cavernosum. Associated with these deep arteries are a number of arteriovenous shunts that receive much of the blood when the penis is in a flaccid state. The shunts are contracted, directing the greater amount of blood to the corpora cavernosa when the muscular walls of the deep arteries are relaxed during erection. On entering the corpora cavernosa, the branches of each deep artery give rise both to small arteries that supply ordinary capillary beds and to thick-walled arteries that provide blood directly to the cavernous spaces. These latter arteries, the *helicine arteries*, are contracted and coiled when the penis is flaccid.

The peripheral position of the veins receiving blood from the sinuses and their greater length in the corpora cavernosa than in the corpus cavernosum urethrae suggest that compression of these vessels may aid retention of blood during erection, or at least slow detumescence. However, hemodynamic studies indicate that the increased flow of blood in the helicine arteries alone should be sufficient to produce erection.

The corpus cavernosum urethrae is filled in a similar manner. However, the albuginea is more elastic, the lacunae are more uniform in size and the outflow of blood is not blocked to the same extent. The spongiosum naturally swells during erection, owing to the increased blood supply, but it always remains compressible and does not assume the rigidity of the paired cavernous bodies.

Lymphatics

Numerous lymphatics are found in the skin of the shaft, prepuce, and glans (superficial plexus) and in the mucosal stroma of the urethra. A deeper lymphatic network in the erectile tissues has also been described. The lymphatics drain chiefly into the inguinal lymph nodes.

Nerves

The penis is abundantly supplied with spinal, sympathetic, and parasympathetic nerve fibers. The sensory spinal fibers terminate in a variety of end organs: free sensory endings, Meissner's corpuscles in the papillae, and Pacinian corpuscles and end bulbs of Krause in the connective tissue.

Sympathetic and parasympathetic motor fibers form extensive networks in the walls of the blood vessels and the smooth muscle of the cavernous trabeculae.

SEMEN

Semen consists of seminal plasma, spermatozoa and usually some cells cast off from the lining of the reproductive ducts and glands. Seminal plasma consists of the secretion of the prostate, seminal vesicles, bulbourethral glands, and epididymis, the chief contribution being from the prostate and seminal vesicles. The seminal plasma serves as an energy source and vehicle for the spermatozoa.

The volume of semen from a normal ejaculation varies greatly among different individuals and in the same individual, as does the number of sperm. A typical ejaculate is about 3 ml, containing 200 to 300 million sperm/ml, but there is a great deal of variation in the amount of ejaculate and in the number of sperm. An individual is not considered to have an excessively low sperm count until the number drops below 200,000,000/ml. In addition, most men have a large number of abnormal sperm, and other factors such as motility may affect fertility.

Testicular or epididymal sperm are inactive but quickly become active in seminal plasma (or saline). They carry little of the energy sources necessary for metabolism but acquire this from the carbohydrates, chiefly fructose, in the seminal plasma. The sugar is reduced to lactic acid, glycolysis being best carried out under nearly anaerobic conditions.

DEVELOPMENT OF THE MALE REPRODUCTIVE SYSTEM

The *gonads* make their first appearance on the mesial surface of the mesonephros as ridge-like thickenings of the coelomic epithelium, the *genital ridges*, which at first extend from the midthoracic to the sacral levels. As development proceeds, the anterior portion retrogresses and the gonads become restricted to the lumbar region. The cells of the ridge proliferate and form a band composed of a large number of small cuboidal cells which stain rather intensely. The source of the cuboidal cells forming the ridge is in doubt. Although it has been suggested that these cells are derived from the coelomic epithelium or from the underlying mesenchymal cells, more recent investigation indicates an origin of cells seeded into the forming genital ridge from mesonephric tubules. Scattered between these somatic cells are larger spherical cells with vesicular nuclei and clearer cytoplasm, the *primitive germ cells*. The primitive germ cells do not arise in situ but migrate in from the yolk sac and are believed to be endodermal in origin.

As the epithelial mass with its contained germ cells continues to proliferate, irregular plugs or strands of epithelial cells, the *medullary* or *sex cords*, extend into the underlying connective tissue. The deepest portions of the cords, which lie closest to the mesonephric tubules, anastomose with

one another and with a cell mass derived from the mesonephros to form the anlage of the *rete*.

Up to about the sixth week, development proceeds similarly in both sexes. This is the so-called "indifferent" period. Although sex is determined by the constitution of the fertilized ovum, histological differences between the male and female cannot be observed during this period.

From the sixth week on, histological changes occur that lead to a definite differentiation of the gonads. In the *testis*, a layer of embryonal connective tissue, the future *tunica albuginea*, grows in between the medullary cords and the epithelial cells immediately adjacent to the coelom. It separates the latter, which persist as the misnamed germinal epithelium, until it gradually is reduced to a single layer of squamous cells that forms the visceral layer of the tunica vaginalis. The medullary cords become more distinct and elongate to form the convoluted *seminiferous tubules*. The deeper portions of the cords develop short connecting segments, the tubuli recti, that communicate with the anastomotic rete testis. This, in turn, communicates with the efferent ductules (from mesonephric tubules) and thence with the ductus epididymis and ductus deferens (both from the mesonephric duct).

At the time of the indifferent stage in gonadal development, there is, in addition to the mesonephric ducts, a pair of lateral *paramesonephric* (*Müllerian*) ducts. From these the female genital ducts are derived, but they degenerate in the male. The differentiation of the duct system is under the influence of the developing testis.

During subsequent development, the larger cells (germ cells) in the seminiferous tubule seem to become temporarily smaller, although still distinct in chromosomal content, before eventually giving rise to spermatogenic cells. The other cells in the cords give rise to Sertoli cells while some of the cells between the cords form interstitial cells (Fig. 19.28 and 19.29). The androgens

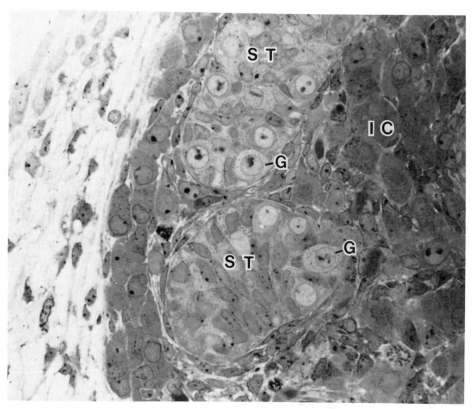

Figure 19.28. Section through the testis of a male fetus. The developing seminiferous tubules (ST) contain primitive germ cells (G) but no spermatogenic stages. They are surrounded by glandular interstitial cells (IC) (×350).

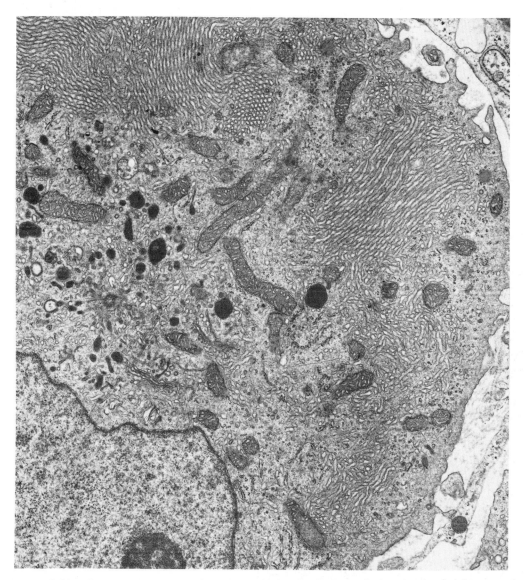

Figure 19.29.   Electron micrograph of a portion of a fetal interstitial cell, showing the Golgi zone and agranular endoplasmic reticulum characteristic of these androgen-producing cells. Male fetus, 10 cm CRL (×15,000).

testosterone and dehydrotestosterone from the interstitial cells promote development of two groups of accessory male structures. The seminal vesicles, ductus deferens and epididymis develop under the influence of testosterone and the prostate and external genitalia respond especially to dehydrotestosterone. A factor from the Sertoli cells, *Müllerian inhibiting factor*, speeds the regression of the Müllerian duct, leaving only a few remnants.

References

Christensen AK: The fine structure of testicular interstitial cells in the guinea pig. *J Cell Biol* 26:911–935, 1965.

Christensen AK: Leydig cells. In Hamilton DW, Greep RO (eds): *Endocrinology*, section 7, vol 5: *Male Reproductive System: Handbook of Physiology*. Washington, D.C., American Physiological Society, 1975.

Christensen AK: Specific contacts between Leydig cells and macrophages in the rat testis. *Anat Rec* 184:377, 1976.

Clermont Y: Kinetics of spermatogenesis in mammals: seminiferous epithelium cycle and spermatogonial renewal. *Physiol Rev* 52: 198–236, 1972.

Dym M, Fawcett DW: The blood-testis barrier in the rat and the physiological compartmentation of the seminiferous epithelium. *Biol Reprod* 3:308–326, 1970.

Dym, M: Morphology of the monkey testis: Comparison with human and with lower mammalian species. In Anand Kumar TC (ed): *Non-Human Primate Models for Study of Human Reproduction*. Basel, S. Karger, 1980, pp 116–128.

Dym, M, Cavicchia, JC: Further observations on the blood-testis barrier in monkeys. *Biol Reprod* 17:390–403, 1977.

Fawcett, DW: Ultrastructure and function of the Sertoli cell. In Hamilton DW, Greep RO (eds): *Endocrinology*, section 7, vol 5: *Male Reproductive System: Handbook of Physiology*. Washington, D.C., American Physiological Society, 1975.

Fawcett, DW, Bedford, JM: *The Spermatozoon: Maturation, Motility, Surface Properties, and Comparative Aspects*. Baltimore, Urban and Schwarzenberg, 1979.

Holstein, AF, Roosen-Runge, EC: *Atlas of Human Spermatogenesis*. Berlin, Gross Verlag, 1981.

Hamilton, DW: Structure and function of the epithelium lining the ductuli efferentes, ductus epididymis, and ductus deferens in the rat. In Hamilton DW, Greep RO (eds): *Endocrinology*, section 7, vol 5: *Male Reproductive System: Handbook of Physiology*. Washington, D.C., American Physiological Society, 1975.

Leblond, CP, Clermont, Y: Definition of the stages of the cycle of the seminiferous epithelium in the rat. *Ann NY Acad Sci* 55:548–573, 1952.

Mann, T: *Biochemistry of Semen and of the Male Reproductive Tract*. New York, John Wiley & Sons, 1964.

Nagano, T, Suzuki, F: Freeze-fracture observations on the intercellular junctions of Sertoli cells and of Leydig cells in the human testis. *Cell Tissue Res* 166:37–48, 1976.

Ross, MH: Contractile cells in human seminiferous tubules. *Science* 153:1271–1273, 1966.

Russell, LD: Sertoli-germ cell interrelations: a review. *Gamete Res* 3:178–202, 1980.

Steinberger, E: Hormonal control of mammalian spermatogenesis. *Physiol Rev* 51:1–22, 1971.

Wartenberg, H: Differentiation and development of the testis. In Burger H, deKretser D (eds): *The Testis*. New York, Raven Press, 1981.

Chapter 20

THE FEMALE REPRODUCTIVE SYSTEM

The female genital organs are composed of the ovaries, the genital ducts—the oviducts, uterus and vagina—and the external genitalia, including the labia majora, labia minora and clitoris. The ovaries are the site of proliferation of the germ cells during fetal life and of the periodic release of these cells in the adult. In addition, they play a dominant role in production of hormones modulating the condition of the reproductive organs. The mammary glands are not genital organs, but are important glands of the female reproductive system.

THE OVARY

The ovaries are somewhat flattened, ovoid bodies, measuring about 4 cm in length, 2 cm in width and 1 cm in thickness, suspended on either side of the uterus (Fig. 20.1). Each is attached to the broad ligament by a peritoneal fold, the mesovarium, and to the uterus by the ligament of the ovary. The ovarian vessels and nerves pass in the suspensory ligament of the ovary (infundibulopelvic ligament) to the hilus, where they enter the inner or medullary portion of the ovary.

At the hilus, the connective tissue of the mesovarium and ovarian ligament passes into the ovary and becomes continuous with the ovarian connective tissue. The mesothelial covering of the mesovarium changes at the hilus to a low cuboidal *surface epithelium* which covers the ovary. Directly underneath the surface epithelium, the connective tissue forms a dense fibrous layer, the *tunica albuginea*, composed of closely packed fibers and few cells.

In sections of the ovary, two zones may be distinguished: a central deeper portion, the *medulla*, and a broad outer layer, the *cortex* (Fig. 20.2). The two zones blend without distinct demarcation. The medulla is composed of a framework of loose connective tissue rich in elastic fibers and containing numerous large blood vessels, lymphatics and nerves. Bundles of smooth muscle fibers are found near the hilus. In some individuals, vestiges of fetal structures, the *rete ovarii*, occur as epithelial strands or tubules in the region of the hilus. The cortex consists of a compact, richly cellular connective tissue in which are scattered the characteristic epithelial structures of the ovary, the *ovarian follicles* (Fig. 20.2).

Ovarian Follicles

The cortex of the ovary of a young adult woman contains a large number of follicles in different stages of growth and of degeneration (*atresia*). The size and complexity of follicles vary with the stage of development, but each is composed of an oocyte surrounded by epithelial cells and, in large follicles, one or two connective tissue coats (Fig. 20.3).

The most abundant and smallest follicles are called *primordial follicles*. They consist of a *primary oocyte* in the stage of arrested meiotic prophase (see Chapter 19), surrounded by a few flattened *follicular cells* (Fig. 20.4). These follicles have remained in this condition since the fifth or sixth month of fetal development, are unresponsive to gonadotropins, and constitute a resting stage. A few follicles are continually leaving this stage; such follicles that have begun growth are designated *primary follicles*. The follicular cells divide and enlarge

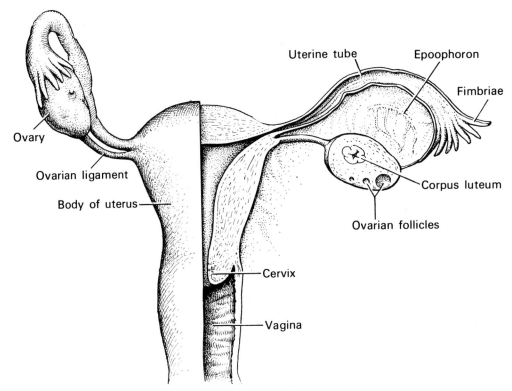

Figure 20.1.   Diagram of the internal organs of the female reproductive system seen from the dorsal side. The ovary and uterine tube are shown in approximately normal position at the *left* and they are drawn apart and away from the uterus at the *right*.

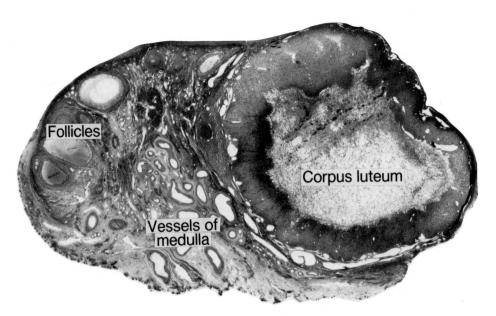

Figure 20.2.   Section of an ovary of a normal adult baboon. The cortex forms a rim around the ovary except in the *lower center*, where vessels from the mesovarium enter the medulla. Fibroblasts have invaded the clot in the center of the corpus luteum (×8.5).

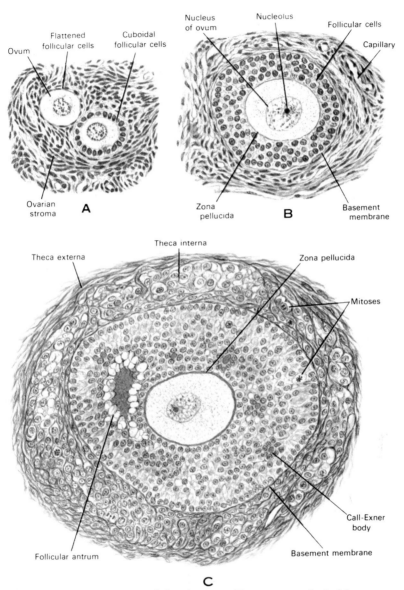

Figure 20.3.   Follicles in various states of development. These were selected from a normal human ovary removed surgically on the 14th day of the cycle and fixed by injection with Bouin's fluid. The patient was 36 years of age. The illustrations are drawn at a uniform magnification (×289). Sections illustrated in *A* and *B* were stained in hematoxylin and eosin, *C* in Masson's trichrome stain without a preliminary application of hematoxylin. *A*, two follicles in early stages of development: primordial (*left*) and primary (*right*). *B*, an early stage of a growing follicle. *C*, a follicle, showing the beginning of the formation of the antrum (early antral follicle).

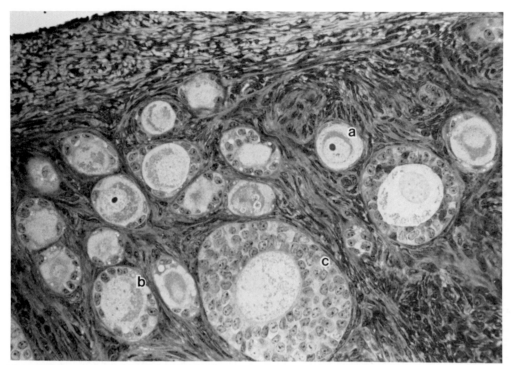

Figure 20.4.   Section through the cortex of a rhesus monkey ovary. The surface epithelium is in the *upper left*. A typical primordial follicle is seen at *a*. As the follicles grow, they form first a continuous cuboidal layer of granulosa cells (*b*), then a solid multilayered follicle (*c*). Only a few of the oocyte nuclei appear in the section (×215).

to form a complete layer of cuboidal cells, the *granulosa cells*. A basal lamina separates these cells from the rest of the ovary. As the oocyte increases in size (while remaining in arrested prophase), a glycoprotein extracellular material begins to accumulate between the oocyte and the granulosa cells. This material forms a thick uniform layer around the oocyte, the *zona pellucida* (Figs. 20.5 and 20.6).

As the solid *preantral follicle* continues to grow the granulosa becomes multilayered, the zona pellucida thickens, and the oocyte grows from about 10 μm to over 100 μm. Before the end of the preantral follicle stage, stromal cells in the connective tissue surrounding the granulosa layers become organized into a distinct layer, the *theca interna*. Some of the cells in this layer become epithelioid and later, as this layer becomes highly vascularized, these rounded cells accumulate lipid droplets and acquire

some of the other characteristics of steroid-producing cells.

The next stage of development of the follicle is that of the *antral follicle*, so-called because a fluid-filled space or *antrum* develops and increases in size within the granulosa layer. The *follicular fluid* originally appears as several small pools of serous material that coalesce to form the antrum (Fig. 20.7). As the antrum enlarges, it separates the cells lining the wall of the follicle, the *mural granulosa*, from those surrounding the oocyte, the *cumulus oophorus*, leaving only a *stalk* of cells connecting the two groups (Figs. 20.8 and 20.9). The layer of cumulus cells immediately adjacent to the zona pellucida is often called the *corona radiata*; processes from these cells extend through the zona pellucida to contact the surface of the oocyte (Fig. 20.6). Occasionally there are small bodies among the granulosa cells called Call-Exner bodies

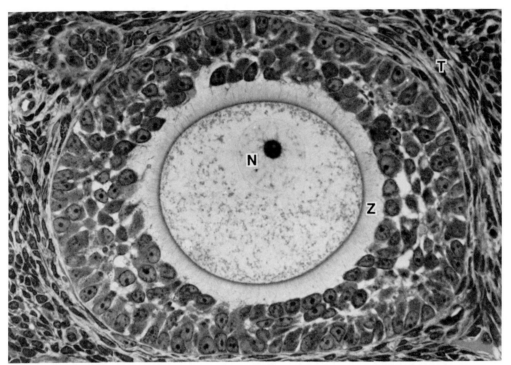

Figure 20.5. Section of a preantral solid follicle from a baboon ovary. The nucleus (N) contains a prominent nucleolus. A pale zona pellucida (Z) is interposed between the oocyte and the granulosa cells; it is traversed by fine processes of granulosa cell cytoplasm. The thecal layers (T) are just beginning to be distinguished (×530).

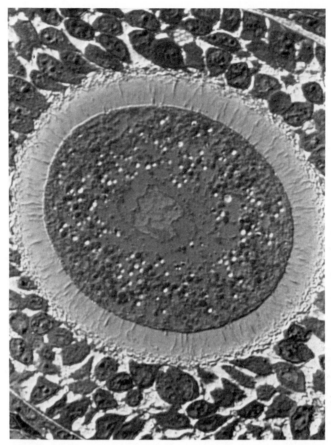

Figure 20.6. A semi-thin section of an oocyte of a rabbit, taken with Nomarski optics. Note the protoplasmic projections traversing the zona pellucida (×900). (Courtesy of Dr. Everett Anderson.)

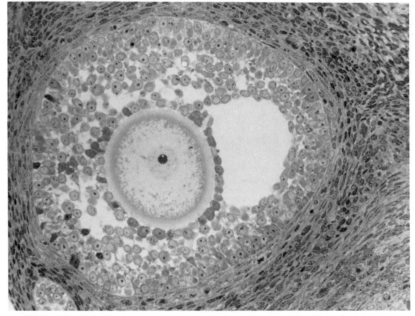

Figure 20.7. Section through a follicle in the early antral stage of development (×225).

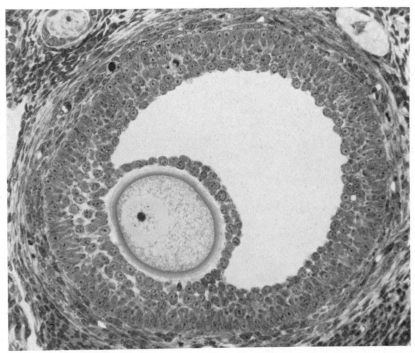

Figure 20.8.   Section through a follicle with a larger antrum. The thin rim of granulosa cells over the ovum is the cumulus; the layers of granulosa cells surrounding the antrum constitute the mural granulosa (×225).

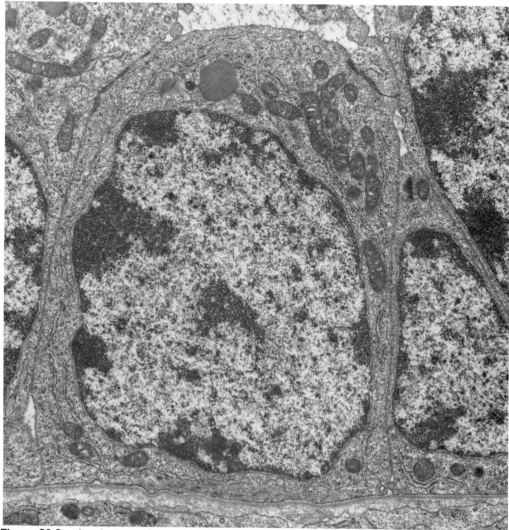

Figure 20.9. An electron micrograph of a section through an ovarian follicle. Note the granulosa cells resting on a basal lamina (×40,000). (Courtesy of Dr. Everett Anderson.)

(Fig. 20.3). These structures have the appearance of isolated pockets of basal laminar material.

The *mature antral follicle* (*Graafian follicle*) contains a large oocyte with a large nucleus and prominent nucleoli. This primary oocyte is still in arrested prophase of the first meiotic division. A very thick zona pellucida separates the oocyte from the innermost layer of granulosa cells, the corona radiata, except for areas where the long slender processes of the granulosa cells penetrate to the oocyte. The coronal cells

share communicating (gap) junctions both with each other and with the oocyte. The surface of the oocyte has numerous microvilli, but they do not extend far into the zona pellucida (Fig. 20.10). The cytoplasm of the oocyte contains a number of large complex Golgi regions, typical dense spherical mitochondria with peripheral septate cristae, annulate lamellae and numerous small, dense peripheral granules called cortical granules. Although RNA synthesis occurs during the early growth period, at this stage there is little protein synthesis, and

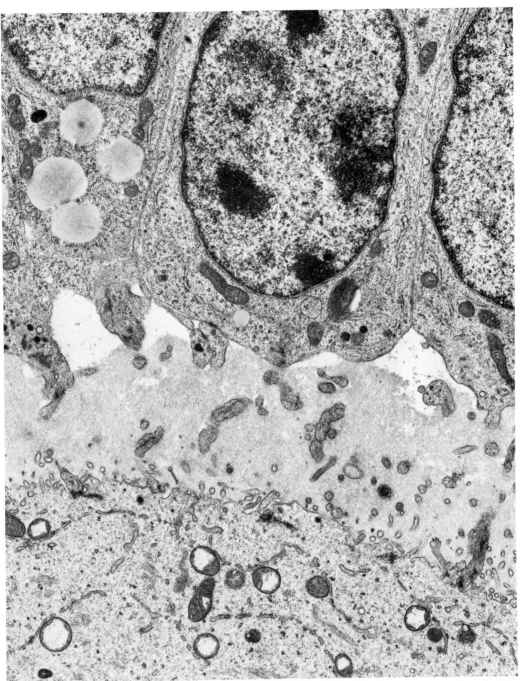

Figure 20.10.   The layer of granulosa cells adjacent to the ovum is called the corona radiata. In this micrograph these cells (*top*) send processes through the zona pellucida to the surface of the oocyte. Note that the small microvilli on the surface of the oocyte project only a short distance into the zona pellucida (×12,000). (Courtesy of Dr. Everett Anderson.)

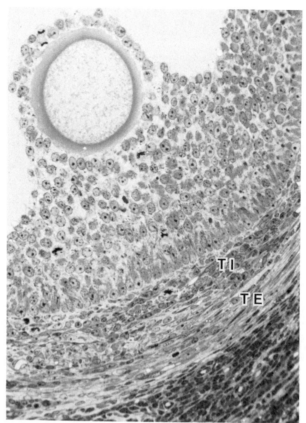

Figure 20.11. Section through the cumulus and stalk of a large antral follicle. A distinct theca interna (*TI*) and theca externa (*TE*) can be distinguished (×250).

granular endoplasmic reticulum is not conspicuous, but ribosomes are abundant in the cytoplasm.

The mural granulosa cells lining the mature follicle constitute a stratified cuboidal epithelium (Fig. 20.11). The basal layer of the mural granulosa cells is low columnar and rests on a prominent basement membrane. The granulosa cells are small, with irregular cell outlines and uniform nuclei. They frequently share junctions, including somewhat unusual annular communicating junctions (Fig. 20.12). The cytoplasm contains a few lipid droplets, strands of rough endoplasmic reticulum with a flocculent intracisternal content, and lysosomes (Fig. 20.13).

The theca interna has become thicker and consists of a network of capillaries with interspersed epithelioid cells (Fig. 20.14). When first seen, the glandular cells of the

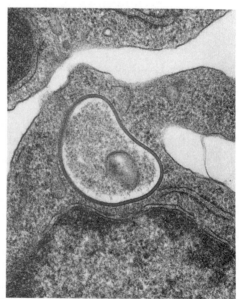

Figure 20.12. Annular gap junction in a granulosa cell from an ovarian follicle of a mouse (×70,000). (Courtesy of Dr. Everett Anderson.)

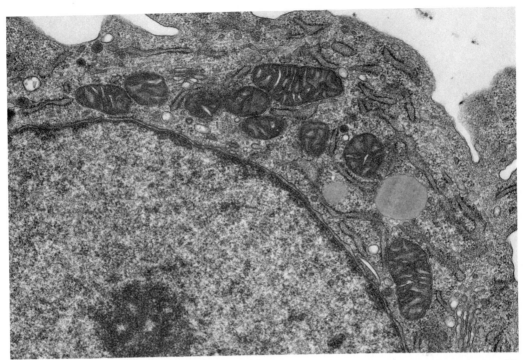

Figure 20.13.   Section through a granulosa cell. Note that the organelles are more consistent with a cell producing small amounts of glycoprotein than with one producing steroids. Mouse (×50,000). (Courtesy of Dr. Everett Anderson.)

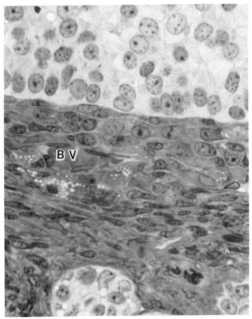

Figure 20.14.   Section through the wall of a large follicle, illustrating the mural granulosa (*top*) and theca interna. Near the blood vessel (*BV*), several of the glandular cells of the theca interna contain pale lipid droplets (×750).

theca interna are among the smallest and least distinctive steroid-producing cells in the body. Even during the antral follicle stage, theca interna cells have only a few lipid droplets and small areas of agranular endoplasmic reticulum. The surrounding connective tissue is less vascular than the theca interna, with a greater number of collagen fibers and an occasional smooth muscle cell. It forms a relatively indistinct external coat, the *theca externa*, of the follicle.

Ovulation

During each menstrual cycle, one large antral follicle undergoes *ovulation*, the release of the oocyte by rupture of the follicle. Ovulation is preceded by a series of preovulatory changes initiated approximately 36 hours prior to release of the ovum. These changes become most pronounced in the last 12 hours. The antral fluid increases in amount and appears less homogenous. The concentration of hyaluronic acid is greater in this secondary follicular fluid than in the original follicular fluid. The increased fluid production tends to disperse the granulosa cells. The basement membrane of the granulosa cells disintegrates and the follicle bulges on the surface of the ovary. Usually a portion of the follicle wall forms a projection, the *stigma*, on the otherwise smooth convexity of the surface of the ovary. The wall of the follicle and the overlying tunica albuginea become progressively thinner. This region blanches, then ruptures, often with a small loss of blood. Some of the slightly gelatinous follicular fluid oozes out, followed after a slight pause by the release of the cumulus oophorus with its contained oocyte. The remaining follicle collapses. The cumulus mass containing the oocyte adheres to the surface of the ovary until the *fimbriae* (folds around the opening) of the oviduct are swept across the ovary by the muscular activity in the ligaments of the ovary and oviduct. The ciliary activity of the fimbriae then moves the cumulus and oocyte into the oviduct.

Maturation of the Oocyte

During all of the follicular growth until the preovulatory changes, the oocytes remain in an arrested stage of the first meiotic prophase. The meiosis that is initiated in the fetal period proceeds through the initial stages of prophase (leptotene, zygotene, pachytene, and diplotene) in the same manner as in spermatogenesis until the prophase is arrested (Fig. 19.9). During preovulatory development, the nucleus of the oocyte completes diakinesis, the nuclear envelope disperses and a metaphase spindle organizes at the margin of the oocyte. The subsequent division separates the homologous chromosomes (reduction division), but the division of cytoplasm is unequal. The cell with the majority of the cytoplasm is the *secondary oocyte*; the small cell with only a little cytoplasm is the *first polar body*, which remains within the zona pellucida adjacent to the secondary oocyte.

The secondary oocyte then proceeds without further synthesis of DNA to the metaphase of the second meiotic division, where it is once again arrested. Only after ovulation and fertilization (or during degeneration) is the second meiotic division completed, and the small *second polar body* formed. Both polar bodies normally degenerate leaving only the fertilized ovum as the viable result of the two divisions of meiosis.

Formation of the Corpus Luteum

After ovulation the collapsed wall of the follicle forms a glandular structure called a *corpus luteum*. At first the corpus luteum has a highly folded wall formed of strands of granulosa and theca interna cells surrounding a central clot composed of retained blood and follicular fluid (Figs. 20.15 and 20.16). As the cells differentiate and enlarge, the corpus luteum becomes more homogeneous in appearance and occupies the greater part of the ovary. The corpus luteum is more massive than the follicle from which it arose, just as the quantity of progesterone it produces is many times greater than that of estrogen produced by the follicle before ovulation. The process of transformation of the follicle, *luteinization*, takes place over a period of several days. It begins even before ovulation in that the granulosa cells produce small but detectable quantities of progesterone several hours before ovulation.

The greatest bulk of the corpus luteum is formed from transformed granulosa cells (Fig. 20.17). These *granulosa lutein* cells undergo some increase in number but more especially they hypertrophy. They become large (30 μm) irregular cells with a folded surface abutting the interstitial space and share communicating junctions with adjacent lutein cells (Fig. 20.18). Agranular endoplasmic reticulum becomes abundant and the mitochondria have more tubular cristae than they did in the follicle (Fig. 20.19). Cells derived from the theca interna undergo somewhat similar modifications to form the *paralutein* or *theca lutein cells*.

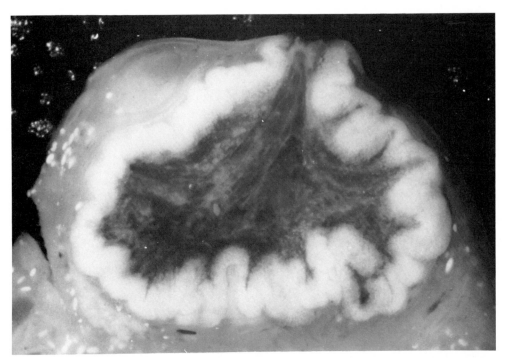

Figure 20.15. Micrograph of a hemisected corpus luteum of a baboon in the first days after ovulation. Note the stigma at the *top*, where the oocyte in its cumulus was released, and the folding of the wall of the follicle (×14).

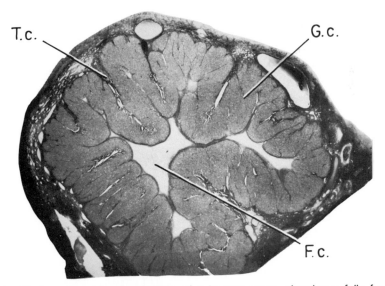

Figure 20.16. Photomicrograph of a section of a human ovary, showing a fully formed corpus luteum of pregnancy. Granulosa lutein cells (*G.c.*) form the major portion of the corpus; theca lutein cells (*T.c.*) surround it and penetrate between folds of granulosa lutein cells; a remnant of the follicular cavity (*F.c.*) contains loose connective tissue (×5).

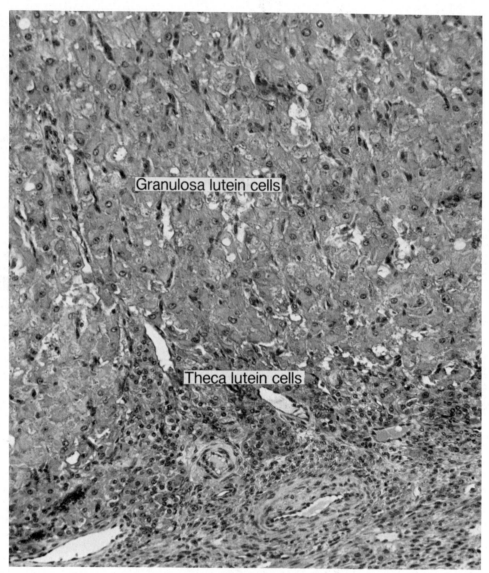

Figure 20.17. Human corpus luteum from the second month of pregnancy. Small dark theca lutein cells are seen near the blood vessels at the margin of the larger granulosa lutein cells (×180).

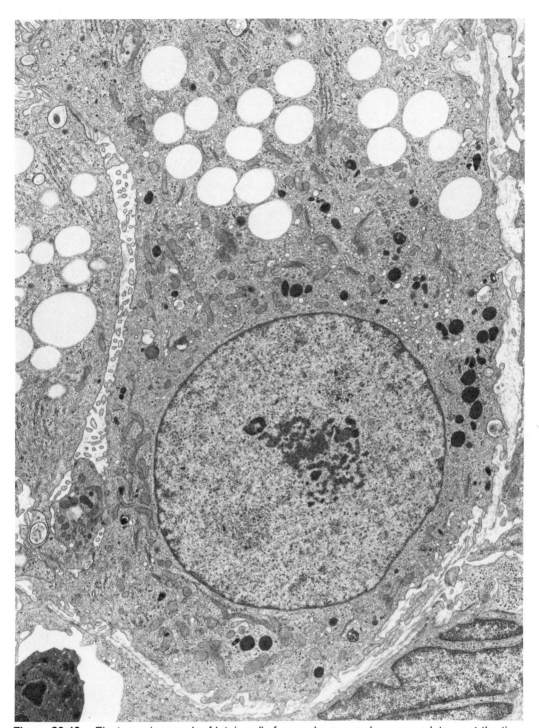

Figure 20.18.   Electron micrograph of lutein cells from a rhesus monkey corpus luteum at the time of implantation. Note the large size of the cell, the numerous lipid droplets, and the irregularity of the cell borders (×9,200).

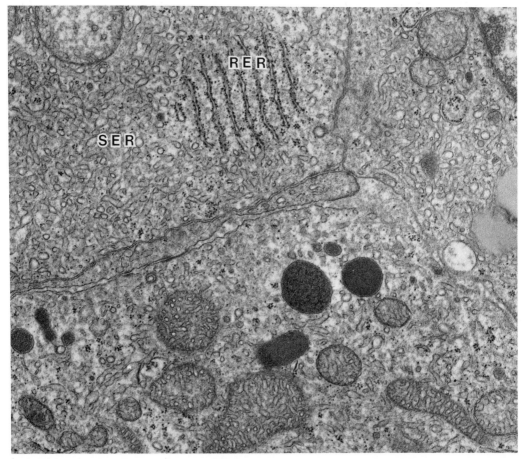

Figure 20.19. Electron micrograph of a human corpus luteum of pregnancy. The abundant smooth endoplasmic reticulum (SER) has a branched tubular form. The mitochondria have tubular cristae. Studies of other steroid-secreting cells suggest that the dense vesicles are both lysosomes and peroxisomes. *RER*, rough endoplasmic reticulum (×23,000).

Theca lutein cells are seen along the folds and periphery of the corpus luteum (Fig. 20.17). These cells remain smaller than the granulosa lutein cells, and their agranular endoplasmic reticulum is less ordered in its arrangement.

Blood vessels from the theca interna grow into the corpus luteum, forming an extensive network of sinusoidal capillaries among the lutein cells. Fibroblasts that accompany the vessels penetrate the central clot and reorganize it into a connective tissue core.

Levels of estrogen and progesterone produced by the corpus luteum reach a peak by six days after ovulation and, if the ovulated ovum is not fertilized, the corpus lu-

teum begins to regress by nine to ten days. If the ovum is fertilized and implants, which is estimated to occur about six days after ovulation, there are only a few days in which to "rescue" the corpus luteum. A gonadotropin produced by the implanted conceptus (*chorionic gonadotropin*) is necessary to replace the diminishing luteinizing hormone and continue the hormonal activity of the corpus luteum. If pregnancy does ensue, the lutein cells continue to hypertrophy and to produce progesterone and estrogen. (In addition, for reasons not yet understood, some of the lutein cells come to contain colloid droplets and high levels of calcium). The steroids produced by the corpus luteum are only necessary for approximately two months, after which the fetal-placental unit becomes the primary source of the steroids supporting pregnancy.

In the later stages of pregnancy or if pregnancy does not occur, the corpus luteum undergoes regression with decrease in cell size followed by autolysis of some cells and invasion by macrophages. The result of this regression is a rather amorphous hyaline residual structure that persists in the ovary for several cycles as a *corpus albicans* (Fig. 20.20).

Follicular Growth, Atresia, and the Menstrual Cycle

Primordial follicles become activated at a relatively constant rate, although there is some suggestion that as the number of primordial follicles is reduced the rate of formation of primary follicles decreases. Sin-

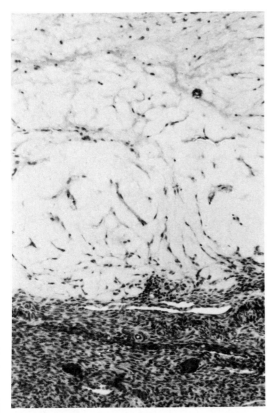

Figure 20.20. Section through a portion of a corpus albicans, the hyaline remnant of a degenerated corpus luteum (×130).

gle layered or multilaminar preantral follicles also can be found at any stage, and it is thought that neither the activation or growth of these developing follicles is dependent on gonadotropins. The late preantral follicle develops appreciable binding capacity for *follicle stimulating hormone* (FSH) which seems to promote cell division, and the antral follicle binds not only FSH, but also, as it becomes larger, *luteinizing hormone* (LH). A number of small antral follicles develop through early life, but until maturation of the hypothalamus prior to *menarche* (the onset of the menstrual cycle) the antral follicles undergo atresia and do not achieve ovulation.

In the adult woman, only preantral and small antral follicles are found at the onset of menstruation. A few antral follicles begin to grow and by about the sixth day after the onset of menstruation one of the follicles begins to grow larger than the others, and can then be recognized as the follicle destined to ovulate. Any other antral follicles over 2 mm in diameter tend to undergo atresia rather than continuing development.

Circulating blood levels of estrogens and progesterone are low at the start of menstruation and increase during the preovulatory period. The principal estrogen in women, 17β-estradiol, then reaches a pronounced peak just before the LH peak that precedes ovulation (Fig. 20.21). Studies of ovarian vein blood demonstrate that the ovary with the largest follicle is responsible for the vast majority of this hormone. Since the follicle destined to ovulate grows from about 6 mm to over 20 mm during the week before ovulation, it is not surprising that it dominates estrogen production. Incubation of slices or isolated components of the follicle also demonstrates the steroidogenic capacity of the follicle. As with most steroid-secreting cells, a variety of compounds are formed, including several androgens, estrogens, and progesterone. It appears that in larger follicles the cells of the theca interna synthesize a number of steroids, including a large amount of androgen. In

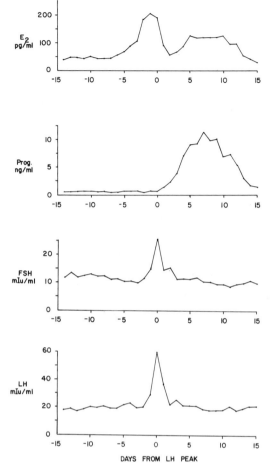

Figure 20.21. Mean values of LH, FSH, progesterone, and estradiol in the same aliquots of daily serum samples obtained from women during ovulatory cycles. The day of the LH maximum value is the reference day.

vitro studies suggest that some of this is converted to estrogens (aromatized) in the theca interna, and the rest is aromatized to estrogens in the granulosa. After the preovulatory estrogen peak, the follicle also produces small amounts of progesterone. Estrogen production first diminishes, then rises after ovulation and plateaus when the corpus luteum is fully formed. The corpus luteum is the source of estrogen as well as progesterone after ovulation.

Atresia can occur at any stage in the cycle of follicular development. The form that this atresia takes varies with both the stage of the cycle and the stage of development of the follicle (Fig. 20.22). Primordial follicles undergo degeneration leaving little trace. After the zona pellucida has developed during growth of preantral follicles it is relatively resistant to degeneration, and larger solid follicles tend to leave it behind as a persistent remnant (Fig. 20.22). Once the antral stage follicle has been achieved the thecal cells tend to undergo hypertrophy during atresia while the granulosa cells autolyze more rapidly (Fig. 20.23). (An exception to this is just after ovulation, when occasionally granulosa cells of some nonovulated follicles may undergo luteinization, forming small accessory corpora lutea).

The persistence of hypertrophied thecal cells contributes glandular cells to the interstitium of the ovary. Such *glandular interstitial cells* are abundant in a number of animals, but are relatively inconspicuous in the human ovary.

There are probably as many as a million oocytes formed during the fetal stage, and around 400,000 are present at the onset of puberty. Since fewer than 400 ova will ever be ovulated, the odds of given oocyte escaping atresia are less than one in 1000, but one can hardly underestimate the importance of those oocytes that escape the common fate.

Occasionally a vesicular follicle in undergoing atresia will leave a thickened basal lamina (Fig. 20.23). This structure is called a "glassy membrane" or later, when its membranous origin is no longer apparent, a "little corpus albicans."

It is generally thought that the estrogen peak from the ovary produces the LH peak from the pituitary by feedback action on the hypothalamus and on *gonadotropin releasing factor*. The elevated progesterone and estradiol levels of the postovulatory phase of the cycle have a negative feedback resulting in a reduction in overall gonadotropin levels and the loss of support of the corpus luteum that leads to menstruation. In addition, it can be shown that follicles produce several nonsteroidal materials.

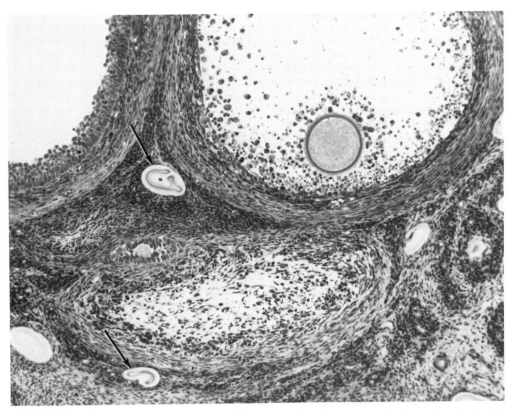

Figure 20.22. Section through the cortex of the ovary of a rhesus monkey. A portion of a healthy follicle is in the *upper left*. In the *upper right*, a follicle undergoing atresia shows extensive degeneration of the granulosa, but the oocyte is intact. In the *lower center* is the granulosal remnant of another atretic follicle. The pale structures (*arrows*) are residual zonas of degenerated oocytes (×120).

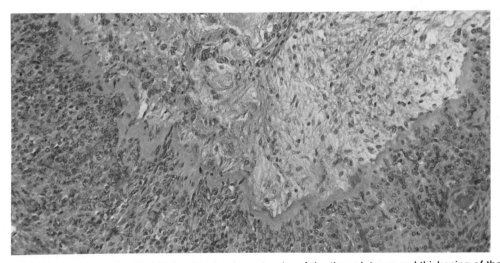

Figure 20.23. Human atretic follicle, showing hypertrophy of the theca interna and thickening of the basement membrane which is forming a glassy membrane. The granulosa cells have been replaced by connective tissue (×200).

Follicular inhibiting factor (*inhibin*) from the granulosa cells of the enlarging follicle apparently acts as a feedback hormone to reduce pituitary output of FSH in response to gonadotropin releasing factor. Another factor (or factors) from follicles inhibits maturation of the oocyte and still another reduces LH binding to ovarian receptors. *Relaxin*, a peptide hormone produced by the corpus luteum, may aid in conditioning the cervix of the uterus at parturition.

Blood Vessels

The major blood supply to the ovary comes from the ovarian artery, which passes medially from the lateral aspect of the mesovarium to anastomose with the ovarian branch of the uterine artery. From this continuous structure, a number of branches enter the ovarian medulla at the hilus where they can be seen as unusually large coiled vessels. At roughly the cortical-medullary junction the vessels ramify and anastomose in plexuses. The branches arising from the plexuses enter the cortex radially and form extensive capillary beds in relationship to the growing follicles. The veins accompany the arteries in the ovary; they also form a plexus in the medulla and exit at the hilus.

Lymphatics

Lymph capillaries begin in the theca externa of the follicles and unite into somewhat larger vessels which pass radially through the medulla and leave at the hilus. There they are collected in a number of lymphatic trunks that drain into the lumbar lymph nodes.

Nerves

Nerve fibers, mostly unmyelinated, enter at the hilus and follow the course of the blood vessels. Many terminate in the muscle fibers of the medullary blood vessels. Others enter the cortex and form delicate plexuses in the thecae but apparently do not penetrate the basement membranes of the follicles. According to some authors, groups of sympathetic ganglion cells are found in the medulla.

THE OVIDUCTS

The *oviducts* (*Fallopian* or *uterine tubes*) are paired structures, each of which is 12 to 15 cm long and 6 to 8 mm in diameter. The oviducts not only act as conduits for sperm but, through the combined muscular contraction of the supporting mesentery (mesosalpinx) and the ciliary action of the epithelium, sweep ova from the surface of the ovary and conduct them into the interior where fertilization occurs.

Four regions of the tubes are usually distinguished. Beginning with the ovarian end, these are: infundibulum, ampulla, isthmus, and uterine or interstitial segment. The *infundibulum* is funnel-shaped and is formed of a number of fan-shaped *folds* or *fimbriae* (Fig. 20.1). The *ampulla* is the longest of the segments and, like the fimbriae, is thin walled. It terminates in a relatively short segment which extends to the uterus, the *isthmus*. This segment is smaller in diameter and thicker walled than the ampulla. The last portion, the *interstitial segment*, is situated in the wall of the uterus. The mucosa of the infundibulum and ampulla is composed of branched folds with correspondingly deep grooves (Figs. 20.24 and 20.25). The lumen thus is very irregular in shape. The folds progressively decrease in height toward the uterus and are low in the isthmus. In the interstitial segment there are only slight folds, and the cavity reaches its smallest diameter, about 1 mm.

The *epithelium* lining the Fallopian tubes is a simple columnar type, some cells of which are ciliated, whereas others are narrow, peg-shaped, and nonciliated secretory cells. (Figs. 20.25 and 20.26). These secretory cells produce glycoprotein-containing granules that release their contents into the lumen. The height of the epithelium and the proportion of ciliated to nonciliated secretory cells, although varying considerably even in neighboring regions of a tube, show changes that correlate with the stages of the menstrual cycle. In the oviduct of the human, cells with forming cilia are appar-

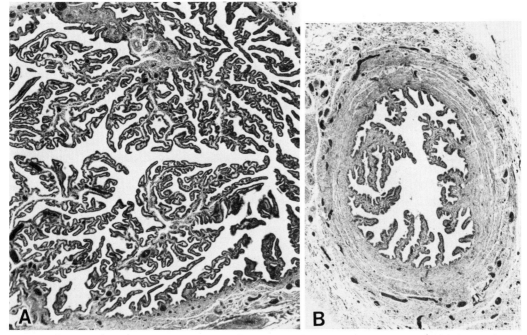

Figure 20.24. *A*, ampulla of a human oviduct, near the infundibulum. The mucosa is elaborately folded, providing extensive surface. *B*, isthmic portion of the same oviduct. The folds are less elaborate and the diameter reduced (×24).

ent in the middle of the follicular phase of the menstrual cycle, and both secretory and ciliated cells are large and fully differentiated at ovulation. Subsequently the number of ciliated cells declines by 10 to 15 per cent, and the height of both cell types is reduced during the luteal phase. During pregnancy, the epithelium is quite low, and there are fewer ciliated cells.

The cilia beat toward the uterus, but the roles of the beating cilia and muscular contraction in transport of the ovum from the ampulla to the uterus have not been clearly delineated.

The connective tissue of the lamina propria is richly cellular; it is quite compact in the isthmus but more loosely arranged in the high folds of the ampulla.

The *muscularis* lies directly adjacent to the mucosa and is composed of an inner circular layer of smooth muscle that grades by individual fiber groups into a thinner outer longitudinal layer. The muscularis is thicker and the longitudinal layer less dis-

continuous in the isthmic, as opposed to the ampullary, portion of the oviduct.

The *serosa* has the usual structure of peritoneum.

The larger *blood vessels* run in the connective tissue along the bases of the folds. They send off branches that give rise to a dense capillary network.

The *lymphatics* arise as relatively large lacunae in the connective tissue of the mucosal folds. These empty into narrower channels that pass through the muscularis and form a rich subserous net. The lymphatics drain into the upper lumbar lymph nodes.

The *nerves* form a rich plexus in the connective tissue, from which fibers pass to the blood vessels and muscular tissue and to the epithelial lining.

THE UTERUS

The uterus serves as the site of nurture of the fetus and also as a conduit for sperm passage, an appropriate environment for

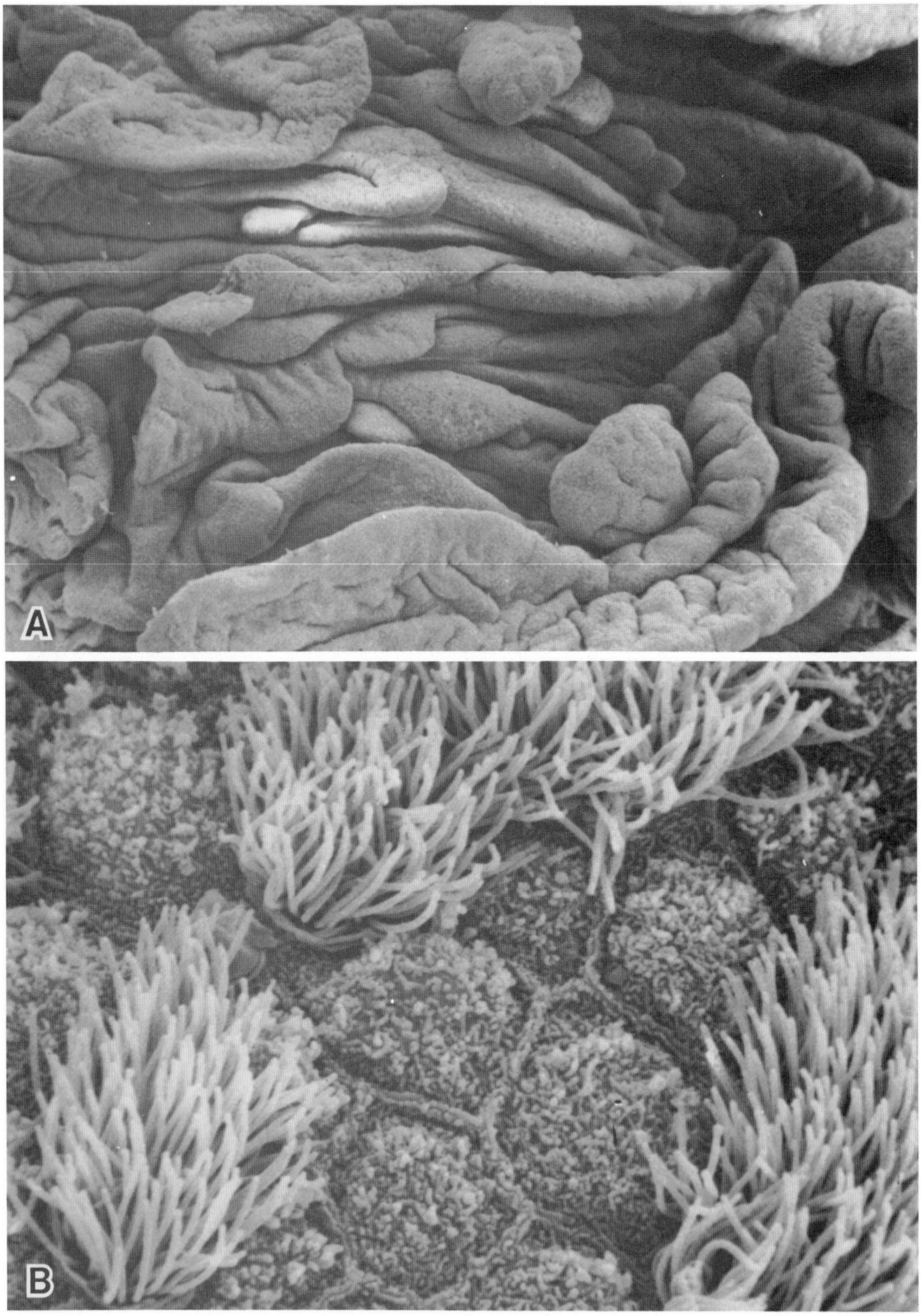

Figure 20.25. *A*, scanning electron micrograph of the fimbriae of the infundibulum of the oviduct of a baboon. Note that these folds converge towards the opening into the oviduct (*right*). *B*, higher magnification of the surface of the same oviduct, illustrating ciliated and nonciliated cells. The latter have prominent cell boundaries. This animal was in the progestational phase of the cycle (*A*, ×50; *B*, ×5,650).

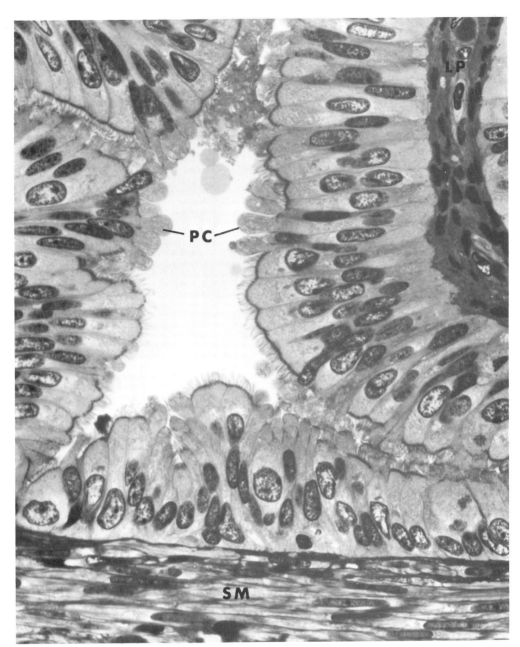

Figure 20.26.   Light micrograph of a portion of the oviduct of a monkey. Peg-shaped (secretory) cells (*PC*) are interspersed with ciliated cells. *SM*, smooth muscle cells of muscularis; *LP*, lamina propria (*upper right*) (×685).

implantation, and a partner in placental formation. It must allow orderly expansion of the *conceptus* (the developing embryo and its extraembryonic membranes) and eventually must expel the fetus.

The uterus is thick walled, pear-shaped, and somewhat flattened dorsoventrally in its upper two-thirds. It varies considerably in size, averaging some 7 cm in length, 5 cm in width at its upper (broadest) part, and 2.5 cm in thickness. The cavity of the uterus is a dorsoventrally flattened slot.

The oviducts open into the broad superior lateral aspect of the lumen, and the caudal portion narrows before entering the vagina.

Anatomically, two main regions of the uterus are distinguished: an upper *body* or *corpus* with its rounded, dome-shaped top, the *fundus*, and a narrower, cylindrical *cervix* whose terminal portion projects into the vagina as the intravaginal portion. The narrow zone of transition between corpus and cervix is known as the *isthmus*.

The wall of the uterus consists of three coats which, from the outermost inward, are the serosa or *perimetrium*, the muscularis or *myometrium* and the mucosa or *endometrium*.

The *perimetrium* is the peritoneal layer of the broad ligament, which covers the corpus and a portion of the cervix. It is firmly attached to the underlying muscularis and has the usual structure of a serous membrane.

Myometrium

The myometrium is a massive muscular coat, about 15 mm in thickness, consisting of bundles of smooth muscle fibers held together by connective tissue. The disposition of the muscle fibers is quite complicated but generally three layers may be distinguished. The inner, muscular layer, the *subvascular stratum*, consists of fibers running longitudinally, i.e., parallel to the long axis of the organ. The middle layer, *vascular stratum*, forms the bulk of the muscularis and is composed mainly of fibers running circularly or spirally. In the interstitial tissue are numerous large blood vessels, especially veins. The outer layer, *supravascular stratum*, is relatively thin and is composed of both circular and longitudinal fibers. The latter predominate and form a fairly distinct subserous layer which becomes continuous with the longitudinal muscle coat of the vagina. In the cervix, the inner longitudinal layer is absent.

The muscle cells of the uterus of a nulliparous woman have a length of 40 to 90 μm, the variations conforming to definite phases of the menstrual cycle. The fibers are shortest in the first week after menstruation and reach their greatest length in the fourth week of the cycle. During pregnancy, the muscle tissue of the uterus is greatly increased. This is due partly to an increase in the number but mainly to the tremendous increase in the size of the muscle fibers, which in the later stages of pregnancy may have a length of over 500 μm.

The interstitial tissue contains numerous blood vessels and consists of loosely arranged collagenous fibers and relatively few connective tissue cells. Elastic fibers are found in considerable amounts in the outer layer of the muscularis and in the subserous connective tissue. The inner portions of the myometrium are relatively poor in elastic tissue. In the cervix, elastic tissue is abundant.

Endometrium

The endometrium is composed of a superficial portion, the *functionalis*, and a deeper portion, the *basalis*. During each menstrual cycle the functionalis undergoes a remarkable series of changes, while the basalis is relatively unaffected. The functionalis is generated by growth from the basalis and is then broken down and sloughed. The passage of endometrial debris, together with some blood, through the cervix into the vagina is known as menstruation, and it is this phenomenon that gives the cycle its name.

At the peak of its development, the endometrium is 4 to 5 mm thick. It is covered by a surface epithelium of simple columnar cells, some of which are ciliated, and has numerous branching coiled tubular glands. The stroma is similar to that of other mucous membranes, except that the fibroblasts are stellate and are more similar to mesenchymal cells than fibroblasts in other locations. The stromal fibroblasts are capable of epithelioid transformation into decidual cells. The vasculature is bipartite in that the basalis portion of the endometrium is supplied by straight branches (basal arteries) and the functionalis portion is supplied by spiral arteries. There is no sub-mucosa and the border between the endometrium and myometrium is irregular.

Menstruation occurs typically at intervals of about 28 days and lasts for 3 to 5 days, but there is great variability in length of the cycle among different individuals and often from one cycle to the next in any one individual. The first day of menstrution is counted as the first day of the menstrual cycle.

The menstrual cycle is considered to have three stages, each of which may be characterized by distinctive structural features (Figs. 20.27 to 20.30). The indicated duration of each stage is based on a 28-day cycle. The *menstrual* stage occupies the first 3 to 5 days of the cycle, during which time there is an external menstrual discharge. The *follicular* or *proliferative* (estrogenic) stage begins with the termination of menstruation and extends to about the middle of the cycle. The *luteal* (*secretory* or progestational) stage extends from the middle to the end of the cycle. Sometimes the late secretory stage is designated the *premenstrual* stage which is terminated by the appearance of external bleeding. The length of the proliferative stage is less constant than that of the others, and variations

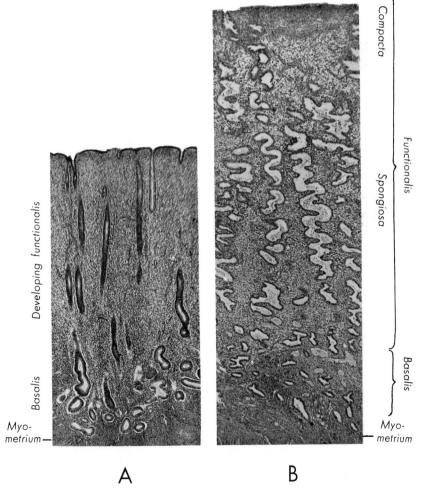

A   B

Figure 20.27.   Human endometria. *A*, proliferative stage, about day 10 of menstrual cycle; *B*, late secretory stage, day 25 of cycle (×30). (Preparations by Dr. Arthur Hertig.)

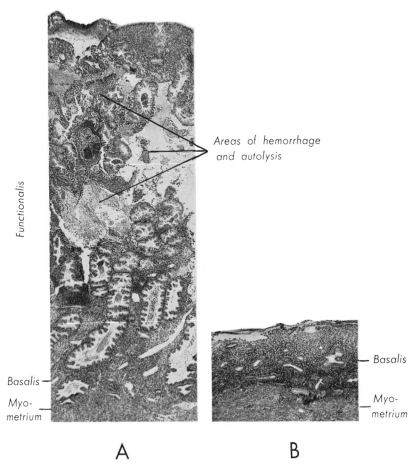

Figure 20.28. Human endometria. *A*, early menstrual phase; *B*, termination of menstruation (×30). (Preparations by Dr. Arthur Hertig.)

in its duration are chiefly responsible for the varying lengths of the menstrual cycles.

By the end of the menstrual flow, the functionalis has been sloughed. The subsequent follicular stage of the cycle is the period in which rapid regeneration of the endometrium occurs under the influence of estrogen from the developing follicle. Epithelial cells from the glands of the basalis spread over the remaining stromal cells to re-establish the luminal epithelium. Subsequently the glands elongate. In the early follicular stage (5–7 days) the glands are relatively short and straight, and the epithelium is simple tall columnar (Figs. 20.27 and 20.29). Only a few mitotic figures are present in the epithelium and stroma. In the middle and late follicular stages the glands become longer and larger, and the

epithelium becomes pseudostratified. Mitoses are particularly abundant in the glandular epithelium in the midfollicular stage. Pseudostratification is maximal in the late follicular stage (11–14 days) just prior to ovulation. Coiled arteries grow into the regenerating tissue and, toward the end of the proliferative stage, a considerable degree of edema develops, although it is not as pronounced as in the luteal stage. During the follicular stage, the endometrium increases from a postmenstrual thickness of 0.5 mm or less to 2 or 3 mm.

Following ovulation, the luteal or secretory stage of the cycle commences. Characteristically the endometrium increases in thickness, the glands become highly coiled, and the endometrium becomes increasingly vascular (Fig. 20.27). In the early luteal

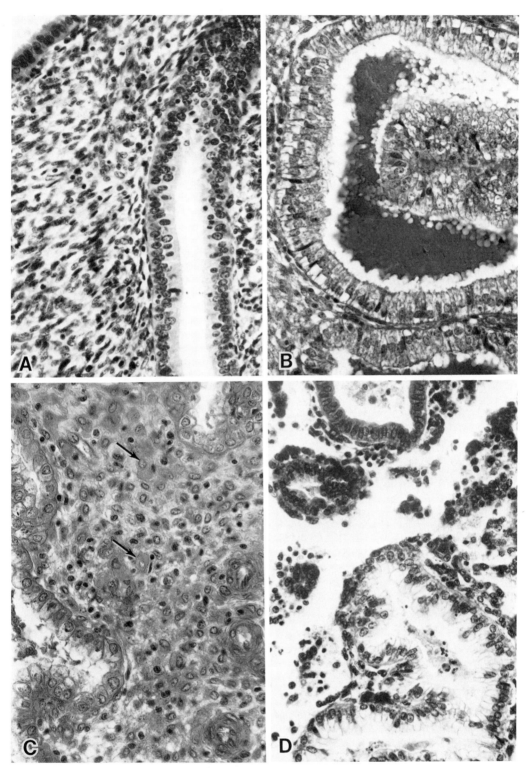

Figure 20.29. Section through the functionalis layer of the human endometrium during different stages of the menstrual cycle. *A*, mid-proliferative stage. The relatively straight uterine glands are beginning to show nuclear crowding. *B*, early secretory stage. The glands show the typical vacuolation beneath the nuclei, due to the extraction of glycogen. *C*, late secretory (premenstrual) phase. Some pseudodecidual cells are forming in the stroma (*arrows*). Several sections of a spiral artery are seen on the right. *D*, early menstrual stage. Leucocytic infiltration has occurred, and the endometrium is beginning to disintegrate (×300).

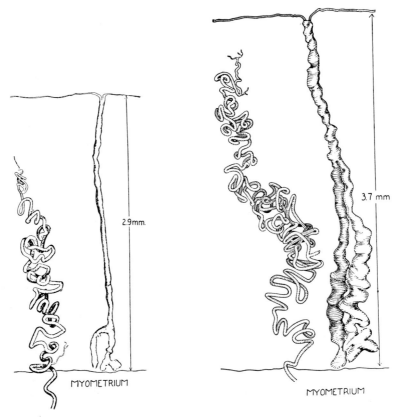

Figure 20.30. Projection reconstructions of the coiled arteries and the glands in the endometrium of rhesus monkey. *Left*, early proliferative stage; *right*, late secretory stage. (After Daron.)

stage the epithelial cells of the glands increase in width, reducing the pseudostratification and increasing the tortuosity of the glands. Shortly after ovulation, glycogen begins to accumulate in the basal portions of the glandular epithelial cells, and the nuclei become more apically situated (Fig. 20.29). By about day 18, glycogen has accumulated to the extent that almost the entire basal portion of the gland cell appears vacuolated in hematoxylin and eosin preparations. As the luteal phase continues, basal glycogen diminishes, the cells become broader, and a glycoprotein secretory material appears in the wide glandular lumina. The glands are now so coiled that in sections they may give a "saw-toothed" appearance. However, it is only the portions of the glands within the functionalis that are undergoing these modifications. In the

basalis, the glands remain relatively straight-walled.

The gland cells take on typical characteristics of glycoprotein-producing cells, with strands of granular endoplasmic reticulum that are slightly dilated with flocculent content. In addition, unusually large mitochondria are found in the base of these cells, and the nucleoli have an unusual canalicular structure of unknown significance.

Within the stroma, edema is beginning to increase to a maximum by about day 22 and the endometrium reaches its greatest thickness (5 to 6 mm). The spiral arteries are now highly coiled and reach nearly to the luminal epithelium (Fig. 20.30). Some of the stromal cells around the spiral arteries begin to enlarge, forming a cuff of epithelioid cells, the *pseudodecidual cells* (Fig. 20.29).

The late portion of the luteal stage (sometimes called the premenstrual stage) concludes the menstrual cycle. It occurs as the corpus luteum is declining and circulating levels of estrogen and progesterone are significantly lowered. Increased decidualization of stromal cells occurs in the more superficial parts of the endometrium. This divides the functionalis into a *stratum compactum* and a deeper *stratum spongiosum*. As menstruation approaches, leukocytes invade the stroma, edema increases, and erythrocytes are released from the vessels into the surrounding connective tissue (Figs. 20.28 and 20.29).

The progressive regression of the corpus luteum leaves the endometrium without the support of either estrogens or progesterone. The spiral arteries undergo periodic episodes of contraction and relaxation. Initially blood leaves the damaged peripheral portion of the vascular system and enters the stroma. As degenerative changes continue, subsequent episodes of vascular engorgement cause the overlying endometrium to lose its integrity, the endometrium breaks down, and menstruation begins. Endometrial debris, consisting of necrotic glandular and stromal cells plus venous blood and traces of arterial blood, flows into the vagina. The process continues until the entire functionalis has been removed. With the development of a new group of antral follicles in the ovary, which begin to restore circulating levels of estrogens (especially estradiol), growth of the endometrium starts again.

The Cervix

The cervix, although a portion of the uterus, is different in a number of ways from the body and fundus. Not only is the inner longitudinal layer of muscle missing, but progressing towards the vagina there is an increasing substitution of fibrous tissue for smooth muscle. The smooth muscle also responds differently from that of the body of the uterus to some physiological conditions.

The mucosa of the cervix does not participate in menstruation, and is somewhat thicker than that of the body of the uterus. It is composed of numerous folds, the palmitate folds, and intervening clefts that end in simple pits. Because these pits or glands are continuous with the clefts and have the same type of epithelium, the cervix is sometimes considered to be aglandular.

The lining epithelium consists mainly of high columnar mucous secreting cells, although a few ciliated cells may also be present (Fig. 20.31). The mucus-secreting cells are uniform in height at any given stage, reaching their greatest height during the secretory stage. The mucus has a low viscoelasticity about the time of ovulation. At other times it may be quite resistant to sperm penetration. Closure of pockets of epithelium frequently occurs, leading to the formation of cysts, the Nabothian follicles. Near the external opening of the cervix, the simple columnar epithelium changes abruptly to a stratified squamous epithelium, and this type of epithelium also covers the external surface of the cervix as it protrudes into the vagina (Fig. 20.31).

Unfortunately, the epithelium of the cervix has a tendency to undergo metaplastic changes, and it is common practice to screen regularly for cervical cancer by sampling cervical cells.

Blood Vessels

Branches from each uterine artery penetrate to the middle (vascular) layer of the uterine muscle and then continue both ventrally and dorsally in this layer to the midline, forming the arcuate arteries. They anastomose with the branches from the other uterine artery. Two sets of branches arise from these arched arteries: (*a*) small branches that course peripherally and supply the supravascular (outer) part of the uterus, and (*b*) larger radial branches that course centrally. Branches from the latter in turn form two systems. One set, which penetrates the endometrium for a variable distance, depending on the stage of the cycle, is extremely coiled (spiral arteries) and terminates in a tuft of arterioles (Fig.

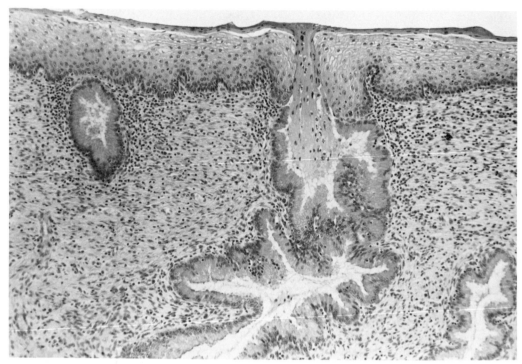

Figure 20.31.   Section through a wall of the human cervix near the external opening. The clefts are lined with a tall columnar (mucous) epithelium, while the surface epithelium in this region is stratified squamous (×350).

20.30). The other set supplies the inner layer of the uterine muscle and the basal part of the endometrium, where branches from it anastomose with the branches of the coiled arteries. The endometrium is thus supplied by a basal and a superficial set of vessels. The basal set, as would be expected, does not undergo modifications with the stages of the cycle, but the spiral arteries show pronounced changes. During the proliferative stage of the cycle, they penetrate only one-half or two-thirds through the thickness of the endometrium, but during the secretory stage they increase in extent, approach the surface and, with the tissue loss at menstruation, may protrude into the uterine lumen. Their peripheral part then undergoes necrosis. The menstrual blood, however, does not come mainly from the arteries but from the veins. With the reparative postmenstrual process, the vessels again grow.

Menstrual fluid is composed of extravasated blood, desquamated tissue and the secretion of the uterine glands. The discharge does not clot, for it is markedly fibrinolytic, unless there is a rather large blood flow.

Lymphatics

The lymph vessels are larger and more abundant in the uterus than in most other organs of the body. They are enlarged during pregnancy. All layers of the uterine wall have lymph vessels except the superficial part of the endometrium (compactum), which is devoid of them. During its cyclical changes, the endometrium exhibits pronounced changes in its water content, and these changes are probably responsible for the unusually extensive lymph drainage.

Nerves

Both myelinated and unmyelinated nerve fibers occur in the uterus. The latter predominate and are connected with minute ganglia found in the upper vaginal wall near its junction with the cervix. These fibers supply the walls of the blood vessels and the muscle tissue of the myometrium. The myelinated fibers apparently run to the mucosa and form a scanty plexus beneath the epithelium.

Fertilization, Cleavage, and Transport

Deposition of sperm occurs in the vagina where, because of the low pH, sperm life is relatively short. From this depot sperm make their way into the cervix. The higher pH of the cervix and body of the uterus is more compatible with sperm motility and survival. The sperm are distributed throughout the uterus, probably by muscular contraction, but orgasm is not essential for this distribution. Some sperm pass through the uterotubal junction and into the oviduct.

During their passage to the site of fertilization the sperm become capable of fertilizing an ovum and retain that capacity for about 24 to 48 hours. The ovulated ovum (secondary oocyte) is thought to be in a condition to be fertilized for 12 to 24 hours. Before contacting the ovum the fertilizing sperm must penetrate through the matrix of the cumulus and corona radiata and then through the zona pellucida surrounding the ovum. During this process sperm undergo the *acrosome reaction*, which is the fusion of the outer acrosomal membrane with the sperm plasma membrane. This fusion results in the release of the acrosomal content and the exposure of the inner acrosomal membrane. It is thought that hyaluronidase aids in penetration of the cumulus matrix, and *acrosin*, a trypsin-like enzyme, probably aids penetration of sperm through the zona pellucida. (Alternatively, acrosin might function in fusion of sperm with the ovum cell membrane.)

Detailed study of laboratory animals reveals that after penetrating the zona, the head of the sperm lies flat against the surface of the oocyte and the sperm loses its motility. Initial fusion of oocyte and sperm plasma membranes occurs near the posterior end of the sperm head (the equatorial segment). The rest of the head is then surrounded by folds of ovum plasma membrane. First the sperm head and only later the midpiece and tail are taken into the ovum. After the sperm fuses with the oocyte plasma membrane the cortical granules in the oocyte are released (by fusion with the surface membrane), and the zona pellucida becomes resistant to sperm penetration.

After fertilization the oocyte completes the second meiotic division, again by uneven cytoplasmic division, and the second polar body is formed. The remaining haploid number of chromosomes forms the female pronucleus. Meanwhile the sperm head swells and the chromatin decondenses to become the male pronucleus. The two pronuclei move toward the center of the ovum, the nuclear membranes disperse, and the chromosomes are organized into a single metaphase plate. Replication of DNA takes place during the pronuclear stage. Consequently when the chromosomes from the two pronuclei come together on a single metaphase plate, the diploid number is restored and daughter chromatids from both sets of chromosomes then pass to the poles at anaphase. Completion of this first mitotic division of the zygote is the beginning of the process of cleavage. Cleavage of the zygote, unlike normal cell division, results in progressively smaller cells (*blastomeres*). No centrioles are present in the early cleavage stages.

Very few cleavage stages of the human have been recovered and studied. However, the current use of in vitro fertilization to alleviate infertility due to blocked oviducts is providing more information on cleavage stages. It is clear from studies of other animals that during the process of cleavage the blastomere cytoplasm is changing, new proteins are synthesized, mitochondria change their characteristics, and centrioles appear. After several divisions a cluster of cells, the *morula*, is formed, still surrounded by a zona pellucida. The outer cells of the morula flatten and then develop junctional complexes. Fluid accumulates between blastomeres, then coalesces to form a single cavity that transforms the morula into a *blastocyst*. The outer layer of the blastocyst constitutes a single epithelial layer, the *trophoblast*; a cluster of blastomeres within this layer at one side of the cavity is called the *inner cell mass*. The blastomeres of the inner cell mass at first have no distinctive features, but in a short time those nearest the cavity flatten and extend beyond the inner cell mass beneath the trophoblast adjacent to the cavity. This layer (*hypoblast*) later differentiates into *endoderm* (see Chapter 3).

The developing embryo enters the uterus, probably as a morula, about 3 ½ days after ovulation. From studies with other primates it is clear that passage through the isthmic and interstitial segments of the oviduct takes only a few hours. Consequently most of cleavage takes place in the ampullary segment of the oviduct. The blastocyst implants in the uterine endometrium 5 ½ or 6 days after ovulation, about two days after entering the uterus.

Implantation and Placentation

During implantation, the blastocyst must come into contact with the luminal surface of the endometrium, adhere to and penetrate the luminal epithelium and its basal lamina, and expand in the underlying stroma. During cleavage and cavity formation, the blastocyst does not directly contact maternal cells because it is still covered by the zona pellucida. Within the uterus, the blastocyst loses the zona pellucida, a process accomplished apparently by shedding. None of the stages between the zona-encased blastocyst until penetration of the stroma of the uterus have been described in the human. These events must be surmised by comparison with other mammals.

At the initiation of implantation the blastocyst of the rhesus monkey is oriented with the inner cell mass adjacent to the uterine surface, to which the overlying trophoblast cells adhere (Fig. 20.32). Some of

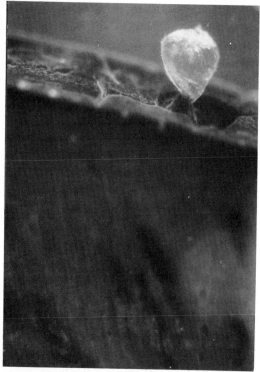

Figure 20.32. The earliest implantation stage seen in primates. The blastocyst has invaded the endometrium only in a restricted spot. A depression in the surface of the endometrium indicates that the blastocyst was held between the dorsal and ventral surfaces. Excised site from rhesus monkey uterus, day 9.5 of gestation (×30).

the trophoblast cells near the inner cell mass fuse so that there are many nuclei in a mass of cytoplasm without intervening cell membranes. This *syncytial trophoblast* adheres to the uterus and penetrates between uterine epithelial cells by extending flange-shaped processes toward the stroma. Rather than destroying the surrounding uterine epithelium, the trophoblast initially shares junctional complexes with the adjacent uterine cells. After further growth of the syncytial trophoblast and proliferation of cellular trophoblast, the blastocyst penetrates into the uterine stroma. Consequently initial invasion is accomplished by infiltration rather than erosion.

The earliest human implantation site is estimated to have been collected about a day after the beginning of implantation, approximately 7½ days after ovulation (Fig.

20.33). In this specimen, syncytial tropho-blast has penetrated through the uterine epithelium and spread in the stroma, form-ing a thickened mass between the inner cell mass and the endometrium.

In penetrating into the endometrium the syncytial trophoblast initially surrounds the subepithelial plexus of maternal capil-laries. When the endothelium is lost from these capillaries, blood-filled *lacunae* are formed within the trophoblast (Fig. 20.34). The blood exposed to syncytial trophoblast does not clot; as a result, when many vessels have been transformed into extensive in-terconnected lacunae within the syncytium, maternal blood begins to circulate through these spaces. By the close of this *previllous stage*, the syncytial trophoblast has changed from a relatively compact mass to a thin layer surrounding lacunae filled with maternal blood.

When the blastocyst begins to implant, the endometrium is in the midprogesta-tional stage. By eight days after ovulation, the implanted blastocyst is making detect-able amounts of chorionic gonadotropin, and by day 12 it has definitely taken over support of the corpus luteum from pituitary gonadotropin. Consequently the endome-trium, under the influence of estrogen and progesterone from the rescued corpus lu-teum, remains highly vascular.

The endometrium grows over the im-planting blastocyst, placing the entire con-ceptus within the endometrium. The en-dometrium that grows over the blastocyst is called the *decidua capsularis*, that be-neath the conceptus the *decidua basalis*, and the remainder is designated the *decidua parietalis*. Soon after invasion of the endo-metrium there is a transitory inflammatory response; numerous leukocytes enter the stroma around the conceptus. Subse-quently the stromal cells become enlarged and *decidualized* and the inflammation re-sponse declines.

Establishment of Placental Villi

At the end of the previllous stage, the periphery of the conceptus consists largely

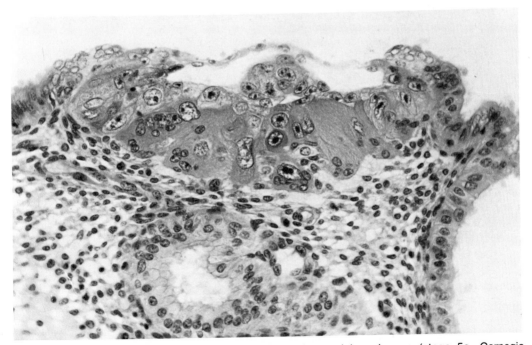

Figure 20.33.   The earliest implantation stage yet observed in a human (stage 5a, Carnegie Collection). Irregular masses of syncytial trophoblast, together with cytotrophoblast cells, form a pad beneath the small central inner cell mass. The uterine epithelium has not yet grown over the abembryonic trophoblast (×300).

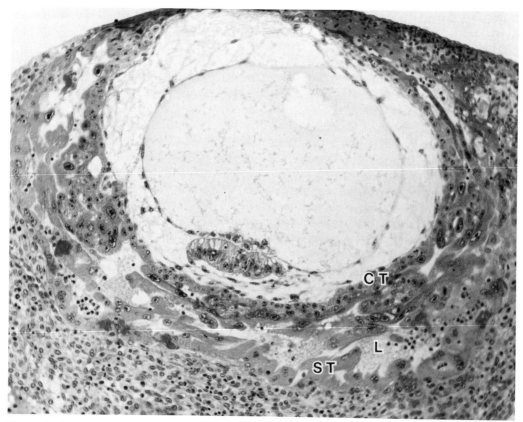

Figure 20.34. With further growth of the conceptus, syncytial trophoblast (*ST*) has tapped maternal vessels, and blood is situated in trophoblastic lacunae (*L*). The cytotrophoblast (*CT*) forms the inner aspect of the trophoblast (stage 5c, Carnegie Collection) (×160).

of spaces or lacunae filled with circulating maternal blood and confined by irregular sheets of syncytial trophoblast. Toward the developing embryo, the syncytial tropho-blast is lined by a continuous layer of *cyto-trophoblast* (cellular trophoblast), which in turn is overlain by forming mesoderm. The association of mesoderm with trophoblast is called *chorion*, and the establishment of this layer converts the implanted blastocyst into a *chorionic vesicle*.

Cytotrophoblast proliferates rapidly, and columns of cells extend radially into the syncytial trophoblast toward the endome-trium. These cell columns of cytotropho-blast covered by syncytial trophoblast are *primary villi*. When the cell columns reach the endometrial surface they spread, form-ing the *cytotrophoblastic shell*, which en-

compasses the conceptus except where ma-ternal blood enters and leaves the devel-oping placenta.

At the same time that cytotrophoblast is proliferating and extending through the syncytium, mesenchyme invades into the base of the primary villi to form a stromal core of the villi and convert them into *secondary villi*. Subsequently fetal vessels develop in the mesenchymal core of the villi and become confluent with vessels forming in the embryo and with blood is-lands in the yolk sac. After the appearance of fetal vessels, the villi are called *tertiary villi*. Contraction of the heart of the embryo begins about 21 days after ovulation, when the total conceptus is about 1 cm in diam-eter.

Tertiary villi initially form over the entire circumference of the chorionic vesicle. As development continues, only the villi with direct access to the maternal blood prosper; these villi become extensive and are called the *chorion frondosum*. It is this portion of the chorionic vesicle that forms the discoidal definitive placenta. The remaining villi (*chorion laeve*) atrophy, forming the avascular or smooth chorion.

The wall of the placenta on the fetal side is the *chorionic plate*. It is composed of the connective tissue in which the fetal vessels ramify, and is covered by the mesothelium of the rapidly diminishing extraembryonic coelom on the side toward the amnion, and by the trophoblast lining the intervillous space on the side toward the endometrium. (Figs. 20.35 and 20.36). The villi arising from the chorionic plate are termed *stem villi*. Some branches of the stem villi pass to and adhere to the decidua basalis, where they are attached by cytotrophoblast and are often embedded in deposits of fibrin and fibrinoid, a glycoprotein secretion. The region of contact between villi and endometrium is the *basal plate*, and the villi that make such contact are called *anchoring villi* (Fig. 20.37). Repeated branching of stem villi into the intervillous space lying between the chorionic and basal plates results in an extensive mass of *free villi* that end in the intervillous space where they are consequently completely surrounded by maternal blood. The various free and anchoring villi derived from a single major stem villus constitute a *fetal cotyledon*.

During the early part of gestation, cytotrophoblast of the anchoring villi forms a nearly continuous layer of the basal plate. Some dispersion of the cytotrophoblast occurs due in part to the formation of a glycoprotein secretion, fibrinoid, between these cells. Many of the cytotrophoblast cells differentiate into large isolated cells in the basal plate, the "X-cells." As fibrin and other debris are added to the fibrinoid, some of the cytotrophoblast cells die and some of the anchoring villi become embedded in infarcted regions.

The growing placenta comes to occupy about 30% of the uterine surface, then enlarges slowly as the uterus expands to accommodate the growing fetus (Fig. 20.38). In the last month there is no net growth of the placenta, and this structure which, in the early stages outweighed the developing embryo, now has only $\frac{1}{7}$ the weight of the fetus.

Structure of Placental Villi

The establishment of tertiary villi and the restriction of villi to a discoidal portion of the chorionic vesicle establishes the general pattern of the placenta. Subsequent changes include increasing abundance of villi and maturation of these structures. The villi of the first trimester are broad, about 70 μm. On the surface of the villus is a rather thick uniform layer of syncytial trophoblast with evenly spaced nuclei. The surface membrane facing the intervillous space has numerous microvilli, between which are caveolae (coated pits) and absorption canaliculi or tubules. Golgi complexes, both rough and smooth endoplasmic reticulum, vesicles, granules, and lipid droplets are prevalent within the syncytium. Beneath the syncytial trophoblast is a continuous layer of cuboidal cellular trophoblast (*Langhans cells*) which share desmosomal junctions with each other and with the syncytium. This cytotrophoblast is apparently the "feeder" population for the syncytium, since only these cells synthesize DNA and undergo mitosis, and fusion of these cells with the syncytial trophoblast has been demonstrated. A thick basal lamina beneath the cytotrophoblast separates the trophoblast layers from the stromal core of the villus. The stroma contains blood vessels that terminate as capillary loops in the smallest villi. The capillaries in the villi are without fenestrae and have extensive bands of intermediate filaments. There are no nerves or lymphatics in placental villi. The fetal stroma in the first trimester is loose, with only a few collagen fibers. Large vacuolated macro-

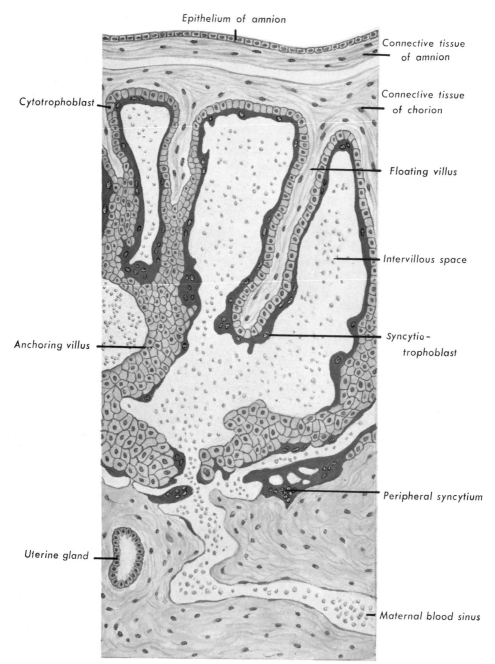

Figure 20.35. Semischematic diagram of structure of fetal and maternal tissues of the placenta (Redrawn and modified after Hamilton, Boyd, and Mossman.)

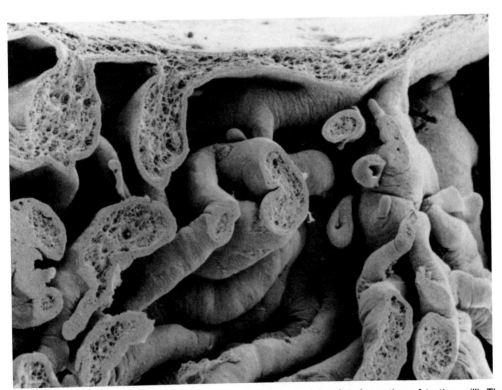

Figure 20.36.   A portion of the periphery of a chorionic vesicle after formation of tertiary villi. The mesoderm of the chorionic plate (*top*) is spongy-looking tissue. Stem villi extend down from the chorionic plate. Note the branching of the stem villus on the right (×97). (Courtesy of Dr. Barry F. King.)

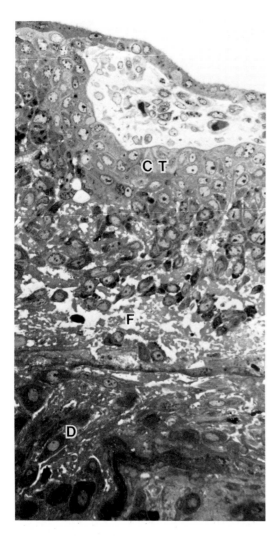

Figure 20.37. Anchoring villi of human placenta at the end of the first trimester. The cytotrophoblast cells (*CT*) beneath the light mesodermal core proliferate and differentiate. Dense maternal decidual cells (*D*) are seen beneath the acellular fibrinoid material (*F*) in the center (×420).

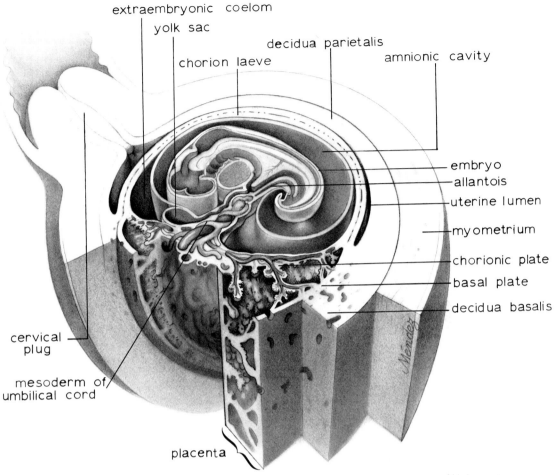

Figure 20.38. Diagram of the pregnant uterus depicting major regions and layers of the placenta and other extraembryonic membranes.

phages called *Hofbauer cells* are abundant and occupy discrete spaces within the connective tissue of the villus (Fig. 20.39).

By the third trimester of gestation, there may be as many as 15 generations of branching villi from the chorionic plate. The major branches contain distributive (nonexchange) vessels. The first order of villi that contain only capillaries are *intermediate villi*. These may branch, but otherwise end in *terminal villi* (Fig. 20.40). Intermediate villi are long (300 to 600 μm), but slender. Even at term, however, some intermediate villi may appear similar to those of early gestation. Terminal villi arise irregularly from intermediate villi, are rel-

atively short, may have a constricted neck region, and contain capillary loops that are often dilated.

As gestation continues, the terminal villi are reduced to about 35 μm in diameter. The cytotrophoblast layer becomes discontinuous, and cytotrophoblast cells are inconspicuous at term. (However, extensive processes from these cells are seen in electron micrographs). An uneven distribution of nuclei within syncytial trophoblast results in clusters of nuclei, *syncytial knots*, and regions where the syncytial trophoblast is very thin (Fig. 20.39). The dilated fetal capillaries become situated close to the surface and even bulge the surface of syncytial

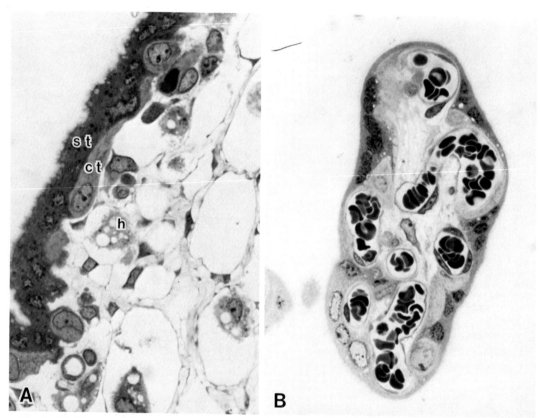

Figure 20.39. *A,* free villus from the end of the first trimester. There is a thick layer of syncytial trophoblast (*ST*) and numerous cytotrophoblast cells (*CT*). Hofbauer cells (*h*) are in apparent spaces within the fetal stroma (×730). *B,* cross section of a villus from a term human placenta. Many of the nuclei in the syncytial trophoblast are aggregated. Capillaries are abundant, and in several areas the syncytial trophoblast is thin over the capillaries (×730).

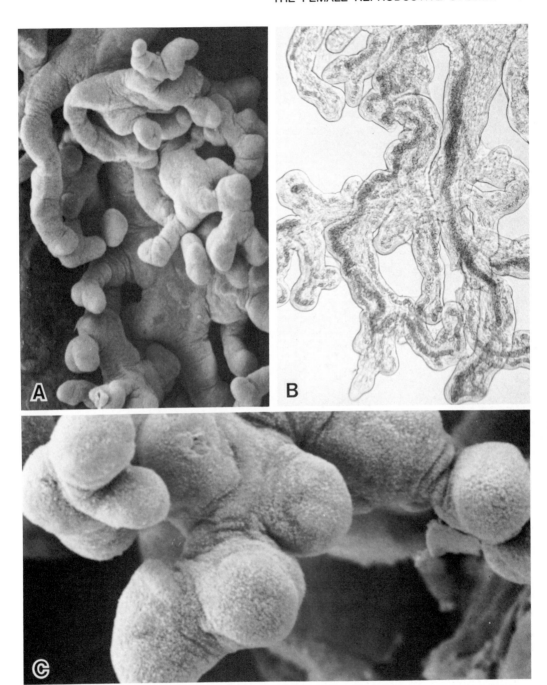

Figure 20.40. Villi from a term placenta, washed free of maternal blood. *A*, scanning electron micrograph showing short terminal villi branching from intermediate villi (×230). *B*, transilluminated villi showing abundant capillary loops in intermediate and terminal villi (×212). *C*, higher magnification scanning electron micrograph of human term placental villi. The numerous microvilli on the surface are barely visible at this magnification (×500). (*C* courtesy of Dr. Barry F. King.)

trophoblast in the thin regions. The total thickness of the layer between maternal and fetal blood (syncytial trophoblast + basement membrane + endothelium of fetal capillaries) approaches 2 μm. Consequently the diffusion distance between maternal blood in the intervillous space and fetal blood in placental capillaries is greatly

reduced in the later placenta, facilitating oxygenation of fetal blood.

It has been estimated that there is roughly 10 m² of villous surface in the term human placenta. In addition, the microvilli of the syncytial trophoblast amplify this area by at least 9 times, increasing the area for diffusion, receptors, and transport systems (Fig. 20.41).

Changes in the Endometrium

As the conceptus grows, it pushes the overlying decidua capsularis against the op- posite surface of the uterus, obliterating the uterine lumen. The endometrium through- out the uterus becomes decidualized. The decidual cells, highly modified stromal cells, are large cells with thin mitochondria, some rough endoplasmic reticulum, many filaments, and charcteristic granules in pe- culiar projections from the periphery of the cells (Fig. 20.42). The decidua basalis grad- ually thins so that at term only a thin layer separates the basal plate from underlying myometrium.

It is not certain what the role of decidual

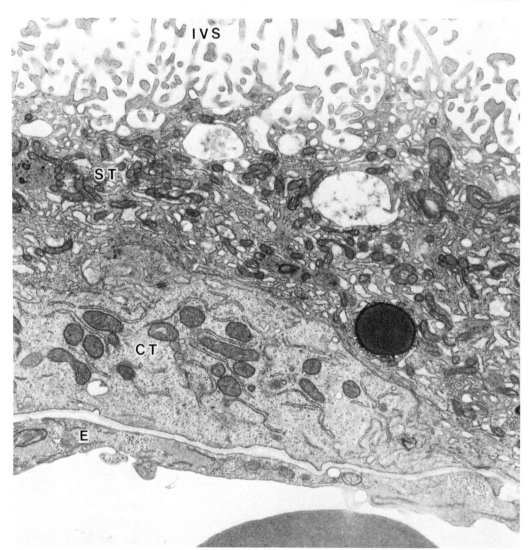

Figure 20.41. Transmission electron micrograph of trophoblast from a term human placenta. The microvilli of the syncytial trophoblast (*ST*) project into the intervillous space (*IVS*). *CT*, cytotrophoblast; *E*, endothelium (×14,000).

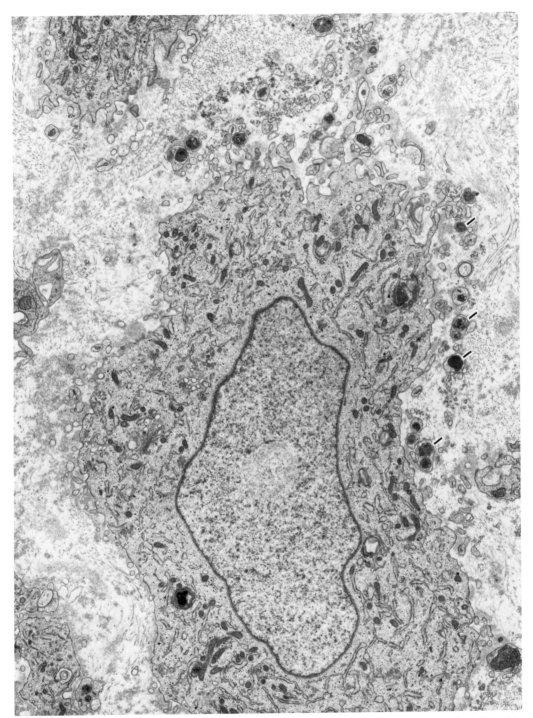

Figure 20.42.   Decidual cell from the parietal decidua of a term human conceptus. The thin mitochondria, branching endoplasmic reticulum, and especially the peripheral processes with granules (lines) are characteristic of these cells (×9,500). (Courtesy of Dr. Barry F. King.)

cells is in pregnancy. Both a protective role in preventing trophoblast from penetrating into the myometrium (*placenta accreta*) and a secretory role have been suggested. Decidual cells can produce prostaglandins and pituitary-type prolactin in vitro, but the significance of this synthetic activity has not been established.

Placental Circulation

After the trophoblast has enlarged the placenta so that the spiral arteries of the endometrium are incorporated into the basal plate, the general pattern of maternal blood flow is established within the placenta. The ends of spiral arteries at the basal plate become reinforced by a cone of cells in their lumen and by trophoblast in the vessel wall. These vessels send a stream of blood into the intervillous space that passes towards the chorionic plate, then spreads among the villi. This highly oxygenated blood then flows laterally among the villi before returning to large veins that pass from the basal plate to the vascular layer of the uterus.

Fetal blood returning to the placenta in umbilical arteries is distributed by vessels that ramify on the surface of the chorionic plate, then enter stem villi. Distributing vessels in the various generations of stem villi eventually terminate in capillaries in intermediate and terminal villi. The terminal villi in particular constitute little more than a syncytial covering of loops of enlarged capillaries. The blood then returns to the chorionic plate to pass via the umbilical vein back to the fetus. Thus the flow of fetal blood in the capillaries is partially crosscurrent and partially countercurrent to the flow of maternal blood in the intervillous space. This directional flow of maternal blood within the intervillous space, coupled with the large flow of maternal blood ($\sim$ 500 cc/min near term) provide for efficient exchange.

Placental Function

The placenta is the major exchange unit between fetal and maternal organisms. Oxygen, carbon dioxide, water, and a number of small molecules and lipid-soluble molecules pass by diffusion from the maternal to the fetal system. In addition the placenta is an active participant in many other exchanges. In later pregnancy the fetus acquires some passive immunity from the maternal system by passage of IgG from maternal to fetal blood (but IgA and IgM do not cross the placenta). The passage of IgG is facilitated by a receptor for the Fc portion of the molecule in the surface membrane of syncytial trophoblast. How this immunoglobulin is protected from mechanisms of protein degradation during transport through the syncytium is not fully understood. Many other receptors are found on syncytial trophoblast (e.g., transferrin, insulin), and the syncytium also has receptors for the different classes of amino acids that it transports. Transport of D-glucose, the major substrate for oxidative metabolism in the fetus, has also been shown to be facilitated by a surface membrane receptor.

The placenta has in addition a major role in synthesis of a number of protein, glycoprotein, and steroid hormones. Of particular importance are *chorionic gonadotropin* (hCG), formed in large amounts early in pregnancy, and *placental lactogen* (hPL), formed in later pregnancy. The chorionic gonadotropin maintains the corpus luteum of pregnancy until placental progesterone levels become elevated. Placental lactogen stimulates milk synthesis in the mammary glands in preparation for lactation.

The placenta, in concert with several fetal organs, forms the *fetal-placental unit* in synthesizing steroids. The placenta *per se* secretes progesterone, and converts dihydroepiandrosterone sulfate formed by the fetal adrenal glands into estrone. The level of estrone in the maternal blood can consequently be used as a test of fetal viability. The steroid hormones produced by the placenta maintain the pregnancy from the later part of the second month until term.

THE VAGINA

The wall of the vagina consists of three coats: mucosa, muscularis, and fibrosa (Fig. 20.43).

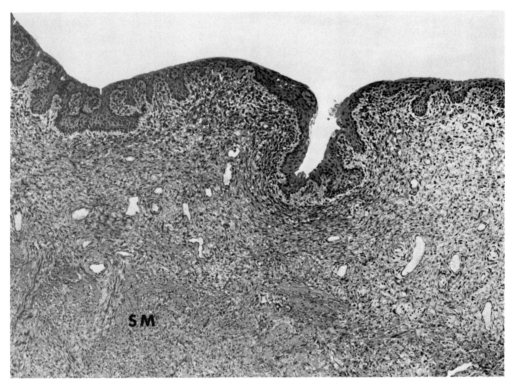

Figure 20.43.   Light micrograph of a portion of the vaginal wall of a monkey. *SM*, smooth muscle (×170).

The *mucosa* shows transverse folds or rugae. It is lined by stratified squamous epithelium which rests on a basement membrane and an underlying lamina propria. Many studies have been made from biopsy specimens in attempts to correlate changes in the epithelium with the menstrual cycle. The findings described, however, are not entirely harmonious, because there are variations in the structure of the epithelium in different parts of the vagina that make it difficult to establish the presence or absence of cyclical changes.

The vaginal epithelium is rich in glycogen which, in the primates, increases with the administration of estrogen. This has also been established in women, and it has been fairly well determined that, in the estrogen phase of the cycle, the vaginal fluid has a lower pH than at other times. This is attributed to the action of the lactic acid-forming bacteria on the carbohydrate from the vaginal epithelium. The bacteria adhere to the microplicae of the superficial cells until just before these cells are desquamated into the lumen (Fig. 20.44).

In the tissue beneath the epithelium, lymphocytes and polymorphonuclear leukocytes are common. These invade the epithelium especially just before, during, and just after menstruation, and they appear as free cells in the lumen of the vagina.

The lamina propria consists of loose connective tissue especially rich in elastic fibers. It also contains polymorphonuclear leukocytes and lymphocytes, as noted above, and it occasionally has aggregations of lymphocytes resembling solitary nodules. A few isolated glands resembling those of the cervix may be found in the uppermost portion of the vagina. Elsewhere the vaginal wall is entirely devoid of glands, and the mucus found in the lumen is derived from the glands of the cervix. In addition, a transudate from the rich mucosal vasculature is believed to add moisture to the vagina, especially during sexual arousal.

The *muscularis* consists mainly of bun-

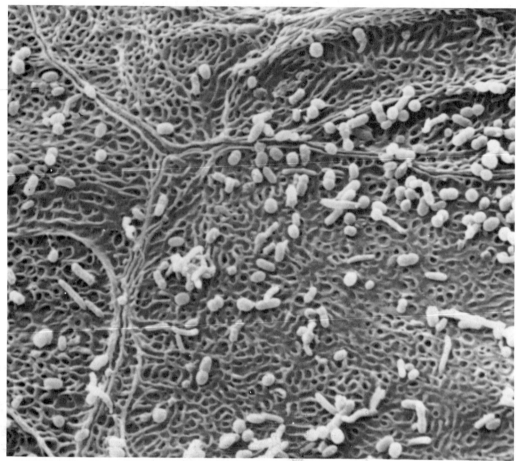

Figure 20.44. Scanning electron micrograph of the surface of the vagina of a rhesus monkey. Note the microplicae and adherent bacteria (×5,000). (Courtesy of Dr. Barry F. King.)

dles of longitudinally disposed smooth muscle fibers that become continuous with the myometrium of the uterus. In the inner portion of the muscularis, circular bundles interlace with the longitudinal ones. the muscle bundles are separated by connective tissue rich in elastic fibers. At the entrance there are skeletal muscle fibers in the vaginal wall.

The *fibrosa* consists of dense connective tissue with many coarse elastic fibers. It serves to connect the vagina with the surrounding structures.

The *hymen* is a thin, transverse semilunar fold at the opening of the vagina into the vestibule. It has the same structure as the vaginal mucosa.

The larger *blood vessels* run in the deeper portion of the mucosa, giving off branches that break up into capillary networks in the stroma and muscularis. These networks have a general direction parallel to the surface. The capillaries empty into the veins that form a plexus of broad venous channels in the muscularis. In the rugae, there are large veins which give the rugae somewhat the character of erectile tissue.

An unusually well developed system of *lymph vessels* is present in the wall of the vagina.

The vagina receives both myelinated and unmyelinated *nerve fibers*. The latter, which are connected with scattered groups of ganglion cells, innervate the muscle tissue and walls of the blood vessels. Sensory myelinated fibers arborize in the mucosa. Their terminals are not fully known.

THE EXTERNAL GENITALIA

The *vestibule*, into which the vagina and urethra open, is lined by a typical stratified squamous epithelium whose superificial layers are cornified. It contains numerous small mucous glands, the minor vestibular glands, placed chiefly near the clitoris and opening of the urethra. They are similar in structure to the glands of Littré of the male reproductive system. The greater vestibular glands or *glands of Bartholin*, analogous to the bulbourethral glands of the male, are situated in the lateral wall of the vestibule, their ducts opening close to the base of the hymen.

The *clitoris* consists mainly of erectile tissue similar to that of the corpora cavernosa of the penis. It is covered with a thin stratified squamous epithelium, underneath which is a papillated stroma rich in blood vessels and containing numerous sensory nerve fibers with highly specialized terminations, such as Meissner's corpuscles and Pacinian corpuscles.

The *labia minora*, which flank the vestibule, are covered with stratified squamous epithelium whose basal layer contains considerable pigment. The underlying, richly vascular connective tissue contains numerous elastic fibers and tall slender papillae that interdigitate with the epithelium. In the stroma are found large sebaceous glands, not associated with hairs, and nerve endings similar to those of the clitoris.

The *labia majora* are folds of skin which cover the labia minora. They have the general structure of skin and consist of a stratified squamous epithelium and an underlying dermis of fibroelastic tissue. On the outer side there are numerous hairs, sweat glands and sebaceous glands. On the inner side the epidermis is thinner and hairs are absent. The interior of the labia are filled with fatty tissue.

THE MAMMARY GLANDS

The mammary glands are cutaneous in origin, developing within the superficial fascia (Fig. 20.45). Each gland consists of 15 to 20 lobes, each of which is a compound gland with a separate lobar duct opening at the apex of the nipple. As compound tubuloalveolar glands they reach full development only during lactation when they are functioning in infant nutrition. The product, milk, is unique in the complexity and specificity of its constituents: fats, proteins, and a sugar (lactose).

A superficial layer of subcutaneous fat covers all but the nipple and the surrounding modified integument, the areola. There is also a deep layer of retromammary fat. Between these is a "mammary parenchymal layer" consisting of (a) the epithelium of the ducts and alveoli forming the lobules, (b) a fine connective tissue surrounding the epithelial components of each lobule, and (c) connective tissue forming interlobar and interlobular septa. Strands of fibers (Cooper's ligaments) anchor the parenchymal layer through the subcutaneous fat to the dermis. The amount of connective tissue varies considerably with the functional state of the glands, being reduced in the lactating gland.

Ducts

There is one main duct for each lobe. These lobar ducts course through the nipple, usually opening independently on the surface. In the resting gland, the openings to the ducts are ordinarily plugged with keratinized cells. Just beneath the nipple there is a local enlargement (lactiferous sinus). The ducts branch as in any compound gland, a terminal duct finally entering each lobule. The epithelium lining the terminal duct is simple cuboidal. It increases in height as the ducts increase in size, and it becomes stratified squamous near the opening onto the surface. Lying within the epithelium basally are myoepithelial cells. These are more readily ob-

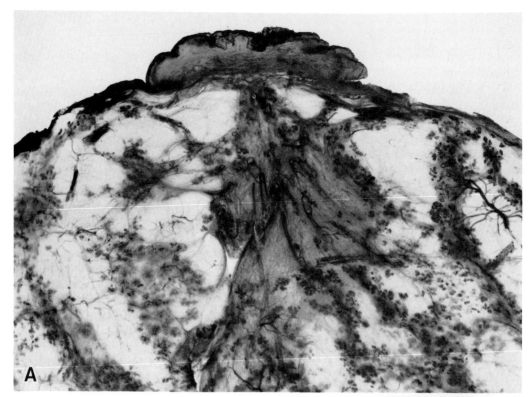

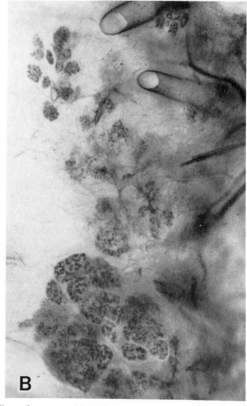

Figure 20.45.   Hematoxylin-stained, cleared thick slice of a normal inactive human mammary gland. The light areas are fatty tissue. *A*, in the center of the picture is a cluster of ducts transsected as they converge toward the nipple in the areola (×3.5). *B*, parts of three ductal lobular units from the preparation above. The branching duct going to the alveoli is particularly clear in the center lobule. Two large ducts and associated vessels are in the upper right (×24). (Photographs from a preparation by Dr. S. R. Wellings and H. M. Jensen.)

served in the larger ducts, where they form a nearly continuous layer.

Nipple and Areola

The skin of the nipple is pigmented and somewhat wrinkled, and it has tall connective tissue papillae. It has many sebaceous but no sweat glands or hairs. The *areola*, an area extending outward from the nipple for 1 to 2 cm, is also pigmented and has modified mammary glands (glands of Montgomery) that produce small elevations on the surface and whose ducts open through the skin of the areola. Sweat and sebaceous glands and a variable number of coarse hairs are also present. The subcutaneous tissue of the nipple and areola contains collagen and elastic fibers attached to the overlying epidermis and radially and circularly coursing smooth muscle fibers. The smooth muscle fibers contract in response to cold, touch, and psychic stimuli producing wrinkling of the areoli and elevating the nipple.

Glandular Epithelium

The epithelium of the mammary gland varies greatly with its functional state and among individuals. The basic functional unit with regard to both response to hormones and pathological conditions is the *terminal ductal-lobular unit*; that is, the terminal duct and its surrounding alveoli.

The Inactive Mammary Gland

The glandular tissue in a nonlactating mammary gland of a sexually mature, nonpregnant woman is sparse and consists of tubules that have the appearance of ducts even within the lobules (Fig. 20.46). Many inactive glands show deviations from this normal structure, however, and a considerable percentage has, without any clinical symptoms, some degree of gross or microscopic cystic disease or other abnormalities. About 8% of the women born in the United States develop cancer of the breast. This is usually (85%) epithelial in origin (carcinoma).

The Mammary Gland during Lactation

Throughout pregnancy, the mammary gland undergoes extensive changes in prep-

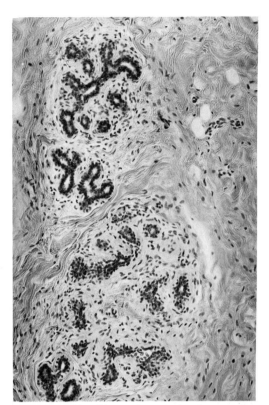

Figure 20.46. Photomicrograph of a section through two lobules of an inactive mammary gland. Woman, 20 years of age (×140).

aration for lactation. The tubules characteristic of the inactive gland form buds that enlarge into alveoli. As this growth of glandular tissue proceeds, the fat and the intralobular and interlobular connective tissue decrease in amount, the latter forming septa in which the ducts are embedded (Fig. 20.47). The alveoli at the termination of pregnancy are large and irregular in shape, although there is frequently great variation in the degree of development among the lobules or even within a lobule (Fig. 20.47). The alveoli are lined by a simple cuboidal epithelium that rests on a delicate basement membrane (Fig. 20.48). Electron micrographs show that the cells have microvilli, relatively large mitochondria, a Golgi complex that enlarges during secretory activity and granular endoplasmic reticulum that increases during milk protein synthesis (Fig. 20.49).

Milk consists of a proteinaceous fluid

Inactive lobule   Active lobule

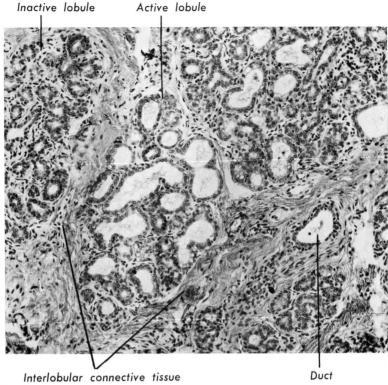

Interlobular connective tissue   Duct

Figure 20.47.   Photomicrograph of a section of mammary gland showing active and inactive glandular tissue. Fourth day postpartum. Woman, 29 years of age. Surgical specimen (×140).

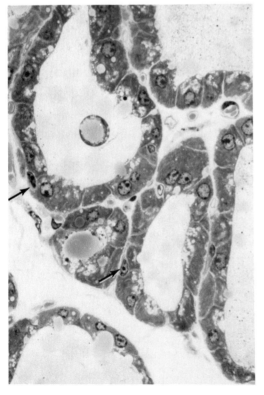

containing salts, casein, lactalbumin, milk sugar (lactose), and suspended fat droplets. The fat is in the form of neutral triglycerides with a relatively high degree of unsaturation. Milk is rich in calcium needed by the growing infant, and in a number of vitamins and ions. However, it is a poor source of vitamin D and iron. It contains plasma proteins, of which IgA is probably the most important, since it may have an antibacterial function in the intestinal lumen of the infant. Some cellular debris is also present.

Colostrum is the secretion formed during the first few days after parturition. It contains appreciable cellular debris including cells of probable leukocytic origin, large fat globules, and more immunoglobulins than milk. The greater resemblance of colostrum

Figure 20.48.   Active mammary gland of the mouse. Milk proteins, lactose, and lipid accumulate in the lumen of the gland. Myoepithelial cells (*arrows*) underlie the glandular epithelium (×690).

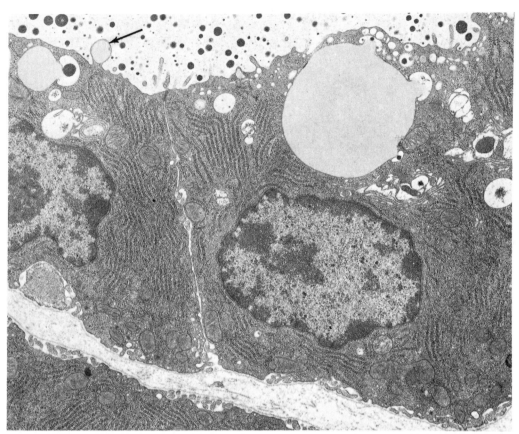

Figure 20.49.   Electron micrograph of an active mammary gland of a mouse. The cells have many of the features of a protein-exporting cell. Note also the lipid droplets, and the lipid being budded into the lumen (*arrow*). Protein granules are abundant within the glandular lumen (×8,800).

to blood serum suggests that it is more of a transudate than is milk.

The secretory process for protein constituents of milk resembles that of other cells which synthesize proteins for export. The proteins are synthesized in association with polyribosomes, packaged in the Golgi complex and then transported in membrane-bounded vesicles to the apical surface, where they are discharged by a merocrine mode of secretion. This is a relatively rapid process, and it has been shown in experimental animals that tritiated leucine incorporated into milk proteins is released into the duct system within 30 min after administration. The disaccharide lactose is synthesized in the Golgi complex, and the initial vesicles released from this area contain both lactose and proteins. The casein is originally dispersed, but aggregates into a number of discrete micelles within each

vesicle before exocytosis. The milk so formed is isotonic to plasma, with half of the osmotic pressure being attributable to lactose. Although esterification of the fatty acids into triglycerides probably occurs in the endoplasmic reticulum, the lipid droplets appear to arise in the cytoplasm outside the Golgi complex and pass to the apical end of the cell. They project outward and are pinched off into the lumen enclosed by a membrane derived from the cell plasmalemma, along with an ultramicroscopic portion of cytoplasm. The amount of cytoplasm lost is small but the process is classified as an apocrine secretion.

The original development of the mammary glands to prominence takes place at puberty under the influence of elevated ovarian steroid levels. The estrogens seem to promote duct development, and progesterone aids alveolar development. During pregnancy not only is there an elevated progesterone level, but in addition the placenta produces a placental lactogen (MPL or mammotropic factor). These hormones together with adrenal corticoids promote development of the mammary glands during pregnancy. After parturition, prolactin is the most important hormone for initiation and maintenance of synthesis of milk. Insulin and adrenal corticoids are necessary, however, and any major disturbance of thyroid function can be deleterious to lactation.

Milk "let-down," the mobilization of milk from the secretory alveoli, is brought about by the release of oxytocin from the posterior pituitary. The oxytocin in turn causes the myoepithelial cells to contract, producing milk expulsion. Oxytocin release is caused by stimulation of the hypothalamus through a variety of external stimuli including suckling, baby crying, or breast distention.

After cessation of lactation, the epithelium of the mammary glands involutes, and the alveoli decrease in size until they become no longer recognizable. The connective tissue and fat again become abundant as the structure of an inactive gland is reassumed.

The mammary glands undergo progressive atrophy after the *menopause.* Some of the lobules and ducts may be obliterated; the connective tissue becomes increasingly dense and frequently hyalinized. Cystic dilation of the ducts frequently occurs.

The Mammary Gland of the Male

There is little agreement as to the normal constitution of the male breast. Some mammary tissue always is present, but it attains its maximal development during early adolescence and then normally undergoes involution. The gland consists of ducts with usually no alveoli or lobulation. Under conditions of abnormal hormonal stimulation, as in some testicular tumors, the male mammary gland may enlarge and develop extensively, a condition designated as gynecomastia.

Blood Vessels

The mammary gland is a cutaneous structure and receives its blood supply, as does much of the integument, from several neighboring vessels. The intercostals, internal mammary and thoracic branches of the axillary arteries provide vessels that subdivide and form a rich capillary plexus around the ducts and alveoli. The richness of the blood supply fluctuates with activity, being much greater in the active than in the inactive or the involuted gland. From the capillaries, veins arise which accompany the arteries.

Lymphatics

The lymph vessels of mammary glands are numerous. An understanding of the course of these vessels is facilitated by keeping in mind the fact that the gland arises from the ectoderm and grows into the underlying mesoderm and that in this underlying tissue there is, over the whole body, a plexus of lymph vessels. Thus, as the developing ducts grow deeply into the connective tissue, lymph vessels accompany them and drain toward the surface into the subcutaneous lymph plexus. This plexus is particularly well formed beneath the areola. From the subcutaneous plexus, vessels pass to the axillary lymphatics and nodes along the pectoral muscles. There are accessory paths of drainage. Some vessels cross the midline, others follow the branches of the internal mammary artery and drain through the sternal nodes, and still others may drain into the abdominal lymph nodes. Because of the frequency of mammary carcinoma, the lymph drainage of this gland is of great importance.

Nerves

Cranial, spinal, and sympathetic nerves supply the gland, the larger trunks following the interlobar and interlobular connective tissue septa. The nerve terminals break up into plexuses that surround the alveoli just outside their basal laminae. From these plexuses, delicate fibrils have been described passing through the basal lamina and ending between the secreting cells. Nonencapsulated, branched, and single sensory fibers are common around the ducts and in the dermis of the nipple, and are less common in association with the ducts of Montgomery's glands. There is a rich sympathetic innervation of the vessels of the mammary glands, but neither the glandular epithelium nor the myoepithelial cells are innervated.

DEVELOPMENT OF THE FEMALE REPRODUCTIVE SYSTEM

Differentiation of the *ovary* begins later and differs considerably from testis development. The medullary cords and rete formed during the indifferent period gradually involute, although vestiges of the rete may remain in the adult ovary. On the other hand, the more superficial cells continue to proliferate forming a thick layered epithelial mass. The masses of cells are partially subdivided by thin strands of connective tissue into clusters of epithelial cells that are destined to become the follicle cells and oogonia (the latter derived from the primordial germ cells that migrated into the ridge from the yolk sac). At first, the clusters consist of several larger cells scattered in a mass of small follicular cells. Later, each cluster is broken up by invading connective tissue into several primordial follicles, each containing a single oogonium surrounded by a layer of flattened follicular cells.

Proliferation of oogonia continues until about the sixth month. By the time of birth all of the germ cells in the ovary are primary oocytes and a dense connective tissue layer the *tunica albuginea* has formed beneath the germinal epithelium which persists as a layer of cuboidal or columnar cells constituting the surface epithelium of the ovary.

As mentioned in the previous chapter the primordia of the female genital ducts are the Müllerian ducts of the embryo. These begin in both sexes as coelomic invaginations into the cranial portions of the meso-nephric ridge which then grow caudally, running parallel and close to the mesonephric duct. Caudally, the two Müllerian ducts approach each other and fuse to form a terminal unpaired tube which ends in the urogenital sinus between the openings of the mesonephric ducts. The paired upper portions become the *uterine tubes* or *oviducts*, while the unpaired terminal portion forms the uterus and a major portion of the vagina. In the meantime, the mesonephric duct and tubules, rather than forming the efferent ductules and epididymis as they do in the male, degenerate, leaving only a few nonfunctional remnants in the broad ligament of the ovary.

Development of Mammary Glands

In animals with numerous pairs of mammary glands, the beginnings of these glands are represented by two ridges of thickened epithelium, the mammary lines, which extend from the axillary to the inguinal regions. At various points on these ridges, epithelial proliferations form the primordia of future glands, while the intermediate portions of the milk lines ultimately disappear. In the human, the mammary line (ridge) is poorly defined and of brief duration, and normally only one pair of glands develops. Each gland appears in the second month as a broad epidermal thickening in the region of the future nipple, produced by a proliferation and downgrowth of the germinative layer. The thickening spreads laterally to form a hemispherical mass whose convex surface is directed towards the dermis. Externally, the circular patch of skin, or mammary area, corresponding to the thickening sinks below the surface as the mammary pit.

About the fifth month, a varying number of secondary sprouts, the future lactiferous ducts and sinuses, grow down into the dermis and there branch repeatedly with the branches ending in terminal swellings. At first the sprouts are solid but, from the seventh month on, lumina appear in various places and finally become confluent.

This process of branching and canalization continues until birth, the histological picture being that of a prepubertal gland. The formation of the glandular alveoli does not take place until adolescence.

Soon after birth, the shallow mammary pit is raised above the surface by the proliferation of connective tissue. The central portion develops into the nipple, which contains the openings of the lactiferous ducts. The remainder of the mammary area forms the areola, which is distinguished from the surrounding skin by its hairlessness, pigmentation and thinness of epidermis.

References

Adams EC, Hertig AT: Studies on the human corpus luteum. I. Observations on the ultrastructure of development and regression of the luteal cells during the menstrual cycle. *J Cell Biol* 41:696–715, 1969.

Amsterdam A, Linder H, Gröschel-Stewart U: Localization of actin and myosin in the rat oocyte and follicular wall by immunofluorescence. *Anat Rec* 187:311–327, 1977.

Anderson E, Albertini D: Gap junctions between the oocyte and companion follicle cells in the mammalian ovary. *J Cell Biol* 71:680–686, 1976.

Blandau RJ, Moghissi K; *Biology of the Cervix.* Chicago, University of Chicago Press, 1973.

Boyd JD, Hamilton WJ: *The Human Placenta.* Cambridge, W. Heffer & Sons, 1970.

Edwards RG: *Conception in the Human Female.* New York, Academic Press, 1980.

Enders AC: The fine structure of the blastocyst. In Blandau RJ (ed): *The Biology of the Blastocyst.* Chicago, The University of Chicago Press, 1971, pp 71–94.

Enders AC: Fine structure of anchoring villi of the human placenta. *Am J Anat* 122:419–452, 1968.

Enders AC, Hendrickx AG, Schlafke S: Implantation in the rhesus monkey. Initial penetration of endometrium. *Am J Anat* 167:275–298, 1983.

Enders AC, King BF: The cytology of Hofbauer cells. *Anat Rec* 167:231–252, 1970.

Enders AC, Schlafke S: Differentiation of the blastocyst of the rhesus monkey. *Am J Anat* 162:1–21, 1981.

Hertig AT, Adams EC: Studies on the human oocyte and its follicle. I. Ultrastructural and histochemical observations on the primordial follicle stage. *J Cell Biol* 34:647–675, 1967.

Hertig AT, Rock J, Adams EC: A description of 34 human ova within the first 17 days of development. *Am J Anat* 98:435–494, 1956.

Huszar G, Roberts JM: Biochemistry and pharmacology of the myometrium and labor: regulation at the cellular and molecular levels. *Am J Obstet Gynecol* 142:25–237, 1982.

Kaufmann P, Sen DK, Schweikkart G: Classification of human placental villi. I. Histology. *Cell Tissue Res* 200:409–423, 1979.

Kelley LK, King BF, Johnson LW, Smith CH: Protein composition and structure of human placental microvillous membrane: external surface, sialic acid containing, extrinsic and intrinsic components. *Exp Cell Res* 123:167–176, 1979.

King BF: Ultrastructure of the nonhuman primate vaginal mucosa: epithelial changes during the menstrual cycle and pregnancy. *J Ultrastruct Res* 82:1–18, 1983.

King BF: Absorption of peroxidase-conjugated immunoglobulin G by human placenta: an in vitro study. *Placenta* 3:395–406, 1982.

Mestwerdt W, Muller O: Morphology and morphometry of human preovulatory follicles collected during LH surge, with emphasis on granulosa cells. In Hafez ESE (ed): *In Vitro Fertilization and Embryo Transfer.* England, MTP Press Limited, 1982, pp. 233–242.

Noyes, RW, Hertig, AT, and Rock, J: Dating the endometrial biopsy. *Fertil Steril* 1:3–25, 1950.

Ockleford CD, Clint JM: The uptake of IgG by human placental chorionic villi: a correlated autoradiographic and wide aperture counting. *Placenta* 1:91–111, 1980.

Richards JS: Hormonal control of ovarian follicular development: A 1978 perspective. *Recent Prog Horm Res* 35:343–368, 1979.

Teasdale F: Gestational changes in functional structure of human placenta in relation to growth. *Am J Obstet Gynecol* 137:560–568, 1980.

Upadahyay S, Luciani JM, Zamboni L: The role of the mesonephrons in the development of indifferent gonads and ovaries of the mouse. *Ann Biol Anim Biochim Biophys* 19:1179–1184, 1979.

Chapter 21

THE ENDOCRINE GLANDS

In the evolution of larger and more complex organisms, specialized control systems have been developed which serve to integrate the functions of the various and often widely scattered organs. One such control system is neural; the other principal mechanism operates through endocrine secretion and response.

An endocrine gland is one whose product passes by way of the blood vascular system to other cells in the body, where it elicits a specific response. Such a product is called a *hormone*, and typically its target cells throughout the body have receptor molecules for this substance. Endocrine glands vary greatly in size, from the small but essential parathyroid glands to the large thyroid gland with which the former are associated. Whether the endocrine cells constitute only a small portion of an organ, like the scattered enteroendocrine cells of the digestive tract, or form the major portion of an endocrine gland, they have a number of features in common. The cells secreting the hormones (parenchyma) are epithelial, epithelioid, or neuronal. The glands are richly vascularized by highly permeable capillaries. Although it is often stated that an endocrine gland is one whose product passes directly into blood vessels rather than into ducts, this is only partially accurate. Endocrine glands either lack ducts or the ducts do not communicate with the endocrine cells. However, the hormones pass from endocrine cells into intercellular spaces and the interstitium, from which they must diffuse to and enter the vascular system. The placenta is an exception, since hormones formed in the syncytial trophoblast can pass directly into maternal blood that surrounds the placental villi.

Embryologically there are a limited number of patterns of development. Secretory cells of major endocrine glands are derived from the central nervous system (neurohypophysis), from neural crest cells (adrenal medulla), as outgrowths of the alimentary tract that subsequently lose their connection with the lumen (adenohypophysis, pancreatic islets, thyroid, parathyroid), or as epithelioid cells from mesoderm of the urogenital ridge (adrenal cortex, Leydig cells, ovarian steroid cells).

A number of recent developments have aided our understanding of endocrine functions. Radioimmunoassay has made possible the assessment of blood levels of different hormones in different parts of the body. Immunohistochemical methods are currently being used to localize not only the major sites of hormone production but also cells that produce more than one hormone or, conversely, cells in different organs that produce the same hormone. For example, many of the peptide hormones originally thought to be unique to the enteroendocrine system are also produced in the brain. Analysis of the molecular structure of individual hormones has shown that portions of the molecule in different hormones are similar; thus the α-chains of three different glycoprotein hormones produced by the pituitary are similar. Molecules are also produced that contain several hormones within their amino acid sequences; for example, pro-opiomelanocortin contains the sequences for several hormones.

When classifying the endocrine glands by the nature of their products, there are three major types of glands: steroid-producing glands, peptide-producing glands, and glands producing hormones related to neurotransmitter substances.

The steroid-secreting glands synthesize

their product from cholesterol, and tend to produce hormones that circulate in association with proteins. The steroid hormones affect the target cells via specific cytoplasmic receptors and, after translocation to the nucleus, affect DNA transcription. Steroid-secreting cells typically have abundant smooth endoplasmic reticulum (where enzymes for several steps in cholesterol synthesis are located, as well as 3β-hydroxysteroid dehydrogenase, the enzyme catalyzing the conversion of pregnenolone to progesterone). They have numerous mitochondria with tubular cristae (where the enzymes for cholesterol side chain cleavage are located, as well as enzymes acting on the 11 and 18 positions of the steroid molecule). These cells often have lipid droplets that contain fatty acids and some cholesterol, but little stored hormone. Although many of the steroid-secreting glands can synthesize cholesterol, most of the cholesterol used by these cells typically comes to them from the vasculature by way of lipoprotein carriers which are endocytized, providing precursor cholesterol for subsequent hormone synthesis. Since steroid hormones are readily soluble in membrane lipids, they can leave the cell of origin by diffusion through the cell membrane rather than by exocytosis of granules.

The products of protein and polypeptide-producing glands are usually synthesized as larger precursor molecules or *prohormones* in the rough endoplasmic reticulum, and are shortened to the active hormone either before storage in a secretory granule or prior to exocytosis of the secretory granule. These cells typically store their product in membrane-bounded secretory granules. Consequently such cells resemble zymogenic cells in having abundant rough endoplasmic reticulum, a moderately large Golgi apparatus, and numerous secretion granules that are released by exocytosis. The molecules released when the granules fuse with the surface membrane must diffuse through the interstitial space, and then pass through or between endothelial cells to reach the blood. Unlike steroid hormones, the peptide hormones bind to specific membrane receptors at the surface of target cells, rather than cytoplasmic receptors, and they activate the cyclic nucleotide system of the receptor cell.

The third type of gland is that producing simple hormones from small precursors using only a few steps. These glands are derived from the nervous system, and have as typical examples the pineal and adrenal medulla. Their hormones, like the protein and peptide type, exert their influence on target cells by binding to specific membrane receptors. However, since the synthesis of their product involves neither the ribosomal system nor steroid synthesis, accumulation of storage granules is the principal cytological characteristic of these cells.

Simply because a substance acts as a hormone does not mean that this is the only way it can function. A substance which, when released from a cell, passes via the blood system to another cell and elicits a response is acting as a hormone. If it diffuses to a local cell and elicits a response it is functioning as a *parahormone* and its secretion is referred to as *paracrine*. In the nervous system, when a substance emitted by a neural ending elicits a response from the postsynaptic membrane, it is acting as a *neurotransmitter*. The same substance may pass to its target cell by diffusion or by transport in the blood. Thus far such substances that act by all three delivery systems are all active amines, but a number of other substances, especially the peptides, have been identified as having both paracrine and endocrine functions.

The morphology of the endocrine cells of the ovaries and testes, the placenta, and pancreatic islets has been considered in the chapters on the systems with which these organs are associated. Consequently the pituitary, thyroid, parathyroid, adrenal, and pineal glands will be described in this chapter.

THE PITUITARY

Organization and Origin

The *pituitary gland* (*hypophysis cerebri*) is derived in part from an evagination of oral ectoderm of the dorsal median region of the *stomodeum* (*Rathke's pouch*) and in part from an evagination of the *infundibular portion* of the diencephalon of the brain, the latter portion maintains its connections in the adult (Fig. 21.1). The major part of the gland (anterior and posterior lobes) lies in a fossa of the sphenoid bone, the *sella turcica*. This part is ensheathed by the dura, a thickened extension of which, the *diaphragma sellae*, roofs over the sella turcica. There is a small aperture in the diaphragm through which the *pituitary stalk* passes. The suprasellar portion of the gland includes the pituitary stalk and that portion of the hypothalamus known as the *median eminence* of the *tuber cinereum*. The *infun-dibular stem* forms the bulk of the pituitary stalk. The smaller component, the *pars tuberalis*, surrounds the infundibular stem and flares out onto the median eminence.

Table 21.1 gives the various parts of the gland, their embryological derivation, and the more common synonyms. Figures 21.2 and 21.3 illustrate their relationships. In addition, there is a persistent remnant of the original stomodeal diverticulum in humans that is called the *pharyngeal hypophysis*.

The *pars nervosa* and *pars intermedia* are intimately fused, forming a single main division, the *posterior lobe*. However, spaces lined by epithelial cells are often present between the *intermediate* lobe and the

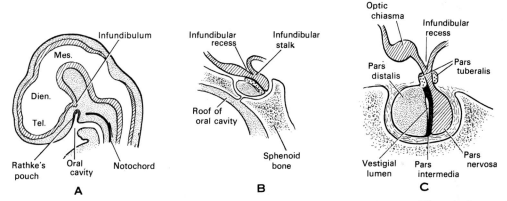

Figure 21.1. Diagrammatic sagittal sections of the human pituitary gland at different stages of develoment. *A*, cephalic region of a six-week embryo showing Rathke's pouch as an outgrowth from the dorsal wall of the oral cavity. The infundibulum is seen as a thickening in the floor of the diencephalon (*Dien.*). *Tel.*, telencephalon and *Mes.*, mesencephalon. *B* and *C*, stages of pituitary development at the end of the third and fourth months, respectively. The interrelationships of the major subdivisions of the gland in the four-month fetus approximate those of the adult. (Redrawn and modified after Langman J: *Medical Embryology*, ed. 4. Baltimore, Williams & Wilkins, 1981, p 341.)

Table 21.1.
Components of the Pituitary and their Derivation

Derivations	Divisions	Components		Lobes of Pituitary Gland Within Sella Turcica
Oral ectoderm	Adenohypophysis	Pars tuberalis Pars distalis—pars anterior Pars intermedia		Anterior lobe
Neural ectoderm	Neurohypophysis	Pars nervosa—infundibular process (neural lobe) Infundibulum (neural stalk)	Infundibular stem Median eminence of tuber cinereum	Posterior lobe

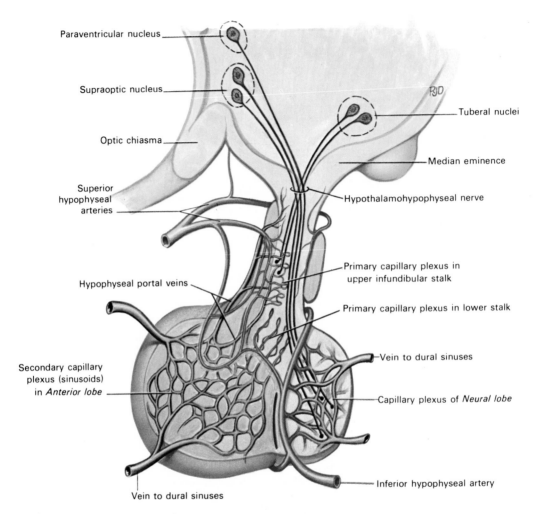

Figure 21.2. Diagram of the blood supply of the pituitary gland as seen from the left side. The infundibular stalk is shown in sagittal section and portions of the left sides of the anterior and neural lobes have been removed in order to show the vessels that penetrate deeply into the glandular tissue. The left inferior hypophyseal artery is shown in its course at the exterior of the gland, above the cut surface of the glandular tissue. The inferior hypophyseal artery joins with its corresponding vessel of the opposite side (not visible from the left) to form an arterial circle around the junction of the neural lobe with the anterior lobe. Branches from the circle penetrate inward, as shown, to supply the neural lobe and the lower portion of the infundibular stalk. Although veins are shown in this diagram that drain the anterior lobe directly, current evidence suggests that the veins draining the anterior lobe are confluent with veins draining the posterior lobe.

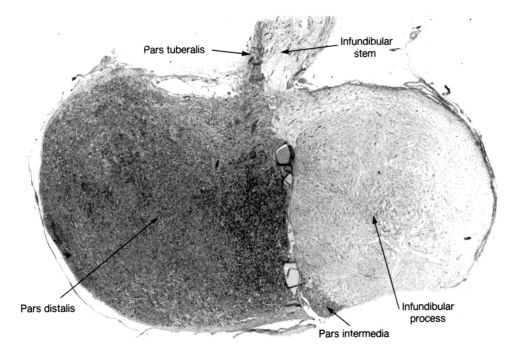

Pars tuberalis

Infundibular stem

Pars distalis

Infundibular process

Pars intermedia

Figure 21.3. Micrograph of a section through most of a human pituitary, stained with hematoxylin and eosin (×11).

neural lobe. They frequently contain some colloid, and they are often described as *Rathke's cysts*; they should not be confused with remnants of Rathke's pouch which rarely persist in the human but are common in some other mammals.

The human pituitary gland measures about 1.2 to 1.5 cm in the transverse plane, about 1 cm in the sagittal plane and about 0.6 cm in height. Both its weight and its dimensions vary considerably. In the human, the weight of the anterior lobe can double with pregnancy and decreases slightly in old age. The average weight of the pituitary in the male is about 0.5 to 0.7 g, being slightly heavier in non-pregnant women and much heavier in pregnant women.

Blood and Nerve Supply

The *blood supply* of the pituitary has unusual features, and is unusually important in that it provides the avenue of control of the *adenohypophysis* by the nervous system. This avenue involves the release of special hormones, or *releasing factors*, from

groups of modified neurons in the hypothalamus. The releasing factors are carried by the blood stream a short distance to the adenohypophysis, where they control the release of various pituitary hormones. Hence, the pituitary is under *neurosecretory* control. It therefore is appropriate to describe the vascular patterns in advance of the microscopic structure (Fig. 21.2). The major features of this blood supply are that the anterior lobe receives no direct arterial supply, but is supplied by vessels from the neurohypophysis, especially the *infundibulum*, and that there are extensive anastomoses of the blood vessels throughout the neurohypophysis.

The pituitary is supplied by *superior hypophyseal arteries*, which usually arise from the circle of Willis (a critical arterial channel which encircles the pituitary stem and supplies both vertebral and carotid blood to this brain region), somewhat variable *middle hypophyseal arteries*, and *inferior hypophyseal arteries* from the internal carotids. The superior hypophyseal vessels supply the infundibulum and thence the anterior lobe by way of a portal system. The middle hypophyseal arteries, which can arise either from the superior hypophyseal arteries or directly from the internal carotids, pass to the infundibular stem and neural lobe. The inferior hypophyseal vessels serve mainly for the blood supply of the neural lobe, although their interlobar branches do give off some vessels that anastomose with branches from the superior hypophyseal vessels to supply the lower portion of the infundibulum and thence, by a short portal system, the anterior lobe. It is to be noted that the anterior lobe is no longer believed to receive direct arterial supply, and it is therefore dependent upon the portal systems from the infundibulum.

There are several superior hypophyseal arteries and their pattern is complex due to numerous variations and anastomoses with each other and vessels of the circle of Willis. The superior hypophyseal arteries form a ring interior to the circle of Willis and send capillaries to the infundibulum.

The arterioles in the median eminence and upper part of the stalk terminate in characteristic patterns of looped sinusoidal capillaries, that form an external (superficial) plexus in a region of the infundibulum rich in nerve endings. Vessels from this plexus (a) unite to form the long portal vessels passing superficially on the infundibular stalk down to the *pars distalis*, and (b) send branches that form the internal (deep) plexus of vessels in the *median eminence* and adjacent to the ventricular recess. These deep vessels also eventually connect to the long portal vessels. The long portal vessels, together with short portal vessels that pass to the pars distalis from the lower part of the infundibulum, constitute the *hypophyseal portal system*. Thus, a pathway is established by which neurosecretory material released from nerves in the median eminence can pass directly to the pars distalis. Because of the small size of the veins draining the anterior pituitary and the high concentration of adenohypophyseal hormones in the portal blood, it has been suggested that there may be ret-

rograde flow through some of the long portals to the median eminence, and through the short portals to the posterior lobe.

The *pars nervosa (neural lobe)* receives its blood supply from the *inferior hypophyseal arteries*, which form an arterial circle near the junction of the anterior and posterior lobes. Numerous arterial branches pass into the neural lobe tissue to enter sinusoidal capillaries. Interlobar arteries from the arterial circle also contribute branches which anastomose with vessels from the superior hypophyseal arteries, as outlined above, to supply the lower (intraglandular) portion of the infundibulum and thence to the sinusoidal capillaries of the pars distalis (Fig. 21.2). The sinusoidal capillaries of the neural lobe have an important function in receiving neurosecretory material conveyed to the neural lobe by nerve fibers from the hypothalamus. The veins from the neural lobe are confluent with veins from the anterior lobe, and drain into the cavernous sinus, forming the major pathway of efflux of blood from the pituitary.

The sinusoidal capillaries of the pars distalis form an elaborate plexus of channels which are wider than the sinusoidal capillaries of the neural lobe. Electron micrographs show a fenestrated type of endothelium in the sinusoidal capillaries of both locations with diaphragms spanning the fenestrae as described in Chapter 12.

The *innervation* of the hypophysis consists chiefly of the *hypothalamo-hypophyseal tracts* of nonmyelinated nerve fibers that extend into the neural lobe from their cells of origin in the *supraoptic* and *paraventricular nuclei* and of tracts from other regions of the hypothalamus to the upper part of the stalk (Fig. 21.2). They serve to carry neurosecretory substances. There are no nerves to the anterior lobe, other than some vasomotor fibers with blood vessels. Although the parenchymal cells of the pars distalis have no nerve supply, there is substantial evidence that they are under nervous control.

Initial indication of the manner in which

the anterior pituitary could be controlled by the nervous system came from the observation that nerve fibers had endings with large numbers of neurosecretory granules in close association with the external capillary plexus in the median eminence. This observation supported the hypothesis that neurohumoral substances could pass through the portal vessels to the pars distalis, and thereby control secretion of anterior pituitary hormones. During the 1970s, three of these hypophysiotropic hormones, called *releasing hormones* or *releasing factors*, were isolated and completely characterized, and several others are in the process of characterization. It has also been found that active amines (especially dopamine and norepinephrine) have effects on the release of adenohypophyseal hormones. The relation of the infundibular recess to the internal capillary bed in the infundibulum also suggests that the third ventricle could be a pathway for substances moving between the pituitary vessels and the brain.

Microscopic Structure and Function

Pars Distalis

About 75% of the pituitary is anterior lobe. The parenchyma of this lobe is formed of anastomosing cords of cells separated from sinusoidal capillaries by only a meager amount of irregularly arranged connective tissue. Small masses of colloid occur within the cell cords only occasionally.

On the basis of staining reactions in routine preparations, early pituitary cytologists divided the parenchymal cells into *acidophils*, *basophils*, and *chromophobes*. In hematoxylin and eosin preparations, the cytoplasmic granules of the acidophils stain well with eosin, but the granules of the basophils do not stain well with hematoxylin. However, the acidophilia was based on the staining of the granules of these cells, and the basophils were given that designation not on the usual basis of numerous ribosomes but rather because the granules were not acidophilic and could be stained with the aniline blue component of Mallory's or Masson's trichrome stains.

The use of different staining methods, coupled with understanding of hormonal negative feedback control of most anterior pituitary hormones, allowed investigators to use augmentation or ablation of end organ hormones to indicate at least six cell types in the pars distalis. More recently, immunohistochemistry has confirmed these findings, and suggested a greater degree of commonality than previously suspected. Only the immunohistochemical localization of hormones in the secretion granules of individual cells provides specific evidence of their synthetic activity. Nevertheless, the routine designations are still used, and the different cell types will be described in relation to these categories.

The *chromophobes* tend to appear in groups near the centers of the cords. Their nuclei are surrounded by a small amount of diffuse, light staining cytoplasm, and cell boundaries are not distinguishable in ordinary preparations. Secretory granules of specific types are usually not seen by light microscopy in cells classified as chromophobes. However, electron microscope studies show relatively few nongranular cells, and it appears that most of the cells counted as chromophobes in routine preparations are acidophils and basophils that have become degranulated in the course of secretory activity.

The *acidophils* (*alpha cells*) stain readily and are easily identified in ordinary preparations (Figs. 21.4 and 21.12). These cells are usually larger than the chromophobes, and their cytoplasm contains secretion granules which take the acid dyes such as eosin, acid fusion and orange G.

The acidophils can be divided into two groups. The most abundant cell type stains strongly with orange G or eosin, tends to be rounded and has abundant granules. This is called the *somatotrope*, because it secretes *somatotropin* (or *growth hormone*). It was originally identified because adenomas of these cells caused the condition of acromegaly in adults. In electron micrographs, these cells have numerous spherical dense granules 300 to 400 nm in diameter,

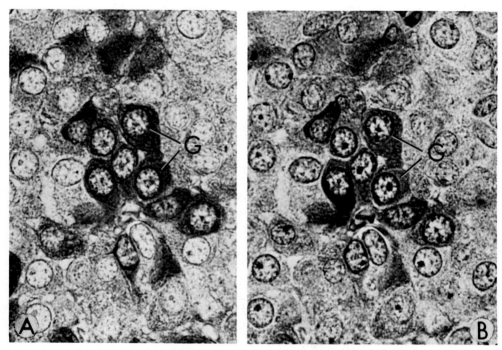

Figure 21.4. Photomicrographs of a section of rat pars distalis. In *A*, the section has been stained immunohistochemically, after application of a rabbit antiserum to human growth hormone. This selectively demonstrates the cells (*G*) whose cytoplasm contains growth hormone. In *B*, the section shown in *A* has been destained and subsequently restained by the Masson's trichrome procedure which shows that these cells stain as acidophils. The growth hormone cells shown in *A* have given the characteristic reaction of cells that are identified as acidophils by routine histological methods. Both figures, ×1000. (Reprinted with permission from Baker, B.L.: *J Histochem Cytochem* 18: 1970.)

and considerable rough endoplasmic reticulum (Fig. 21.5). They are typical of a polypeptide-producing endocrine cell, and consequently similar to the alpha cells of the pancreatic islets and the C cells of the thyroid gland.

The second type of acidophil is the *mammotrope*, which secretes *prolactin*. This polyhedral cell type was difficult to identify with certainty until immunohistochemistry was used, and care must be taken since there is substantial homology between the somatotropin and prolactin molecules. In electron micrographs, the granules in mammotropes vary greatly in size. Although they are usually not as abundant as the granules in somatotropes, they may be bigger or, if they are in the process of lysosomal degradation, smaller and irregular in

shape (Fig. 21.5). Almost all of the increase in size of the pituitary in pregnancy is the result of proliferation of mammotropes.

The *basophils* show considerable variation in their staining properties, both within an individual gland and from one species to another. The cytoplasmic granules also vary in size in a given cell and in different species; they measure up to about 200 nm in the rat (Figs. 21.5 and 21.6). Thus, the granules are definitely smaller than in the acidophils. The granules stain poorly with hematoxylin, well with the aniline blue of the trichrome methods (Fig. 21.12) and excellently with the periodic acid-Schiff (PAS) technique. It is to be noted that the granules of all of the basophils of the pars distalis stain by the PAS method because of their content of glyco-

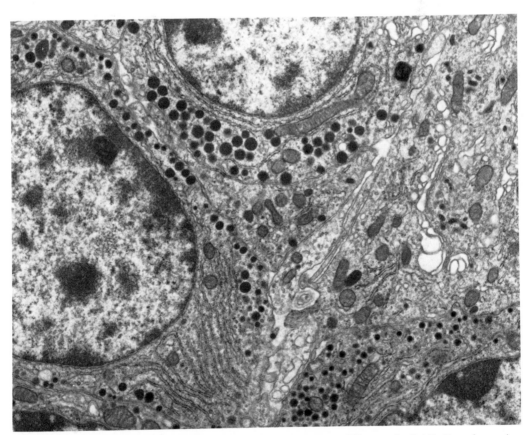

Figure 21.5. Pars distalis from a mouse pituitary, illustrating the difference in distribution of granules in different cell types. The cell at *top center* is a typical somatotrope (GH-producing) cell; the cell to the *upper right* is probably a mammotrope (prolactin-producing) cell; the others are basophils (×12,000).

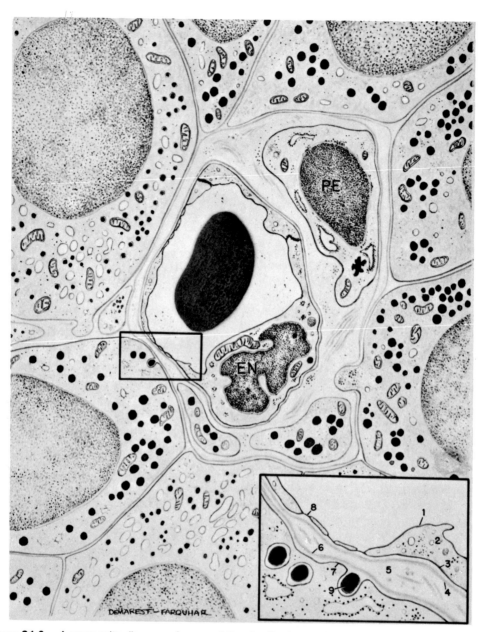

Figure 21.6.   A composite diagram of some of the details observable in electron micrographs of the pars distalis. The cytoplasm of the capillary endothelial cell is generally attenuated except in the region around the nucleus (*EN*). The perivascular space may be narrow as seen at the *left* of the capillary or it may be relatively broad as shown at the *right*. It contains collagen and connective tissue cells; a perivascular macrophage (*PE*) is included in the diagram. The parenchymal cells also rest on a basal lamina. The area enclosed by the rectangle is enlarged at the *lower right*. Structures between the lumen of the capillary and the cytoplasm of a parenchymal cell are numbered in sequence. *1*, plasma membrane of luminal surface of endothelial cell; *2*, endothelial cell cytoplasm; *3*, membrane of basal surface of endothelial cell; *4*, basal lamina of endothelial cell; *5*, perivascular space; *6*, basal lamina of parenchymal cell; and *7*, the plasma membrane of a parenchymal cell. In some areas, *8*, the endothelial cells have fenestrae closed only by thin diaphragms. At *9*, the membrane around a secretion granule is shown in continuity with the parenchymal cell membrane. ×12,000; *inset*, ×40,000. (Reprinted with permission from Farquhar, M.G.: *Angiology 12:* 1961.)

proteins, and that none of the acidophils stain with PAS.

Originally only two types of basophils could be identified: a population staining with aldehyde fuchsin and responding to thyroidectomy called *thyrotropes*, and a population that did not stain with aldehyde fuchsin and was known to include *gonadotropes*, which secrete gonadotropins. It is now known that the latter population also includes the *corticotropes*. The thyrotropes are angular cells with small granules (<100 nm). They constitute only 6% of the anterior lobe cells. The gonadotropes are more rounded than the thyrotropes, and have a slightly dilated endoplasmic reticulum and granules that are uneven in density.

The proportion of each of the cell types present in the cell cords varies greatly, not only in different regions of the anterior lobe but even in adjacent cords. In the human hypophysis, the basophils are most numerous in the region of the midsagittal plane and anterolateral margin of the gland. The acidophils are most numerous in the central and posterior part of each lateral half of the gland. A survey of much of the gland is necessary in order to determine the percentages of the various cell types.

Recent studies have documented stages in the formation and depletion of granules in the different cell types. The mature secretory granules are released from the cells by exocytosis, similar to that observed for exocrine glands (Fig. 21.6). The released products must then pass from the interstitium into the sinusoidal capillaries.

Function of the Pars Distalis

The multiplicity of the functions of the anterior hypophysis is shown by the disabilities that result from its surgical removal or destruction by disease.

After hypophysectomy, there is a cessation of general body growth and an involution of the gonads, the thyroid and the cortex of the adrenal glands. Numerous secondary effects also result. For instance, the inactivation of the gonads with loss of their endocrine function is followed by involution of the accessory reproductive organs. Involution of the thyroid gland brings about a lowering of the basal metabolic rate. The involution of the adrenal cortex results in a lowering of resistance to stress and a disturbance in carbohydrate metabolism. Because of the multiple hormones produced the pars distalis was called the master gland of the endocrine system. However it is now clear that the pituitary is not only under direct and indirect feedback control by its target organs, but also under control by the central nervous system. Consequently it constitutes a major homeostatic gland integrating nervous system and non-nervous system endocrine relationships.

The pars distalis secretes six well-recognized hormones as well as several others, some of which have not yet been shown to be physiologically significant (see Table 21.2). The hormones receive their names in most cases, from the name of the target organ plus the suffix *trophic* or *tropic*. The two suffixes are often used interchangeably.

The hormones are polypeptide in nature and can be divided into three groups. The first of these is the somatomammotropin group, composed of single-chain proteins with disulfide loops, and including somatotropin and prolactin. The second is the glycoprotein group, in which the active hormone is formed of two subunits synthesized separately (α and β) with most of the difference between hormones being in the β subunit. This group includes *luteinizing hormone* (LH), *follicle stimulating hormone* (FSH) and *thyroid stimulating hormone* (TSH). The third group is derived from a single molecule, *pro-opiomelanocortin*, and includes the amino acid sequences of *adrenocorticotropic hormone* (ACTH) as well as *melanocyte-stimulating hormone* (MSH), *β-lipotropin* (β-LPH), *β-endorphin*, and others.

Somatotropin (Somatotropic Hormone, STH; Growth Hormone, GH)

Somatotropin stimulates body growth, particularly growth of long bones by promoting the proliferation of cartilage cells

Table 21.2.
Classification of Pars Distalis and Comparable Placental Hormones

Class	Members	Molecular Weight	Amino Acids	Action
I. Simple peptide derivatives of pro-opiomelan-ocortin	ACTH	4,500	39	Stimulates adrenal cortex
	α-MSH	1,800	13	Stimulates melano-cytes
	β-Lipotropin	11,200	91	Mobilizes fatty acids
	β-MSH	2,000	18	Stimulates melano-cytes
	β-Endorphin	4,000	31	Analgesic effects
II. Glycoproteins with α and β subunits, the latter conferring biological specificity	LH	29,000	α subunit: 89 β subunit: 115	Promotes sex steroid secretion
	FSH	29,000	α subunit: 89 β subunit: 115	Promotes follicle growth and Sertoli cell synthesis of ABP
	TSH	29,000	α subunit: 89 β subunit: 112	Stimulates thyroid
	Chorionic gonadotropin	46,000	α subunit: 92 β subunit: 139	Maintains corpus luteum of pregnancy
III. Simple proteins with disulfide loops	Growth hormone	21,800	191	Promotes bone elongation
	Prolactin	22,500	198	Promotes mammary growth and milk production
	Placental lactogen	21,800	191	Promotes milk production

in the epiphyses. Hypophysectomy of growing animals brings about a cessation of growth, which can be restored by administration of the hormone. In the human, anterior lobe tumors produce gigantism when they occur before closure of the epiphyses; when they occur after epiphyseal closure, they produce acromegaly, i.e., an increase in thickness of the mandible and of the bones of the calvaria, hands, and feet.

Although GH produces an increase in incorporation of sulfate into cartilage matrix in vivo, it has been determined that the effect comes from a secondary hormonal mediator, *somatomedin*, found in the serum after GH release. Somatomedin has not yet been fully characterized, but several growth factor molecules rather similar to proinsulin have been shown to be somatomedin peptides.

The regulation of GH secretion is mediated by a hypothalamic releasing factor (GHRF) and by an inhibiting factor, the surprisingly widely distributed peptide hormone *somatostatin*. Less than 5% of the stored GH is released per day. Human GH is somewhat different from nonprimate GH, which does not show biological activity in the human. Consequently the use of genetic engineering to produce primate-type GH has been encouraging.

Prolactin (Mammotropin, Luteotropic Hormone, LTH)

This hormone stimulates the synthesis of milk proteins, lipids, and carbohydrates. Its action is on mammary glands that have hypertrophied during pregnancy under the influence of estrogen and progesterone. Control of prolactin secretion is largely negative. There is a hypophyseal inhibiting factor (PIF) and both dopamine, which binds to specific receptors on the mammotropes, and norepinephrine have inhibitory effects on secretion. Experimental work suggests that there is also a stimulating factor influenced by serotonergic mechanisms.

Adrenocorticotropin (Adrenocorticotropic Hormone, ACTH; Corticotropin)

The atrophy of the adrenal cortex which follows hypophysectomy can be prevented by injections of ACTH. Administration of ACTH to normal animals produces hypertrophy and hyperplasia of the adrenal cortex, particularly of the zona fasciculata and zona reticularis, and increased secretion of glucocorticoids, mineralocorticoids, and androgens. Since ACTH is derived from the same molecule as β-LPH, and the latter includes the β-endorphin sequence, it is not surprising that these molecules have been localized to the same cells in the anterior pituitary. ACTH secretion is under the feedback control of the glucocorticoid cortisol. High levels of cortisol in the blood both suppress the release of the hypothalamic peptide *corticotropin releasing factor* (CRF) and inhibit the response of the pituitary to this factor. CRF in turn stimulates both synthesis and release of ACTH.

Thyrotropic Hormone (TSH)

Thyrotropic hormone stimulates the thyroid gland by binding to specific membrane receptors on the follicular cells, stimulating adenylate cyclase, and enhancing iodine transport and binding, thyroglobulin synthesis, the proteolysis of thyroglobulin and subsequent release of thyroid hormones, and cell growth. Thyrotropes are stimulated to secrete by a hypothalamic factor (*thyrotropic releasing hormone* TRH). There is a negative feedback loop in that thyroid hormones both inhibit TRH release and the response of thyrotropes to this factor. The complexity of control of TSH

release is shown by the fact that, in addition to the previously mentioned controls, estrogen increases the response of thyrotropes to TRH, while somatostatin decreases this response. Also cold increases TRH release.

Follicle-Stimulating Hormone (FSH)

Follicle-stimulating hormone promotes growth of antral follicles in the ovary in the female, and growth of the testes and spermatogenesis in the male. Immunocytochemistry demonstrates overlap in the distribution of gonadotropes containing anti-FSH-reactive granules with gonadotropes containing anti-LH-reactive granules, as well as populations of these cells that contain only one or the other granule type. FSH secretion is stimulated by *gonadotropin releasing hormone* (GnRH) from the hypothalamus, and is inhibited by estradiol and by inhibin, but the feedback effects involve actions at different levels within the brain and pituitary.

Luteinizing Hormone (LH)

Luteinizing hormone is necessary for ovulation and promotes progesterone production by the ovary and testosterone production by the Leydig cells of the testis. Like FSH, its release is stimulated by GnRH. The preovulatory peak of LH, however, is a response to increasing estradiol levels, although the pulsatile release of GnRH (under the influence of the arcuate nucleus) is apparently permissive. LH is under negative feedback control of progesterone.

The major hormones of the pars distalis generally act on their target tissues by binding to specific receptor molecules on the cell membrane, and usually stimulate a second messenger in the cyclic nucleotide system. They are all under both nervous system and hormonal feedback control. However, the feedback of the hormones elicited from the target organ can be complex, having different effects at different concentrations, interacting with other hormones, affecting different areas in the brain, or directly affecting the tropic cells in the pituitary.

Pars Intermedia

The pars intermedia of most mammals consists of several layers of epithelial cells located, as the name implies, between the pars distalis and the pars nervosa. This lobe is rudimentary in man and consists of a relatively thin zone of cells that are often grouped around vesicles that contain a small amount of colloid. The zone blends with the pars distalis anteriorly and some of its cells migrate posteriorly into the contiguous neural lobe (Fig. 21.7). Some of the cells stain deeply with basic dyes, whereas others are small and pale staining.

In mammals with a well-developed pars intermedia and in the human fetus, proopiomelanocortin is processed almost entirely to *melanocyte-stimulating hormone* (MSH) and β-*endorphin* in the pars intermedia. In amphibians, MSH controls the dispersal of melanin granules within the cytoplasmic branches of the melanocytes and thus alters skin color. The normal function of this hormone in mammals is obscure, but its injection does increase pigmentation, probably by stimulating melanin synthesis.

β-Endorphin, like the enkephalins, binds to what were originally called the opiate receptors in the CNS. Its analgesic effects

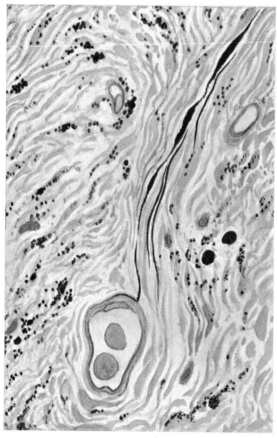

Figure 21.7. Posterior hypophysis. A section from the pars nervosa, human, age 26. Nerve fibers containing neurosecretory material (*deep blue*) are cut in both cross and longitudinal sections. One of the longitudinal sections shows three bulging masses of neurosecretory material; it appears to terminate on the surface of a small blood vessel (*lower center of field*). Larger accumulations of neurosecretion (Herring bodies) appear at *right*. Nuclei of pituicytes are stained *red*. A 4-μm section, stained with chrome hematoxylin and phloxine (×1200).

in the brain and effects on peripheral tissues are currently being explored.

Neurohypophysis

The *neurohypophysis* includes the infundibular process (neural lobe) and the infundibulum which, in turn, includes the infundibular stem and the median eminence of the tuber cinereum (Fig. 21.2). The neurohypophysis consists of unmyelinated nerve axons from the hypothalamo-hypophyseal tract, its blood vasculature and a few cells related to neuroglia, the *pituicytes* (Fig. 21.7). Many of the axons come from nerve cells with their large cell bodies located in the supraoptic and paraventricular nuclei of the hypothalamus (Fig. 21.8). Most of these axons pass as the infundibular stem to the neural lobe, where they terminate as dilated nerve endings containing large neurosecretory granules as well as some small vesicles (Figs. 21.9 and 21.10). A few of the

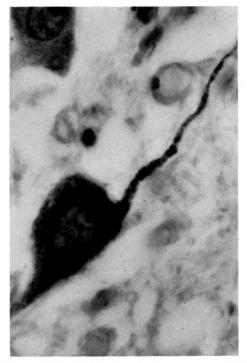

Figure 21.8. Photomicrograph of a neuron from the human supraoptic nucleus. Both the nerve cell body and its axon contain granular neurosecretory material. Chrome hematoxylin stain. (×1200). (Courtesy of Dr. S. L. Palay.)

axons from the supraoptic and paraventricular nuclei terminate in the superficial region of the median eminence, as do those from other areas of the hypothalamus that are believed to provide the hypophysiotropic hormones (releasing factors).

In routine histological preparations, the neural lobe is rather undistinguished, since the individual axons and endings cannot be discerned. However larger accumulations of neurosecretory material and occasional degradative products are seen as *Herring bodies*. Histochemical methods, especially those demonstrating sulfide groups (e.g. aldehyde fuchsin) localize neurosecretory material not only in the enlarged endings, but also in some of the axons. Most easily seen in the substance of the neurohypophysis are the nuclei of the pituicytes and the numerous capillaries.

In some respects, the pituicytes resemble the neuroglia cells found elsewhere in the central nervous system, i.e., they are small cells with ramifying processes but without the distinctive features of nerve cells. Unlike neuroglia cells, many of the pituicytes contain variable numbers of refractile droplets or granules in their cytoplasm. Some of the pituicytes also contain yellow-brown pigment granules, the number of which increases with age.

The nuclei of the pituicytes (Fig. 21.7) are round or oval with a fine chromatin network. The cytoplasm is drawn out into a variable number of processes which often end either on the walls of blood vessels or on connective tissue septa of the gland. In routine preparations, the cytoplasm surrounding the nucleus is barely discernible, and the processes cannot be followed. Between the cell bodies, the meshwork of interweaving processes stains faintly.

The secretory substances released into the blood vessels of the neural lobe are formed in cell bodies of the nerve cells of the supraoptic and paraventricular nuclei located in the hypothalamus of the brain, and they pass by way of the unmyelinated fibers of the cell bodies to the neural lobe.

There are two octapeptides stored and

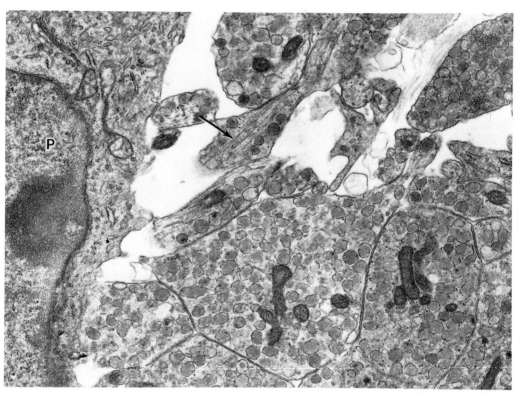

Figure 21.9.   Infundibular process of the guinea pig. A pituicyte (*P*) appears at the *left.* Neurotubules of two axons are seen in the *middle* (*arrow*). The nerve terminals have numerous neurosecretory granules (×16,800).

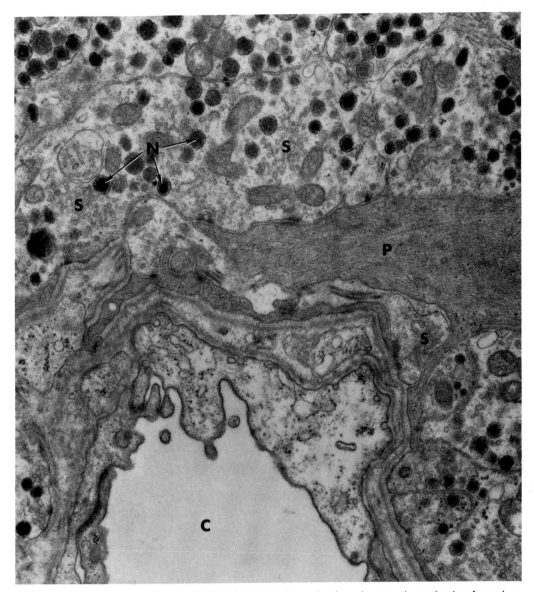

Figure 21.10. Electron micrograph showing axonal terminations in neurohypophysis of monkey. The axonal terminals contain both dense neurosecretory granules (*N*) and small clear vesicles (*S*) resembling synaptic vesicles. *C*, capillary; *P*, pituicyte process. The basal laminae are obvious (×24,000).

released from the neural lobe. *Oxytocin* produces contraction of the myoepithelial cells of the alveoli of the mammary gland, and, because of its effect on the smooth muscle of the uterus, can be used to induce labor at term. *Antidiuretic hormone* (ADH, *vasopressin*) increases water retention by modifying the permeability to water of collecting tubules of the kidney. These hormones are synthesized in different cells in both the paraventricular and the supraoptic nuclei. They are non-covalently linked to polypeptides, the *neurophysins*, both during their transport down the hypothalamo-hypophyseal tract and in the neurosecretory granule. The two neurophysins are specific and contain cystine groups (which facilitate their visualization by staining).

Release of the hormones from the nerve endings occurs with appropriate stimulation of the CNS. Suckling, or even crying by a mother's infant, stimulates oxytocin release and consequently milk let-down.

Pars Tuberalis

Like the parenchyma of the pars distalis and intermedia, the tuberalis takes its embryonic origin from Rathke's pouch epithelium. It continues to form a layer of cuboidal cells that covers the anterior portion of the neural stalk and part of the tuberal area of the brain (Fig. 21.1c). The cytoplasm of the cells is faintly basophilic. In contrast with the pars intermedia, the pars tuberalis is quite vascular. The cells frequently form follicles which contain colloid. In the pars tuberalis, especially at its upper and lower poles, groups of squamous cells have been described which probably are "remnants" from the craniopharyngeal duct. Although small amounts of pars distalis-type hormones (LH, FSH, TSH) have been found here by immunocytochemistry, no significant physiological role has yet been determined.

Pharyngeal Hypophysis

A small body of tissue which resembles that of the anterior lobe is generally present in the vault of the human nasopharynx, but not in other species. It is located near the position where the anterior lobe develops, and it is described as a structure measuring 3.5 to 7 mm in length by 1 mm or less in width. The cells appear to be structurally identical to those of the anterior lobe by light microscopy and have been shown to contain prolactin. It is not known whether or not it can serve as an accessory gland.

THE THYROID GLAND

Structure and Origin

The adult thyroid gland consists of two lateral lobes and a connecting part, the isthmus. The lobes lie lateral to the superior part of the trachea and the inferior part of the larynx. The isthmus crosses anterior to the trachea at the level of the second to fourth tracheal cartilages. A me-dian process, the pyramidal lobe, is present in a number of individuals, extending upward from the left side of the isthmus. The thyroid has a connective tissue sheath formed by the deep cervical fascia. Beneath this is a delicate stratum of connective tissue, the true capsule of the gland. Delicate trabeculae and septa penetrate the gland, indistinctly dividing the lobes and lobules which in turn are composed of follicles.

The thyroid is an extremely labile gland and varies in size and structure in response to a large number of factors, among which are sex, nutrition, temperature, age, season and the iodine content of the food.

The structural unit of the thyroid is the *follicle* (Fig. 21.11). These units are usually of microscopic dimensions but may become sufficiently large, as in colloid goiter, to be visible macroscopically. Follicles vary greatly in shape as well as in size, but they are usually irregularly spheroidal. In highly activated glands they become extremely irregular in shape (Fig. 21.12). A follicle consists of a layer of simple epithelium enclosing a cavity, the follicular cavity, which usually is filled with a gel-like material, *colloid*.

The parenchyma of the embryonic thyroid gland presents a classic example of a follicular pattern of epithelial differentiation (discussed in Chapter 4). The endodermal primordium of the gland is a single, midventral diverticulation of the pharyngeal floor which originates at about the level of the second branchial arch in most vertebrates. The relative posterior migration of this rudiment, occasioned by differential growth of the head and other organs, results in its eventual positioning far caudal to its origin. The rudiment proliferates, at first as loose strands and clusters which interact inductively with surrounding mesenchyme during the migration, and it undergoes a series of buddings, the smallest of which pinch off to form isolated follicles. Surrounding mesenchyme differentiates into the connective tissue framework and rich vascular network characteristic of the gland. Isolated, aberrant groups of thyroid

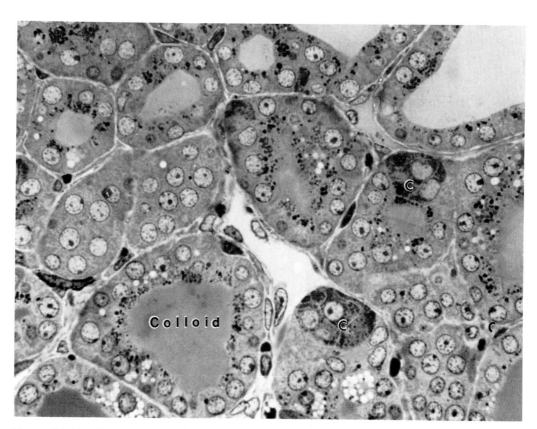

Figure 21.11.   Normal thyroid of the cat, illustrating the typical pattern of follicles in this active thyroid gland. The dark granules in the apical ends of follicular cells are phagolysosomes. The clusters of darker cells at the periphery of two follicles in the *right center* are calcitonin cells (*C*). (×900).

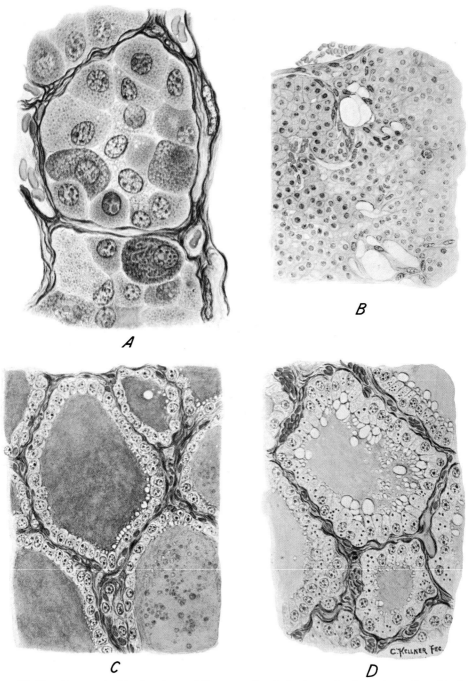

Figure 21.12. Camera lucida drawings of the normal anterior hypophysis and parathyroid of man (*upper*) and the normal and activated thyroid of the rhesus monkey (*lower*). *A*, anterior hypophysis of an executed man, 38 years old. Cords of cells are from the central part of the gland. In three of the acidophils (*pink*), the Golgi area is stained *bluish.* In the basophil in the lower cord, a negative picture of the Golgi apparatus is shown as clear canals. Chromophobes are present in the middle of the central cord. The rather large amount of connective tissue shown in the drawing is characteristic of the human anterior hypophysis. A colloid mass (*blue*) is shown at the lower part of the inferior cell cord. Modified Masson stain (×1250). *B*, parathyroid of normal human adult. The oxyphils are pink and the chief cells are *bluish purple.* The spaces shown were filled with fat. Hematoxylin-eosin stain (×350). *C*, thyroid of a normal adult rhesus monkey. A few peripheral and central colloid vacuoles are shown. Modified Masson stain (×570). *D*, activated thyroid of a normal adult rhesus monkey. The thyroid was activated by injections of an anterior hypophysis extract. The epithelium is high and many absorption vacuoles are present. Colloid droplets and vacuoles are present in the thyroid epithelium. Modified Masson stain (×570).

tissue may be scattered along the migratory pathway and at the point of origin near the base of the tongue.

The thyroid gland produces *thyroxine* (*tetraiodothyronine*) and *triiodothyronine*, is necessary for normal growth in the child, and is a major regulator of metabolism in the adult. Thyroxine increases oxidative activity and protein synthesis in many organs. Although tetra- and triiodothyronine are not steroids, they behave somewhat similarly in that in the circulation they are highly bound to serum proteins (especially thyroid-binding globulin and thyroid-binding prealbumen). Also, they exert their effects on those target cells bearing the appropriate intracellular receptor.

The thyroid gland is large, typically 15 to 20 g. This large size is a result of the unusual nature of the synthesis and storage of a hormone (thyroxine) as only a small part of a very large glycoprotein molecule (thyroglobulin). Furthermore, typical blood levels of thyroid hormones are high (5 to 11 μg/dL for thyroxine and 75 to 200 ng/dL for T_3). A separate population of cells within the thyroid gland produces a very different hormone, *calcitonin*, a polypeptide hormone that decreases the calcium level in the blood by interfering with the activity of parathyroid hormone (parathormone) in bone resorption.

The *follicular* or *chief cells* have their apical ends facing inward, i.e., toward the follicular cavity, and their basal ends resting on the basal lamina. In addition to the follicular cells, there are cells which are found singly or in small groups in the follicle. Those within the follicle are wedged between the follicular cells and the basal lamina; they generally do not extend to the colloid cavity. These cells were originally called parafollicular because of their position, but with the discovery that they produce calcitonin, they are now called *calcitonin* cells or simply C cells (Fig. 21.11).

The calcitonin cells are apparently of different embryonic origin from the follicular cells. It has been suggested that in higher vertebrates they may be derived from neural crest cells. They are often considered part of the amine precursor uptake and decarboxylation (APUD) system, since in many species they contain serotonin as well as calcitonin. In the adult, the calcitonin cells are generally larger than the follicular cells, and they have a more eosinophilic cytoplasm due to the staining of the granules. They are relatively sparse in humans compared to many other mammals, and are most common as single cells deep in the center of the two lateral lobes (Fig. 21.13). As might be expected with the final product a 32 amino acid polypeptide (the calcitonin monomer), the fine structure of the cells is rather similar to the growth hormone producing cells of the pituitary, with strands of rough endoplasmic reticulum, moderate Golgi complex, and many small granules (Fig. 21.13). Although calcitonin can prevent bone resorption, the importance of this role in normal humans is not clear, since increased blood calcium levels not only trigger calcitonin release but also reduce parathormone production.

The follicular cells are generally cuboidal in the normal gland (Fig. 21.13) but become low cuboidal or even squamous in the relatively inactive gland. They enlarge and become tall columnar cells during periods of increased activity (Figs. 21.12*D*). The intercellular boundaries are distinct and fairly obvious under the light microscope. Typical junctional complexes provide cell adhesion and prevent paracellular passage of colloid from the follicle.

The nuclei are generally rounded in shape, and the cytoplasm is lightly basophilic. The mitochondria are rod-shaped or filamentous and vary in number with the activity of the cell. The Golgi complex is located on the apical side of the nucleus. The cytoplasm also contains a few lipid droplets and numerous PAS-positive droplets (colloid resorption droplets). An additional type of cell is occasionally seen in the follicle, the colloid cells of Langendorff. They are slender cells with darkly staining cytoplasm that often appear to be filled with colloid, and they have pyknotic nuclei

(Fig. 21.13). They are degenerating cells and may be sloughed into the lumen of the follicle, adding their contents, including nucleoproteins and proteolytic enzymes, to the colloid.

The fine structure of the follicular cells reflects both the synthesis of glycoprotein and its resorption. An active follicular cell has abundant dilated rough endoplasmic reticulum. In addition to small secretory vesicles that transport thyroglobulin to the apical surface, lysosomes also bud off the Golgi membranes.

The apical end of the follicular cell has short, irregularly distributed microvilli which are more numerous on the columnar (hyperactive) cells than on the lower, relatively inactive cells.

On stimulation with TSH, large flanges of cytoplasm engulf some of the colloid in the follicles, and large phagosomes are formed which quickly become phagolysosomes (Fig. 21.14). With progressive digestion of the thyroglobulin, tetra- and triiodothyronine are liberated (about 90 min after elevation of TSH) to enter the circulation. Mono- and diiodothyronine are dehalogenated within the follicular cells, making the iodine again available and much of the thyroglobulin is broken down to amino acid constituents.

Although the thyroglobulin is the storage

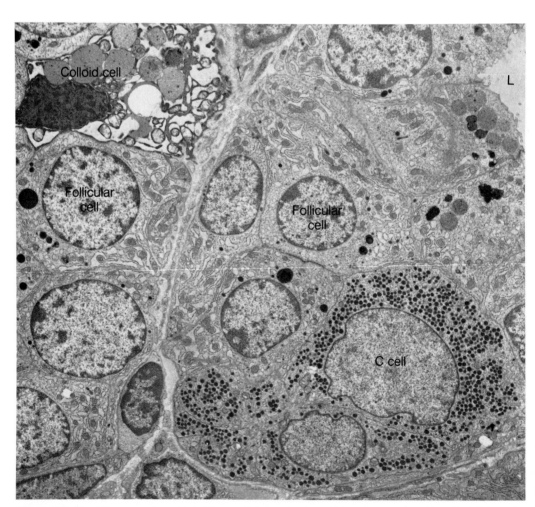

Figure 21.13. Electron micrograph of a partially tangential section through two thyroid follicles of a cat. The lumen (*L*) of the follicle with the C cells in its wall is in the *upper right* (×4,200).

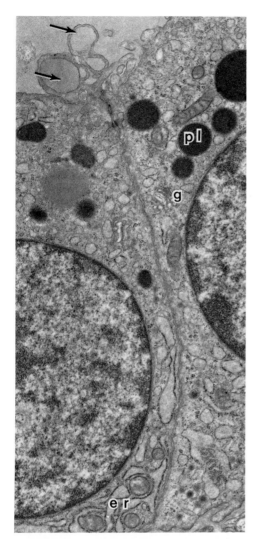

Figure 21.14. Active thyroid follicular cells of the cat. Flanges of cytoplasm (*arrows*) surround colloid from the follicular lumen at the margin of the cells. Several phagolysosomes (*pl*) are present in the apical cytoplasm. Rough endoplasmic reticulum (*er*) is seen throughout the cell but is particularly abundant basally. Golgi elements (*g*) are lateral and apical to the nuclei (×16,000).

form of thyroid hormones within the follicle, the extent of its iodination can vary with the availability of iodine in the diet. Thyroglobulin is a large glycoprotein (~660,000 daltons) with over 100 tyrosyl groups and 23 oligosaccharide side chains. The follicular cells actively transport iodide from the interstitium, then oxidize it to "active iodine" at the apical end of the cell.

In this form it can iodinate the tyrosyl group on the already formed thyroglobulin. Some of the mono- and diiodinated groups are coupled to form tri- and tetraiodothyronine within the follicle.

A series of excellent studies using isotopically labeled precursors has demonstrated that the polypeptide "backbone," the short chain oligosaccharides and proximal sugars of the longer oligosaccharides of the thyroglobulin molecule, are formed in the rough endoplasmic reticulum (Fig. 21.15). The more distal sugars and terminal sugars are incorporated after the nascent protein has been transported to the Golgi. It is this uniodinated product that is transported to the apical end of the cell in small vesicles. At the apical end of the cell or at the cell surface, iodination occurs. This surface has small microvilli, pinocytotic processes and micropinocytotic vesicles. Both of the latter two structures participate in endocytosis. The pinocytotic processes give rise to large phagosomes filled with colloid. The micropinocytotic vesicles probably participate in membrane recycling as well as colloid uptake. The studies on incorporation indicate that synthesis of thyroglobulin takes approximately 2 hr. Synthesis and hydrolysis of thyroglobulin can occur simultaneously.

Thyroid-stimulating hormone (TSH) not only stimulates endocytosis and lysosomal hydrolysis of colloid to release the active portions of the molecule, but also stimulates thyroglobulin synthesis and growth of the thyroid. Since TSH is under feedback inhibition from the thyroid hormones, a drop in tetra- and triiodothyronine in the circulation leads to increased TSH release from the pituitary. If the thyroglobulin in the follicles is inadequately iodinated, then little hormone will be released, TSH stimulation will continue, the amount of colloid will increase, and the size of the gland will increase. The increase in mass provides the gland with more iodine-trapping potential in the event of a temporary iodine deficiency. However, when there is a chronic shortage of iodine in the diet, the continual stimulation of the thyroid results in

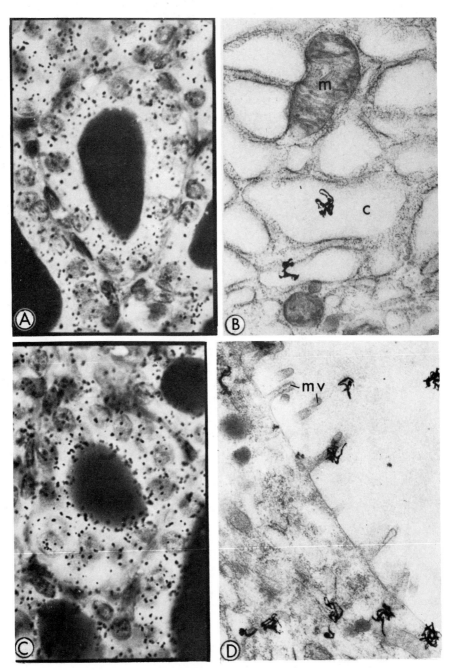

Figure 21.15. Light and electron micrographs of radioautographic preparations of thyroids from rats sacrificed at different intervals of time after injection of leucine-³H. *A*, radioautograph of a periodic acid-Schiff and hematoxylin stained preparation from an animal sacrificed at 30 min after injection of labeled leucine. Radioactivity is seen rather diffusely over the cytoplasm in the light micrograph. *B*, electron micrograph of a radioautographic preparation from an animal sacrificed at 1 hr after injection. Irregularly shaped silver grains, indicating the location of the incorporated leucine, are seen over the cisternae (*c*) of the endoplasmic reticulum. *m*, mitochondrion. *C*, radioautograph of tissue fixed at 4 hr after injection of labeled leucine. The labeled material is present chiefly in the adluminal ends of the cell. *D*, electron micrograph of a radioautograph at 3½ hr after injection of labeled leucine. Silver grains are seen in the adluminal cytoplasm and also in the colloid. *mv*, microvilli. *A* and *C*, ×1200; *B* and *D*, ×30,000. (Reprinted with permission from Nadler, N. J., Young, B., Leblond, C. P., and Mitmaker, B. O.: *Endocrinology 74:* 1964.)

crowded follicles, cystic follicles and a compromised vasculature. This condition of *colloid goiter* produces an enlarged thyroid with many regions that are no longer capable of normal function. In addition to storage in colloid, the binding of thyroid hormones to plasma proteins also has a saving effect since only the fraction of a percentage of molecules that is unbound is active, and consequently the half life of thyroxine (the hormone with the greater affinity for the carriers) is relatively long.

Blood Vessels

The thyroid has a rich plexus of blood and lymph capillaries, which are in intimate relation to the follicular epithelium. The capillaries around the follicles are of the more permeable type and have many endothelial fenestrae. The arteries, at the places where they branch, frequently have localized pad-like thickenings beneath the intima. These do not encircle the vessels. They may assist in shunting the blood to different parts of the gland as the arteries contract, and they may also serve to reduce the pulse wave. Arteriovenous anastomoses are common. The architecture of the blood vessels, as well as the fact that all of the follicles do not show the same degree of activity at any one time, indicates that there are fluctuations in the amount of blood received by different parts of the gland.

Nerves

A large number of nonmyelinated nerve fibers are present in the walls of the thyroid arteries. Most of these terminate in plexuses around the blood vessels.

Function

The main effect of the thyroid hormone is on the rate of metabolism of tissues in general. The ramifications of this effect are very extensive, however, extending to activities as diverse as the rate of absorption in the intestine, carbohydrate metabolism, the rate of the heart beat, mental activity, general body growth and many other effects. In the adult, *hypothyroidism* causes a syndrome called *myxedema*, characterized by a low basal metabolic rate. The opposite condition, *hyperthyroidism*, is likewise characterized by a high basal metabolic rate. It can be caused by an autoimmune defect in which antibodies develop against the TSH receptor (Graves' disease). These antibodies mimic TSH binding, resulting in over-stimulation of the gland. However, hyperthyroidism may also be idiopathic.

Hypothyroidism in the infant can cause developmental abnormalities including mental retardation. The administration of thyroid hormone to deficient infants will allow normal development; in recognition of this fact, some states in the United States require that all newborns have their thyroid hormone levels tested.

The thyroid is not essential to life, although in early work the close topographical association of the parathyroids with it caused confusion on this point.

THE PARATHYROID GLANDS

Structure and Origin

There are normally two pairs of parathyroids in mammals. Because of the origin of their parenchymal cells from the endodermal epithelium of the third and fourth pharyngeal pouches, respectively, they are sometimes designated as parathyroids III and IV.

The parathyroids from the third pouch are associated with the thymus during the first part of its caudal migration, before detaching from the thymus and becoming associated with the dorsal surface of the thyroid. The parathyroids from the fourth pouch detach from the rest of the pharyngeal epithelium and become associated with the thyroid later. As a consequence the parathyroids III become the inferior parathyroids, and parathyroids IV become the superior parathyroids. Parathyroid "rests" may be found anywhere along the migration route of the thymus, from the neck to the mediastinum.

In man, a member of each pair lies on the posterior surface of each lateral lobe of the thyroid, near the arterial anastomosis of the inferior and superior thyroid arteries.

These glands, which are somewhat flattened, measure some 6 mm in length and about half this in width. In man they are brown, but in some species they are white or only faintly colored. A connective tissue capsule separates them from the thyroid. Delicate connective tissue septa partially divide the gland into poorly defined lobules, and still finer septa tend to separate the epithelial cells into anastomosing cords and groups (Fig. 21.16). The separation of epithelial cell groups by connective tissue becomes particularly obvious in the adult as a result of an increase in fat cells that continues progressively throughout life.

The parathyroid glands are small glands with an aggregate weight of only about 120 mg. They secrete a polypeptide hormone, *parathormone*, which plays a vital role in the regulation of blood calcium levels. Like other peptide hormones, it is originally synthesized as a larger pre-prohormone, the

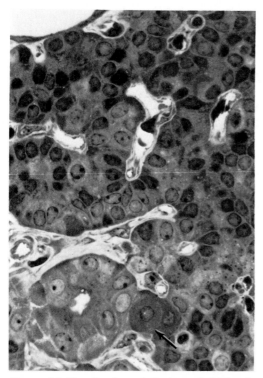

Figure 21.16. Cords and clusters of chief cells are seen in this parathyroid of an adult baboon. The scant connective tissue is highly vascular. An apparent oxyphil cell is seen (*arrow*) (×675).

115-amino acid pre-proparathormone. This peptide is rapidly cleaved to proparathormone in the endoplasmic reticulum, and then cleaved to the 84 amino acid polypeptide parathormone in the Golgi apparatus.

The epithelial parenchyma retains a cord-like epithelial character reminiscent of its endodermal origin. It is composed of two types of cells: the *principal* or *chief cells* and the *oxyphil cells* (Fig. 21.12*B*). The chief cells are of constant occurrence, while the oxyphil cells do not appear in man until near the end of the first decade and are not abundant until puberty. They have been observed in only a few other species, including monkeys.

The chief cells are polyhedral in shape and have round nuclei with loosely arranged chromatin giving a vesicular appearance.

It has been estimated that in the normal adult only about a third of the chief cells are actively synthesizing and secreting parathormone. The synthetically active cells usually stain a little darker in light microscopy. Cytologically they can be seen to contain small membrane-bounded secretory granules, a patch of rough endoplasmic reticulum, a relatively large Golgi complex, filamentous mitochondria and little glycogen (Figs. 21.17 and 21.18). The less active cells have a smaller Golgi complex, few or no secretory granules, considerable glycogen and lipofuscin pigment. Because the glycogen is leached in routine histological preparations, the cells have a relatively light or clear appearance. There is some evidence that when circulating levels of calcium are high, the secretory granules are degraded within the chief cells.

The oxyphil cells are larger than the chief cells, but they usually have smaller and darker staining nuclei (Fig. 21.17). Their cytoplasm stains well with eosin and contains fine granules. The cytoplasm of the oxyphil contains an abundance of mitochondria, a factor that is apparently responsible for their acidophilic staining in light microscopy. The function of these cells is unknown. It has been suggested that

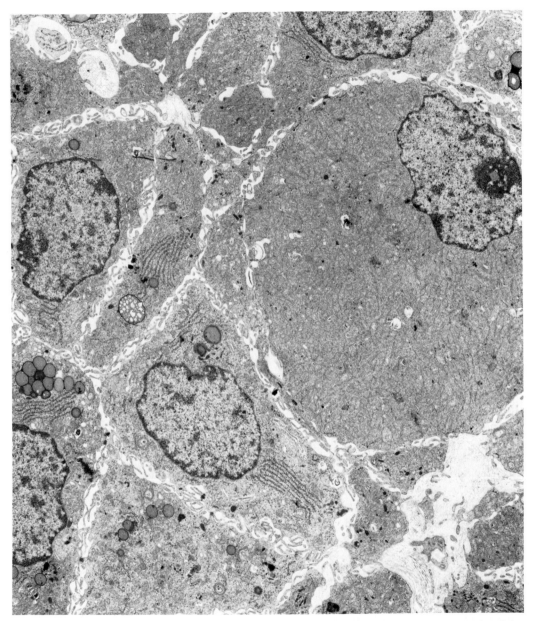

Figure 21.17. Parathyroid from a rhesus monkey, showing a single large oxyphil cell on the *right*, surrounded by smaller chief cells. Note the lipid and clusters of endoplasmic reticulum in the chief cells. Most of the cytoplasm of the oxyphil cell is occupied by unusual mitochondria (×5,500). (Courtesy of Dr. Barry F. King.)

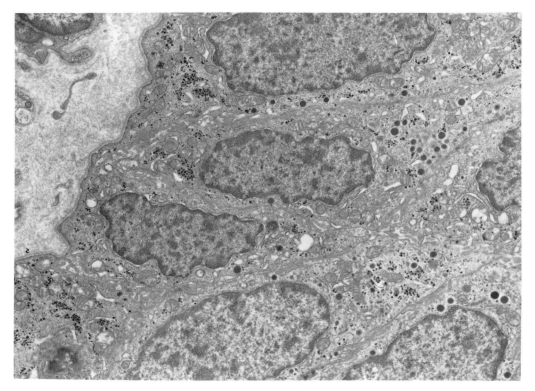

Figure 21.18. Chief cells of a cat parathyroid, showing small amounts of glycogen and several small but distinct secretion granules (×8,800).

they may represent a stage in the life cycle of the chief cells because transitional forms between the cell types are often seen in preparations for light microscopy.

Hyperparathyroidism is relatively common, usually as the result of a benign chief cell tumor (adenoma) of one of the glands. In addition, parathyroid glands consisting almost exclusively of oxyphil cells have been removed from hyperparathyroid patients and removal has successfully reduced the circulating levels of parathormone, indicating that oxyphil cells may also be active in parathormone production. However, such oxyphil cells have more rough endoplasmic reticulum than do those in normal parathyroids.

Small colloid follicles are of frequent occurrence in the parathyroid. This colloid has no relation functionally to that of the thyroid. In contrast with the thyroid, the parathyroid contains no more iodine than do other tissues of the body.

Blood Vessels and Nerves

The parathyroids have an abundant blood supply, but in vascular injections the capillaries, although of the highly permeable fenestrated type, do not appear to be as numerous as in the thyroid. In man there is said to be a plexus of veins at the periphery of the gland.

Unmyelinated nerves in small numbers occur in the parathyroid. They are probably vasomotor.

Function

The parathyroid glands regulate calcium concentration, primarily by stimulating resorption of bone and reabsorption of calcium ions from the ultrafiltrate of the kidney and, with the aid of vitamin D, by absorption of calcium from the gut. Removal of the parathyroids causes a fall in blood calcium, nervous hyperexcitability and spasms, leading to death. Calcium administration relieves these symptoms, and the injection of parathyroid extract or parathyroid hormone maintains the animals in good health. Such injections in normal animals raise the blood calcium, and excessive doses will cause death.

Removal of one or more of the parathyroids does not cause a compensatory hypertrophy of those which remain. In rickets the parathyroids enlarge. The parathyroids readily "take" in autotransplantation.

The marked differences in function of the parathyroid and thyroid glands are emphasized by comparison of gland sizes and size fluctuations. The parathyroids respond directly to blood calcium levels and are not under control of other endocrine glands or the nervous system. Parathormone is effective at low concentrations in the blood, and since calcium is readily available from bones as well as the diet, the blood levels of this ion do not ordinarily fluctuate widely. This means that the demands for parathormone production remain fairly constant. Furthermore, there are no unusual dietary substances, such as iodine, in

the parathormone molecule and no specialized storage or mobilization requirements for this hormone. Therefore, the parathyroid chief cells are remarkable cytologically only in the sense that they are relatively inactive in appearance as compared to the principal cells of other endocrine organs.

THE ADRENAL GLANDS
Structure and Origin

The adrenal glands are paired organs, one being situated close to the cranial pole of each kidney in the retroperitoneal tissue. Both are somewhat flattened, the left adrenal gland is crescentic, the right one more pyramidal in shape. The combined weight of the two glands is 10 to 12 g, the left usually being somewhat heavier than the right one.

The adrenal glands are composite organs consisting functionally and structurally of two distinct parts, the *cortex* (*interrenal tissue*) and the *medulla* (*chromaffin tissue*) (Fig. 21.19). The cortex produces a number of steroids, of which the most physiologically significant in the human are the mineralocorticoid *aldosterone* and the glucocorticoid *cortisol*. The medulla produces epi-

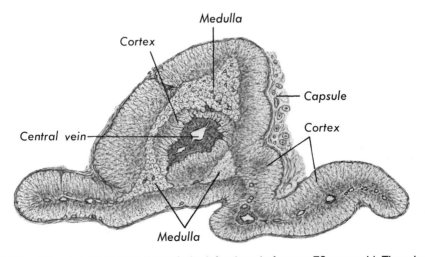

Figure 21.19. A transverse section through the left adrenal of a man 72 years old. The adrenal was surgically removed in an attempt to give relief in prostatic carcinoma with metastases. The central vein has a thick wall containing bundles of smooth muscle. Camera lucida drawing (×6).

nephrine and, in lesser amounts, norepinephrine. The principal secretory cells of medulla and cortex have differing embryonic origins; those of the medulla are derived from neural crest cells whereas those of the cortex differentiate from mesodermal cells in the nephrogenic ridge.

The *fetal cortex* arises in the fourth to sixth week of pregnancy, becomes quite large and participates in the "*fetal-placental unit*" (See Chapter 20). Its cells have the abundant smooth endoplasmic reticulum and mitochondria with tubular cristae typical of steroid secreting cells (Fig. 21.20). In addition, their large Golgi zones have numerous associated granules and are probably responsible for sulfation of the steroid product. The dehydroepiandroste-

rone sulfate produced by the fetal cortex is converted to estrogen (estrone) by the placenta. The level of estrone produced has been used as a test of fetal viability. A few small cells that will form much of the definitive cortex first appear superficial to the fetal cortex several weeks after its origin. After parturition, the fetal cortex involutes over a period of months, and the *definitive cortex* is derived from the superficial cells and probably in part from the fetal cortex. Shortly after the fetal adrenal forms, neural crest cells migrate into the forming cortex where they first form isolated clusters, then coalesce to form the medulla.

The adrenal gland in the adult is covered by a thick capsule of connective tissue composed chiefly of collagenous fibers and fi-

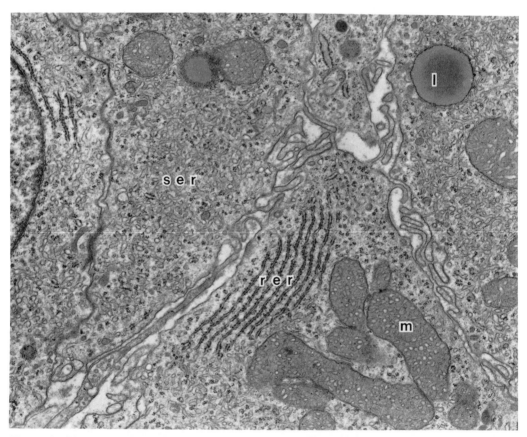

Figure 21.20. Human fetal adrenal corticular cells. In addition to rough endoplasmic reticulum (*rer*) the cells have abundant branched tubular smooth endoplasmic reticulum (*ser*), lipid droplets (*l*), and mitochondria (*m*) with tubular cristae. These features are characteristic of active steroid-producing cells (×15,800).

broblasts. Vessels and nerves course in the capsule. Delicate connective tissue trabeculae composed of collagenous and reticular fibers extend inward from the capsule. Arterioles also extend into the gland in a characteristic pattern described below under "Blood Supply."

The hilus is situated ventromedially (toward the vena cava) and is chiefly marked by the emerging thick walled adrenal vein.

The arrangement of the cortex and medulla in the human does not have the uniformity characteristically found in laboratory animals. This may be due in part to the irregularity in shape of the human adrenal. The line of separation between the cortex and medulla is frequently very irregular and, in single sections, clumps of cortical cells may appear to be surrounded by medulla, but studies of serial sections show that these clumps are connected with the cortical zone. The distribution of the medulla also varies in different adrenal glands. It often is absent from the "wings" of the glands and then the two sides of the cortex abut against each other, separated only by connective tissue and small veins (Fig. 21.19).

Cortex

The cortex is classically divided into three zones according to differences in the cordlike arrangement of its cells: an outer zone, the *glomerulosa*; a middle zone, the *fasciculata*; and an inner zone, the *reticularis* (Fig. 21.21). The fasciculata is by far the broadest of the three but is not uniform in structure throughout. Primarily because of differences in the lipid content of its cells and the consequent differences in staining, the fasciculata may be divided into outer and inner zones, but there is no sharp demarcation between these zones.

The *zona glomerulosa* is a relatively narrow zone in which the arrangement of the cords is such that the cells are in ovoid groups (Fig. 21.22). There is no central cavity within a cell group as in exocrine glands, but there is a rich network of blood vessels just outside. The cells tend to be columnar, and they have spherical nuclei that stain rather heavily. A few lipid droplets may be found in the cytoplasm, but they are sparse in comparison with the droplets in the zona fasciculata. The cytoplasm has a well developed smooth endoplasmic reticulum and the Golgi complex is often on the side of the nucleus facing toward the blood vessel. The mitochondria of this region generally have shelf-like cristae similar to those of most other organs.

The zona glomerulosa produces *aldosterone* in response to plasma *angiotensin II*. Aldosterone is a potent mineralocorticoid, causing Na^+ retention in exchange for K^+ in the kidney. Typical circulating levels of aldosterone are about 10 ng/dL. The cells of the zona glomerulosa lack 17α-hydroxylase, an enzyme necessary for one of the steps in the sequence of formation of cortisol from cholesterol. Consequently, the glomerulosa does not participate in the formation of this steroid.

The *zona fasciculata*, the broadest zone, is composed of cell cords coursing parallel to one another in a radial direction toward the medulla (Figs. 21.21 and 21.22). The cords are usually only one or two cells in width. In three-dimensional reconstructions, it is seen that each cord is enclosed by a longitudinally oriented meshwork of sinusoidal capillaries. The secretory cells are generally cuboidal or polyhedral in shape, and they are sometimes binucleate. The nuclei appear more vesicular than those of the glomerulosa, with less dense chromatin. The cells are relatively large, and their cytoplasm contains an abundance of lipid droplets composed of cholesterol, fatty acids and neutral fat (Fig. 21.23). Since the lipids are dissolved by the usual technical procedures, the cytoplasm has a spongy appearance. Electron microscopy confirms the presence of numerous lipid droplets and shows that most of the endoplasmic reticulum is of the smooth-surfaced type (Figs. 21.23 and 21.24). Mitochondria are numerous and are characterized by having tubular rather than shelf-like cristae.

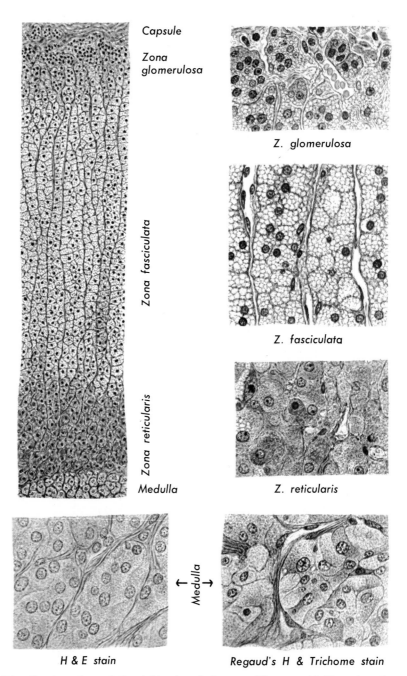

Capsule

Zona glomerulosa

Z. glomerulosa

Zona fasciculata

Z. fasciculata

Zona reticularis

Z. reticularis

Medulla

Medulla

H & E stain

Regaud's H & Trichome stain

Figure 21.21. Sections through the right adrenal of a man 35 years old. The adrenal was removed in an attempt to give relief from a testicular tumor with metastases. The tissue was fixed in Helly's fluid (formol Zenker). The section used for all of the drawings, except the *lower left*, was stained with Regaud's hematoxylin and Masson's trichrome. The low power (*upper left*) is ×205; the others, ×535.

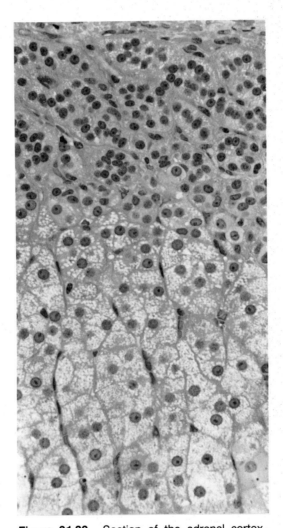

Figure 21.22. Section of the adrenal cortex, showing the smaller cells of the zona glomerulosa *above*, and the larger cells of the zona fasciculata *below*. The vacuolar appearance of the cells of the fasciculata is due to the presence of many small lipid droplets (×350).

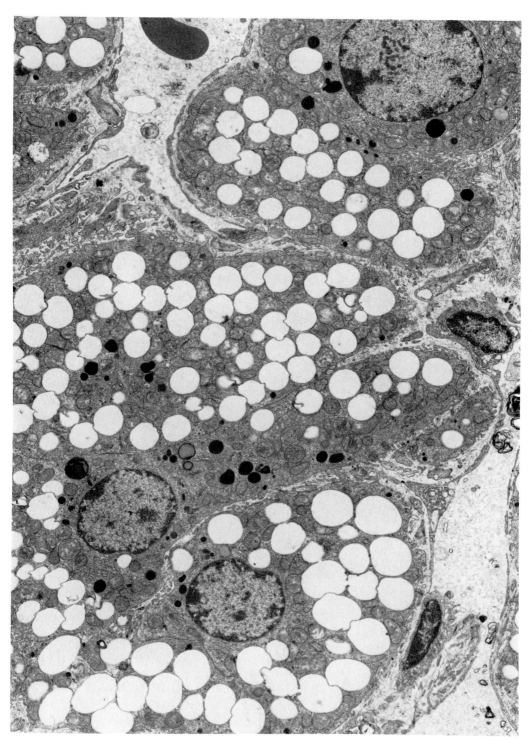

Figure 21.23. Cells of the zona fasciculata from a rhesus monkey adrenal cortex. Note the sinusoidal capillaries adjacent to the parenchymal cells. The pale lipid droplets are a conspicuous feature of these cells and function in storage of fatty acids and cholesterol (×5,800). (Courtesy of Dr. Barry F. King.)

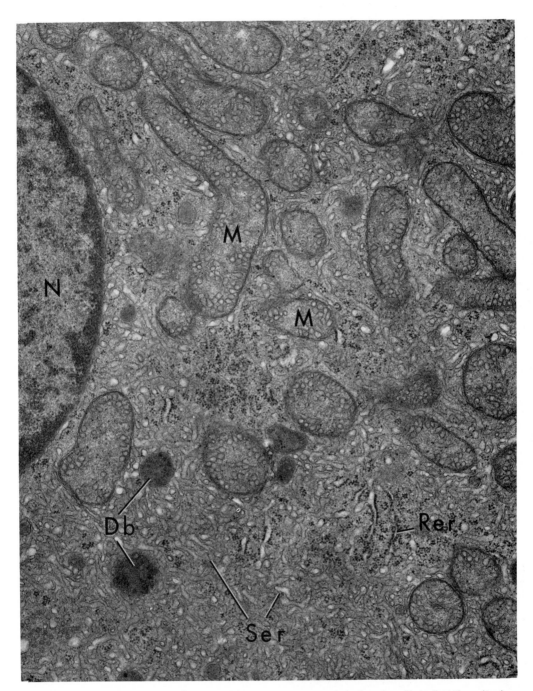

Figure 21.24. Section of the zona fasciculata of the human adrenal cortex. Note that the mitochondria (*M*) have tubular rather than shelf-like cristae. Smooth endoplasmic reticulum (*Ser*) is abundant, although some rough endoplasmic reticulum (*Rer*) is present. *Db*, dense bodies, probably lysosomes; *N*, nucleus (×22,000). (Courtesy of Drs. J. A. Long and A. L. Jones.)

The *zona reticularis* is composed of a network of cell cords. The cells are generally smaller than those of the fasciculata, and they frequently have deeply staining nuclei (Fig. 21.25). The cytoplasm has relatively few lipid droplets in comparison with the fasciculata, and the droplets vary greatly in size. In addition many cells of the reticularis have large numbers of lipofuscin granules (Fig. 21.26). The cells of the reticularis, like those of the fasciculata, have extensive smooth endoplasmic retic-

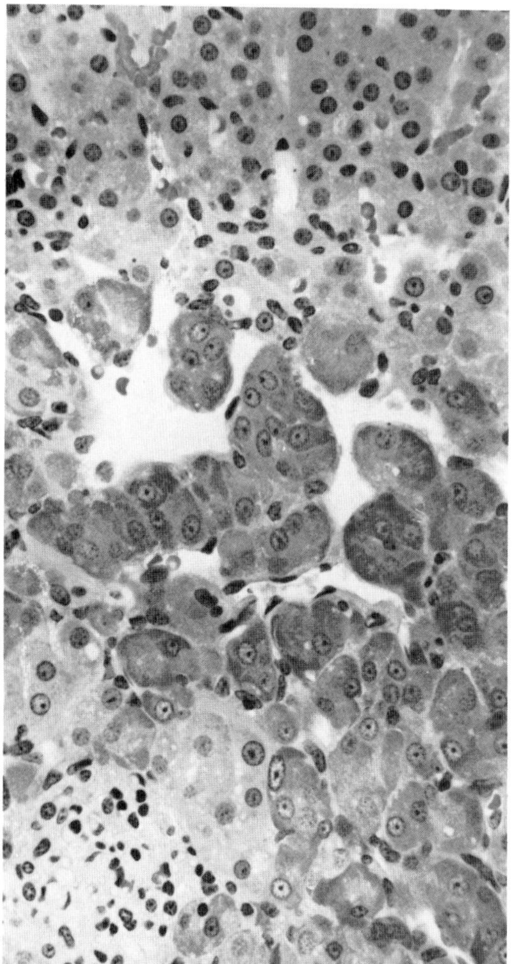

Figure 21.25. Section of the zona reticularis *above*, and medulla *below*, of the same monkey adrenal as that in Figure 21.22. The chromaffin cells of the medulla are larger and more darkly stained than the cells of the reticularis. The pale region in the *lower left* is a nerve bundle (×350).

ulum. It should be noted that the secretory cells form continuous cords through the zones and that the change in cytology from one zone to the next is gradual rather than abrupt.

The major products of the fasciculata and reticularis are *cortisol* and *dehydroepiandrosterone*. Cortisol, the most important glucocorticoid in humans, has a protein-wasting effect and promotes gluconeogenesis (formation of glucose from amino acids). It shows a marked diurnal fluctuation. Normally it is present in the blood in much larger amounts (10 μg/dL) than aldosterone and is bound to transcortin, the steroid-binding globulin, and to albumen. Only about 10% is free. Free cortisol is rapidly cleared by the liver. ACTH produced in corticotropes of the pars distalis causes secretion of cortisol and temporary loss of some of the lipid from the cells of the zona fasciculata.

In chronic stimulation both zona fasciculata and part of the reticularis hypertrophy. When the cortex is destroyed, as by tuberculosis of the adrenal, the hypofunctional condition is known as Addison's disease. Hyperfunction leads to Cushing's syndrome.

Although it is probable that the outer portion of the fasciculata produces much of the cortisol in the unstressed individual, the source of hormone is broadened with stimulation. The androgenic hormone dehydroepiandrosterone in normal levels has little effect. However, because of the common pathways in steroid synthesis, dysfunctional states can result in production of large amounts of sex steroids by the adrenals, which, in some cases leads to virilization in women or, more rarely, feminization in men.

Medulla

The secretory cells of the medulla are found in anastomosing groups in close association with blood vessels (Figs. 21.21 and 21.25). The cells tend to be polygonal to columnar in shape, and contain fine cytoplasmic granules which become brown

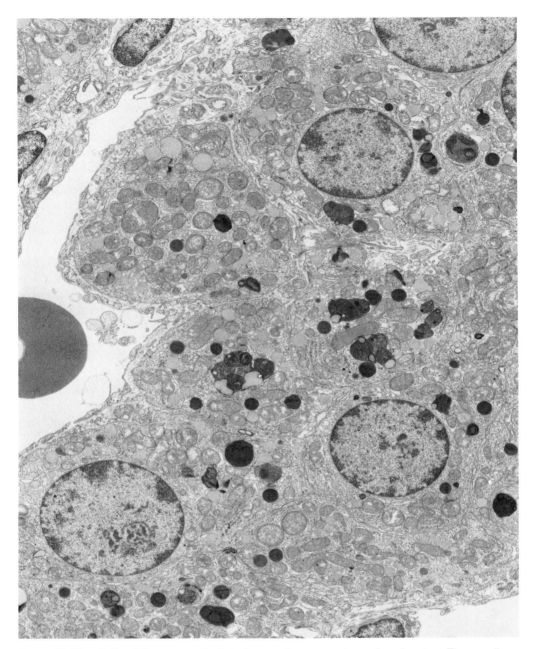

Figure 21.26. Cells of the zona reticularis from a rhesus monkey adrenal cortex. These cells are smaller, have fewer lipid droplets and more lipofuscin than do the cells of the fasciculata (×5,800). (Courtesy of Dr. Barry F. King.)

when oxidized by potassium bichromate. They are therefore known as *chromaffin cells* (Fig. 21.21). The granules also "stain" by other oxidizing agents. Thus, they become green with ferric chloride, yellow with iodine and brown with osmium tetroxide.

The chromaffin reaction of the granules is due to their content of *catecholamines*, derivatives of tyrosine. Two types of catecholamines are present in the medulla: *epinephrine* and *norepinephrine*. In many mammals, two types of cells can be identified on the basis of their "staining reactions" with solutions of substances such as silver and iodide and on the basis of differences in autofluorescence; the norepinephrine secreting cells give much stronger reactions than do the epinephrine secreting cells. By electron microscopy the granules of both cell types are similar in size but those of the norepinephrine type are more electron dense. Chromaffin cells have a well developed Golgi complex, an average number of mitochondria and a moderate amount of rough endoplasmic reticulum. However, they are principally characterized by large numbers of dense-cored (chromaffin) granules (Fig. 21.27).

In the human, the granules are more heterogeneous, and there is only a tendency toward two cell types.

The production of catecholamines uses tyrosine from the liver, forming DOPA, then dopamine in the cytoplasm. Current evidence suggests that dopamine is converted to norepinephrine within the chromaffin granules (almost all of the dopamine oxidase is situated in the granule or granule membrane) and that the conversion of norepinephrine to epinephrine again takes place in the cytoplasm. Both products are secreted by exocytosis of the chromaffin granules. The conversion of norepinephrine to epinephrine depends on phenylethanolamine N-methyltransferase, an enzyme catalyzing the addition of a terminal methyl group to norepinephrine. This enzyme is induced in the chromaffin cells by glucocorticoids from the cortex.

The secretory cells of the adrenal medulla have many similarities to postganglionic neurons: both are derived from neural crest in the embryo, both are innervated by preganglionic sympathetic fibers and both secrete norepinephrine. However, medullary cells differ from postganglionic neurons in that the neurons cannot convert norepinephrine into epinephrine and neurons secrete at nerve endings, whereas medullary cells secrete into the interstitium from which the hormone enters the blood vessels.

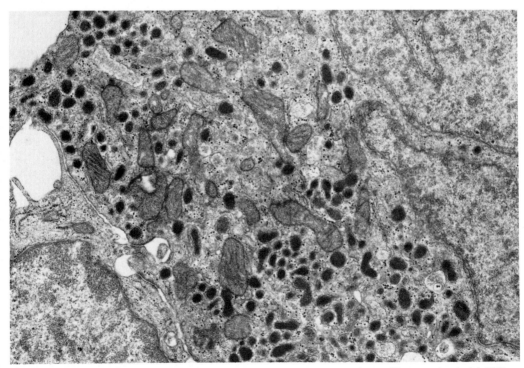

Figure 21.27. Monkey adrenal medulla, showing the numerous chromaffin granules (×14,000).

Catecholamines are quickly inactivated or sequestered, and stimulation of the preganglionic sympathetic fibers to the medulla results in temporary circulating levels as much as 1000 times the resting amount. The effects of elevated epinephrine are very widespread, resulting in elevated blood pressure, increased heart rate, accelerated blood clotting, and other changes generally associated with increasing the ability of the organism to respond by the extensive muscular activity that might be involved in an emergency situation.

Blood Supply

The adrenal glands are highly vascular organs. The arterial supply is subject to great individual variation in the human, but there is always a number of small arteries to each gland. These commonly arise from the inferior phrenic, celiac and renal arteries. The adrenal arteries usually branch before entering the gland so that there are small branches entering the cap-

sule at intervals over most of its surface. From arteries that enter and course in the capsule, three sets of branches arise (Fig. 21.28). One set supplies capillaries to the capsule and the blood from these is collected in the veins of the capsule. The second set supplies sinusoidal capillaries to the cortex which then empty into veins within the medulla. Consequently, the chromaffin cells in the medulla are exposed to high levels of corticular steroids. The third set sends arteriolar branches directly through the cortex to the capillary plexus of the medulla (Fig. 21.28). The venules arising from the second and third sets drain into the vena cava through the central medullary vein, which is unusually thick walled for a vein with many longitudinally directed smooth muscle fibers. In both the cortex and medulla, the terminal network from the arterioles is in close relationship to the secretory cells. Electron micrographs show that the sinusoidal capillaries have a fenestrated type of endothelium and they are

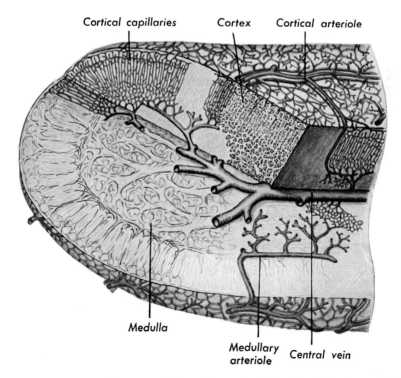

Figure 21.28. Blood supply of adrenal of dog. One end of the adrenal is shown. (After Flint JM: *Johns Hopkins Hosp Reports* 9:153–230, 1900.)

physiologically "leaky," facilitating exchanges between the interstitium surrounding the endocrine cells and the lumen of the vessel. Lymph vessels have not been described in the adrenal gland except in relation to the larger blood vessels.

Nerves

The adrenals are abundantly supplied with nerves. Most of these are derived from the sympathetic division of the autonomic nervous system and course through the splanchnic nerves. Some of the fibers are distributed to the cortex. The majority, however, pass to the medulla; these have been described as being preganglionic. A few ganglion cells are present in the medulla.

Stimulation of the splanchnic nerves causes an outpouring of epinephrine. Cutting the splanchnics inhibits the secretory activity of the medulla.

Postnatal Involution of Human Adrenal Glands

The adrenal glands at birth in the human are relatively large bodies about one-third the size of the kidneys, whereas in the adult they are about $1/28$ the size of the latter organs. Following birth, the adrenals undergo a pronounced involution. In the first 14 days of postnatal life, this decrease amounts to one-third their birth weight, and in the first four months it amounts to one-half. The loss in weight is due to the degeneration of the inner part of the cortex. At birth the cortex consists of a narrow, outer zone, which will proliferate and form the cortex of the adult, and a massive inner zone, the "fetal cortex," which is destined largely to degenerate.

The adrenal glands attain their large prenatal size by a steady growth throughout intrauterine life. Their growth in this period is proportionate to general body growth.

THE PARAGANGLIA

Under the heading of *paraganglia* are included groups of cells that are closely associated both anatomically and embryologically with the sympathetic nervous system. They are largely retroperitoneal, occurring in association with sympathetic ganglia. In shape, staining reaction, and neural crest origin, the cells are similar to those composing the adrenal medulla. They are clear when unstained, become yellow with chromic acid and its salts and turn dark with osmic acid. The cells are oval or polyhedral and have a cordlike arrangement. They lie in close contact with capillaries. Because they are embryologically and structurally similar to the chromaffin cells composing the medulla of the adrenal and have the same staining reaction, it is assumed that they secrete norepinephrine.

The *aortic chromaffin bodies* (lumbar paraganglia) are relatively large, irregularly paired masses formed by a fusion of paraganglia. They are located retroperitoneally and lie ventrolaterally to the aorta at about the level of the origin of the inferior mesenteric artery.

THE PINEAL BODY

The pineal body or pineal gland (*epiphysis cerebri*) in man is a slightly flattened, cone-shaped appendage of the brain measuring 8 to 12 mm in length and 5 to 8 mm in width. Its base is constricted to form a hollow penduncle by which it is attached to the roof of the third ventricle with a narrow prolongation of the third ventricle (the pineal recess) extending up into it. Pia mater covers the pineal body except at its attachment and forms a capsule from which connective tissue trabeculae invaginate the epithelially derived parenchyma of the organ, partially dividing it into poorly defined lobules. The capsule and trabeculae carry numerous blood vessels and nerves (Fig. 21.29).

In all vertebrates that have pineal systems, a saccular organ is present during embryonic stages as the primordium evaginates from the roof of the diencephalon. However, in all mammals, in some reptiles (snakes and turtles) and in some birds, there is a rapid proliferation of secondary, tertiary and subsequent evaginations which

Interlobular trabecula   Blood vessels

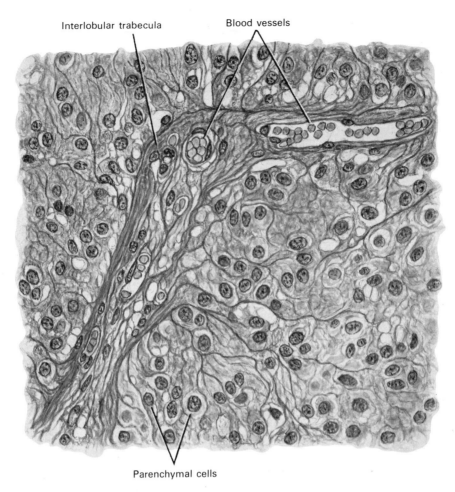

Parenchymal cells

Figure 21.29. Section through the pineal gland of a woman 37 years of age. Hematoxylin and eosin (×535).

converts the sac into cords and follicles of *pinealocytes* (principal pineal cells) interwoven with *glial cells* within the parenchyma of the organ.

The *pinealocytes* have relatively large nuclei with prominent nucleoli, and their nuclei often have an irregular contour because of infoldings of the nuclear envelope. The cytoplasm usually stains lightly in hematoxylin and eosin preparations. The cells have an irregular shape which can be demonstrated after the del Rio-Hortega silver method (Fig. 21.30) or when traced in serial electron micrographs. They have cytoplasmic processes with club-shaped terminations near other principal cells and slightly

larger, flattened terminations in the vicinity of perivascular spaces.

The endoplasmic reticulum of the pinealocytes is mostly smooth surfaced and ribosomes and polysomes are dispersed. The Golgi complex consists of flattened sacs and rounded vesicles of the usual pattern. The mitochondria are fairly large and have the usual shelf-like cristae. The cytoplasm is characterized particularly by numerous microtubules of indefinite length. The cytoplasm also has lipochrome pigment and lysosomes, and most importantly, abundant, dense-cored, membrane-bounded granules, particularly in the pinealocyte processes.

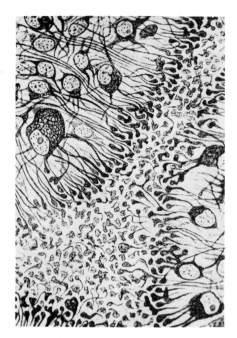

Figure 21.30. Section of a pineal gland of a boy. The parenchymal cells and their processes were impregnated with silver. The processes are shown extending into an interlobular septum. Collagenous tissue and glia are not shown with this technique. Semidiagrammatic. (After Del Rio-Hortega P: Pineal gland. In *Cytology and Cellular Pathology of the Nervous System*, vol 1. Baltimore, Williams & Wilkins, 1932, pp 637–703.)

The *glial cells* provide a network surrounding and pervading the cords and follicles (Figs. 21.31 and 21.32). They are less numerous than the pinealocytes, and their nuclei are smaller and darker staining. Their cytoplasm is also more basophilic. The cells are usually elongated, and they have long cytoplasmic processes seen best after special silver techniques. They are usually considered a type of astrocyte. The glial cells are characterized by numerous fine filaments, 5 to 6 nm in diameter, that are not nearly so abundant in pinealocytes, and their mitochondria have unusually electron-dense matrices. The cristae also have a different arrangement, with some oriented longitudinally and some transversely. The endoplasmic reticulum is rough surfaced and is unevenly distributed in compact masses. The cytoplasm also has numerous single membrane-bounded bodies of varying diameter, which are probably responsible for the fine granulation seen under the light microscope; these are probably lysosomes.

Sand granules (corpora arenacea, acervuli) are generally present in the human pineal body. They are mulberry-shaped concretions which show concentric zones in sections (Fig. 21.32) and are largely hydroxyapatite. They are found in the capsule and also within the organ, usually surrounded by or adjacent to areas rich in glia. They are not present in many species, and their significance is not understood.

The pineal body reaches its maximal development in man by the middle of the first decade or shortly thereafter. It shows regressive changes later in life, but these are quite variable in time of appearance.

The pineal system of some of the *lower vertebrates* (e.g., many lizards) consists of two bodies: a *parietal (or parapineal) organ,* which is placed in or above an opening in the roof of the skull as a "third eye," and a

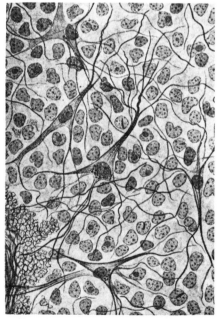

Figure 21.31. Pineal gland, showing the glial cells and their processes. The nuclei of the parenchymal cells are also shown. Silver preparation. (After del Rio-Hortega.)

Glia   Parenchyma

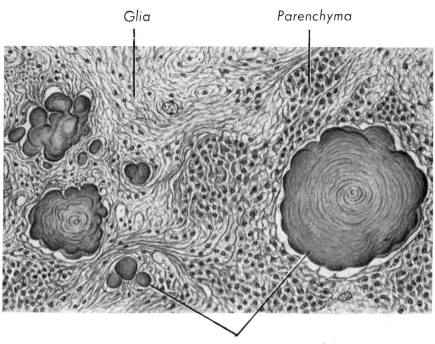

Calcareous granules (acervuli)

Figure 21.32. Section through a region of the pineal gland of a woman 37 years old, showing calcareous granules. Hematoxylin and eosin (×240).

deeper lying intracranial *epiphysis*. Cytological studies show that many of the cells lining the lumina of these structures have characteristics similar to the cones of the retina. The pineal organs of mammals, birds and some reptiles lack such photoreceptor elements and differ markedly from the pineals of the lower vertebrates. However, there is reason to believe that the mammalian pinealocyte is homologous to the pineal photoreceptor of lower vertebrates because both display synaptic ribbons in their cytoplasm and because pineal photoreceptors in some lower vertebrates also contain dense-cored membrane-bounded vesicles suggestive of secretory activity.

Although there have been a number of divergent opinions regarding the *functions of the pineal body* in mammals, it is generally agreed that it is an endocrine or neuroendocrine organ and not a useless vestige. There is considerable evidence that it has an inhibitory action on the development and maturation of the gonads. This was suggested first by clinical observations that boys having tumors of pineal-supporting elements (which presumably crowd out the pinealocytes) show precocious development of the gonads. This view has been supported by experimental studies which show that pinealectomy of young rats results in early maturation of the gonads in both sexes.

The pineal has a high level of *serotonin* and of *melatonin* (5-hydroxyindole) and an enzyme, hydroxyindole O-methyltransferase (HIOMT) that has a role in the synthesis of melatonin from serotinin. It is known that melatonin produces blanching of melanophores in amphibians, having an effect opposite to that of the melanocyte-stimulating hormone of the pituitary gland.

In several mammals with a seasonal breeding cycle, it has been shown that the pineal has a modulating influence on reproduction, tending to suppress premature gonadal development, inhibit reproduction during the off-season, and synchronize the diurnal cycle with the light cycle. Diurnal variation in melatonin production also occurs in the human, but no clear-cut role in normal physiology has been discerned.

In addition to melatonin and serotonin, a number of hypothalamic-hypophyseal peptides are found in the pineal, but their levels are substantially lower than in regions of the hypothalamus.

The mammalian pineal body is supplied by *postganglionic sympathetic nerve fibers* which have their cells of origin in the superior cervical ganglion. This is one of the rare instances in which a portion of the central nervous system receives a sympathetic supply. The pineal also has a *rich vascular supply.* Studies on the rat show that substances such as intravital colloidal dyes diffuse into the pineal body. This is not true of brain tissue in general, in which there is a hematoencephalic or blood-brain barrier.

The responses of the pineal gland to light are abolished by extirpation of the superior cervical ganglion, the source of the postganglionic nerve fibers to the pineal. On the basis of the various findings, it has been proposed that the pineal gland is part of a neuroendocrine mechanism regulating the gonads, and perhaps other organs, in response to light.

Eventually, the pineal organ may be found to have other important products and functions in addition to those suggested by the evidence concerning melatonin and serotonin. It has recently been shown experimentally that melatonin increases rod disc membrane turnover in mammals (see Chapter 22).

Whereas in many lower vertebrates the pineal itself seems to be a photoreceptor, in higher forms the photic input to the organ seems to have been assumed by the lateral eyes. The sensory input is relayed to the pineal via fibers that course in the optic nerves and the median forebrain bundle to make apparent connection with the sympathetic fibers supplying the gland. Pineal function is a subject of active investigation, and additional information is anticipated with further utilization of newer techniques.

References

Pituitary

Baker BL: Studies on hormone localization with emphasis on the hypophysis. *J Histochem Cytochem* 18:1–8, 1970.

Baker BL: Functional cytology of the hypophysial pars distalis and pars intermedia. In Knobil E, Sawyer WH (eds): *Handbook of Physiology*, section 7: Endocrinology, vol 4, part 1. Washington, D.C., American Physiological Society, 1974, pp. 45–80.

Bergland RM, Page RB: Pituitary-brain vascular relations: a new paradigm. *Science* 204:18–24, 1979.

Brownstein MJ, Russell JT, Gainer H: Synthesis, transport, and release of posterior pituitary hormones. *Science* 207:373–378, 1980.

Childs GV, Ellison DG: A critique of the contributions of immunoperoxidase cytochemistry to our understanding of pituitary cell function, as illustrated by our current studies of gonadotropes, corticotropes and endogenous pituitary GnRH and TRH. *Histochem J* 12:405–418, 1980.

Doughaday WH: *Endocrine Control of Growth.* New York, Elsevier, 1981.

Flerko B: The hypophysial portal circulation today. *Neuroendocrinology* 30:56–63, 1980.

Krieger DT, Martin JB: Brain peptides. *N Engl J Med* 304:876–885, 1981.

Marx JL: Synthesizing the opioid peptides. *Science* 220:395–397, 1983.

Nakane PK: Classification of anterior pituitary cell types with immunoenzyme histochemistry. *J Histochem Cytochem* 18:9–20, 1970.

Page RB, Munger BL, Bergland RM: Scanning microscopy of pituitary vascular casts. *Am J Anat* 146:273–302, 1976.

Pelletier G, Robert F, Hardy J: Identification of human anterior pituitary cells by immunoelectron microscopy. *J Clin Endocrinol Metab* 46:534–547, 1978.

Severinghaus AE: The cytology of the pituitary gland. In *The Pituitary Gland.* Baltimore, Williams & Wilkins, 1938, pp 69–117.

Walker AM, Farquhar MG: Preferential release of newly synthesized prolactin granules is the result of functional heterogeneity among mammotrophs. *Endocrinology* 107:1095–1104, 1980.

Wislocki GB: The vascular supply of the hypophysis cerbri of the rhesus monkey and man. In *The Pituitary Gland.* Baltimore, Williams & Wilkins, 1938, pp 48–68.

Zuereb GP, Prichard MML, Daniel PM: The hypophyseal portal system of vessels in man. *Q J Exp Physiol* 39:219–229, 1954.

Thyroid Gland

Andros G, Wollman SH: Autoradiographic localization of iodine[125] in the thyroid epithelial cell. *Proc Soc Exp Biol Med* 115:775–777, 1964.

Austin LA, Hunter H: Calcitonin: physiology and pathophysiology. *N Engl J Med* 304:269–278, 1981.

Ekholm R, Wollman SH: Site of iodination in rat thyroid gland deduced by electron microscopic autoradiography. *Endocrinology* 97:1432–1444, 1975.

Klinck GH, Oertel JE, Winship I: Ultrastructure of normal human thyroid. *Lab Invest* 22:2–22, 1970.

Nadler NJ, Young BA, Leblond CP, Mitmaker B: Elaboration of thyroglobulin in the thyroid follicle. *Endocrinology* 74:333–354, 1964.

Nunez EA, Gershon MD: Cytophysiology of thyroid parafollicular cells. *Int Rev Cytol* 52:1–80, 1978.

Tice LW, Wollman SH, Carter RC: Changes in tight junctions of thyroid epithelium with changes in thyroid activity. *J Cell Biol* 66:657–663, 1975.

Wollman SH: Structure of the thyroid gland. In De Visscher M (ed): *The Thyroid Gland.* New York, Raven Press, 1980, pp 1–19.

Parathyroid Glands

Aurbach GD, Marx SJ, Spiegel AM: Parathyroid hormone, calcitonin and the calciferols. In Williams RH (ed): *Textbook of Endocrinology.* Philadelphia, W.B. Saunders, 1981, pp 922–1031.

Chertow BS: The role of lysosomes and proteases in hormone secretion and degradation. *Endocr Rev* 2:137–173, 1981.

Gaillard PJ, Talmage RV, Budy AM (eds): *The Parathyroid Glands.* Chicago, University of Chicago Press, 1965.

Greep RO: Parathyroid glands. In von Euler US, Heller H (eds): *Comparative Endocrinology,* vol 1. New York, Academic Press, 1963, pp 325–370.

Munger BL, Roth SI: The cytology of the normal parathyroid glands of man and Virginia deer. A light and electron microscopic study with morphologic evidence of secretory activity. *J Cell Biol* 16:379–400, 1963.

Roth SI: Anatomy of the parathyroid glands. In DeGroot LJ, Carhill GF Jr, Martini L, Nelson DH, O'Dell W, Potts JIJ, Steinberger E, Winegrad AI (eds): *Endocrinology.* New York, Grune & Stratton, 1979.

Adrenal Glands

Black VH, Mierlak J, Katz T, Miao P, Huima T, McNamara N: Isolated guinea pig adrenocortical cells in vitro: morphology and steroidogenesis in control and ACTH-treated cultures. *Am J Anat* 165:225–248, 1982.

Gwynne JT, Strauss JF: The role of lipoproteins in steroidogenesis and cholesterol metabolism in steroidogenic glands. *Endocr Rev* 3:299–329, 1982.

Jaffe RB, Serón-Ferré M, Crickard K, Kortinok D, Mitchell BF, Huhtaniemi IT: Regulation and function of the primate fetal adrenal gland and gonad. *Recent Prog Horm Res* 37:41–96, 1981.

Long JA, Jones AL: Observations on the fine structure of the adrenal gland of man. *Lab Invest* 17:355–370, 1967.

Long JA, Jones AL: Alterations in fine structure of the opossum adrenal cortex following sodium deprivation. *Anat Rec* 166:1–26, 1970.

Motta P, Muto M, Fujita T: Three dimensional organization of mammalian adrenal cortex. A scanning electron microscopic study. *Cell Tissue Res* 196:23–38, 1979.

Winkler H, Westhead E: The molecular organization of adrenal chromaffin granules. *Neuroscience* 5:1803–1823, 1980.

Pineal Body

Axelrod J: The pineal gland: a neurochemical transducer. *Science* 184:1341–1348, 1974.

Kelly DE: Pineal organs: photoreception, secretion, and development. *Am Sci* 50:597–625, 1962.

Reiter RJ: The pineal. In Horrobin DF (ed): *Ann Res Review,* vol 3. Montreal, Eden Press, 1978.

Reiter RJ, Fraschini F: Endocrine aspects of the mammalian pineal gland: a review. *Neuroendocrinology* 5:219–255, 1969.

Vollrath L: The pineal organ. In *Handbuch der Mikroskopische Anatomie des Menschen,* vol 6, Berlin, Springer Verlag, 1981, pp 1–475.

Wolstenholme GEW, Knight J (eds): The pineal gland. In *Ciba Foundation Symposium.* Edinburgh, Churchill-Livingstone, 1971.

Wurtman RJ: The pineal as a neuroendocrine transducer. *Hosp Pract* 15:82–92, 1980.

Chapter 22

THE ORGANS OF SPECIAL SENSES

Vertebrate animals display a remarkable degree of *cephalization*—the concentration of major neural, feeding, and sensory organs in the anteriormost parts of the body. While, as noted in discussion of neural tissue, sensory information is provided from all regions, specialized organs providing input related to sight, smell, taste, hearing, and equilibrium are highly evolved and have come, in higher vertebrates, to be localized in the head. These organs are among the most intricate and delicate mechanisms of the body. Interestingly, the signals they provide in response to external stimuli are initiated in specialized epithelial cells. And in each case, these sensory epithelial cells are characterized by elaborately modified and expanded apical surfaces, usually in the form of uniquely differentiated microvilli or cilia.

THE EYE

The *eyeball* (*bulbus oculi*) is essentially a spherical structure, lightproof except for its transparent anterior surface (the *cornea*), which contains a system of refracting media with convex surfaces. These transmit light rays reflected from outside objects and focus them as an inverted image on the *neural retina* which contains photosensitive cells (*rods* and *cones*). Rods and cones initiate nervous activity which, when amplified, coordinated and integrated by other excitable cells of the retina, is relayed over fibers of the optic nerve to the brain. There the sensation of vision is experienced. Accommodation for distance (focus) occurs through change of curvature of one of the refracting bodies (the *lens*) promoted by alteration of the tension exerted on it by

the mechanism from which it is suspended (the *ciliary body*). In front of the lens and perpendicular to the optic axis (direction of light transmission) is an adjustable diaphragm (the *iris*), the aperture of which (the *pupil*) regulates light admitted.

The eye is suspended by a series of ligaments in the bony *orbit*. The orbit also contains the *extrinsic ocular muscles* (which control movements of the eyeball), the *lacrimal gland* (which moistens the anterior surface), the nerves and blood vessels supplying the eye and orbital structures, and a considerable amount of connective tissue and fat. Also associated with the eye are the lids and a duct system which drains the tears from the eye into the nasal cavity.

In form, the eyeball (Fig. 22.1) is more accurately described as consisting of the segments of two spheres, unequal in radius. The larger sphere forms the posterior five sixths of the eyeball. The cornea constitutes a segment of the smaller sphere and hence, displays greater curvature. The two segments are structurally continuous.

Ocular Development

A brief insight into the embryonic origins of the components parts of the eye is essential to understanding their interrelationships in the fully developed organ. Basically, there are three sites of origin for these parts: (*a*) the lateral neuroectodermal walls of the embryonic brain in the region of the diencephalon; (*b*) the surface ectoderm of the head; and (*c*) the mesenchyme (much of it neural crest-derived) interposed around and between the above two epithelial components. Shortly after neural tube closure (Chapter 3), lateral outpocketings on left and right sides of the diencephalon

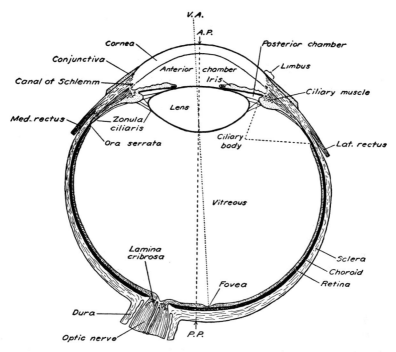

Figure 22.1. Schematic horizontal meridional section of right eye. *A. P.*, anterior pole; *P.P.*, posterior pole; *V.A.*, visual axis (×3). (Redrawn and modified from Salzmann M: *The Anatomy and Histology of the Human Eyeball in the Normal State*. Chicago, 1912.)

result in the formation of two neuroepithelial *optic vesicles*, each remaining attached to the brain wall via a hollow *optic stalk*. Each optic vesicle comes to underlie closely the surface ectoderm of the head and at the point of approximation induces that ectoderm to undergo an inward invagination to form a *lens vesicle*. As the lens vesicle pinches off from the surface ectoderm, its basal surface and that of the nearby optic vesicle are totally surrounded by mesenchyme. A concomitant change now occurs in the configuration of the optic vesicle; an invagination of its distal (anterior) half, much like a depression on the side of a tennis ball, results in a conversion of the single walled optic vesicle into a double walled hemispheric *optic cup*. The invagination is particularly pronounced along the ventral surface of the lens vesicle and along the optic stalk where it produces a transient groove termed the *optic fissure* (or *choroid fissure*). Within the newly formed optic cup, the apical surfaces of the two layers

are brought into contact or close proximity. The outermost layer of the optic cup will remain a simple, but highly pigmented layer, the *pigment epithelium*, whereas the inner layer undergoes profileration and stratification not unlike that encountered in other parts of the neural tube wall. It becomes the highly complex photoreceptive *neural retina*. The mesenchyme which occupies the invagination of the optic cup will eventually occupy the *vitreous chamber* of the eye. The lens vesicle becomes partially enveloped by the free margins of the optic cup and the mesenchyme surrounding all these components begins its differentiation to form nourishing, protecting and supportive tunics.

Hence, in its basic structure, the wall of the eyeball consists of two epithelial layers (derived from the neuroectodermal cup) and two mesodermally derived connective tissue tunics which taken together enclose the lens and the transparent media through which light is transmitted to a sensitive retina. The overlying surface epithelium differentiates into *conjunctival* epithelium and, in conjunction with underlying mesenchyme, into the transparent *cornea*. The posterior wall of the lens vesicle thickens with the development of its highly specialized cells and the whole vesicle becomes the solid, biconvex and highly transparent *lens*.

The outermost connective tissue tunic is the *tunica fibrosa*, comprising the stroma of the *cornea* and *slcera*. The cornea forms the anterior portion of this tunic and is transparent. A fact not commonly appreciated is that most of the refraction of light takes place at the air-cornea interface rather than in the lens, the refractive power of the cornea being about 2½ times that of the lens. The remainder of the outer tunic is the sclera, a tough grayish-white collagen-rich coat, a part of which is seen through the overlying transparent conjunctiva as the "white" of the eye. The tendons of the extrinsic ocular muscles insert into the sclera.

The inner connective tissue tunic of the eye is the *tunica vasculosa*, or *uvea*, which includes the *choriod*, *ciliary body* and the stroma of the *iris*. All three regions of this tunic are laid down upon the outer epithelium of the optic cup. Each is characterized by vascularity and pigmentation. In addition, the ciliary body and iridial stroma contain smooth muscle. The latter muscle fibers, interestingly, have originated by differentiation of optic cup ectodermal epithelial cells. These regulate pupil diameter. The ciliary body contains the muscle of accommodation; by its contraction, the tension on the zonular fibers of the *suspensory ligament* supporting the lens is relaxed and the lens assumes a greater curvature to bring the image of near objects into correct focus on the retina (Figs. 22.2 and 22.3).

The epithelial optic cup derivatives enclosed by those tunics include the photosensitive *neural retina* and the *pigment epithelium* layer. The forward extension of both of these epithelial layers forms the double internal lining layers of the ciliary body and iris (Fig. 22.3).

With growth in diameter of the eye, new cells are added to the sensory retina by proliferation near its optic cup margins. There is progressive central to peripheral differentiation of the new cells as they assume definitive positions along the expanding retinal circumference. The cells may differentiate into photoreceptors, several varieties of interneurons, glial cells (*Müller cells*), or *ganglion cells*. The latter are the most basal in location (near the vitreal surface) and they sprout axons which are the pathways for impulses generated from all parts of the retina. Eventually these axons converge at the optic stalk where, still following the basal epithelial surface, they course along the walls of the optic fissure toward the brain. As their numbers increase, the optic stalk epithelium becomes filled with nerve fibers and is then recognizable as the optic "nerve." Closure of the optic fissure along the optic nerve and ventral surface of the optic cup normally completes enclosure of the *central artery and vein* which nourish the retina from its vitreal surface. In the adult eye, the retinal axons converge into the optic nerve about 3 mm medial to the posterior pole of the eye. Since this disc of convergence consists almost entirely of nerve fibers, this area constitutes a *blind spot*. Almost at the posterior pole is a small area of the retina known as the *macula lutea*, in the center of which is a depression—the *fovea centralis*. This is the region of most acute vision.

Certain commonly used descriptive terms facilitate discussion of the histology of the eyeball. Thus, the *anterior pole* of the eye is coincident with the midpoint of the cornea. A point diametrically opposite is the *posterior pole*. A line connecting the anterior and posterior poles is the *geometric axis* of the eye. This must be distinguished from the *visual axis*, which is a line joining the fovea centralis and the *nodal point* of the optic system. This latter point, which is the optical center, lies in the posterior part of the lens.

A section of the eyeball passing through

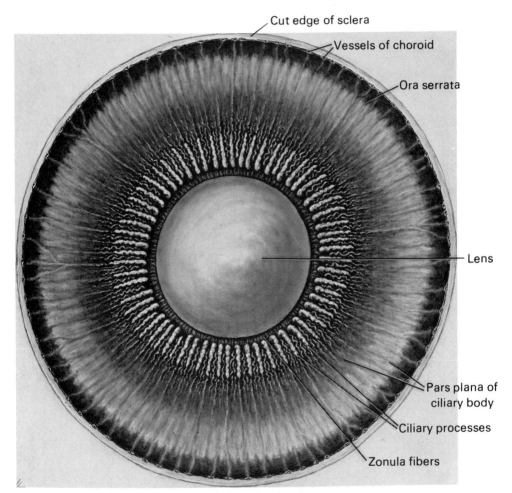

Figure 22.2. Ora serrata, ciliary body, zonula ciliaris and lens viewed from behind after removal of the vitreous body and the posterior hemisphere (including the sensory retina) (×4.6). (Courtesy of Dr. S. R. Detwiler.)

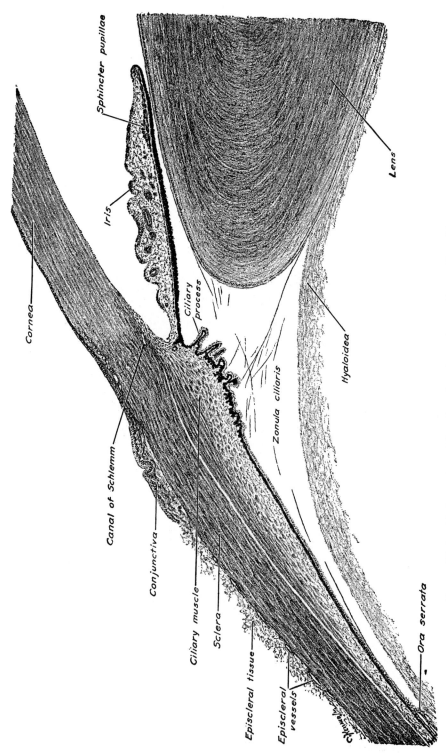

Figure 22.3.   Horizontal meridional section through anterior portion of human eye.

the anterior and posterior poles is designated a *meridional section*. Most instructive of the various meridional sections is that which passes through the horizontal meridian. At an angle of 90° to this plane is the vertical meridian, dividing the eyeball into a medial, or nasal, half and a lateral, or temporal, half. The equator of the eye is a circle taken equidistant from the two poles; sections parallel to this plane are called equatorial sections.

The term "outer" (or external) refers to that which is nearer the surface of the eyeball; "inner" (or internal) refers to that which is nearer the midpoint of the bulb.

As can be seen from its embryology, the optic cup-derived parts of the eye constitute an appendage of the brain, and the optic "nerve" is really a fiber tract of the CNS. By similar logic, the mesenchymally derived ocular tunics relate to the neural parts of the eye in a manner similar to the relationships of the meninges to the brain and spinal cord.

Tunica Fibrosa

The Sclera

The sclera (Figs. 22.1, 22.3, and 22.9), which forms the opaque posterior five-sixths of the protective outer tunic, is composed of dense fibrous connective tissue, thickest at the posterior role (about 1 mm) and gradually thinner until it is only 0.3 mm thick at the insertion of the recti muscles. It is pierced by three sets of apertures, or *emissaria*, through which pass nerves, blood vessels and lymphatics. Across the head of the optic nerve, connective tissue fibers continuous with the sclera form a sieve-like plate. These fibrous components have developed in such a way as to infiltrate among the optic nerve axons which leave the retina there. This region is termed the *lamina cribrosa*.

Although the sclera and corneal stroma are structurally continuous, their junction is marked externally by a slight circular furrow, the *external scleral sulcus*. On the inner surface of the sclera, there is also an *internal scleral sulcus*. The posterior margin

of this furrow projects slightly as the *scleral spur* (scleral roll), to which the muscles of the ciliary body are attached (Figs. 22.3 and 22.9). The furrow itself is filled by the *trabecular meshwork*. At the base of the furrow lies the *canal of Schlemm*.

Three layers of tissue may be designated in the sclera but they are not sharply delimited. The outermost is the *episcleral tissue*, composed of loose collagenous and elastic fibers. Superficially, it is continuous with loose orbital adventitia (*Tenon's space*); inwardly, it merges with the sclera proper; anteriorly, it attaches the conjunctiva to the sclera. It is distinguished by its relatively large number of blood vessels.

The *sclera proper* is a dense feltwork of collagenous fiber bundles running parallel to the surface. Near the cornea and around the optic nerve the bundles of fibers are disposed chiefly in an equatorial direction; elsewhere, they cross and interlace. Numerous delicate elastic fibers are interspersed with the collagenous fibers, particularly at the periphery of the bundles. The cellular component consists of flattened fibroblasts between the fiber bundles.

The tendons of the extrinsic ocular muscles resemble the sclera in structure except that the fiber bundles are all parallel and there are many thick elastic fibers. At their insertions, the tendon bundles continue into the sclera, spreading among those of the sclera.

The *lamina fusca*, the third zone, represents a transition between the sclera and the choroid. Here elastic fibers increase in number and thickness, the collagenous bundles become smaller and branched pigment and other cells appear (see discussion below).

The Cornea

Viewed from in front, the cornea appears slightly elliptical, with a horizontal diameter of about 12 mm and a vertical diameter of about 11 mm. Viewed from behind, it is circular, the difference in the two aspects being due to the fact that the sclera overlaps the anterior surface of the cornea above and below more than it does laterally and medially. The zone of transition between the cornea and sclera, known as the *limbus*, is about 1 mm in width and has histological features differing from the remainder of the cornea (Figs. 22.3 and 22.9).

The *corneal epithelium* is stratified squamous, five or six cell layers in thickness (50 to 100 μm). The deepest cells are columnar, each resting on a basal lamina that is part of the thick Bowman's (basement) membrane. The cells of the remaining layers range from polyhedral to very flat. Although the surface cells are thickened in the regions of their nuclei, the thickenings are directed toward the deeper cell layers. This accounts for the smooth surface characteristic of the cornea.

None of the corneal cells lose their nuclei or normally undergo keratinizaton. They are attached to each other by desmosomes.

Bowman's membrane appears homogenous under the light microscope. Electron micrographs show that it contains an irregular network of relatively fine collagenous fibers. The fibers of the posterior border blend with the superficial lamellae of the corneal stroma.

The *substantia propria* (*corneal stroma*) forms about 90% of the thickness of the cornea and is composed of connective tissue fibers and cells. The characteristic transparency of the cornea is related, in part, to the pattern of its collagenous fibrils arranged in layers, or lamellae, which course parallel with the surface of the cornea. The fibrils within any one lamella are strictly parallel to one another but those of adjacent lamellae differ in direction (Fig. 22.4). Some fibrils also course from one lamellae to another, anchoring the lamellae together. The fibrils within each lamella, as well as the different lamellae themselves, are also held together by a glycosaminoglycan matrix rich in chondroitin sulfate A, keratosulfate and hyaluronic acid. These macromolecules apparently contribute to corneal transparency. Continual loss of water from the corneal surface, which prevents turgescence of the tissue, is an addi-

tional important factor in maintaining corneal transparency.

Most connective tissue cells of the corneal stroma are flat fibroblasts located between and parallel to the lamellar collagenous fibers. In sections cut tangential to the corneal surface it can be seen that the fibroblasts have branching processes that often come into close apposition with neighboring cell processes.

During formative stages of the corneal stroma, the earliest collagen is actually secreted by the corneal epithelial cells. Thereafter mesenchymal cells invade the region between lens and corneal epithelium and contribute further to the building of collagenous lamellae. This sequence is significant also in that a cavitation occurs in the mesenchyme between the corneal stromal layers and the margins of the optic cup and the lens, leading to the formation of the fluid-filled *anterior ocular chamber*. This chamber is lined over its anterior (corneal) margin by simple low cuboidal epithelium which by tradition has been termed the *corneal "endothelium"* (more accurately a mesenchymal epithelium or mesothelium). The endothelium is continuous at the margins of the anterior chamber with a less tightly knit epithelium that forms a network over the pillars of the trabecular meshwork and the anterior surface of the mesenchymally derived iris stroma (Fig. 22.3).

The prominent basement membrane of the endothelium separates the latter from the corneal stroma. Traditionally, it has been termed *Descemet's membrane*. It appears homogeneous under the light microscope. It has resiliency and elasticity, and while it stains, to some extent, with elastic tissue dyes (e.g., resorchin-fuchsin) it is doubtful that elastic fibers are present. It consists of a basal lamina and reticular fibers of a collagenous type lacking typical 64 nm cross bands.

The cornea proper is entirely devoid of blood vessels, deriving its nutrition from the anterior chamber and the superficial

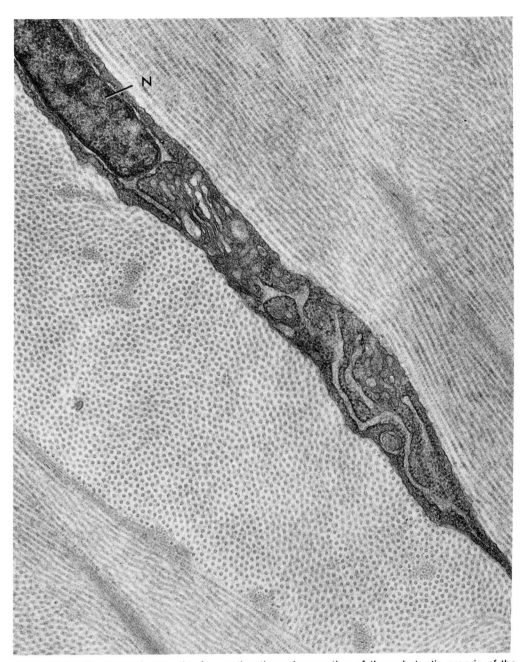

Figure 22.4. Electron micrograph of a section through a portion of the substantia propria of the cornea. A portion of a stromal cell, with its nucleus (*N*), is seen between lamellae of collagenous fibrils. Note the precise alignment of collagenous fibrils at right angles to each other in adjacent lamellae. The endoplasmic reticulum of the stromal cell is not as prominent in the cornea of an adult as it is in the case illustrated, a chicken 5 days after hatching (×34,000). (Reprinted with permission from E.D. Hay and J. P. Revel: *Monographs in Developmental Biology*, vol. 1, 1969.)

marginal plexus of vessels (discussed below under "The Limbus").

The cornea has a rich sensory nerve supply derived from the ophthalmic division of the trigeminal nerve. Small branches of this nerve enter at the periphery and branch extensively in the substantia propria as they course toward the surface and the center of the cornea. Near Bowman's membrane, this *plexus proprius* ends in a terminal net from which fibers, both individually and in bundles, pass as the corneal *rami perforantes* through pores in Bowman's membrane. There they break up into finer branches which extend forward and terminate between the epithelial cells. Other nerve endings are found in the stroma and just under the epithelium at the limbus.

The Limbus

This is a transitional zone about 1 mm wide between the cornea and the adjacent sclera and conjunctiva (Figs. 22.1 and 22.3). The corneal epithelium, as it passes over into the limbus, increases in thickness up to 10 or more cells. The surface cells retain the characteristics of those of the cornea, but the basal cells become smaller and the basal border becomes irregular in contour. These are characteristics of the conjunctival epithelium with which the epithelium of the limbus is continuous. Here also the corneal stroma loses its regular lamellar arrangement, the fiber bundles becoming irregular like those of the sclera. Some elastic fibers are also found.

The only blood vessels which nourish the cornea are found in the limbus, where they form a marginal plexus in the superficial stroma and a series of meridonally directed loops which extend to the border of Bowman's membrane. These vessels are derived from the anterior ciliary artery, a derivative of the ophthalmic division of the internal carotid.

Descemet's membrane and the corneal endothelium become thinner as they approach the *trabecular meshwork* of the iris angle. The surface over the meshwork has an irregular contour and numerous spaces extending inward toward the canal of Schlemm (see "The Iris Angle").

Tunica Vasculosa (Uvea)

This tunic is composed of the *choroid*, *ciliary body* and *iridial stroma* and is characterized by the presence of numerous blood vessels, interstitial spaces, fibroblasts, and pigment cells. After removal of the overlying sclera and cornea, it greatly resembles a grape (uva); hence the synonym *uvea*.

The Choroid

The term choroid (chorioid) is derived from the resemblance of this layer, in vascularity, to the chorion serving the fetus. It forms the posterior part of the uvea. Superficially, it often appears after fixation as separated from the sclera by a space, the so-called *perichoroidal space*, across which delicate lamellae of the choroid pass obliquely to blend with the lamina fuscia of the sclera.

Internally, the choroid is intimately related to the pigment epithelium layer of the retina. When the retina is detached, the pigment epithelium frequently remains adherent to the choroid. The choroid extends anteriorly to the smooth muscle bundles of the ciliary body. However, in at least one species (hamster), a highly cellular and compacted region separates it from the ciliary muscle at the level of the ora serrata. Recent evidence suggests that this compact zone as well as several layers of epithelioid fibroblasts just within the lamina fusca provide a barrier which may inhibit movement of intercellular materials between the inner choroid and sclera. Since the pigment epithelium also presents a formidable barrier to paracellular movement, the possibility is now suggested that interstitial fluids of the choroid may to some extent be isolated from the retinal and scleral layers which border it.

Histologially, the choroid has traditionally been divided into four layers. The *suprachoroid* (*lamina suprachoroidea, epichoroid*), the superifical layer of the choroid, consists of loosely arranged collagenous and elastic fibers which course obliquely backward from choroid to sclera, bridging the perichoroidal space. Within the meshwork of fibers, there are fibroblasts, some macrophages, and numerous chromatophores that contain black-brown melanin granules.

The *vessel layer* (*stratum vasculosa*) is, in thicker portions of the choroid, sometimes subdivided into an outer layer of large vessels (*Haller's layer*) and an inner layer of medium-sized vessels (*Sattler's layer*). In the region of the fovea, only smaller vessels are present; anterior to the equator, the small vessels often seem to merge with the capillary layer.

The veins of the vessel layer converge to

form four whorl-like patterns—the *vortices*. In each vortex, the veins unite in an ampulla from which a single vortex vein arises. The vortex veins (*vena vorticossae*) leave the eye through emissaria in the sclera, two superiorly and two inferiorly. Choroidal stroma occupies the spaces between the vessels. Its stellate chromatophores have slender processes.

The *capillary layer* (*lamina choriocapillaris*), a remarkably rich vascular layer clearly not continued forward into the ciliary body, supplies the outer layers of the retina (Fig. 22.5). Its capillaries form a cavernous, sinusoidal network which almost directly overlies the lamina vitrea (the elaborate basement membrane of the pigment epithelium). The endothelium is

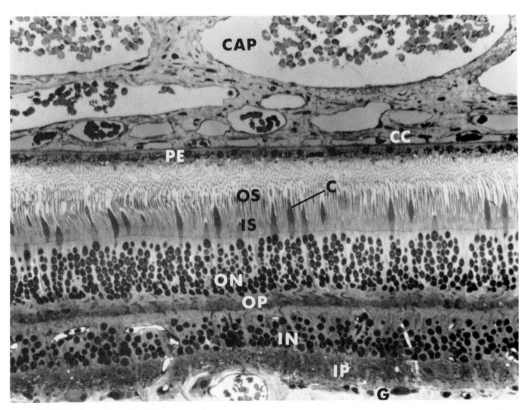

Figure 22.5. Light micrograph of a section through a human neural retina (*bottom*), pigment epithelium (*PE*), and choroid (*top*). *CAP*, choroid capillaries; *CC*, choriocapillaris; *OS*, outer segments of photoreceptor layer; *IS*, inner segments of photoreceptor layer; *ON*, outer nuclear layer; *OP*, outer plexiform layer; *IN*, inner nuclear layer; *IP*, inner plexiform layer; *G*, ganglion cell layer. Note that cone photoreceptors (*C*) are scattered but prominent compared to numerous thin rod photoreceptors (×200). (Courtesy of Dr. Donald Minckler.)

highly fenestrated on the side facing the pigment epithelium. The highly interconnected vascular passages serve a high rate of blood flow and volume.

The interspaces are filled by a stroma of delicate collagenous and elastic fibrils which is continuous with that of the vessel layer. Toward the vessel layer, pigment cells are lacking. On the inner aspect of the capillary layer, a condensation of elastic fibrils forms the outer lamella of the lamina vitrea.

The *lamina vitrea (Bruch's membrane)* has been considered as the innermost layer of the choroid. In fact, it is a prominent basement membrane of the pigment epithelium, and hence primarily of optic cup derivation. It is about 2 to 2.5 μm thick with a thin outer lamella composed of slender collagenous fibers and a plexus of elastic fibers, likely of mesenchymal origin.

The ciliary nerves course in the suprachoroid and give off fine branches which form plexuses in the choroidal stroma. Multipolar ganglion cells associated with the plexuses are probably concerned with autonomic innervation of blood vessels.

In certain teleost fishes a silvery layer (*argentea*) is found between the suprachoroid and the vessel layer. It is formed by specialized cells containing crystals of guanine and extends into the iris, giving a characteristic silvery luster.

In most mammals, but not in man, a reflecting layer, the *tapetum lucidum*, is developed in the posterior region of the choroid. Lying between the choriocapillaris and the vessel layer, it consists either of

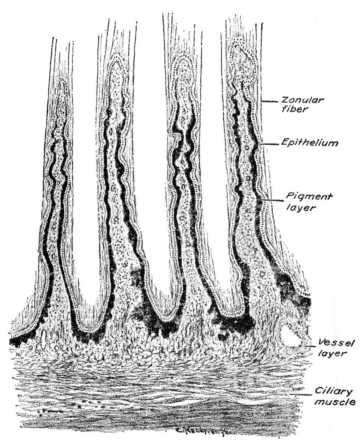

Figure 22.6. Drawing illustrating an equatorial section through the ciliary body of the human eye.

several layers of flattened cells, the *cellular tapetum* (carnivores) or fine fibers, the *fibrous tapetum* (herbivores).

The Ciliary Body

The choroid extends anteriorly as far as the *ora serrata*, which is the anterior margin of the sensory portion of the retina (Figs. 22.1 and 22.2). In front of the ora serrata, the uvea is thickened to form the *ciliary body*, a plicated ring to which the *suspensory ligament* of the lens is attached and from which the iris extends. In meridional section, the ciliary body is triangular in shape (Fig. 22.3). Its outer aspect blends

into the sclera. Its inner surface faces the vitreous body and lens, and when viewed macroscopically from behind, it displays two zones (Fig. 22.2). The posterior two-thirds appears darkly pigmented and is relatively smooth. This is the *orbiculus ciliaris* or *pars plana*. The anterior one-third bears some 70 to 80 radially arranged pale ridges, the *ciliary processes*; this region is the *corona ciliaris* (*pars plicata*) (Figs. 22.6 and 22.7).

The anterior aspect of the ciliary body continues into the stroma of the iris, its outer edge is attached to the scleral spur, and between these two parts the ciliary

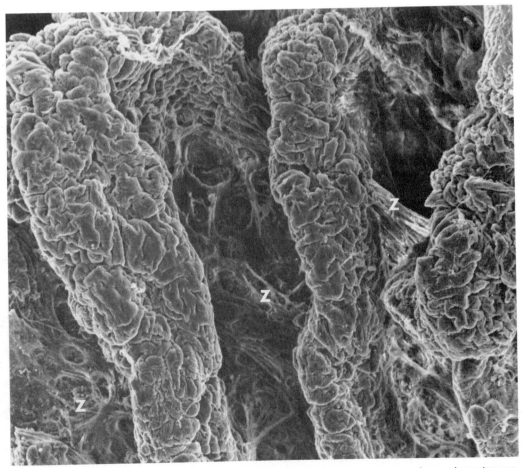

Figure 22.7. Scanning electron micrograph showing several ciliary processes from a hamster eye. The surfaces of these processes face the posterior chamber, into which they secrete ocular fluid. In life they are covered by a basal lamina, to which collagenous zonular fibers (Z) (suspensory ligament of the lens) are attached. These have collapsed in preparation (compare to Fig. 22.6) (×620). (Micrograph in collaboration with Dr. Gregory S. Hageman.)

body blends into the trabecular meshwork approaching the iris angle.

The ciliary body represents a forward continuation of the choroid except for its capillary layer, plus a double-layered internal epithelial lining, the *pars ciliaris retinae*. This latter is an anterior continuation of the neural retina and pigment epithelium beyond the ora serrata. It is interesting to note, considering its optic cup origin, that the two layers of the pars ciliaris retinae lie apex-to-apex. Hence, basal lamina coats the epithelial surfaces facing the posterior

and vitreous chambers on the one side and the ciliary vessels and musculature on the other.

In the outer ciliary body, smooth muscle forms a mass of appreciable bulk (Figs. 22.3 and 22.8). According to the directions in which they are disposed, three sets of fibers are distinguished.

The *meridional fibers* (longitudinal fibers, *Brücke's muscle*) are outermost. They begin in the relatively sparse star-shaped groups near the suprachoroid and, increasing in number, form bundles which run

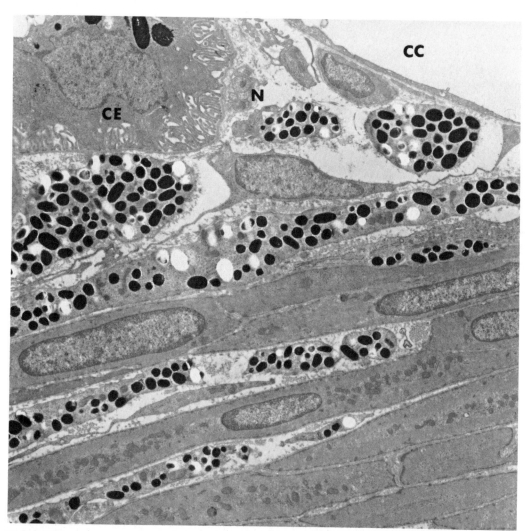

Figure 22.8. Electron micrograph of ciliary musculature (*lower half* of figure) and a small portion of the ciliary epithelium (*CE*) (hamster eye). Numerous pigment cell processes are also seen as well as a ciliary capillary (*CC*) and a small nerve (*N*). The smooth muscle cells control accommodation for distance (×6,500). (Micrograph in collaboration with Dr. Gregory S. Hageman.)

anteriorly to insert into the scleral spur (Fig. 22.3).

The *radial fibers* lie internal to the meridional fibers. They are intermingled with connective tissue elements which become continuous anteriorly with the meshwork of the iris angle.

The *circular fibers* (*Müller's muscle*) are continuous with the radial fibers and lie at the inner edge of the ciliary body. These course in a circular direction around the ciliary body just posterior to the root of the iris. Immediatley anterior to them is the *circulus arteriosus iridis major,* source of the arterial supply to the iris and ciliary processes.

The blood vessels of the ciliary muscle run in the interstitial tissue and are of small caliber. They are branches of the *long posterior ciliary* and *anterior ciliary arteries.*

The ciliary muscle is innervated by parasympathetic fibers of the oculomotor nerve. Preganglionic fibers reach the ciliary ganglion by way of the short motor root; the postganglionic fibers are axons of ganglion cells in the ciliary ganglion and course to the ciliary muscle through the short ciliary nerves. These fibers are myelinated, an exception to the rule that postganglionic fibers are nonmyelinated.

The collective contraction of the ciliary muscles relaxes tension in the suspensory ligament of the lens, thus allowing the normally elastic lens to assume a more convex form (accommodation for near-focus).

The *vessel layer* underlying the muscles is similar in structure to that of the choroid, except that there are fewer chromatophores, more collagenous fibers, and the vessels are mostly veins. The arteries supplying this region enter through the ciliary muscle.

In the pars plana, the vessels are arranged almost in a single layer. Further forward in the pars plicata, the vessels are disposed in several layers. The ciliary processes are formed by localized thickenings of the vessel layer (Fig. 22.6).

The *lamina vitrea* of the ciliary body is a continuation of the vitreous lamina of the choroid and it contains the same structures: an outer elastic lamella and an inner basement membrane of the pigment epithelium. In the ciliary region, however, an added layer of connective tissue is interposed between the two. The elastic lamella fades out at about the middle of the pars plicata and the intermediate zone of collagenous fibers merges with the stroma of the vascular layer. The basement membrane continues onto the iris.

The *pigment epithelium* of the ciliary body is a forward continuation of the pigment epithelium layer of the retina. Its cells are filled with round melanin granules and their plicated cell borders are difficult to distinguish by light microscopy, except on the summits of the ciliary processes, where the cells are more cuboidal and have less pigment (Fig. 22.6). This accounts for the characteristic white appearance of the ciliary processes.

The *ciliary epithelium* represents a continuation of the neural retina. Over the inner (vitreal) surface of the ciliary body, this becomes a single layer of columnar epithelial cells, unpigmented except in the region of the iris root, where they acquire pigment and together with the pigment epithelium continue over the back surface of the iris. Over the summits of the ciliary processes, the ciliary epithelial cells become cuboidal in shape. Electron micrographs show cytological characteristics commonly found in epithelial cells that are active in transport, such as numerous infoldings of the basal plasma membranes of both epithelial layers (e.g., in Fig. 22.8) and the presence of a fenestrated type of endothelium in the capillaries of the ciliary processes.

The *aqueous humor* (intraocular fluid) is not only a fluid refractive medium in the eye; its circulation is also essential for the nutritive support of the retina and other refractile elements. Maintenance of proper intraocular fluid pressure ensures the physical stability of the eye and the functional interrelationship of its refractile components. Aqueous humor is constantly secreted into the posterior chamber and, after circulating through the chamber as well as percolating through the interstices of the vitreous body and iridial stroma, it is drained at a balanced rate at the angle of the anterior chamber. Formation of aqueous humor involves activity by the ciliary epithelium and its numerous ciliary processes. A filtrate from the ciliary capillaries passes through the epithelial cells where some proteins, glucose and urea are subtracted and other substances, such as ascorbic acid, sodium chloride and bicarbonate are added.

When different substances are injected into the blood, some reach the aqueous humor in amounts approaching that in plasma whereas many others such as protein, inulin and trypan blue do not. The lack of passage from the blood to the aqueous humor is regarded as due to a *blood-aqueous barrier.* A principal barrier against paracellular passage seems to be the occluding junctions of the ciliary epithelium. The cells of the epithelium probably determine which substances pass via an intra- or transcellular route.

The *internal limiting "membrane"* of the retina is a thin layer that is actually the basal lamina and reticular lamina of the optic cup. It continues over the inner (vitreal) side of the ciliary epithelium.

The Iris

The *iris* is a thin circular diaphragm placed directly in front of the lens. It forms a distensible aperture, the *pupil,* located slightly to the nasal side of its center. Its peripheral border (*ciliary border, iris root*) extends from the anterior aspect of the ciliary body (Fig. 22.3); its *pupillary border* rests on the lens. The iris divides the space between the cornea and the lens into the *anterior chamber* ahead and the *posterior chamber* behind. The two communicate through the pupil.

The anterior surface of the iris shows a division into two regions, an inner *pupillary zone* and an outer *ciliary zone,* which differ in structure and frequently also in color. The irregular circular line (about 1.5 mm from the pupillary margin) which forms the junction between these two zones is known variously as the *collarette, iris frill* or *angular line.* It marks the position of an underlying system of arteriovenous anastomoses, the *circular vasculosus iridis minor.*

The pupillary zone is radially striated and, near the collarette, shows a number of depressions, the *pupillary crypts,* which may also occur in the neighboring part of the ciliary zone. At the pupillary margin is a dark border which represents the limit of the pigmented double-layered posterior epithelium (*pars iridica retinae*).

The ciliary zone is marked by a series of fine radial striations formed by blood vessels. In its outer half are a number of concentric circular *contraction furrows.* Near the ciliary border, *ciliary crypts* are seen. These are smaller than the pupillary ones.

Like the ciliary body, the iris contains structural continuations from the tunica vasculosa (uvea), including an *endothelium, anterior border layer* and a *vessel layer* (stroma). These parts are lined on their posterior aspect by *dilator pupillae* muscles and a double-layered pigmented pars iridica retinae. This latter is an optic cup-derived anterior continuation of the pars ciliaris retinae, and like it is covered by basal lamina on both anterior and posterior basal surfaces (Fig. 22.9).

The endothelium of the anteior surface of the iris is continuous with the endothelium of the iris angle and, in turn, with that of the cornea (Fig. 22.3). It is a thin discontinuous and delicate layer that is difficult to demonstrate in sections prepared for light microscopy (Fig. 22.9).

The anterior border layer is a stromal region immediately beneath the endothelium. By virtue of the leakiness of the endothelium, intraocular fluid has direct access to its components. It is the layer which determines the color of iris. It has few collagenous fibers, no blood vessels, is formed principally of *chromatophores—* branched connective tissue cells containing granules of yellowish-brown pigment. The layer is lacking over the crypts and is thin on the contraction furrows.

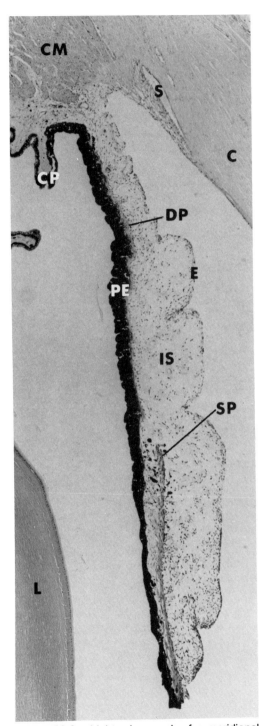

Figure 22.9. Light micrograph of a meridional section through a human iris and nearby ocular tissues. *L*, lens; *CP*, ciliary processes; *CM*, ciliary muscle; *S*, Schlemm's canal; *C*, corneal stroma; *PE*, iridial pigmented epithelium; *IS*, iridial stroma; *E*, iridial endothelium; *DP*, dilator pupillae muscle; *SP*, sphinctor pupillae muscle (×50). (Preparation by Dr. Donald Minckler.)

The color of the iris depends upon the thickness of the anterior border layer and the degree of pigmentation of its cells. In the brown iris, the layer is thick and the cells heavily pigmented. In the blue iris, the layer is thin with a mininum of pigment. Light striking it, therefore will pass through this layer and the underlying stroma and be reflected as blue from the darkly pigmented posterior epithelium.

The vessel layer consists of a great number of blood vessels imbedded in a loose stroma of delicate collagenous fibrils, with some elastic fibers and a number of stromal cells. Most of the latter are pigmented (chromatophores).

The arteries of the iris are branches of the *greater arterial circle*, located at the root of the iris and supplied by the anterior and posterior ciliary arteries. Within the stroma of the iris, the arteries course radially and spirally. Arteries of the iris have a poorly developed intima, a relatively thin muscular layer and an unusually thick collagenous adventitia. The spiral patterns and firm connective tissue walls permit the vessels to straighten or coil without stretching or kinking; modifications well suited to the changes in the radial dimensions of the iris.

In the stroma of the pupillary zone there is a circular band of smooth muscle fibers, the *sphincter pupillae* (Figs. 22.3 and 22.9). Their contraction reduces the diameter of the opening. Curiously, this smooth muscle is of *ectodermal origin*, derived from the pigment epithelium layer by a transformation of epithelial cells into smooth muscle fibers, a fact now firmly established by electron microscopic studies. The muscle cells are clearly separated from mesenchyme by a basal lamina through all stages of differentiation. Contraction of the *dilator pupillae* muscle (Figs. 22.3, 22.9, and 22.10) produces dilation of the pupil. It too seems to be derived from pigment epithelial cells. Because both groups of the iridial smooth muscle cells retain some characteristics of epithelial cells they are sometimes described as "*myoepithelial cells.*"

Together with the ciliary muscle, the

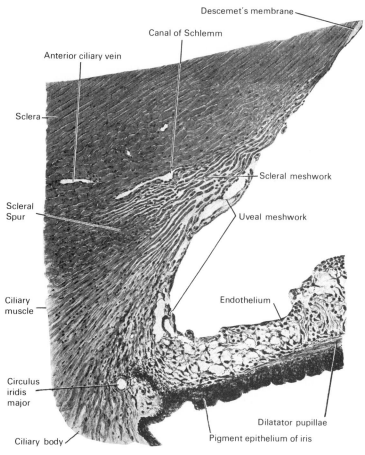

Figure 22.10. Light micrograph showing a meridional section through the iris angle of a human eye.

sphincter and dilator pupillae comprise the *intrinsic muscles* of the eye. The sphincter is innervated by parasympathetic fibers of the oculomotor nerve. These follow the same course as those described for the ciliary muscle. The dilator pupillae is innervated by the sympathetic division of the autonomic nervous system, receiving nonmyelinated postganglionic fibers from the superior cervical ganglion. These travel in the internal carotid nerve to the cavernous plexus, thence to the Gasserian ganglion and ophthalmic division of the trigeminal nerve and finally by way of the nasociliary nerve and long ciliary nerves to reach the dilator muscle.

The ciliary epithelium, as it nears the root of the iris, acquires increasing amounts of pigment. From the ciliary body, it is continued over the posterior surface of the iris juxtaposed to and indistinguishable from the pigment epithelium (Figs. 22.9 and 22.10). So densely pigmented is this layer that neither cell boundaries nor nuclei can be distinguished in routine preparations for light microscopy. If the pigment is bleached out, however, the cells of both layers can be seen as columnar or prismatic elements with round nuclei. At the pupil, these two remnants of the embryonic cup margin become confluent, bending slightly forward around the pupillary border as the *pigment seam*. There they join the single-layed and discontinuous endothelium lacing over the anterior surface of the iris.

The Iris Angle

The lateral borders of the anterior chamber have, in meridional section, an angular shape. This *iris angle,* or *angle of the anterior chamber,* is occupied by loose spongy tissue, the *trabecular* (or *uveal*) *meshwork* which fills in the scleral furrow and extends behind to the ciliary body (Fig. 22.10). In section, the apex of the triangle formed by the meshwork is continuous with Descemet's membrane and the posterior lamellae of the cornea. Its base merges with the anterior ciliary body, its outer border adjoins the tissues of the adjacent sclera and cornea, and, its inner border bounds the anterior chamber.

The trabecular meshwork forms as a result of elaborate folding of the anterior chamber "endothelium" over numerous pillars and lamellae of connective tissue. A labyrinth of intraocular fluid-filled channels are thus developed which course around and through the pillars and lamellae. The spaces of the meshwork, known as the *intertrabecular spaces (of Fontana),* are in direct communication with the anterior chamber. (Fig. 22.11). They narrow with distance from the anterior chamber, and their endothelial linings become increasingly difficult to distinguish from fibroblasts and smooth muscle cells of the ciliary body, even at ultrastructural levels of resolution.

Each pillar or lamella contains a core of collagenous and elastic fiber bundles, the latter being especially prominent (Fig. 22.11). Unmyelinated axons are also found, though rarely in humans. A variety of experiments has shown that the endothelial coverings of the pillars and lamellae are not continuous, and that considerable fluid exchange occurs between the connective tissue and intertrabecular spaces (discussed below).

Along the inner border of the scleral meshwork, there is a thin layer of trabeculae that lack elastic fibers and that are round. In some species, the trabeculae along the inner border form a well-defined structure known as the *pectinate ligament.* This name is sometimes used for the similarly located, but poorly developed, trabeculae in the human eye.

The *angular aqueous plexus (canal of Schlemm)* also lies in the scleral furrow, close to its bottom. In meridional sections, it appears as one or more endothelial lined oval spaces, just in front of the scleral spur and adjacent to the trabecular meshwork (Figs. 22.3 and 22.10). Actually, it encircles the eye as a canal which irregularly divides and recombines into two or more branches. It communicates peripherally by means of 20 to 30 small branches with the anterior ciliary veins in the neighboring scleral tissue. The outer borders of the endothelial cells of Schlemm's canal are in contact with the lining cells of some of the intertrabecular spaces.

Together with the meshwork of the angle, Schlemm's canal provides one mode of exit from the eye for the intraocular fluid. Although the exact mechanism remains obscure, much evidence demonstrates that intraocular fluid passes readily through the intertrabecular spaces to reach the canal. Particulate matter appears to be entrapped within the meshwork and engulfed by macrophages, or by endothelial cells of the intertrabecular spaces of the canal itself. The latter aspect is the subject of considerable current debate. Under normal conditions, only aqueous humour is found in Schlemm's canal. It has been suggested that the action of the ciliary muscle on the scleral spur provides a pumping mechanism for the canal.

Schlemm's canal, however, is probably not the only route for intraocular fluid drainage. Increasing evidence suggests that considerable amounts of the fluid (or its components) course across the trabecular endothelium to reach interstitial connective tissue from which it apparently has access to nearby episcleral vessels and perhaps lymphatic channels. This rather diffuse drainage is formed through the *"uveoscleral"* outflow in distinction to the *"conventional"* outflow via Schlemm's canal.

The aqueous humour, secreted by the ciliary epithelium, carries nutrients, substrates and metabolites. As outlined previously, it also maintains an intraocular pressure which is higher than that in the surrounding tissues and thus, together with

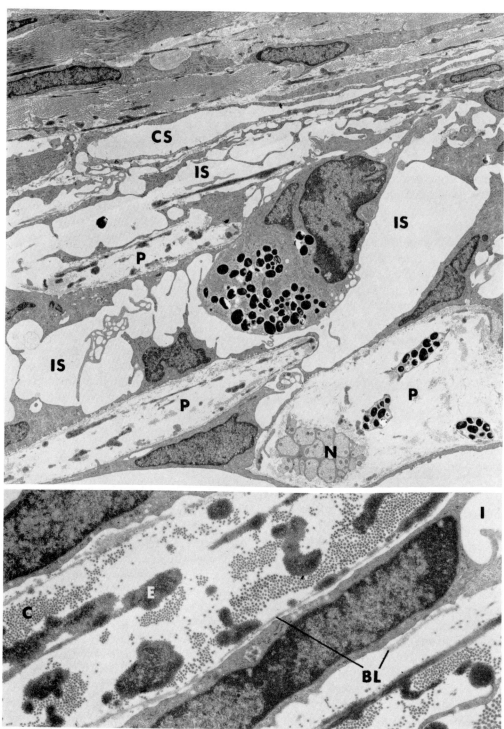

Figure 22.11. *Top*, electron micrograph of a meridional section through the trabecular meshwork of a hamster eye. Note three connective tissue pillars (*P*), intertrabecular spaces (*IS*), canal of Schlemm (*CS*), overlying sclera (*top*), and a small nerve (*N*). A large pigment-containing cell is seen at center (×4,100). *Bottom*, higher magnification view of portions of two meshwork pillars. Note concentrations of collagen fibers (*C*) as well as elastic fiber beams (*E*). An intermittent, but frequently prominent, basal lamina (*BL*) separates lining cells of the intertrabecular spaces (*I*) from the connective tissues of the pillars (×14,000). (Both micrographs in collaboration with Dr. Gregory S. Hageman.)

the fibrous tunics, it plays an important role in maintaining stability of optical dimensions. A normal intraocular pressure is present when the aqueous humour is formed and drained at normal rates. An increase in intraocular pressure, known as *glaucoma*, occurs when there is defective drainage by the outflow channels at the iris angle.

The Retina

The retina (*pars optica retinae*) is the part of the eye which transduces the stimulus of light into nerve impulses, resulting in the sensation of vision. Thus it might be considered that all other parts of the eye assist the retina in the proper performance of its highly specialized function.

The retina, having arisen from the optic cup, consists of two epithelial layers lying with their apical surfaces in apposition. These are an outer *pigment epithelium*, and an inner *neural retina*. In pathological detachment of the retina, or as often occurs in fixed specimens, the two parts of the retina separate, the pigment epithelium remaining adherent to the choroid.

The neural retina is firmly attached to underlying structures at only two regions—at its scalloped anterior margin, the *ora serrata* (Fig. 22.1), and at the *optic disc*, where the nerve fibers exit the wall of the bulb to form the optic nerve (Fig. 22.25). Detached from the pigment epithelium, it is a delicate layer which in life is transparent.

Except at the optic disc (optic papilla), the fovea centralis and the extreme periphery, the neural retina consists of nine layers (Figs. 22.5, 22.18, and 22.19), which from without inward, are arranged as follows: (*a*) layer of rod and cone outer and inner segments; (*b*) external limiting "membrane" (outer zone of intercellular attachments); (*c*) outer nuclear layer; (*d*) outer plexiform layer; (*e*) inner nuclear layer; (*f*) inner plexiform layer; (*g*) ganglion cell layer; (*h*) nerve fiber layer; and (*i*) internal limiting membrane (basal lamina).

The nature and significance of the layers of the neural retina will be better under-

stood if it is realized that the stratification depends upon the location and interrelationships of the photoreceptor cells and the intraretinal neurons of the afferent pathway. Considered in order of initiation and conduction of an impulse, the photoreceptor portions of the *rod* and *cone cells* occupy the layer of that name. The *outer nuclear layer* consists of the nuclei and cell bodies of the photoreceptor cells, and the *outer plexiform layer* is where axon-like photoreceptor cell processes make synaptic junctions with dendrites of *bipolar neurons* and with processes of *horizontal cells*. The nuclei of the bipolar cells lie in the *inner nuclear layer*, their axons pass into the *inner plexiform layer*, where they synapse with the dendrites of the ganglion cells. The relatively large cell bodies of the latter form the *ganglion cell layer*; their long axons course in the *nerve fiber layer* to the optic disc, where all the axons converge to form the optic nerve. These fibers are continuous to the brain, where the great majority end in the lateral geniculate body, from which another neuron system carries the nerve impulse to the visual areas in the occipital cortex.

The true photoreceptive elements, the rods and cones, lie furtherest removed, facing the pigment epithelium, and oriented *away* from the light stimulus, which to affect them must first pass through all the intervening layers and their organelles (except at the fovea). These are all maintained in a remarkably transparent state. Also, the nervous pathway at first travels directly toward the source of the stimulus before turning to course toward the brain. This seemingly *inverted* retina is characteristic of all vertebrates.

The Rod Cells

In all vertebrates, rod cells are elongate and oriented perpendicular to the retinal epithelium. They possess apical protrusions, each divided into parts, the *inner* and *outer segments*. Together these are slender cylindrical elements, 40 to 60 μm in length and about 2 μm in diameter. Rod outer and inner segments vary in length and width in different species (Fig. 22.12). The outer segment is the most distal part and is the receptor that "traps" light. It is made up of hundreds of flattened membranous sacs piled in a stack of uniform diameter (Figs. 22.13 to 22.17). The membranes of the sacs contain molecules of visual pigment (*rhodopsin*) which absorb the light and undergo steric chemical conformational changes (*transduction*) that lead to the production of a generator potential by the photoreceptor cell. The compact stacked arrangement of the flattened sacs orients and increases enormously the membrane surface over which photic absorption and transduction can occur.

The base of the outer segment is connected with the inner segment by a slender ciliary stalk which contains nine peripheral doublet microtubules that emanate from a centriole or basal body. Striated ciliary rootlets extend from the centriole into the inner segment cytoplasm. Thus, the outer segment is a specialized cilium that differs from the cilia of most other types of epithelium (Chapter 4) mainly in the lack of a central pair of microtubules and in the unique and massive development of the surrounding cell membrane to form the flattened sacs. The outer portion of the inner segment contains mitochondria, in some species quite closely packed. The inner portion of each inner segment contains the Golgi complex and rough and smooth endoplasmic reticulum. In the retinas of some lower vertebrates, filamentous elements in the inner segment are contractile, serving to advance or retract the outer segment with reference to the pigment epithelium in response to light or dark.

Radioautographic and immunocytochemical studies of retinas show that rod cells synthesize new membrane-bound proteins in the inner segments. These proteins are transported to the cell membrane of the inner segment as Golgi-derived vesicles. After fusion of the vesicle membranes with the cell membrane, the new membrane and protein (especially rhodopsin) are conducted along the ciliary stalks to the bases of the outer segments where groups of new sacs are formed by infoldings of the cell membrane. The older sacs are displaced outward as new sacs are built below, and they are eventually shed from the tips of the rods into the region of the pigment epithelium. In the human rod outer segment, it is estimated that ten days are required for a given sac to be transported from its formation at the base to its shedding site at the tip. Thus, the outer segment membranes and proteins of the rod cells are continually renewed, and during their life spans, held in register with their massive membrane surfaces perpendicular to the direction of incoming light rays (Fig. 22.17). (See additional discussion regarding this pattern in relation to the pigment epithelium.)

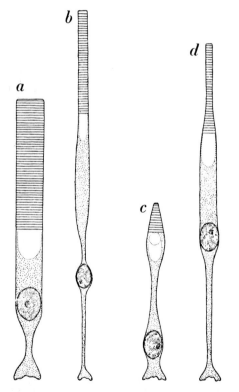

Figure 22.12. Diagrams of rod and cone cells. Although the retinal photoreceptors differ somewhat in different species, they have a similar general organization in all vertebrates. *Left*, typical rod cells from the frog retina (*a*) and the human retina (*b*); *right*, typical cone cells from the frog (*c*) and human (*d*). (After R. W. Young: *Sci Am* 223: 1970.)

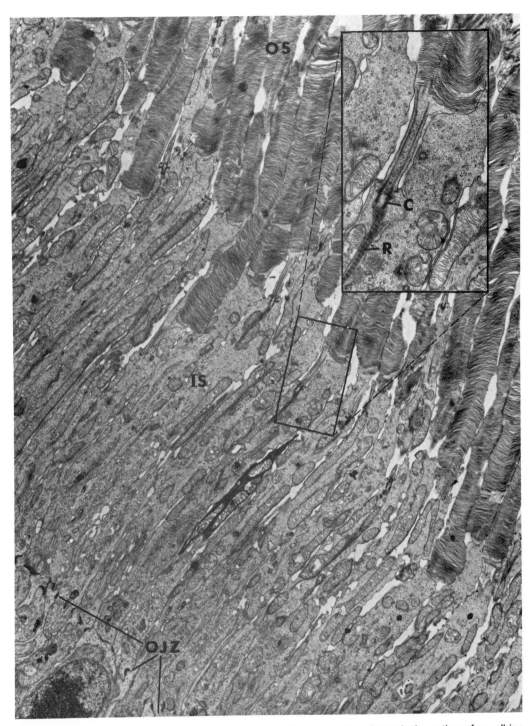

Figure 22.13. Low magnification electron micrograph of a section through the retina of an albino rat (a pure rod retina). The region of outer segments (*OS*) and inner segments (*IS*) covers most of the field.The outer junctional zone (*OJZ*) separates the above region from the outer nuclear layer (*lower left corner*). Details of the connection between outer and inner segments of one rod cell are shown at higher magnification in the *inset*. The outer segment begins as a narrow ciliary stalk with a centriole (*C*) at its base. A ciliary rootlet (*R*) extends from the centriole into the inner segment cytoplasm (×6000; *inset* ×15,000). (Courtesy of Dr. David Chase.)

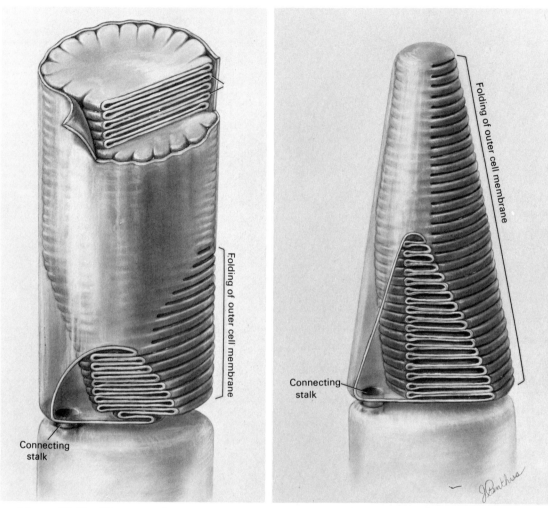

Figure 22.14. Diagrammatic representation of the ultrastructure of amphibian rod and cone cell outer segments. In the rod, there is a continual formation of new sacs by repeated infolding of the cell membrane. As the older sacs are displaced away from the base of the outer segment, they lose their attachment to the cell membrane, and they are eventually cast off. The sacs of the cone outer segment are also continually replaced, but in a less obvious sequential fashion. (Courtesy of Dr. Richard W. Young.)

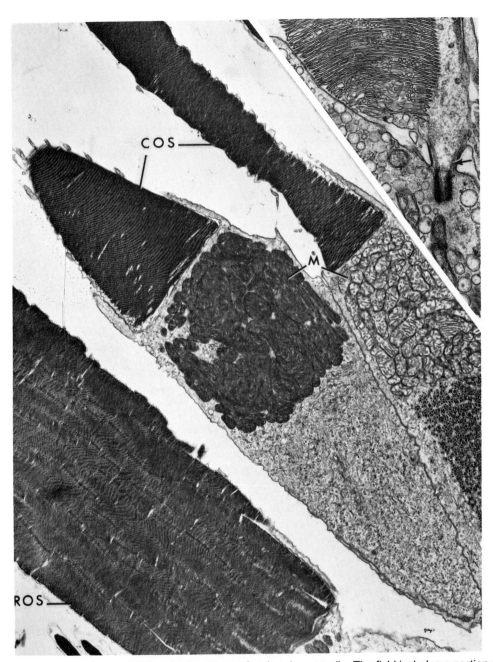

Figure 22.15. Electron micrograph of portions of rod and cone cells. The field includes a portion of the outer segment of a rod (*ROS*) and the outer segments of a double cone (*COS*). The field also includes cone inner segments, showing closely packed mitochondria (*M*) in the outer portion of the inner segment. Endoplasmic reticulum is found chiefly in the inner portion of the inner segment. The electron-dense granules seen in the inner segment of one of the cones represent glycogen. *Inset, upper right,* junction of outer and inner segments of a photoreceptor cell at higher magnification. *Arrow,* connecting stalk. The electron-dense material subjacent to the stalk is the basal body. *Lower figure,* from a newt, *Taricha torosa* (×7200); *inset,* a photoreceptor cell from the same species at higher magnification (×16,450). (*Lower figure* courtesy of Dr. Anita Hendrickson.)

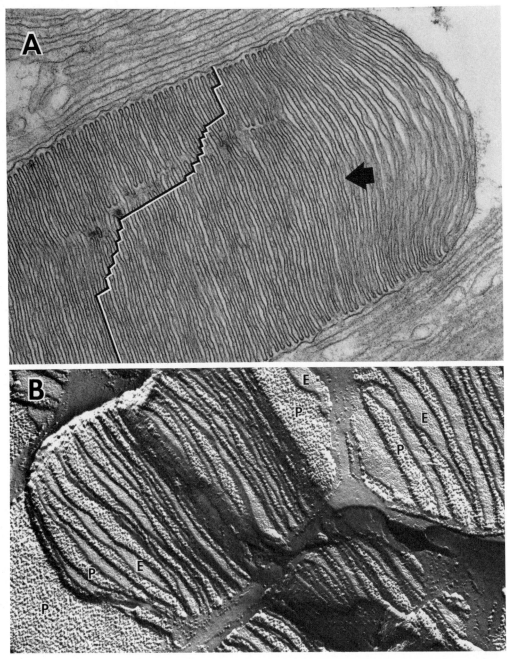

Figure 22.16. *A,* high magnification electron micrograph showing vertical section through the distal tip of a rod outer segment. The flattened membranous sacs, or disks, are packed within the plasma membrane. The *zig-zag line* denotes the approximate plane of fracture which occurred during freeze-fracture preparation of the replica seen in *B.* If, after fracture, the tip of the outer segment is lost and the exposed stump (*zig-zag line*) is replicated and viewed from the direction of the *arrow,* alternating layers of exposed disk membrane P and E faces are revealed. The tightly congregated particles on the P faces are believed to mark the location of rhodopsin molecules (×65,000). (Both micrographs in collaboration with Dr. Gregory Hageman.)

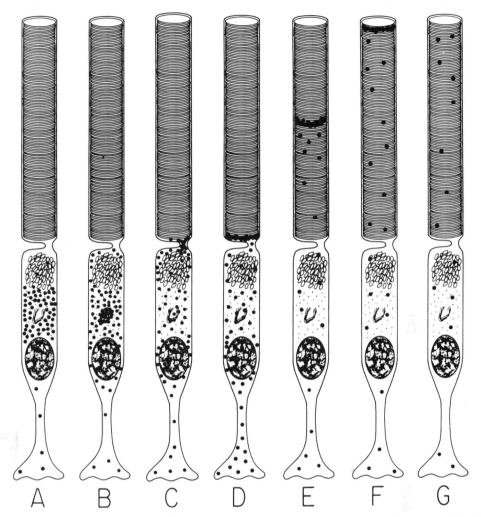

A   B   C   D   E   F   G

Figure 22.17.   Diagrammatic representation of the results of radioautographic studies of frog retinae fixed at different intervals of time after injection of labeled amino acids. Labeled material in newly synthesized protein (*dots*) is found in the region of the endoplasmic reticulum and the Golgi complex within 10 min after the injection (*A* and *B*). At later intervals, the newly formed protein passes around the mitochondria of the outer segment and reaches the connecting stalk (*C*). The synthesized protein is found in a newly formed basal disc of the outer segment in about 1 week (*D*), then moves outward (*E*) and reaches the end of the outer segment in about 8 weeks (*F* and *G*). (Courtesy of Dr. Richard W. Young.)

When the retina is removed from the fresh eye of an animal which has been kept in the dark, it appears purplish-red in color. The color fades rapidly when the preparation is exposed to light. Rod pigment, *rhodopsin* or *visual purple*, consists of vitamin A aldehyde, now known as *retinal* (formerly called retinene) combined with a protein known as *rod opsin*. When a pigment molecule is exposed to light, there is a steric change in the form of the retinal (from *cis* to *trans*) and the relationship between retinal and its combined protein is broken. This leads to a change in electrical potential in the cell that results in the formation of a membrane generator potential (signal). This signal is transmitted through the rod cell and along a basally directed process known as the *rod spherule*. This is the site of synaptic contact of rod basal process and the dendrites of a bipolar cell. After light stimulation, the visual purple is rapidly reconstituted.

Animals that are particularly active at night (e.g., rats and mice) have many rods and few or no cones. Animals active only in daytime have retinas composed almost entirely of cones (e.g., diurnal lizards and turtles). The respective roles of the mixed population of rods and cones in the human eye are well-established. The rods have a low threshold of stimulation by light, are particularly important in intensity (dark and light) discrimination and are active in night vision.

The Cone Cells

Except in the region of the fovea centralis and its immediate vicinity, the cones are flask-shaped, having a relatively short and conical outer segment and a relatively broad and bulbous inner segment. The region that connects the cone inner segment to the cone body is short and it is not constricted as it is in the rods (Fig. 22.12). Cone outer segments are composed of sacs somewhat like those of the rods. The cone sacs differ, however, in that they remain attached to the enveloping ciliary plasma membrane from which they arise, are less closely packed, and they become progressively smaller in diameter along the length of the cone (Figs. 22.14 through 22.16). The cone outer segment is attached to the cone inner segment by a ciliary stalk that is similar in structure to that in the rod.

In some species, the inner segment often contains a characteristic oil droplet or accumulations of glycogen just beneath the connecting cilium. Otherwise it resembles the rod inner segment in having a region of closely packed mitochondria followed by a region containing the Golgi complex and smooth and rough endoplasmic reticulum.

The basal regions of cone cells broaden into an extensive synaptic apparatus known as the *cone pedicle.*

Radioautographic studies of retinas sacrificed at intervals subsequent to injection of labeled amino acids show that new pro-teins are also synthesized in the inner segments of the cones (i.e., in the regions of the rough endoplasmic reticulum and Golgi complex) just as in the rods. The new proteins, however, are transported more rapidly into and along the cone outer segments by comparison to the longer sequential pattern in the rods. However, there is no doubt that the cone is renewed by the progressive formation of new sacs. When sacs form during the cyclic regeneration of a cone outer segment, each newly formed sac at the base of the stack is larger than the preceding one, and thus the cone becomes tapered or conical in shape. The functional significance of this fact and mechanism by which it is achieved remain mysteries.

The visual pigments of the cones are associated with the sacs of the outer segment, as in rods. However, in the cones, the pigment consists of retinal (retinene) combined with one of *three* different cone opsins, depending upon the type of cone and its particular wavelength (color) sensitivity. The basic steps in light absorption and in the generation of an impulse are similar to those of rods, but cones respond to light of relatively high intensity, and they function for visual acuity and for color perception, especially under daylight intensity. Detection of different colors apparently depends upon the presence of the different pigments in the cones, each absorbing light most efficiently at red, blue or green wavelengths. Rods, on the other hand, apparently have only one type of pigment.

Plexiform and Nuclear Layers

These are shown in Figs. 22.18 and 22.19. The external limiting "membrane" is really not a discrete membrane, but rather a region of junctional complexes between the microvillous outer ends of the supporting retinal neuroglial cells (*Müller's cells*) and the adjoining photoreceptor cells. It is more accurately termed the *outer junctional zone.*

The outer nuclear layer consists of rod and cone cell bodies containing their nuclei. The cone nuclei are located close to the outer junctional zone, and with the exception of the region of the fovea, they are limited to a single row. The rod nuclei are more numerous than cone nuclei, except in the fovea, and are distributed in several layers.

The outer plexiform layer is composed chiefly of the basally directed processes (*spherules* and *pedicles*) of rod and cone cells, the dendrites of bipolar cells, and processes of horizontal cells (see below). These are in synaptic relationship with the spherules or pedicles acting as presynaptic components in transferral of the photoreceptor generator potential to the bipolar cells where it is converted to a membrane potential. Synaptic contacts with the horizontal cells and between spherules and pedicles themselves integrate and modify the photoreceptor input. The spherules of rods are indented, enclosing the dendrites of one or more bipolar cells and several horizontal cells in an enclosed synaptic cleft (Figs. 22.19 and 22.20). The presynaptic (photoreceptor) element is characterized by typical hollow synaptic vesicles plus a *synaptic ribbon*, an unusual organelle common to several types of receptor cells. Synaptic ribbons are dense proteinaceous plaques oriented perpendicular to the synaptic surface and bounded by numerous vesicles (Fig. 22.21). Cone pedicles are much larger in their dimensions, contain several synaptic indentations incorporating the processes of many bipolar and horizontal cells and display multiple synaptic ribbons (Figs. 22.20 and 22.21).

The *inner nuclear layer* is thinner than the outer nuclear layer but resembles it in general appearance. It contains the nuclei of the *bipolar neurons*, nuclei of association neurons known as *horizontal cells* and *amacrine cells*, nuclei of the supporting *Müller's cells*, and nuclei of other astrocyte-like glial cells. In general, the nuclei of this layer are arranged in three zones: an outer one of horizontal cell nuclei; a middle one of bipolar cell nuclei; and an inner one in which amacrine cell nuclei predominate (Fig. 22.20). The morphology and interrelationships of these cells are discussed below.

Müller's cells are the most obvious glial population of the neural retina. Their distribution and relationships resemble to some degree the fibrous astrocytes of the central nervous system (CNS). The Müller's cell processes course among receptor and other cell bodies and processes, extending from the inner to outer limiting "membranes."

The *inner plexiform layer* consists of the processes of the amacrine cells, the axons of the bipolar cells and the profusely branched dendrites of the *ganglion cells*. An intricate array of synaptic interconnections of all these cells provides an appropriately integrated and controlled input to the ganglion cells. The axonal terminals of bipolar cells are unusual for neurons in that they contain synaptic ribbons.

The *ganglion cell layer* is composed of multipolar ganglion cells, among which are scattered neuroglial cells. Branches of the retinal blood vessels are also present. The several types of ganglion cells are variable in size (11 to 30 μm) with clear round nuclei containing one or more prominent nucleoli.

The *nerve fiber layer* consists of the axons of the ganglion cells. These nonmyelinated fibers are arranged in bundles which run parallel to the inner surface of the retina and converge at the optic disk to form the optic nerve. Between the bundles are numerous fibrous astrocyte-like cells (*spider cells*) and rows of Müller's cell processes. Also present in this layer are the retinal blood vessels, indented into the retinal epithelium much in the manner seen for vessels supplying the central nervous system.

The *"internal limiting membrane"* is formed by the apposition of the expanded inner processes of Müller's cells, their basal lamina, and their relation to the basal (vitreal) surface; a situation homologous to the glia limitans externa of the CNS.

Retinal Modification in the Maculae Lutea and Fovea Centralis

Near the posterior pole of the eye, the human neural retina shows a funnel-shaped

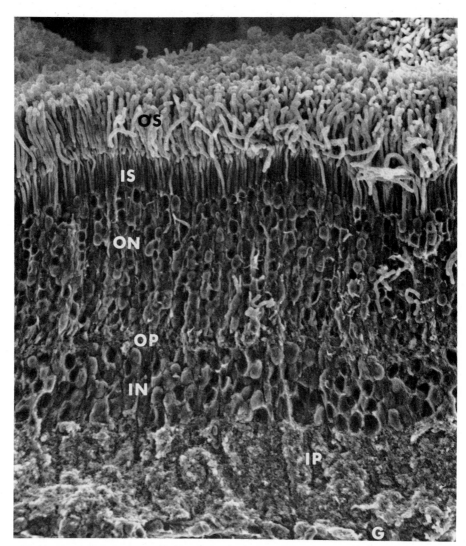

Figure 22.18. Scanning electron micrograph of a cross-fractured hamster neural retina. The pigment epithelium has been removed, exposing photoreceptor outer segments (*OS*). Other visible layers include inner segments (*IS*), outer nuclear layer (*ON*), outer plexiform layer (*OP*), inner nuclear layer (*IN*), inner plexiform layer (*IP*), and a portion of the ganglion cell layer (*G*) (×800). (Micrograph in collaboration with Dr. Gregory S. Hageman.)

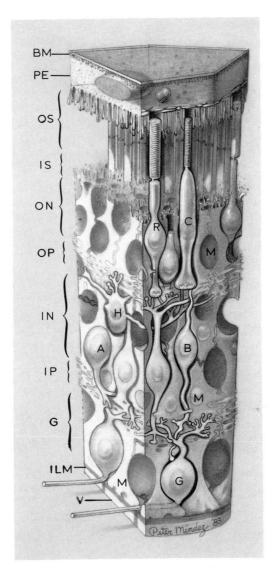

Figure 22.19. Principal layers and component cell types within the neural retina and pigment epithelium (*PE*). Retinal layers are labeled as in Figure 22.18. Also shown are Bruch's membrane (*BM*), the inner limiting membrane (*ILM*), and the edge of the vitreous body (*V*). The basic relationships among rod (*R*) and cone (*C*) photoreceptors and also bipolar (*B*), horizontal (*H*), amacrine (*A*), and ganglion (*G*) neurons are depicted. Müller cells (*M*) and their processes occupy nearly all non-neuronal, non-photoreceptor space.

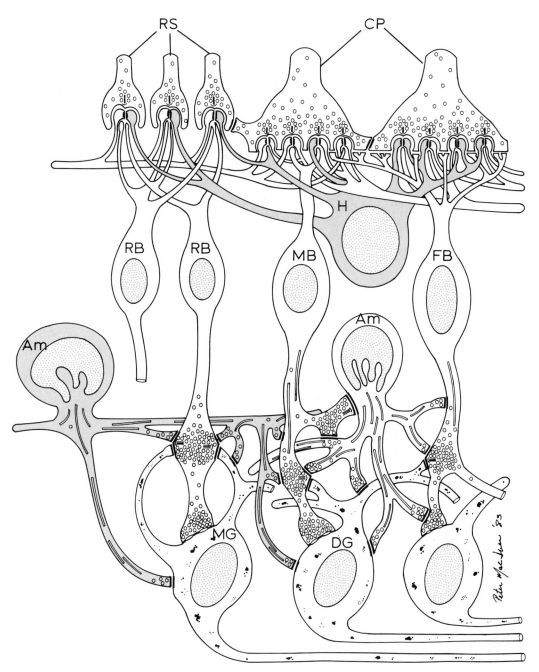

Figure 22.20. Major synaptic circuitry known to exist among photoreceptor and neuronal cells of the neural retina. Rod spherules (*RS*) have synaptic contacts with rod bipolar cells (*RB*) and horiziontal cells (*H*). Cone pedicles (*CP*) display contacts with midget bipolar cells (*MB*), flat bipolar cells (*FB*) and horizontal cells. Amacrine cells (*AM*) make synaptic contact with midget ganglion cells (*MG*) and diffuse ganglion cells (*DG*) as well as with bipolar cells. The most direct synaptic path from photoreceptor to ganglion cell is via bipolar cells. Other pathways and cell types than shown are being elucidated by current investigations. (Adapted from M. J. Hogan, J. A. Alvarado, and J. E. Weddell: *Histology of the Human Eye. An Atlas and Textbook.* Philadelphia, W. B. Saunders, 1971. After J. E. Dowling and B. B. Boycott: *Proc R Soc Lond (Biol)* 166:80–111, 1966.)

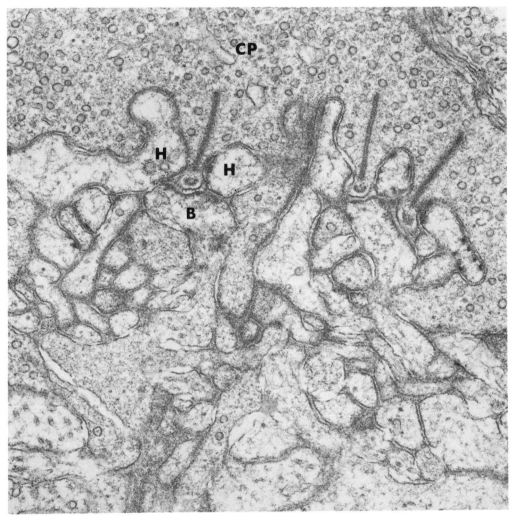

Figure 22.21. High magnification electron micrograph of the outer plexiform layer in a goldfish retina. A cone pedicle (*CP*) is seen with numerous synaptic vesicles distributed in its cytoplasm. Three synaptic ribbons occupy positions juxtaposed to areas of synaptic contact along the basal surface of the indented pedicle. Bipolar (*B*) and horizontal (*H*) cell processes make synaptic contact with the pedicle at these points (×48,750). (Courtesy of Dr. Dean Bok.)

depression of its layers. This region has a yellowish color when viewed in gross specimens; hence, it is named the *macula lutea*, or yellow spot. The inner layers of the retina are deviated from the center of the region, leaving a small pit known as the *fovea centralis* (Fig. 22.22). There the photoreceptors consist only of cones. In the center of the fovea, in an area which is about 0.5 mm in diameter, the cones are extremely slender and closely packed. This appears to explain partly the high visual acuity of the fovea.

Peripheral to the foveal region, rod receptors gradually increase among the cones until three to four rods intervene between individual cones in areas peripheral to the macula. It has been estimated that there are about 7,000,000 cones in the retina; of this number, about 13,000 are said to be in the macular region and about 4,000 in the fovea centralis. Estimates of the number of rods range from 75,000,000 to 170,000,000.

Retinal Interneuronal Associations and Functions

The chief interneuronal relationships in the retina, as currently described and interpreted from electron microscopic studies, are shown schematically in Figure 22.20. The cone pedicles make separate synaptic contacts with dendrites of two types of bipolar cells: *midget bipolars* and *flat bipolars*. It seems, in the fovea at least, that a single midget bipolar cell is in synaptic contact with a single cone. This appears correlated with the high visual acuity of the central part of the fovea. Contact of the midget bipolar cell dendrite with the cone cell terminal forms a part of a triadic synaptic complex, with the dendritic ending of the bipolar cell located between endings of

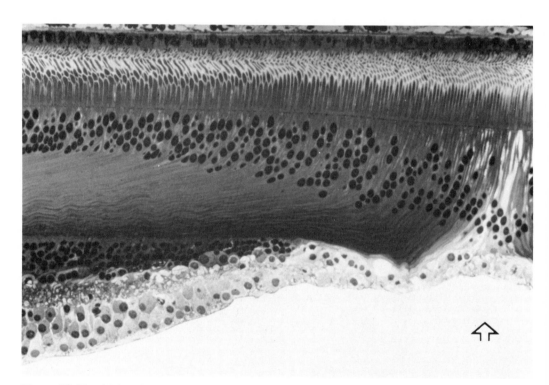

Figure 22.22. Light micrograph of a section through the fovea centralis (*arrow*) of a human retina. Note thinning and lateral displacement of nuclear, plexiform, and ganglion cell layers, as well as abundance of cone photoreceptors. Compare with Figure 22.5 (×200). (Courtesy of Dr. Donald Minckler.)

two separate horizontal cells. Contacts between rod and cone cell terminals are present also, but the significance of some of these contacts is not fully understood.

Each *rod bipolar* cell synapses with several rod cells (only two are included Fig. 22.20). This correlates with the finding that rods generally function as groups. Rod cell terminals are also in contact with processes of the horizontal cells.

The cell bodies of the amacrine cells, located in the inner cell layer of the retina, have processes that extend into the inner plexiform layer where they make contact with axon terminals of all types of bipolar cells and with the dendrites of both types of ganglion cells. They also make contact with each other; i.e., amacrine to amacrine contact.

Two types of ganglion cells have been identified: *midget ganglion cells*, with each cell dendrite in contact with the axon of a single midget bipolar cell, and *diffuse ganglion cells* which make contact with all types of bipolar cells. The synapses of the bipolar cells with the diffuse ganglion cells are both axodendritic and axosomatic in type.

The above retinal interneuronal relationships are significant in relation to the arrangement of retinal visual fields. The *visual field* of a particular ganglion cell is defined as that area of the retina which, upon stimulation, affects the ganglion cell. Each visual field consists functionally of a central region and a peripheral region; in light-adapted retinas, these two concentric fields function antagonistically. For example, if a given ganglion cell is excited when light is applied to the center of its visual field it will be inhibited when light is applied to the periphery of its field. When light is applied to the periphery and center of the field of the particular ganglion cell at the same time, there is a summation of effects and the ganglion cell gives a weak response. In color vision, it appears that the center of a field responds maximally to light of another wavelength. In other words, the antagonistic central and peripheral zones of a field may be color coded.

The diameters of visual fields, particularly the diameters of the central portions of the fields, differ in different parts of the retina. In visual fields of the fovea, the diameter of the center of the field may be within the magnitude of the diameter of a single cone. This is another factor underlying the greater visual acuity of the foveal region.

The antagonistic responses to stimulation of "central" and "surround" regions of visual fields appear to correlate with the arrangement of neurons shown in Figure 22.20. A change in light intensity at the center of a field sets up a stimulus which is probably transmitted by direct receptor-bipolar-ganglion cell contacts. In cone vision, this is by cone cell-midget bipolar cell-midget ganglion cell. On the other hand, a change in light intensity in the peripheral portion of the visual field of a ganglion cell sets up a stimulus which reaches the ganglion cell by a circuitous route that is apparently mediated by amacrine-amacrine cell contacts along the way.

The intricate circuitry of bipolar, ganglion, horizontal, and amacrine cells undoubtedly underlies many more modulating, feedback and coordinating processes in this first level of visual integration. Some of these are beginning to be uncovered with newer methods. Functional understanding of the system is further complicated by recent reports of *efferent* fibers coursing from the brain to the retina, presumably performing some feedback or modulating task. Additionally, new neuronal cell types are being described as essential parts of the circuitry. For example, an *interplexiform cell* has recently been noted in the inner nuclear layer of several species. It apparently establishes synaptic contact among several amacrine cells. Much is yet to be learned before the circuitry of this cell gains functional understanding.

Blood Vessels of the Retina

The layer of rod and cone outer and inner segments, the outer nuclear layer, and the outer plexiform layer are devoid of blood vessels. Their nourishment comes from the choriocapillaris of the choroid. The remaining layers of the retina are supplied by a system of retinal vessels derived from the central *retinal artery*, which enters the eye in the optic nerve (into which it gained entrance via the embryonic optic fissure). The larger arteries lie indented into the nerve fiber layer, with finer branches looping into the ganglion cell and inner plexiform layers. Two capillary networks are formed, one in the nerve fiber layer and another which extends as far as the outer border of the inner nuclear layer. Like capillaries of the CNS epithelium, those of the neural retina are continuous (nonfenestrated). The retinal veins follow the course of the arteries.

The Ora Serrata

The scalloped anterior border of the neural retina is the ora serrata (Figs. 22.1 and 22.2), its margin forming a step which may be rounded, angular or even overhanging. Approaching this region, the rods and cones become shorter and thicker, the nuclear layers thinner and the ganglion cell and nerve fiber layers are lacking. There is a corresponding increase in the number of glial cells.

The Pigment Epithelium

The function of the pigment epithelium is beginning to be elucidated coincident with experiments cited above concerning membrane protein turnover in photoreceptor inner and outer segments. The thin apical processes of the pigment epithelial cells surround and interdigitate with the outer segments. Hence, it has been suspected that they might serve a role of physical and/or metabolic support for the photoreceptors. In many lower vertebrates the processes are rich in pigment granules, and these migrate up and down each process in response to illumination, seemingly masking to a degree the outer segments in conditions of bright light and, conversely, exposing them in dim light or darkness. The processes are also present and closely associated with outer segments in the human

retina, but they are not highly pigmented, so dim/bright retinal accommodation occurs chiefly through other mechanisms. However, tracer experiments with labeled vitamin A and studies of hereditary and vitamin A deficiency induced retinal dystrophy suggest that the epithelium, via its processes, serves as a storage site in the continual cyclic supply of this vitamin to the outer segment membranes. As new flattened membrane sacs are being added to the bases of rod and cone outer segments bunches of them are released at the distal tips. These cast-off membranes are phagocytized by the nearby pigment epithelial cells (Figs. 22.23 and 22.24) and their components are either degraded and removed or recycled to the photoreceptors. The shedding of photoceptor membranes follows a diurnal rhythm related to periods of maximum activity for each type of receptor. Packets of rod sacs are shed after the onset of daylight in experimental animals and cone sacs are shed either after light onset or well after dark onset. Replenishment of rod outer segment membranes clearly follows the period of greatest demand for rod vision (dim light), but replenishment of cone outer segment membranes appears to be less restricted in time.

It appears that the membrane recycling accounts for sequential and progressive renewal of rod and cone opsins into the outer segments. Vitamin A, however, may be recycled from the pigment epithelium by another mechanism which reinserts it more generally over the whole outer segment.

The Optic Nerve

The nerve fibers of the retina converge at the optic disc and turn outward to pass through the sieve-like *lamina cribrosa* as the optic nerve (Fig. 22.25). In this intraocular portion, the nerve has a structure similar to that of the nerve fiber layer; i.e., bundles of nonmyelinated fibers surrounded by glial cell processes.

Immediately behind the lamina cribrosa, the nerve fibers acquire myelin sheaths, with a consequent increase in diameter of the entire nerve. Since the optic nerve actually is a tract of the brain rather than a true peripheral nerve, it is not surprising that it should resemble the CNS in its coverings and its histological characteristics.

The myelinated orbital portion of the optic nerve is surrounded by three connective tissue sheaths: an outer *dura*, an inner *pia* and an intermediate *arachnoid*, which houses a *subarachnoid space*. These sheaths are continuous with the corresponding meninges of the brain; at the bulb, the arachnoid and pia blend with the choroid and the sclera. The subarachnoid space is not detectable by light microscopy as the nerve nears the lamina cribrosa.

From the pial sheath, connective tissue trabeculae invaginate with basal laminae into the nerve and in conjunction with the arrangement of neuroglial elements form a system of septa which enclose groups of nerve fiber bundles. Between the bundles are glial cells whose processes and fibers penetrate between the individual nerve fibers.

For a distance of about 12 mm behind the eye, the septa are united to a central core of connective tissue, the *central supporting tissue strand* (a remnant of the fused embryonic optic fissure). This carries the *central artery* and *central vein* of the retina. Small branches from these vessels course in the septal system to supply the nerve itself.

The Lens

The lens (Fig. 22.26) is a transparent and somewhat plastic biconvex epithelial body situated between the iris and the vitreous body. Its posterior surface has a greater convexity than the anterior surface (Fig. 22.1). Three structural components make up the lens, a *capsule*, an *anterior epithelium* and the *lens "substance."*

The capsule consists of a basal lamina and reticular lamina ensheathing the lens. Actually, it is the basement membrane that has surrounded the lens since its emergence as an epithelial lens vesicle. It is of varied thickness in different parts of the lens but always thinnest at the posterior pole. A zone concentric with the equator serves for the insertion of the *zonular fibers* of the *suspensory ligament* (Fig. 22.3).

The anterior epithelium is a single layer of cuboidal cells on the anterior lens surface, just under the capsule. The posterior epithelial cells have been greatly modified to form the primitive *lens fibers* during embryonic development. At the equator, or margin, the cells are elongated and arranged meridionally in rows (Fig. 22.27). This is the region where new lens fibers are constantly being formed during lens growth, and the cells themselves may be regarded as young lens fibers.

The lens substance consists of elongated prismatic lens fibers. The first fibers that form during embryonic development arise by elongation and differentiation of the posterior epithelial cells of the lens vesicle, and they are oriented in an anteroposterior direction. Succeeding fibers are formed superficially by mitosis, elongation and differentiation of epithelial cells at the equator of the lens. Consequently, these fibers are arranged meridionally in concentric layers. The older and deeper fibers lose their nuclei but the epithelial cells near the equator continue to multiply and differentiate into new lens fibers. As a result, the concentric layers show varying degrees of differentiation. Individual fibers can be identified more readily in the outer part of the lens, known as the *cortex*, than in the inner part, sometimes called the *nucleus*, where the fibers are condensed and more homogeneous. The regions of the lens where cortical fibers from opposite sectors converge and make contact are known as lens *sutures*.

Ultrastructurally the epithelial cells of the equatorial region have numerous interdigitations and occasional desmosomes. The lens fibers also show interdigitations, particularly in the so-called sutures. Both epithelial cells and fibers are remarkable in the extent to which their adjacent cell surfaces are occupied by communicating (gap) junctions. The functional significance of this high degree of apparent coupling remains unclear. However, the lens, like the

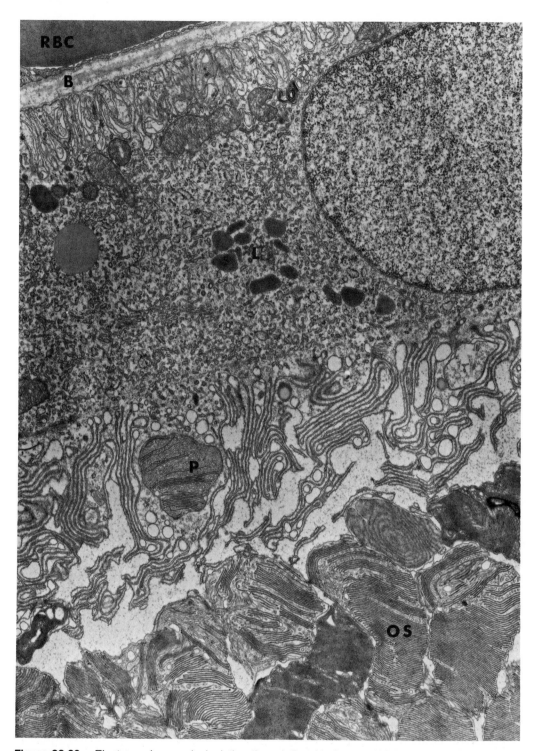

Figure 22.23. Electron micrograph depicting the relationship between the pigment epithelium and retinal rod outer segments (*OS*) in an albino rat. A pigment epithelial cell is seen with its nucleus (*upper right*), lysosomes (*L*) and numerous pleated apical processes extending toward the disorganized tips of the outer segments. Unlike normally pigmented animals the albino rat does not possess pigment granules in its pigment epithelial cells. A portion of one outer segment tip (*P*) has been phagocytized by the pigment epithelial cell.Bruch's membrane (*B*) is seen to consist of the epithelial basal lamina, connective tissue and the basal lamina of a capillary in the choroid. A red blood cell (*RBC*) occupies the choriocapillaris whose endothelial wall is richly fenestrated. Note the folded basal surface of the pigment epithelial cell (×14,000). (Courtesy of Dr. David Chase.)

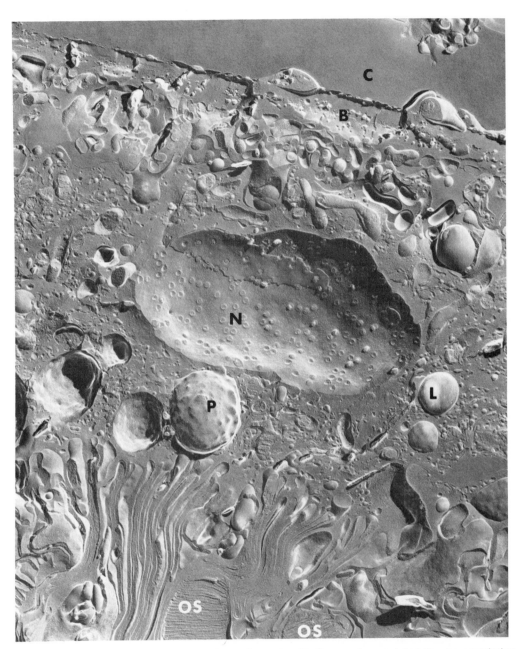

Figure 22.24. Freeze-fracture replica of the pigment epithelium and associated tissues correlating to that seen in Figure 22.23. Note photoreceptor outer segments (*OS*) and their relation to pleated apical processes of the pigment epithelium. A phagosome (*P*) containing shed outer segment material is visible as well as several lysosomes (*L*), nuclear envelope (*N*), folded pigment epithelium basal surface adjacent to Bruch's membrane (*B*), and the fenestrated endothelium of the choriocapillaris (*C*) (×15,800). (Micrograph in collaboration with Dr. Gregory S. Hageman.)

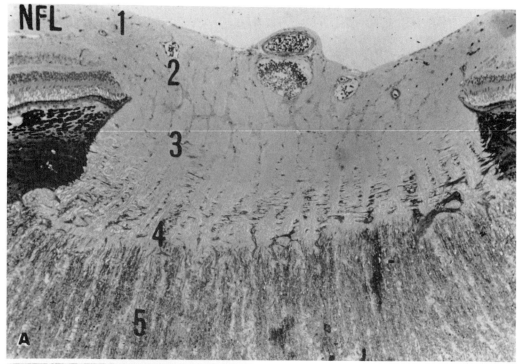

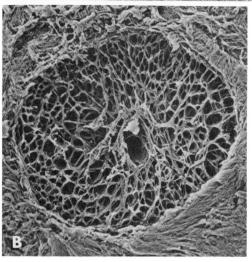

Figure 22.25. *A,* light micrograph showing a horizontal section through a human optic nerve head. The central artery is seen bordering the vitreous chamber at top center. The axons of the retinal nerve fiber layer (*NFL*) converge at *1* and *2,* descend past the choroid at *3,* penetrate the lamina cribrosa at *4,* and become myelinated within the optic nerve at *5* (×100). (Courtesy of Dr. Donald Minckler.) *B,* scanning electron micrograph of an optic nerve head, viewed from the vitreous chamber after the retinal components, axons, myelin, and glial elements have been corrosion digested to reveal the lacy collagenous network of the lamina cribrosa (×33). (Courtesy of Dr. Jeh Chin.)

cornea, is avascular and totally dependent for its nutrition upon the circulating intraocular fluid and transport by its own cells.

The Zonula Ciliaris

The *zonula ciliaris* (*zonule of Zinn, suspensory ligament*) is a system of delicate collagenous fibers which form a fairly thick band radiating from the equatorial zone of the lens capsule to the inner surface of the ciliary body, thereby fixing the lens in place (Fig. 22.3). Many of the fibers arise from the orbiculus ciliaris and sweep forward over the surface of the ciliary body to the lens capsule. Others come from the corona ciliaris. They arise from the basement membrane in the valleys between the ciliary processes (Figs. 22.6 and 22.7) and are closely applied to the sides of the latter as they course radially inward to the lens.

The zonular fibers are inserted on the lens capsule in two main zones: in front of the equator and just behind it. Those inserting in front are thicker.

Recalling the arrangement of the smooth muscle fibers of the ciliary muscle and its

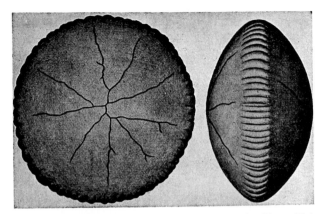

Figure 22.26. The lens, viewed from behind and from the side. (From Eisler, after Rabl.)

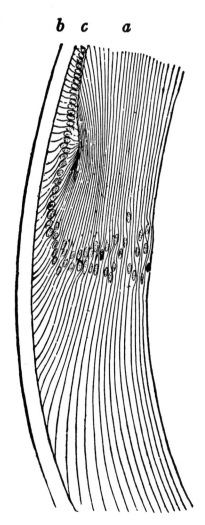

b c a

Figure 22.27. Drawing illustrating a section through the margin of lens, showing longitudinal sections of lens fibers and transition from epithelium to lens fibers. *a*, lens fibers; *b*, capsule; *c*, epithelium. (Merkel-Henle.)

attachment anteriorly to the scleral spur, it becomes evident that contraction of this muscle will cause the ciliary body and choroid to be pulled forward, while the ciliary processes will at the same time be displaced toward the equator of the lens. The result of both actions will be to relax the tension normally maintained on the zonular fibers. The highly elastic lens capsule, released from tension, is thus enabled to compress the plastic lens cortex to a more spherical form. This constitutes the process of *accommodation*, by which images of near objects are brought to correct focus on the retina. It should be noted that in a state of rest, the ciliary muscle is relaxed and the zonula ciliaris and lens are under tension.

The Vitreous Body

The *vitreous body* occupies the space between the lens and the retina. (This space is not the posterior chamber.) In the fresh condition, the vitreous body is a transparent, firm jelly-like body (actually a form of connective tissue). The molecular meshwork provided by its fibers and ground substance molecules provides for percolation of the intraocular fluid (aqueous humor) during its normal circulation through anterior, posterior and vitreous chambers. The vitreous body is particularly adherent to the retina in the region of the ora serrata and at the optic disc. On its anterior surface is a broad shallow depression, the *patellar fossa*, which accommodates the posterior convexity of the lens. From the optic disc to the patellar fossa, runs the *hyaloid canal*, which marks the site of the fetal hyaloid artery. In electron micrographs, the vitreous body appears to have a dispersed collagenous fibrillar structure, somewhat condensed along anterior and posterior margins.

The Eyelids

The eyelids are movable folds which protect the eye from injury and excessive light. Each lid is covered by a thin skin, which on the posterior surface is modified to form a transparent mucous membrane, the *conjunctiva*. This lines the lid as the *palpebral conjunctiva* and is reflected onto the anterior surface of the eye up to the cornea as the *bulbar conjunctiva*. The reflection forms a deep recess known as the *fornix*. The form of the lid is maintained by a tough fibrous *tarsal plate*. In the connective tissue between this and the anterior surface are the palpebral fibers of the *orbicularis oculi muscle*. Associated with the free margin of the lid are the *eyelashes* and certain small glands (Fig. 22.28).

The upper and lower lid are similar in all main respects. The skin is thin. It is provided with many fine downy hairs, with which are associated small sebaceous glands. Numerous small sweat glands and pigment cells are also present. The subcutaneous layer is a loose connective tissue, rich in elastic fibers, containing no fat, and loosely adherent to underlying muscle.

The *orbicularis oculi* is a thin oval sheet of concentrically disposed skeletal muscle, innervated by the facial nerve, and loosely united to the underlying tarsel plate by submuscular connective tissue. Its action is to bring the lids together. Tendon fibers of the *superior levator palpebrae* muscle pass through the connective tissue either to insert on the lower anterior surface of the tarsal plate or to attach to the skin of the lid. This muscle acts to raise the lid.

The *tarsal plate*, or *tarsus*, is a curved plate of dense fibrous connective tissue with some elastic fibers. Its lower free border extends to the lid margin and its upper border serves for attachment of the invol-

untary *superior palpebral muscle* (muscle of Müller). Embedded in the tarsal plate are simple branched alveolar *tarsal* or *Meibomian glands*. These sebaceous glands are arranged in a single row with their long axes perpendicular to the lid margin. Each gland consists of a long straight central duct into which numerous alveoli open. The ducts are lined by simple cuboidal epithelium and open onto the lid margin by a series of minute orifices. Their fatty secretion lubricates the lids, preventing them from sticking and forming a seal when closed.

The eyelashes, arranged in two or three irregular rows in the lid margin, are short heavy curved hairs. Their follicles extend obliquely up to the tarsal plate. They lack arrector pilori muscles. Large sebaceous glands are associated with them as well as large spiral sweat glands.

The *conjunctiva* consists of an epithelium and a connective tissue substantia propria Fig. 22.29. At the lid margin, the epithelium has the stratified squamous character of the epidermis with which it is continuous. Over the tarsal plates (palpebral conjunctiva), it is reduced to two layers of cells; the surface cells are tall columnar and the deeper ones, low cuboidal. In the fornix a third layer of cells appears. Toward the limbus, the bulbar conjunctival epithelium is thickened, the superficial cells becoming flatter and the deep cells cuboidal. At the limbus it is stratified squamous. Throughout the conjunctiva, but particularly in the fornix and bulbar region, goblet cells occur.

The substantia propria consists of a thin layer of fine connective tissue fibers in which a profuse infiltration of lymphocytes occurs, especially in the region between the upper border of the tarsal plate and the fornix. Over the tarsal plate, the substantia propria firmly anchors the epithelium; elsewhere, it merges with the richly elastic subconjunctival connective tissue.

In the subconjunctival tissue above the upper border of the tarsal plate are several small tubuloalevolar glands. Their ducts open on the conjunctival surface. Small accessory lacrimal glands lie in the loose

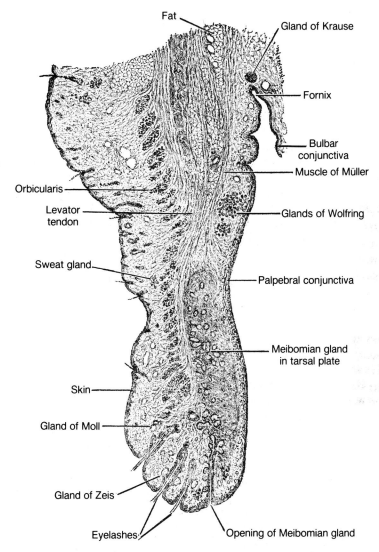

Figure 22.28. Drawing illustrating a vertical section through a human upper lid.

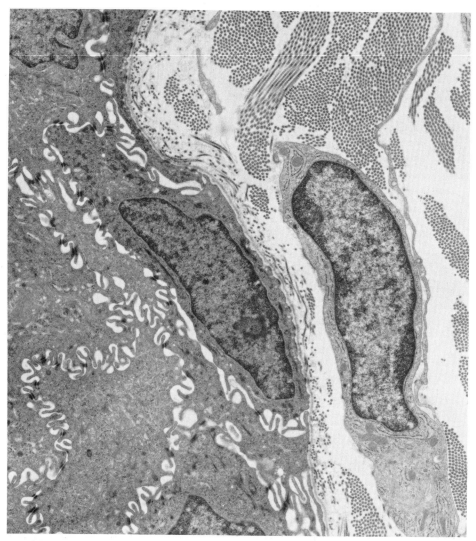

Figure 22.29. Electron micrograph of the basal portion of bulbar conjunctiva. Part of the stratified squamous epithelium is seen at *left*. Connective tissue of the mucosa seen at *right* merges with the sclera to the right of the field of view (×9,100). (Micrograph in collaboration with Dr. Gregory S. Hageman.)

connective tissue beneath the fornix conjunctivae and open into the margin of the fornix.

The Lacrimal Glands

The lacrimal gland lies in the superior temporal region of the orbit, just within the orbital margin. It is divided into a *superior* and an *inferior lobe*, which are continuous around the lateral horn of the aponeurosis of the levator muscle. It secretes the tears, which empty into the conjunctival sac through 10 or 12 ducts opening just in front of the superior fornix.

The lacrimal gland is a serous compound tubuloalveolar gland. It resembles the parotid gland. There are numerous myoepithelial cells at the base of the epithelium. The smaller secretory ducts are lined by a single layer of cuboidal cells; the larger ducts have a double-layered epithelium.

The stroma consists of loose connective tissue which blends with surrounding structures. In the adult, considerable lymphatic tissue occurs in the stroma.

THE EAR

The ear contains a series of receptors specialized for hearing and also for the perception of the position of the head and head movement. The receptors for these diverse functions are housed within the same organ because each employs the same basic cytological mechanism—an epithelial cell surmounted by a group of projections called cell "hairs" (actually modified microvillar and ciliary projections). When its hairs are bent in a particular plane and to a given degree, the hair-carrying cell generates signals at a specific frequency and transmits these to afferent axonal endings along the basal surface of that cell. The afferent axons conduct the signals to the brain. Hair cells accomplish these diverse functions by three remarkable adaptations: (*a*) certain cells have minute weights positioned near the end of their projecting hairs; *gravity or linear movement* will variously bend these hairs and provide the basis for a series of nerve signals to the brain; (*b*) other groups of hair cells are surmounted by a gelatinous keel which is displaced by fluid flowing through a narrow channel; by evolving such devices in each of three body planes the amount and direction of any *angular movement* of the head can be signaled by the subjacent nerve endings; (*c*) still other hair cells are mounted between two flexible membranes so that their hairs are bent as the membranes are displaced in response to hydraulic movement induced by sound waves impinging on the eardrum; the signals sent to the brain from the nerve endings on these cells form the basis for *hearing*.

The apparatus for each of these types of reception is mounted within fluid-filled spaces deep within the petrous portion of the temporal bone of the skull. The complex of interconnecting channels containing these receptors is called the *inner ear*. The receptors for position and motion need no access to the external environment, but the mechanism for hearing requires a chamber, the *middle ear*, across which sound waves from the air are transmitted to the fluid spaces of the inner ear. In addition, a channel is required for the passage of sound waves from the external environment to the middle ear; the passageway is part of the *external ear*.

The sound waves collected by the external ear produce vibrations of the *tympanic membrane*, also known as the *ear drum* (Fig. 22.30). The latter forms the outer wall of the *tympanic cavity*, which, with the *auditory (Eustachian) tube*, comprises the middle ear. The tympanic cavity contains three articulated bones, the *auditory ossicles*. By movement of the ossicles, vibrations produced by the sound waves reach the inner ear. The inner ear consists of a complex of fluid-filled membranous chambers and canals known as the *membranous labyrinth* (Fig. 22.30). Localized areas of neuropeithelium in the membranous labyrinth supplied by the eighth cranial nerve comprise the sensory mechanisms discussed above (Fig. 22.31). The membranous labyrinth is, in turn, suspended within a

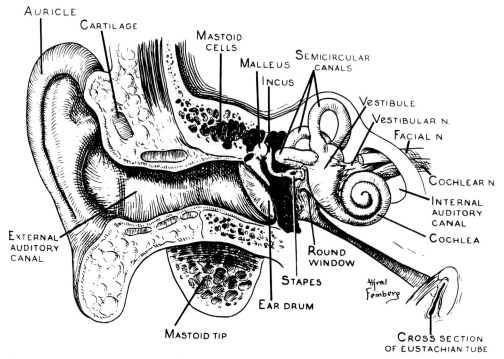

Figure 22.30. Diagram of the external ear (extending from the auricle to the eardrum), the middle ear (containing the middle ear ossicles, malleus, incus, and stapes and communicating with the pharynx via the Eustachian tube) and the inner ear (formed by the three semicircular canals, the vestibule, and the cochlea). The nerve signals arising from the inner ear travel to the brain via the cochlear and vestibular divisions of the eighth cranial nerve. (Reprinted with permission from H. Davis (ed): Hearing and Deafness: A Guide for Laymen. New York, Holt, Rinehart & Winston, 1947.)

fluid-filled cavity lined by layers of particularly hard bone, the *osseous labyrinth.* The osseous and membranous labyrinths of the inner ear lie in close proximity to the middle ear at two small membrane-covered apertures known, respectively, as the *oval window* and the *round window* (Figs. 22.30 and 22.34). The membrane of the former houses the base of one of the ossicles, the stapes; the membrane of the latter is known as the *secondary tympanic membrane.*

Otic Development

The membranous labyrinth is an evolutionary derivation of the anterior parts of a much simpler and superficial segmented system of vibratory sensing organs known in lower swimming vertebrates as the *lateral line system.* Concurrently, the middle ear ossicles have evolved from some of the articulating bones of more primitive jaws.

This evolution is reflected in the patterns of embryonic development of the mammalian ear, a pattern which also helps to clarify the adult morphology.

The membranous labyrinth is derived embryonically as an invaginating saccule, *the otocyst,* budded inward from the ectodermal epithelium on each side of the head. Through a series of epithelial outgrowths, constrictions, and coiling, it is shaped into its delicate *saccular* and *macular* parts plus three *semicircular canals* and the *cochlea.* Surrounding mesenchyme encases these in a fluid-filled casket of bone, while nearby the three ossicles take form by intramembranous ossification. All this development is occurring in the upper reaches of the first and second branchial arches. The first pharyngeal pouch will also be a major contributor. The rapidly expanding pouch engulfs the region of ossicle formation and extends well beyond, forming the large endodermal epithelium-lined tympanic cavity within the developing temporal bone. The ossicles remain articulated with each other, suspended across the tympanic cavity. Each is left enshrouded with a thin coat of mesenchyme and an endodermal epithelial covering that is continuous with that covering the walls of the cavity. The tympanic cavity similarly overgrows two muscles, the *stapedius* and *tensor tympani*, and a branch of the facial nerve, the *chorda tympani*. Concomitantly, the first branchial groove has deepened to form the *external auditory meatus* (*canal*). Its close relationship to the pouch is maintained so that the endodermal lining of the tympanic cavity remains closely adherent to the ectoderm of the meatus (with only scant intervening mesenchyme) in the area of the future *tympanic membrane* (eardrum). After the outermost ossicle, the *malleus*, is positioned on the tympanic surface of the eardrum, and the most medial one, the *stapes*, is similarly situated on the membrane of the oval window, the adult relationships of the ear have been established.

The External Ear

The external ear consists of the *auricle* or *pinna*, plus the external auditory canal. The auricle contains an irregularly shaped plate of elastic cartilage except in the *lobule*. The skin of the auricle is thin and contains numerous hairs and sebaceous glands; the posterior surface also has some sweat glands.

The external auditory canal (meatus) is a slightly S-shaped channel leading to the middle ear and separated from the latter by the tympanic membrane. The outer wall of the canal contains elastic cartilage while that of the inner portion is formed by a part of the temporal bone (Fig. 22.30). Both portions are lined by skin which is continuous with that of the auricle.

The skin which lines the cartilaginous portion of the auditory canal contains stiff hairs which guard against the entrance of foreign objects. It also contains sebaceous glands associated with the hairs. Simple coiled tubular glands are present and these open directly to the surface of the skin by long narrow ducts; these are known as *ceruminous glands* because they contribute to the ear wax, or *cerumen*, which consists of secretion from both types of glands plus desquamated epithelial cells. The cells of the ceruminous glands are columnar and contain numerous brown pigment granules and fat droplets.

The skin of the bony portion of the auditory canal is thinner and adheres closely to the periosteum. The hairs of this portion are fine; they and the sebaceous glands are present only on the superior wall of the canal.

The Middle Ear

The middle ear consists of an extensive series of air-filled spaces in the temporal bone, the main one being the *tympanic cavity*; this cavity is ventilated by the *auditory* (*Eustachian*) *tube* which, as a remnant of the first pouch, leads to the pharynx. The tympanic cavity is composed of a laterally compressed chamber, the *atrium*, and an *epitympanic recess*, the *attic*, above the level of the tympanic membrane. The cavity is continuous posteriorly, via the *tympanic antrum* with the *mastoid cells* which are air-filled spaces in the mastoid process of the temporal bone.

The lateral wall of the middle ear cavity is formed almost entirely by the *tympanic membrane*. The periphery of the membrane is fixed firmly by fibrocartilage in a groove (the *tympanic sulcus*) in the surrounding bony ring. Superiorly, the bony ring is notched, so that a small area of the membrane, the *pars flaccida* remains lax; the greater part is the *pars tensa*.

The bone-supported inner wall of the middle ear cavity bears a rounded eminence, the *promontory*, which marks the position of the first, or basal, coil of the underlying cochlea. Somewhat above and behind this is an oval aperture, the *oval window* onto the membrane of which fits the base of the stapes. Behind and below the promontory is a funnel-shaped recess which leads to a second aperture in the bone, the *round window* which is closed by the thin *secondary tympanic membrane.*

Extending across the tympanic cavity is the chain of three small bones, the *auditory ossicles* (Fig. 22.30). These, from without inward, are the *malleus* (hammer), the *incus* (anvil) and the *stapes* (stirrup). The *manubrium* (handle) of the malleus is attached to the tympanic membrane. Its head lies in the epitympanic recess, where it articulates with the head of the incus. The long process of the latter bends sharply near its end to articulate with the head of the stapes. The base of the stapes is fixed to the border of the oval window by a ring of elastic fibers.

Associated with the auditory ossicles are several ligaments and two small muscles, the *tensor tympani* and *stapedius* muscles.

Lining the tympanic cavity, and investing all the structures contained within, is the *tympanic mucosa.* This mucosa also lines the air-filled spaces of the mastoid bone and covers the inner surface of the tympanic membrane. Its thin connective tissue layer is covered in part by a simple squamous epithelium and in part by pseudostratified epithelium composed of ciliated columnar cells interspersed with secretory cells. The secretory portion is thought to be the source of fluid in middle ear infections; the cilated cells may play a part in removal of this fluid.

The *tympanic membrane* is a thin, rather rigid, semitransparent structure, the outer cutaneous layer of which is composed of thin skin. This epithelium is reduced to a thin stratum germinativum and a thin stratum corneum. The inner layer consists of a single layer of squamous epithelial cells on a sparse lamina propria. Between these two epithelia is the substantia propria, the main mass of the tympanic membrane, containing two layers of tendon-like collagenous fiber bundles. The outer fibers are disposed in a radial manner from the manubrium of the malleus outward to the fibrocartilaginous ring. The inner fibers are circular and most numerous near the periphery. Both layers are lacking in the upper, pars flaccida portion of the membrane.

The malleus, incus, and stapes, are com-pact bone. Their articular surfaces and patches of the stapes, manubrium and malleus are hyaline cartilage. The stapes alone contains a marrow cavity.

The *tensory tympani* and the *stapedius* are striated skeletal muscles. The tensor tympani lies in a canal just above the auditory tube and it ends in a tendon inserted into the upper malleus. When this muscle contracts, it draws the malleus inward and thus tenses the tympanic membrane. It is innervated by the fifth cranial (trigeminal) nerve.

The stapedius lies within a small conical bony projection, the *pyramidal eminence,* on the posterior wall of the tympanic cavity. Its tendon passes through a minute aperture in the summit of the eminence and is inserted into the stapes. It is innervated by the seventh cranial (facial) nerve.

The middle ear mechanism functions to amplify the force of sound waves that move the eardrum. It does so in such a way that the vibrational force per unit area is increased at the foot plate of the stapes in the oval window. This amplification necessitates no added energy, because the eardrum is about 18 times as large as the opening in the oval window. Therefore, the movements transmitted through the ossicle chain have enough force to move the stapes against the fluid of the inner ear. Thus the eardrum and the membrane covering the oval window move together, their impedance (the amount of resistance to movement) being well-matched.

In addition to impedance matching, the middle ear provides adjustment of the responsiveness of the ossicle chain. It was previously thought that the tensor tympani and stapedius muscles functioned primarily to dampen ossicle movement and thus protect the delicate inner ear structures from excessive vibrations. Their contraction is now also thought to set the degree of tension in the tympanic membrane facilitating transmission of moderate intensity sounds through the middle ear, improving hearing in a noisy environment and preventing hearing of our own voices too loudly.

The *auditory (Eustachian) tube* is a flattened canal leading from the anterior wall of the tympanic cavity to the nasopharynx (Fig. 22.30). In its upper extent, near the middle ear, it is surrounded by a bony wall. Below this osseous part, the reinforcing wall is formed partly by hyaline cartilage. In its lower portion, patches of elastic fibers occur in the matrix.

The auditory tube mucosa consists of a lamina propria covered by a low ciliated columnar epithelium. In the bony part, the mucosa is thin and firmly united to the underlying bony wall. In the cartilaginous part, the mucosa is loose and the epithelium becomes a pseudostratified ciliated variety. Goblet cells occur near the pharyngeal opening, as well as tubuloacinar mucous glands.

The auditory tube serves to ventilate the middle ear. Normally collapsed, the tube is opened during chewing and swallowing to allow pressure equilibration. Unfortunately, it also serves as a route for the spread of infection.

The Internal Ear

The internal ear is an interconnected series of bony-walled chambers and passages containing similarly shaped membraneous sacs and canals (Figs. 22.30 and 22.34). These are the *osseous labyrinth* and the *membranous labyrinth*, respectively. Intervening between the two is a space, the *perilymphatic space* (actually a highly fluid connective tissue space) which contains the fluid *perilymph*. Within the membranous labyrinth there is also a fluid, the *endolymph*.

The Osseous Labyrinth

Although the osseous labyrinth is not a separate entity, its bony wall is harder than that of the surrounding bone from which it can be freed by careful dissection. Seen thus, it consists of an ovoid central chamber, the *vestibule*, from which are given off the three *semicircular canals* and the *cochlea*.

The osseous vestibule of the inner ear is separated from the osseous middle ear by a plate of bone which is pierced by the *oval window* and the *round window*. A narrow canal known as the *vestibular aqueduct* extends from the vestibule to the posterior surface of the petrous portion of the temporal bone and houses the membranous *endolymphatic duct* (Fig. 22.31).

The three osseous semicircular canals are arranged with their respective planes perpendicular to each other. Thus, there are two vertical canals and one horizontal canal. The two vertical ones are *superior* (anterior) and *inferior* (posterior) canals; the horizontal one is known as the *lateral*, or external canal. The lateral canals of the two sides lie in the same horizontal plane. The orientation of the vertical canals is such that the plane of the superior canal on one side is approximately parallel to the plane of the inferior canal of the opposite side. Just after leaving the vestibule, each canal has a dilation known as the *ampulla*.

The central chamber of the osseous vestibule of each ear is continuous anteriorly with a spiral cavity which constitutes the bony *cochlea*. The latter is a spiral chamber which houses the *organ of Corti* (Fig. 22.31). In man, the apex of the cochlear canal is directed forward, outward and downward (Fig. 22.34).

The Membranous Labyrinth

The *membranous labyrinth* is a connected series of sacs and canals whose walls are formed of a fibrous connective tissue lined internally by simple squamous epithelium of ectodermal origin. In general, the membranous labyrinth has the same form as the osseous labyrinth in which it is contained. However, that part enclosed within the osseous vestibule is divided into two sacs (compare Figs. 22.30 and 22.31). The larger of these, the *utricle*, is an elliptical sac from which the membranous semicircular canals extend. In front of the utricle is the smaller spherical *saccule* which connects by a short and narrow canal, the *ductus reuniens*, with the membranous cochlea, or *cochlear duct*. The utricle and the saccule are connectd by the *utriculosaccular duct*, the two parts of which converge and continue backward through the vestib-

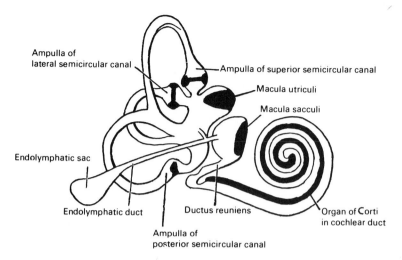

Figure 22.31. Outline of cavities of the left membranous labyrinth viewed from the medial aspect. Receptor regions of the neuroepithelium are sketched in *black*. (Redrawn from Schaffer.)

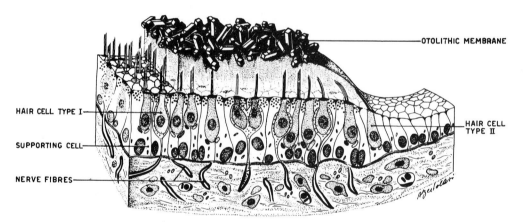

Figure 22.32. Schematic drawing of the macula, as found either in the saccule or in the utricle of the vestibule. (Reprinted with permission from S. Iurato: Submicroscopic Structure of the Inner Ear. New York, Pergamon Press, 1967, p 18.)

ular aqueduct as the slender *endolymphatic duct*. Under the dura of the posterior surface of the temporal bone, this duct terminates in a blind enlargement, the *endolymphatic sac* (Fig. 22.31).

The membranous labyrinth only partially fills the space within the osseous labyrinth. At places, it lies close to the periosteum of the osseous wall, with which its connective tissue layer then blends. For the most part, however, it lies suspended in the perilymph by a number of connective tissue

trabeculae which pass from the periosteum to the membranous wall.

In certain definite regions, the wall of the membranous labyrinth is considerably modified to form the true sensory areas. In these, the epithelium takes on a special complexity and among its cells the fibers of the vestibulocochlear (eighth cranial) nerve terminate. There are six such neuroepithelial areas in each labyrinth: two are macular, lying in the utricle (*macula utriculi*) and saccule (*macula sacculi*) respectively;

one lies in each ampulla, the *cristae ampullares*; and one in the cochlear duct, the *organ of Corti* (Fig. 22.31). The maculae and cristae ampullares (concerned with position and motion sense) are within the vestibule of the osseous labyrinth and are supplied by the vestibular portion of the eighth nerve; the organ of Corti (concerned with hearing) is located in the cochlea and is supplied by the cochlear division of the eighth nerve.

The Vestibule

The *maculae* represent local thickenings of the membranous walls, each about 3 mm by 2 mm in extent, forming an elevation into the endolymphatic space. The epithelium is composed of *supporting* (sustenacular) and *hair cells* (Fig. 22.32).

The supporting cells are tall columnar elements with their bases resting on the basal lamina and with their apical portions extending to the lumen and forming a support for the hair cells. Their lateral borders are irregular. The nuclei are oval, and they stain rather densely (Fig. 22.32). The cytoplasm contains the usual organelles plus numerous "secretory" granules and an abundance of microtubules. The latter join a dense terminal web (Fig. 22.33). At the edge of the macula, the supporting cells show a gradual transition into the simple squamous epithelium characteristic of the remainder of the membranous labyrinth.

The hair cells occupy the apical part of the epithelium. Two types have been described (Fig. 22.33). The first is a flask-shaped cell embraced over its entire inferior aspect by a single large chalice-like nerve terminal. The second is a cylindrical cell contacted by a series of nerve endings only around its base. Some of these nerve endings are afferent and receive signals from the hair cell while others are considered to be efferent and deliver signals from the brain to the hair cell. Both the afferent and efferent nerve fibers belong to the vestibular branch of the eighth cranial nerve and both types are myelinated. They lose their myelin in the lamina propria, just prior to contacting the hair cells (Fig. 22.33).

In the apical portion of each hair cell, there is a dense terminal web which, combined with the terminal webs of the adjacent supportive cells, is usually described as a *cuticular plate* (Fig. 22.33). The "hairs" of the hair cells are in reality groups of processes each containing a number of nonmotile microvillous projections (called *sterocilia*) and one cilium (a *kinocilium*). The

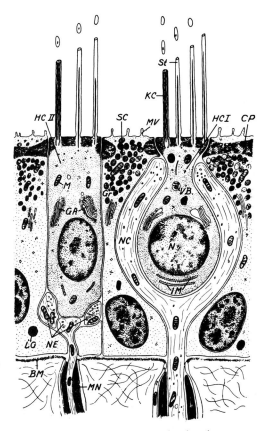

Figure 22.33. This schematic drawing represents a section through the specialized sensory epithelium found in the maculae of the saccule and utricle and in the crista ampullaris of each semicircular canal. *HC I*, hair cell of type *I*; *HC II*, hair cell of type *II*, *SC*, supporting cell; *St*, stereocilia; *KC*, kinocilia; *N*, nucleus; *GA*, Golgi apparatus; *IM*, intracellular membranes; *VB*, multivesicular body; *NC*, nerve chalice; *CP*, cuticular plate; *M*, mitochondrion; *NE*, nerve endings, both afferent and efferent; *BM*, basement membrane; *MN*, myelinated nerve fiber; *LG*, lipid granule; *MV*, microvilli. (Reprinted with permission from J. Wersall: *Acta Otolaryngol (Suppl) (Stockh)* 126:1, 1956.)

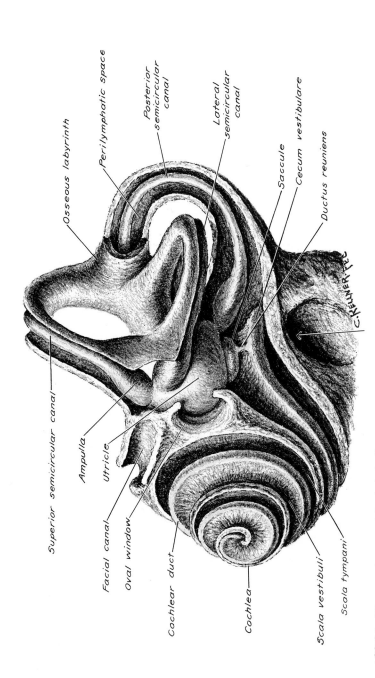

Figure 22.34 The membranous labyrinth (*yellow*) is shown within the channels of the bony labyrinth. The outer and lateral walls of the bony labyrinth have been removed in order to show the membranous labyrinth. Perilymph fills the spaces around the membranous labyrinth; endolymph is within the cavities of the membranous labyrinth. Compare with Figure 22.31. (Based on a model by Tramond but considerably modified.)

sterocilia are arranged in regular hexagonal patterns and together with the kinocilium they extend outward from the epithelium for 20 to 25 μm in a tapering group to penetrate a peculiar deposit which covers the surface of the macula.

This deposit, the *otolithic "membrane,"* consists of a gelatinous substance containing a great number of minute crystals composed chiefly of calcium carbonate—the *otoconia* or *otoliths* (Fig. 22.32).

The hair cells transduce a deformation of the hairs into a generator potential when their hairs are bent in a given azimuth and to a given degree by the action of linear movement or of gravity on the overlying otolithic membrane. This evokes an action potential in the underlying afferent nerve endings. This cytological mechanism provides the brain with information both on the position of the head in space and on linear head movements.

Each *semicircular canal* forms an arc which is slightly more than a semicircle. It does not occupy the center of the osseous canal but lies against the periosteum of the outer border to which it is attached (Fig. 22.34). Connective tissue trabeculae from the wall of the osseous canal also serve to anchor it in the perilymphatic space.

Certain special features are present in the structure of the *cristae ampullares,* the sensory areas which are found in each ampulla. Here the membranous wall is thickened to form a ridge, placed tranversely to the long axis of the canal. This ridge consists of the tunica propria, containing many nerve fibers and blood vessels, surmounted by a specialized columnar epithelium.

The epithelium of the cristae consists of *sustenacular cells* and *hair cells* that are remarkably similar to those of the maculae. A rounded and longitudinally striated gelatinous mass, the *cupula,* is spread over the surface of the cells (Fig. 22.35), separated from the epithelium by a narrow space containing endolymph. The long tapering hairs of the cells pass through this space and penetrate for some distance into the cupula, each hair occupying a narrow

canal filled with endolymph. The hairs in the middle of the crista stand perpendicular to its surface, whereas those at the border are inclined toward the median plane of the cupula.

Fibers of the vestibular nerve terminate in the epithelium of the crista. The naked axons pierce the basement membrane and form contacts around each of the two types of hair cells similar to those in the maculae.

Because the cupula has a flexible attachment to the crista ampullaris, it can be swayed by flow of endolymph within the semicircular canals. Rotation of the head will cause a deflection of the cupula in two or more of the semicircular canals resulting

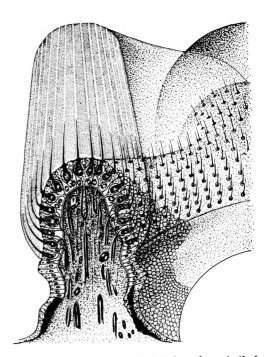

Figure 22.35. Schematic drawing of one-half of a crista ampullaris, showing innervation of its epithelium. Thick nerve fibers form nerve calyces around type I hair cells at the summit of the crista, medium caliber fibers innervate type I hair cells on the slope of the crista, and medium caliber and fine nerve fibers from a nerve plexus which innervates hair cells of type II. The gelatinous mass surmounting the hair cells is the cupula, which is pushed to and fro by the flow of the endolymph in the semicircular canal. (Reprinted with permission from J. Wersall: *Acta Otolaryngol (Suppl) (Stockh)* 126:1, 1956.)

in movement of the hairs embedded in its base. The underlying nerve endings are then signaled and the brain thus receives information regarding both speed and direction of movement.

The Cochlea

The osseous cochlea consists of a conical axis of spongy bone, the *modiolus*, or hub, around which a spiral bony canal is wound (Fig. 22.34). This canal makes about two and one-half turns in man. The base of the modiolus forms the bottom of the internal auditory meatus, through which fibers of the cochlear nerve enter (Figs. 22.36 and 22.37). These fibers are processes of the bipolar ganglion cells of the spiral ganglion, which is lodged in the *spiral canal of the modiolus.*

Projecting from the modiolus partly across the osseous canal of the cochlea is a shelf of bone, the *osseous spiral lamina*, which follows the spiral turns of the cochlea. Along the outer wall of the canal, opposite the osseous spiral lamina, is a projection of thickened periosteum, the *spiral ligament* (Figs. 22.37 and 22.38). A connective tissue membrane, the *membranous spiral lamina*, bridges the space intervening between the spiral ligament and the osseous spiral lamina. Thus, the osseous canal of the cochlea is divided into two spirally parallel parts, an upper *scala vestibuli* and a lower *scala tympani** (Fig. 22.37).

A thin membrane, the *vestibular membrane (membrane of Reissner)*, extends obliquely outward from the thickened periosteum covering the upper surface of the osseous spiral lamina, to the upper part of the spiral ligament. This membrane forms the roof of a triangular-shaped membranous labyrinth canal known as the *cochlear duct (scala media)* (Fig. 22.37).

The scala vestibuli and scala tympani course parallel with the cochlear duct in-

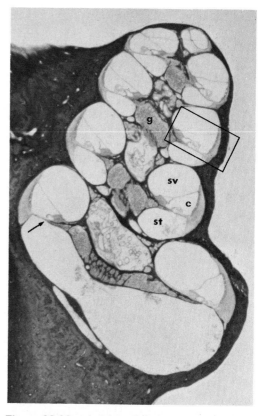

Figure 22.36. Axial section through the cochlea of a guinea pig. In the spaces of the bony core are the ganglia (*g*), which contain sensory neurons supplying the hair cells of the organ of Corti. The cochlear duct (*c*), scala tympani (*st*) and scale vestibuli (*sv*) are marked in one turn of the cochlea. The area outlined in black is the region depicted in Figure 22.38. In this guinea pig, a portion of the hair cells in the basal turn was damaged before death by exposure to excessive sound. In this region, the hair cells are absent (*arrow*). Note the increasing length of the basilar membrane toward the apex of the cochlea. (Courtesy of Dr. W. Marovitz.)

---

* The terms "upper" and "lower" are here used arbitrarily as if the cochlea were oriented with its base downward and its apex upward. "Inner" and "outer" are used to designate directions with respect to the axis of the cochlea, the modiolus.

terposed between them. The scala vestibuli extends from the vestibule and is in close relation to the oval window whereas the scala tympani has its base at the round window; the two communicate directly only at the apex of the cochlea through a small canal, the *helicotrema.*

The cochlear duct is a narrow tube in which the organ of hearing is located (Figs. 22.37 and 22.38). Its closed apex is the *cecum cupulare.* The cochlear duct is tri-

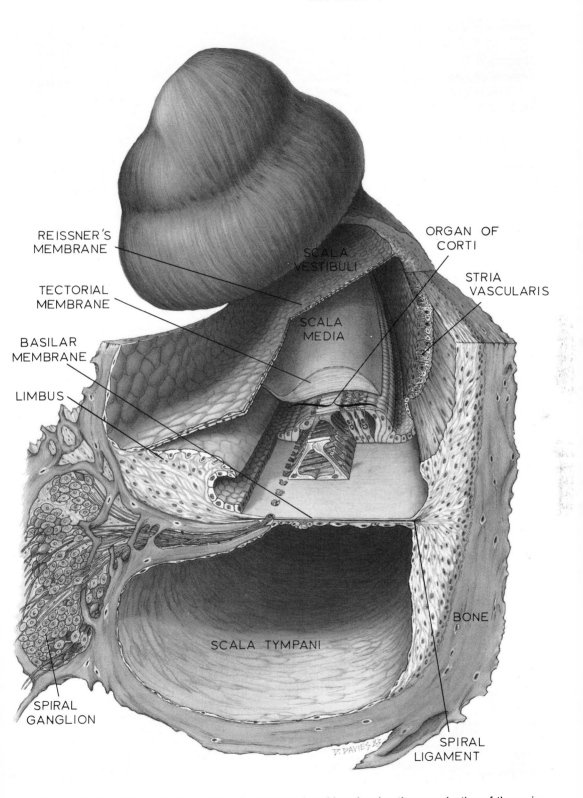

REISSNER'S
MEMBRANE

TECTORIAL
MEMBRANE

BASILAR
MEMBRANE

LIMBUS

SPIRAL
GANGLION

SCALA
VESTIBULI

SCALA
MEDIA

SCALA TYMPANI

ORGAN OF
CORTI

STRIA
VASCULARIS

BONE

SPIRAL
LIGAMENT

D. DAVIES 83

Figure 22.37. Schematic illustration of a dissected cochlea showing the organization of the major compartments and structures surrounding the organ of Corti.

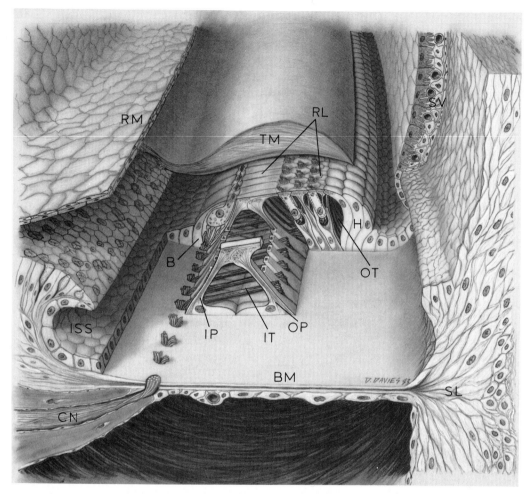

Figure 22.38. Higher magnification view of a dissected cochlea. The area included is approximately equal to that outlined in Figure 22.36. Structures visible include the basilar membrane (*BM*), cochlear nerve (*CN*), spiral ligament (*SL*), stria vascularis (*SV*), tectorial membrane (*TM*), Reissner's membrane (*RM*), and the inner spiral sulcus (*ISS*). The outer tunnel (*OT*) and inner tunnel (*IT*) of the organ of Corti are open to view. These are surrounded by the inner pillar cells (*IP*), outer pillar cells (*OP*), cells of Hensen (*H*), and border cells (*B*). The reticular lamina (*RL*) is composed of the apices of several supportive cells of the organ of Corti, detailed in Figure 22.39.

angular in transverse section, thus allowing a division of its walls into upper, outer and lower.

The upper or vestibular wall, formed by the vestibular (Reissner's) membrane, consists of a thin central lamina of connective tissue covered on either side by simple squamous epithelium. The epithelium on the upper surface is continuous with a mesenchymal epithelium lining the scala vestibuli whereas the lower surface epithelium

is that of the cochlear duct and is of ectodermal origin.

The outer wall of the cochlear duct is formed by the *spiral ligament*, a thickening of the periosteum which appears triangular in cross section (Figs. 22.37 and 22.38). The outer portion of the ligament, adjacent to the osseous wall, is dense fibrous connective tissue while the inner portion is more loosely arranged. The portion of the ligament along the lateral border of the scala media is known as the *stria vascularis* due to the numerous capillaries in its subepithelial connective tissue. The cochlear duct epithelium of this region is relatively thick and pseudostratified.

The vascular stria is thought to be active in the production of endolymph and the regulation of ion content. The endolymph, unlike extracellular fluids in any other part of the body (and unlike perilymph), has a high potassium (144 mEq/liter) and a low sodium (15 mEq/liter) content. It thus resembles intracellular fluid. Reabsorption of endolymph may also take place in the stria vascularis (and perhaps in the endolymphatic sac).

The complex lower or tympanic wall of the chochlear duct is formed by the outer osseous spiral lamina, the whole membranous spiral lamina, and special modifications of their epithelial and connective tissue layers.

A firm, cellular thickening of periosteal connective tissue along the upper border of the osseous spiral lamina forms an elevation known as the *limbus* (Figs. 22.37 and 22.38). The limbus has upper and lower projections known, respectively, as the *vestibular lip* and the *tympanic lip*. They partially enclose a groove, the *internal spiral sulcus*. Lateral to its attachment to the vestibular membrane, the limbus is covered by columnar epithelium bearing a cuticular formation. This extracellular structure extends laterally as the *tectorial membrane* (Figs. 22.38 and 22.39).

The tympanic lip projects slightly farther outward than the vestibular lip. Its upper surface forms the floor of the internal spiral sulcus lined by a single layer of clear flat cuboidal cells, which continue to the vestibular lip. The lower surface of the tympanic lip is covered by the thin layer of mesenchymal epithelium lining the scala tympani.

The *basilar membrane* extends from the tympanic lip outward to the *crista basilaris* of the spiral ligament. It consists of fine straight unbranched fibers, the *basilar fibers* or *auditory strings*, embedded in a sparse homogeneous ground substance.

The basilar membrane varies in breadth along the turns of the cochlea. It is greatest at the apex, diminishing toward the base to its narrowest extent in the proximal end of the basal coil.

The Organ of Corti

On the upper surface of the basilar membrane, the cochlear duct epithelial cells form a complex, spirally disposed *organ of Corti*—the organ of hearing. This cochlear receptor has three principal components: (*a*) a framework which supports the receptive hair cells and provides a mechanism for transformation of acoustic energy into the proper stimulus for the hair cells; (*b*) the hair cells, which transduce mechanical stimuli into generator potentials; and (*c*) the nerve endings which receive afferent signals from the hair cells and provide efferent input to them. The hair cells are intimately related to the endings of the cochlear division of the vestibulocochlear nerve.

The organ of Corti extends the entire length of the cochlear duct with the exception of a short distance at either end. A variety of specialized cells provide the components listed above. All except the hair cells may be considered as sustentacular cells (Figs. 22.38 and 22.39).

The *border cells* are slender columnar elements which rest on the tympanic lip and form a single row along the inner side of the inner hair cells. Their surfaces are provided with a cuticle.

The *inner hair cells* are larger than the outer hair cells, being broader and longer. They form a single row occupying the upper part of the epithelial layer. The rounded base of each cell rests on the adjacent supporting cells. The surface of this cell has a number of processes (traditionally described as hairs) in contact with the tectorial membrane. The processes and other features of the inner hair cells resemble those of the outer hair cells described in detail below.

The *inner phalangeal cells* are aligned along the inner surface of the inner pillar cells. Their bases rest on the cochlear basal

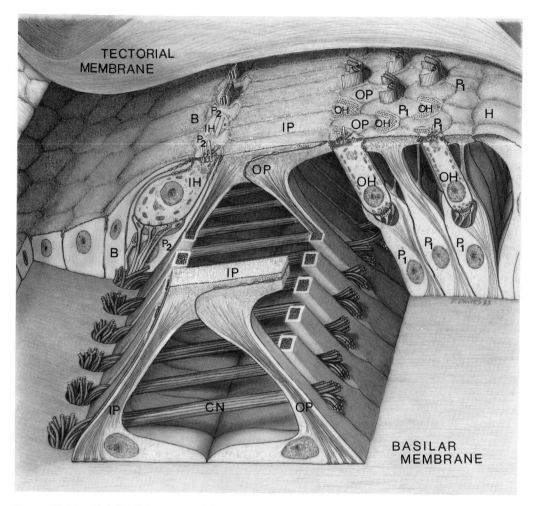

Figure 22.39. Details of the organ of Corti. In addition to the cells shown in Figure 22.38, the outer hair cells (*OH*), inner hair cells (*IH*), outer phalangeal cells (or Deiter's cells) (P_1) and inner phalangeal cells (P_2) are depicted. Phalangeal and pillar cells are characterized by massive bundles of filaments and microtubules. The apical parts of these cells comprise the rigid reticular lamina which forms a supportive framework around apices of the hair cells. Numerous gap junctions and occluding junctional networks interconnect phalangeal and pillar cells. Fibers of the cochlear nerve (*CN*) provide afferent and efferent endings on inner and outer hair cell bodies.

lamina (a component of the basilar membrane). The nucleus lies in the lower portion of the cell, which is continued as a slender process to the surface. Here it ends in a small cuticular plate.

The *inner and outer pillar cells* each consist of a broad curved base which contains the nucleus, and an elongated body or pillar which contains a stout bundle of closely packed microtubules. The thickened end of the pillar away from the base is known as

the head. Its cytoplasm contains a dense "cuticular plate" into which the microtubules are attached. The head of the outer pillar presents a convexity on its inner side, which fits a corresponding concavity on the head of the inner pillar, the heads of opposite pillars thus "articulating" with each other. From their articulation, the pillars diverge, so that their bases, on the cochlear basal lamina, are widely separated. A series of arches is thus formed which encloses a

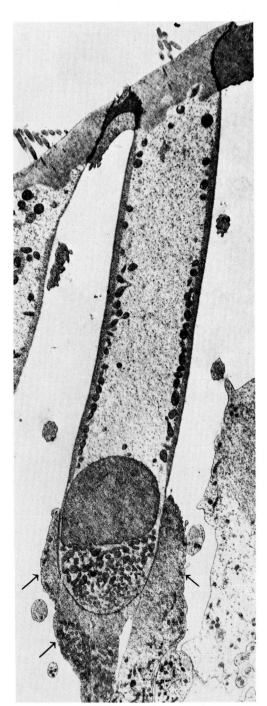

triangular canal, the *inner tunnel* or Corti's tunnel. This is crossed by delicate nerve fibers.

The *outer phalangeal cells (cells of Deiters)* are the supporting elements for the outer hair cells, one for each cell. Like the hair cells, their number varies along the cochlear duct. They form three rows in the basal coil, four in the middle coil and five in the apical coil. Between the innermost of the outer phalangeal cells and the outer pillar there is a space, the *space of Nuel.*

Each outer phalangeal cell is elongated with its basal portion resting on the basal lamina and its slender apical portion extending between the hair cells. The nucleus is rounded and is located within the basal portion of the cell. Each phalangeal cell has a facet in its lateral wall which supports the base of the neighboring hair cell.

The cytoplasm of each phalangeal cell contains bundles of microtubules which divide into two groups at the level of the neighboring hair cells. One group terminates in the cup-shaped facet which houses the hair cell and the other continues to the surface where it spreads out into a flat "cuticular plate." Adjacent plates interdigitate and are collectively known as the *reticular lamina.* The cuticular plates of each row of phalangeal cells interdigitate with those of the next row and also with the outer ends of the hair cells (Figs. 22.40 and 22.41).

The *outer hair cells* are columnar in shape and their apical surfaces bear short sensory hairs which contact the tectorial membrane. The base of each cell, supported by a phalangeal cell, contains the nucleus and a granular, mitochondria-rich cytoplasm (Fig. 22.40).

Electron micrographs show that the hairs are straight microvilli with internal longitudinal filaments similar to those accumulated in the neighboring cuticular plates of

Figure 22.40. Electron micrograph showing two outer hair cells from the organ of Corti of the chinchilla. One of the hair cells is shown in its entirety. At its base, this cell contains a nucleus and numerous mitochondria and receives several nerve endings (*arrows*). The middle portion is relatively empty. The apical portion is closely associated with surrounding cuticular plates. Note the extensive extracellular space between hair cells and the apical portions of the outer phalangeal cells (×3500). (Reprinted with permission from C. Smith: *Adv Sci* 24:419, 1968).

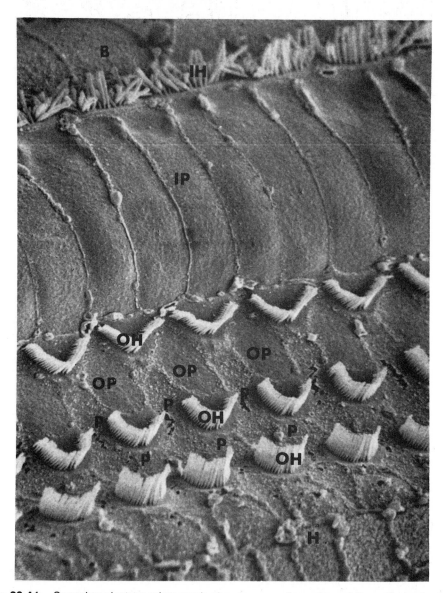

Figure 22.41. Scanning electron micrograph showing a surface view of the reticular lamina of a cat's organ of Corti after removal of the tectorial membrane. Three rows of outer hair cells (*OH*) and one row of inner hair cells (*IH*) are visible. Border cells (*B*) and Hensen cell (*H*) apical surfaces are also seen. The interdigitating cuticular plates formed by the apices of inner pillar (*IP*), outer pillar (*OP*) and outer phalangeal (*P*) cells is well demonstrated in this view (×2800). (Courtesy of Dr. Masayuki Miyoshi.)

the phalangeal cells. The apical lateral border of each hair cell contacts its supporting cells by occluding junctions which effectively separate endolymph from perilymph. In freeze-fracture images, these junctions resemble those seen between neighboring epithelial cells in a number of locations where paracellular flux is known to be blocked.

Freeze-fracture preparations of the cochlea show special patterns of intramembranous particles on the cytoplasmic faces of the nonjunctional, lateral borders of the hair cells indicating that the inner and outer hair cells may differ in their functions. They also suggest that the nonjunctional portions of the membranes play an important role in transduction.

The hairs project from the surface in a regular pattern, with three rows forming a W (or in some mammals a V) shape facing the modiolus (Fig. 22.41). The hairs are in contact with, but apparently not firmly embedded in, the tectorial membrane. As is the case for the outer phalangeal cells, there are three rows of outer hair cells in the basal coil of the cochlea (Fig. 22.41), four rows in the upper end of the basal coil and in the middle coil and five rows in the apical coil.

The *cells of Hensen* are tall columnar elements lateral to the outer phalangeal cells. They form the outer border of the organ of Corti. The space between the outer phalangeal cells and the cells of Hensen is known as the *outer tunnel.*

The *cells of Claudius* are cuboidal in shape and have a clear cytoplasm. They line the outermost portion of the basilar membrane.

The extracellular *tectorial membrane* is continuous with the cuticle-like covering apparently formed by cells of the limbus region (Fig. 22.37). Beyond the limbus it becomes thickened into a striated gelatinous structure which overhangs the internal spiral sulcus and extends outward to the cells of Hensen. The upper surface is more convex than the lower one.

The tectorial membrane is particularly susceptible to distortion in fixed preparations. In the living condition it is in contact with the processes of the hair cells.

The organ of Corti is innervated by the cochlear division of the auditory nerve which enters the axis of the modiolus from the internal auditory meatus and divides into a number of branches. From these, numerous fibers radiate to the osseous spiral lamina, in the base of which they enter the *spiral ganglion* (Figs. 22.36 and 22.37).

The cells of the spiral ganglion are peculiar, in that they maintain their embryonic bipolar condition throughout life.

Their myelinated central processes course through the modiolus and the internal auditory meatus to their terminal nuclei in the medulla. Their peripheral processes, also myelinated, pass outward in bundles in the osseous spiral lamina. Branches from these enter the tympanic lip of the limbus, where they lose their myelin and pass through the *foramina nervosa* (minute apertures in the tympanic lip) to their terminations in the organ of Corti. In the latter, the fibers run in three bundles parallel to the inner tunnel. One bundle lies just inside the inner pillar beneath the row of inner hair cells. A second bundle runs in the tunnel to the outer side of the inner pillar. The third bundle crosses the inner tunnel (*tunnel fibers*) and turns at right angles to course between the outer phalangeal cells. From all of these bundles of fibers, delicate terminal fibers are given off which end in branching telodendria around the bases of the hair cells.

Apparently not all of the nerve fibers serving the hair cells are afferent (transmit impulses from the hair cells). Electron microscopy of the endings around the hair cells (Figs. 22.40 and 22.42) discloses that some harbor large populations of synaptic vesicles. This suggests that they convey efferent or feedback input to the hair cells, but the functional significance of this finding remains unclear.

Physiology of the Auditory Mechanism

Sound waves reaching the tympanic membrane cause it to vibrate at the same frequency. The movement consequently imparted to the auditory ossicles moves the base of the stapes in and out of the oval window at the same frequency. Since the fluid perilymph on the other side of the oval window lies in a chamber with rigid bony walls and is itself incompressible, the inward movement of the stapes produces a pressure wave within the perilymph which can be relieved only by a compensating outward movement of the secondary tympanic membrane covering the round window.

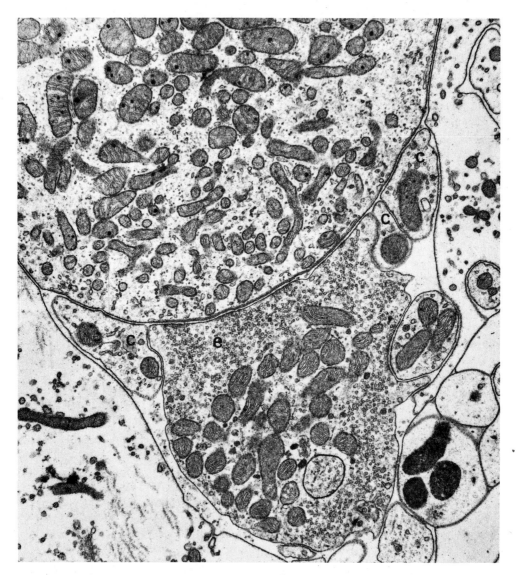

Figure 22.42. Electron micrograph of the nerve endings on the basal part of the outer hair cell of the chinchilla organ of Corti. One large efferent (*e*) and three small afferent (cochlear) (*c*) nerve endings terminate on the hair cell. Note the large number of mitochondria in this portion of the hair cell (×31,500). (Reprinted with permission from C. Smith and G. Rasmussen: *J Cell Biol* 26:63, 1965.)

Two avenues for the transfer of a pressure wave are available. It could travel the length of the scala vestibuli and pass by way of the slender helicotrema to the perilymph of the scala tympani, thence to the round window, or it could be transmitted across the vestibular membrane to the endolymph of the cochlear duct. This would cause displacement of the basilar membrane toward the scala tympani; conse-

quently, the pressure wave would be transmitted to the perilymph of the scala tympani and released at the round window. Thus a sound of a given frequency would cause movements of the basilar membrane of equal frequency.

The hair cells are firmly supported within a framework (the reticular lamina) mounted on the basilar membrane, their hairs contact the overlying tectorial membrane, and these membranes are "hinged" to maintain a parallel relationship when the basilar membrane is distorted. Such distortion thereby imparts a shear force between the tectorial and basilar membranes that results in bending of the hairs to a proportional degree (Fig. 22.43). The hair cells transduce the bending into generator potentials which stimulate appropriate signals in the afferent nerve endings.

This chain of events does not readily account for the fact that the auditory mechanism is capable of differentiating between vibrations of different frequencies—in other words, pitch or tone. Damage to structures at the base of the cochlea leads to a loss of hearing for high tones and damage near the apex affects reception of lower tones. Because the breadth of the basilar membrane is less near the base of the cochlea and greater near the apex, it has been assumed that the basilar membrane vibrates in a specific region for different sound frequencies.

It is now known, however, that large regions of the basilar membrane vibrate for all frequencies, but the waves that travel up to the cochlear spiral produce maximum displacement of the membrane at different sites depending on the tone of the incident sound. The lower the frequency of the sound waves, the farther from the oval window the maximum displacement of the basilar membrane occurs. Central nervous system mechanisms sort out the input signals

so that the site of maximum basilar membrane displacement (as well as vibratory patterns in adjacent regions) and thus the pitch and quality of a sound are discerned. The loudness of a tone is thought to be determined by the amount of basilar membrane set into maximum motion. It has been suggested that the outer hair cells are particularly concerned with determining the intensity of sound and the inner hair cells with pitch discrimination. Moreover, the nerve endings on hair cells are arranged not only for the reception of excitation but also for inhibition. Efferent innervation brings to the organ of Corti central nervous system mechanisms of inhibition which may aid in pitch and loudness discrimination.

The total hair cells in man is probably less than 20,000. These cells are damaged or destroyed by sounds of exceptionally high intensity and are not replaced if lost. One cannot lose many cells from the extraordinarily delicate and sensitive organ of Corti without suffering significant hearing loss. The protection of the ear against excessive noise must be taken seriously.

THE ORGAN OF SMELL

The sense of smell is perceived in a restricted specialized portion of the mucosa in the upper part of each nasal cavity. This *olfactory mucosa* contains unusual epithelial nerve cell bodies which provide the mechanism for olfactory reception on their

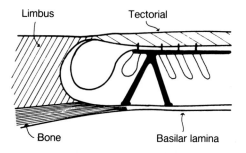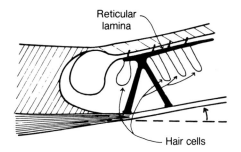

Figure 22.43. Diagram showing how the shearing action between two stiff structures, the tectorial membrane and the basilar lamina, bends the hairs of the hair cells. (Reprinted with permission from H. Davis: In *Physiological Triggers and Discontinuous Rate Processes*, edited by T. Bullock. Washington, D.C., American Physiological Society, 1957.)

exposed ends and send an axon from their basal end to the first olfactory way station in the brain—the *olfactory bulb*.

The olfactory mucosa can be distinguished with the naked eye by its brownish-yellow color which contrasts with the reddish tint of the surrounding respiratory mucosa. The epithelium is psueodstratified columnar, and is considerably thicker than that of the respiratory region. The epithelial cells are of at least three kinds: basal cells, sustentacular cells, and olfactory cells (Figs. 22.44 and 22.45).

The *basal cells* are probably supportive in function, line nearly all the epithelial basal surface, and are the only cells not reaching the apical surface. They relate closely to the sustentacular cells.

The *sustentacular cells* are more numerous. Each cell consists of: a superficial portion which is shaped like a stout cylinder and contains pigment and granules arranged in longitudinal rows; a middle portion which contains an oval nucleus; and a thin filamentous process which extends from the nuclear portion down between the cells of the deeper layers. The luminal surface of the cell is covered with microvilli. Desmosomes bind the apical portion of the cell to the adjacent olfactory cells.

The *olfactory cells*, the epithelial neurons, lie between the sustentacular cells. Their nuclei are spherical, lie at different levels, but most more deeply placed than those of the sustentacular cells. From the nuclear portion of each cell a delicate process extends to the surface, where it is expanded in a minute knob (sometimes called the olfactory vesicle). From this terminal knob several cilia arise, each from a typical basal body. Near their base these are typical cilia, but more distally their long, narrow extensions contain only two microtubules. The cilia do not project vertically but are flattened against the mucosal surface; they are thought to be the portion of the olfactory cell that reacts with odor-producing chemicals. The mucosal surface and the cilia are constantly bathed by the product of special

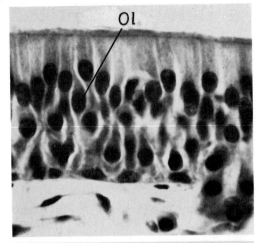

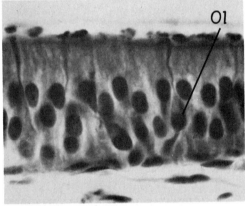

Figure 22.44. Photomicrographs of the olfactory mucosa showing the olfactory cells (*Ol*) between the sustentacular cells. The *upper figure*, stained with hematoxylin and eosin, also shows part of a gland of Bowman (*lower right*); the *lower figure* is a silver-stained preparation which demonstrates the bipolar nature of the olfactory neurons (×1100). (From preparations by Dr. G. Hamlett.)

tubular serous glands (the *glands of Bowman*) which underlie the olfactory mucosa and deliver their products to its surface.

From the opposite pole of the olfactory cell a single fiber extends to join one of the olfactory nerves that pass centrally through the cribriform plate of the ethmoid bone to terminate in the olfactory bulb. The olfactory cell is thus a bipolar ganglion cell with a short peripheral and a long central process. This is the only example in man of sensory ganglion cells occupying a surface epithelium, a common situation in certain lower animals.

A fourth type of cell, the *microvillar cell*, has recently been reported in human olfactory epithelium. Its nucleus lies close to the apical surface, where it displays short microvilli. Since it also projects a basally directed process, it is suspected of being a bipolar neuron, similar to the olfactory cell.

The basement membrane supporting this epithelium is not well developed. The underlying *stroma* consists of loosely arranged collagenous fibers, delicate elastic fibers and connective tissue cells. Embedded in the stroma are the numerous simple branched tubular glands (of Bowman). Each consists of a duct, a body, and a fundus. The secreting cells are large, irregular, and contain a yellowish pigment which, with that of the sustentacular cells, is responsible for the peculiar color of the olfactory mucosa.

The paired *olfactory bulbs* of man are small extensions of the cerebral hemispheres; in some lower animals these constitute a much more substantial portion of the brain. They consist of both gray and white matter arranged in six distinct concentric layers.

The superficial *layer of olfactory fibers* consists of a dense plexiform arrangement of the axons of the olfactory cells. From this layer the axons pass deeper to a layer containing discrete fiber nests, the *olfactory glomeruli*. Here the olfactory cell axons make contact through a *plexiform layer* with the dendritic terminals of the main relay neurons of the bulb, the *mitral cells* and the *tufted cells* which occupy the next layer. These are large neurons; their axons leave the bulb along a *longitudinal fiber layer* to form the *olfactory tract* which carries signals to the central parts of the brain.

This direct relay path is influenced by several other neurons in the bulb, especially the prominent *granule cells*. These have cell bodies in a *granule cell layer* and dendrites extending into the overlying *plexiform*

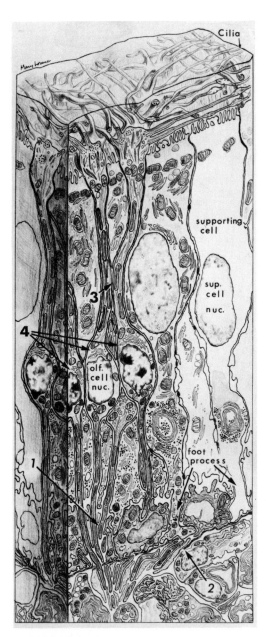

Figure 22.45. Schematic drawing showing the olfactory mucosa with the sensory cells terminating in apical expansions from which many modified cilia arise and lie on the mucosal surface. The supporting cells are surmounted by microvilli. *1*, axons arising from olfactory neurons; *2*, basement membrane; *3*, apical portion of olfactory neuron; *4*, cell bodies of olfactory neurons. (Reprinted with permission from D.Frisch: *Am J Anat* 121:87, 1967.)

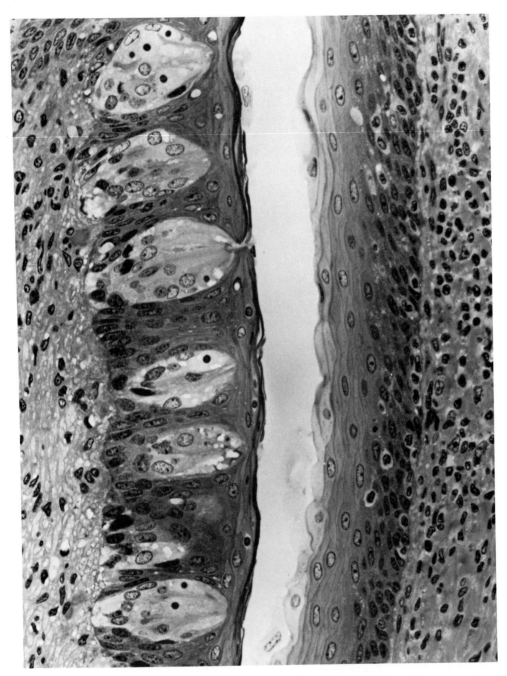

Figure 22.46. Light micrograph of taste buds in the wall of a vallate papilla from Rhesus monkey. The taste bud at the *upper center* shows a taste pore. At least three types of nuclei can be seen within the taste buds, suggesting at least three different cell types. Lymphocytes can be seen within the stratified squamous epithelium (×400).

layer. The granule cell is a form of anaxonic interneuron, distinguished by having no definitive axon and both providing and re-

ceiving synapses on adjacent regions of its dendritic surfaces (reciprocal synapses). The granule cells are thought to provide inhibitory activity for the initial processing of olfactory information that occurs in the olfactory bulb.

It is clear that the olfactory cells are akin to sensory ganglion cells in the dorsal root ganglion. These cells receive chemical stimuli, provide transduction to a nervous impulse and conduct this signal to a region of the central nervous system. The olfactory stimuli must be volatile and at least slightly soluble in both water and lipid. Olfactory cells have extraordinary sensitivity; certain substances can be detected at concentrations lower than most methods of chemical analysis. The sense of smell is closely related to the sense of taste, but of the two, olfaction is by far the more sensitive.

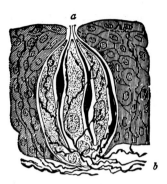

Figure 22.47. An early drawing illustrating sustentacular (*light*) sensory (*dark*) cells in a taste bud from side wall of circumvallate papilla. *a*, taste pore; *b*, nerve fibers, some of which enter the taste bud while others end freely in the surrounding epithelium. (Merkel-Henle.)

THE ORGAN OF TASTE

The "organ" of taste is rather diffuse, consisting of specialized *taste buds* located in the mucosa of the tongue, parts of the palate, and the pharynx. Taste buds are concentrated in the tongue, especially in the side walls of the *circumvallate papillae* (Fig. 22.46), in some of the *fungiform papillae* and in folds (*foliate papillae*) which occur along the posterolateral margin of the tongue.

Taste buds (Figs. 22.46 and 22.47) are ovoid epithelial structures embedded in the epithelium and connected with the surface by means of minute canals called *taste pores*. In well-fixed tissues, one can distinguish three varieties of cells: (*a*) a few relatively small cells scattered along the basal and lateral borders of the taste bud, (*b*) columnar cells with fairly dark round or oval nuclei, and (*c*) columnar cells with oval nuclei and light cytoplasm. The *light cells* have been described as the taste receptor elements and the *dark cells* as supporting (sustentacular) cells although there has been disagreement on this. Electron microscope studies indicate that there are several types of cells which are designated as types I to IV. Type IV is the basal cell of light microscopy and it apparently functions as a stem cell which divides and differentiates into the other categories. Type II is distin-

guished from type I by the presence of the considerable rough endoplasmic reticulum. Type III has less rough endoplasmic reticulum and more smooth reticulum and it has microvilli (commonly described as hairs) which project into the taste pore. These types may be merely different developmental or functional stages; the cells have a relatively short life span with a fairly rapid turnover.

After transection of the nerves to the taste buds in rabbits, the first degenerative change appears in about 12 hr and the buds disappear completely within 10 days. However, taste buds regenerate rapidly after they become reinnervated. The type IV cell (basal cell) apparently survives and serves as a stem cell.

Sensory fibers of the seventh, ninth, and tenth cranial nerves end within the taste buds. An efferent, presumably feedback or inhibitory, input to the taste buds has also been reported. Because the sensory nerve endings are related to more than one cell type, it is not certain which cell or cells may act as the taste receptor and excite the related nerve endings. Different taste buds are specialized for the perception of salty, sweet, sour or bitter tastes, and these tastes are better perceived on certain parts of the tongue than on others. Substances must be in solution to be tasted, and the amounts required to stimulate sensation are much greater than for the sense of smell. The acuteness of the sense of taste declines with age.

References

The Eye

Basinger S, Bok D, Hall M: Rhodopsin in the rod outer segment plasma membrane. *J Cell Biol* 69:29–42, 1976.

Besharse JC, Hollyfield JG: Turnover of mouse photoreceptor outer segments in constant light and darkness. *Invest Ophthalmol Vis Sci* 18:1019–1024, 1979.

Besharse JC, Pfenninger KH: Membrane assembly in retinal photoreceptors. I. Freeze-fracture analysis of cytoplasmic vesicles in relationship to disc assembly. *J Cell Biol* 87:451–463, 1980.

Bill A: Basic physiology of the drainage of aqueous humor. *Exp Eye Res* 25:291–304, 1977.

Bok D, Heller J: Transport of retinal from the blood to the retina: an autoradiographic study of the pigment epithelial cell surface receptor for plasma retinal-binding protein. *Exp Eye Res* 22:395–402, 1976.

Bok D, Young RW: The renewal of diffusely distributed protein in the outer segments of rods and cones. *Vision Res* 12:161–168, 1972.

Bunt AH, Klock IB: Comparative study of ³H-fucose incorporation into vertebrate photoreceptor outer segments. *Vision Res* 20:739–748, 1980.

Burns-Bellhorn M, Bellhorn RW, Bellhorn JV: Anterior segment permeability to fluorescein-labeled dextrans in the rat. *Invest Ophthalmol Vis Sci* 17:857–862, 1978.

Carter-Dawson LD, La Vail MM: Rods and cones in the mouse retina. I. Structural analysis using light and electron microscopy. *J Comp Neurol* 188:245–262, 1979.

Carter-Dawson LD, La Vail MM: Rods and cones in the mouse retina. II. Autoradiographic analysis of cell generation using tritiated thymidine. *J Comp Neurol* 188:263–272, 1979.

Cooper NGF, McLaughlin BJ: Gap junctions in the outer plexiform layer of the chick retina—thin section and freeze-fracture studies. *J Neurocytol* 10:515–529, 1981.

Davson H: *Physiology of the Eye*, ed 4. New York, Academic Press, 1980.

Dowling JE: The site of visual adaptation. *Science* 155:273–279, 1967.

Dowling JE: Organization of vertebrate retinas. *Invest Ophthalmal* 9:665–680, 1970.

Dowling JE: Vertebrate retina. In Tower DB, Brady RO (eds): *The Nervous System*, vol 1: *The Basic Neurosciences*. New York, Raven Press, 1975, pp 91–100.

Dowling JE, Boycott BB: Organization of the primate retina: electron microscopy. *Proc R Soc Lond (Biol)* 166:80–111, 1966.

Duke-Elder S, Gloster J: The physiology of the eye and vision. In Duke-Elder S (ed): *System of Ophthalmology*, vol 4. St. Louis, CV Mosby, 1968.

Duke-Elder S, Wybar KC: The anatomy of the visual system. In Duke-Elder S (ed): *System of Ophthalmology*, vol 2. St. Louis, CV Mosby, 1961.

Gartner J: The fine structure of the zonular fibre of the rat. Development and aging changes. *Z Anat Entwickl* 130:129–152, 1970.

Hama K, Mizukawa A, Kosaka T: Fine structure of the Müller cell revealed by high voltage electron microscopy. *Sens Processes* 2:296–299, 1979.

Hay ED, Revel J-P: Fine structure of the developing avian cornea. In *Monographs in Developmental Bi-*

Heller J, Bok D: Transport of retinal from the blood of the retina: involvement of high molecular weight lipoproteins as intracellular carriers. *Exp Eye Res* 22:403–410, 1976.

Hogan MJ, Alvarado JA, Weddell JE: *Histology of the Human Eye. An Atlas and Textbook*. Philadelphia, WB Saunders, 1971.

Hollyfield JG: Phagocytic capabilities of the pigment epithelium. *Exp Eye Res* 22:457–468, 1976.

Hollyfield JG, Rayborn ME: Membrane assembly in photoreceptor outer segments: progressive increase in "open" basal discs with increased temperature. *Exp Eye Res* 34:115–120, 1982.

Hollyfield JG, Rayborn ME, Verner GE, Maude MB, Anderson RE: Membrane addition to rod photoreceptor outer segments: light stimulates membrane assembly in the absence of increased membrane biosynthesis. *Invest Ophthalmol Vis Sci* 4:417–427, 1982.

Kelly DE, Hageman GS, McGregor JA: Uveal compartmentalization in the hamster eye revealed by fine structural and tracer studies: implications for uveo-scleral outflow. *Invest Ophthalmol Vis Sci* 24:1288–1304, 1983.

La Vail MM: Rod outer segment disc shedding in relation to cyclic lighting. *Exp Eye Res* 23:277–281, 1976.

Mann I: *The Development of the Human Eye*. New York, Grune & Stratton, 1950.

O'Connor P, Burnside B: Actin-dependent cell elongation in teleost retinal rods: requirements for actin filament assembly. *J Cell Biol* 89:517–524.

O'Rahilly R: The prenatal development of the human eye. *Exp Eye Res* 21:93–112, 1975.

Pappas GD, Smelser GK: The fine structure of the ciliary epithelium in relation to aqueous humor secretion. In Smelser GK (ed): *The Structure of the Eye*. New York, Academic Press, 1961, pp 453–467.

Polyak SL: *The Retina*. Chicago, University of Chicago Press, 1941.

Rasmussen KE: A morphometric study of the Müller cell cytoplasm in the rat retina. *J Ultrastruct Res* 39:413–429, 1972.

Raviola E: Intercellular junctions in the outer plexiform layer of the retina. *Invest Ophthalmol* 15:881–895, 1976.

Raviola E, Gilula NB: Intramembrane organization of specialized contacts in the outer plexiform layer of the retina. A freeze fracture study in monkeys and rabbits. *J Cell Biol* 65:192–222, 1975.

Raviola G: The fine structure of the ciliary zonule and ciliary epithelium. *Invest Ophthalmol* 10:851–869, 1971.

Raviola G: The structural basis of the blood-ocular barriers. *Exp Eye Res* 25:27–64, 1977.

Raviola G, Raviola E: Paracellular route of aqueous outflow in the trabecular meshwork and canal of Schlemm—a freeze-fracture study of the endothelial junctions in the sclerocorneal angle of the macaque monkey eye. *Invest Ophthalmol Vis Sci* 21:52–72, 1981.

Rohen JW: Das Auge und seine Hilfsorgane. In von Möllendorff W, Bargmann W (eds): *Handbuch der Mikroskopischen Anatomie des Menschen*, vol 3, part 4. Berlin, Springer-Verlag, 1964.

Shimiizu K, Ujiie K: *Structure of Ocular vessels*. Tokyo, New York, Igaku-Shoin, 1978.

Thomas DD, Stryer L: Transverse location of the retinal chromophore of rhodopsin in rod outer segment disc membranes. *J Mol Biol* 154:145–158, 1982.

Tonosaki A, Kelly DE: Fine structural study of the origin and development of the sphincter pupillae muscle in the West Coast newt (Taricha torosa). *Anat Rec* 170:57–74, 1971.

Tripathi RC: Uveoscleral drainage of aqueous humor. *Exp Eye Res* 25:305–308, 1977.

Usukura, J, Yamada E: Molecular organization of the rod outer segment. A deep-etching study with rapid freezing using unfixed frog retina. *Biomed Res* 2:177–193, 1981.

Wald G: The molecular organization of visual systems. In McElroy WD, Glass B (eds): *Light and Life*. Baltimore, Johns Hopkins University Press, 1960, p 724.

Wald G: The receptors of human color vision. *Science* 145:1007–1016, 1964.

Wald G: Visual pigments and photoreceptors—review and outlook. *Exp Eye Res* 18:333–343, 1974.

Walls GL: *The Vertebrate Eye and Its Adaptive Radiation*. Bloomfield Hills, Mich., Cranbrook Institute of Science, 1942.

Westfall JA (ed): *Visual Cells in Evolution*. New York, Raven Press, 1982.

Yamada E: Electron microscopy of photoreceptive membranes—recent progress and future problems. *J Electron Microsc (Tokyo)* 28:579, 1979.

Young RW: Visual cells. *Sci Am* 223:80–91, 1970.

Young RW: Visual cells and the concept of renewal. *Invest Ophthalmol* 15:700–725, 1976.

Young RW: Daily rhythm of shedding and degradation of rod and cone outer segment membranes in chick retina. *Invest Ophthalmol Vis Sci* 17:105–116, 1978.

Young RW, Bok D: Autoradiographic studies on the metabolism of the retinal pigment epithelium. *Invest Ophthalmol* 9:524–536, 1970.

The Ear

Bagger-Sjöbäck D, Gulley RL: Synaptic structures in the type II hair cell in vestibular system of the guinea pig. *Acta Otolaryngol (Stockh)* 88:401–411, 1979.

Bast TH, Anson BJ: *The Temporal Bone and the Ear*. Springfield, Ill., Charles C Thomas, 1949.

Bredberg G: SEM studies of Corti's organ with special reference to its innervation. *Biomed Res* 2:403–414, 1981.

Engstrom H, Angelborg C: Supporting elements in the organ of Corti. Fibrillar structures in the supporting cells of the organ of Corti of mammals. *Acta Otolaryngol (Stockh)* 75:49–60, 1973.

Flock Å: Transduction in hair cells. In Lowenstein WR (ed): *Handbook of Sensory Physiology, vol I: Principles of Receptor Physiology*. Berlin, Springer-Verlag, 1971, p 396.

Flock Å: Electron probe determination of relative ion distribution in the inner ear. *Acta Otolaryngol (Stockh)* 83:239–244, 1977.

Fujimoto S, Yamamoto K, Hayabuchi I, Yoshizuka M: Scanning and transmission electron microscope studies on the organ of Corti and stria vascularis in human fetal cochlear ducts. *Arch Histol Jpn* 44:223–226, 1981.

Gulley RL, Bagger-Sjöbäck D: Freeze-fracture studies on the synapse between type-I hair cell and the calyceal terminal in the guinea pig vestibular system. *J Neurocytol* 8:591–604, 1979.

Gulley RL, Reese TS: Intercellular junctions in the reticular lamina of the organ of Corti. *J Neurocytol* 5:479–507, 1976.

Gulley RL, Reese TS: Regional specializations of the hair cell plasmalemma in the organ of Corti. *Anat Rec* 189:109–124, 1977.

Gulley RL, Reese TS: Freeze-fracture studies on the synapses in the organ of Corti. *J Comp Neurol* 171:517–544, 1977.

Hama K: Fine structure of the afferent synapse and gap junctions on the sensory hair cell in the saccular macula of goldfish—freeze-fracture study. *J Neurocytol* 9:845–860, 1980.

Hentzer H: Histologic studies of the normal mucosa in the middle ear, mastoid cavities and Eustachian tube. *Ann Otol Rhinol Laryngol* 79:825–833, 1970.

Hudspeth AJ: The hair cells of the inner ear. *Sci Am* 248:54–64, 1983.

Igarashi Y: Ontogeny of the inner ear: a scanning electron microscope study. *Biomed Res* 2:427–432, 1981.

Iurato S (ed): *Submicroscopic Structure of the Inner Ear*. New York, Pergamon Press, 1967.

Jahnke K: The fine structure of freeze-fractured intercellular junctions in the guinea pig inner ear. *Acta Otolaryngol (Suppl) (Stockh)* 336:1–40, 1975.

Kimura RS: Ultrastructure of the organ of Corti. *Int Rev Cytol* 42:173–222, 1975.

Meier S: Development of the embryonic chick otic placode. I. Electron microscopic analysis. *Anat Rec* 191:447–458, 1978.

Meier S: Development of the embryonic chick otic placode. II. Electron microscopic analysis. *Anat Rec* 191:459–477, 1978.

Nadol JB, Mulroy MJ, Goodenough DA, Weiss TF: Tight and gap junctions in the vertebrate inner ear. *Am J Anat* 147:281–302, 1976.

Saito K: Fine structure of the sensory epithelium of the guinea pig organ of Corti: afferent and efferent synapses of hair cells. *J Ultrastruct Res* 71:222–232, 1980.

Smith CA: The inner ear: its embryological development and microstructure. In Towers DB (ed): *The Nervous System*, vol 3: *Human Communication and Its Disorders*. New York, Raven Press, 1975.

Ilberg C, Vosteen K-H: Permeability of the inner ear membranes. *Acta Otolaryngol (Stockh)* 67:165–170, 1969.

von Békésy G: *Experiments in Hearing*. (Wever EG, trans.) New York, McGraw-Hill, 1960.

Wersall J: Vestibular receptor cells in fish and mammals. *Acta Otolaryngol (Suppl) (Stockh)* 163:25–29, 1961.

Organs of Smell and Taste

Arstila A, Wersall J: The ultrastructure of the olfactory epithelium of the guinea pig. *Acta Otolaryngol (Suppl) (Stockh)* 64:187–204, 1967.

Beidler LM, Smallman RL: Renewal of cells within

taste buds. *J Cell Biol* 27:263–272, 1965.

Bradley RM, Stern IB: Development of the human taste bud during the foetal period. *J Anat* 101:743–752, 1967.

Farbman AI: Electron microscopy study of the developing taste bud in rat fungiform papilla. *Dev Biol* 11:110–135, 1965.

Frisch D: Ultrastructure of the mouse olfactory mucosa. *Am J Anat* 121:87–119, 1967.

Fujimoto S, Murray RG: Fine structure of degeneration and regeneration in denervated rabbit vallate buds. *Anat Rec* 168:393–414, 1970.

Gray EG, Watkins KC: Electron microscopy of tastebuds of the rat. *Z Zellforsch* 66:583–595, 1965.

Jourdan MF: Ultrastructure de l'épithélium olfactif du rat: polymorphisme des récepteurs. *CR Acad Sci Paris* 280:443–446, 1975.

Mendoza AS, Breipohl W: The cell coat of the olfactory epithelium proper and vomeronasal neuroepithelium of the rat as revealed by means of the ruthenium-red extraction. *Cell Tissue Res* 230:139–146, 1983.

Moran DT, Rowley JC III, Jafek BW: Electron microscopy of human olfactory epithelium reveals a new cell type: the microvillar cell. *Brain Res* 253:39–46, 1982.

Murray RD, Murray A: Fine structure of taste buds of rabbit foliate papillae. *J Ultrastruct Res* 19:327–353, 1967.

Oakley B, Benjamin RM: Neural mechanism of taste. *Physiol Rev* 46:173–211, 1966.

Zotterman Y (ed): *Olfaction and Taste*. New York, Macmillan, 1963.

INDEX

A band, skeletal muscle, 267, 283
A (alpha) cell, pancreas, 588–589
Absorption, small intestinal epithelium, 558, 561
Absorptive cell
  colon, 565
  small intestinal epithelium, 544
Accessory pancreatic duct, 582
Accomodation, eye, 861
Acetylcholine
  cardiac muscle, 296
  neurotransmitter, 327, 329, 361
Acetylcholinesterase, synapse, 329
Acid
  phosphatase, histochemical study, 4
  secretion, 53–538
  tissue staining, 4
Acidophils, hypophysis, 783
Acinar cell, pancreatic, protein synthesis, 36, 583
Acinar unit, liver, 597
Acinus
  glands, 141
  pancreas, 582, 583
Acquired immunity, 241
Acromegaly, 783
Acrosin, 753
Acrosomal cap, 701
Acrosome, 699, 701
  reaction, 753
ACTH (see Adrenocorticotropic hormone)
Actin
  cardiac muscle fiber, 288
  intestinal epithelium, 552
  microfilaments, 60, 128, 552
  skeletal muscle, 262–263, 276
  smooth muscle, 254
  terminal web, 128
α-Actinin, 133, 274
Action potential
  neuron, 299, 302, 331, 348
  skeletal muscle, 283
Active immunity, 241
Addison's disease, 812
Adenohypophysis (see also Pituitary), 781
Adenoids, 451, 526
Adenosine diphosphate (ADP), 283
Adenosine triphosphate (ATP)
  formation, 57
  skeletal muscle contraction, 283–284
ADH (antidiuretic hormone), 676
Adipocytes, 162, 171
Adipose tissue
  brown, 188
  white, 183–188
Adrenal gland, 805–807
  cortex, 807–812
    fetal, 806

medulla, 812–816
Adrenergic synapse, 327
Adrenocorticotropic hormone (ACTH) (see Adrenocorticotropin)
Adrenocorticotropin, 787, 789
  stimulation of adrenal, 812
Adventitia (see Tunica adventitia)
Agglutination
  of erythrocytes, 236
  of platelets, 249–251
Aggregation, cellular, 80
Agranulocyte (see also specific kind), 238–243
Air cells (see Alveolus, pulmonary and Alveolar cells)
Aldehyde fixation, 6, 327–328
Aldosterone, 667, 675, 805, 807
Alimentary tract, general features, 506–507
Alkaline phosphatase, bone formation, 213
Allantoic stalk, 110
Allantois, 99, 108
Allocortex, 383
Alpha motor neuron, 371
Alveolar cells, 638, 640
Alveolar ducts, lung, 633, 635
Alveolar macrophage, 640
Alveolar membrane, 640
Alveolar pores, 638
Alveolar sac, 635
Alveolus
  mammary gland, 771
  mucous, 152, 574
  pulmonary, 633, 635
  serous, 152, 574
  teeth, 513
Amacrine cells, 849, 855
Ameboid movement, 75
Ameloblast, 514, 522, 525
Amino acid, structure, 15
γ-Amino-butyric acid, neurotransmitter (GABA), 329–330
Amnion, 99
Ampulla
  ductus deferens, 710
  oviduct, 742
Amylase, pancreatic secretion, 589
Anabolism, 64
Anal canal, 568
Anal sphincter, internal and external, 570
Anal valve, 568
Anaphase, 89, 92–96, 698, 699
Anaphylactic sensitivity, mast cell, 171
Anastomoses, arteriovenous, 410
Anaxonic neuron, 313
Anchoring filament, lymph vessels, 422
Androgen(s)
  aromatization, 694, 740
  adrenal, 812

891